Phillips' Science *of* Dental Materials

Phillips' Science *of* Dental Materials

SECOND SOUTH ASIA EDITION

US Editors

Chiayi Shen PHD

Associate Professor
Department of Restorative Dental Sciences
College of Dentistry
University of Florida
Gainesville, Florida

H. Ralph Rawls PHD

Professor of Biomaterials
Research Division
Department of Comprehensive Dentistry
University of Texas Health Science Center at San Antonio
San Antonio, Texas

Josephine F. Esquivel-Upshaw DMD, MS, MS-CI, FACD

Associate Professor
Department of Restorative Dental Sciences
College of Dentistry
University of Florida
Gainesville, Florida

South Asia Adaptation Editors

Arvind Shenoy MDS

Professor, Department of Conservative Dentistry
Bapuji Dental College, Davangere, INDIA
Member, Board of Studies, Rajiv Gandhi University of Health Sciences
Reviewer, Journal of Indian Dental Association, Journal of Conservative Dentistry, World Dental Journal and Journal of Contemporary Dental Practice

K. Chandrasekharan Nair MDS

Professor Emeritus, Sri Sankara Dental College
Akathumuri, Trivandrum, INDIA
Former Professor Emeritus, Vishnu Dental College
Bhimavaram, INDIA
Former Professor, Department of Prosthodontics
AECS Maaruti College of Dental Sciences and Research
Bangalore, INDIA
Former Chairman, Board of Studies (Dentistry)
Kerala University
Former Member, Faculty of Dentistry, Kerala and Calicut Universities
Former Member, Board of Studies (Dentistry) RGUHS
Bangalore, INDIA

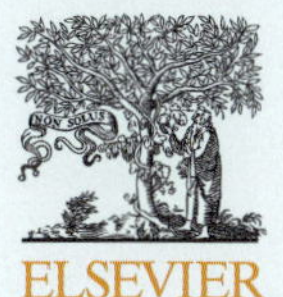

ELSEVIER

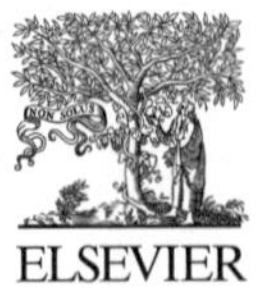

ELSEVIER

RELX India Pvt. Ltd.

Registered Office: 818, Indraprakash Building, 8th Floor, 21, Barakhamba Road, New Delhi-110001
Corporate Office: 14th Floor, Building No. 10B, DLF Cyber City, Phase II, Gurgaon-122 002, Haryana, India

Phillips' Science *of* Dental Materials, 13th Edition, Chiayi Shen, H. Ralph Rawls and Josephine F. Esquivel-Upshaw

ISBN: 978-0-323-69755-2

This adaptation of **Phillips' Science *of* Dental Materials, 13th Edition,** by **Chiayi Shen, H. Ralph Rawls and Josephine F. Esquivel-Upshaw** was undertaken by RELX India Private Limited and is published by arrangement with Elsevier Inc.

Phillips' Science *of* Dental Materials: Second South Asia Edition, Arvind Shenoy, K. Chandrasekharan Nair

Adaptation ISBN: 978-81-312-5611-4
eISBN: 978-81-312-5612-1

First Printed in India 2022, Reprinted 2023 (twice), 2025

Content Strategist: Ruchi Mullick
Content Project Manager: Anand K Jha
Sr *Production Executive:* Dhan Singh Rana

Printed in India by Sanat Printers, Kundli, Haryana

Contributors

William A. Brantley, PhD
Professor Emeritus
Graduate Program in Dental Materials Science
Division of Restorative, Prosthetic and Primary Care Dentistry
College of Dentistry
The Ohio State University
Columbus, Ohio
Chapter 2 Structure of Matter, General Classes of Materials, and Principles of Adhesion
Chapter 9 Metals

Charles F. Defreest, DDS
Dental Laboratory Director
59th Dental Laboratory
Wilford Hall Ambulatory Surgical Center
San Antonio, Texas
Chapter 16 Materials and Processes for Cutting, Grinding, Finishing, and Polishing

Josephine F. Esquivel-Upshaw, DMD, MS, MS-CI, FACD
Professor
Department of Restorative Dental Sciences
College of Dentistry
University of Florida
Gainesville, Florida
Chapter 10 Ceramic-Based Materials
Chapter 12 Dental Implants
Chapter 19 Clinical Research on Restorations

Saulo Geradeli, DDS, MS, PhD
Associate Professor
Department of General Dentistry
School of Dental Medicine
East Carolina University
Greenville, North Carolina
Chapter 1 Overview of Dental Materials

Lawrence Gettleman, DMD, MSD
Professor Emeritus of Biomaterials & Prosthodontics
School of Dentistry
University of Louisville
Louisville, Kentucky
Chapter 11 Prosthetic Polymers and Resins
Chapter 14 Casting Investments and Casting Procedures
Chapter 20 Emerging Technologies

Jason A. Griggs, PhD
Associate Dean for Research
Professor and Chair, Department of Biomedical Materials Science
School of Dentistry
University of Mississippi Medical Center
Jackson, Mississippi
Chapter 18 In Vitro Research on Dental Materials

Jack E. Lemons, PhD
Professor
Department of Prosthodontics
School of Dentistry
University of Alabama at Birmingham
Birmingham, Alabama
Chapter 12 Dental Implants

Jacob G. Park, DDS
Professor of Dentistry/Clinical
School of Dentistry
University of Texas Health Science Center at San Antonio
San Antonio, Texas
Chapter 15 Digital Technology in Dentistry

Rodney D. Phoenix, DDS, MS
Associate Dean for Dental Research
Postgraduate Dental College
Uniformed Services University of the Health Sciences
JBSA-Fort Sam Houston
San Antonio, Texas
Chapter 11 Prosthetic Polymers and Resins

Carolyn M. Primus, PhD
Consultant
Primus Consulting
Bradenton, Florida
Chapter 7 Dental Cements
Chapter 20 Emerging Technologies

H. Ralph Rawls, PhD
Professor of Biomaterials
Research Division
Department of Comprehensive Dentistry
University of Texas Health Science Center at San Antonio
San Antonio, Texas
Chapter 2 Structure of Matter, General Classes of Materials, and Principles of Adhesion
Chapter 3 Physical and Chemical Properties of Solids
Chapter 5 Resin-Based Composites
Chapter 6 Bonding and Bonding Agents
Chapter 15 Digital Technology in Dentistry
Chapter 20 Emerging Technologies

Gottfried Schmalz, DDS, DMD, PhD, Dr.h.c
Professor
Department of Conservative Dentistry and Periodontology
University Hospital
University of Regensburg
Regensburg, Germany
Chapter 17 Biocompatibility

Chiayi Shen, PhD
Courtesy Associate Professor
Department of Restorative Dental Sciences
College of Dentistry
University of Florida
Gainesville, Florida
Chapter 1 Overview of Dental Materials
Chapter 2 Structure of Matter, General Classes of Materials, and Principles of Adhesion
Chapter 4 Mechanical Properties of Solids
Chapter 8 Dental Amalgams
Chapter 13 Auxiliary Materials
Chapter 14 Casting Investments and Casting Procedures

Kyumin Whang, PhD
Professor/Research
Department of Comprehensive Dentistry
University of Texas Health Science Center at San Antonio
San Antonio, Texas
Chapter 5 Resin-Based Composites
Chapter 6 Bonding and Bonding Agents
Chapter 20 Emerging Technologies

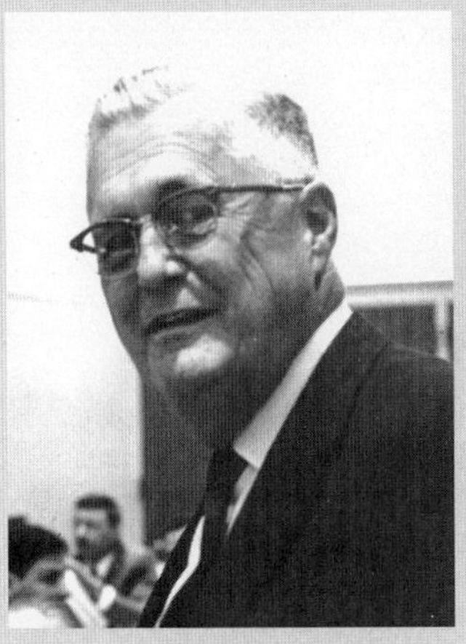
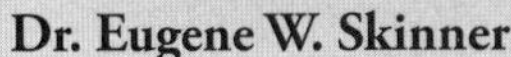

Dr. Eugene W. Skinner

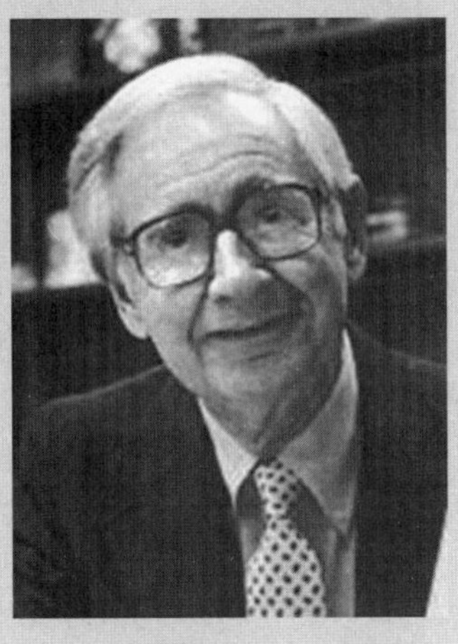

Dr. Ralph W. Phillips

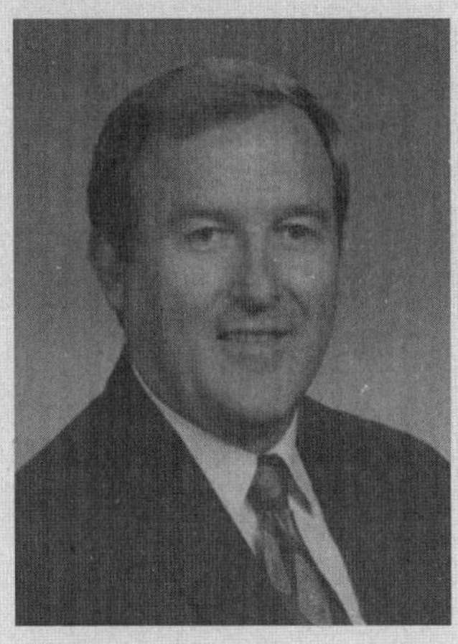

Dr. Kenneth J. Anusavice

We would like to dedicate this edition to the first three editors of this book.
Dr. Eugene W. Skinner *(I–VI),* **Dr. Ralph W. Phillips** *(V–IX),* **Dr. Kenneth J. Anusavice** *(X–XII)*

Dr. Eugene Skinner, a professor of physics at Northwestern University School of Dentistry in Chicago, published the first edition of *The Science of Dental Materials* in 1936. Dr. Skinner introduced Ralph Phillips as a coauthor of the 5th edition of the book in 1960. Dr. Skinner died during the proof-page-reviewing stage of the 6th edition in 1966. He is honored with the "Eugene W. Skinner Memorial Lecture" at Northwestern University. The lecture series was renamed "Eugene W. Skinner and Eugene P. Lautenschlager Memorial Lecture" in the Department of Biomedical Engineering, Northwestern University.
Dr. Phillips renamed the book *Skinner's Science of Dental Materials* in the 7th through 9th editions. After the death of Dr. Phillips in 1991, the book has been subsequently renamed as *Phillips' Science of Dental Materials* since the 10th edition.

Throughout an eminent career that spanned five decades, Dr. Ralph Phillips was recognized as one of the world's foremost leaders in the field of dental materials science. He was one of the first dental scientists to investigate the relationship between laboratory tests and clinical performance. He initiated clinical investigations designed to analyze the effect of the oral environment on restorative materials and to determine the biocompatibility of restorative materials and the efficacy of newer material formulations and techniques of use. Over his many years of service, he remained firmly committed to his original focus on the clinical relevance of laboratory findings, an approach that dominated both his style of teaching and his research activities. Among his main contributions to dentistry, Dr. Phillips pioneered studies of fluoride's influence on the solubility and hardness of tooth enamel and its anticariogenic potential when included in restorative materials. In the 1960s, he coordinated the first workshop on adhesive dental materials, which brought together research experts in the fields of adhesion, polymer science, and tooth structure. During his career, he published more than 300 scientific papers and books and organized more than 40 symposia and conferences related to biomaterials and dental research.

Dr. Kenneth Anusavice is a Distinguished Professor Emeritus at the University of Florida and is one of the leading dental materials scientists in the field. Among his many awards, the Wilmer Souder Award for Research in Dental Materials, awarded by the International Association for Dental Research (IADR) in 1996, was one that he was most proud of. Dr. Anusavice served as the chairman of the International Organization for Standardization (ISO)/Technical Committee (TC) 106/SC 2: Prosthodontic Materials from 1999–2014 and was elected chairman of ISO/TC 106—Dentistry in 2014 until his retirement in 2016. Dr. Anusavice fostered many collaborations with different dental scientists worldwide. He was on the editorial board of numerous journals, most notably *Dental Materials and Journal of Dentistry*. He edited several books, contributed numerous book chapters, and published over 180 peer-reviewed manuscripts and is recognized as the foremost authority in dental materials and ceramic science. Perhaps his most significant contribution to dental materials science is his mentorship of countless students and graduate students who are now respected leaders in the research field. He received the Irwin D. Mandel Distinguished Mentoring Award, awarded by the American Association for Dental Research (AADR) in 2016, which is a true testament to his dedication to fostering the career development of students and junior faculty in the area of research in dental materials.

Dedication

"A mentor is someone who sees more talent and ability within you, than you see in yourself, and helps bring it out of you." — Bob Proctor

As you make your way through life, one is lucky to find people who will help, guide and mentor you. It's even rarer to find people who encourage you and enable you to develop your talents and reach heights you yourself never felt possible.

I have been lucky to have four such individuals, who reposed their faith in me. I remain eternally grateful to all of them. I wish to dedicate this book to them.

Late Dr S V Bhagwat
Dr Surendra Shetty
Dr Sadashiva Shetty
Late Dr Premananda Kamath

—Arvind Shenoy

This book is dedicated to the present and future generations of students of dental profession and to the teachers who are engaged in the noble task of inspiring young professionals

—K. Chandrasekharan Nair

Preface to the Second South Asia Edition

Evolution and development of the dental profession has always been synchronous with that of dental material science. One of the earliest restorative material that caught the attention of the dental profession is dental amalgam which still remains to be practised in many parts of the world. In a meeting of dental professionals, convened by WHO at Geneva in the year 2009 'on the future use of materials for dental restorations' it was recognised that dental caries remains to be a major global public health problem and the demand for dental restorations has not diminished despite much effort in health promotion and disease prevention. It is estimated that only one out of ten needy individuals get restorative treatment. Countries do not follow a uniform pattern in the selection of restorative materials. However, dental amalgam restorations are still taught in the dental curriculum, but much emphasis is placed on tooth-colored restorative materials, leading to an increasing trend in using more composite resins and glass ionomers. Research is being encouraged to find out new restorative materials so that they become readily accessible and cost effective.

It is of paramount interest for the dental professional to be well versed with the science of materials, which are used to restore missing tooth structure. As technological and scientific advancements progress at a breakneck speed, it is imperative that this premier treatise on dental materials should do the same. This is evident from the continuous changes in the text over the years. The original book underwent an evolutionary process in the past years under the able stewardship of Phillips and Anusavice. The 13th edition of Phillips Science of Dental Materials edited by Chiayi Shen, H. Ralph Rawls and Josephine Esquivel-Upshaw has taken the legacy forward.

This, the Second South Asian Edition represents a comprehensive overview of the composition, biocompatibility, physical properties, mechanical properties, manipulative variables, and performance of direct and indirect restorative materials and auxiliary materials used in dentistry. The book is intended as a textbook for dental students, dental hygiene students, laboratory technicians, and dental materials scientists. It is also designed as an authoritative reference book for dentists, dental assistants, dental hygienists, and corporate marketing staff. Although the scientific concepts presented in some chapters are somewhat advanced, the text information in most chapters can be readily understood by individuals with a general college education.

Like the previous edition, this book while maintaining the current and authoritative nature, has incorporated certain features, which would make it more valuable to students and clinicians in the Indian context.

Clinical and practical aspects of various materials have been highlighted in special boxes to enable easy reference without having to go through the entire text. Similarly, Summary has been provided at the end of each chapter in a bulleted format. This provides the chapter at a glance and would be valuable to students just prior to an examination when they would be able to glance over the salient aspects of the chapter. A cumulative list of Review Questions given in each chapter. These have been culled from the question papers of different universities over the last 10 years and would be a useful reference for undergraduate students.

Dental materials available in the developed countries find their way to the Indian user without much delay and, in fact, many materials are developed with a view to keep them within the reach of the common man living in the developing and the underdeveloped countries. This book would give an insight into the characteristics and standards to be maintained by the dental materials, which are used in the Indian clinics. Students, clinicians and researchers would find this book highly readable mainly because of its structure.

Phillips' Science of Dental Materials, 2nd South Asian Edition provides comprehensive, up-to-date information on the materials used in cosmetic and restorative procedures in dentistry. It introduces the physical and chemical properties that are related to selection and use of dental biomaterials, including their composition, mechanical properties, manipulative variables, and the performance of dental restorations and prostheses. This edition adds two new chapters and hundreds of new full-color photographs. In addition several new clinically relevant tips have been provided in most chapters to enable the student to clinically correlate the concepts.

Two new chapters are added: Digital Technology in Dentistry and Clinical Research on Restorations.

Digital technology is being introduced and adapted at a frightening pace and it is more imperative than ever that the astute clinician adapts to the same. A new chapter on Digital Technology helps the reader to grasp the present and future implications of technology in dentistry.

As a clinician it is not only important to understand the physics and chemistry of dental materials but also appreciate their usefulness in clinical practice. Throughout the text we have tried to provide this relevance to the reader. We have also introduced a chapter on the Clinical Research on Restorations and its relevance to clinical dentistry.

This book has been reorganised and divided into five broad parts. Each part is devoted to one aspect of dental materials. The first part deals with the General Properties of Materials, presenting an overview and a detailed discussion on the physical, chemical, mechanical and optical properties of restorative materials.

The second part deals with Direct Restorative Materials, while the third part deals with Indirect Restorative Materials.

The fourth part combines some of the chapters in older editions, based on synergies to provide a simplified overview on the actual fabrication of the prosthesis and also the role that digital technology plays in the same.

The last part provides a comprehensive review of materials evaluation including Biocompatibility and Clinical Research on Restorations, while also looking forward at emerging technologies.

It is our sincere hope that this book will play as productive a role in the understanding and application of dental materials to the current generation, as previous editions have to earlier generations of dentists.

Arvind Shenoy
K Chandrasekharan Nair

Acknowledgments

A work of this magnitude is always a labor of love and can never be completed without the help and support of many individuals who played a pivotal role in this book coming to fruition. Working as we did through the pandemic added different layers of complexities to the project. Collaborating across continents with lock downs and the general panic that the pandemic brought about was challenging and taxing. The lay reader would often not be aware of the sheer magnitude and complexities in bringing out a text such as this.

I would like to place on record my sincere gratitude to all the people who made this possible.

The thirteenth international edition is co-edited by Chiayi Shen, H. Ralph Rawls and Josephine Esquivel-Upshaw. I would like to sincerely thank them for giving us the opportunity to work on this seminal text. Considering the amount of hard work, they would have put into the 13th edition, it is incredibly magnanimous on their part to provide the text for adaptation. I sincerely appreciate the trust placed in us.

This work is also based on the 12th edition by Anusavice, Shen, and Rawls and we would like to acknowledge the pivotal role played by the major contributors to that edition. These include Dr William Brantley, Dr Carolyn Primus, Dr Jack Lemons. We would also like to acknowledge Jeannie Robertson and Dr José dos Santos, Jr for the artwork. I would also like to acknowledge the role played by the contributors to the previous editions. These contributors include Drs Charles F DeFreest, Jack Ferracane, J Rodway Mackert, Jr, Miroslav Marek, Victoria A Marker, Robert Neiman, Barry K Norling, Karl-Johan Söderholm, Grayson Marshall, Sally Marshall, Atul Sarma, Harold R Stanley, and John Wataha, and Mr Paul Cascone.

In the context of the South Asian adaptation Dr K Chandrasekharan Nair has been the bedrock of support and his active cooperation, collaboration, insight and patience have played a substantial role in ensuring the success of this book.

I don't think I could have completed one, let alone two editions of this book without the help and support of my wife Dr Nina Shenoy. Her unflinching support and dedication have been crucial not just to this project, but to everything in our lives. Research, proofreading, or just tolerating a temperamental husband, she has been there through it all! I don't know what I would have done without her!

My parents have been there from the beginning helping, guiding and encouraging me. Their blessings and guidance have helped me at every stage in my life.

I have had a great bunch of graduate students over the years who have always risen to the occasion and helped make my job easier.

Drs Rakshita N, Nikhisha Naik, Archie Khera, Sucharita Vishwakarma, Saleem Ilkal, have all helped me in this project, my sincere thanks to all of them.

Finally, this book would not have come to fruition without the active collaboration of the dedicated people at Elsevier India. The amount of effort they have put in, working across continents to make it happen, is a true lesson in perseverance. A special thanks to Mr Anand K Jha and Ms Nimisha Goswami, for the infinite patience they have shown in balancing deadlines and expediting things to meet with our schedules, and finally producing a world class textbook.

—Arvind Shenoy

I joined Government Dental College, Thiruvananthapuram, as a BDS student, in the year 1967. Those days we were asked to procure Skinner's Science of Dental Materials which was a rare commodity. With great efforts, a local book shop could procure the second edition from Bombay. It was a price possession and I tried to read certain chapters whenever I had a doubt on the notes dictated in the class. My first words of gratitude go to that great author whose magnificent contribution has made me learn the subject of Dental Materials and decades later provided me an opportunity to associate with the same title as an editor.

Prof Jacob Hyson and Prof George Paulose (former Joint Directors of Medical Education, Kerala) were great teachers who have taught me the science of dental materials and molded my vision to make this book attractive primarily to the undergraduate students.

Prof. Satyanarayana Raju M who is heading the Implantology Department of Vishnu Dental College, Bhimavaram, Andhra Pradesh has significantly contributed while revising the chapter (12) on dental implants by way of making critical revisions and additions. Prof. T Mohan Kumar, former Professor of Prosthodontics, Azeezia Dental College, Kollam, Kerala has been a passionate teacher of the science of dental materials for more than two decades has provided significant contributions while editing chapters 4 and 5 of the first south Asia edition of this book. I would like to place on record my great appreciation to these professors.

Prof Arvind Shenoy deserves great appreciation for the timely intelligent interventions made during the making of the second edition.

I would like to thank my former postgraduate students for their open expressions on the expectations of the students about a textbook and that had positive influence while revising the chapters.

I owe a great deal to my father who practiced dentistry in a remote village of Kerala in the late 1940s. Perhaps he has put in me the unknown spark that made me a dentist later. My mother's solid insistence to make me follow the footsteps of my father also deserve a mention. My working environment was always ensured by my wife, Smt. Supriya and as always, stood as a pillar of support. My son, Raman C Nair has encouraged me with his knowledge of information technology in accessing many valuable internet resources. Prof Pradeep C Dathan, my head of the department, has graciously allowed me time to associate with this project.

Shri Anand K Jha, Managing Editor was so patient and at the same time greatly efficient in visualising and executing the work of the second SA edition of Phillips Science of Dental Materials. His erudite team also deserve great appreciation for the keen observation and bringing possible errors to my attention.

The publishers Elsevier India have been kind to us in bestowing this editorial job.

—K. Chandrasekharan Nair

Contents

PART I

General Classes and Properties of Dental Materials

1 Overview of Preventive and Restorative Materials

CHAPTER OUTLINE

KEY TERMS

Auxiliary dental material—Substance used in the construction of a dental prosthesis that does not become a part of the prosthesis.

Preventive dental material—Cement, coating, or restorative material that either seals pits and fissures or releases a therapeutic agent, such as fluoride and/or mineralizing ions, to prevent or arrest the demineralization of the tooth structure.

Restorative dental material—Metallic, ceramic, metal-ceramic, or resin-based substance used to replace, repair, or rebuild teeth and/or enhance esthetics. A direct restorative material is placed in the tooth preparation and is transformed to be a restoration. An indirect restorative material is fabricated extraorally to produce prostheses.

Temporary restorative material—Cement or resin-based composite used for a period ranging from a few days to several months to temporarily restore or replace missing teeth or tooth structure until a definitive, lasting prosthesis or restoration can be placed.

This chapter defines what dental materials are and discusses their role in clinical dentistry. The chapter first describes the function of the oral cavity, the interaction between opposing teeth, and the structure of the tooth. There are potential issues involving teeth that necessitate intervention to restore their function. Some treatment options require the fabrication of devices in the process, and if there is a loss of tooth structure after successful treatments, restorations are required. The materials needed can be categorized as preventive, restorative, and auxiliary materials, as defined by their applications. Some of these materials are expected to be in the oral cavity for an extended period of time. As a result, these materials must not only perform well but also integrate with the tooth structure over time. This chapter discusses the obstacles dental materials are facing and the future challenges for dental biomaterials; it also provides a brief description of the structure of the book.

The Oral Cavity

As an anatomical space and part of the head and neck, the oral cavity consists of the lips, cheeks, minor salivary glands, gingiva, tongue, hard palate, and teeth. As part of human evolution, the oral cavity developed to allow humans to ingest food, chew, swallow, breathe, and speak.

In addition, the oral cavity is a food processor for the body. The presence and colonization of bacteria, along with distinct teeth anatomy, saliva, and chewing (motion), begin the breakdown of food and initiate the digestive process. Therefore, humans are able to obtain the nutrients necessary for survival. Furthermore, both biting and chewing require upper and lower jaws, muscles, and teeth working in unity to achieve this goal. A distinctive component required in this interaction (Fig. 1.1A) to

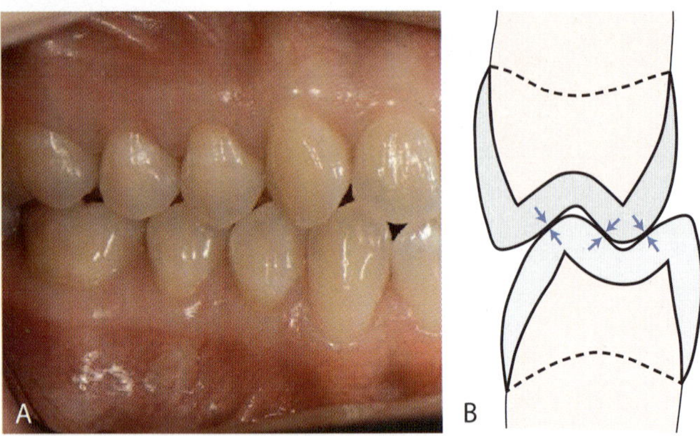

• **Fig. 1.1** Interaction between teeth. **(A)** Natural human dentition of an adult patient showing upper and lower teeth in full-occlusion contact. **(B)** Forces acting on teeth at occlusion.

cut and grind food is force. You will find throughout this book that the term *force* is often used, so a proper presentation of the term is warranted.

Structure of Teeth

In the oral cavity, teeth are firmly joined to the upper and lower jaws by tooth-supporting connective tissues (cementum and periodontal ligament). This assembly of tissues ensures enough flexibility to withstand the forces of mastication and act as thermal and chemical insulators. Teeth perform important functions in the oral cavity. The front teeth can grab and cut food to a size that is suitable for the mouth (bite-size). They also have a role in speech and contribute to facial esthetics. The posterior teeth's morphology is designed to grind the bite-size food into smaller sizes, which facilitates food passage from the throat to the stomach.

At the teeth's full formation and physiological capacity, they will have the following structures: Enamel, dentin, enamel–dentin junction, pulp, and cementum (Fig. 1.2).

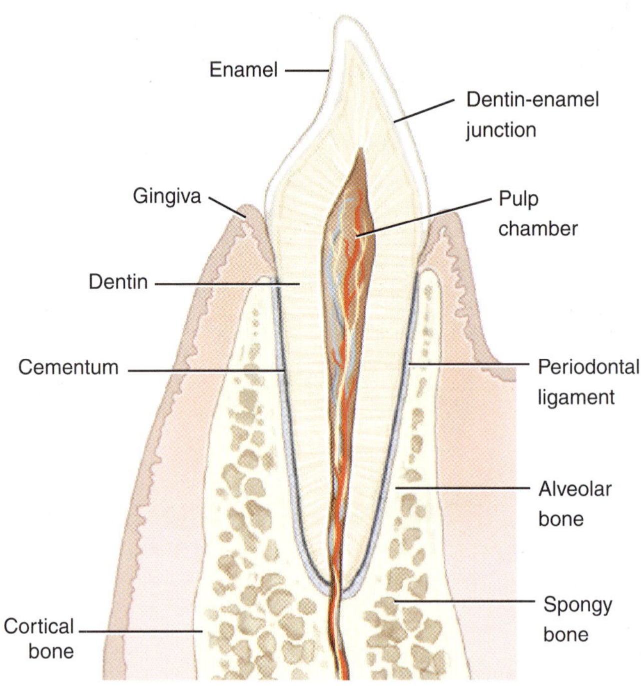

• **Fig. 1.2** Schematic cross-sectional view of a natural anterior tooth and supporting tissues.

Enamel

Dental *enamel* is a biologically ceramic composite made of precisely arranged 20-nm-diameter fibrous apatite crystals (92–94 vol%). The meaning of *composite* will be discussed in Chapter 2. The remaining 2–4 wt% nonmineral content is represented by water, lipids, and several peptides. This small amount of nonmineral components, along with its hierarchical anisotropic structure, regulates the mechanical properties of enamel to respond to the tooth's functional needs, such as strength and resistance to wear upon loading. On a micrometer scale, enamel contains rod and interrod structures (Fig. 1.3), beginning at the enamel–dentin junction and extending to the tooth surface. The ability of the

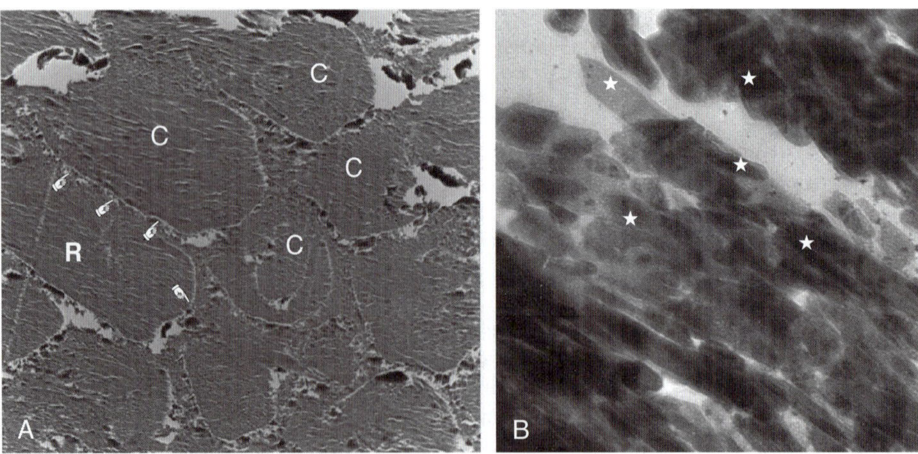

• **Fig. 1.3** Transmission electron microscope images of sound enamel. **(A)** High-resolution image of enamel depicting the structural organization between rods (R) and interrods (C) (33000). **(B)** Ultrahigh-resolution image showing the distribution of crystal in one rod *(white star)*. The semiwhite spaces between crystals are porosities (3200,000).

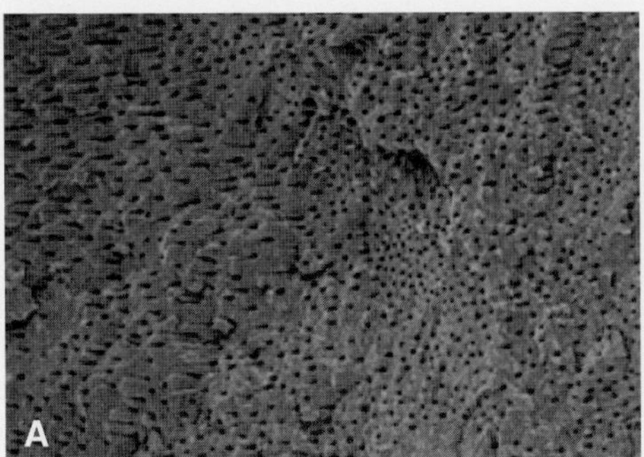

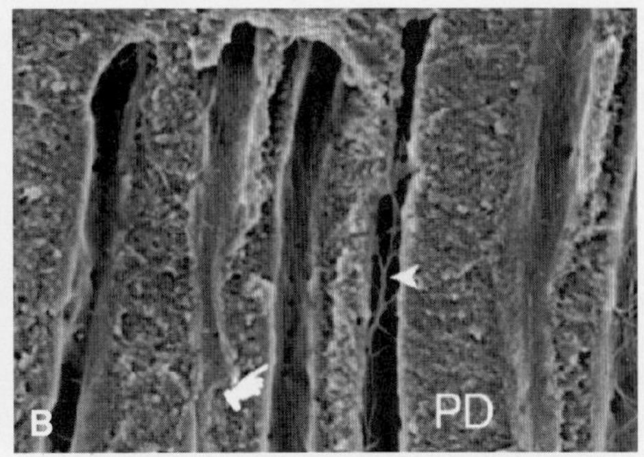

• **Fig. 1.4** Scanning electron microscopy images of fractured sound dentin specimens. **(A)** Massive presence of open tubules (×400). **(B)** Higher magnification of a longitudinal fracture allowing the visualization of intertubular dentin (PD), peritubular dentin *(white index)*, and the organic structure lying free within the dentinal tubule know as *lamina limitans (white arrow)* (×4000).

rigid rod structure, along with the organic interrod component, to weaken the stress concentration at the crack tip, if present, improves the resistance of the enamel to fracture from the stress generated at the surface contact.

Dentin

Dentin is a composite mineralized tissue that contains less mineral than enamel and is composed of nanocrystalline carbonated hydroxyapatite (Fig. 1.4). The organic content (30 vol%) is almost exclusively type I collagen fibrils plus noncollagen proteins, such as proteoglycans. In addition, this tissue has a peculiar morphological feature: The presence of tubules extending from the enamel−dentin junction to the pulp. These tubules have diameters varying from 2.5 μm near the pulp tissue to 0.8 μm at the enamel−dentin junction. They also run transverse to the root or in an S-shape in the crown. This anisotropic, hierarchically oriented, and less mineralized microstructure serves as a foundation, shapes the roots, and protects the pulp. When loaded intraorally and force is applied parallel to the tubules, dentin responds better mechanically than when loads are applied perpendicularly.

Dentin-Enamel Junction

Between the harder, brittle enamel and the softer, durable (tough) dentin, a functionally graded junction, the dentin-enamel junction (DEJ), is present, allowing a smooth transition of loads from the enamel to the dentin (Fig. 1.5). This interface inhibits the propagation of cracks from the enamel to the dentin, thus supporting the tooth's integrity during masticatory actions. Even though fracture lines between enamel and dentin appear as a result of continuous masticatory action and/or occasional impact loading, enamel infrequently debonds from dentin, making the DEJ highly resistant to damage.

Cementum

Cementum is a mineralized tissue covering the entire root surface of the tooth. Cementum is composed of water, organic matrix, and mineral. About 50% of the dry mass is inorganic and consists of hydroxyapatite crystals. The remaining organic matrix is largely made up of collagen and, to a lesser degree, glycoproteins and proteoglycans. The main function of cementum is to support or anchor the tooth, together with the principal periodontal fibers and alveolar bone.

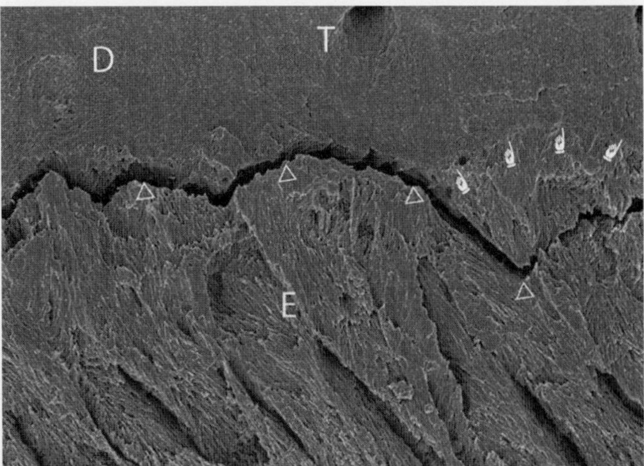

• **Fig. 1.5** Scanning electron microscopy image of the dentin-enamel junction region of sound human tooth showing dentin (D), enamel (E), and dentinal tubule (T). The pointers depict the smooth transition between the enamel and dentin. Because of the structural difference between the enamel and the dentin, cohesive separation at the interphase, indicated by Δ, is an artifact from sample preparation.

Pulp

The dental pulp is centrally located in the pulp cavity and quite often resembles the external surface of the tooth. This specialized, loose, fibrous connective tissue is composed of collagen fibrils and organic ground substance composed of 75% water and 25% organic material. As an organ, the pulp fulfills key physiological functions, namely, formative or developmental (generates dentin), nutritive (supplies nutrients and moisture through the vascular system), protective (responds to injury and noxious stimuli), and sensory (nerve fiber network transmits afferent pain). Whenever possible, especially while using dental materials, preserving the health of such vital tissue is highly desired.

Historical Use of Restorative Materials

Dentistry as a specialty is believed to have begun about 3000 BCE. Gold bands and wires were used by the Phoenicians (after 2500 BCE). Around 700 BCE, the Etruscans carved ivory or bone for the construction of partial dentures that were fastened to natural teeth by means of gold wires or bands, which were used to position extracted teeth in place of missing teeth.

Inscriptions on Egyptian tombstones indicate that tooth doctors were considered to be medical specialists, and they were not known to have performed restorative dentistry. However, some teeth found in Egyptian mummies were either transplanted human teeth or tooth forms made of ivory. The earliest documented evidence of tooth implant materials is attributed to the Etruscans as early as 700 BCE (Fig. 1.6). Around CE 600, the Mayans used implants consisting of seashell segments that were placed in anterior tooth sockets. Hammered gold inlays and stone or mineral inlays were placed for esthetic purposes or traditional ornamentation by the Mayans and later the Aztecs (Fig. 1.7). The Incas performed tooth mutilations using hammered gold, but the material was not placed for decorative purposes.

Cavities in teeth have been replaced or restored from ancient times up into the 18th century with a variety of materials including stone chips, ivory, human teeth, turpentine resin, cork, gums, and metal foils (lead and tin). More recently, gutta-percha, cements, metal-modified cements, unfilled synthetic resin, composites, other metals (gold leaf, amalgam, and a variety of cast metals and alloys), ceramics, and metal-ceramics have been used for tooth restoration. Paré (1509–1590) (Fig. 1.8), a surgeon to four kings, used lead or cork for tooth fillings. Queen Elizabeth I (1533–1603) used cloth fragments to fill the cavities in her teeth. Fauchard (1678–1761) (Fig. 1.9), the father of modern dentistry, used tin foil or lead cylinders to fill tooth cavities. Wealthy patients preferred to have teeth that were made of agate, mother of pearl, silver, or gold. Modern dentistry began in 1728, when Fauchard published a treatise describing many types of dental restorations, including a method for the construction of artificial dentures made of ivory.

Gold foil has also been employed for dental restorative purposes. Pfaff (1715–1767), the dentist of Frederick the Great of Prussia, used gold foil to cap the pulp chamber. Bull began producing beaten gold in Connecticut for dental applications in 1812. Arculanus recommended gold-leaf dental fillings in 1848. Sponge gold was introduced in 1853 in the United States and England to replace gold leaf. In 1855, Arthur promoted the use of cohesive gold in the United States. In 1897, Philbrook described the use of metal fillings made from wax patterns of the tooth cavity.

Using filings from silver coins mixed with mercury, Taveau, in France, developed what was likely the first dental amalgam in 1816. The Crawcour brothers, who emigrated from France to the

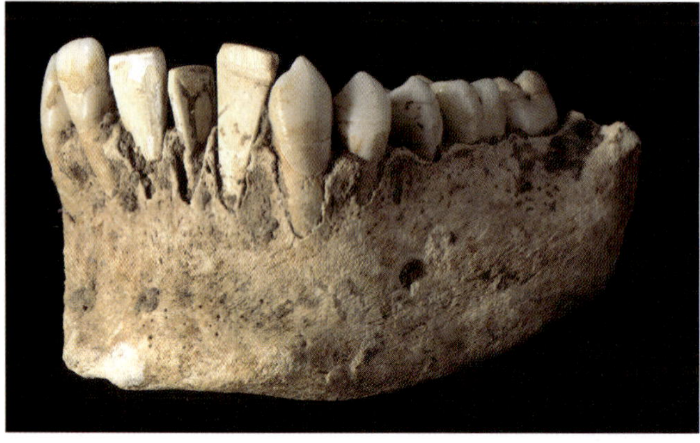

• **Fig. 1.6** This mandible, dated CE 800, was found in Honduras. It shows three implanted incisors made of carved seashells. Calculus formation on these three implants indicates that they were not made solely for a burial display but served as fixed, functional, and esthetic tooth replacements. (Image © President and Fellows of Harvard College, Peabody Museum of Archaeology and Ethnology, 33-19-20/254.0.)

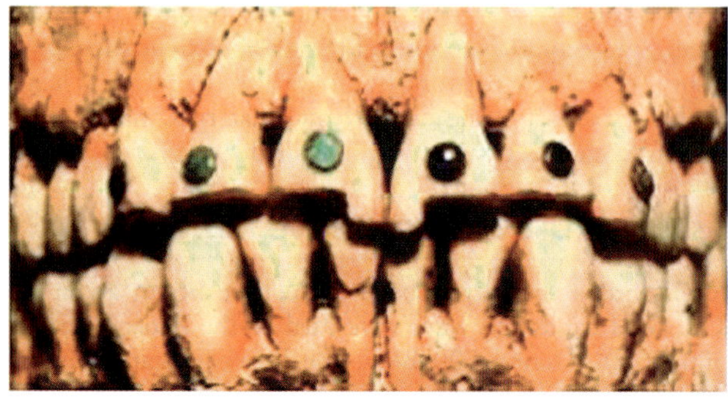

• **Fig. 1.7** Mayan jaw with stones and metal inlay decorations still intact on the teeth.

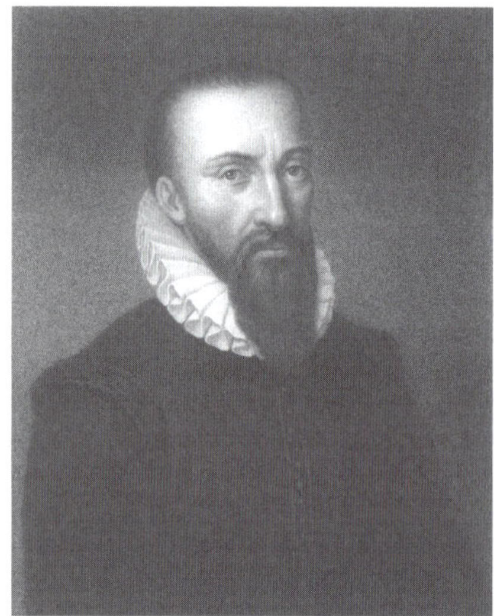

• **Fig. 1.8** Ambroise Paré (1509–1590) was the royal surgeon for Kings Henry II, Francis II, Charles IX, and Henry III.

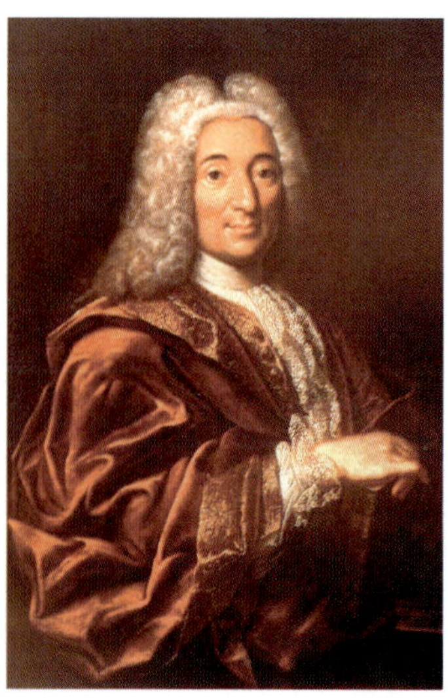

• **Fig. 1.9** Pierre Fauchard (1678–1761), known as the father of modern dentistry.

United States, introduced Taveau's amalgam fillings in 1833; however, graduates of the Baltimore Dental College subsequently took an oath not to use amalgams in their practices. Many dentists criticized the poor quality of the early amalgam restorations. This controversy led to the "amalgam war" from 1840 to 1850, during which heated debates occurred over the benefits and drawbacks of dental amalgam. Research on amalgam formulations from the 1860s through the 1890s greatly improved the handling properties and the clinical performance of amalgam filling materials. In 1895, Black proposed standardized cavity preparations and manufacturing processes for dental amalgam products.

Gold shell crowns were described by Mouton in 1746, but were patented by Beers in 1873. In 1885, Logan patented a porcelain fused to a platinum post, replacing the unsatisfactory wooden posts previously used to build up intraradicular (within the tooth root) areas of teeth. In 1907, the detached-post crown was introduced, which was more easily adjustable.

In 1756, Pfaff described a method for making impressions of the mouth in wax, from which he constructed a model with plaster of Paris. Pfaff's use of plaster of Paris allowed dentists to make impressions of the patient's edentulous jaws in the mouth. Duchateau, a French pharmacist, and de Chemant, a dentist, designed a process in 1774 for producing hard, decay-proof porcelain dentures. In 1789, de Chemant patented an improved version of these "mineral paste" porcelain teeth. The porcelain inlay was introduced soon thereafter, in the early 1800s. However, porcelain bonding to metals was not fully refined for metal-ceramic crowns until the mid-1900s.

The dentures of George Washington (1732–1799) fit poorly, and he suffered terribly throughout his presidency (1789–1797). Washington never wore wooden teeth, as has been reported; he wore dentures made of some of his own teeth, bovine or hippopotamus teeth, ivory, or lead. Prior to his first term as president, he had worn partial dentures that were fastened to his remaining teeth. During the inauguration for his first term as president in 1789, Washington had only one natural tooth remaining; he wore his first full set of dentures, which were made by John Greenwood. The base of these dentures was made of hippopotamus ivory carved to fit the jaw ridges. The upper denture contained ivory teeth and the lower one consisted of eight human teeth fastened by gold rivets that screwed into the denture base. The two dentures were secured in Washington's mouth by spiral springs.

In 1808, Fonzi, an Italian dentist, developed an individual porcelain tooth form that was held in place with an embedded platinum pin. Planteau, a French dentist, first introduced porcelain teeth in the United States in 1817. In 1822, Charles Peale, an artist, fired mineral teeth in Philadelphia, and Samuel Stockton began the commercial production of porcelain teeth soon thereafter, in 1825. Ash further developed an improved porcelain tooth in England around 1837.

Evans (1836) refined the method of making accurate measurements in the mouth. However, it was not until 1839 that Charles Goodyear's invention of a low-cost vulcanized rubber allowed dentures to be molded accurately to fit the mouth. Vulcanized rubber denture bases that held denture teeth accelerated the demand for accurately fitting dentures at a reasonably low cost. Since 1839, denture bases have advanced in quality through the use of acrylic resins and cast metals. In 1935, polymerized acrylic resin was introduced as a denture base material to support artificial teeth.

Up to this point, we have focused primarily on the historical evolution of direct filling materials and some rather crude indirect materials. Prior to the 20th century, because of inadequate technology and lack of electricity, fillings were of rather poor quality and did not fit well within the teeth. However, in 1907, Taggart developed a more refined method for producing cast inlays using the lost wax technique. Cast alloys were introduced later in the 20th century, further developing this technology. Commercially pure titanium, noble alloys, and base metal alloys of nickel–chromium, cobalt–chromium, or cobalt–nickel–chromium are now available for use in the production of cast inlays, onlays, crowns, and frameworks for fixed all-metal or metal-ceramic dentures and for removable dentures. Few major improvements in the construction of multiple-unit fixed dental prostheses (FDPs; bridges) occurred until the early 1900s. Mason developed a detachable facing to a crown to hold an artificial tooth in place for an adjacent missing tooth. Thomas Steele (1904), a colleague of Mason, introduced interchangeable facings, which solved the problem of fractured facings.

Even though the practice of dentistry antedates the Christian era, comparatively little historical data exist on the science of dental materials. The use of fluoride to prevent tooth demineralization originated from observations in 1915 of low decay rates among people in areas of Colorado whose water supplies contained significant concentrations of fluoride. Controlled water fluoridation (1 ppm) to reduce tooth decay (demineralization) began in 1944, and the incidence of tooth decay in children who had access to fluoridated water has decreased by 50% since then. The use of pit and fissure sealants and fluoride-releasing varnishes and restorative materials has reduced the caries incidence even further.

Little scientific information about dental restorative materials has been available until recently. Prior to this knowledge, the use of these materials was entirely an art, and the only testing laboratory was the mouth of the patient. Today, despite the availability of sophisticated technical equipment and the development of standardized testing methods for evaluating the biocompatibility of preventive and restorative materials, this testing still sometimes occurs in the mouths of patients. The reasons for this situation are diverse. In some instances, products are approved for human use without being tested in animal or human subjects. In other instances, dentists use materials for purposes that were not indicated by the manufacturer; for example, a ceramic product may be used for posterior FDPs when the product has been recommended only for inlays, onlays, crowns, and anterior three-unit FDPs.

The first significant scientific interest arose during the middle of the 19th century, when research studies on amalgam began. At about the same time, some reports appeared in the literature of studies on porcelain and gold foil. These sporadic advances in knowledge finally culminated in the investigations of G.V. Black, who began his research studies in 1895. Hardly a phase of dentistry exists that was not explored and advanced by this pioneer in restorative dentistry.

Categories of Dental Materials

Dental materials may be fabricated using any of the four classes of materials: Metals, ceramics, polymers, or composites (Chapter 2). From the viewpoint of intended applications, they are classified as preventive, restorative, and auxiliary (Table 1.1).

Preventive Materials

Preventive dental materials usually include polymer-based materials that seal susceptible surfaces of the tooth (i.e., pits and fissures)

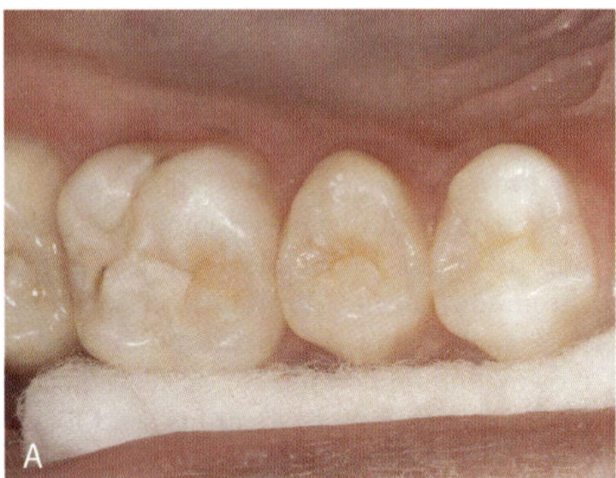
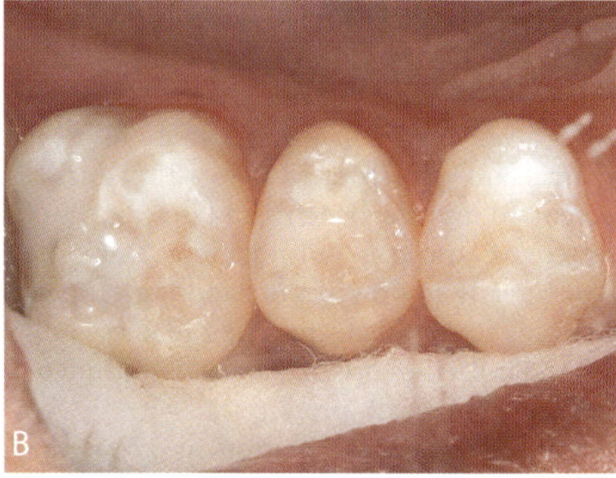

• **Fig. 1.10** Preventive sealant. **(A)** One sealant *(dashed white arrow)* that needs repair and an area of a deep groove planned to receive sealant *(pointer)*. **(B)** Sealant repaired a new one placed.

against caries (Fig. 1.10A and B) and/or release fluoride or other therapeutic agents to prevent or inhibit the progression of tooth decay (dental caries). The service life of restorative materials may be limited to a short-term application (up to several months) or moderately long time periods (1−4 years) when they are used to release therapeutic agents. This is because either the materials deteriorate as they release the therapeutic agents, or they lose their preventive capability as the release rates fall below the therapeutic limit.

Restorative Materials

After successful treatment of the disease and removal of the infected tissue, the obvious loss of the tooth structure needs restoration. Depending on the amount of tooth structure loss, the restoration can be a filling, inlay/onlay, full crown, bridge, implant, or denture.

Restorative dental materials consist of synthetic components that are used to repair or replace tooth structure. They are grouped by composition, specific function, the type of tooth structure they are replacing, or method of fabrication. This section focuses on the method of fabrication, which is classified into direct and indirect restorative materials. However, a temporary restoration is often needed before the final definitive restorations are delivered, especially for indirect restorations.

Direct Restorative Materials

Direct restorative materials are a group of materials placed directly into a designed tooth preparation that go through a phase transformation from a flowable or moldable state to a functional, solid state while they are being adapted to the preparation. Pure gold in foil form, for example, can be used to make dental restorations ("fillings") directly on the teeth, but this technique is rarely used today (Chapter 9). Amalgam alloy is a metallic powder containing silver, tin, and copper, which generates a condensable (moldable) mixture that allows placement and carving at the intraoral temperature within a reasonable working time when mixed with mercury. Once this mixture hardens, the solid exhibits enough strength to perform duties as a tooth-replacement material (Chapter 8).

In a similar way, glass or ceramic particles of different sizes (micron to nano), shapes, and compositions are incorporated into a variety of liquid monomers to generate the so-called resin-based composite materials. As a result, composite materials of different viscosities and compositions are formulated. Clinically, this group of materials can be transformed from moldable to a solid state within a short period of time when two components are mixed or when a single component, as received, is exposed to a high-intensity blue light (Fig. 1.11). The mechanism of transformation of the former is called *chemical polymerization,* and the latter is called *photopolymerization,* giving dental practitioners timeless control when manipulating, inserting, or sculpting the material intraorally (Chapter 5). One unique aspect that characterizes these materials is their capacity to micromechanically adhere to the teeth and other dental material substrates via bonding mechanisms. This aspect fostered the concept of minimally invasive dentistry. Their capacity to mimic or reproduce tooth color is highly relevant.

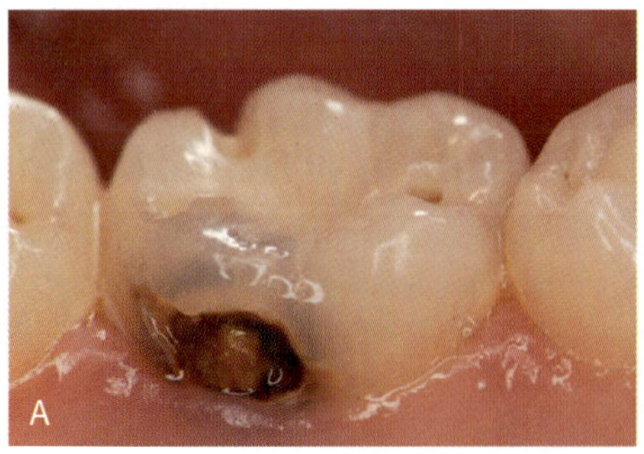
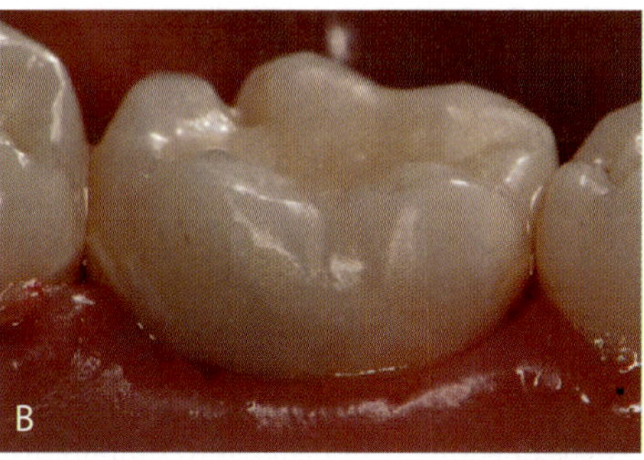

• **Fig. 1.11** Direct composite restoration. **(A)** An active/arrested carious lesion at the lingual surface on a lower molar tooth. **(B)** After surgical removal of the infected carious tissues, a direct restorative material was placed.

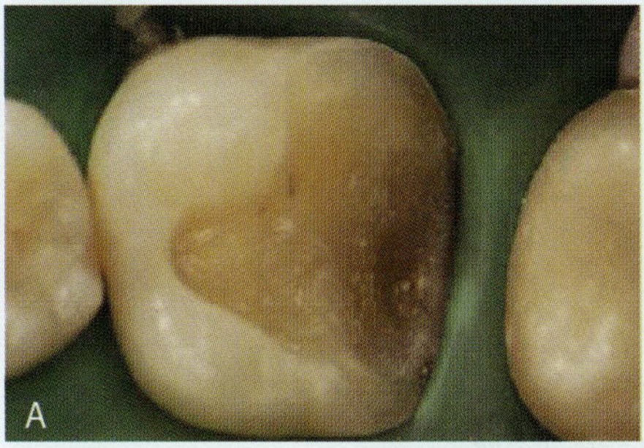

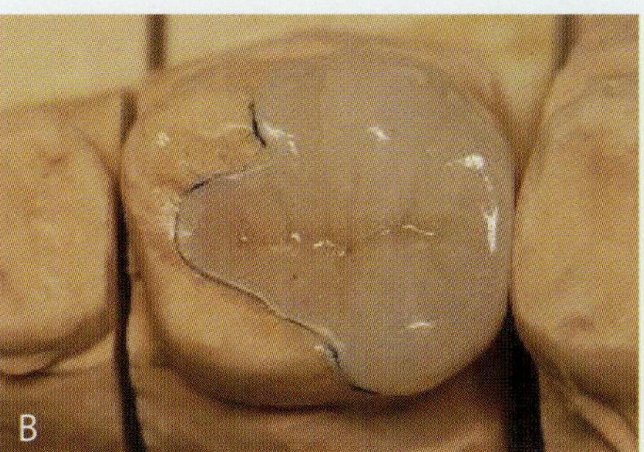

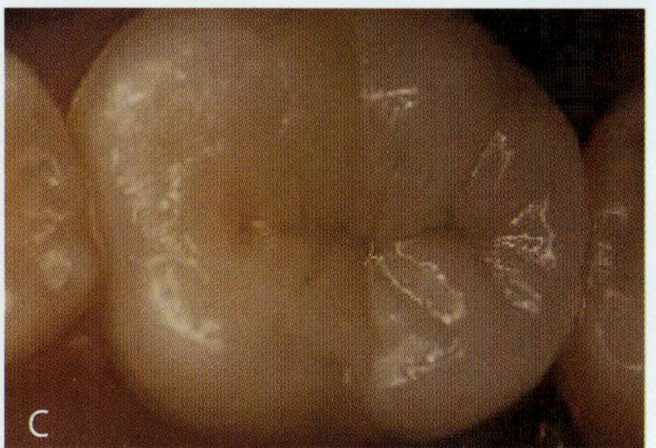

• **Fig. 1.12** Indirect ceramic restoration. **(A)** Tooth preparation isolated with rubber dam. **(B)** Indirect ceramic restoration made and adapted to a stone cast. **(C)** Clinical view of the tooth/ceramic assembly after finishing the adhesive luting steps. (Courtesy: Dr Karine Barizon.)

Indirect Restorative Materials

During their assembly, some restorations and prostheses undergo intra- and extraoral steps before placement in the oral cavity (Fig. 1.12A and B). These materials and techniques are meant to replace large areas of lost tooth structure, in addition to actual teeth. They are generally called *indirect restorative materials* and can be fixed by cementation (Fig. 1.12C) or remain removable, like a partial denture held by friction (Fig. 1.13), or a complete denture (Fig. 1.14), which is held to soft tissue by wetting. The issue of wetting is discussed in Chapter 2.

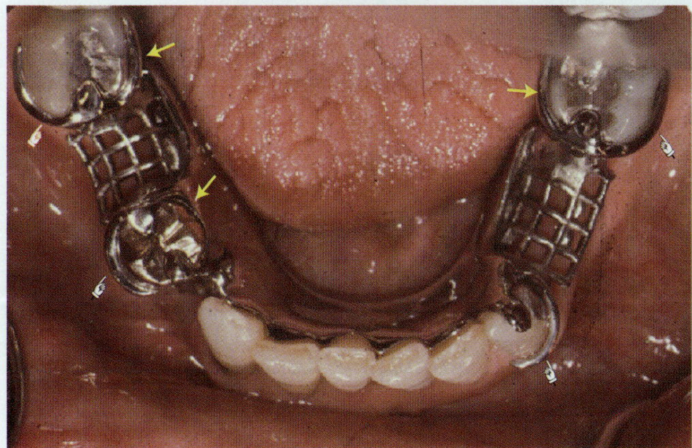

• **Fig. 1.13** A removable partial denture framework in place. The pointers indicate the retentive clasps, and the arrows indicate the reciprocal clasps. The wire mesh area between teeth provides sites for retaining artificial teeth with tissue-colored denture resin.

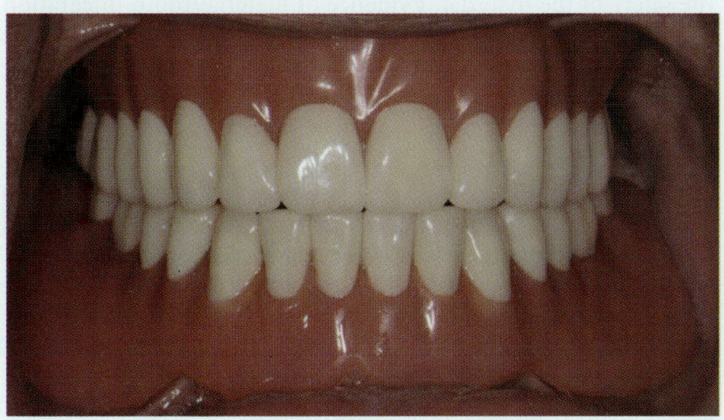

• **Fig. 1.14** A set of complete removable dentures.

Metals and alloys, because of their mechanical properties, have been used for making indirect dental prosthetic restorations that include inlays/onlays, crowns and bridges, removable partial frameworks, and implants. A metal-ceramic or porcelain fused to metal (PFM) system is one in which esthetic ceramics are fused with metal substrates, where the metal functions as a coping, supporting substructure (Fig. 1.15A). This allows the combination of metal's strength and ceramic's esthetics. Metals are crucial components of corrective orthodontic devices, helpful when aligning crooked teeth, and are used as a base for the placement of artificial plastic and ceramic teeth (partial denture framework) and for retentive features (clasps) in partial denture frameworks (Fig. 1.13).

Ceramics, because of their esthetic appearance, have also been used to restore lost tooth structure partially (inlays/onlays) or completely (crowns) or to completely replace a missing tooth or teeth (multiple-unit FDPs or bridges). However, because of the need for high fracture resistance and esthetic appeal, ceramic prostheses are constructed in multiple layers. The ceramic–ceramic or all-ceramic structure is similar to that shown in Figure 1.15B, except that the metal coping is replaced with a thicker and tougher ceramic core and one or two thin layers of translucent veneering esthetic ceramic (Chapter 10).

Temporary and Provisional Restorative Materials

Temporary restorative materials, also known as *provisional restorative materials,* are products used for dental restorations that are not intended for moderate- or long-term applications. Indirect prostheses can take some time to be created and delivered, so temporary restorations are applied to protect the prepared tooth by covering any enamel, dentin, or pulp exposed to the buccal environment. These provisional restorations enable patients to speak and eat normally. Examples include cements for luting provisional prosthetic restorations; other restoratives used for fillings; orthodontic wires; and acrylic resins used when making provisional inlays, onlays, crowns, and FDPs that span two or more tooth positions. Depending on the dental procedures needed, a temporary/provisional restoration may be in service for several months and up to a year (Fig. 1.16A and B).

Auxiliary Materials

Several different substances are needed to fabricate dental prostheses, appliances, and direct restorations. These substances, however, do not constitute part of these devices or restorations and, as a result, are called *auxiliary materials.* Among these are impression-making materials, gypsum cast materials to make dies, dental waxes to make wax patterns (Fig. 1.17) (Chapter 13), investments

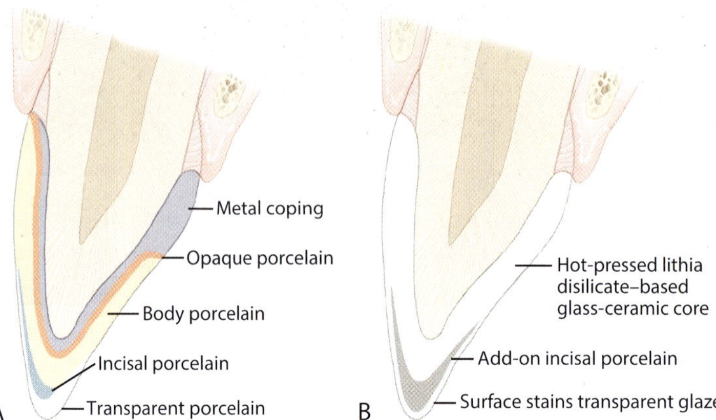

• **Fig. 1.15** Schematic illustration of two crown prostheses. **(A)** A metal-ceramic crown. The gray region is the metal coping. The remaining color regions represent various types of ceramics used to render esthetic appearance. **(B)** A lithium disilicate all-ceramic crown. The thin metal coping is replaced with a thick ceramic core, and the multilayer ceramics are replaced with incisal porcelain.

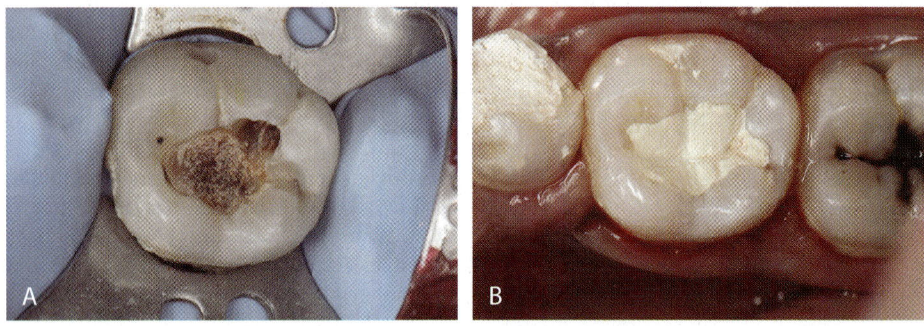

• **Fig. 1.16** (A) Caries excavation completed in a deep carious lesion and an interim restoration will be placed to induce remineralization of dentin. (B) Interim restoration completed with bioactive material to seal the activity and encourage remineralization.

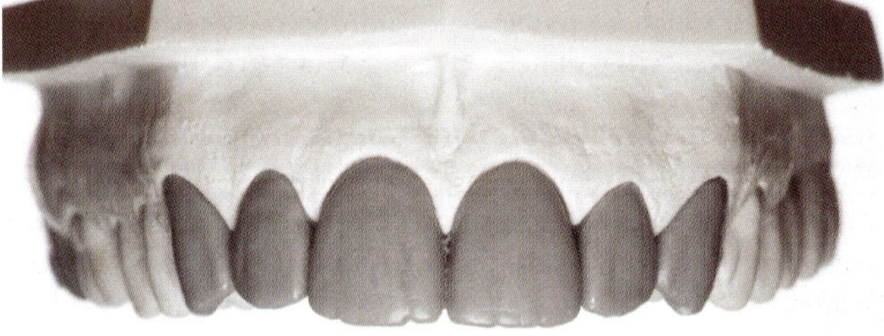

• **Fig. 1.17** Wax-up of anterior teeth on a gypsum cast. This approach is an important step in the decision-making process between the patient and the clinician for the esthetic outcome and surface stains.

for metal casting (Chapter 14), and finishing and polishing abrasives for shaping and esthetics (Chapter 16). Additional materials are used in the auxiliary capacity but are not discussed as auxiliary materials in this book, such as plastic matrix for composites (Chapter 5), acid-etching solutions for enhancing bonding of direct restorations (Chapter 6), metal matrix for amalgam (Chapter 8), and acrylic resins used to make customized impressions and bleaching trays (Chapter 11).

Challenges of Dental Materials in the Oral Cavity

The overriding goal of dentistry is to maintain or improve the quality of life of the patient. This goal can be met by preventing disease, relieving pain, improving the efficiency of mastication, enhancing speech, and improving appearance after tooth and bone loss. However, dental restorations and appliances, compared with the natural dentition, endure additional challenges to withstand the oral environment. For example, as a replacement or addition to the tooth structure, they need to be retained in place. A strong and durable tooth/material interphase is desirable. They should resist repeated loading during occlusion. Both factors dictate the longevity of the restoration. They should be manipulated following very specific instructions in order to ensure their intraoral performance. The patient's acceptance of the restoration is determined by the esthetic appearance, cost, and the safety of the material. Evidence of material/tooth integration through the formation of hydroxyapatite also brings the possible need for tissue repair. These aspects are discussed in the following sections.

CRITICAL QUESTION

Retention of restorations can be achieved by mechanical or adhesive means; what are the advantages and disadvantages of these approaches?

Retention of Restorations

Retention, that is, the action of absorbing and continuing to hold a substance or material, is a highly relevant interfacial mechanism.

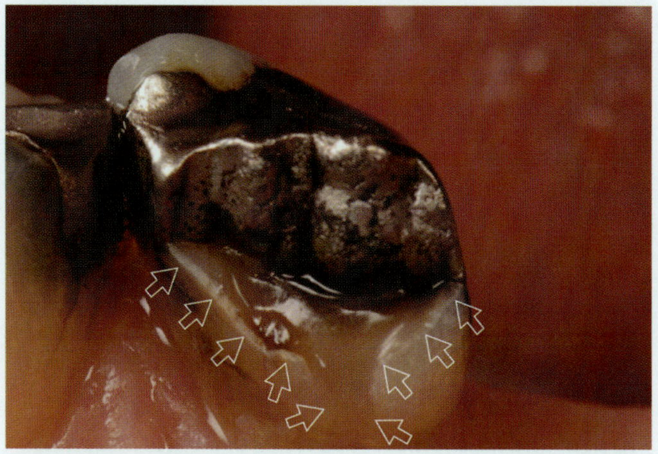

• **Fig. 1.18** Fracture of the buccal cusp of a lower first premolar with an extensive intraorally serviced amalgam restoration. Open arrows delineate the area of fracture. Even though the amalgam remained firmly retained by the remaining tooth structure without the support of the lost cusp, it is considered a failed restoration and needs replacement.

Enamel and dentin, for instance, are two different biological materials held together by a graded interphase varying smoothly between the two adherent phases. Restorative materials must be secured to their intended location to be functional. However, there was no similar interphase available to hold restorative materials to the tooth structure in the beginning of dentistry.

The early approach was to remove the tooth structure, mainly to provide a location for macromechanical retention and create resistance to dislodgement of the restorations. The drawback with this approach is the common clinical observation of cusp fractures resulting from structural flaws of the tooth structure left by the surgical removal of decayed tissue (Fig. 1.18), tooth pain caused by dentin hypersensitivity, and root canal therapy to remove hyperemic or necrotic pulp. Although restorations were retained satisfactorily by mechanical means, the nonadhesive dental materials of the time often left a discontinuity between the mechanically prepared surface and the restorative material used, which could lead to new carious lesions and pulp pathologies. This scenario led to the development of several pulp-protective philosophies and materials aimed at minimizing the penetration of bacteria and their by-products into the pulp, in addition to thermal insulation.

The acid-etching of enamel, combined with fluid resinous materials adopted in the 1950s, marked the first step toward generating a continuous interphase between the restoration and tooth structure. Technically, the process merely transforms macromechanical to micromechanical retention, with minimal tooth reduction beyond the removal of decayed tissue. Much later, etching of dentin with the same agent was accepted, and our knowledge of the dentin surface structure after etching expanded. New strategies of bonding, along with the introduction of new materials, have brought the idea of generating a stable and strong tooth/restoration interphase one step closer. Although progress has been made, the durability of this interphase remains a challenge. Adhesion and bonding are discussed in Chapter 6.

Restoration Longevity in Terms of Mechanical Integrity

From both a patient's and a clinician's perspective, a restoration should last a lifetime. Although some materials are expected to last more than a lifetime, in a real-world scenario, the longevity of restorations is shorter than expected, especially for direct restorations. According to research, dentists spend more than 50% of their time replacing failed direct restorations. As a result, the longevity of dental biomaterials used in restorations is extremely relevant to the profession and to patients.

One of the major advances in the knowledge of dental materials and their manipulation began in 1919, when the US Army requested the National Bureau of Standards (now known as *the National Institute of Standards and Technology* [NIST]) to establish specifications for the evaluation and selection of dental amalgams for use in federal service. The dental profession enthusiastically received these specifications, and similar specifications were subsequently requested for other dental materials. In 1928, dental research at the National Bureau of Standards was taken over by the American Dental Association (ADA).

Standards for dental materials have been developed to aid producers, users, and consumers in the evaluation of the safety and effectiveness of dental products. The ADA's Standards Committee on Dental Products (SCDP) develops specifications for dental materials, oral hygiene products, infection-control products, dental equipment, and dental instruments. Many countries have a dental standards organization that is charged with the development of test standards to ensure product reliability and safety. In addition, TC 106 of the International Organization for Standardization (ISO) develops international standards. These international standards often require information about composition; information about physical properties, as obtained by standard test methods; biocompatibility data; and data covering every provision of the official specification.

From a material standpoint, meeting the specification for mechanical properties means the material possesses enough strength to withstand occlusal loading, but this does not guarantee durability. As mentioned earlier, the placement of dental materials, or restorations, over tooth structures leads to an interplay between solid materials and a series of linked and/or nonlinked, complex joints. The interfacial position at or within the tooth and the physical quality of the dental materials involved in this complex assembly have great effects on the longevity of the restoration. Other factors, such as the selection of materials, clinical indication, patient awareness of their oral hygiene, and manipulation of and compliance with the dental material manufacturer's guidelines, will undoubtedly affect the long-term clinical performance of the restorations. These aspects are discussed in more detail in the chapters following.

Esthetic Appearance

Another important objective of dentistry is to restore or improve esthetics—the color and appearance of natural dentition—such as teeth bleaching with whitening agents. In recent decades, esthetic considerations in restorative and prosthetic materials have increasingly gained greater emphasis, making the development of general-purpose, technique-insensitive, tooth-colored, and color-stable restorative materials a mainstream of dental materials research. Resin-based composite (Chapter 5) and ceramics (Chapter 10) are the two most notable examples.

Even though esthetic materials that mimic natural dentition in color, texture, and reflectance allow the clinician to achieve outstanding esthetic and functional results, they also require strong artistic abilities. For example, knowledge of the underlying scientific principles of color and other optical effects on the appearance of the restorative material is essential in order to master esthetic results. Additionally, effective communication among the clinician, technician, and patient is important to achieve the proposed goal and avoid unrealistic expectations.

Safety of Dental Materials

Standards for dental materials have been developed to aid producers, users, and consumers in the evaluation of the safety and effectiveness of dental products. As mentioned previously, national dentistry standards/specifications have been implemented by the ADA's SCDP, and international standards have been implemented by the ISO's TC 106. Manufacturers can choose between testing their materials according to either national or international standards. However, for a manufacturer to market its product in certain European countries, a European Conformity (CE) marking must be obtained based on the product's ability to meet one or more national or international standards for performance and quality. A CE marking indicates that the product complies with European guidelines for health, safety, and environmental protection legislation.

The existence of material evaluation standards does not prevent the manufacturing, marketing, purchase, or use of dental or medical devices that do not meet these standards. However, producers or marketers of products and devices are expected to meet the safety standards established for those products in the countries in which they are sold. Thus, a producer may be given premarket approval in the United States by the US Food and Drug Administration (FDA) to sell a dental device or restorative material without that product being tested by the ADA or any other agency to determine whether the product is in accordance with the material's specifications. Nevertheless, these agencies are becoming increasingly dependent on one another to ensure that all products marketed worldwide are safe and effective.

For a dental material to be used in the oral cavity, this material should be harmless to all oral tissues and contain no toxic, leachable, or diffusible substance that can be absorbed into the circulatory system, causing systemic toxic responses, including teratogenic or carcinogenic effects. The material must also be free of agents that could elicit sensitization or an allergic response in a sensitized patient. These are considered general characteristics of biocompatibility.

Because safety is relative, no dental device (including restorative materials) is completely safe. The selection and use of dental devices or materials assume that the benefits will far outweigh the known biological risks. However, there is always the possibility that a patient will experience adverse effects from dental treatment. The conceptual aspects of biocompatibility, with specific emphasis on the solid and liquid materials of greatest relevance to dentistry, are presented in Chapter 17.

Capability of Initiating Tissue Repair or Regeneration

Although restorative dental materials primarily focus on replacing missing tooth structure or missing teeth with synthetic materials, evidence shows that certain materials have triggered healing or repair of tooth structure. For example, fluoride ions released in slightly acidic conditions, along with calcium phosphate, can promote the formation of hydroxyapatite within demineralized enamel matrix or become incorporated into the crystal lattice as fluorapatite, resulting in a lower solubility of enamel. The newly formed hydroxyapatite, however, lacks the structure and mechanical properties of natural enamel. As a result, the challenge is to develop biomimetic approaches in re-creating the hierarchical structure on the surface of the damaged enamel. Another example is when there is deep cavitation where dental pulp exposure has occurred, and a pulp capping agent is used. The response of the pulp to these materials is a biological healing process leading to the formation of reparative dentin that protects the remaining healthy pulp.

Understanding the underlying mechanisms of this "natural healing" biological process enables the clinician to pharmacologically trigger this event for promoting reparative dentin formation. As restorative dentistry is gradually transforming toward biology-driven repair strategies, replacement, and regeneration, the goal is regeneration of the entire tooth. The current progress in regenerative dentistry is presented in Chapter 19.

Physical and Mechanical Properties of Dental Materials

The science of dental materials covers a broad range of terminology, composition, microstructure, and properties used to describe or predict the performance of preventive and restorative biomaterials. Of greatest importance is the potential of this information to predict clinical performance and to allow us to analyze the causes of structural degradation and failure of these materials when they no longer serve their intended functions.

Most properties of biomaterials can be grouped into one of the broadest categories, i.e., physical properties. This book has been designed to separate material properties into subcategories that allow a clearer visualization of the variables that are most likely to influence the success or failure of preventive and restorative dental materials.

- Chemical properties generally comprise the behavior of materials in a chemical environment with or without any other external influences.
- Mechanical properties are related primarily to the behavior of materials in response to externally applied forces or pressures.

Of course, in a clinical environment, the behavior of dental materials may be dependent on several variables simultaneously, but a general understanding of a material's performance will be controlled by our ability to differentiate primary from secondary factors or properties. Lists of the most relevant chemical, manufacturing, mechanical, optical, and thermal properties are presented below. Separate chapters are devoted to more detailed descriptions: Chapter 3, "Chemical and Physical Properties of Solids," and Chapter 4, "Mechanical Properties of Dental Solids." Because of the dramatic increase in the use of digital technology and computer-aided design/computer-aided manufacturing (CAD−CAM) technology, an entire chapter (Chapter 15) has been devoted to this (Chapter 15).

General Categories of Biomaterials Properties

Chemical properties and parameters

- Corrosion
- Hygroscopy
- Solubility
- pH sensitivity
- Reactivity
- Surface energy
- Surface tension

Properties of importance in manufacturing or finishing processes

- Castability

TABLE 1.1 Comparative Applications and Durability of Preventive and Restorative Dental Materials

Material Type	Applications of Products	Potential Preventive Benefits	Durability
Resin adhesive	A	F (certain products)	M
Resin sealant	S	S	M
Resin cement	L	F (certain products)	M
Compomer	B, L, R	F	M
Hybrid ionomer	B, L, R	F	M
Glass ionomer (GI)	A, B, L, R, S	F, S	L, M
Metal-modified GI	R	F	L, M
Zinc oxide–eugenol	B, L, T	—	L, M
Zinc phosphate	B, L	—	M
Zinc polycarboxylate	B, L	—	M
Zinc silicophosphate	B, L	F	M
Resin composite	R	F (certain products)	H
Dental amalgam	R	—	H
Ceramic	R	—	H
Metal-ceramic	R	—	H
Metal-resin	R	—	M, H
Temporary acrylic resin	T	—	L
Denture acrylic	R	—	H
Cast metal	R	—	H
Wrought metal	R	—	H

Applications: A, adhesive; B, base; L, luting agent; S, pit/fissure sealant; R, restorative; T, temporary restorative.
Potential preventive benefit: F, fluoride-releasing material; S, sealing agent.
Durability: L, low; M, moderate; H, high.

Brittleness
Creep resistance
Hardness
Melting temperature or melting temperature range
Flowability under hot isostatic pressing (HIP) temperature and pressure conditions
Machinability
Polishability

Mechanical properties

Brittleness
Compressive strength
Ductility
Elastic modulus
Fatigue strength
Fracture toughness
Hardness
Microtensile strength
Poisson's ratio
Proportional limit
Shear strength
Tensile strength
Work or stain hardening
Yield strength

Optical properties and parameters

Absorptivity
Color
Fluorescence
Luminescence
Opacity
Photosensitivity
Reflectivity
Refractive index
Translucency
Transmittance

Thermal properties and parameters

Coefficient of thermal expansion or contraction
Eutectic temperature
Fusion temperature
Glass transition temperature
Heat of vaporization
Heat of fusion
Liquidus temperature
Melting point
Softening point
Solidus temperature
Specific heat
Thermal conductivity
Thermal diffusivity
Vapor pressure
Viscosity

Physical Properties

A physical property is any measurable parameter that describes the state of a physical system. The changes in the physical properties of a biomaterial can serve to describe the changes or transformations of the material when it has been subjected to external influences such as force, pressure, temperature, or light. Because these properties may include other properties listed above, a more detailed description of their characteristics is presented in Chapter 3, "Chemical and Physical Properties of Solids." In contrast to physical properties, chemical properties define the ways in which a material behaves during a chemical reaction or in a chemical environment.

Several properties listed above may fall into more than one category. For example, the optical properties can simply be grouped under physical properties. However, because of the importance of esthetics in dentistry, optical properties have been placed in a separate category. There are many other properties to be considered in a dental setting. However, this book focuses on those most relevant to the biomaterials and auxiliary materials designed for use in dental clinics and dental laboratories.

Applications of Dental Materials

The directions taken by the dental profession will affect the future of dental materials, although the practice of dentistry will depend on current and future developments in dental materials science. Dentistry will continue to focus on the preservation and enhancement of oral health through the prevention of caries and periodontal disease and the rehabilitation of missing, damaged, and/or destroyed hard and soft tissues. A cure for dental caries will have a dramatic impact on the use of **restorative materials** to improve the form and function of teeth with cavitated lesions. The need to restore teeth will always exist because of the time-dependent failure or degradation of restorative materials and oral tissues. The decision on which biomaterials to use for a given clinical situation will be controlled by the known benefits of each choice compared with the known risks. There has been a conscious change toward a preventative, minimally invasive approach to dentistry with an increasing use of bioactive materials.

Why Do Dental Students, Dentists, and Dental Educators Need to Understand the Principles of Dental Materials Science?s

Dentists and engineers have similar long-range objectives in their professions—that is, to design, construct, and evaluate devices or structures that can be subjected to a wide range of environmental conditions. In 1936, E.W. Skinner described the need for the principles of physics and chemistry to be applied in restorative dentistry in a similar manner as they were applied to structural engineering.

Although many technological advances have been proposed since 1936 to improve the quality of dental materials used in dentistry, a challenge remains for end users to critically evaluate the claims made on the reported performance of dental materials and to relate these claims carefully to well-established physical principles for the specific classes of materials. The current era of evidence-based dentistry is consistent with this need to understand cause-and-effect relationships that allow us to predict with reasonable certainty the time-dependent behavior of preventive, restorative, and auxiliary materials.

The Future Need for Dental Biomaterials

Future developments in dentistry and the need for optimal oral health care will dictate the future of dental materials science. Dentistry will continue to focus on the preservation and enhancement of oral health through the prevention of caries, periodontal disease, and their sequelae and the rehabilitation of missing, damaged, or destroyed hard and soft tissues. A cure for dental caries will have a dramatic impact on the use of restorative materials to restore form and function to teeth with cavitated lesions. However, there will still exist a continuous need to repair or restore time-dependent failure or degradation of restorations and a need for the treatment of noncarious-related issues. As a result, deciding which materials to use for a given clinical condition or situation will depend on the known benefits of each treatment choice compared with the known risks.

Because a cure for caries and the development of processes for root or tooth regeneration are probably several decades away, most of the restorative materials employed today will likely remain in use for the foreseeable future. Materials like dental amalgam (Chapter 8), for example, have made reliable restorations for centuries. The use of amalgam has been declining rapidly, not because there are more durable and technique-insensitive restorative materials available in the market but because of concerns regarding the impact of mercury release into the environment. Furthermore, the world has moved into an era of high esthetic demand at the expense of durability and cost. In contrast to the treatment for dental caries, the demand for esthetic enhancement will continue well into the future. Development and research for direct restorative biomaterials that are less technique-sensitive, especially the existing esthetic resin-based composite brands, still have great room for improvement. In addition, strategies that aim to increase the hardness, toughness and resistance to wear, and impact of these materials is relevant to the field. An interesting approach relies on creating composites with tailored microstructures, or bio-inspired platelet-reinforced composites created by magnetic manipulation of alumina platelets.

The benefits of caries prevention have led to a reduction in the need for complete and removable dentures. Minimally invasive concepts have led to the sealing of defective or leaking restorations with preventive resins rather than continuing to use more destructive replacement procedures. Thus, the development of effective bio-inspired remineralizing agents for acid-damaged enamel and dentin repair and the development of smart materials that lead to self-repair of defective joints or of a material's internal flaws, as well as dental pulp regeneration, will be critical challenges to the future of dental materials. In addition, the need for replacement of restorations should decrease over the next several decades, in lieu of the minimally invasive philosophy. However, this reduction will be offset by the increased demand for esthetic restorations (discussed in Chapter 19).

CRITICAL QUESTION

Which factors determine when dental material products become obsolete?

Technology has advanced tremendously over the past 40 years, resulting in innovations such as laser applications, imaging procedures, three-dimensional (3D) printing technology, low-shrinkage composites, smart ceramics, and minimally invasive dental procedures, which have generated benefits for several fields. CAD−CAM technology for making indirect restorations, for example, has reduced the demand for both impression materials and some indirect auxiliary materials that were used by laboratory technicians to fabricate indirect prostheses (discussed in Chapter 15).

Subsequently, one question has accompanied the dental profession for centuries: When does a restorative material become obsolete? For example, silicate cement (Chapter 7) was used to restore anterior esthetic restorations because the color perception resembled tooth structure, and there was a serendipitous ability to release fluoride. Although the latter is beneficial in preventing recurrent caries, fluoride release occurs at the expense of surface degradation, discoloration, and marginal breakdown over time, resulting in defective and stained margins (Fig. 1.19) and loss of anatomical contour. Furthermore, more durable resin-based composites and improved micromechanical bonding procedures made silicate cements virtually obsolete by the mid-1970s.

Therefore we can conclude that some restorative materials became obsolete for the following reasons: (1) Their drawbacks overall far outweighed their known advantages; (2) material degradation led to undesirable margin adaptation and esthetics; (3) metallic appearance was generally unacceptable to patients; (4) alternative restoratives exhibit superior performance, mimic the physiology of the tooth, and are less technique-sensitive; (5) alternative materials led to cheaper treatment for patients; and/or (6) improvements in material microstructure occur as a result of technological advances. In short, restorative materials become obsolete when an alternative material is able to provide a better balance among all the previously mentioned diverse requirements and expectations.

Organization of the Book

In 1936, Dr Skinner, the author of the first edition of this book, expressed significant concerns regarding the need for knowledge of dental materials

> *Unfortunately, there are too many unscrupulous dental manufacturers who make impossible claims for inferior products, thus deceiving the dentist. There have been actual cases of highly advertised dental materials, which have been made extremely popular among dentists simply by clever advertising methods, whereas careful laboratory tests have shown products to be distinctly inferior. The well-informed dentist will be able to discriminate between fact and propaganda and will refuse to be duped in this manner.*

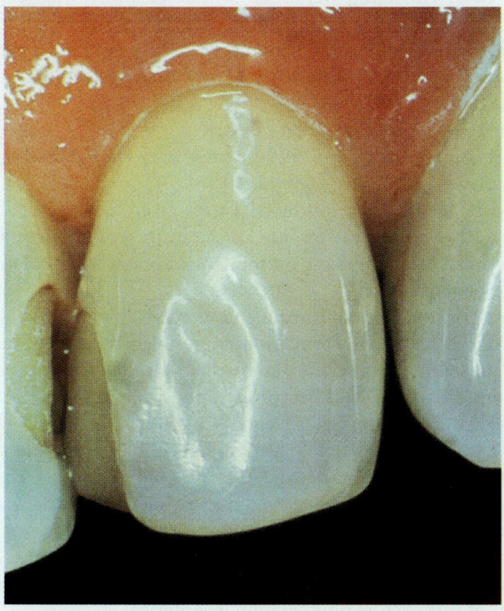

• **Fig. 1.19** Anterior class III silicate cement restorations exhibiting severe surface degradation, marginal staining, and general discoloration.

He emphasized the need for the principles of physics and chemistry to be applied in restorative dentistry in a similar manner as they were applied to structural engineering. The current era of evidence-based dentistry is consistent with our aims of presenting fundamental principles of materials and understanding cause-and-effect relationships that allow us to predict, with reasonable certainty, the time-dependent behavior of dental materials.

To achieve these aims, this book is organized into five parts: (I) General Classes and Properties of Dental Materials; (II) Direct Restorative Materials; (III) Indirect Restorative and Prosthetic Materials; (IV) Fabrication of Prostheses; and (V) Assessing Dental Restorations.

Following the overview of dental materials in this chapter, Part I focuses on the structure and properties of materials. Chapter 2 explains how the molecular or crystalline structure determines the classes of materials and renders each class its unique properties. This chapter also discusses the origin of adhesion, an important feature of dental restorations. Chapter 3 discusses the physical and chemical properties relevant to dental applications, and Chapter 4 examines the mechanical properties of dental materials.

The chapters in Part II focus on direct restorative materials, including resin-based composites (Chapter 5), bonding agents (Chapter 6), dental cements (Chapter 7), and metallic restorations (Chapter 8). As stated earlier, these materials share the same feature of being manipulated chairside and applied to the oral cavity before they reach their full functional state. Therefore, preventive materials are discussed with direct restorative materials.

The chapters in Part III discuss the use of indirect restorative materials, such as dental casting alloys and wrought metals (Chapter 9), ceramic-based materials (Chapter 10), denture base resins (Chapter 11), and dental implants (Chapter 12).

Chapters 13 through 16 in Part IV describe the materials and technologies needed to fabricate indirect prostheses. Chapter 13 discusses auxiliary materials, which include impression materials, gypsum products, and dental waxes, which are used to fabricate the wax patterns needed for final prostheses. The process of making metal castings using the lost wax method is discussed in Chapter 14, and Chapter 15 discusses the use of digital technology for making dental prostheses without using traditional auxiliary materials but instead relying on digital imaging and CAD−CAM technology. Finally, all restorations, direct or indirect, require certain degrees of surface modification to improve their clinical performance. The procedures and the essential instruments used for finishing and polishing restorations are discussed in Chapter 16.

The goal of dentistry is to maintain or improve the quality of life of the patient. The restorations involved must prevent disease, relieve pain, improve the efficiency of mastication, enhance speech, improve appearance, and most importantly, last for a long time. Part V aims to address the question of how we assess restorations. As stated, all materials undergo some sort of interaction with the oral tissue. The biological considerations, known as *biocompatibility,* are covered in Chapter 17. Clinical evaluations of a dental restoration represent a different level of assessment for restorations. Chapter 18 discusses the components of clinical studies, using one to illustrate how variables can be collected from the study. Finally, although new materials that address the particular needs of restorative dentistry are emerging and alternative treatment philosophies are being adopted, the advancement of new technologies in other disciplines has benefited dental materials science in a variety of ways. Chapter 19 analyzes potential future technologies in dentistry and describes both recently emerged technologies and those anticipated in the coming decades.

Acknowledgment

The authors acknowledge Dr Kenneth J. Anusavice for his contribution to the earlier editions of this chapter.

Summary

- Dentists must select a material, or materials, for either direct or indirect applications aiming to restore the patient's intraoral functions.
- Properties of materials can be categorized into chemical and physical properties.
- Chemical properties are generally composed of the composition and behavior of materials in a chemical environment, regardless of any interaction with other external influences.
- Physical properties are measurable variables that describe how an object looks, feels, or acts when the object is probed by external agents, such as heat, light, moisture, or force.
- Dental materials may be fabricated by using any of the four classes of materials: Metals, ceramics, polymers, or composites.
- From the viewpoint of intended applications, they are classified as preventive, restorative, and auxiliary.
- Newer innovations such as laser applications, imaging procedures, three-dimensional (3D) printing technology, low-shrinkage composites, smart ceramics, and minimally invasive dental procedures, have generated benefits for several fields.

Selected Readings

ADA Standards Committee on Dental Products (ADA SCDP) ADA, website: http://www.ada.org/280.aspx; This website provides details on ANSI/ADA specifications for dental materials, instruments, and equipment and the working groups of the ADA Standards Committee on Dental Products.

Borcic J, Anic I, Urek MM, *et al:* The prevalence of non-carious cervical lesions in permanent dentition. *J Oral Rehabil* 31:117-123, 2004.

Coleman R.L. Physical Properties of Dental Materials (Gold alloys and accessory materials). Research Paper No. 32 US Government Printing Office: Washington, DC; This publication represents the first major effort to relate the physical properties of dental materials to the clinical situation. The American Dental Association specification program was established based on this historical review of the philosophy and the content of the facility created at the National Bureau of Standards.

Erb RM, Libanori R, Rothfuchs N, *et al:* Composites reinforced in three dimensions by using low magnetic fields. *Science* 335:199-204, 2012.

Federal Register: Medical Devices; Dental Device Classification; Final Rule and Withdrawal of Proposed Rules, 1987, 30082; A listing of the dental materials and devices classified in Category III by the Food and Drug Administration as of that date.

Food and Drug Administration (FDA), website: http://www.fda.gov

FDA Center for Devices and Radiological Health, website: http://www.fda.gov/cdrh/consumer/c-products.shtml

Gallo M.A.; Doull J. History and scope of toxicology. In: Casarett and Doull's Toxicology. Pergamon Press: New York, pp. 3–11.

Hensten-Pettersen A.; Jacobsen N. Perceived side effects of biomaterials in prosthetic dentistry. J Prosthet Dent 65 138 (1991).

International Organization for Standardization (ISO), website: http://www.iso.org

International Organization for Standardization (ISO) TC 106–Dentistry website: http://www.iso.org/iso/en/stdsdevelopment/techprog/workprog/TechnicalProgrammeTCDetailPage.TechnicalProgrammeTCDetail?COMMID=2916

He LH, Swain MV: Understanding the mechanical behaviour of human enamel from its structural and compositional characteristics. *J Mech Behav Biomed Mater* 1:18–29, 2008.

Hensten-Pettersen A, Jacobsen N: Perceived side effects of biomaterials in prosthetic dentistry. *J Prosthet Dent* 65:138-144, 1991.

Jäger I, Fratzl P: Mineralized collagen fibrils: A mechanical model with a staggered arrangement of mineral particles. *Biophys J* 79:1737–1746, 2000.

Kallus T.; Mjör I.A. Incidence of adverse effects of dental materials. Scand J Dent Res 99 236 (1991).

Klaassen C.D.; Eaton D.L. Principles of toxicology. In: Casarett and Doull's Toxicology. Pergamon Press: New York, pp. 12–49.

Munksgaard E.C. Toxicology versus allergy in restorative dentistry. In: Advances in Dental Research. International Association for Dental Research: Bethesda, pp. 17–21.

Phillips R.W. Changing trends of dental restorative materials. Dent Clin North Am 33 (2) 285 (1989); A review of the trends in biomaterials that are influencing dental restorative procedures, particularly in esthetic dentistry. Emphasis is on bonding technology and its application.

Additional References on Dental History

American Dental Association. 125th anniversary commemoration. J Am Dent Assoc 108 (4) 473–586 (1984).

Asbell M.B. Dentistry, a Historical Perspective. Torrence & Co: Bryn Mawr, PA; A historical account of the history of dentistry from ancient times, with emphasis on the United States from colonial times to the present period.

Bennion E. Antique Dental Instruments. Sotheby's Publishing: New York.

Black C.E.; Black B.M. From Pioneer to Scientist. Bruce Publishing: St. Paul, MN; The life story of Greene Vardiman Black, "Father of Modern Dentistry," and his son Arthur Davenport Black, late Dean of Northwestern University Dental School.

Carter W.J.; Graham-Carter J. Dental Collectibles and Antiques. ed 2 Dental Folklore Books: Bethany, OK.

Gardner P.H. Foley's Footnotes: A Treasury of Dentistry. Washington Square East Publishing: Wallingford, PA.

Glenner R.A.; Davis A.B.; Burns S.B. The American Dentist. Pictorial Histories Publishing: Missoula, MT; A pictorial history with a presentation of early dental photography in America.

Guerini V. A History of Dentistry, from the Most Ancient Times Until the End of the Eighteenth Century. Milford House: Pound Ridge, NY.

Hoffmann-Axthelm W. History of Dentistry. Quintessence Publishing: Chicago.

Koch C.R.E. History of Dental Surgery. National Art Publishing: Chicago.

Lobbezoo F, Ahlberg J, Raphael KG, *et al:* International consensus on the assessment of bruxism: Report of a work in progress. *J Oral Rehabil* 45:837-844, 2018.

Lufkin A.W. A History of Dentistry. Lea & Febiger: Philadelphia.

McCluggage R.W. A History of the American Dental Association, A Century of Health Service. American Dental Association: Chicago.

Munksgaard EC: Toxicology versus allergy in restorative dentistry. *Adv Dent Res* 6:17–21, 1992.

Nanci A: Ten Cate's oral histology: development, structure, and function. 9th ed. St. Louis, Elsevier, 2018.

Ring M.E. Dentistry: An Illustrated History. Harry N Abrams Inc: New York.

Souder W.H.; Peters C.G. An investigation of the physical properties of dental materials. Bur St Tech Paper (1920). 157, Dent Cos 62:305 (March).

Stock SR, Vieira AE, Delbem AC, *et al:* Synchrotron micro Computed Tomography of the mature bovine dentinoenamel junction. *J Struct Biol* 161:162-171, 2008.

Thompson VP, Watson TF, Marshall GW Jr, *et al: Outside-the-(cavity-prep)-box thinking. Adv Dent Res* 25:24-32, 2013.

Volponi1 AA, Zaugg LK, Neves V, *et al: Tooth Repair and Regeneration. Curr Oral Health Rep* 5:295–303, 2018.

Weinberger B.W. An Introduction to the History of Dentistry. Mosby: St Louis; Includes medical and dental chronology and bibliographic data (2 volumes).

Weinberger B.W. Pierre Fauchard, Surgeon-Dentist. Pierre Fauchard Academy: Minneapolis, MN; A brief account of the beginning of modern dentistry, the first dental textbook, and professional life 200 years ago.

Wynbrandt J. The Excruciating History of Dentistry: Toothsome Tales and Oral Oddities from Babylon to Braces. St Martin's Press: New York.

2

Structure of Matter, General Classes of Materials, and Principles of Adhesion

CHAPTER OUTLINE

KEY TERMS

Adhesion—A molecular or atomic attraction between two contacting surfaces promoted by the interfacial force of attraction between the molecules or atoms of two different species; adhesion may occur as chemical adhesion, mechanical adhesion (structural interlocking), or a combination of both.

Adhesive and adherend—Substance that promotes adhesion of one substance or material to another. An adherend is a material substrate bonded to another material by means of an adhesive.

Alloy and alloy system—An alloy is a crystalline solid with metallic properties that is composed of two or more chemical elements, at least one of which is a metal and all of which are mutually soluble in the molten state. Alloy systems are all possible alloyed combinations of two or more elements, at least one of which is a metal. For example, the binary gold–silver system includes all possible alloys of gold and silver, varying from 100% gold and 0% silver to 100% silver and 0% gold.

Bonding—The action of joining objects or particles together by means of adhesive or force of attraction.

Ceramic—Solid-phase compounds of metallic and nonmetallic elements.

Cohesion—Bonding between molecules or atoms of the same species.

Composite—A material made of two or more constituent components with significantly different physical or chemical properties that, when combined, produce a material with characteristics different from the individual components.

Contact angle—Angle of intersection between a liquid and a surface of a solid that is measured from the solid surface through the liquid to the liquid/vapor tangent line originating at the terminus of the liquid/solid interface; used as a measure of wettability, whereby no wetting occurs at a contact angle of 180° and complete wetting occurs at an angle of 0°.

Copolymer—Polymer made of two or more types of monomers. A *random copolymer* is when there is no sequential order of monomer types along the polymer chain. A *block copolymer* is when groups of each type of monomer appear in the same polymer chain. A *graft or branched copolymer* is when a sequence of one type of mer unit is grafted onto the backbone of a second type of monomer to form a branched structure.

Crosslink—A difunctional or multifunctional monomer that forms a link between two growing polymer chains during polymerization that results in a three-dimensional interconnected polymer network.

Curing—Chemical reaction in which low-molecular-weight monomers are converted into high-molecular-weight materials through polymerization to attain desired properties.

Elastic recovery—The shape of objects changes under an applied force. When the force is removed, the object will recover to its original shape instantly if it is an *elastic* solid, or the recovery process occurs over a period of time if it is a *viscoelastic* material. The greater the viscous nature of a material, the less complete the recovery.

Glass-transition temperature (Tg)—(1) The temperature above which a sharp increase in the thermal expansion coefficient occurs, indicating increased molecular mobility. (2) The temperature at which macromolecule molecular motion begins to force the polymer chains apart. Thus, polymeric materials soften when heated above this temperature.

Grain and grain boundary—A grain is a single crystal in the microstructure of a metal. Metals and alloys are solids consisting of many individual grains, and the interface between adjacent grains is the grain boundary.

Metal—(1) An element or alloy whose atoms readily lose electrons to form positively charged ions. (2) A metallic material composed of one or more chemical elements, which is opaque, ductile, relatively malleable, a good conductor of electricity, a good thermal conductor, and usually lustrous when light is reflected from its polished surface.

Microstructure—Structural features of a metal, including grains, grain boundaries, phases, and defects such as porosity, revealed by microscopic imaging of the chemically or electrolytically etched surface of a flat, polished specimen.

Micromechanical bonding—Mechanical adhesion associated with bonding of an adhesive to a roughened adherend surface.

Monomer and mer—A monomer is a chemical compound that is capable of reacting to form a polymer; each monomer becomes a *mer* of a polymer.

Phase and phase diagram (constitution diagram)—A graph of equilibrium phases and solubility limits for an alloy system as a function of composition and temperature.

Polymer—Large molecules (aka *macromolecules*) formed by the union of many simple repeating units (mers); the chemical process is known as *polymerization.*

Primary bond—Bonding between atoms that include ionic, covalent, and metallic bonds.

Resin or synthetic resin—Blend of monomers and/or macromolecules with other components, which form a material with a set of useful properties.

Solid solution (metallic)—A solid crystalline phase containing two or more elements, at least one of which is a metal and whose atoms share the same crystal lattice.

Strain—Magnitude of deformation (stretching, compression, or shear) occurring in response to an applied force.

Stress—The perpendicularly directed force, exerted as pressure or tension, on a material that causes the object to deform (strain), measured in units of force per unit area.

Surface energy—The excess energy of attraction that the surface of a material (liquid and solid) has compared with the bulk of the material because molecules or atoms at the surface are not surrounded by their fellows as those in the bulk. It can be treated as the work (energy) required to build an area of a particular surface and has the unit of mN/m^2.

Surface tension—The tendency of fluid surfaces to contract to the smallest surface area by an inward force caused by the imbalance of mutual attraction between molecules on the liquid surface. The very inward force also keeps the molecules of the surface constantly under tension. The cohesive force keeping molecules bonded on the surface is known as the *surface tension* of the liquid, with the unit of mN/m.

Thermoplastic polymer—Macromolecule material made of linear and/or branched chains, which softens when heated above the glass-transition temperature (Tg); it can then be molded to a new shape and cooled below the Tg to retain the new configuration.

Thermoset polymer—Polymeric material that retains a crosslinked structure during polymerization; the acquired structure results in a rigid polymer that, upon heating, does not soften enough to be molded to a new configuration.

van der Waals forces—Short-range force of physical attraction that promotes adhesion between molecules of liquids or molecular crystals; also known as *secondary bond.*

Wetting and wetting agent—Wetting is the ability of a liquid to maintain contact with a solid surface; it reflects the intermolecular interactions when the two are brought in intimate contact. A wetting agent is a surface-active substance that can be applied to a solid substrate to reduce the surface tension of the liquid to be placed on the solid; the purpose is to promote wetting or adhesion.

CRITICAL QUESTION

When the state of material (vapor, liquid, and solid) changes, what happens between atoms or molecules that make up the material?

Around 460 BCE, the Greek philosopher Democritus proposed that all matter was composed of indivisible particles called *átomos* (*á* = "un"; *temno* = "to cut"; meaning "uncuttable"), which is the origin of the name *atoms*. We know that an atom consists of a nucleus surrounded by a cloud of negatively charged electrons, as depicted in the electron cloud model of an atom (Fig. 2.1). Except for the hydrogen atom, where there are no neutrons, the nucleus contains a mix of positively charged protons and electrically neutral neutrons. The electrons of an atom exist in different clouds at various energy levels. An atom becomes a negative ion when it gains electron(s) and a positive ion when it loses electron(s).

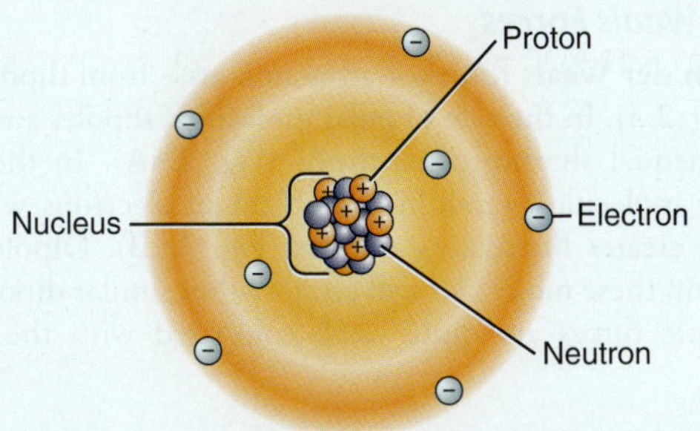

• **Fig. 2.1** Electron cloud model of an atom. The neutrons (blue spheres) and protons (spheres with "+") occupy a dense central region called the nucleus. The orange cloud formation illustrates the trace of electrons (spheres with "–") as they move around the nucleus.

Two or more atoms can form an electrically neutral entity called a molecule. Attraction between atoms and between molecules result in materials we can see and touch. Consider water as an example. Chemically, the basic unit of water is a molecule made of two hydrogen atoms and one oxygen atom. If each molecule attains a kinetic energy that is higher than the attraction between these molecules, they appear in vapor form. As the surrounding temperature decreases, the level of kinetic energy within individual molecules decreases and the attraction between them becomes more prominent, so that they condense to a liquid form. Further cooling yields a solid called ice, where the kinetic energy is so low that the molecules are immobilized by the attraction between them.

The transformation between vapor, liquid, and solid is called the change of state. A change from the solid to the liquid state will require additional energy—kinetic energy—to break loose from the force of attraction. This additional energy is called the **latent heat of fusion**. The temperature at which this change occurs is known as the **melting temperature** or fusion temperature. When water boils, energy is needed to transform the liquid to vapor, and this quantity of energy is known as the **heat of vaporization**. It is possible for some solids to change directly to a vapor by a process called sublimation as seen in dry ice; this, however, has no practical importance as far as dental materials are concerned.

CRITICAL QUESTION

Which types of primary bonds control the properties of dental resins and cast alloys?

Interatomic Bonds

The preceding brief focus on change of state raises a question concerning the types of forces holding these atoms and molecules together. The electronic structure of an atom is relatively stable if it has eight electrons in its outer valence shell, as noble gases do, except for helium, which has only two electrons. Other atoms must lose electrons to, acquire electrons from, or share electrons with yet other atoms to achieve a stable configuration—that is, eight electrons in the outer shell. These processes produce strong or primary bonds between atoms. The bonding of atoms within a molecule also creates new but much weaker forces holding the molecules together. These are often called secondary bonds.

Primary Bonds

The formation of primary bonds depends on the atomic structures and their tendency to assume a stable configuration. The strength of these bonds and their ability to re-form after breakage determine the physical properties of a material. Primary atomic bonds (Fig. 2.2), also called chemical bonds, may be of three different types:

1. Ionic
2. Covalent
3. Metallic

Ionic Bonds

The classic example of ionic bond is the bond between the Na^+ and Cl^- of sodium chloride (Fig. 2.2A). Because the sodium atom contains one valence electron in its outer shell and the chlorine atom has seven electrons in its outer shell, the transfer of the sodium valence electron to the chlorine atom results in the stable compound Na^+Cl^-. In dentistry, ionic bonding exists in some dental materials, such as in gypsum structures and phosphate-based cements.

Covalent Bonds

In many chemical compounds, two valence electrons are shared by adjacent atoms (Fig. 2.2B). By virtue of sharing electrons, the two atoms are held together by covalent bonds to form a molecule that is sufficiently stable, and electrically neutral in a definite arrangement. The hydrogen molecule, H_2, exemplifies covalent bonding. The single valence electron in each hydrogen atom is shared with that of the other combining atom, and the valence shells become stable. Covalent bonding occurs in many organic compounds, such as in dental resins, where they link to form the backbone structure of hydrocarbon chains (Chapter 6).

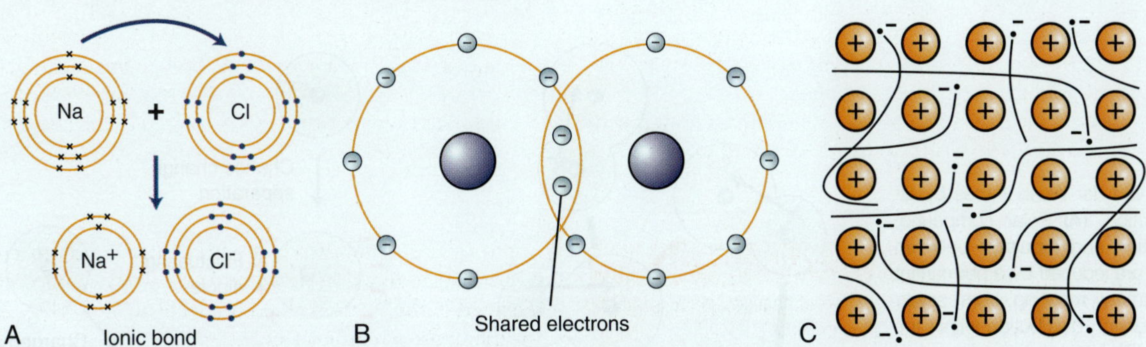

• **Fig. 2.2** Primary bonds. **(A)** Ionic bond, characterized by electron transfer from one element (Na) to another (Cl). **(B)** Covalent bond, characterized by electron sharing and very precise bond orientations. **(C)** Metallic bond, characterized by electron sharing and formation of a "cloud" of electrons that bonds to the positively charged nucleus in a lattice.

Metallic Bonds

The third type of primary atomic interaction is the **metallic bond** (Fig. 2.2C). The outer-shell valence electrons can be removed easily from metallic atoms and positive ions can be formed. The free valence electrons can move about in the metal space lattice (Chapter 4) to form what is sometimes described as an electron "cloud" or "gas." The electrostatic attraction between the electron cloud and the positive ions in the lattice provides the force that bonds the metal atoms together as a solid.

The free electrons give the metal its characteristically high thermal and electrical conductivity. These electrons absorb light energy, so that all metals are opaque to transmitted light. The metallic bonds are also responsible for the ability of metals to deform plastically. The free electrons can move through the lattice, whereas their plastic deformability is associated with slip along crystal planes. During slip deformation, electrons easily regroup to retain the cohesive nature of the metal.

Combination of Primary Bonds

Although we can describe the three primary bonds separately, it is also possible to find more than one type of primary bond existing in one material. Consider calcium sulfate ($CaSO_4$), the main ingredient of gypsum products (Chapter 13), as an example (Fig. 2.3). In the sulfate ion (SO_4^{2-}), the sulfur and oxygen atoms are held together covalently but they are short of two electrons. Calcium has two electrons in the outer orbit, which are easily removed and transferred to the SO_4. The result is a Ca^{2+} ion with attraction for an SO_4^{2-} ion.

CRITICAL QUESTION

Is hydrogen bonding controlled by a van der Waals force?

Secondary Bonds

In contrast with primary bonds, secondary bonds do not share electrons. Instead, charge variations among atomic groups of the molecule induce dipole forces that attract adjacent molecules or parts of a large molecule.

$$Ca^{2+}\left[O{=}S(=O)_2{-}O \right]^{2-}$$

• **Fig. 2.3** Combination of primary bonds. Ionic bond between Ca^{2+} and $[SO_4]^{2-}$, covalent bonds between S and O.

van der Waals Forces

These **van der Waals** forces of attraction arise from dipole attractions (Fig. 2.4). In the case of polar molecules, dipoles are induced by an unequal sharing of electrons (Fig. 2.4A). In the case of nonpolar molecules, random movement of electrons within the molecule creates fluctuating dipoles (Fig. 2.4B). Dipoles generated within these molecules will attract other similar dipoles. Such interatomic forces are quite weak compared with the primary bonds.

Hydrogen Bond

The hydrogen bond is a special case of dipole attraction of polar compounds. It can be understood by studying a water molecule (Fig. 2.5). Attached to the oxygen atom are two hydrogen atoms. These bonds are covalent. As a consequence, the protons of the hydrogen atoms pointing away from the oxygen atom are not shielded efficiently by the electrons. They become positively charged. On the opposite side of the water molecule, the electrons that fill the outer shell of the oxygen provide a negative charge. The positive hydrogen nucleus is attracted to the unshared electrons of neighboring water molecules. This type of bond is called a hydrogen bridge. Polarity of this nature is important in accounting for the intermolecular reactions in many organic

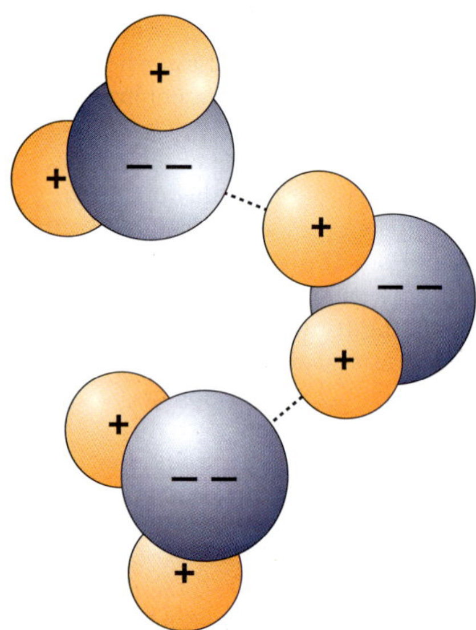

• **Fig. 2.5** Hydrogen bond formation between water molecules. The polar water molecule bonds to adjacent water molecules via an H (*orange*)–O (*blue*) interaction between molecules.

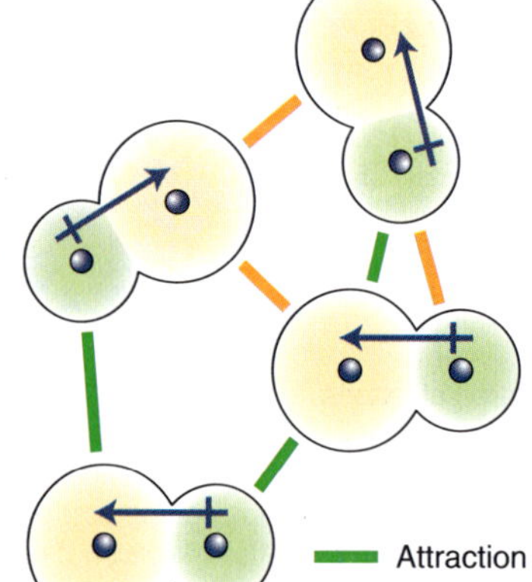

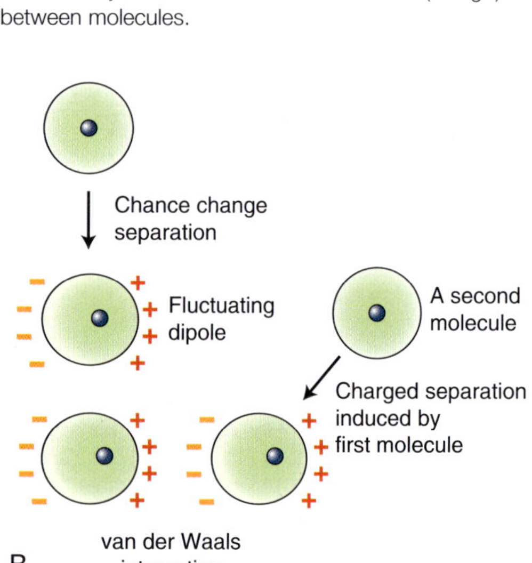

• **Fig. 2.4** van der Waals forces by dipole attraction. **(A)** Polar compound; the attraction and repulsion between molecules are induced by a permanent dipole moment resulting from asymmetrical electron distribution within the molecule. **(B)** Nonpolar compound; a temporary dipole (fluctuating dipole) occurs when the symmetrical distribution of electrons in a molecule becomes asymmetrical temporarily; it then attracts the dipole to adjacent molecules, resulting in the eventual interaction.

compounds—for example, the sorption of water by synthetic dental resins.

Atomic Arrangement

All materials we use consist of trillions of atoms. As described earlier, they are attracted to each other and retain a particular physical appearance. The question is in which configuration they are held together. In 1665, Robert Hooke (1635–1703) explained crystal shapes in terms of the packing of their component parts, like stacking musket balls in piles. This is an exact model of the atomic structure of many familiar metals, with each ball representing an atom.

In the solid state, atoms combine in a manner that ensures minimal internal energy. For example, sodium and chlorine share one electron at the atomic scale. In the solid state, like grains of salt, they do not exist in individual pairs; in fact, each sodium ion is attracted to six chlorine ions and vice versa (Fig. 2.6). They form a regularly spaced configuration (long-range repetitive space lattice) known as a crystal. A space lattice can be defined as any arrangement of atoms in space in which every atom is situated similarly to every other atom.

There are structures where regularly spaced configurations do not occur in the solid state. For example, the molecules of some of the waxes used by a dentist or laboratory technician are distributed at random when solidified. This noncrystalline formation is also known as an amorphous structure.

CRITICAL QUESTION

Which dental substances are examples of crystalline materials, noncrystalline materials, and combinations of crystalline and noncrystalline materials?

Crystalline Structure

There are 14 possible lattice types. The type of space lattice is defined by the length of each of three unit cell edges (called the axes) and the angles between the edges. The simplest and most regular lattice is a cubic, as shown in Figure 2.7A; it is characterized by axes that are all of equal length and meet at 90° angles, representing the smallest repetitive volume of a crystal, which is called a unit cell. Each sphere represents the positions of the atoms. Their positions are located at the points of intersection of three planes, each plane (surface of the cube) being perpendicular to the other two planes. These planes are often referred to as crystal planes. However, the simple cubic arrangement shown in Figure 2.7A is hypothetical, as it leaves enough space to fit additional atoms per unit cell. Most crystalline lattices of atoms also contain sites of missing atoms. Each missing atom site is called a vacancy.

Most metals used in dentistry belong to the cubic system. For example, iron at room temperature has an atom at each corner of the cube and another atom at the body center of the cube (Fig. 2.7B). This crystal form is called a body-centered cubic cell. Copper, on the other hand, has additional atoms at the center of each face of the unit cell but none at the center of the cube. This form is called a face-centered cubic cell (Fig. 2.7C).

Other types of space lattices of dental interest are shown in Figure 2.8. The hexagonal close-packed arrangement (Fig. 2.8G) observed in titanium, zinc, and zirconium has become an important crystalline structure in dentistry. Note that each unit cell consists of three layers of atoms.

All metallic-based dental materials are crystalline. Some pure ceramics, such as alumina and zirconia core materials, are entirely crystalline.

Noncrystalline Structure

Glass is a typical noncrystalline solid of SiO_2 because its atoms tend to be arranged in nonrepeating units (Fig. 2.9). The ordered arrangement of glass is more or less locally interspersed with a considerable number of disordered units. Because this arrangement is also typical of liquids, such solids are sometimes called **supercooled liquids**. Because of the complexity of the physical configuration of polymer chains (Chapter 6), the molecules of resins are not favored to arrange in orderly repeating patterns. Therefore, polymeric-based materials used in dentistry are usually noncrystalline.

The structural arrangements of the noncrystalline solids do not represent such low internal energies as do crystalline arrangements of the same atoms and molecules. They do not have a definite

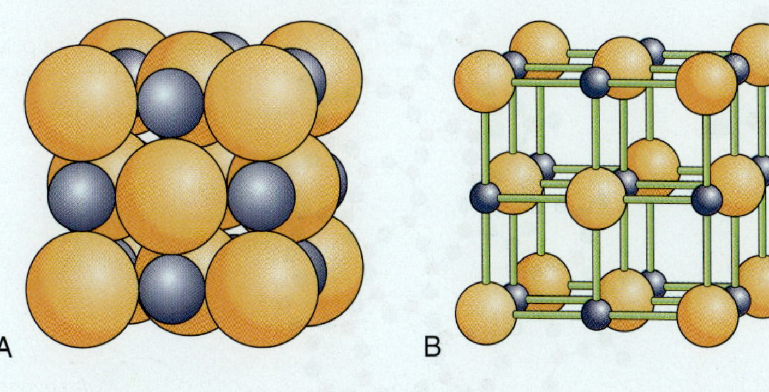

• **Fig. 2.6** The atomic arrangement of table salt. **(A)** Sphere model showing that atoms are actually closely packed together. **(B)** Ball-and-stick model displaying the three-dimensional position of the atoms and bonds between them. The orange spheres are chlorine ions and the blue spheres are sodium ions.

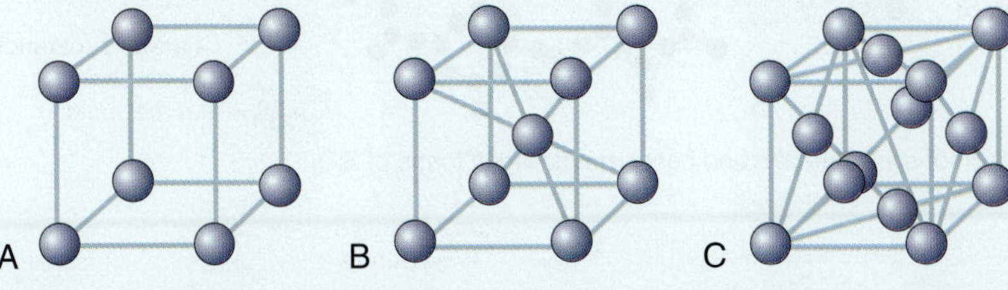

• **Fig. 2.7** Unit cells of the cubic space lattices: **(A)** Simple cubic; **(B)** body-centered cubic; **(C)** face-centered cubic.

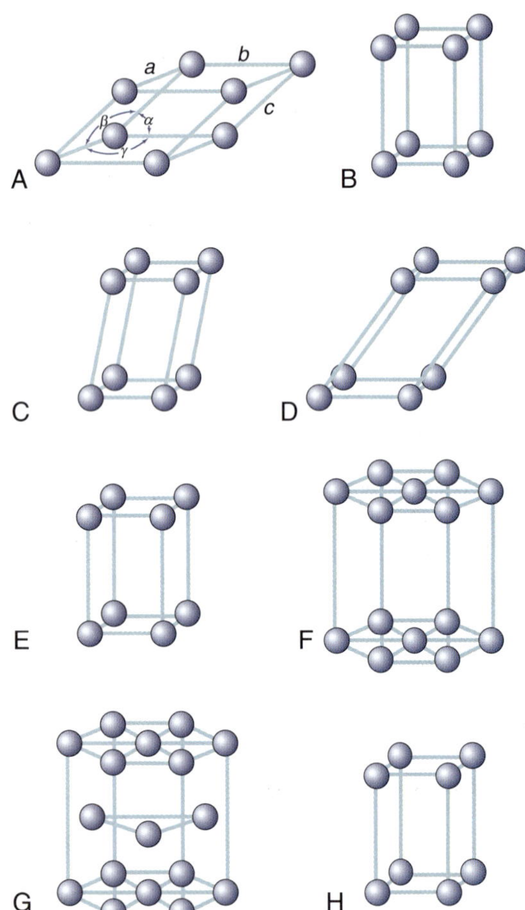

• **Fig. 2.8** Other lattice types of dental interest. **(A)** Rhombohedral; a = b = c; α = β = γ ≠ 90°. **(B)** Orthorhombic; a ≠ b ≠ c; α = β = γ = 90°. **(C)** Monoclinic; a ≠ b ≠ c; α ≠ β = γ = 90°. **(D)** Triclinic; a ≠ b ≠ c; α ≠ β ≠ γ ≠ 90°. **(E)** Tetragonal; a = b ≠ c; α = β = γ = 90°. **(F)** Simple hexagonal; a = b ≠ c; α = β = 90°; γ = 120°. **(G)** Close-packed hexagonal; a = b ≠ c; α = β = 90°; γ = 120°. **(H)** Rhombic; a = b ≠ c; α = β = 90°; γ = 120°.

melting temperature but rather gradually soften as the temperature is raised. The temperature at which there is an abrupt increase in the **thermal expansion coefficient**, indicating increased molecular mobility, is called the **glass-transition temperature (Tg)**; it is characteristic of the particular glassy structure. Below Tg, the material loses its fluid characteristics and gains significant resistance to shear deformation. When set, synthetic dental resins are examples of materials that often have glassy structures with a Tg greater than body temperature.

Many dental materials often consist of a noncrystalline glassy matrix and crystalline inclusions (filler phase). Crystalline inclusions provide desired properties including color, opacity, increased thermal expansion coefficients, and, in some dental ceramics, increased radiopacity (Chapter 10). The filler phase of resin-based composite (Chapter 5), on the other hand, can be crystalline, such as quartz particles or noncrystalline glass spheres.

CRITICAL QUESTION

How does the interatomic bond distance affect the thermal property of materials?

Interatomic Bond Distance and Thermal Energy

We can treat an atom as a discrete particle with definite boundaries and volume established by the electrostatic fields of the electrons. Between any two atoms, there are forces of attraction drawing them together and forces of repulsion pushing them apart. Both forces increase as the distance between the atoms decreases. The force of repulsion increases much more than the force of attraction as the atoms get closer (Fig. 2.10A). The balance between these two forces is essentially attractive when the two atoms are far apart, and becomes repulsive only when the atoms are much closer.

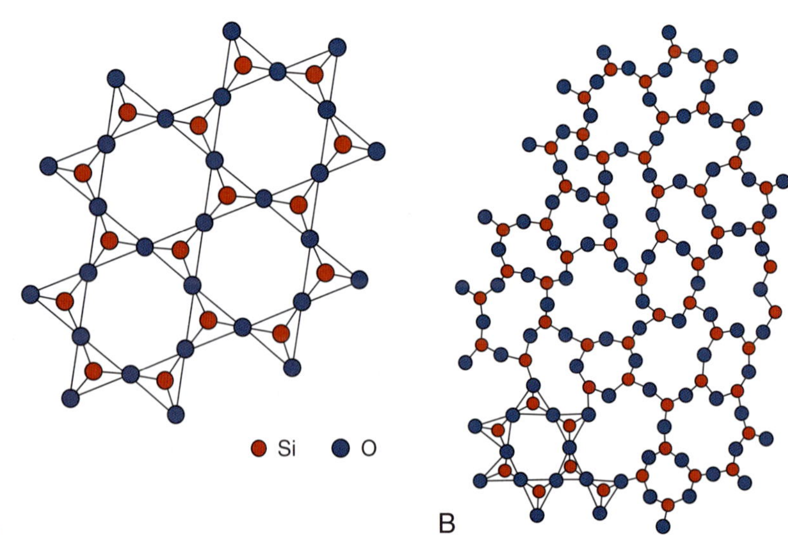

• **Fig. 2.9** Two-dimensional illustration of crystalline (*left*) and noncrystalline (*right*) forms of SiO_2.

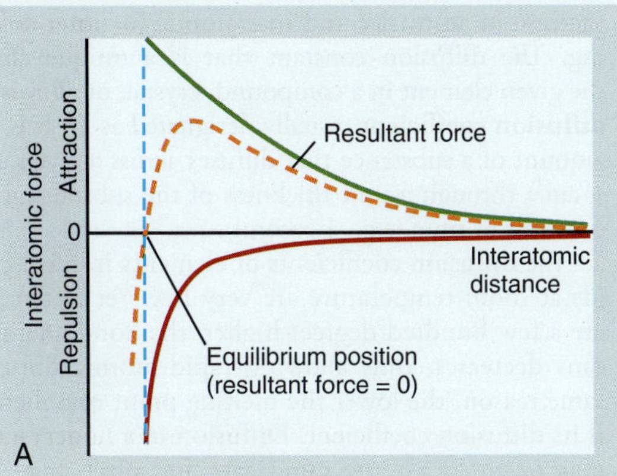

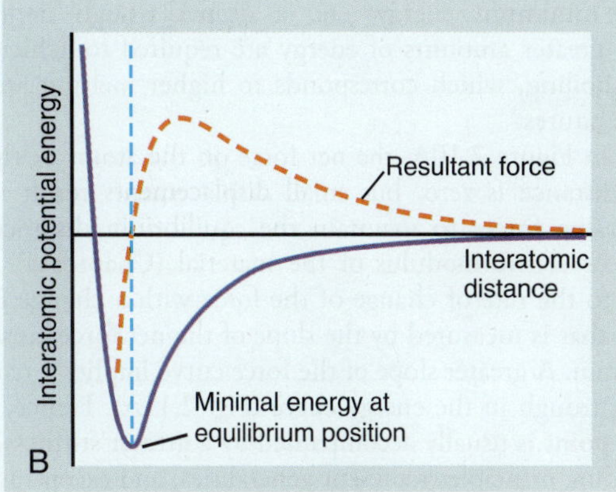

• **Fig. 2.10** Interaction between two atoms. **(A)** Relation of interatomic forces to interatomic distance. The resultant force (– –) is the sum of attraction (—) and repulsion (—) forces. At the equilibrium position (– –), either a negative (repulsive) or a positive (attractive) force is required to move the atom out of its equilibrium position. **(B)** Integration of the interatomic force (– –) shown in **A** over the interatomic distance yields the interatomic energy (—). Note that the potential energy is at minimum when equilibrium (– –) is reached.

Bond Distance

The position at which both forces are equal in magnitude (but opposite in direction) is considered the equilibrium position of the atoms (Fig. 2.10A). The interatomic distance at equilibrium represents the distance between the centers of the two adjacent atoms.

Bonding Energy

Since the conditions of equilibrium are more nearly related to the energy factor than to interatomic distance, the relationships in Figure 2.10A can be more logically explained in terms of interatomic energy. Energy is defined as the product of force and distance. Integration of the interatomic force (dashed line in Fig. 2.10A) over the interatomic distance yields the interatomic energy (Fig. 2.10B). In contrast with the resultant force, the energy needed to keep them far apart does not change much initially as two atoms come closer together. As the resultant force approaches zero, the energy needed to keep them apart decreases as the repulsion force becomes significant (Fig. 2.10B). The energy finally reaches a minimum when the resultant force becomes zero. Thereafter, the energy increases rapidly because the resultant repulsive force increases rapidly with little change in interatomic distance. The minimal energy corresponds to the condition of equilibrium and defines the equilibrium interatomic distance.

Thermal Energy

The atoms in a crystal at temperatures above absolute zero are in a constant state of vibration, and the average amplitude is dependent on the temperature: The higher the temperature, the greater the amplitude and, consequently, the greater the kinetic or internal energy. For a certain temperature, the bottom of the trough in Figure 2.10B denotes the minimal energy required to maintain equilibrium. As the temperature increases, the amplitude of the atomic (or molecular) vibration increases. It follows also that the mean interatomic distance increases (Fig. 2.11) as well as the internal energy. The overall effect is the phenomenon known as thermal expansion.

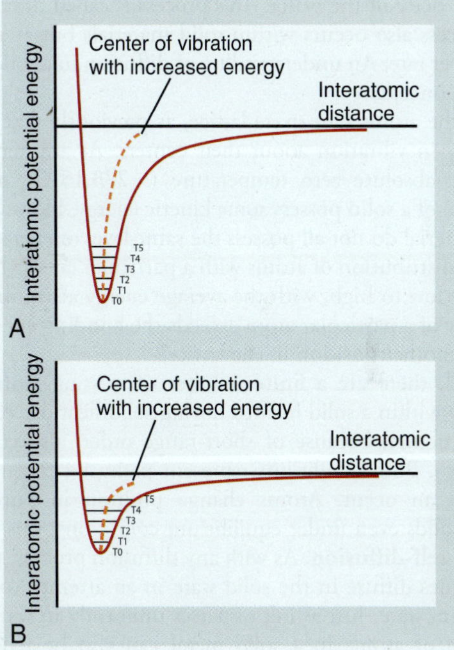

• **Fig. 2.11** Thermal energy and bonding energy. As the temperature rises from T_0 to T_5, the interatomic distance increases. For the solid with a deeper potential energy trough **(A)**, the actual increase in distance is less than that of the solid with a shallower potential energy trough **(B)**. Therefore, less thermal expansion and a higher melting temperature are expected for **A**. In addition, a high melting temperature usually is accompanied with a greater stiffness.

As the temperature increases from T_0 to T_5 in Figure 2.11, the mean interatomic distance increase is less with the deeper energy trough (Fig. 2.11A) than that in shallower energy trough (Fig. 2.11B). This means that the linear coefficient of thermal expansion (α) of materials with similar atomic or molecular structures tends to be inversely proportional to the melting temperature. If the temperature continues to increase, the increase of interatomic distance will result in change of state. A solid melts to a liquid, and the liquid subsequently vaporizes to a gas. For a solid with greater minimum energy, i.e., a deeper trough depth (Fig. 2.11A), greater amounts of energy are required to achieve melting and boiling, which corresponds to higher melting and boiling temperatures.

As shown in Figure 2.10A, the net force on the atoms at the equilibrium distance is zero, but small displacements result in rapidly increasing forces to maintain the equilibrium distance. The stiffness or elastic modulus of the material (Chapter 4) is proportional to the rate of change of the force with a change in displacement that is measured by the slope of the net force curve near equilibrium. A greater slope of the force curve implies a narrower, deeper trough in the energy curve (Fig. 2.11A). Hence, a high melting point is usually accompanied by a greater stiffness.

The preceding principles represent generalities, and exceptions do occur. Nevertheless, they allow one to estimate the influence of temperature on the properties of most of the dental materials discussed in subsequent chapters.

Diffusion

When we place a drop of ink in a bowl of water, we observe the spread of the ink in the water. It will eventually disperse through the entire body of the water. This process is called diffusion. The same process also occurs within solid materials but at a substantially slower rate. An understanding of diffusion in a solid requires two new concepts.

First, the atoms in a space lattice, as previously described, are constantly in vibration about their centers. At any temperature above the absolute zero temperature (−273.15°C), atoms (or molecules) of a solid possess some kinetic energy. However, atoms in the material do not all possess the same level of energy. Rather, there is a distribution of atoms with a particular energy that varies from very low to high, with the average energy at equilibrium. If the energy of a particular atom exceeds the bonding energy, it can move to another position in the lattice.

Second, there are a finite number of missing atoms (called vacancies) within a solid formed during solidification. A noncrystalline structure, because of short-range order, also contributes some space. Both conditions represent pathways through which diffusion can occur. Atoms change position in pure, single-element solids even under equilibrium conditions; this process is known as **self-diffusion**. As with any diffusion process, the atoms or molecules diffuse in the solid state in an attempt to reach an equilibrium state. Just as ink disperses uniformly in water, a concentration of atoms in a solid metal can also be redistributed through the diffusion process.

Diffusion may also occur in the other direction to produce a concentration of atoms in a solid. For example, if the sugar in the water becomes supersaturated, the molecules of sugar diffuse toward each other and the sugar crystallizes out of solution. In the same manner, a solid copper–silver alloy with higher copper concentration may cause supersaturation of copper in silver, which forces diffusion of copper atoms to increase the concentration of copper locally, causing them to precipitate.

CRITICAL QUESTION

Why are mercury and gallium of interest as components of direct restorative materials?

Diffusion rates for a given substance increase as temperature, the chemical potential gradient, concentration gradient, or lattice imperfections increase. The diffusion rate will decrease with an increase in atom size and interatomic (or intermolecular) bonding. The diffusion constant that is a unique characteristic of the given element in a compound, crystal, or alloy is known as the **diffusion coefficient**, usually designated as D. It is defined as the amount of a substance that diffuses across a given unit area (e.g., 1 cm^2) through a unit thickness of the substance (e.g., 1 cm) in one unit of time (e.g., 1 second).

The diffusion coefficients of elements in most crystalline solids at room temperature are very low. Yet at temperatures that are a few hundred degrees higher, the bond energy between atoms decreases, thus allowing rapid atomic diffusion. For the same reason, the lower the melting point of a metal, the greater is its diffusion coefficient. Diffusion in a noncrystalline material may occur at a more rapid rate and often may be evident at room or body temperature. The disordered structure enables the molecules to diffuse more rapidly with less activation energy. Both mercury and gallium are liquid at room temperature because of their melting points at –38.36°C (–7.05°F) and 29.78°C (85.60°F), respectively. When either liquid metal is mixed with a suitable metal alloy, atoms in the alloy dissolve and diffuse rapidly within the liquid metal at intraoral temperature. The result is a new solid metal compound. This process has been utilized in dentistry for making metallic direct restorative materials (Chapter 8).

Metals

Metals, by their appearance and usage, have several characteristics. A clean, polished metallic surface exhibits a luster that cannot be duplicated by other classes of solids. Most metals emit a metallic sound ("ring") when they are struck by another metal. They are generally excellent thermal and electrical conductors. Metals are more resistant to deformation or rupture from external forces and denser than nonmetallic structures. Most metals are also far more ductile and malleable than nonmetals, which are generally brittle. The significance of strength, ductility, malleability, and brittleness will be discussed in the chapter on mechanical properties (Chapter 4). Only a few metals are resistant to tarnish and corrosion in air at room temperature.

Pure metals, in common with other chemical elements, can be identified by their specific melting and boiling points and by their basic physical and chemical properties. Some relevant properties for metals of dental interest are listed in Table 2.1. Information about the atom size, crystal structure, and chemical properties of these elements is provided in Table 2.2. Note that several important elements have more than one crystal structure (polymorphic forms), depending on the temperature, and have multiple valences.

Of the 118 elements currently listed in the periodic table (Fig. 2.12), about 88 can be classified as metals. One common feature in the atomic structure of metal elements is that the outermost electrons (valence electrons) around the neutral metallic atoms are easily given up. This property constitutes the basis of the metallic bond, where a "cloud" of valence electrons becomes the "glue" for the positively charged ionic cores made of the nuclei and the balance of the bound electrons. The bond is nondirectional, allowing the ionic cores to break interatomic bonds easily and establish new bonds with other ionic cores at different positions. This property enables metals to undergo distortion before fracturing (properties of ductility and malleability) under mechanical stresses. It should be noted that many metals of importance for dental alloys are transition elements that have incomplete inner electron shells.

TABLE 2.1 **Physical Properties of Elements in Dental Alloys**

Element	Symbol	Atomic Weight	Melting Point (°C)	Density (g/cm³)	Thermal Expansion Coefficient (10^{-6}/K)
Aluminum	Al	26.98	660	2.70	23.6
Carbon	C	12.01	630	2.22	6.0
Chromium	Cr	52.00	271	7.19	6.2
Cobalt	Co	58.93	1495	8.85	13.8
Copper	Cu	63.54	1083	8.96	16.5
Gold	Au	196.97	1063	19.32	14.2
Indium	In	114.82	156	7.31	33.0
Iridium	Ir	192.20	2454	22.50	6.8
Iron	Fe	55.85	1527	7.87	12.3
Magnesium	Mg	24.31	650	1.74	25.2
Mercury	Hg	200.59	−39	13.55	40.0
Molybdenum	Mo	95.94	2619	10.22	4.9
Nickel	Ni	58.71	1453	8.90	13.3
Palladium	Pd	106.40	1552	12.02	11.8
Platinum	Pt	195.09	1769	21.45	8.9
Rhodium	Rh	102.91	1966	12.44	8.3
Silicon	Si	28.09	1410	2.33	7.3
Silver	Ag	107.87	961	10.49	19.7
Tin	Sn	118.69	232	7.30	23.0
Titanium	Ti	47.90	1668	4.51	8.5
Tungsten	W	183.85	3410	19.30	4.6
Zinc	Zn	65.37	420	7.133	0.4

Data from Lyman T, editor: *Metals Handbook*, vol 1, ed 8, Cleveland, OH, 1964, American Society for Metals.

CRITICAL QUESTION

Why are the general physical and mechanical properties of metallic dental materials different from those of ceramic and polymeric dental materials?

What important metals for dental alloys are transition elements? What special chemical and physical properties are possessed by transition metals?

Pure metals have limited uses in dental and engineering applications because they are too soft to resist deformation from external forces. It has been found that mixtures of two or more metallic elements or mixtures of one or more metals and nonmetallic elements often result in improved properties beyond what the individual elements can provide. This combination of elements is called an alloy. An alloy system refers to all possible combinations (weight percentage or atomic percentage) of elements in the system. Alloys are generally prepared by fusion of the elements above their melting points. In this book, the term "metal" is used all-inclusively to include alloys and pure metals. If the phenomenon discussed does not apply to both alloys and pure metals, a distinction will be made. The mechanisms for property improvement, and the effects on physical and chemical properties of alloys, are discussed in some detail in Chapter 9.

To make a metal prosthesis, an exact wax or plastic pattern of the prosthesis is prepared initially. Using a dental investment, an expanded mold is prepared from the pattern, into which the molten alloy is filled under pressure (Chapter 14). When the alloy solidifies, it shrinks to the intended dimensions. The mechanical properties of the final cast prosthesis can often be manipulated by regulating the cooling procedure. In this chapter segment, we will first discuss how a solid emerges from the molten (liquid) state and the resultant microstructure of pure metals. We then will discuss the criteria for forming different types of alloys, the interpretation of phase diagrams, and refinement of the properties of alloys by controlled heating and cooling.

CRITICAL QUESTION

Why do dental alloys begin freezing by heterogeneous nucleation rather than by homogeneous nucleation?

Solidification and Microstructure of Metals

If a pure metal is melted and cooled to room temperature under very clean laboratory conditions, a graph of its temperature-versus-time

TABLE 2.2 **Atom Size, Crystal Structure, and Chemical Properties of Elements in Dental Alloys**

Element	Symbol	Atom Radius (nm)	Crystal Structure	Oxidation States	Electronegativity
Aluminum	Al	0.118	Face-centered cubic	+3	1.61
Carbon	C	0.067	Hexagonal (graphite) Diamond cubic (diamond)		
Chromium	Cr	0.166	Body-centered cubic	+2, +3	1.66
Cobalt	Co	0.152	Hexagonal close-packed (≤450°C) Face-centered cubic (>450°C)	+2	1.88
Copper	Cu	0.145	Face-centered cubic	+1, +2	1.9
Gallium	Ga	0.136	Orthorhombic	+3	1.81
Gold	Au	0.174	Face-centered cubic	+1, +3	2.54
Iron	Fe	0.156	Body-centered cubic (≤911°C) Face-centered cubic (>911°C)	+2, +3	1.83
Mercury	Hg	0.171	(Liquid above –39°C)	+2	2
Molybdenum	Mo	0.190	Body-centered cubic	+6	2.16
Nickel	Ni	0.149	Face-centered cubic	+2, +3	1.91
Platinum	Pt	0.177	Face-centered cubic	+2, +4	2.28
Palladium	Pd	0.169	Face-centered cubic	+2, +4	2.2
Silver	Ag	0.165	Face-centered cubic	+1	1.93
Tin	Sn	0.145	Body-centered tetragonal	+4	1.96
Titanium	Ti	0.176	Hexagonal close-packed (≤880°C) Body-centered cubic (>880°C)	+2, +3, +4	1.54
Zinc	Zn	0.142	Hexagonal close-packed	+2	1.65

Values for atom radius and electronegativity were obtained from http://periodictable.com/.

behavior would look similar to that in Figure 2.13. The temperature decreases steadily from point A to point B′. An increase in temperature then occurs from point B′ to point B, at which time the temperature remains constant until the time indicated at point C is reached. Subsequently, the temperature of the metal decreases steadily to room temperature (D). The temperature, Tf, indicated by the "plateau" portion of the curve at BC, is the solidification temperature of the pure metal. This is also the melting point or fusion temperature.

During the initial cooling, the molten metal remains in the liquid state to point B′, which is below the solidification temperature; this process is termed supercooling or undercooling. During the supercooling stage, crystallization of the pure metal begins. Once the crystals begin to form, the release of latent heat from liquid changing to solid causes the temperature to rise to Tf, where it remains until crystallization is completed at point C. Supercooling of pure metals occurs only in clean, inert containers under circumstances in which heterogeneous nucleation of metal crystals is not possible.

Nucleus Formation

Solidification of a metal requires nuclei of crystallization. The liquid state can be imagined as one of a multitude of random atoms surrounding numerous unstable atomic aggregates or clusters that are attempting to form crystal nuclei. These temporary nuclei are called embryos. On approaching the solidification temperature, these embryos increase in number and size, but they are still unstable and tend to dissolve into the liquid matrix. However, once the supercooled process is completed, there is a tendency for some of these embryos to survive and thus become solidification nuclei. This method of nucleus formation is called homogeneous nucleation, and the formation of nuclei in the molten metal is a random process with equal probability of occurring at any point in the melt.

CRITICAL QUESTION

What are the contributions of the surface free energy and the volume free energy to the overall free energy of these embryos as a function of the embryo size? What is meant by the term critical nucleus size?

Another method of forming stable embryos is for the atoms in the molten metal to contact some surface, particles in the melt, or particles in the container. Such a process is known as heterogeneous nucleation because a foreign body "seeded" the nucleus. The distribution of these foreign bodies is not necessarily random. Under dental casting conditions, heterogeneous nucleation occurs at the mold wall (investment) or in the molten alloy at impurity particles or particles of special grain-refining elements.

It should be noted that supercooling is not necessary for heterogeneous nucleation. In fact, heterogeneous nucleation should

Periodic Table

Period	1 IA	2 IIA	3 IIIB	4 IVB	5 VB	6 VIB	7 VIIB	8 VIIIB	9 VIIIB	10 VIIIB	11 IB	12 IIB	13 IIIA	14 IVA	15 VA	16 VIA	17 VIIA	18 VIIIA
1	1 Hydrogen **H**																	2 Helium **He**
2	3 Lithium **Li**	4 Beryllium **Be**											5 Boron **B**	6 Carbon **C**	7 Nitrogen **N**	8 Oxygen **O**	9 Fluorine **F**	10 Neon **N**
3	11 Sodium **Na**	12 Magnesium **Mg**											13 Aluminum **Al**	14 Silicon **Si**	15 Phosphorus **P**	16 Sulfur **S**	17 Chlorine **Cl**	18 Argon **Ar**
4	19 Potassium **K**	20 Calcium **Ca**	21 Scandium **Sc**	22 Titanium **Ti**	23 Vanadium **V**	24 Chromium **Cr**	25 Manganese **Mn**	26 Iron **Fe**	27 Cobalt **Co**	28 Nickel **Ni**	29 Copper **Cu**	30 Zinc **Zn**	31 Gallium **Ga**	32 Germanium **Ge**	33 Arsenic **As**	34 Selenium **Se**	35 Bromine **Br**	36 Krypton **Kr**
5	37 Rubidium **Rb**	38 Strontium **Sr**	39 Yttrium **Y**	40 Zirconium **Zr**	41 Niobium **Nb**	42 Molybdenum **Mo**	43 Technetium **Tc**	44 Ruthenium **Ru**	45 Rhodium **Rh**	46 Palladium **Pd**	47 Silver **Ag**	48 Cadmium **Cd**	49 Indium **In**	50 Tin **Sn**	51 Antimony **Sb**	52 Tellurium **Te**	53 Iodine **I**	54 Xenon **Xe**
6	55 Cesium **Cs**	56 Barium **Ba**	57-71 Series of Lanthanide Elements	72 Hafnium **Hf**	73 Tantalum **Ta**	74 Tungsten **W**	75 Rhenium **Re**	76 Osmium **Os**	77 Iridium **Ir**	78 Platinum **Pt**	79 Gold **Au**	80 Mercury **Hg**	81 Thallium **Tl**	82 Lead **Pb**	83 Bismuth **Bi**	84 Polonium **Po**	85 Astatine **At**	86 Radon **Rn**
7	87 Francium **Fr**	88 Radium **Ra**	89-103 Series of Actinide Elements	104 Rutherfordium **Rf**	105 Dubnium **Db**	106 Seaborgium **Sg**	107 Bohrium **Bh**	108 Hassium **Hs**	109 Meitnerium **Mt**	110 Darmstadtium **Ds**	111 Roentgenium **Rg**	112 Copernicium **Cn**	113 Nihonium **Nh**	114 Flerovium **Fl**	115 Moscovium **Mc**	116 Livermorium **Lv**	117 Tennessine **Ts**	118 Oganesson **Og**

Series of Lanthanide Elements	57 Lanthanum **La**	58 Cerium **Ce**	59 Praseodymium **Pr**	60 Neodymium **Nd**	61 Promethium **Pm**	62 Samarium **Sm**	63 Europium **Eu**	64 Gadolinium **Gd**	65 Terbium **Tb**	66 Dysprosium **Dy**	67 Holmium **Ho**	68 Erbium **Er**	69 Thulium **Tm**	70 Ytterbium **Yb**	71 Lutetium **Lu**
Series of Actinide Elements	89 Actinium **Ac**	90 Thorium **Th**	91 Protactinium **Pa**	92 Uranium **U**	93 Neptunium **Np**	94 Plutonium **Pu**	95 Americium **Am**	96 Curium **Cm**	97 Berkelium **Bk**	98 Californium **Cf**	99 Einsteinium **Es**	100 Fermium **Fm**	101 Mendelevium **Md**	102 Nobelium **No**	103 Lawrencium **Lr**

• **Fig. 2.12** Periodic chart of the elements.

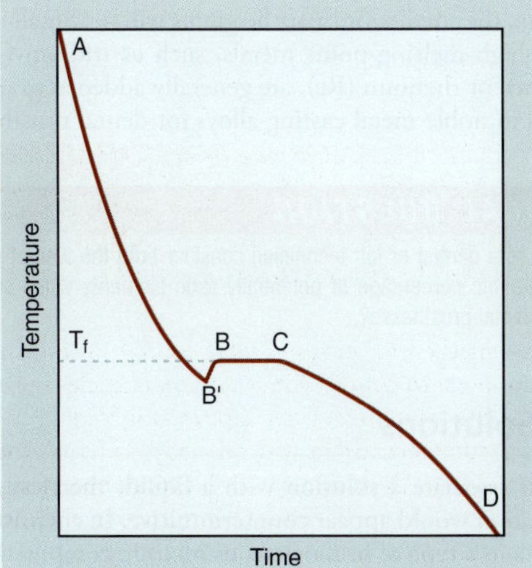

• **Fig. 2.13** A time–temperature cooling curve for a pure metal, illustrating supercooling.

account for most of the nucleation that occurs during dental casting. The uniformity of distribution of heterogeneously formed nuclei is difficult, in principle, to control because the distribution of the different types of "seeds" is not likely to be uniform.

CRITICAL QUESTION

Why might the rates of cooling and solidification affect the grain size of a dental casting?

Liquid-to-Solid Transformation of Cast Metals

As a liquid metal cools and solidifies, crystals are formed by diffusion of atoms from the molten metal to existing nuclei of crystallization. The crystals extend along certain favored crystallographic directions and form dendrites. The heat released by the solidifying metal (in extending the arms of dendrites) reduces supercooling around the arm, which impedes solidification in affected regions and results in highly elongated extension of the arms. Subsequently, secondary extension arms of the dendrites branch off the primary arms, and tertiary arms off the secondary arms, resulting in a three-dimensional dendritic structure. Dendrites can also grow perpendicular to the walls of the mold cavity toward the center of the casting. Numerous dendritic crystals form and grow until they eventually become large enough to impinge upon each other. Solidification is completed when the liquid metal in the interdendritic spaces between the dendrite arms freezes to yield crystals. Each crystal within the solidified metal is called a grain. Thus, a grain is a microscopic single crystal that has a different orientation from that of the adjacent grains. The interface between adjacent grains is called a grain boundary. The solidified metal is also called polycrystalline.

The grain boundaries in a solidified metal are revealed when examining the microstructure of a polished surface that has been etched. When a highly polished metal surface is subjected to a chemical or an electrolytic etching solution, the atoms near grain boundaries are preferentially removed, creating microscopic grooves that scatter light because these atoms have higher energy compared with atoms in the interiors of grains. An as-cast dendritic pattern may be present, like the Pd-based alloy shown in Figure 2.14, or a dendritic microstructure may not exist, such as for the high-palladium alloy having an equiaxed grain structure shown in Figure 2.15. The term equiaxed means that the three dimensions of each grain are similar, in contrast to the elongated shape and size of the dendrites in Figure 2.14.

Figure 2.16 is a schematic illustration of the coalescence of individual grains to form an equiaxed grain structure. Solidification starts from isolated nuclei in the molten metal, and these crystals gradually grow by the clustering of atoms and extend toward each other. When the adjacent crystals are eventually in contact, their growth stops, as shown in Figure 2.16E. The final polished and etched microstructure depicting grain boundaries is shown in Figure 2.16F. The grain boundary regions are the last portions of the molten metal to solidify and can serve as sites for precipitate formation and sinks for impurity atoms.

CRITICAL QUESTION

How does the grain size affect the properties of cast dental alloys?

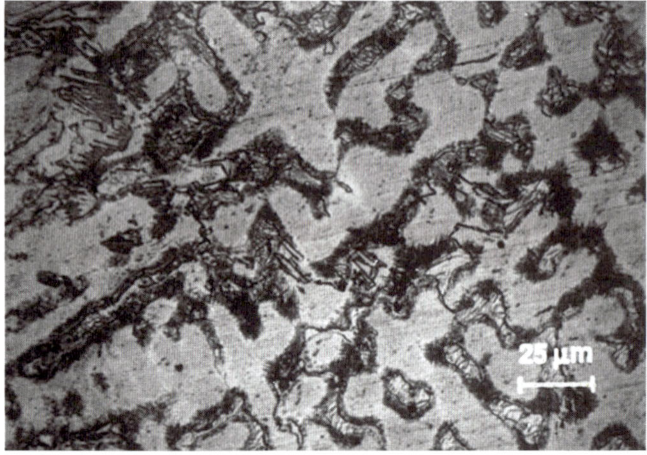

• **Fig. 2.14** Optical microscopic image of a polished and etched palladium-based alloy with a dendritic as-cast microstructure. Higher magnification scanning electron microscope (SEM) images reveal that the complex interdendritic regions can contain a eutectic constituent. (From Carr AB, Brantley WA: New high-palladium casting alloys: part 1. Overview and initial studies. *Int J Prosthodont* 4:265, 1991. Reproduced with permission from Quintessence Publishing Company, Inc.)

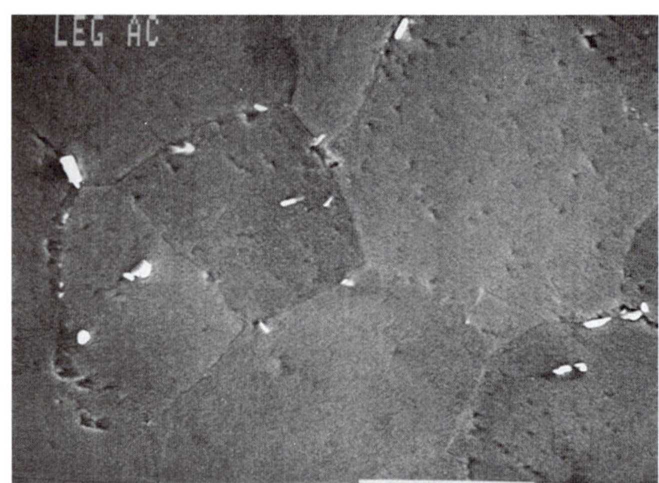

• **Fig. 2.15** Scanning electron microscope (SEM) image of a polished and etched high-palladium alloy with an equiaxed fine-grain as-cast microstructure. The white-appearing particles are ruthenium-rich and arise from the use of ruthenium as a grain-refining element. (From Brantley WA, Cai Z, Foreman DW, et al: X-ray diffraction studies of as-cast high-palladium alloys. *Dent Mater* 11:154, 1995. Reproduced with permission.)

Grain Refinement and Grain Size

In general, the smaller the grain size of the metal, the better are its physical properties. For example, the yield strength of many metals has been found to vary inversely with the square root of the grain size. Consequently, obtaining a small grain size during casting is an advantage.

There are two variables that can reduce the grain size during solidification: Number of nuclei of crystallization and rate of crystallization. A greater number of nuclei will yield a greater number of grains, and thus the size of each grain is reduced. As pointed out previously, the formation of nuclei of crystallization can be increased by the amount of supercooling and the rate of cooling. If the crystals grow more rapidly than the formation of nuclei of crystallization, the grains will be larger than if the reverse condition prevails. Conversely, if the formation of nuclei occurs faster than the growth of crystals, a small grain size will be obtained. Consequently, slow cooling results in large grains. In other words, the more rapidly the liquid state can be changed to the solid state, the smaller or finer the grains will be. Small concentrations of high-melting-point metals, such as iridium (Ir), ruthenium (Ru), or rhenium (Re), are generally added as grain-refining elements to noble metal casting alloys for dental prostheses.

CRITICAL QUESTION

Why should a dentist or lab technician consider both the weight percentage and the atomic percentage of potentially toxic elements when selecting an alloy for dental prostheses?

Solid Solutions

We often associate a solution with a liquid; therefore, the term solid solution would appear counterintuitive. In chemistry, a solution refers to a type of homogeneous mixture composed of two or more substances. That means we could have a solution in the solid, liquid, or vapor state. The key word is homogeneous. Consider the palladium–silver (Pd–Ag) alloy system, which is relevant

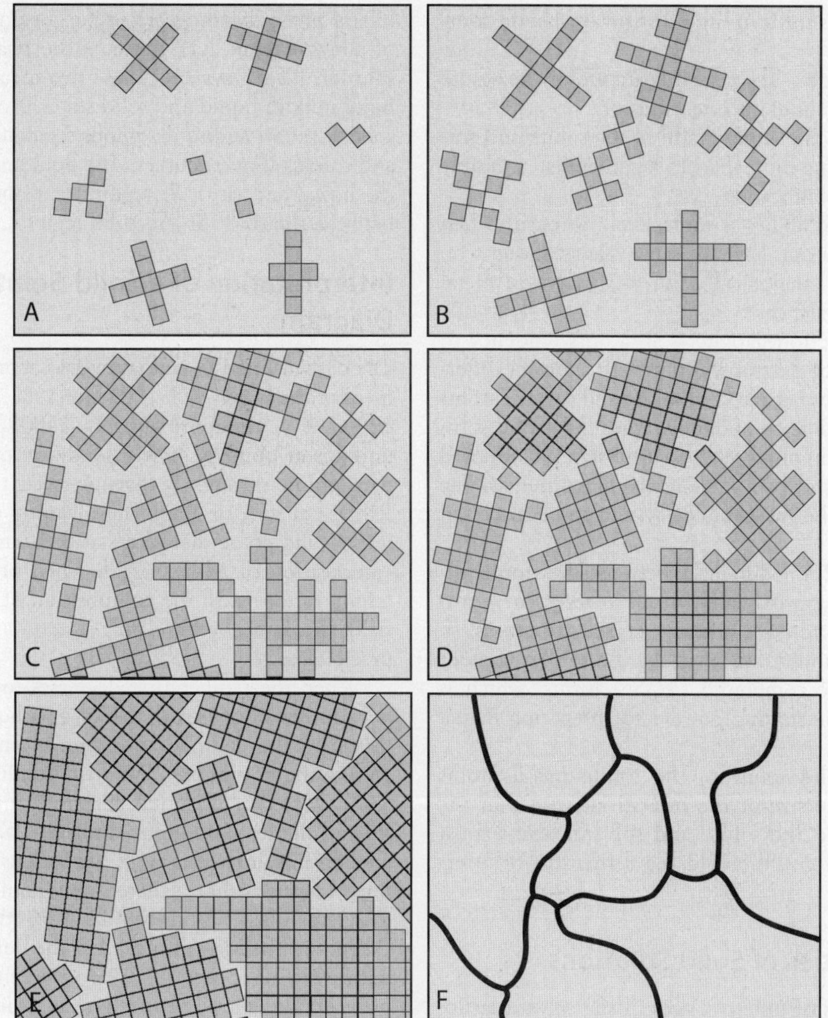

• **Fig. 2.16** (A–F) Stages in the formation of metallic grains during the solidification of a molten metal. (From Rosenhain W: *Introduction to Physical Metallurgy*, ed 3, London, 1935, Constable and Co. Reproduced with permission.)

for an important group of metal–ceramic alloys (Chapter 9), as an example. When an alloy in this system is solidified, the silver atoms are distributed randomly in the space lattice of the palladium atoms, thereby forming a solid solution. Because the silver atoms become integrated into the crystal structure of palladium, no microstructural evidence of a mechanically removable phase exists because there is only one phase. The term phase in chemistry is defined as a physically distinctive and homogeneous region of matter. If the binary Pd–Ag alloy appears to be inhomogeneous as a result of improper cooling, it can be heat-treated at elevated temperatures for sufficiently long time to promote solid-state diffusion that ensures the uniform distribution of silver atoms in the palladium lattice.

Solutes and Solvents

In liquid solutions, the substance present in the greater amount is the solvent, and the substance of the lesser amount uniformly dispersed in the solvent is the solute. The same principle applies in solid solutions, where the solute atoms are uniformly dispersed in the crystal structure of the solvent atoms. There are two principal atomic arrangements for solid solutions.

The first type is the substitutional solid solution in which the atoms of the solute occupy the positions in the crystal structure that are normally occupied by the solvent atoms in the pure metal. For a Pd–Ag alloy, the crystal structure of both elements is FCC, and Ag atoms replace Pd atoms randomly in the crystal structure of Pd; Ag is the solute, and Pd is the solvent. The second type is the interstitial solid solution, in which the solute metal atoms are present in random positions (interstices) between the atoms in the crystal structure of the solvent metal. This type of solid solution requires that the solute atoms be much smaller in diameter than the solvent atoms, and these solid solutions are usually limited to relatively small concentrations of solute. The family of carbon steels is an example of an interstitial solid solution of carbon in iron. Another example is commercially pure titanium (CP Ti), an alloy for implants and restorative dentistry (Chapter 9), which consists of high-purity (≥99 wt%) titanium, with oxygen, carbon, nitrogen, and hydrogen atoms dissolved interstitially.

Conditions for Solid Solubility

According to the four Hume–Rothery rules discussed in textbooks on engineering materials science, the conditions that dictate solubility of metals for forming substitutional solid solutions are as follows:

1. Type of crystal structure—The crystal structure of the solute and the solvent metals should be identical.
2. Atom size difference—The atomic radii of the solute and solvent atoms must differ no more than 15%; otherwise, multiple phases occur during solidification.
3. Valence—Maximum solubility is more likely to occur when the solvent and solute atoms have the same valence; otherwise, metal atoms of lower valence will tend to dissolve in metal with atoms of higher valence.
4. Electronegativity—Electronegativity is an atom's tendency to attract a bonding pair of electrons. Alloys with a greater difference in electronegativity between the solute and solvent atoms tend to form intermetallic compounds rather than solid solutions. Intermetallic compound refers to a substance composed of definite proportions of two or more elemental metals, like AuCu and $AuCu_3$ in the Au–Cu alloy system to be discussed later.

According to Table 2.2, the difference between the atomic diameters for Ag and Sn is approximately 4%. However, these two metals differ in valence and have different crystal structures, so there is limited solid solubility for Sn in Ag. As the Sn content increases, an intermetallic compound (Ag_3Sn) forms, which is an important phase in the starting powder for preparing dental amalgams (Chapter 8).

For an interstitial solid solution, the solute metal atoms must be smaller than the size of the interstitial spaces in the solvent metal lattice, and the solute and solvent atoms must have similar electronegativity to avoid the formation of intermetallic compounds.

Mechanical Properties of Solid Solutions

Substituting solute atoms of different sizes in the solvent lattice causes localized distortion, which is known to improve the mechanical properties of alloys, such as greater force or pressure required for deformation of the material. For example, although pure gold in the cast condition is too soft for restorations, adding only 5 wt% of copper will provide adequate strength and hardness to the Au–Cu alloy that are sufficient for the casting to be used for small inlays. Mechanisms of strengthening metals through alloying will be discussed later in this chapter and in Chapter 9.

CRITICAL QUESTION

Why is the study of binary phase diagrams important, even though dental alloys contain more than three elements and the conditions during solidification and cooling after casting are far removed from equilibrium?

Equilibrium-Phase Diagrams

A phase diagram shows conditions (pressure, temperature, volume, etc.) at which thermodynamically distinct phases occur and coexist at equilibrium. The phase diagrams in this book are temperature–composition graphs showing the boundaries of phase transformation in two-element alloy systems under atmospheric pressure. For three-component alloy systems, a three-dimensional (3D) phase diagram is needed to include the third element but would be much more complex. (Two-dimensional portrayals of important ternary phase diagrams for three-component alloy systems are provided in engineering reference texts.) Nevertheless, binary phase diagrams are useful for understanding the structure of alloys. Figure 2.17 presents the phase diagram for the solid solution Pd–Ag system. These two metals exhibit complete solubility in both liquid and solid states. Note the liquid, liquid-plus-solid (L + S), and solid regions separated by the liquidus (upper) and solidus (lower) curves. The liquidus is the boundary between the liquid and (L + S) regions, and the solidus is the boundary between the (L + S) and solid regions.

Interpretation of a Solid-Solution Phase Diagram

The dashed line PO in Figure 2.17 represents cooling of a liquid metal containing 65% Pd and 35% Ag from 1500°C (P) to 800°C (O). At approximately 1400°C, line PO intersects the liquidus at point R, where solidification begins. We can draw a parallel line through R that intersects the solidus at M. The line RM is called a tie line. The meaning of the tie line is that the initial solid phase that forms at that temperature should have the composition of M, 77% Pd, when projected to the horizontal (composition) axis; the composition of the liquid remains essentially the same because only a very small amount of solid has precipitated.

When the temperature decreases to point S (~1370°C), the new compositions of the solid and liquid phase may be determined by the tie line YW, a parallel line drawn through S intersecting the liquidus at Y and the solidus at W. Projecting points Y and W to the horizontal axis shows that the solid formed is 71% Pd and the remaining liquid phase is 57% Pd. When the vertical cooling line intersects with the solidus at T (~1340°C), the tie line NT shows that if there is any liquid left at this temperature, the remaining liquid should have the composition of 52% Pd (point N). Most if not all of the liquid has converted to solid with 65% Pd (point T). When the temperature decreases below point T, the alloy is entirely solid, with a composition of 65% palladium.

It should be reemphasized that the phase diagram describes the equilibrium state of the alloy for different composition–temperature conditions. The cooling process would have to be held at each of the foregoing temperatures for a prolonged time sufficient for atomic diffusion to enable the approach to equilibrium conditions for both the liquid and solid phases.

CRITICAL QUESTION

Why is the development of microsegregation in cast alloys more pronounced when there is a greater difference between the liquidus and solidus temperatures?

Coring and Homogenization Heat Treatment

In practice, cooling of a casting does not allow phases in the alloy to reach equilibrium at each temperature before solidification is completed. For example, the first stable nucleus that forms at the temperature R (or slightly below) in Figure 2.17 is richer than 65% Pd. As the solidification continues with temperature decreasing, the Pd content in the liquid decreases so that each succeeding "layer" that solidifies on this nucleus will have reduced Pd content and increased Ag content than the previous layer. Before reaching the solidus temperature (T) in Figure 2.17, the composition (point N) of the remaining liquid to solidify between the outermost layers of the adjacent solid particles would have Ag richer than 35%. The

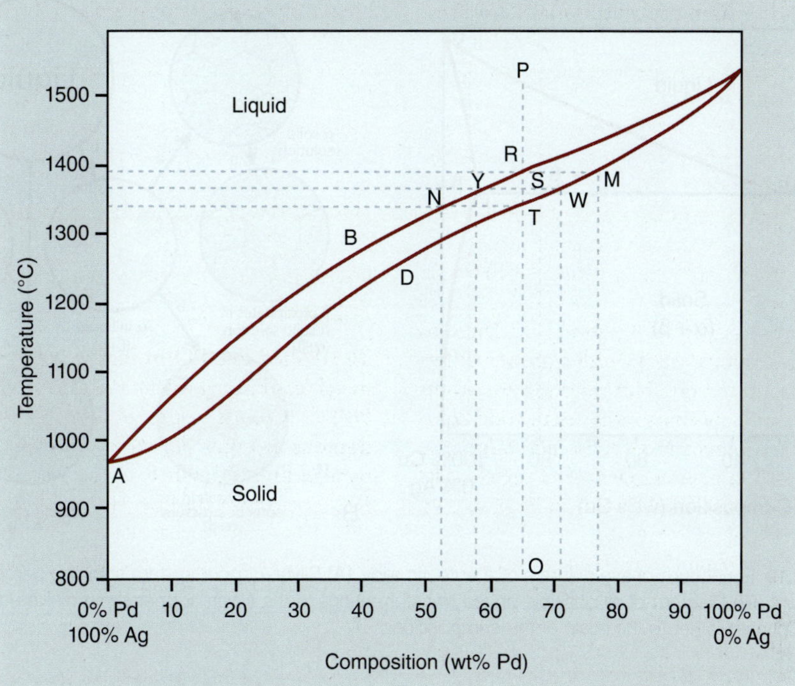

• **Fig. 2.17** Equilibrium-phase diagram for the palladium–silver system showing percentages by weight. Only the percentage composition for palladium is given; the percentage composition for silver is determined by subtracting the palladium composition from 100.

solid particles (dendrites or grains) have what is termed a cored structure, with the composition varying from the center (containing more Pd) to the outer surface (containing less Pd). Thus, the central portion of each particle contains larger amounts of the component with the higher solidification temperature (Pd), and the outer portions contain larger amounts of the component with the lower solidification temperature (Ag). It follows, because more atomic diffusion would be required to achieve near-equilibrium compositions, that the larger the temperature range between liquidus and solidus, the greater is the tendency toward coring.

A cored structure represents an inhomogeneous microstructure, making alloys more prone to tarnish and corrosion (Chapter 3). For Pd–Ag alloys, it is necessary to have Pd dispersed uniformly for providing tarnish and corrosion resistance in the oral environment (which causes silver to tarnish). Alloys with heterogeneous microstructures have greater resistance to permanent deformation than alloys with homogeneous microstructures, as discussed in Chapter 9. The ductility of an alloy that is single phase under equilibrium conditions increases after a homogenization heat treatment that eliminates nonequilibrium secondary phases.

CRITICAL QUESTION

What are the advantages and disadvantages of eutectic alloys? How do the alloy compositions of binary eutectic systems affect their properties?

Eutectic Alloys

When the two metals in a binary system have the same crystal structure but limited mutual solid solubility, the phase diagram may include two solid solutions, one rich in the first metal and the other rich in the second metal. Figure 2.18 shows a phase diagram for the Ag–Cu system and a schematic microstructure of each phase. Three phases can be observed: A liquid phase (L), a silver-rich substitutional solid-solution phase (α) containing a small percentage of copper atoms, and a copper-rich substitutional solid-solution phase (β) containing a small percentage of silver atoms. The solidus curve is the boundary line ABEFD, and the liquidus curve is AED. In the α + β region (CBEFG), both solid solutions exist. Note that the alloy composition represented by E has the lowest melting point of the alloy system. The composition of point E is known as the eutectic composition, 28% Cu and 72% Ag, for the Ag–Cu alloy system. Because point E is also on the solidus curve, the eutectic composition should solidify completely at a single temperature (the eutectic temperature) that is referred to as an invariant point.

Phase Changes of Eutectic Alloys

The Ag–Cu phase diagram (Fig. 2.18A) represents a typical binary eutectic phase diagram and is used in the following discussion of the phase changes that can occur during cooling. Line ABC (termed a solvus line) shows the solid solubility of Cu in silver for the α solid solution as the temperature changes; this solid solubility reaches a maximum at point B (~9% at 780°C). Solvus line DFG shows that the solid solubility of Ag in Cu reaches a maximum at point F (~8% at 780°C) but has a very low value at 300°C (point G).

The eutectic liquid composition solidifies at a single temperature to a solid phase comprising two phases (α and β). A lamellar structure with alternating layers of the α and β phases typically forms, such as shown in Figure 2.18B, because a minimal amount of diffusion is required to produce the needed segregation of the two different atom species.

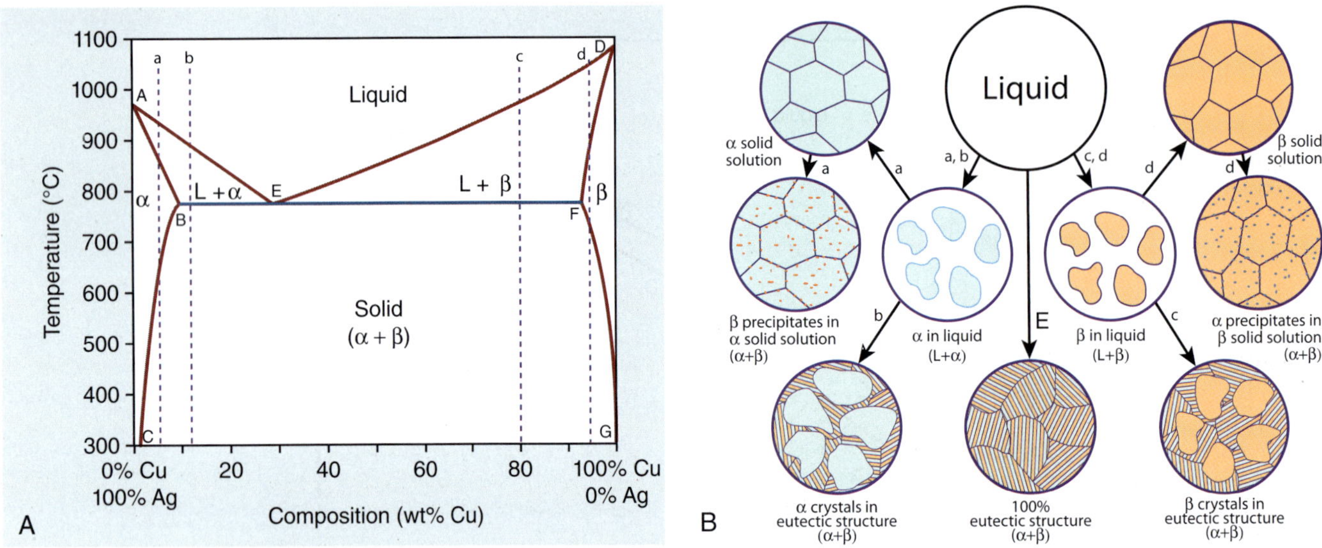

• **Fig. 2.18** Equilibrium-phase diagram of a eutectic alloy. **(A)** Silver–copper system showing percentages by weight. **(B)** Diagram of all possible phase transformations in the silver–copper system. Note that the ratio of phases is not to the scale of the composition.

Figure 2.18B illustrates phase-transformation equilibrium cooling of five different alloy compositions in the Ag–Cu system. For the molten 5% Cu alloy (line a), cooling to the (L + α) region causes precipitation of α crystals within the liquid. Further cooling past line AB results in complete solidification of the alloy to α solid solution. As the alloy is cooled further, the solubility limit at BC forces precipitation of β solid solution within α, typically at grain boundaries or interdendritic regions. There is no eutectic microstructure for this alloy composition because the cooling (vertical dashed line) does not cross the eutectic isotherm line (BEF). When the cooling of a liquid-phase (line b) alloy containing 12% Cu crosses AE, crystals of α emerge in the liquid. When this alloy cools past line BEF, the remaining liquid forms a lamellar eutectic structure around existing α crystals. The amount of the eutectic constituent in the microstructure of the solid alloy depends on how close the alloy composition is to the eutectic composition. For the alloy containing 80% Cu (line c), the changes in composition during cooling are similar as in line b, except that now the first solid to form as crystals in the liquid phase is the β solid solution. At a temperature below BEF, this alloy will have β crystals surrounded by the lamellar eutectic structure. For the molten 94% Cu alloy (line d), the sequence of phase transformation is the same as in line a, except that it forms β solid solution instead.

Physical Properties and Application of Eutectic Alloys

Alloys that contain the eutectic constituent in their microstructures are relatively brittle, whereas alloys with microstructures lacking the eutectic constituent are ductile. Alloy embrittlement occurs because the alternating lamellae of the α and β phases inhibit the movement of dislocations (Chapter 9), which increases strength and hardness but decreases ductility. The tarnish resistance of these alloys without the eutectic constituent is superior to that of the alloys containing this constituent.

Eutectic alloys have several important applications in dentistry because they correspond to a composition with the lowest melting point in an alloy system. They are used in joining metal components through processes of brazing or soldering (Chapter 9). The Ag–Cu eutectic composition is also used to produce spherical particles that are combined with Ag_3Sn lathe-cut particles to be reacted with mercury to form a dispersed-phase dental amalgam (Chapter 8).

Peritectic Alloys

Like the eutectic transformation, the peritectic reaction is an invariant reaction that occurs at a particular composition and temperature. Figure 2.19 is the phase diagram for the Ag–Pt alloy

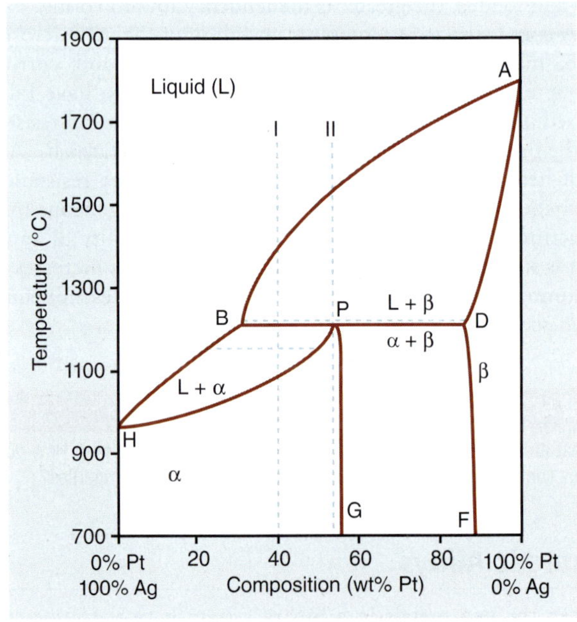

• **Fig. 2.19** Equilibrium-phase diagram of the platinum–silver system showing percentages by weight.

system, which is useful for instructional purposes, although there is no Ag–Pt dental alloy. The pure metals Ag and Pt have the FCC structure. Rather than the difference in atomic radii, the dominant factor is the considerably greater difference in melting temperature for Ag and Pt compared with Ag and Cu. The α phase in the Ag–Pt system is silver-rich, the β phase is platinum-rich, and the two-phase (α + β) region results from the limited solid solubility of less than approximately 12% Ag in Pt at 700°C (point F). Figure 2.19 also shows that the equilibrium solid solubility of Pt in Ag is approximately 56% at 700°C (point G). The peritectic transformation occurs at point P (alloy II), where the liquid (composition at point B) and the platinum-rich β phase (composition at point D) transform into the platinum-rich α phase (composition at point P). For a composition, such as exists for alloy I, cooling through the peritectic temperature results in the transformation of the liquid and β phase (L + β) to the α phase, with some of the liquid phase remaining (L + α). For both of these transformations, the α phase forms at the interface between the liquid and β phase. Because extensive diffusion is required in these phases for the transformation to occur, peritectic alloys are highly susceptible to coring during rapid cooling. This cored structure has inferior corrosion resistance and is more brittle than the homogeneous solid-solution phase. The peritectic reaction in the Ag–Sn system is of great importance for the alloy that reacts with mercury to form dental amalgam for restorations, as discussed in Chapter 8.

Solid-State Reactions in High-Noble and Noble Alloy Systems

The strength and hardness in some metal alloys may be manipulated by the presence or absence of uniformly dispersed fine particles or certain phases within the original matrix phase. The process can be achieved via a solid-state reaction (i.e., a controlled heating and cooling protocol, also called heat treatment) without changing the configuration of the object. The best-known example is the ordering of Au–Cu alloys.

CRITICAL QUESTION

By which two mechanisms does copper provide strengthening and hardening of gold casting alloys?

Gold–Copper System

Figure 2.20 presents the Au–Cu phase diagram, where both weight and atomic percentages are shown. The melting range

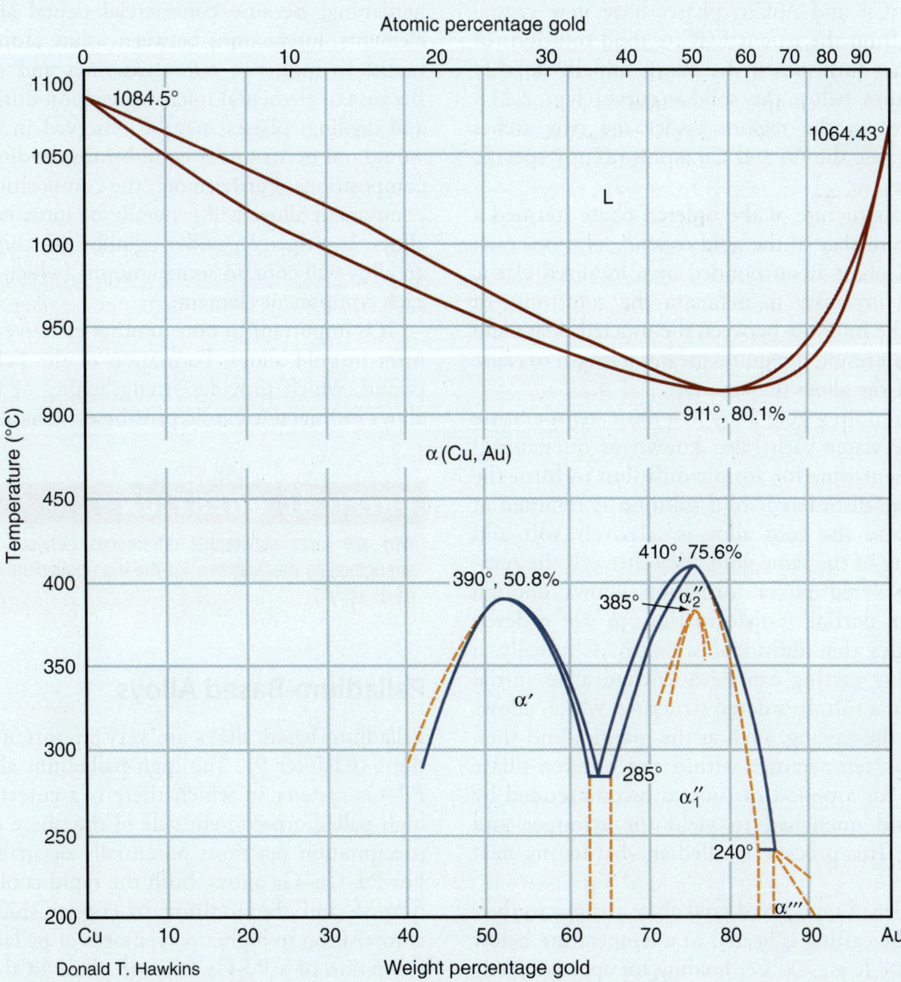

• **Fig. 2.20** Equilibrium-phase diagram for the gold–copper system. (The temperature range between 450°C and 900°C has been condensed.) (With permission from *Metals Handbook*, ed 8, vol 8, Metals Park, OH, 1973, American Society for Metals, p. 267.)

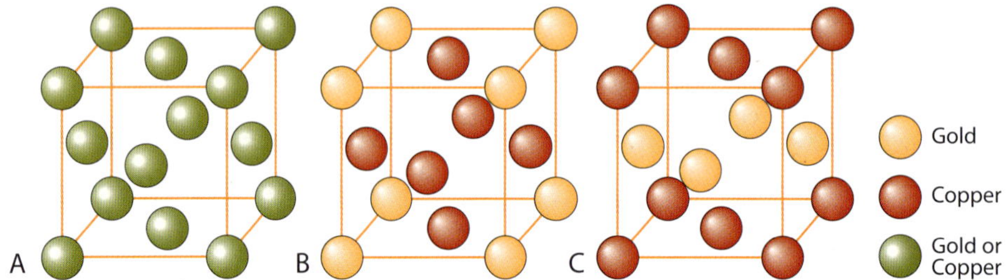

• **Fig. 2.21** Structure of Au–Cu alloy. **(A)** Disordered substitutional solid solution. **(B)** Superlattice of $AuCu_3$. **(C)** Superlattice of AuCu.

between the solid and liquid phases is narrow for all compositions, and the liquidus and solidus curves meet at 80.1 wt% Au. At the lower half of the diagram, there are two arch-shaped regions. One arch spans the composition range between 40 and 65 wt% Au and peaks at 390°C with 50.8 wt% Au (α'). The atomic ratio of Au to Cu at the peak is 1:3, indicating the formation of the intermetallic compound $AuCu_3$ in this region. The second arch spans the composition range between 65 and 85 wt% Au and peaks at 410°C with 75.6 wt% Au ($\alpha 2''$). The atomic ratio of Au to Cu at this peak is 1:1, indicating the formation of intermetallic compound AuCu in this region. The α solid solution that forms when the alloys initially solidify has a disordered structure in which the Au and Cu atoms randomly occupy the lattice sites (Fig. 2.21A). The AuCu and $AuCu_3$ phases have new crystal structures that differ from the parent FCC α solid solutions of Au and Cu atoms that form when the alloys initially solidify at elevated temperatures below the solidus curve (Fig. 2.21B and C). These phases in the regions under the two arches are called ordered because the Au and Cu atoms occupy specific locations in the lattices.

Because the crystal structure of the ordered phase (termed a superlattice) differs from that of the gold α solid solution, each region of the ordered phase is surrounded by a localized elastic strain field, which is necessary to maintain the continuity of atomic bonds across the interface between the ordered phase and the matrix α phase. As a result, it requires greater strength to cause plastic deformation of the alloys (Chapter 9).

Rapid cooling of a molten gold alloy in a room-temperature water bath or an ice-water bath (also known as quenching) does not allow sufficient time for atomic diffusion to form the ordered structure. The disordered solid solution is retained at room temperature, and the gold alloy is relatively soft and ductile. Bench cooling of the same gold alloy through the temperature range of ordered phase formation allows enough atomic diffusion for partial transformation to an ordered structure that provides the additional strength. Clinically, a type 3 or 4 gold alloy casting can be quenched after initial solidification to retain a soft disordered structure, which allows easier adjustment of the casting, such as the margin, and then reheated to a specific temperature within the ordered-phase region (e.g., 400°C) for a period of time as recommended by the manufacturer and quenched to yield the stronger and harder ordered alloy. This process is called age-hardening heat treatment.

To reverse the hardened type 3 or 4 gold alloy castings to their softened condition, the casting is heated to a temperature below the solidus temperature (e.g., 700°C), holding for approximately 10 minutes to convert the alloy to the disordered substitutional solid solution, and then quenched to retain the disordered phase. The process is called a solution heat treatment.

It should be noted that the quenched, softened condition for types 3 and 4 gold alloys is metastable, and slow increases in hardness and strength will occur with time under room-temperature or intraoral conditions as a result of low-temperature ordering. This behavior was shown in an elegant study by Watanabe et al. (1994), who also described a high-gold alloy containing gallium that is capable of rapid intraoral ordering.

Other Noble Alloys for Dental Applications

Dental gold casting alloys may contain solute metals (Cu, Pd, and Pt), which provide solid-solution strengthening, along with minor amounts ($< 1\%$) of Zn or Ir forming precipitates, leading to age hardening. Because commercial dental alloys contain multiple elements, interactions between solute atom species have the potential to influence microstructures and mechanical properties. Because of elemental microsegregation during rapid solidification and cooling, phases may be observed in cast dental alloys that would not occur under equilibrium conditions for the same alloy compositions. Furthermore, the compositions of phases in multicomponent alloys will generally be more complex than in binary alloys. In principle, under equilibrium conditions, each phase in an alloy will contain some amount (which may be minuscule) of each component element.

It is important to note another effective age-hardening mechanism in gold alloys: Formation of the $FePt_3$ intermetallic compound, which provides strengthening of the original high-gold alloys for metal–ceramic prostheses (Chapter 9).

CRITICAL QUESTION

Why are there substantial differences between the microstructures and strengthening mechanisms for the high-palladium alloys and the palladium–silver alloys?

Palladium-Based Alloys

Palladium-based alloys are very important for ceramic applications (Chapter 9). The high-palladium alloys are based on the Pd–Ga system, in which there is a eutectic composition at the high-palladium-content side of the phase diagram, and complex precipitation reactions potentially occur at lower temperatures. For Pd–Cu–Ga alloys, both the rapid cooling rate during solidification and the addition of copper shift the Pd–Ga eutectic composition to higher percentages of palladium that result in the formation of a Pd_2Ga eutectic phase in the cast microstructure. Both Pd–Cu–Ga and Pd–Ga alloys have a fine submicron "tweed" structure that can be observed by transmission electron microscopy. This structure appears to form by a martensitic phase transformation in the FCC structure of the palladium solid-solution matrix and remains stable during the firing cycles for dental porcelain. Strengthening of these alloys occurs by the solid-solution mechanism and by the formation of Pd_5Ga_2 precipitates in some Pd–Cu–Ga alloy compositions. In contrast, the Pd–Ag alloys are based on the binary alloy system discussed earlier in this chapter and have much simpler microstructures than the high-palladium alloys, with secondary phases forming in the Pd solid-solution matrix because of the solute atoms in the alloy compositions. Heat treatment of these alloys can cause microstructural changes that significantly affect mechanical properties.

Multicomponent Dental Alloy Systems

Various age-hardening mechanisms have been employed (often empirically) by alloy manufacturers, and these may vary depending on the alloy composition. There are many possible ternary alloys, quaternary alloys, and higher order multicomponent alloy systems that can be used for restorative dentistry. Such systems are complex, and the phase-diagram data available are extremely limited. Thus, binary phase diagrams are often used to estimate the effect of individual elements on the phases formed, along with the resulting microstructures of these cast alloys. However, such equilibrium diagrams should be interpreted carefully because actual casting and cooling processes reflect nonequilibrium conditions.

Ceramics

Ceramics are solid-phase compounds of metallic and nonmetallic elements. Recall that the valence electrons of metallic atoms can be transferred to nonmetallic atoms or groups of atoms with outer shells that are nearly complete with electrons to form stable compounds by ionic bonds, and that nonmetallic atoms may also share electrons to form another kind of compound by covalent bonding. Both scenarios deprive compounds of free electrons, thus making them poor conductors of heat and electrical current. Even though they comprise metallic elements but lack characteristics of metal substance, ceramics are considered nonmetallic, inorganic structures.

In the search for the ideal restorative material, dental ceramics have become attractive because of their biocompatibility, long-term color stability, chemical durability, wear resistance, and ability to be formed into precise shapes, although in some cases, ceramics require costly processing equipment and specialized training for lab technicians. In this segment, we will discuss the general structure of ceramics and how the structure affects the mechanical properties of ceramics. Further information on the structure, properties, benefits, and drawbacks of specific ceramic materials used for crown and bridge prostheses will be provided, along with recent developments in dental ceramics.

Structure of Ceramics

Like metals, ceramics have 3D crystalline structures, but they are much more complicated than those of metals because they need to accommodate different kinds of atoms, maintain electric charge neutrality within the unit cell, and achieve high packing efficiency. Normally, the metallic elements lose their original crystalline structure and adopt a new one. Consider magnesium oxide (MgO), a significant ingredient in investment materials (Chapter 14) and modern dental ceramics (Chapter 10); Mg in metallic crystal has a hexagonal structure (Fig. 2.8F), and the structure of MgO, which is the same as NaCl (Fig. 2.6B), shows that anions O^{2-} (large orange spheres) retain an FCC structure, whereas Mg^{2+} ions (small blue spheres) are in the interstitial locations because they are smaller in size. Current dental ceramics are based on silicate ($[SiO_4]^{4-}$ tetrahedron), alumina (Al_2O_3), and zirconia (ZrO_2).

Soda–lime glass is a silicate-based material commonly used for windowpanes, glass containers (bottles and jars), and artworks. It is manufactured by melting raw materials, which are silica, soda, lime, and small quantity of varieties of metallic oxides. It has all the ingredients needed to form crystalline structures, but the composition used in soda–lime glass yields short-range, repetitive-order structures. Therefore, ceramic materials with a short-range repetitive order of their structural units are usually called glasses or glassy phase, which are also transparent to the light. Glassy phases of ceramic melt at lower temperature. They play an important role in the fabrication of ceramic-based prostheses (Chapter 10).

The complexity of crystalline and the strong bonds holding the atoms together make the solid-state reactions of ceramic sluggish. At a normal cooling rate, the ceramic does not have enough time to arrange itself into the complicated crystalline structure it could achieve. We, nonetheless, can subject these materials to a heat treatment like that of Au–Cu system by nucleation and growth of crystals in the glass-matrix phase. This type of material is used in dentistry to balance the translucency and opacity of the prostheses. They are called glass-ceramics.

Most metal-forming operations depend on the casting of molten metal and/or mechanical forming of the metal (Chapter 9). These operations are rarely used in ceramic-forming operations because of the high melting point and almost extreme brittleness (no ductility) of ceramics. We will learn in Chapter 10 that fabricating dental ceramics into prosthetic shapes and configurations is conducted through one of the three categories of processes: Sintering, hot isostatic pressing, and computer-aided design/computer-aided manufacturing (CAD−CAM) (see also Chapter 15). A prosthesis is first sculpted out of dental ceramic powder with the help of a binder, which is followed by a heating process called sintering. During sintering, the packed ceramic particles are densified and agglomerate to the intended form. Primary bonding occurs between the particles by liquid-phase sintering with a glassy phase, or solid-state sintering. The preparation of hot isostatic pressing is like metal casting, except that dental ceramic is not melted but softened enough to be pressed into a mold with a cavity of the shape of the prosthesis. CAD−CAM comprises all processes that require the use of a computer to control the making of prostheses. Each of the three structures of the ceramics discussed earlier can be formulated to facilitate each of the three fabrication processes.

Mechanical Properties of Ceramics

Most ceramic materials are described as brittle; that is, they are incapable of large deformations without fracture (Chapter 4). Let us examine the deformation of a metal (Au) and a ceramic (MgO) in terms of atoms' movement between two rows of atoms (Fig. 2.22) in response to a pair of forces pushing the top row right and bottom row left. In the case of metal, every atom in the top row must break a metallic bond with one atom and reconnect with another one in the bottom row. For example, atom 2 breaks a metallic bond with atom 3 and then reconnects with atom 5. The coordination arrangement is the same as before (Fig. 2.22A). This kind of movement is called slip, and the interphase where it occurs is called a slip plane. In the case of ceramic, which consists

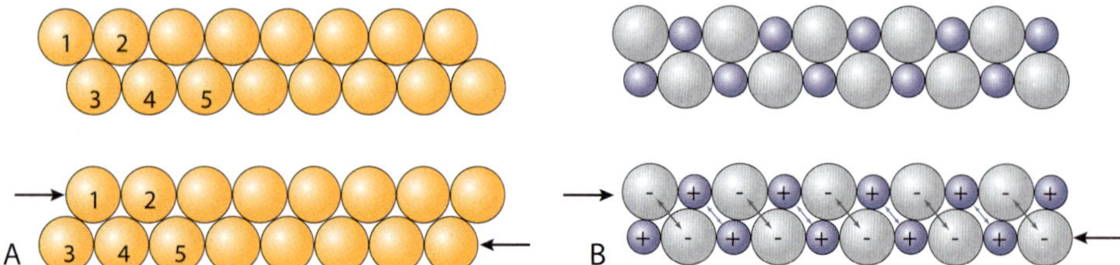

• **Fig. 2.22** Comparison of slip. **(A)** Monoatomic metals of Au. **(B)** Biatomic ceramic of MgO; Mg is shown by the blue spheres, and oxygen is shown by the gray spheres. More force is required to displace atoms because of attraction between different atoms and repulsion between similar atoms.

of Mg^{2+} and O^{2-} ions, a similar movement necessitates the breaking of strong ionic bonds, like the gold atoms need to break metallic bonds. Before the ions complete the transition to restore the original atomic arrangements, they must overcome the high-energy positive–positive and negative–negative repulsion forces when they encounter ions of the same charge (Fig. 2.22B). The entire process requires a tremendous expenditure of energy. This requirement restricts the mechanism of slip in ceramic materials.

Thus, slip restriction makes ceramic materials brittle and more resistant to fracture under compression but not under tension. In practice, defects such as pores within the bulk and cracks on the surface are often introduced during processing, production, and handling (Chapter 10). These irregularities produce stress concentrations in a material (Chapter 4). For ductile materials such as gold, the stress concentration can be relieved by atomic slippage. For brittle materials, the stress concentration cannot be relieved and can easily exceed the tensile strength of the materials, causing fracture. Under compression, defects like cracks do not accentuate the stress. Thus, ceramic materials are much stronger in compression than in tension. The role of defects in the longevity of ceramic-based prostheses and means of minimizing the impact of these defects are discussed in Chapter 10.

Polymers

Polymers are a class of natural or synthetic substances composed of very high-molecular-weight molecules with repeating units, called macromolecules. For synthetic polymers, each repeating unit is called mer in the polymer and a monomer before becoming part of the macromolecule by a chemical reaction called polymerization. The main chain of a macromolecule is called the backbone. Generally, resin is a solid or highly viscous substance of plant or synthetic origin that is typically convertible into polymers. For our purpose, resins are compositions of either monomers or macromolecules blended with other components to provide a material, after polymerization, with a useful set of properties.

Synthetic resins polymerize randomly from activated local sites. Thus, depending on the ability of the chains to grow from their local activation sites, the molecular chains that form within a polymeric material will vary in length, shape, and structure. Although the primary bonds are holding the atoms within a polymer chain, there may be secondary bonds and/or hydrogen bonds between polymer chains. In addition, polymer chains often become entangled, adding complexity to the structure. As a result, many physical and mechanical properties are determined largely by intermolecular forces. In this section, we will discuss the nature of polymers, their physical and mechanical properties, and polymerization. Restorative, bonding, and prosthodontic applications of polymers are discussed in Chapters 5, 6, and 11, respectively.

Fundamental Nature of Polymers

Polymerization is a repetitive intermolecular chain-growth reaction that can proceed almost indefinitely, sometimes reaching molecular weights as high as 50 million. The two most significant features of polymers are very large macromolecules and virtually limitless chain configurations and conformations.

Molecular Weight

Because of the difference in the length of chains in the polymer, a method of expressing an "average" molecular weight of a heterogeneous polymer is needed for the overall molecular weight of polymers. The number-average molecular weight ($\bar{M}n$) is the total weight of a polymer divided by the overall number of molecules present in the material. The number of molecules can be obtained by measuring the osmotic pressure of the polymer solution. The weight-average molecular weight ($\bar{M}w$), which can be obtained by light scattering of the same polymer solution, is the sum of molecular weight multiplied by the respective weight fraction. The International System (SI) unit for the molecular weight of polymers is the same as that of nonpolymer compounds; it is g/mol and is also known as Dalton (Da).

Considering the concepts just discussed, the ratio $\bar{M}w/\bar{M}n$ (called the polydispersity) of a polymer is a measure of the range and distribution of chain sizes. Polymers with an equal value of $\bar{M}w$ but different values of polydispersity will exhibit somewhat different properties. For example, polymers of higher polydispersity will begin to melt at a lower temperature and have a larger temperature range of melting.

Chain Branching and Crosslinking

It is possible for a growing polymer chain to branch and lose its linear form (Fig. 2.23). Branching is analogous to extra arms growing out of a backbone polymer chain; thus, the probability of entangled chains increases. When a monomer has more than one site for growing a chain, it can chemically connect two or more growing chains (Fig. 2.24). Because of the interlinking of many chain backbones, a highly crosslinked polymeric material can consist of just a few giant molecules or even a single giant molecule.

Copolymer Structures

Polymers that have only one type of repeating unit (mer) are homopolymers; those with two or more types of mer units are known as copolymers. There are three different types of copolymers by the arrangement of repeating units:

Random copolymer—No sequential order exists among the two or more mer units along the polymer chain.

AAAAAABBBBBAAAABBBBBBAAAAABBB

Block copolymer—Identical monomer units occur in relatively long sequences (blocks) along the main polymer chain.

AAAAAABBBBBAAAABBBBBBAAAAABBB

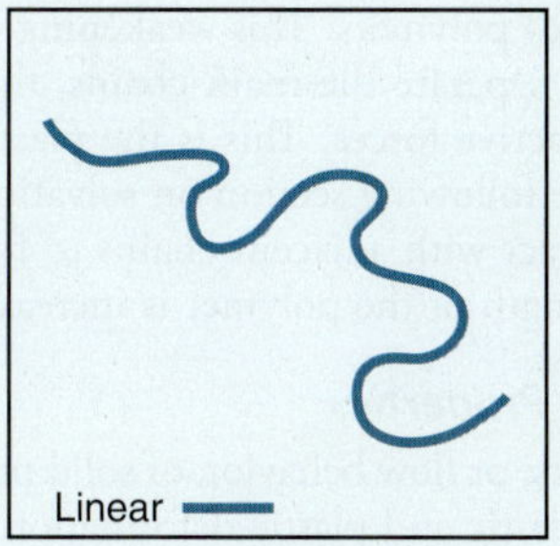

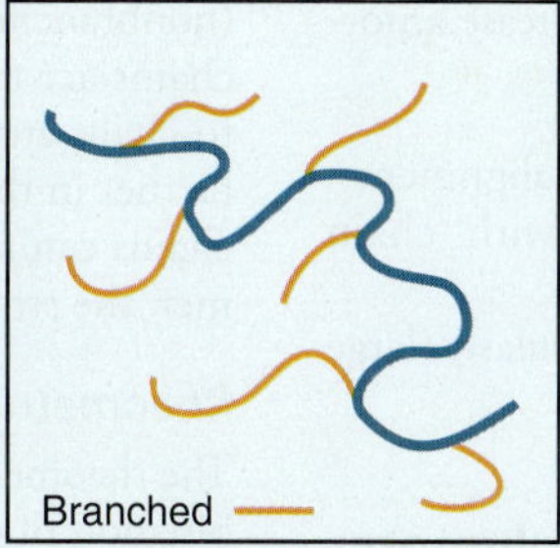

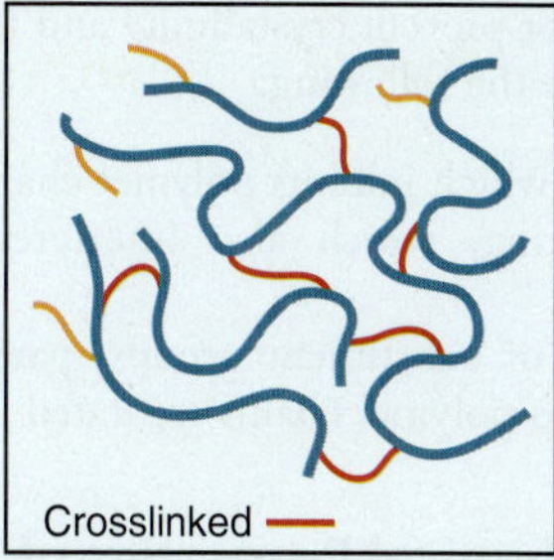

• **Fig. 2.23** Schematic diagrams of linear, branched, and crosslinked polymers.

methyl methacrylate

Crosslinking

ethylene glycol dimethacrylate

Crosslinked methacrylate copolymer

• **Fig. 2.24** A crosslinked structure is formed by copolymerization, where at least one comonomer is multifunctional. Here methylmethacrylate is copolymerized with ethylene glycol dimethacrylate.

Graft or branched copolymer—Sequences of one type of mer unit (B) are "grafted" onto a backbone chain of a second (A) type of mer unit to form a branched configuration (see Fig. 2.23).

```
AAAAAAAAAAAAAAAAAAA
   B      B      B
   B      B      B
   B      B      B
   B      B      B
                 B
```

Molecular Organization

In most polymers, the chains are coiled and entangled in a very random pattern known as an amorphous structure (Fig. 2.25, *left*). In others, the chains align themselves to form a highly ordered region, like that of crystalline structures (Fig. 2.25, *right*). Most polymeric materials combine these two forms of organization in greater or lesser proportions. Characteristically, the dental polymers are predominantly amorphous, with little or no crystallinity. The polymer chains form a tangled mass, analogous to cooked spaghetti, in which each spaghetti string is a mile or so long. Such polymer segments have little chance to migrate and are immobile in the solid state.

However, many linear polymers have regions of long-range ordering that produce a degree of crystallinity depending on the secondary bonds that can be formed, the structure of the polymer chain, the degree of ordering, and the molecular weight. Polymer crystallinity usually increases strength, rigidity, hardness, and melting temperature, but at the price of reduced ductility—that is, increased brittleness.

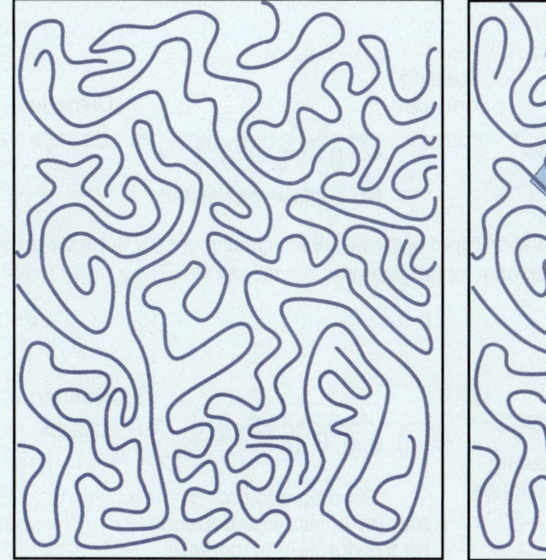

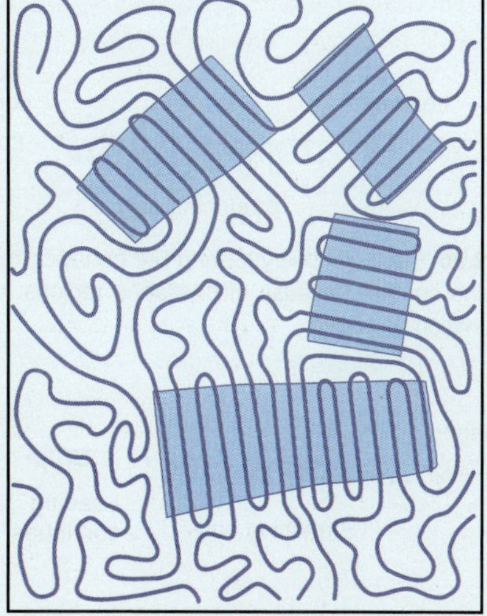

• **Fig. 2.25** Schematic diagram of polymers that contain only amorphous intermolecular and intramolecular organization *(left)* and combinations of both amorphous and crystalline regions *(shaded areas on right)*.

Factors that reduce or prevent crystallinity and increase amorphous character include the following:

Copolymer formation, which inhibits polymer chain alignment
Polymer-chain branching, which also interferes with chain alignment
Random arrangement of substituent groups, particularly large side groups that keep polymer chains separated

Physical and Mechanical Properties of Polymers

The performance of polymers depends on the interaction between polymer chains and their response to external stimuli. These properties can be grouped into three interrelated categories: Mechanical, dissolution, and thermal.

Mechanical Properties—Deformation and Recovery

In the absence of crosslinking, only relatively weak interpolymer-chain bonds (van der Waals and hydrogen bonds) are available to hold the polymer chains together in a solid state. Chain slippage decreases as chain length increases because the bonds between chains, together with chain entanglements, resist dislodgment of the individual chains. At a certain chain length, the resistance provided by interchain bonds and entanglements becomes strong enough to exceed the covalent bond strength of the carbon–carbon bonds along the backbone chains. At this critical chain length, an applied force can rupture chains rather than dislodge them and cause one chain to slide past another. This balance between the strength of the interchain bonds and the covalent bonds along the backbone chains explains why the physical and mechanical properties of polymers increase with increased molecular weight up to a certain point. Subsequently, increased molecular weight becomes less important.

Although dependent on its type, a resin generally develops mechanical strength only when its degree of polymerization is relatively high, in the range of approximately 150–200 recurring mer units. Above this molecular weight, there is very little increase in strength with further polymerization. Likewise, the molecular-weight distribution of the polymer plays an important role in determining physical properties. In general, a narrow distribution of molecular weight yields the most useful balance among required properties.

Long side chains extending from the main backbone chain (i.e., chain branching) generally produce a weaker resin with a lower softening temperature in comparison with linear-chain (nonbranched) polymers. This weakening occurs because the side chains act to separate the main chains, thus reducing the chain-to-chain attractive forces. This is the plasticizing effect discussed further in the following section on solvation. However, if the side chains can react with adjacent chains to form a crosslinked polymer, the strength of the polymer is increased.

Rheometric Properties

The rheometry, or flow behavior, of solid polymers involves a combination of elastic and plastic deformation, followed by elastic recovery after the stresses are eliminated. The chain length, number of crosslinks, temperature, and rate of force application (fast impact versus slow extension or extrusion) determine which type of behavior dominates. A force applied to polymers for an extended period causes the material to undergo all of the following deformations: Elastic strain, plastic strain, and viscoelastic strain.

1. Elastic strain is reversible deformation and will be quickly and completely recovered when the force is eliminated, as the result of polymer chains uncoiling and then recoiling (Fig. 2.26).
2. Plastic strain is irreversible deformation that cannot be recovered and results in a new, permanent shape as a result of slippage among polymer *chains* (Fig. 2.27).
3. Viscoelastic strain consists of both elastic and plastic deformation in addition to those mentioned in 1 and 2. The elastic portion of the viscoelastic strain will recover when the force is removed, but the recovery takes time to complete because the elastic recovery process is impeded by the viscous flow resistance among chains. The amount of deformation that is not recovered within the viscoelastic strain will be additional to 1.

Solvation and Dissolution Properties

When a polymer is immersed in a liquid solvent, it can absorb the solvent, swell, soften, and even dissolve in the solvent. If the polymer–solvent interactions are higher than the polymer–polymer attraction forces, the polymer chain segment starts to absorb solvent molecules, increase the volume of the polymer matrix, and become solvated in the solvent. It, however, is a slow process. The longer the chains extend, the more slowly the polymer dissolves. Crosslinking provides enough bridges between linear chains to form a 3D network that decreases solvent sorption, making the polymer nonsoluble. Elastomer, a rubber-like material that is lightly crosslinked, can swell more easily and to a greater extent than do plastics but does not dissolve. Crystalline regions having higher polymer–polymer interaction act as physical

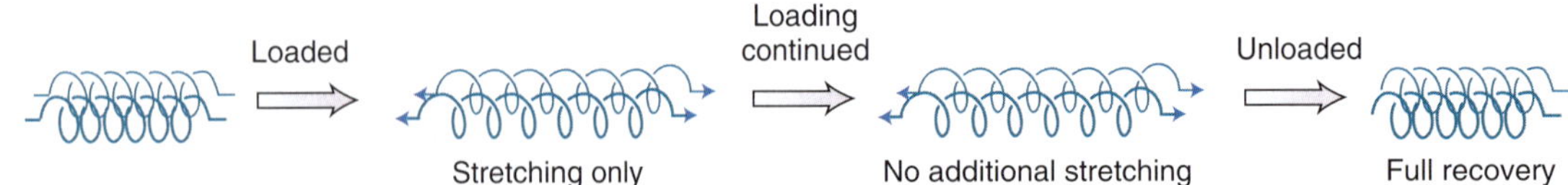

• **Fig. 2.26** Elastic recovery: Spring-like behavior (rapid and reversible). Chains uncoil, but they do not slip past one another because of crystalline regions, entanglements, or crosslinks. Thus, they recoil completely when unloaded.

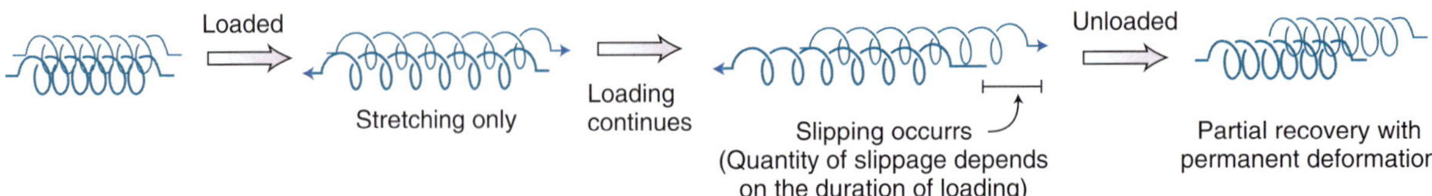

• **Fig. 2.27** Viscoelastic recovery: Chains stretch and uncoil and also slip past one another, producing plastic, irreversible, permanent distortion, and partial recovery when unloaded.

crosslinks, reducing swelling and solubility. Chain branching should increase solubility.

The ability to absorb low-molecular-weight compounds makes it possible to modify the properties of polymers by a process called plasticization. Low-molecular-weight compounds, known as plasticizers, are often added to resins to lower their softening or melting/fusion temperatures, making a resin that is normally hard and stiff at room temperature, flexible, and soft. For example, polyvinylchloride (PVC) pipe is hard and rigid, whereas PVC water-line tubing is soft and elastic and contains a very high level of plasticizer. In recent years, certain plasticizers, particularly phthalates, have received public attention as a potential ingestion hazard in the soft plastics used in infants' and children's toys.

A plasticizer acts to partially neutralize the secondary bonds or intermolecular attractions that normally prevent the resin chains from slipping past one another (i.e., undergoing plastic flow) when the material is stressed. In some cases, this action is analogous to that of a solvent, with the plasticizing agent penetrating between the chains and increasing the intermolecular spacing. This type of plasticizer is referred to as an external plasticizer because it is not a part of the polymer's structure. Its molecular attraction to the polymer should be high to avoid volatilization or leaching out during the fabrication or subsequent use of the resin.

Plasticizing can also be accomplished by copolymerization with a suitable comonomer. In this case, the plasticizing agent becomes part of the polymer and acts as an internal plasticizer. Plasticizers usually reduce the strength, hardness, and softening temperature of the resin. For example, both internal and external plasticizers are used to help form soft, cushioning liners for dentures.

Thermal Properties

Polymers can be reshaped into many configurations, depending on whether the polymeric material is a "thermoset" or a "thermoplastic."

Thermoplastic polymers soften when heated above Tg, the temperature where secondary bonds weaken, and the resin softens and becomes ductile or rubbery (Fig. 2.28). Above the Tg, the resin can then be shaped and molded and, upon cooling, retains the new configuration. This process can be repeated almost indefinitely. Thermoplastic resins are made of linear and/or branched chains. Without crosslinking, covalent bonds holding chains together, they can soften (and eventually melt) above Tg and are usually soluble in organic solvents.

In contrast, thermoset polymers are formed by heating a precursor mixture, which initiates polymerization, and the ensuing chemical changes render it rigid after cooling. Resins are crosslinked in this state, and thus, they are insoluble and will not melt when heated beyond their glass-transition temperature but instead become rubbery (Fig. 2.28). In this manner, the chains are rendered more flexible when heated, and the crosslinks prevent chain slippage and reshaping. Thermoset resins decompose if heated to a high enough temperature.

If two otherwise-similar linear polymers are compared, the one with the higher molecular weight will also have a higher Tg. This is because as the length of the linear-polymer chain is increased, the number of bond sites increases along that chain. In addition, the longer length of the chain increases the chance for chain entanglements. The number-average molecular weight ($\bar{M}n$) is indicative of both Tg and the strength of the polymer. As the temperature increases, thermally induced rotations and vibrations among polymer segments increase. This molecular motion forces chains apart, breaks bonds, increases thermal expansion, and facilitates chain disentanglement. These factors, in turn, induce chain slippage and explain the thermoplastic behavior of a resin

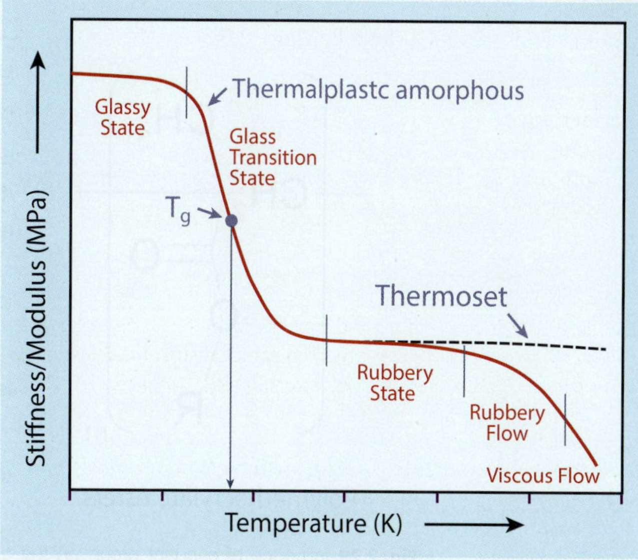

• **Fig. 2.28** Effect of temperature on the stiffness of amorphous thermoplastic and thermoset polymers. Both materials exhibit glass-transition and rubbery states. The structure of thermoplastic polymer turns to rubbery and then viscous liquid, whereas thermoset polymer remains rubbery and then burns. An amorphous polymer takes on characteristic glassy-state properties, such as brittleness, stiffness, and rigidity.

when the temperature exceeds Tg. As the degree of crosslinking increases, slippage is progressively reduced, and the material becomes progressively more resistant to thermal softening.

Figure 2.29 illustrates the effect of the size and configuration of pendant groups on the Tg of poly(methacrylate) ester compounds. The figure shows that Tg decreases from 125°C for the shorter methyl group to 33°C for the longer n-butyl group. The isomer of respective groups, because of compact configuration, results in a smaller reduction of Tg.

Chemistry of Polymerization

Traditionally, there are two classes of polymers as determined by the polymerization mechanism: Addition and condensation polymers. Addition polymers contain the same atoms as the monomer in their repeating units, whereas condensation polymers contain fewer atoms because of the formation of by-products during the process. Emphasis, however, has changed to classify polymerization as to whether the process occurs between the functional groups of polymer chains in steps or by propagating of a growing chain by taking in monomers sequentially. Condensation polymers usually are formed by a stepwise intermolecular reaction of reactive functional groups of monomers with multiple functional groups, also known as step-growth polymerization. Addition polymers occur by propagation from active growing chains where monomers are sequentially added to one end of the chain, also known as chain-growth polymerization. Note that the classification by growth mechanism disregards the existence of by-products; therefore, step-growth polymerization does not always produce by-product, and chain-growth polymerization can yield by-products, depending on the monomers involved.

Addition Polymerization (Chain-Growth Polymerization)

For addition polymerization to occur, monomers must contain an unsaturated bond, which may exist in a double carbon-to-carbon

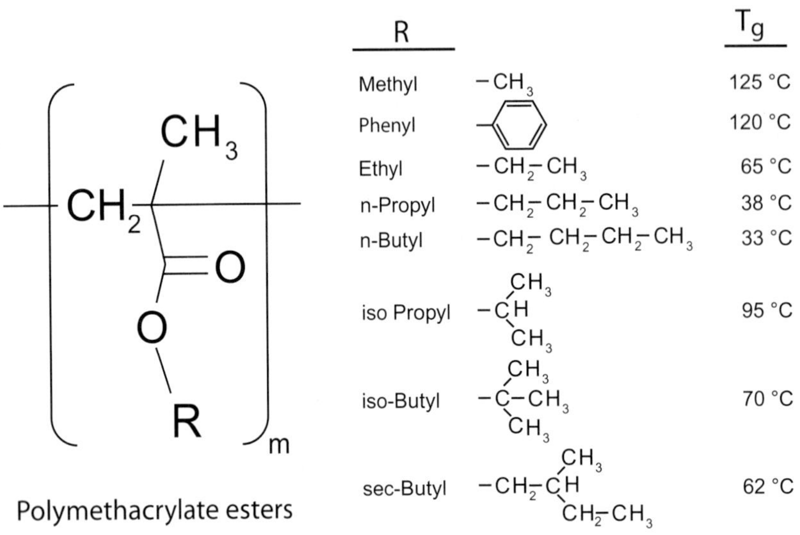

Polymethacrylate esters

R		Tg
Methyl	$-CH_3$	125 °C
Phenyl	(phenyl ring)	120 °C
Ethyl	$-CH_2-CH_3$	65 °C
n-Propyl	$-CH_2-CH_2-CH_3$	38 °C
n-Butyl	$-CH_2-CH_2-CH_2-CH_3$	33 °C
iso Propyl	$-CH(CH_3)CH_3$	95 °C
iso-Butyl	$-C(CH_3)(CH_3)-CH_3$	70 °C
sec-Butyl	$-CH_2-CH(CH_3)CH_2-CH_3$	62 °C

• **Fig. 2.29** Influence of pendant group on the glass-transition temperature of polymethacrylate esters. *R* represents ester radicals.

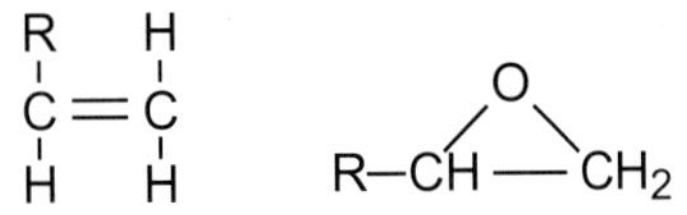

• **Fig. 2.30** Unsaturated functional groups for chain-growth polymerization: Vinyl *(left)* and epoxy ring *(right).*

bond or in a ring structure, as shown in Figure 2.30. Carbon–carbon double-bond units are known as vinyl groups and are most often exemplified in dentistry by methacrylate monomers ($H_2C{=}CR{-}COOCH_3$). Ring-opening monomers are represented by imine rings found in polyether impression materials (Chapter 13) and by epoxy rings found in silorane-based restorative resins (Chapter 5).

An initiator is also needed to start chain-growth polymerization. The initiator could be a free radical, that is, a substance containing one unpaired electron but that carries no net charge for polymerizing vinyl base monomers (R•), or an ionic compound that carries charges but maintains electrical neutrality as a catalyst for polymerization of monomers comprising rings. Stages of addition polymerization by free radicals are discussed in the following section, using methyl methacrylates, a vinyl monomer, as the model materials. The process occurs rapidly, almost instantaneously, and the reactions are exothermic, with considerable heat evolved.

Stages in Addition Polymerization of Vinyl Monomers

There are four stages in the addition polymerization chain reaction: Induction, propagation, termination, and chain transfer.

- Induction

  The induction stage comprises two processes: Generation of free radicals (activation) and initiation of polymerization. Benzoyl peroxide, which is commonly used in dental resins, can be activated rapidly between 50°C and 100°C or by a second compound, such as amine, to release free radicals (Fig. 2.31). The third method is light-activated initiation, which allows control of polymerization with precision by varying light intensity. The latter has become the preferred method of curing resin-based composites (Fig. 5.15). The stage of curing remains the same regardless of the method of activation. Induction is the period during which initiator molecules become energized and break down into free radicals, followed by these radicals reacting with monomer molecules to initiate chain growth (Fig. 2.32). This period is greatly influenced by the purity of the monomer. Any impurities present that are able to react with activated groups can increase the length of this period by consuming the activated initiator molecules. However, the higher the temperature, the more rapid is the formation of free radicals, and consequently, the shorter is the induction period.

  When a free radical approaches a monomer with a high-electron-density double bond, an electron is extracted, and it pairs with

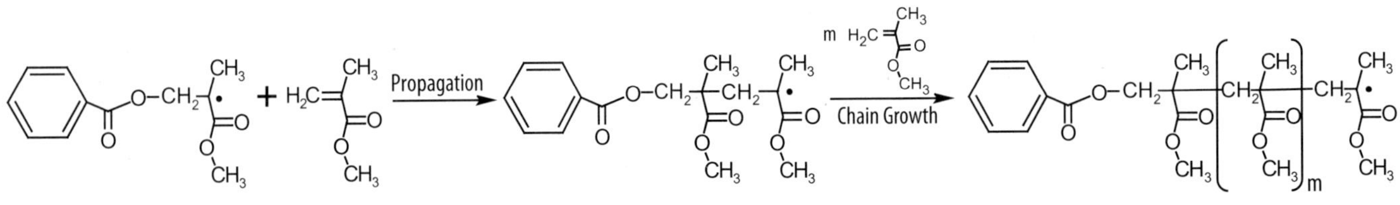

Propagation

Chain Growth

• **Fig. 2.31** Activation (heat or chemical) of benzoyl peroxide (BPO). During activation, the bond between the two oxygen atoms indicated by the hollow arrow is broken, and the electron pair is split between the two fragments. The dot adjacent to the oxygen atom symbolizes the unpaired electron of the free radical.

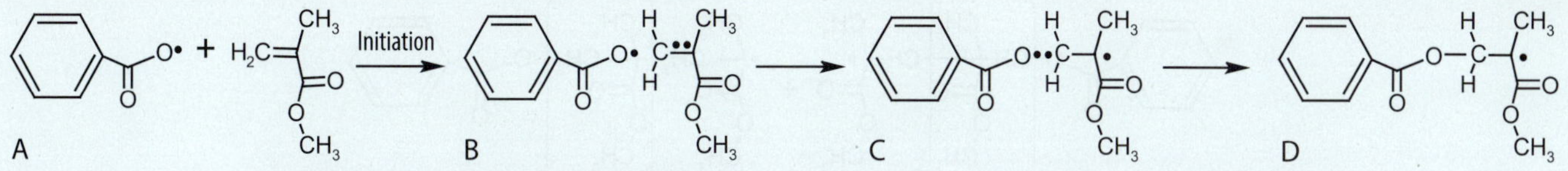

• **Fig. 2.32** Initiation of a methylmethacrylate molecule by free radical. As the unpaired electron of the free radical approaches the methylmethacrylate molecule (**A** and **B**), one of the electrons in the double bond is attracted to the free radical to form an electron pair and a covalent bond between the free radical and the monomer molecule (**C** and **D**). When this occurs, the remaining unpaired electron makes the new molecule a free radical **(D)**.

the R• electron to form a bond between the radical and the monomer molecule, leaving the other electron of the double bond unpaired. Thus, the original free radical bonds to one side of the monomer molecule and forms a new free radical site at the growing end of the chain (Fig. 2.32).

- Propagation
  The resulting free radical–monomer complex then acts as a new free radical center when it approaches another monomer to form a dimer, which also becomes a free radical. This reactive species, in turn, can add successively to a large number of methyl-methacrylate molecules so that the polymerization process continues through the propagation of the reactive center. Propagation reactions are further illustrated in Figure 2.33. Because little energy is required once chain growth begins, the process continues with the evolution of heat and leads to large polymer molecules within seconds.
- Termination
  The chain reactions should continue until all the monomer has been converted to polymer chains. However, there is a strong tendency of growing radicals to react and cause termination of chain growth. The probability increases as the monomer concentration decreases. The termination step can occur in two ways: Coupling and disproportionation. Coupling is by a direct combination of two free radical chain ends that deactivates the radicals with the formation of a covalent bond (Fig. 2.34). Disproportionation involves the transfer of a hydrogen atom from one growing chain to another (Fig. 2.35). The free radical donates the hydrogen and becomes unsaturated while the other receives the hydrogen and becomes saturated. Therefore, there are always unsaturated functional groups remaining in resin-based composite restorations (Chapter 5) and denture bases (Chapter 11).
- Chain transfer
  The process of chain transfer involves transferring the reactivity of a radical to another species, along with the termination of the donating radical. The example in Figure 2.36 shows a monomer being activated without the initiator (BPO). Because the terminated chain gained an unsaturated functional group, it could be reactivated by another chain transfer and continue to grow again.

CRITICAL QUESTION

What are the stages of activation and free radical initiation and curing? Which three activation processes are used for dental polymers?

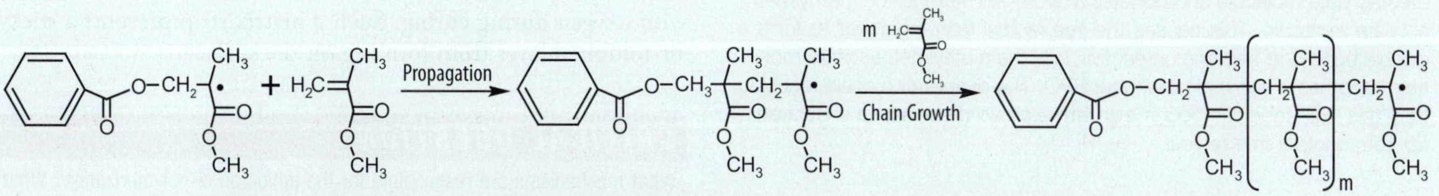

• **Fig. 2.33** Propagation and chain growth. As the initiated molecule approaches other methylmethacrylate molecules, the free electron interacts with the double bond of the methylmethacrylate molecule and incorporates the molecule to the growing chain, and a new, longer free radical is formed.

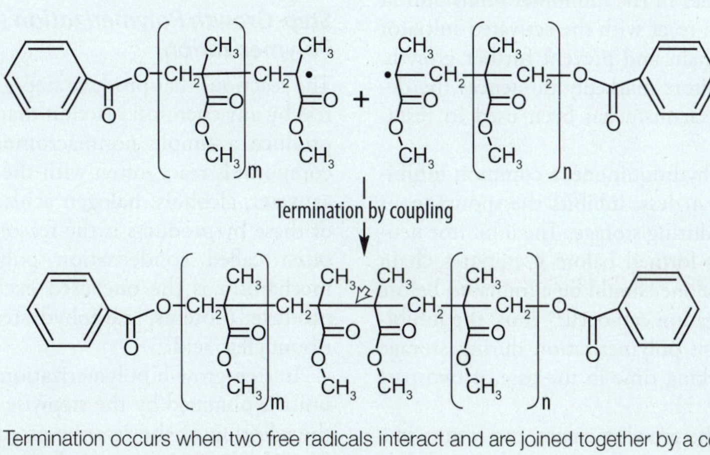

• **Fig. 2.34** Termination occurs when two free radicals interact and are joined together by a covalent bond *(hollow arrow)* but lose their reactivities.

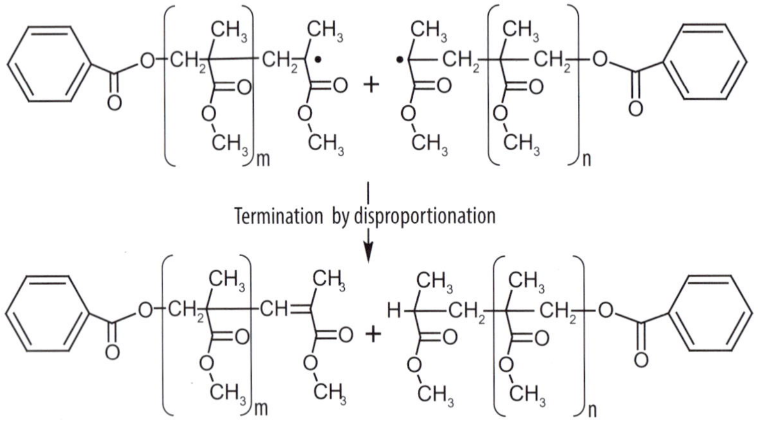

Termination by disproportionation

• **Fig. 2.35** Disproportionation occurs when two growing free radicals approach each other; one radical becomes unsaturated end group *(left)* after it donates a hydrogen atom to the other free radical, which becomes a saturated molecule *(right)*. The end group that becomes saturated is the passivated segment of the polymer chain.

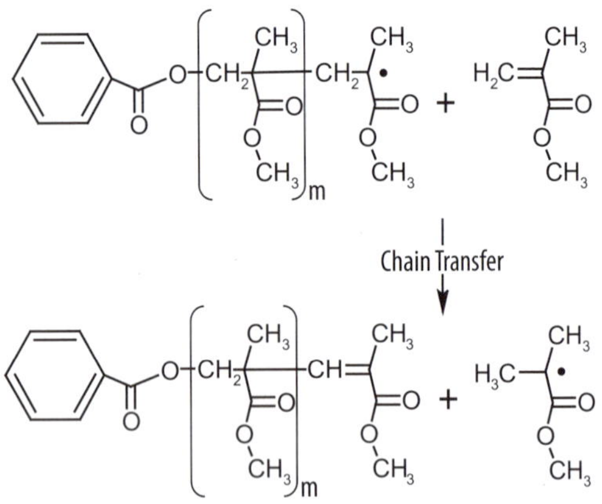

Chain Transfer

• **Fig. 2.36** Chain transfer occurs when a free radical approaches a methylmethacrylate molecule and donates a hydrogen atom to the methylmethacrylate molecule. This causes the free radical rearrangement to form a double bond and become unreactive, and the methylmethacrylate monomer becomes a free radical without BPO. The deactivated chain resulting from this exchange can become an active growing chain by a chain transfer from another free radical.

Inhibition of Addition Polymerization

The polymerization reactions are not likely to result in a complete exhaustion of the monomer, nor do they always form polymers of high molecular weight. Impurities in the monomer often inhibit such reactions. An impurity can react with the activated initiator or with an activated growing chain and prevent further growth. Although the presence of inhibitors markedly influences the degree of polymerization, the mechanism has been used in resin-based dental materials.

Addition of methyl ether of hydroquinone, a common inhibitor, in the amount of 0.006% or less, inhibits the spontaneous polymerization of dental resins during storage. The inhibitor neutralizes any free radical as it is formed before it initiates chain growth. Therefore, all hydroquinone should be eliminated before polymerization by chain propagation can occur. Thus, the inhibitor not only prevents premature polymerization during storage but also provides adequate working time in the case of two-part (self-cure) systems.

Oxygen reacts readily with the growing chains and results in a radical of low reactivity that does not attract monomers and thus inhibits chain growth. Oxygen inhibition mostly affects the surface exposed to ambient air and produces a greasy film of unpolymerized resin on newly placed sealants and resin-based restorations. The oxygen-inhibited layer generally is unfavorable but can be beneficial in building up a light-cured composite restoration. When new composite is placed over the oxygen-inhibited surface and light-cured, the once-inhibited resin is now shielded from oxygen and exposed to fresh free radicals activated by the light curing. The process promotes bonding between layers of composites. Drawbacks with oxygen inhibition are the higher release of poorly cured material to the adjacent tissues, softer resin (composite) surfaces that are more susceptible to wear and discoloration, and a weaker bond to a tooth surface if the material shrinks away from the oxygen-inhibited layer during curing.

A common clinical practice is to use a matrix material, which helps to shape the resin and acts as a barrier to prevent contact with oxygen during curing. Such a matrix strip prevents a sticky, air-inhibited layer from forming on the surface.

CRITICAL QUESTION

What mechanisms are responsible for the inhibition of polymerization? What are the benefits of inhibitors in dental resins? What role does O_2 play as an inhibitor?

Step-Growth Polymerization (Condensation Polymerization)

The reactions that produce step-growth polymerization can progress by any chemical reaction that joins two or more molecules to produce a simple nonmacromolecular structure. The primary compounds react, often with the formation of by-products such as water, alcohols, halogen acids, and ammonia. The formation of these by-products is the reason step-growth polymerization is often called condensation polymerization. This step-growth mechanism is the one used exclusively in biological tissues to produce proteins, carbohydrates, deoxyribonucleic acid, and ribonucleic acid.

In step-growth polymerization, a linear chain of repeating mer units is obtained by the stepwise intermolecular condensation or the addition of the reactive groups in which bifunctional or trifunctional monomers are all simultaneously active, as opposed to the activation of one monomer at a time of a growing chain in chain-growth addition polymerization. There are two approaches to form condensation polymers: One having both reactive functional groups in one molecule and the other having two types of difunctional monomers. The following example is for the polymerization of one type of diol:

$$\text{HO}-(\text{silicone})-\text{OH} + \text{n HO}-(\text{silicone}) - \text{OH} \rightarrow \text{H(O}-\text{silicone)n}+1-\text{OH} + \text{n } H_2O\uparrow \quad (1)$$

Very often a catalyst is needed to accelerate the reaction, and the resultant molecular weight increases as the duration of the reaction increases. If a monofunctional impurity is present, the reaction will limit the growth of the polymer chain by rendering a chain end inactive.

There are two more examples related to stepwise polymerization in Chapter 13. In one, water is removed in the process of joining one type of monomer (trimercaptan) to form a polysulfide rubber with an oxidizing agent; in the other case, ethanol is removed in the process of joining siloxane molecules to form silicone rubber involving two types of monomers.

The formation of polymers by step growth is comparatively slow because the reaction proceeds in a stepwise fashion from monomer to dimer to trimer, and so forth, until large polymer molecules containing many mer units are eventually formed. Such a polymerization process tends to stop when the chains have grown to certain sizes that are less mobile and with few functional groups left to react.

CRITICAL QUESTION

What are the practical benefits of using copolymer resins for dental applications?

Copolymerization

Resin-based materials used in dentistry that require polymerization at chairside or in the laboratory usually comprise more than one type of monomer. In many of the polymerization reactions described previously, the macromolecule is formed by the polymerization of a single type of structural unit. However, two or more chemically different monomers, each with some desirable property, can be combined to yield specific physical properties of a polymer. As defined earlier, the polymer formed is a copolymer, and the process of formation is known as copolymerization.

Composite Materials

A composite is a material made of two or more constituent components with significantly different physical or chemical properties that, when combined, produce a material with characteristics different from the individual components.

Most importantly, the combination is designed to achieve specific functional properties. The individual components remain separate and distinct within the finished structure, differentiating composites from mixtures and solid solutions.

Microstructure of Composite

The discontinuous phase is usually harder and stronger than the continuous phase and is called the reinforcement or reinforcing material, whereas the continuous phase is named the matrix or binder. Each class of materials discussed so far can be either the matrix or the reinforcement phase of a composite, or both phases of the composite. The reinforcement phase, which is discontinuous, can be in the form of particles, short fibers in random direction, unidirectional long fibers, woven fabrics, laminates, or honeycomb. The reinforcement phase of the composite materials used in dentistry is mostly glass or ceramic particles and some short fibers. Often the term filler is used to represent the reinforcement phase of the particles and short fibers.

Benefit of Composite Structure

The most cited benefits of adding harder, stronger, or tougher fillers to a matrix are the improvement in the stiffness, strength, or toughness of the resulting materials. By the rule of mixtures, the final properties of the material will be between those of the two constituent materials. Strength enhancement alone would not necessarily satisfy the clinician's need at chairside. Clinicians need to prepare materials at chairside, adapt them to the tooth structure, shape them while they are still soft, and then allow the material to set to the hardened stage capable of withstanding the occlusal load (Chapter 1). The most noted composite used in modern dentistry is resin-based composite made of a polymeric resin matrix embedded with glass or ceramic particles (Chapter 5). The matrix phase alone can be fluid enough to adapt to tooth surfaces and set to a solid. The addition of filler particles to the matrix can increase the viscosity of the mixture, providing the bulk for shaping the matrix phase and rendering much-needed strength. Filler particles, on their own, would have no ability to form a firm solid, but with the help of the matrix phase, fillers can form a useful solid structure. In dentistry, the term composite has been used exclusively for resin-based composite materials.

Composite Materials Used in Dentistry

In addition to resin-based composites (Chapter 5), the following chapters show that most dental materials, if examined in detail, are composed of dissimilar subunits as in composites. For example, aqueous dental cements are the result of reactive filler particles mixed with an acid solution. The product of reaction becomes a continuous phase, and unreacted particulates are the discontinuous phase (Chapter 7). Dental amalgam is the result of the partial dissolution of alloy particles in mercury, where new mercury-rich phases emerge as the matrix holding the unreacted portion of the alloy particles together (Chapter 8). Multiphase metal alloy can have precipitates dispersed in the microstructure (Chapter 9). Keep in mind that metal alloys are not treated as composites, but they do possess structures of a composite nature. Dental porcelain consists of a glassy matrix and a ceramic filler particle phase for strengthening purposes (Chapter 10). Denture-base resins incorporate polymer beads in the monomer to make the mixture easily workable for processing. Those beads dissolve partially, and the remaining portion is dispersed within the polymerized matrix (Chapter 11). Impression materials have a wide range of filler contents facilitating the specific requirements of impression making (Chapter 13). Various allotropic forms of silica (SiO_2) are incorporated in investment material for metal casting to induce fracture resistance at elevated temperatures and provide thermal expansion of the mold during heating to compensate for metal casting shrinkage (Chapter 14). For abrasive instruments, hard abrasive grits use resin (or rubber), metal, and glass (or ceramic) as the binder to make instruments for various surface-reduction and finishing processes (Chapter 16). Not all composite materials mentioned are made with strengthening in mind but, rather, to fulfill other goals, such as the ability to manipulate the material. Nonetheless, adjusting the filler phase to improve the strength of the final material has been done in some of those materials.

Factors Influencing Properties of Composites

The properties of particle-filled resin composites are influenced by three major factors: Component properties, filler content by volume, and interfacial interaction between filler and matrix. The matrix phase is characterized by the stiffness and the fillers by particle size, size distribution, specific surface area, and particle shape. The strength of the composite increases with the filler-volume fraction, up to a limit. Both factors are discussed in Chapter 5. Interfacial interaction can considerably affect properties. For the filler in the resin composite to be effective, a good bonding between the filler and the matrix is essential to enable the matrix to transfer the load to the filler to resist fracture. This means that the filler becomes an integral part of the matrix phase.

Recall from the section on types of bonds that both primary and secondary bonds hold materials together. These bonds occur within the same material; for example, metallic bonds form within metals after melting and solidification. Ceramic powders are packed together and sintered into a solid object. Solid polymer blends can be made by melting two thermoplastics together and solidifying. How do the fillers bond to the matrix? In dental amalgam, there is a chemical reaction between the mercury and metal alloys, where the bonding between filler and matrix is likely the primary bond. It is the same with the aqueous-based dental cements.

For the other materials, the matrix is usually a resinous fluid phase before solidifying, and there is often no chemical reaction between the two components. There must be some sort of interaction between the liquid and the solid keeping them together after the liquid phase solidifies. In the next section, the interactions between the solid surface and the liquid phase in holding these materials together are examined.

CRITICAL QUESTION

Why does a liquid that can adhere to one material not necessarily adhere to another material of a different composition?

Adhesion and Bonding

So far, we have been exploring the attraction between atoms and molecules. Although we do not expect to observe a similar attraction between two nonmagnetized solid objects, we do notice that two solids can adhere to each other with or without the help of a third substance or device. As examples, an artificial denture stays attached to the soft tissue when saliva is present, plaque or calculus adheres to tooth structure, and a transmucosal abutment is fixed to the implant root by a screw (Fig. 2.37). The first two examples involve bonding at the molecular scale and the last is achieved first by mechanical means and then by osseointegration (Chapter 12). Some of the dental materials you will be learning about are bonded to the hard tissue to replace the missing part of the tooth structure to restore its functions. Therefore, an understanding of the fundamental principles associated with bonding is important to the dentist.

When the molecules of one substrate adhere or are attracted to molecules of the other substrate, the force of attraction is called **adhesion** when unlike molecules are attracted and **cohesion** when the molecules involved are of the same kind. The material that is used to cause bonding is known as the **adhesive** and the material to which it is applied is called the **adherend**. In a broad sense, adhesive bonding is simply a surface attachment process, which is usually qualified by specifying the type of intermolecular attraction that may exist between the adhesive and the adherend.

CRITICAL QUESTION

Why is the potential energy of the atom on the surface higher than that of atoms within the bulk of the material?

Surface and Surface Energy

A surface is defined as the outermost layer of an object. We know that solids or liquids are made up of a finite number of atoms or molecules bonded by primary and/or secondary bonds. This means that their surface is populated by atoms or molecules,

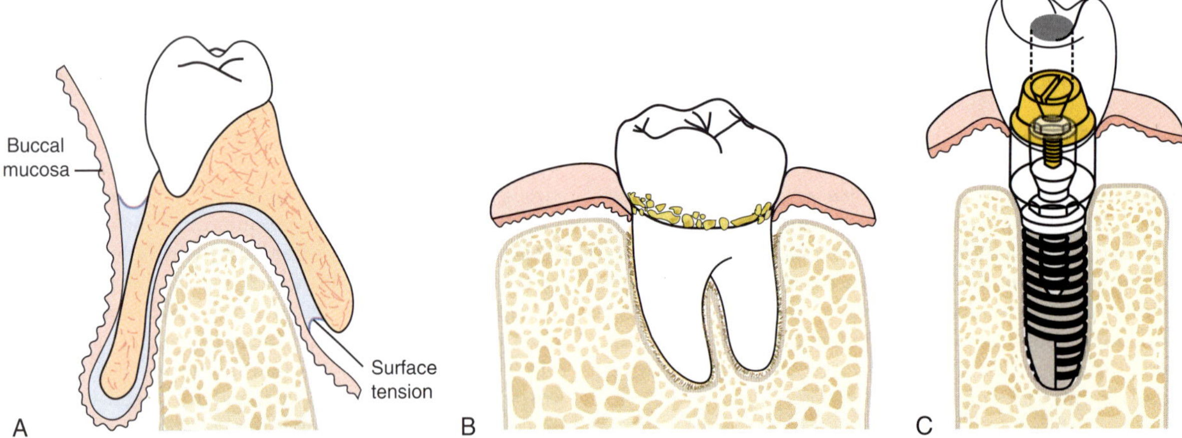

• **Fig. 2.37** Examples of solid adhering to solid in dentistry. **(A)** Retention of denture base; saliva fills in the space between the denture and soft tissue, providing retention through capillary attraction (see Fig. 2.39). The space between the denture and the soft tissue is exaggerated to show the capillary attraction. **(B)** Plaque formation on the enamel surface, which converts to calculus by calcification. **(C)** The implant root is first retained by the bone mechanically, followed by osseointegration for long-term implant stability. (Courtesy: Dr InchanKo.)

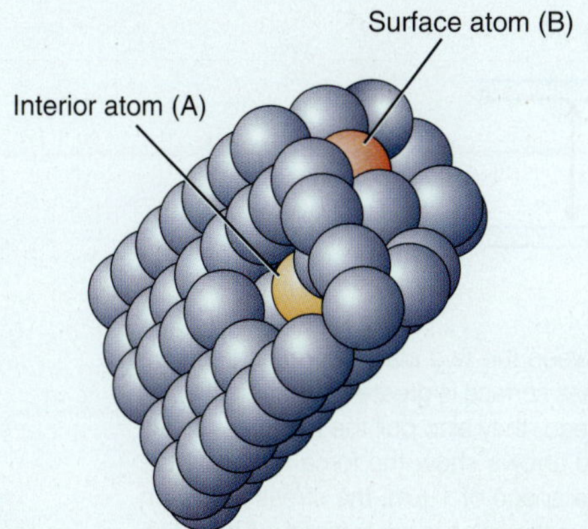

• **Fig. 2.38** Comparing an atom under the surface **(A)** with one on the surface **(B)** reveals that a bond balance exists around the interior atom **(A)**, while the surface atom **(B)** is free to develop bonds to atoms or molecules approaching the surface.

which are ready to attract other atoms or molecules approaching the surface. It is the secondary bond formed between water molecules and the glass surface that makes a drop of water spread on a clean glass slide and keeps it from flowing when the glass slide is tilted. We can explain this phenomenon of attraction between atoms by the potential energy discussed in Figure 2.10. Consider the space lattice shown in Figure 2.38. Inside the lattice, all the atoms are equally attracted to each other. The interatomic distance for atom "A" has a balanced array of neighbors surrounding it and the energy is minimal. At the surface of the lattice, atom "B" is not equally attracted in all directions and the energy is greater. This energy quantifies the work needed to disrupt intermolecular bonds resulting in a new surface. Thus, it is called the **surface energy**. The functional chemical groups available or the type of crystal plane of a space lattice present at the surface may affect the surface energy.

Molecules in air may be attracted to the surface and become adsorbed on the material surface. Initially the attraction between them is secondary bonding (van der Waals force). As the distance between the molecules from air and the surface diminishes, primary bonding may occur. Silver, platinum, and gold adsorb oxygen readily. Neither gold nor platinum forms stable oxides at room temperature; therefore, the bond between oxygen and metal remains secondary. In the case of silver, silver oxide may form as oxygen becomes bonded to silver by covalent bonding. This process is called chemisorption and is limited to the monolayer of oxide present on the surface. Both phenomena constitute adhesion, where oxygen is the adhesive and metals are the adherends.

The energy on the surface per unit area is referred to as the surface energy (in mJ/m^2) or **surface tension** (in mN/m). Falling liquid drops form spherical shapes, which have the smallest surface area of all known shapes, and they maintain the state of the lowest energy. Any acquired surface impurity—such as an adsorbed gas, an oxide, or human secretions—can cause a reduction in the surface energy and adhesive qualities of a given solid as these impurities constitute the new surface. Table 2.3 lists the surface energy of selected solids and liquids.

CRITICAL QUESTION

What conditions are necessary to achieve the strongest level of bonding?

TABLE 2.3 Surface Energy of Selected Materials

Material	Surface Energy (mJ/m^2)
Solids	
Enamel[a]	92
Dentin[a]	87
Teflon[b]	20
Gold alloy[c]	51–54
Ni–Cr[c]	48
Commercial pure titanium[c]	50
Acrylic denture resinsd	46–54
Liquids	
Water[e]	72 @ 25°C
Mercury[e]	486 @ 25°C
Saliva[f]	53 @ 25°C
Dentin bonding agent[g]	34–55

Note: Depending on the measuring methods and the materials used, the values obtained are likely to be different among studies. The table is intended to give readers a general idea of surface energies of selected materials.
[a]Data from Weerkamp et al (1988), *J Dent Res* 67:1483.
[b]Data from Janczuk (1999), *J Colloid Interface Sci* 211(1):96–103.
[c]Data from Sardin et al (2002), *J Oral Rehab* 31:140.
[d]Data from Sipahi et al (2001), *J Dent* 29:197.
[e]Data from *Handbook of Chemistry and Physics* (2011), 91st Edition, pp. 6–127.
[f]Data from Glantz (1970), *Odontol Rev* 21:119.
[g]Data from Gonçalves et al (1997), *Braz Dent J* 8:43.

Wetting

When an impurity-free polished glass plate is placed on top of another similar plate and pressed together, they exhibit no tendency to adhere. Regardless of how smooth these glass surfaces may appear to be, they are likely to be rough on an atomic or molecular scale. Consequently, when they are placed in apposition, only the "hills" or high spots are in contact. Even if primary or secondary bonding occurs at these points of contact, these areas usually constitute only an insignificant portion of the total surface, and no perceptible adhesion takes place. In addition, no attraction is expected when the surface molecules of the attracting substances are separated by distances greater than 0.7 nm (0.0007 μm).

The examples of adhesives bonding to solid surfaces given earlier involved either a gas or liquid. It is obvious that gas and liquid can adapt to a solid surface by flowing into surface irregularities to provide contact over a greater part of the surface of the solid. If a drop of water is introduced between the same two glass plates before they are pressed together, considerable difficulty is encountered in separating the two plates (Fig. 2.39). This is a result of the capillary action from intermolecular attractive forces between water and the glass plates.

To produce adhesion on any targeted surface, the liquid must flow easily over the entire surface and adhere to the solid. This characteristic is known as **wetting**. If the liquid does not wet the surface of the adherend, adhesion between the liquid and the adherend will be negligible or nonexistent. The ability to wet the substrate is the dominating contributor to the adhesive bond when the adhesive sets from liquid to solid.

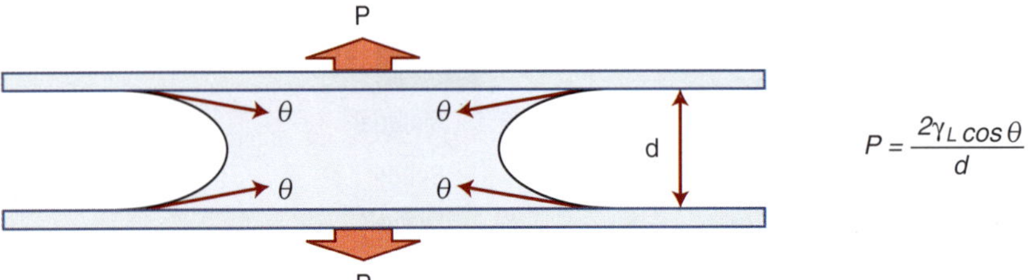

• **Fig. 2.39** Two glass plates and water film. The liquid (water) between the two plates spreads because of good wetting. The attraction between the water molecule and glass surface is greater than the cohesive force between water molecules. Therefore, as water molecules spread, they also pull the two glass slides closer. Small arrows show the vector of surface tension and broad arrows show the force that pulls the slides apart. The surface tension of water is about 72 mN/m. For a space of 1 μm, the stress acting on the slide will be 140 kN/m^2 (0.14 MPa). You will learn in Chapter 4 that the value is relatively low. Therefore, if the glass slides cannot be separated in pure tension by hand it is likely that the water film (d) is only nanometers in thickness.

The ability of an adhesive to wet the surface of the adherend is influenced by a number of factors. The cleanliness of the surface is of particular importance. Impurities on the solid surface often yield a surface of lower energy than the clean surface and prevent any wetting by the adhesive, such as epoxy glue. A surface's surface energy can be so low, such as that of dental wax or Teflon (polytetrafluoroethylene), that it cannot be wet satisfactorily by most dental adhesives (Chapter 13). Impurity-free metal surfaces, on the other hand, because of their high surface energy, interact vigorously with liquid adhesives.

In general, the comparatively low surface energies of organic and inorganic liquids permit them to spread freely on solids of high surface energy. This is a prerequisite of good wetting and strong adhesive joints.

CRITICAL QUESTION

Why does the wetting increase (higher wettability) if the adhesive attraction at the liquid/solid interface is greater than the cohesive attraction of the liquid molecules?

Contact Angle of Wetting

How can we tell if a liquid can wet a solid satisfactorily for bonding, especially when the surface to be bonded is covered by that very liquid? When we place one drop of water on a clean glass slide and others on an acrylic plate and a sheet of Teflon, we will observe that the water drop on the acrylic plate does not spread out as much as the one on the glass slide and the water drop on the Teflon surface appears to bead up. If we observe this at the level of solid substrate, we will see the symmetrical profile of the former water drop resting on a flat surface (Fig. 2.40). Both ends of the profile depict where three phases—vapor (air), liquid (water), and solid (glass, acrylic, or Teflon)—converge. We can draw a tangent relative to the curvature of the liquid profile from the vapor/liquid interface. The tangent line and the solid surface constitute an angle that defines the shape of the liquid; this is called the **contact angle**.

If the force of attraction between molecules of the adhesive and molecules of the substrate is stronger than the attraction between molecules of the adhesive, the liquid adhesive will spread much more broadly over the solid surface and result in a smaller contact angle (Fig. 2.40A). Thus, a small contact angle indicates that the adhesive forces at the interface are stronger than the cohesive forces holding the molecules of the adhesive together. If the adhesive beads up, it means that the force of adhesion is weaker than the cohesive force of the adhesive. Because the tendency for the liquid to spread increases as the contact angle decreases, the contact angle is a useful indicator of spreadability or wettability (Fig. 2.40D). Complete wetting occurs at a contact angle of 0° and no wetting occurs at an angle of 180°. Thus, smaller the contact angles between an adhesive and an adherend, the better the ability of the adhesive to flow into and fill in irregularities within the surface of the adherend. The fluidity of the adhesive influences the extent to which these voids or irregularities are filled.

If oil drops or liquids other than water have been used instead, the observed contact angle will be different. Therefore, it is important to know the identity of the liquid that has been used to determine the contact angles. If none is identified, it is likely that distilled water has been used.

The profile of the liquid on a flat surface shows that there are three distinct interfaces: Vapor/liquid, liquid/solid, and solid/vapor, and that each interface is characterized by an interfacial energy, γ_{VL}, γ_{LS}, and γ_{SV}, respectively. At equilibrium, the chemical potential in the three phases should be equal (Fig. 2.40D). It is important to point out that the Young's equation shown in Figure 2.40 assumes a perfectly flat surface at the molecular level, and any surface roughness and impurities can cause a deviation in the equilibrium contact angle from the contact angle predicted by Young's equation.

CRITICAL QUESTION

How can you prevent the lack of hard tissue details in a gypsum model made from a hydrophobic impression material? What steps can be taken to eliminate this problem when you are using this impression material in the future?

When gypsum products (Chapter 13) are mixed with water to pour dental models in various types of impressions, wetting must occur between gypsum and the impression to ensure good surface quality of the gypsum model. The basic ingredient of the most popular silicone-based elastomeric impression material today is considered to be hydrophobic, because a contact angle of greater than 90° is observed when an aqueous medium is poured into this elastomeric mold. To improve the wettability of the set impression material by a gypsum–water mixture, the operator usually sprays a surfactant (also called debubblizer). The most direct approach by the manufacturer is to incorporate a **wetting agent** (also known as a surfactant) in the impression material during the

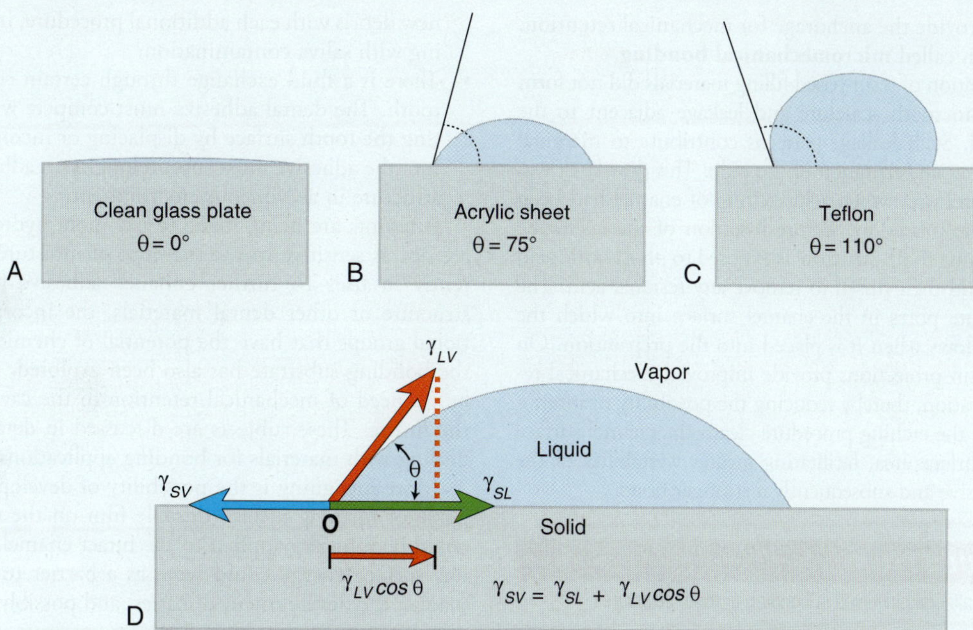

• **Fig. 2.40** Contact angles of distilled water on three surfaces and relationship among interfacial energy. **(A)** Water spreads freely on a flame-cleaned glass slide (good wetting). The profile depicted here is considered having 0° contact angle. **(B)** Water on an acrylic surface. **(C)** Water on a Teflon surface (poor wetting). **(D)** Relationships between the interfacial energies at vapor/liquid (γ_{VL}), liquid/solid (γ_{LS}), and solid/vapor (γ_{SV}) interfaces with respect to contact angle at equilibrium; the relationship is also known as Young's equation.

manufacturing process (Chapter 13). The wetting agent migrates to the solid surface and accommodates surface wetting by the aqueous gypsum-forming mixture. Table 2.4 lists contact angles of probing liquids on selected materials.

CRITICAL QUESTION

Micromechanical bonding of resin sealant to tooth enamel is usually quite effective in preventing pit and fissure areas from tooth decay. However, many factors can reduce the bonding effectiveness, resulting in partial or total loss of the sealant. Which of these factors are possible causes of debonding?

TABLE 2.4 Contact Angles of Probing Liquids on Solid Surfaces

Solid	Contact Angle (°)	Probing Liquid
Amalgam[a]	145	Mercury
Amalgam[b]	77	Water
Acrylic denture resins[b]	75	Water
Dental ceramic (feldspathic core)[c]	71	Water
Dental ceramic (feldspathic core)[c]	54	Bonding resin
Teflon[b]	110	Water
Commercial pure titanium[d]	54	Water
Impression materials		
Polyether[e]	30–44	Water
Polysulfide[f]	76–85	Gypsum solution (0.2 g/mL)
Addition silicone[e]	34–105	Water
Addition silicone (hydrophilic)[e]	20–78	Water
Condensation silicone[e]	82–103	Water

Note: Depending on the measuring methods and the materials used, the values obtained are likely to be different among studies. The table is intended to give readers a general idea of contact angle of various dental materials.
[a]Data from Baran & O'Brien (1977), *JADA* 94:898.
[b]Data from O'Brien (1967), PhD Dissertation, University of Michigan.
[c]Data from Oh et al (2002), *J Prosthet Dent* 88:616.
[d]Data from Ponsonnet et al (2003), *Mat SciEng C-Bio S* 23:551.
[e]Data from Cullen et al (1991), *J Prosthet Dent* 66:261.
[f]Data from Pratten & Craig (1989), *J Prosthet Dent* 61:197.

Mechanical Bonding

Strong attachment of one substance to another can also be accomplished by mechanical means rather than by molecular attraction. Such structural retention may be gross in nature, as evidenced by some nondental applications involving the use of screws, bolts, or undercuts. Similar procedures that involve more subtle mechanisms are also used in restorative dentistry and called mechanical bonding or micromechanical retention.

Before resin-based adhesives were introduced to dentistry, various type of fluids or slightly viscous materials, like zinc phosphate cement (Chapter 7), were being used to retain cast gold alloy crowns or base metal endodontic posts and cores. These materials do not form a strong attraction to the substrate surface, but they provide the needed retention to hold the prostheses in place. In this scenario, the luting medium penetrates into irregularities that exist on the intaglio of the casting and those that are present on the adjoining tooth structure. Upon hardening, the numerous cementing material projections embedded in the adherend surface provide the anchorage for mechanical retention. This process is often called **micromechanical bonding**.

The early formulation of resin-based filling materials did not form a strong attraction to tooth structure and leakage adjacent to the restoration occurred. Such leakage patterns contribute to marginal stain, secondary caries, and irritation of the pulp. This drawback was brought under control only when acid etching of enamel had been accepted as a routine procedure. Before insertion of the resin, the enamel of the adjoining tooth structure is exposed to phosphoric acid for a short period and then rinsed to remove any residual acid. The acid produces minute pores in the enamel surface into which the resin subsequently flows when it is placed into the preparation. On hardening, these resin projections provide improved mechanical retention of the restoration, thereby reducing the possibility of interfacial leakage. In fact, the etching procedure cleans the enamel surface and creates more surface area, facilitating greater wettability of the enamel by the adhesive and subsequently a stronger bond.

CRITICAL QUESTION

What are the main challenges involved in bonding to tooth structure?

Bonding to Tooth Structure

Adhesive bonding to tooth structure and other dental materials has become a major component of restorative dentistry. So far, we have used an ideal adherend that has a clean surface with uniform composition and certain surface irregularities in our discussion of bonding. Bonding to tooth structure is a complex process for the following reasons:

- Tooth composition is not homogeneous. Both organic and inorganic components are present in different amounts in dentin as compared with enamel.
- A material that can adhere to the organic components may not adhere to the inorganic components, and an adhesive that bonds to enamel may not adhere to dentin to the same extent.
- The instruments used to prepare the tooth for bonding leave a rough surface and debris, which promote air entrapment at the interface.
- We routinely treat prepared surfaces with appropriate agents to remove this debris and continue to face the task of removing new debris with each additional procedure, in addition to dealing with saliva contamination.
- There is a fluid exchange through certain components of the tooth. The dental adhesive must compete with water for wetting the tooth surface by displacing or incorporating it. Then, too, the adhesive must sustain long-term adhesion to the tooth structure in an aqueous environment.

Attempts are being made to use more hydrophilic resins that are not as sensitive to the presence of moisture as materials currently in use. To further enhance adhesive bonding to tooth structure or other dental materials, the incorporation of functional groups that have the potential of chemically reacting with the bonding substrate has also been explored. Perhaps there will be no need of mechanical retention in the cavity preparation in the future. These subjects are discussed in detail in the chapters dealing with materials for bonding applications.

More intriguing is the possibility of developing a material capable of forming a thin, durable film on the tooth surface that could be topically applied to the intact enamel. Such a film with low surface energy could serve as a barrier to the formation of plaque, the development of caries, and possibly the deposition of calculus.

Bonding to Restorative Materials

Advances in material science are leading to the development of new materials at a very rapid pace. Concurrently we now understand the importance of creating bonded and sealed interfaces which are impervious to microleakage. In order to achieve this, we need to bond not only to tooth structure but also to the plethora of restorative materials. For example, if we were planning a post and core restoration in a badly mutilated tooth, we would have a post, a core buildup, and a crown, all made of different materials, which would need to bond to each other and to the tooth structure. In addition, we would prefer to have one single bonding system or cement which could bond efficiently to all the substrates, a multi-mode or Universal adhesive. Is this a realistic expectation and is this within the realm of possibility? Current research seems to suggest that not only is this possible, but we may have long-term stable bonds as well.

Summary

- **Interatomic bonds**
  - **Primary bonds**
    - Primary atomic bonds, also called chemical bonds, may be of three different types:
      - Ionic
      - Covalent
      - Metallic
    - **Combination of primary bonds**
  - **Secondary bonds**
    In contrast with primary bonds, secondary bonds do not share electrons. Instead, charge variations among atomic groups of the molecule induce dipole forces that attract adjacent molecules or parts of a large molecule.
    - **van der Waals forces**
    - **Hydrogen bond**
- **Atomic arrangement**
  - **Crystalline structure**
    - There are 14 possible lattice types. The type of space lattice is defined by the length of each of three unit cell edges (called the axes) and the angles between the edges.
    - Most metals used in dentistry belong to the cubic system.
    - All metallic-based dental materials are crystalline. Some pure ceramics, such as alumina and zirconia core materials, are entirely crystalline.
  - **Noncrystalline structure**
    - Glass is a typical noncrystalline solid of SiO_2 because its atoms tend to be arranged in nonrepeating units.
    - Polymeric-based materials used in dentistry are usually noncrystalline.
    - The structural arrangements of the noncrystalline solids do not represent such low internal energies as do crystalline arrangements.
    - Many dental materials often consist of a noncrystalline glassy matrix and crystalline inclusions (filler phase).
    - Crystalline inclusions provide desired properties including color, opacity, increased thermal expansion coefficients, and in some dental ceramics, increased radiopacity.

- **Interatomic bond distance and thermal energy**
  Between any two atoms, there are forces of attraction drawing them together and forces of repulsion pushing them apart.
- **Bond distance**
  The position at which both forces are equal in magnitude (but opposite in direction) is considered the equilibrium position of the atoms.
- **Bonding energy**
  Energy is defined as the product of force and distance. Integration of the interatomic force over the interatomic distance yields the interatomic energy.
- **Thermal energy**
  The atoms in a crystal at temperatures above absolute zero are in a constant state of vibration, and the average amplitude is dependent on the temperature. The higher the temperature, the greater the amplitude and, consequently, the greater the kinetic or internal energy.
- **Diffusion**
  When we place a drop of ink in a bowl of water, we observe that it spreads in the water. It will eventually disperse through the entire body of the water. This process is called diffusion.
- **Metals**
  - Pure metals, in common with other chemical elements, can be identified by their specific melting and boiling points and by their basic physical and chemical properties.
  - One common feature in the atomic structure of metal elements is that the outermost electrons (valence electrons) around the neutral metallic atoms are easily given up.
  - Solid **solutions**
  - In chemistry, a *solution* refers to a type of homogeneous mixture composed of two or more substances. That means we could have a solution in the solid, liquid, or vapor state. The key word is *homogeneous.*
  - The term **phase** in chemistry is defined as a physically distinctive and homogeneous region of matter.
- **Equilibrium-phase diagram**—A **phase diagram** that shows conditions (pressure, temperature, volume, etc.) at which thermodynamically distinct phases occur and coexist at equilibrium.
- Ceramics: Ceramics are solid-phase compounds of metallic and nonmetallic elements.
- Ceramics have 3D crystalline structures, but they are much more complicated than those of metals.
- Current dental ceramics are based on silicate ($[SiO_4]^{4-}$ tetrahedron), alumina (Al_2O_3), and zirconia (ZrO_2).
- Polymers: Polymers are a class of natural or synthetic substances composed of very high-molecular-weight molecules with repeating units, called *macromolecules.* For synthetic polymers, each repeating unit is called **mer** in the polymer and a **monomer** before becoming part of the macromolecule by a chemical reaction called *polymerization.*
- ***Chemistry of polymerization:*** *Traditionally, there are two classes of polymers as determined by the polymerization mechanism: Addition and condensation polymers.*
  - *Addition polymers contain the same atoms as the monomer in their repeating units, whereas condensation polymers contain fewer atoms because of the formation of by-products during the process.*
- **Adhesion and bonding**
  - When the molecules of one substrate adhere to or are attracted to molecules of the other substrate, the force of attraction is called **adhesion** when unlike molecules are attracted and the force of attraction is called **cohesion** when the molecules involved are of the same kind.
  - The material that is used to cause bonding is known as the **adhesive** and the material to which it is applied is called the **adherend.**
- **Surface and surface energy**
  - A surface is defined as the outermost layer of an object.
  - The energy on the surface per unit area is referred to as the surface energy (in mJ/m^2) or **surface tension** (in mN/m).
- **Wetting**
  To produce adhesion on any targeted surface, the liquid must flow easily over the entire surface and adhere to the solid. This characteristic is known as **wetting**. If the liquid does not wet the surface of the adherend, adhesion between the liquid and the adherend will be negligible or nonexistent. The ability to wet the substrate is the dominating contributor to the adhesive bond when the adhesive sets from liquid to solid.
- **Contact angle of wetting**
  When we place one drop of water on a clean glass slide and others on an acrylic plate and a sheet of Teflon, we will observe that the water drop on the acrylic plate does not spread out as much as the one on the glass slide and the water drop on the Teflon surface appears to bead up. We can draw a tangent relative to the curvature of the liquid profile from the vapor/liquid interface. The tangent line and the solid surface constitute an angle that defines the shape of the liquid; this is called the **contact angle**.
- **Mechanical bonding**
  Strong attachment of one substance to another can also be accomplished by mechanical means rather than by molecular attraction.
- **Bonding to tooth structure**
  - Tooth composition is not homogeneous. Both organic and inorganic components are present in different amounts in dentin as compared with enamel.
  - A material that can adhere to the organic components may not adhere to the inorganic components, and an adhesive that bonds to enamel may not adhere to dentin to the same extent.
  - The instruments used to prepare the tooth for bonding leave a rough surface and debris, which promote air entrapment at the interface.
  - There is a fluid exchange through certain components of the tooth. The dental adhesive must compete with water for wetting the tooth surface by displacing or incorporating it. Then, too, the adhesive must sustain long-term adhesion to the tooth structure in an aqueous environment.

Review Questions

1. Discuss in detail interatomic bonds.
2. Discuss in brief ionic bonding.
3. Discuss in brief metallic bonds.
4. Discuss in detail differences between crystalline and noncrystalline materials.
5. Discuss in brief van der Waals forces.
6. Discuss in detail atomic arrangement and crystalline structure.
7. Draw diagrams of three common types of space lattices found in dental materials.
8. What is wettability and contact angle?

9. Write a short note on surface energy and factors affecting the same.
10. Discuss in detail adhesion and mechanical bonding.
11. What are interatomic bonds? Discuss in detail secondary bonds.
12. Discuss in detail factors affecting adhesion.
13. Classify primary bonds and add a note on covalent bonds.
14. Discuss in brief covalent bonds.
15. Discuss in brief hydrogen bonds.

Selected Readings

Abbaschian R, Abbaschian L, Reed-Hill RE: Physical Metallurgy Principles, 4th ed, Stamford CT, Cengage Learning, 2009. An excellent textbook on physical metallurgy that discusses the solidification of metals and alloys and the formation of equiaxed polycrystalline and dendritic microstructures.

Brantley WA, Cai Z, Carr AB, et al: Metallurgical structures of as-cast and heat-treated high-palladium dental alloys. *Cells Mater* 3:103-114, 1993. High-palladium alloys with equiaxed polycrystalline and dendritic microstructures are described. Careful study of the micrographs is useful for comparing the potential structural integrity and some properties of these alloys.

Buonocore M.G. The Use of Adhesives in Dentistry. Charles C Thomas: Springfield, IL; The problems associated with dental adhesives are nicely illustrated. It is of interest that many of the procedures using bonding technology discussed in this text have become commonplace.

Callister W.D. Jr.; Rethwisch D.G. Materials Science and Engineering: An Introduction. ed 8 John Wiley & Sons: Hoboken, NJ; An excellent text on materials science for a more in-depth coverage of materials structure and properties.

CowieJMG, Arrighi V: Polymers: Chemistry and Physics of Modern Materials, 3rd ed, Boca Raton, FL, CRC Press, 2007. Emphasizes structure/property relationships in polymers. Written for nonchemists who require a brief, readable introduction to polymer chemistry.

Glantz P. On wettability and adhesiveness: a study of enamel, dentin, some restorative dental materials, and dental plaque. Odontol Revy20(Suppl 17)1–132 (1969); The author proposed that the reduction of dental caries by topical fluorides resulted from lowering the surface energy of the tooth structure and thereby reducing plaque accumulation over a given interval.

Good R.J. Contact angle, wetting, and adhesion: a critical review. J AdhesSciTechnol61269–1302 (1992); An excellent review on the fundamentals of contact angle and wetting and their relationship to adhesion.

Gordon J.E. The New Science of Strong Materials, or Why You Don't Fall Through the Floor?. ed 2 Princeton University Press: Princeton, NJ; A general discussion of the strength of materials from a fundamental base. The sections on biological structural materials, timber, cellulose, teeth, and bone are particularly interesting.

In: (editors: Phillips R.W.; Ryge G.) Proceedings on Adhesive Restorative Dental Materials. Owen Litho Service: Spencer, IN; The recommendations for critically important areas of research have provided an impetus for investigations in this area.

Habib E, Wang R, Wang Y, et al: Inorganic Fillers for Dental Resin Composites: Present and Future."*ACS BiomaterSciEng* 2:1-11, 2016.

Pampuch, R: An Introduction to Ceramics. Lecture Notes in Chemistry, Vol 86, Springer International Publishing, 2014.

Rueggeberg FA: From vulcanite to vinyl, a history of resins in restorative dentistry. *J Prosthet Dent* 87:364–379, 2002. A comprehensive review of the introduction and evolution of polymeric materials in modern dentistry.

Söderholm K-JM: Coatings in Dentistry—A Review of Some Basic Principles. *Coatings* 2:138-159, 2012. This paper reviews fundamental principles of surface properties/adhesives since these topics form the foundation for most coating procedures used in dentistry.

Van Vlack LH: Elements of Materials Science and Engineering, 6th ed, Reading, MA, Addison-Wesley, 1989. An excellent primer on materials science. Chapter 5 describes phase diagrams, and Chapters 8 and 9 present deformation and strengthening mechanisms for alloys.

Zisman W.A. Influence of constitution on adhesion. Ind Eng Chem 5518–38 (1963); One of the pioneers in surface phenomena discusses parameters that influence wetting.

3

Physical and Chemical Properties of Solids

CHAPTER OUTLINE

KEY TERMS

RHEOLOGY

Dilatant—Resistance to flow increases as the rate of deformation (shear strain rate) increases. The more rapidly dilatant fluids are stirred or forced through a syringe, the more viscous (thicker) and more resistant to flow they become.

Pseudoplastic—Viscous character that is opposite from dilatant behavior in which the rate of flow decreases with increasing strain rate until it reaches a nearly constant value. Thus, the more rapidly pseudoplastic fluids are stirred or forced through a syringe, the less viscous (thinner) and more easily they flow.

Rheology—Study of the deformation and flow characteristics of matter (see *viscosity*).

Thixotropic—Property of gels and other fluids to become less viscous and flow when subjected to steady shear forces through being shaken, stirred, squeezed, patted, or vibrated. When the shear force is decreased to zero, the viscosity increases to the original value over a short time delay.

Viscosity—Resistance of a fluid to flow (see *rheology*).

STRUCTURAL RELAXATION

Creep—Time-dependent plastic strain of a solid under a static load or constant stress.

Sag—Irreversible (plastic) deformation of metal frameworks of fixed dental prostheses in the firing temperature range of ceramic veneers.

COLOR AND OPTICAL EFFECTS

Absorption—The extent to which light is absorbed by the material in an object.

Chroma—Degree of saturation of a particular hue (dominant color).

Color—Sensation induced from light of varying wavelengths that reaches the eye.

Esthetics—Principles and techniques associated with the development of the color and appearance required to produce a natural, pleasing effect in the dentition.

Hue—Dominant color of an object (e.g., red, green, or blue).

Metamerism—Phenomenon in which the color of an object under one type of light source (e.g., room light) appears to change when illuminated by a different light source (e.g., sunlight).

Opacity—The extent to which light does not pass through a material. No image and no light can be seen through an opaque object.

Reflection—The amount of light that reflects from the surface of an object.

Refract/Refraction—The degree to which light is bent when it passes from one medium to another. This makes a spoon appear bent in a glass of drinking water when light passes from air through glass into water, reflects from the spoon, and then passes back through water and glass into air. The index of refraction is a measure of this effect.

Translucency—Property of an object in which light is scattered as it passes through, revealing a diffuse image.

Transmit/Transmission—The amount of light passing through an object.

Transparency—The extent to which light passes through a material and to which an undistorted image can be seen through it.

Value—Relative lightness or darkness of a color. Also known as *luminous reflectance* and the *gray scale*.

THERMAL PROPERTIES

Coefficient of thermal expansion (linear coefficient of expansion)—Change in length per unit of the original length of a material when its temperature is raised by 1 K.

Kelvin (K)—The kelvin (K) temperature scale extends the degree Celsius scale such that zero degrees K is defined as absolute zero (= −273.15°C). Temperatures on this scale are called "kelvins," *not* "degrees kelvin," kelvin is *not* capitalized, and the symbol (capital K) stands alone with *no* degree symbol; 1 K = 1°C, K = °C + 273.15.

Thermal conductivity (coefficient of thermal conductivity)—Property that describes the thermal energy transport in watts per second through a material 1 cm thick with a cross-sectional area of 1 cm^2 when the temperature differential between the surfaces of the material perpendicular to the heat flow is 1 K.

Thermal diffusivity—Measure of the speed with which a temperature change will proceed through an object when one surface is heated.

ELECTROCHEMICAL PROPERTIES

Concentration cell—Electrochemical corrosion cell in which the potential difference is associated with the difference in concentration of a dissolved species, such as oxygen, in solution along different areas of a metal surface. Pitting corrosion and crevice corrosion are types of concentration cell corrosion.

Corrosion—Chemical or electrochemical process in which a solid, usually a metal, is attacked by an environmental agent, resulting in partial or complete dissolution.

Electromotive series—Arrangement of metals by their equilibrium values of electrode oxidation potential. Used to judge the tendency of metals and alloys to undergo electrochemical (galvanic) corrosion.

Galvanic corrosion (electrogalvanism)—Accelerated attack occurring on a less noble metal when electrochemically dissimilar metals are in electrical contact within a liquid-corrosive environment.

Galvanic shock—Pain sensation caused by the electrical current generated when two dissimilar metals are brought into contact in the oral environment.

Stress corrosion—Degradation caused by the combined effects of mechanical stress and a corrosive environment, usually exhibited as cracking.

Tarnish—Process by which a metal surface is dulled or discolored when a reaction with a sulfide, oxide, chloride, or other chemical causes surface discoloration through the formation of a thin oxidized film.

MAGNETIC MATERIALS

Magnet—Metallic material in which the component atoms are so ordered that it attracts iron-containing objects or aligns itself in an external magnetic field.

Tesla—Unit of flux density (T) of the magnetic field produced by a magnet.

Every dentist in the process of making or delivering a restoration must select various materials to complete the task. In making the choice, the dentist must have a thorough knowledge of the properties and behavioral characteristics of the materials chosen, namely, the physical and chemical properties.

- *Physical properties* are based on the laws of mechanics, acoustics, optics, thermodynamics, electricity, magnetism, radiation, atomic structure, and nuclear phenomena. Hue, value, and chroma relate to **color** and perception and are physical properties based on the laws of optics, which is the science that deals with the phenomena of light, vision, and sight. Thermal conductivity, diffusivity, and expansion are physical properties based on the laws of thermodynamics. Mechanical properties, a subset of physical properties based on the laws of mechanics, are discussed in Chapter 4.
- *Chemical properties* are based on the ways in which substances interact, combine, and change, as governed by their outer orbital electrons. The outer electrons are responsible for binding atoms together in molecules and for the electrical, thermal, optical, and magnetic properties of solids.

As examples, the physical properties of color and thermal expansion are of particular importance to the performance of dental ceramics (Chapter 10). Flow and viscosity (the resistance of a fluid to flow) are essential properties of impression materials (Chapter 13). Creep (slow deformation under a static load) is relevant to the clinical performance of amalgam (Chapter 8). Tarnish and corrosion are electrochemical properties that strongly affect the performance of metals and their alloys.

From the categories of dental materials and challenges discussed in Chapter 1, there are specific behaviors of the materials during processing and use that dentists should consider, such as the flowability (or formability), esthetic appearance, thermal expansion, chemical durability, and magnetism of the materials. As examples, flow and viscosity (the resistance of a fluid to flow) are essential properties for mixing direct restorative materials (Chapters 5 through 8) and gypsum products and impression materials (Chapter 13). Creep (slow deformation under a static load) is relevant to the clinical performance of amalgam (Chapter 8) and the fabrication of metal-ceramic prostheses (Chapter 10). The physical properties of color and thermal expansion are of particular importance to the performance of all restorations, especially for dental ceramics (Chapter 10). Tarnish and corrosion are electrochemical properties that strongly affect the performance of metals and their alloys (Chapters 8 and 9). Magnetisable prostheses materials are often used for retaining implant-borne prostheses and for orthodontic tooth movement in place. Mechanical properties, a subset of physical properties based on the laws of mechanics, are discussed in Chapter 4.

These phenomena will be discussed in greater detail in later chapters. However, having a firm grasp of the underlying principles that govern the properties is critical.

Rheology

Rheology is the study of the deformation and flow characteristics of matter, whether liquid or solid. Viscosity is the resistance of a fluid to flow. Dental professionals must manipulate a wide variety of dental materials in a fluid state in order to achieve successful clinical outcomes. Moreover, the success or failure of a given material may be as dependent on its manipulation and handling properties in the liquid state as it is on its performance properties as a solid. Most dental materials are initially in a fluid state so that they can be placed and shaped as required; then they undergo transformation to a solid state, in which they are durable and perform their function. Cements and impression materials undergo a fluid-to-solid transformation in the mouth. Gypsum products used in the fabrication of models and dies are transformed extraorally from fluid slurries into solids (see Chapter 13). Amorphous materials such as waxes and resins appear solid but actually are supercooled liquids that can flow plastically (irreversibly) under sustained loading or deform elastically (reversibly) under small stresses (see Chapters 13 and 11). The ways in which these materials flow or deform when subjected to stress are important to their use in dentistry. The study of flow characteristics of materials is the basis for the science of rheology.

Although a liquid at rest cannot support a shear stress (shearing force per unit shearing area), most liquids, when placed in motion, resist imposed forces that cause them to move. This resistance to fluid flow (viscosity) is controlled by internal frictional forces within the liquid. Thus, **viscosity** is a measure of the consistency of a fluid and its resistance to flow. A highly viscous fluid flows slowly. Dental materials have different viscosities depending on their intended clinical application. In everyday life we find wide differences in viscosities among such fluids as water, syrup, ketchup, moisturizing cream, and toothpaste.

This concept is illustrated in Figure 3.1. A liquid occupies the space between two flat surfaces, as, for example when a spatula is moved through a pasty fluid such as a dental cement to blend two components on a mixing pad. The mixing surface is fixed, and the upper surface (e.g. a spatula blade) moves to the right at a given velocity (V). A force (F) is required to overcome the frictional resistance within the fluid (i.e. the viscosity) and cause the fluid to flow. As discussed in Chapter 4, stress is the force per unit area that develops within a structure when an external force is applied. This stress causes a deformation, or strain, to develop. Strain is calculated as a change in length divided by the initial reference length. If the two surfaces have an area (A) in contact with the liquid, a shear stress (τ) can be defined as $\tau = F/A$. The shear strain rate, or rate of change of deformation, is $\epsilon = V/d$, where d is the shear distance of the upper surface relative to the fixed lower surface and V is the velocity of the moving surface. As the shear force F increases, V increases, and a curve can be obtained for force versus velocity.

Curves depicting shear stress versus shear strain rate are used to characterize the viscous behavior of fluids. The rheologic behaviors of four types of fluids are shown in Figure 3.2. An "ideal" fluid produces a shear stress proportional to the strain rate. That is, the greater the force applied, the faster the fluid flows and the plot is a straight line. This is known as Newtonian viscosity.

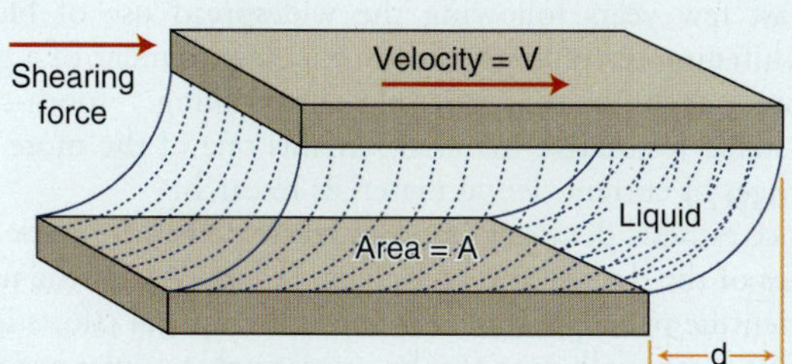

• **Fig. 3.1** Shear strain, ϵ(V/d) of a viscous liquid between two plates caused by translation of the top plate at a velocity, V, relative to the rigid lower plate (i.e. a spatula blade mixing dental cement on a mixing pad).

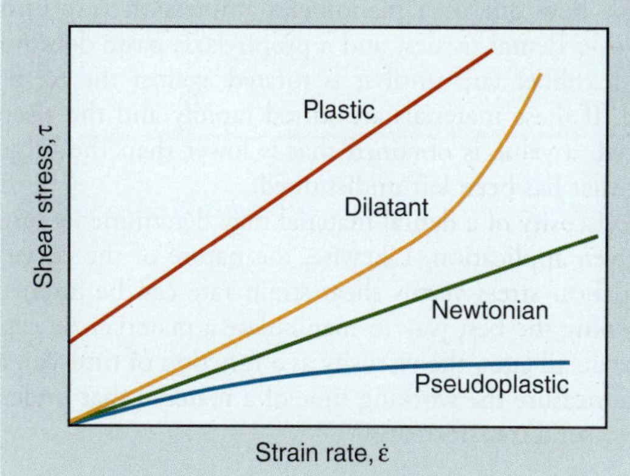

• **Fig. 3.2** Shear stress versus shear strain rate for fluids exhibiting different types of rheologic behaviors.

Because viscosity (h) is defined as the shear stress divided by the strain rate, τ/ϵ, a Newtonian fluid has a constant viscosity and exhibits a constant slope of shear stress plotted against strain rate, as seen in Figure 3.2. The plot is a straight line and resembles the elastic portion of a stress–strain curve (see Chapter 4), with viscosity the analog of the elastic modulus (elastic stress divided by elastic strain). Viscosity is measured in units of megapascals (MPa) per second, or centipoise (cP). Pure water at 20°C has a viscosity of 1.0 cP, whereas the viscosity of molasses is approximately 300,000 cP. This value is similar to that of tempered agar hydrocolloid impression material (281,000 cP at 45°C). Of the elastomeric impression materials, light-body ("thin" consistency) polysulfide has a viscosity of 109,000 cP, compared with 1,360,000 cP for heavy-body ("thick" consistency) polysulfide at 36°C.

Pseudoplastic, Dilatant, and Plastic Behavior

- The viscosity of many dental materials decreases with increasing strain rate until it reaches a nearly constant value. That is, the faster they are stirred, forced through a syringe, or squeezed, the less viscous and more fluid they become. This is pseudoplastic viscosity and is illustrated by the change in slope of the plot in Figure 3.2.
- Liquids that show the opposite behavior are dilatant and become more rigid as the rate of deformation (shear strain rate) increases. That is, the faster they are stirred, the more viscous and resistant to flow they become.
- Finally, some classes of materials behave like a rigid body until some minimum value of shear stress is reached. This is represented by the offset along the shear–stress axis. These fluids, which exhibit rigid behavior initially and then attain constant viscosity, are referred to as "plastic." Ketchup is a familiar example—a sharp blow to the bottle is usually required to produce an initial flow.

Thixotropic Behavior

The viscosity of most fluids decreases rapidly with increasing temperature. Viscosity may also depend on previous deformation of the liquid. Such fluids become less viscous and more flowable upon repeated applications of pressure and are termed **thixotropic**. Dental prophylaxis pastes, plaster of Paris, resin cements, and some impression materials are thixotropic. The thixotropic nature of impression materials is beneficial because the material does not flow out of a mandibular impression tray until it is placed over dental tissues, and a prophylaxis paste does not flow out of a rubber cup until it is rotated against the teeth to be cleaned. If these materials are stirred rapidly and the viscosity is measured, a value is obtained that is lower than the value for a sample that has been left undisturbed.

The viscosity of a dental material may determine its suitability for a given application. Likewise, the nature of the curve representing shear stress versus shear strain rate can be important in determining the best way to manipulate a material. As explained in more detail later, the viscosity as a function of time can also be used to measure the working time of a material that undergoes a liquid-to-solid transformation.

Structural Relaxation

Stress Relaxation

After a substance has been permanently deformed (plastic deformation), there are trapped internal stresses. For example, in a crystalline substance such as a metal, the atoms in the crystal structure are displaced and the system is not in equilibrium. Similarly, in amorphous structures, some molecules are too close together and others too far apart when the substance is permanently deformed.

The displaced atoms are not in equilibrium positions and are therefore unstable. Through a solid-state diffusion process driven by thermal energy, the atoms can slowly return to their equilibrium positions. The result is a change in the shape or contour of the solid as the atoms or molecules change positions. The material warps or distorts. Such stress relaxation is a problem with elastomeric impression materials and can lead to distortions in the impression and subsequent lack of fit, as discussed in Chapter 13.

The rate of relaxation increases with an increase in temperature. For example, if a wire is bent, it may tend to straighten out if it is heated to a high temperature. At room temperature, any such relaxation caused by rearrangement of metal atoms may be negligible. On the other hand, there are many noncrystalline dental materials (such as waxes, resins, and gels) that, when manipulated and cooled, can then undergo relaxation (with consequent distortion) at an elevated temperature. Considerable attention is given to this phenomenon in succeeding chapters because such dimensional changes by relaxation may result in an inaccurate fit of dental appliances.

Creep and Flow

If a metal is held at a temperature near its melting point and is subjected to a constant applied stress, the resulting strain will increase over time.

Creep is defined as the time-dependent plastic strain of a material under a static load or constant stress. The related phenomenon of sag occurs in the permanent deformation of long-span metal bridge structures at porcelain-firing temperatures under the influence of the mass of the prosthesis. For a given thickness, a greater bridge mass is related to greater flexural stress and greater flexural creep. Metal creep usually occurs as the temperature increases to within a few hundred degrees of the melting range. Metals used in dentistry for cast restorations or substrates for porcelain veneers have melting points (for pure metals) or melting ranges (for alloys) that are much higher than mouth temperatures, and they are not susceptible to creep deformation intraorally. However, some alloys used for metal-ceramic prostheses can creep at porcelain veneering temperatures. This phenomenon is discussed further in Chapter 10.

Dental amalgams contain from 42% to 52% of mercury by weight and begin melting at temperatures only slightly above room temperature. (The melting range of an alloy is discussed in Chapter 9.) Because of its low melting range, dental amalgam can undergo creep at a restored tooth site under periodic sustained stress, such as would be imposed by patients who clench their teeth. Because creep produces continuing plastic deformation, the process can, over time, be very destructive to a dental amalgam filling. The relationship of this property to the behavior of amalgam restorations is discussed in Chapter 8. A creep test is required in American National Standards Institute/American Dental Association Specification No. 1 for amalgam alloy and in International Organization for Standardization (ISO) standard No. 1559.

Creep is defined as the time-dependent plastic strain of a material under a static load or constant stress.

The term *flow*, rather than *creep*, has generally been used in dentistry to describe the rheology of amorphous materials such as waxes. The flow of wax is a measure of its potential to deform under a small static load even that associated with its own mass. Although creep or flow may be measured under any type of stress, compression is usually employed in the testing of dental materials. A cylinder of prescribed dimensions is subjected to a given compressive stress for a specified time and temperature. The creep or flow is measured as the percentage decrease in length that occurs under these testing conditions. Creep may cause unacceptable deformation of dental restorations (such as low-copper dental amalgam) made from a material that is used clinically at a temperature near its melting point for an extended period. Creep may also lead to an unacceptable fit of fixed dental prosthesis frameworks when a cast alloy with poor creep (**sag**) resistance is veneered with porcelain at relatively high temperatures (about 1000°C; see Chapter 10).

The term *flow* is used in dentistry to describe the rheology of amorphous materials.

Color and Optical Effects

The preceding sections have focused on those properties that are necessary to permit a material to restore the function of damaged or missing natural tissues. Another important goal of dentistry is to restore or improve **esthetics**—the color and appearance of natural dentition. Esthetic considerations in restorative and prosthetic dentistry have received increasingly greater emphasis in recent decades, and the challenges have grown even greater in the past few years following the widespread use of bleaching and whitening technologies. Thus, the development of a general-purpose, technique-insensitive, direct-filling, tooth-colored, color-stable restorative material remains one of the more serious challenges of current dental materials research.

Since esthetic dentistry imposes severe demands on the artistic abilities of the dentist and technician, knowledge of the underlying scientific principles of color and other optical effects is essential. This is especially true for the increasingly popular restorations that involve ceramic materials (see Chapter 10). More comprehensive treatments of this subject can be found in the "Selected Readings" at the end of this chapter.

Nature of Light and the Role of Human Vision

Light is electromagnetic radiation that can be detected by the human eye. The eye is sensitive to wavelengths from approximately 400 nm (violet) to 700 nm (dark red), as shown in Figs 3.3 and 3.4. The reflected light intensity and the combined intensities of the wavelengths present in incident and reflected light determine the appearance properties of hue, value, and chroma, which are shown in Figure 3.5 and discussed in the next section. For an object to be visible, it must reflect or **transmit** light incident on it from an external source. The incident light is usually polychromatic; that is, a mixture of the various wavelengths, commonly known as "white" light. Incident light is selectively absorbed or scattered (or both) at certain wavelengths. The spectral distribution of the transmitted or reflected light resembles that of the incident light, although certain wavelengths are reduced in magnitude.

- Light is a form of electromagnetic energy that is visible to the human eye.
- The human eye is sensitive to wavelengths from approximately 400 nm (violet) to 700 nm (dark red).
- Goldfish can see infrared radiation that is invisible to us.
- Bees, birds, and lizards have eyes that pick up ultraviolet.

The phenomenon of vision, and certain related terminology, can be illustrated by considering the response of the human eye to light reflected from an object. Light from an object that is incident on the eye is focused in the retina and is converted into nerve impulses, which are transmitted to the brain. Cone-shaped cells in the retina are responsible for color vision. These cells have a threshold intensity required for color vision and respond to wavelengths as shown in Figure 3.4 for both normal color vision and color-deficient vision. Someone with normal vision has maximum sensitivity in the green-yellow region at about 550 nm and is least sensitive in the red and blue-violet regions of the spectrum.

The signals from the retina are processed by the brain to produce the psychophysiological perception of color. Because a neural response is involved in color vision, constant stimulation by a single color may result in color fatigue and a decrease in the eye's response. Defects in certain portions of the color-sensing receptors result in the different types of color blindness; thus, humans vary greatly in their ability to distinguish colors. The eye is highly sensitive in comparing two colors seen side by side, whether on rough, smooth, flat, or curved surfaces.

Nature of the Object Under View

Esthetics is critically important in dealing with dental restorative materials. For good esthetics, the interaction of light with restorative materials must mimic the interaction of light with natural teeth. The nature of the restorative material, or that of any object under view, determines how that object will appear.

Electromagnetic radiation in the visible region interacts with an object through

- **Reflection** from its surface,
- **Absorption**,
- **Refraction**, or
- **Transmission** (i.e. by passing through unchanged).

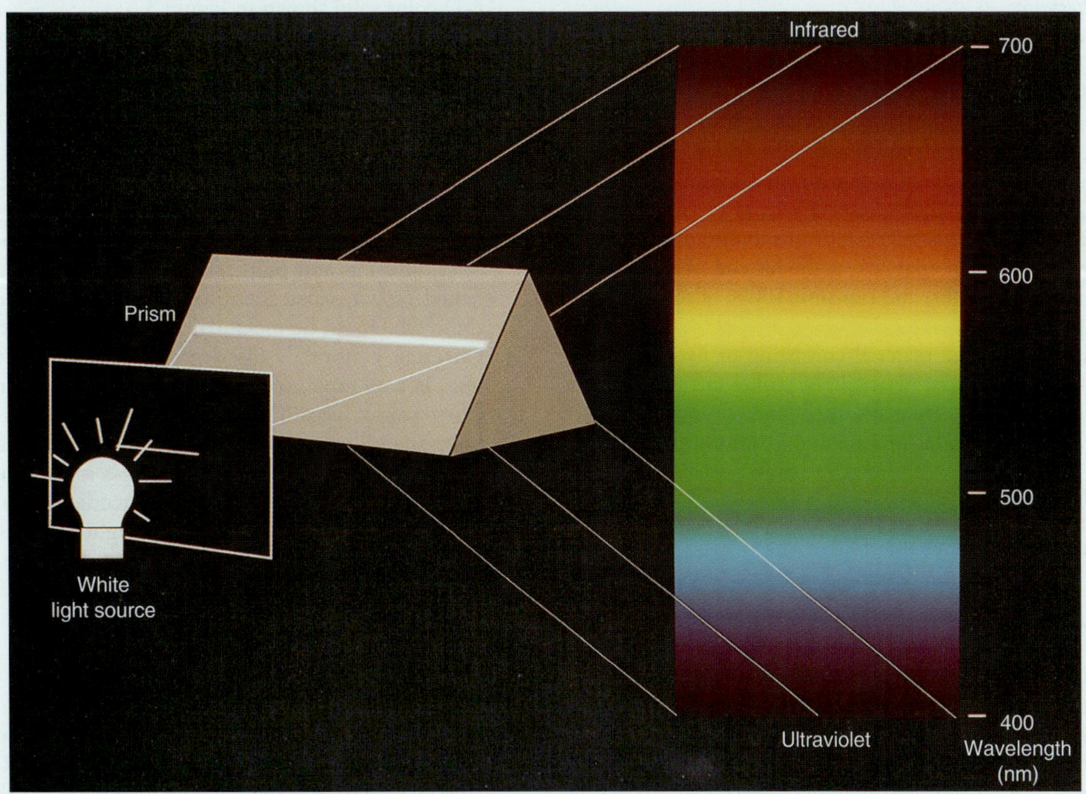

• **Fig. 3.3** Spectrum of visible light ranging in wavelength from 400 nm (violet) to 700 nm (red). The most visually perceptible region of the equal energy spectrum under daylight conditions is between wavelengths of 540 and 570 nm, with a maximum value of visual perceptibility at 555 nm (see Figure 3.4).

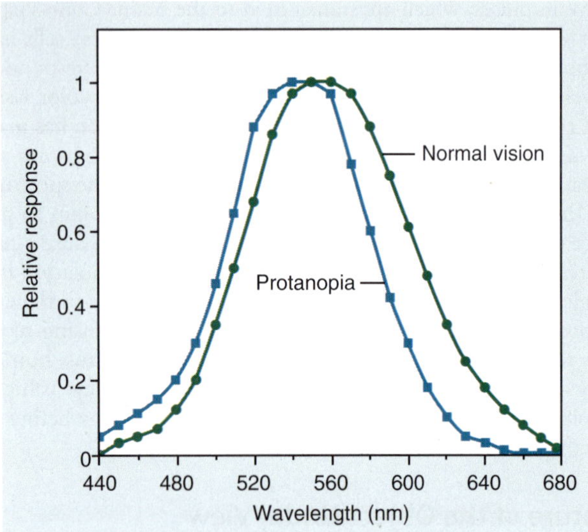

• **Fig. 3.4** Relative visual response of humans to wavelength of light for a normal observer and one with protanopia (red-green) color blindness. Protanopia is experienced by 1% of the male population and 0.02% of the female population.

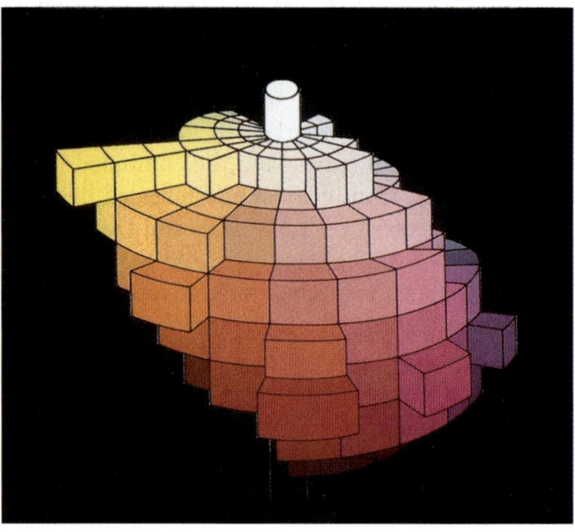

• **Fig. 3.5** The three dimensions of color space. Value increases from black at the bottom center to white at the top center. Chroma increases from the center radially outward, and changes in hue occur in a circumferential direction. (Courtesy of Minolta Corporation, Instrument Systems Division, Ramsey, NJ.)

These phenomena determine the **opacity, translucency**, or **transparency** of an object. Light reflected from rough surfaces *scatters* in many directions because it is reflected at many angles by the uneven surface.

- A perfectly smooth surface gives a mirror-like finish termed *specular reflectance.*
- A flat, surface such as chalk gives a dull appearance termed *diffuse reflectance.*

This influences the appearance of resin composite restorations, which should mimic the reflective pattern of surrounding natural tooth structure.

The opacity of a material is related to the amount of light it can absorb and/or scatter. The opposite of opacity is translucency (transparency). For example, if 1 mm thicknesses of each of two materials absorb 20% and 50%, respectively, of the light passing through them, the former is less opaque or more translucent than the latter. Transparent materials are at the far end of the translucency scale, absorb no light, and transmit 100% of the light that passes through them.

Enamel is a composite material consisting of hydroxyapatite crystals in a protein matrix. When light strikes enamel, some is reflected, some refracted, some absorbed, and some transmitted. Enamel has a refractive index of 1.65 and is translucent.

CRITICAL QUESTION

How is color described objectively and quantitatively?

Three Dimensions of Color

Verbal descriptions of color are not precise enough to describe the appearance of teeth. For example, the definition of *puce* is "a brilliant purplish-red color," according to Microsoft's *Encarta World English Dictionary*, while *Webster's Third New International Dictionary* defines it as "a dark red that is yellower and less strong than cranberry, paler and slightly yellower than average garnet, bluer, less strong, and slightly lighter than pomegranate, and bluer and paler than average wine." These definitions are too variable, complex, and imprecise to describe a desired color of a dental crown to a laboratory technician. Such a written description is subjective and does not clearly and unambiguously allow one to perceive the color. To overcome this problem, color perception is described by three objective variables: hue, value, and chroma. These three parameters constitute the three dimensions of "color space," as shown in Figure 3.5.

- **Hue**: The dominant color of an object, for example red, green, or blue. This refers to the dominant wavelengths present in the spectral distribution. The continuum of these hues creates the 3-D color solid shown in Figure 3.5.
- **Value**: Value is also known as the gray scale. It is the vertical, or Z-axis, of Figure 3.5. Value increases toward the high end (lighter) and decreases toward the low end (darker). Value is also expressed by the "lightness" factor (L^* in Fig. 3.6), with varying levels of gray between the extremes of white and black. Teeth and other objects can be separated into lighter shades (higher value) and darker shades (lower value). For example, the yellow of a lemon is lighter than the red of a cherry. For a light-diffusing and light-reflecting object such as a tooth or dental crown, value identifies the lightness or darkness of a color, which can be measured independently of the hue.
- **Chroma**: Chroma is the degree of saturation of a particular hue. For example, red can vary from "scarlet" to light pink, where scarlet has a high saturation and pink has a low saturation. The yellow color of a lemon is a more saturated, "vivid," color than that of a banana, which is a less saturated, "dull" yellow. Chroma varies radially, perpendicular to the value/L^* axis (see Fig. 3.6A, near the bottom right). Colors in the center are dull (gray). In other words, the higher the chroma, the more intense the color. Chroma is not considered separately in dentistry. It is always associated with the hue and value of dental tissues, restorations, and prostheses.

- Color is produced in different ways, viz. selective reflection, selective absorption, diffraction, scattering, and interference of light.
- Color is not an inherent property of a material but results from multiple factors like the composition, thickness, surface roughness, and the nature of illuminating light.
- The dominant wave length gives **hue**, intensity or saturation gives **chroma**, and the level of brightness provides **value** for the color.

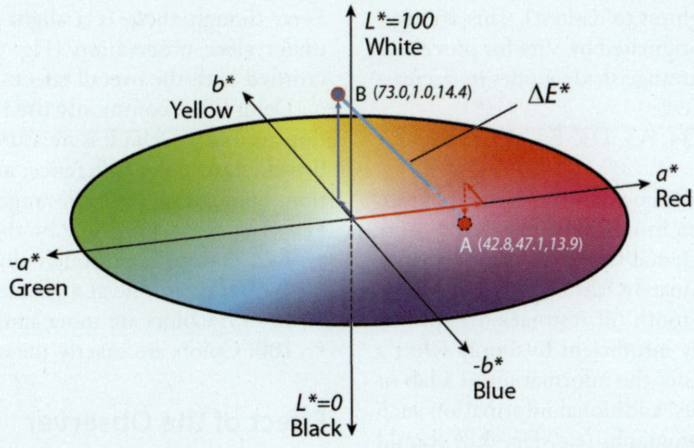

• **Fig. 3.6** Lab color chart showing the color of a red apple at point A (*top and bottom*). For this chart, the appearance is expressed by L* (value) = 42.83; a* (red–green axis) = 45.04; and b* (yellow–blue axis) = 9.52. In contrast, the color of shade A2 porcelain can be described by L* = 72.99; a* = 1.00; and b* = 14.41. (Courtesy of Minolta Corporation, Instrument Systems Division, Ramsey, NJ.)

The components of a color space can be more easily visualized by its individual parts in Figure 3.5B, here seen as discs stacked along the value axis (lightness, L*) on a scale of 0–10 from black to white. Around the periphery are 10 basic hues (dominant wavelength/color). Chroma (strength, saturation) radiates out from the value axis like the spokes of a wheel (illustrated by green).

Figure 3.6 represents a horizontal plane, perpendicular to the L* (value) axis, through the color solid in Figure 3.5. This color chart is based on the Commission Internationale de l'Éclairage L*a*b* color space, in which L* represents the value of an object, a* is the measurement along the red–green axis, and b* is the measurement along the yellow–blue axis. The color of a red apple is shown by the letter A in the upper and lower charts. Its color appearance can be expressed by L* = 42.83, a* = 45.04, and b* = 9.52. In comparison, a dental body (gingival) porcelain of shade A2 can be described by a higher (lighter) L* of 72.99, a lower a* of 1.00, and a higher b* of 14.41.

Color Matching

In dental practice, color matching is most often performed with the use of a shade guide, such as the one shown in Figure 3.7, to select the color of ceramic veneers, inlays, or crowns. Shade guide tabs are used in much the same way as paint chips to match the color of house paint. The individual shade tabs shown in the upper portion of Figure 3.7 are grouped according to hue

- A = Red-brown
- B = Red-yellow
- C = Gray
- D = Red-gray

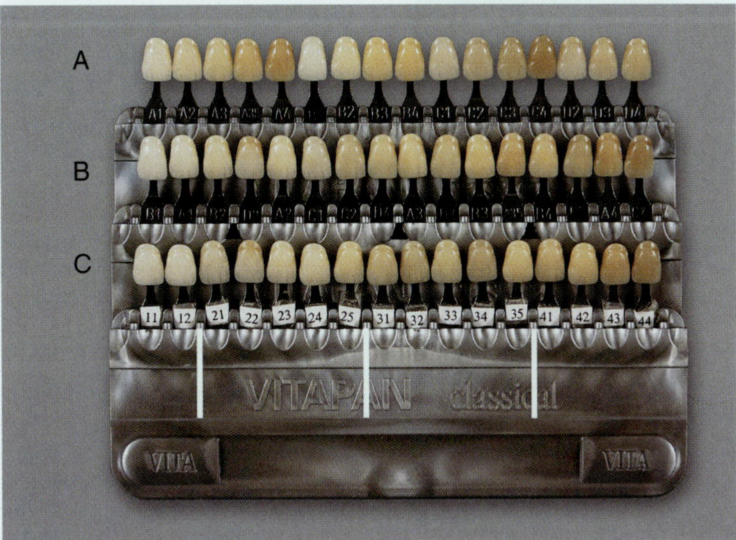

• **Fig. 3.7** Tab arrangements of the Vitapan classical shade guide. **(A)** Manufacturer's arrangement No. 1: group division according to hue. **(B)** Manufacturer's arrangement No. 1: "value scale," no group division. **(C)** Alternative arrangement: according to color difference in relation to the lightest tab, group division. (From Paravina RD, Powers JM: *Esthetic Color Training in Dentistry*, St. Louis, Mosby, 2004.)

followed by value (1 to 4, or lightest to darkest). This arrangement follows the "classical" order originated by Vita for porcelain. Recently, however, the trend is to arrange shade guides in decreasing order of value (lightest to darkest):

B1, A1, B2, D2, A2, C1, C2, D4, A3, D3, B3, A3.5, B4, C3, A4, C4

Matching tooth shades is simplified by the arrangement of tabs by value; this arrangement has been found to be easier and more reliable to use (see RD Paravina, Dental Color Matcher, listed in the "Selected Readings"). Unfortunately, although a reasonable match can be achieved between a tooth (or restoration) and one of the shade guide tabs, it is usually insufficient to simply select a shade from a shade guide and transfer the information to a lab or technician. To ensure esthetic results, additional information such as drawings, descriptions, and photographs (e.g. Fig. 3.8) should also be sent. Obviously if the technician can see the actual teeth, the probability of achieving an acceptable color match will be even greater.

3D master shade guide is gaining popularity with Indian Labs. It gives more accurate shade matching. The resource for further details can be had from the website which is included in the further reading section of this chapter.

Further, the subjective preference of the patient must be taken into account. An exact match between a crown or bridge and the remaining sound teeth is not always sufficient. Patients usually prefer a lighter shade (higher value) in a restoration as compared with the color of the natural teeth. Figure 3.8A shows the result of shade matching in which the two central incisor crowns were selected to be somewhat higher in value than the lateral incisors.

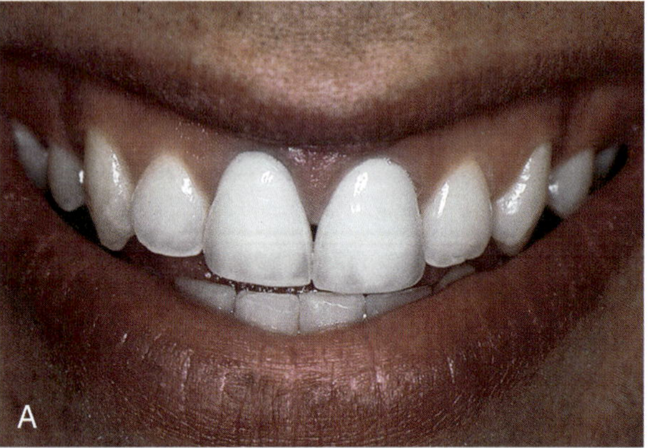

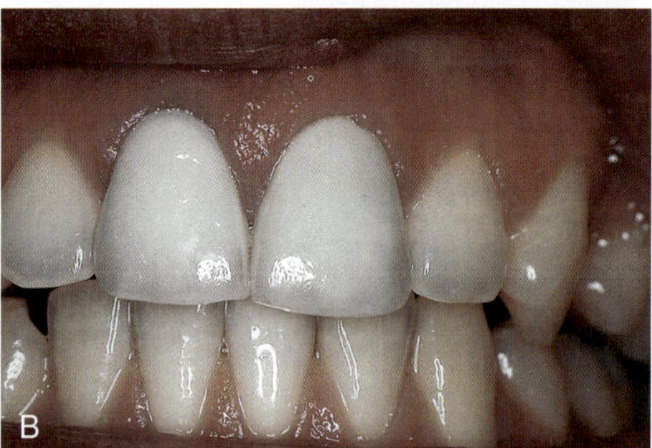

• **Fig. 3.8 (A)** Two central incisor metal-ceramic crowns with porcelain margins. The value (L*) of these crowns is higher than that of the adjacent lateral incisor teeth. **(B)** Close-up view of the metal-ceramic crowns.

Even though there is a slight mismatch, it is perceptible only under close observation (Fig. 3.8B) and the patient was quite satisfied with the overall effect.

Delta E is a commonly used measure to evaluate color perception accuracy. Delta E is measured on a scale from 0 to 100, where 0 is the least color difference, and 100 indicates complete distortion. Standard perception ranges are as follows:

- ≤1.0: Not perceptible by the human eye
- 1–2: Perceptible through close observation
- 3–10: Perceptible at a glance
- 11–49: Colors are more similar than the opposite
- 100: Colors are exactly the opposite

Effect of the Observer

Signals of color are sent to the human brain from three sets of receptors in the retina called cones, which are especially sensitive to red, blue, and green. Factors that interfere with the true perception of color generally include low or high light levels, fatigue of the color receptors, sex, age, memory, and cultural background. According to a 1995 study (Anusavice and Barrett, 1995), there appears to be no effect related to observer age, gender, or clinical experience relative to the accuracy of dental shade matching. However in 2009, a study performed in 9 countries across 15 universities showed that females achieved significantly better shade matching results than males, indicating that gender plays an important role in shade matching.

The level of experience was not found to be a significant factor in shade matching.

At low light levels, the rods in the retina of the human eye are more dominant than the cones, and color perception is lost. As the brightness becomes more intense, color appears to change (Bezold–Brucke effect). Also, if an observer looks at a red object for a reasonably long time, receptor fatigue causes a green hue to be seen when he or she then looks at a white background. For this reason, if a patient is observed against an intense-colored background, the dentist or clinician may select a tooth shade with a hue that is shifted somewhat toward the complementary color of the background color. For example, a blue background shifts color selection toward yellow, and an orange background shifts the color selection toward blue-green. Unfortunately, 8% of men and 0.5% of women exhibit color blindness (see Fig. 3.4). Most commonly, these people cannot distinguish red from green because of the lack of either green-sensitive or red-sensitive cones. However, this deficiency may not affect the shade selection of natural teeth.

CRITICAL QUESTION

Why are some objects color-matched under one type of illumination but mismatched under another illumination source?

Effect of the Light Source

Because the spectral distribution of the light reflected from or transmitted through an object is dependent on the spectral content of the incident light, the appearance of an object is dependent on the nature of the light in which the object is viewed. Daylight, incandescent, and fluorescent lamps are common sources of light in the dental operatory or laboratory, and each of these has a different spectral distribution. Objects that appear to be color-matched under one type of light may appear different under another type. This phenomenon is called **metamerism**.

Thus, if possible, color matching should be done under two or more different light sources, one of which should be daylight, and the laboratory shade-matching procedures should be performed under the same lighting conditions.

CRITICAL QUESTION

Why do some tooth-colored restorations appear to be missing when viewed under "black light" illumination, such as that used in nightclubs and at rock concerts?

Fluorescence

In addition to the processes already discussed, natural tooth structure absorbs light at wavelengths too short to be visible to the human eye. These wavelengths between 300 and 400 nm are referred to as near-ultraviolet radiation. Natural sunlight, photoflash lamps, certain types of vapor lamps, and ultraviolet lights used in decorative lighting ("black lights") are sources containing substantial amounts of near-ultraviolet radiation. The energy that the tooth absorbs is converted into light with longer wavelengths, in which case the tooth actually becomes a light source. This phenomenon is called fluorescence. The emitted light, a blue-white color, is primarily in the 400–450 nm range. Fluorescence makes a definite contribution to the brightness and vital appearance of a human tooth. As an example, ceramic crowns or composite restorations that lack a fluorescing agent appear as missing teeth when viewed under a black light.

A more detailed discussion of color and color perception, the use of shade guides, and other aspects of the science of color matching and its use in the art of restoring a natural, pleasing dentition, can be found under Color and Optical Effects in the "Selected Readings" section.

Radiopacity

X-rays, a form of electromagnetic radiation, lie at the high-energy end of the spectrum. Hence the interaction of dental biomaterials with X-radiation may be classified as an optical property. There are numerous circumstances where it is necessary to be able to distinguish a dental material radiographically from the surrounding tissue. For example, sufficient radiographic contrast is required in an X-ray image in order to assess restorations for marginal defects or breakdown, help differentiate composite restorations from dental caries, and detect microleakage. In case of accidental ingestion or traumatic impaction of dentures or other appliances, a delay in the detection, location, and removal of the appliance and its fragments may be life-threatening. A significant number of foreign bodies of dental origin, with many injuries and deaths, are reported each year, particularly among the elderly.

The amount of X-ray energy absorbed by an object depends on the density and thickness of the material and the energy of the radiation. Generally, the higher the atomic number of the component atoms, the greater the X-ray absorbance and the larger the contrast produced. Polymers and resins are inherently radiolucent, whereas metals with atomic numbers above about 19 (potassium) are inherently radiopaque. To impart radiopacity, restorative resins often utilize strontium- or barium-containing glass-reinforcing particles (see Chapter 5); denture polymers may (but rarely) contain barium sulfate or other heavy-metal compound additives to render them radiopaque. Radiopacity similar to that of hard tissue provides the optimal contrast for dental restorations. When radiopacity is too low, the resin will not be visible on an X-ray image; when it is too high, it may block out and obscure details of adjacent anatomy. Dentin has approximately the same radiodensity as that of aluminum, while enamel has approximately twice the radiodensity of dentin and aluminum. To claim that a composite is radiopaque, the American Dental Association requires commercial dental restorative resins to have a radiopacity at least equal to that of aluminum. To be adequately detectable on medical chest X-ray images, it has been found that a denture resin fragment of 2 mm should have a radiopacity equal or greater than that of 0.2 mm of copper. This requires the resin to have sufficient additive to produce a radiopacity about three times that of aluminum.

Thermal Properties

When restorative materials are placed in deep cavities, the heat transmitted to vital dental pulp must be limited so as to prevent thermal shock and trauma. In other circumstances, as with denture bases in contact with mucosal surfaces, the transmission of a certain amount of thermal energy is desirable to convey the sensations of heat and cold associated with food and beverages. Such attributes are governed by the properties of thermal conductivity and thermal diffusivity. Another category of thermal behavior is the expansion when heated and contraction when cooled. If, for example, a dental restoration expands and contracts at a rate different from that of the adjacent hard tissues, marginal failures and leakage can result. This attribute is governed by the coefficient of thermal expansion.

Thermal Conductivity

Thermal conductivity (κ) is the physical property that governs heat transfer through a material by conductive flow. The conduction of heat within a solid involves the transfer of thermal energy from one part of a material to another across a temperature gradient. It is defined as the quantity of heat in calories per second passing through a material 1 cm thick with a cross section of 1 cm^2 having a temperature difference of 1 K (1°C) and is measured under steady-state conditions in which the temperature gradient does not change. According to the second law of thermodynamics, heat flows from points of higher temperature to points of lower temperature. The International System (SI) unit or measure for thermal conductivity is watts per meter per kelvin ($W \times m^{-1} \times K^{-1}$). In general, thermal conductivities increase in the following order: *polymers* < *ceramics* < *metals*, although there are exceptions.

Materials that have a high thermal conductivity are called *conductors*, whereas materials of low thermal conductivity are called *insulators*. The higher its thermal conductivity, the greater the ability of a substance to transmit thermal energy, and vice versa. If the thermal gradient does not change (i.e. heat is supplied at one end and withdrawn at the other end at a steady rate), the thermal conductivity is a measure of the heat transferred. If, however, the temperature gradient does change with time, which is invariably the case in the mouth, thermal diffusivity will determine the amount of heat transferred and, consequently, the change in temperature experienced.

CRITICAL QUESTION

What is the difference between thermal conductivity and thermal diffusivity, and why does it matter in dentistry?

Thermal Diffusivity

Thermal diffusivity is a measure of the speed with which a temperature change will spread through an object when one surface is heated. It is calculated from the thermal conductivity divided by the product of density and heat capacity:

(1)

$$h = \frac{\kappa}{C_p \times \rho}$$

where h the is thermal diffusivity, κ is the thermal conductivity, c_p is the heat capacity at constant pressure, and ρ is the temperature-dependent density in grams per cm^3 (c_p is numerically equal to the more commonly used term, *specific heat*, which is the quantity of heat needed to raise the temperature of a unit mass by l C).

A material with a high density and high specific heat will likely have a low thermal diffusivity. Such a material changes its temperature very slowly. Low heat capacity and high thermal conductivity lead to high diffusivity, and temperature changes transmit rapidly through the material. As shown in Table 3.1, gold has about one-tenth the heat capacity of dentin, about 500 times the thermal conductivity, and about 600 times the thermal diffusivity. Thus, a pure gold filling would provide the tooth pulp with very little protection against thermal shock as compared with natural dentin.

When the product of heat capacity and density ($c_p \times \rho$) is high, the thermal diffusivity may be low, even though the thermal conductivity is relatively high. Therefore, both thermal conductivity and thermal diffusivity are important parameters in predicting the transfer of thermal energy through a material. Because of the rapid changes in temperature that can occur during ingestion of hot or cold foods and liquids, the thermal diffusivity of a dental restorative material may be more important than its thermal conductivity. Enamel and dentin are effective thermal insulators, as shown in Table 3.1. The thermal conductivities and thermal diffusivities of cementing materials (glass ionomer, zinc phosphate, and composite) compare favorably with these tissues, in contrast with the markedly higher values for metallic restorative materials. Thus, when the remaining dentin between the cavity and the pulp is too thin to provide sufficient thermal protection, an additional layer of an insulating base material should be placed, as discussed in Chapter 7 on Dental Cements.

Coefficient of Thermal Expansion

When materials undergo a temperature increase, the vibrational motion of atoms and mean interatomic (bond) distances increase. This results is an increase in volume—an expansion. The increase is described by the **coefficient of thermal expansion, α**, which is defined as the change in length per unit of the original length of a material when its temperature is raised 1°C (1 K) (see the discussion of thermal energy in Chapter 2):

(2)

$$\alpha = \frac{\Delta L}{L \times \Delta T}$$

where L is the original length, ΔL is the change in length and ΔT is the temperature change. Values for α of some materials of interest in dentistry are presented in Table 3.2. The units are typically expressed as either mm/m K or ppm/K.

This parameter is extremely important in dental applications as broad ranging as producing cast restorations that fit and maintaining the seal at a restoration margin. Its influence often dictates the procedures that have been developed for using wax patterns, casting metal crowns, placing amalgam and composite resin restorations, and preparing metal-ceramic crowns and bridges. A tooth restoration may expand or contract more than the tooth during a change in temperature; thus, there may be marginal microleakage adjacent to the restoration, or the restoration may debond from the tooth. According to the values in Table 3.2, direct restorative materials may change in dimension up to 4.4 times more than the tooth enamel for every degree of temperature change.

The high thermal expansion coefficient of inlay wax is also important because it is highly susceptible to temperature changes. For example, an accurate wax pattern that fits a prepared tooth contracts significantly when it is removed from the tooth or a die in a warmer area and then stored in a cooler area. This dimensional change is transferred to a cast metal restoration that is made from the lost-wax process. Similarly, denture teeth that have been set in denture base wax in a relatively warm laboratory may shift appreciably in their simulated intraoral positions after the denture base is moved to a cooler room before the processing of a denture.

Thermal stresses produced from a thermal expansion or contraction difference are also important in the production of metal-ceramic restorations. Consider a porcelain veneer that is fired to a metal substrate (coping). It may contract to a greater extent than

TABLE 3.1 Density and Thermal Properties of Water, Enamel, Dentin, and Dental Materials

Material	Density (g cm^{-3})	Specific Heat (cal g^{-1} K^{-1})	Thermal Conductivity (W m^{-1} K^{-1})	Thermal Diffusivity (cm^2 s^{-1})
Water	1.00	1.00	0.44	0.0014
Dentin	2.14	0.30	0.57	0.0018–0.0026
Glass ionomer	2.13	0.27	0.51–0.72	0.0022
Zinc phosphate	2.59	0.12	1.05	0.0030
Composite	1.6–2.4	0.20	1.09–1.37	0.0019–0.0073
Enamel	2.97	0.18	0.93	0.0047
Amalgam	11.6	0.005	22.6	0.96
Pure gold	19.3	0.03	297	1.18

TABLE 3.2 Coefficients of Thermal Expansion (α) of Dental Materials Compared with those of Tooth Enamel and Dentin

Material	α (ppm K^{-1})	$\alpha_{material}/\alpha_{tooth\ enamel}$
Aluminous porcelain	6.6	0.58
Dentin	8.3	0.75
Commercially pure titanium	8.5	0.77
Type II glass ionomer	11.0	0.96
Tooth enamel	11.4	1.00
Gold–palladium alloy	13.5	1.18
Gold (pure)	14.0	1.23
Palladium–silver alloy	14.8	1.30
Amalgam	25.0	2.19
Composite	14–50	1.2–4.4
Denture resin	81.0	7.11
Pit and fissure sealant	85.0	7.46
Inlay wax	400.0	35.1

the metal during cooling and induce tangential tensile stresses or tensile hoop (circumferential) tensile stresses in the porcelain, which may cause immediate or delayed crack formation. Although these thermal stresses cannot be eliminated completely, they can be reduced appreciably by selection of materials whose expansion or contraction coefficients are matched fairly closely (within 4%). This is discussed more fully in Chapter 10 on ceramics.

CRITICAL QUESTION

Which factors in the oral environment promote the corrosion of metallic dental restorations and prostheses?

Electrochemical Properties

Dentistry uses a wide variety of metals for restorations and prosthetic devices, the successful clinical performance, and long-term durability of which require adequate corrosion resistance in the oral environment. **Corrosion** is an electrochemical process and is dependent on the ability to conduct electrical current, either by means of free electrons in metals or via ions in solution. Corrosion and its influence on durability and appearance are the major ways in which electrochemistry affects oral well-being. Pulpal pain caused by an electrical current produced when two dissimilar metals are brought into contact, known as galvanic shock, is another. The most important electrochemical effects are toxic and allergic responses to metal ions released by corrosion, which may affect both nearby tissues and distant organs. In most cases corrosion is undesirable. However, a limited amount of corrosion at the margins of dental amalgam restorations may be beneficial, since the corrosion products tend to seal the marginal gap and inhibit the ingress of oral fluids and bacteria.

The oral environment is highly conducive to electrochemical action. It is warm, moist, and subjected to wide fluctuations in temperature and pH. Thus, an understanding of corrosion and the underlying electrochemical properties is essential in order to control electrochemical effects and thereby minimize corrosion and corrosion-induced problems in dentistry.

Tarnish and Corrosion

- **Tarnish** is a surface discoloration on a metal or a slight loss or alteration of the surface finish or luster. In the oral environment, tarnish often occurs from the formation of deposits on the surface of a restoration. Tarnish also arises from the formation of thin films, such as oxides, sulfides, or chlorides. The latter phenomenon may be only a simple surface deposit, and such a film may even be protective, as discussed subsequently. However, it is often an early indication and precursor of corrosion.
- **Corrosion** is a process whereby deterioration of a metal is caused by reaction with its environment. In due course, corrosion can cause severe and catastrophic disintegration of metals. Even if highly localized, corrosion may cause mechanical failure of a structure even though the actual volume of material lost is quite small. Corrosive disintegration can take place through the action of moisture, atmosphere, acid, or alkaline solutions, and certain chemicals. Various sulfides, such as hydrogen or ammonium sulfide, initially tarnish and eventually corrode silver, copper, tin, mercury, and other metals present in their alloys. Also, water, oxygen, and chlorine ions are present in saliva and contribute to the corrosive attack. Various acidic solutions such as phosphoric, acetic, and lactic acids are present at times and, at the proper concentration and pH, can promote corrosion.

Fundamental Basis of Corrosion

Corrosion occurs because most commonly used metals and alloys are not in their lowest energy state (thermodynamically the most stable state). For example, iron (Fe) is not available in nature as pure Fe. Instead, it exists in the form of various oxides of iron, from which metallic Fe is extracted by metallurgical techniques. Similarly, aluminum (Al) is extracted from aluminum oxide (Al_2O_3), and copper (Cu) from Cu sulfides. Oxidized compounds such as Fe_3O_4, Al_2O_3, or CuS (commonly classified as minerals) are thermodynamically stable and consequently occur in nature in these fully reacted forms. Thus, pure metals spontaneously convert to a highly reacted, oxidized state by reacting with, for example, oxygen, sulfur, or chlorine in order to revert to their lowest energy state. This, in essence, is the process of corrosion. Gold is unique: it does not corrode and is available in nature in pure forms. Ceramics, on the other hand, do not corrode because they are already fully oxidized and in their lowest energy states. However, glass-phase ceramics and feldspathic porcelains and glazes can dissolve in acidic and basic media.

Corrosion of a metal is either a chemical or an electrochemical process, in each of which the first step is the loss of an electron.

- *Chemical corrosion* is the direct combination of metallic and nonmetallic elements to yield a chemical compound through oxidation reactions. A good example is the discoloration of silver by sulfur, where silver sulfide forms by chemical corrosion. It can also be a corrosion product of dental gold alloys that contain silver. This mode of corrosion is also referred to as dry corrosion, since it occurs in the absence of water or another fluid electrolyte. Another example is the oxidation of silver–copper alloy particles that are mixed with mercury to prepare certain dental amalgam products. These alloy particles contain a silver–copper eutectic phase; oxidation limits their reactivity with mercury, thereby affecting the setting reaction of the dental amalgam product. This is why it is prudent to store the alloy in a cool, dry location to ensure an adequate shelf life.

- *Electrochemical corrosion*, also known as **galvanic** corrosion, requires the presence of water or some other fluid electrolyte and a pathway for the transport of electrons (i.e. an electrical current). It is also referred to as wet corrosion, since it requires a fluid electrolyte. Electrochemical corrosion is seldom isolated and almost invariably is accompanied by chemical corrosion. However, the electrochemical mode of corrosion is more important for dental materials and is the focus in this chapter.

CRITICAL QUESTION

Which mechanisms of electrochemical corrosion are possible for metallic dental restorations and prostheses?

Electrochemical Mechanism of Corrosion

When a metal is in contact with a fluid electrolyte, the chemical potential causes enough ions to dissolve to form a saturated solution and produce an equal number of free electrons. The loss of electrons by a metal is known as oxidation and is the initial electrochemical event in the corrosion process. The ease with which a metal gives up electrons in solution and oxidizes can be expressed in terms of the *oxidation potential*. An electrochemical cell is illustrated schematically in Figure 3.9.

ISO 10271:2020 (en)

Tarnish—Surface discoloration due to the chemical reaction between a metallic material and its environment.

Corrosion—Physicochemical interaction between a metallic material and its environment that results in a partial or total destruction of the material or in a change of its properties.

An electrochemical cell is composed of three essential components: an anode, a cathode, and an electrolyte; it is a battery, since it produces a voltage and current between the two electrodes. In this example, the anode could be an amalgam restoration and the cathode a gold alloy restoration, with saliva serving as the electrolyte.

The *anode* is the surface or site on a surface where positive ions (M^+) are formed (i.e. the metal surface that is undergoing an oxidation reaction and corroding) with the production of free electrons, as illustrated by the following anodic/oxidation reaction:

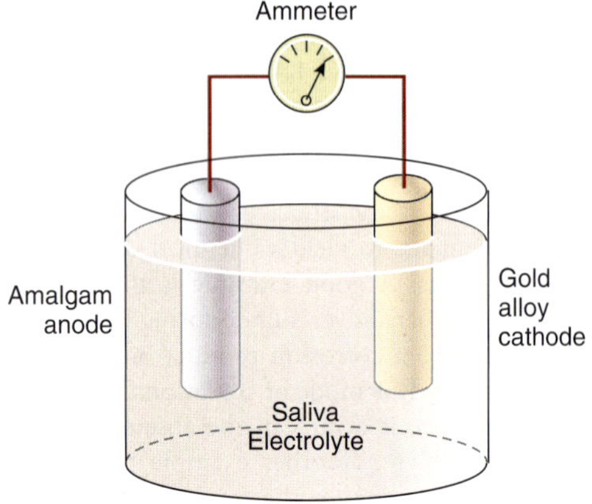

• **Fig. 3.9** Diagram of an electrochemical cell consisting of a simulated amalgam anode, a gold alloy cathode, and saliva as the electrolyte.

(3)

$$M^\circ \rightarrow M^+ + e^-$$

Once the solution is saturated with metal ions, the reverse reaction, reduction, can occur. The *cathode* is the surface or sites on a surface where metal ions are deposited from a saturated solution and consume free electrons produced at the anode. Several reduction reactions can take place, depending on the environment. For example, metal ions may be removed from the solution to form metal atoms (reaction 4) as occurs in metal plating; hydrogen ions may be converted to hydrogen gas (reaction 5); or hydroxyl ions may be formed (reaction 6).

Cathodic/reduction reaction:

(4)

$$M^+ + e^- \rightarrow M^\circ$$

(5)

$$2H^+ + 2e^- \rightarrow H_2\uparrow$$

(6)

$$2H_2O + 4e^- \rightarrow 4(OH)^-$$

The electrolyte supplies the ions needed at the cathode and carries away the corrosion products at the anode. The external circuit serves as a conduction path to carry electrons (the electrical current) from the anode to the cathode. An electrical potential difference that is, a voltage (V), can be measured, which has considerable importance in that it is capable of producing a physiological sensation such as pain. This difference in electrical potential is also known as electromotive force (EMF).

In order for electrochemical corrosion to be an ongoing process, the production of electrons by the oxidation reactions at the anode must be exactly balanced by the consumption of electrons in the reduction reactions at the cathode. Often the cathodic reactions can be considered to be the primary driving force for electrochemical corrosion. This is a very important consideration in determining the rate of a corrosion process, and it can be used advantageously in order to reduce or eliminate corrosion.

Different metals have different tendencies for oxidation because of their differences in electronic structure; this tendency to oxidize (ionize) is measured by the *electrode potential* expressed in volts or millivolts. The more negative the electrode potential, the easier it is for any particular metal to ionize and oxidize, and the more susceptible it is to tarnish and corrosion. The more positive its electrode potential, the less the metal's susceptibility to tarnish and corrosion. Recall that noble metals have their full complement of eight outer electrons and that they have very low tendencies to give up electrons and oxidize. Therefore, noble metals have a very positive electrode potential and are highly resistant to corrosion. Noble metals include gold, platinum, palladium, iridium, rhodium, osmium, and ruthenium. Their presence in alloys can confer varying levels of corrosion resistance.

The basis for judging the tendency of metals and alloys to undergo electrochemical corrosion is the **electromotive (or galvanic) series**, which arranges metals by their equilibrium values of electrode potential. Table 3.3 presents an electromotive series useful for dental metals and alloys in water at 25°C. Each of these standard half-cell potentials may be considered as the voltage of an electrochemical cell in which one electrode is the hydrogen electrode (reaction 5), designated arbitrarily as zero potential, and the other electrode is the element of interest. The sign of the electrode potential in Table 3.3 indicates the polarity in such a cell. Metals with a more positive potential have a lower tendency to dissolve and are therefore more resistant to becoming oxidized and corroded in aqueous environments.

If two pure metals are immersed in an electrolyte and connected by an electrical conductor to form a galvanic cell, the metal with the lower (more negative) electrode potential in Table 3.3 becomes the anode and undergoes oxidation, that is, its ions go into solution.

Corrosion in the mouth is typically an ongoing process. Many types of electrochemical corrosion are possible in the oral environment because saliva, with the salts it contains, is a weak electrolyte. The electrochemical properties of saliva depend on the concentrations of its components, pH, surface tension, and buffering capacity. Each of these factors may influence the strength of any electrolyte. Thus, the magnitude of the resulting corrosion process will be controlled by these variables.

In an environment in which a metal is corroding, both anodic and cathodic reactions take place simultaneously on the surface of the metal. Metal ions go into solution or form corrosion products because of the anodic reactions and other ions are reduced in the cathodic reactions. These two reactions may occur at randomly distributed sites on the metal surface or, more frequently, there are anodic areas at which mostly the metal dissolves and cathodic areas at which mostly other ions are discharged. Several forms of electrochemical corrosion are based on the mechanisms that produce these inhomogeneous areas; they are discussed below.

TABLE 3.3 Electromotive Series of the Metals

Metal	Ion	Electrode Potential (V)
Gold	Au^{+}	+1.50
Gold	Au^{3+}	+1.36
Platinum	Pt^{2+}	+0.86
Palladium	Pd^{2+}	+0.82
Mercury	Hg^{2+}	+0.80
Silver	Ag^{+}	+0.80
Copper	Cu^{+}	+0.47
Bismuth	Bi^{3+}	+0.23
Antimony	Sb^{3+}	+0.10
Hydrogen	H^{+}	−0.00
Lead	Pb^{2+}	−0.12
Tin	Sn^{2+}	−0.14
Nickel	Ni^{2+}	−0.23
Cadmium	Cd^{2+}	−0.40
Iron	Fe^{2+}	−0.44
Chromium	Cr^{2+}	−0.56
Zinc	Zn^{2+}	−0.76
Aluminum	Al^{3+}	−1.70
Sodium	Na^{+}	−2.71
Calcium	Ca^{2+}	−2.87
Potassium	K^{+}	−2.92

Dissimilar Metals

An important type of electrochemical reaction occurs when combinations of dissimilar metals are in direct physical contact. This happens in adjacently placed metal restorations where the metal surfaces have different compositions. The alloy combinations that may produce galvanic corrosion or electrogalvanism through the flow of galvanic currents may be in either continuous or intermittent contact. An example would be a dental amalgam restoration placed on the occlusal surface of a tooth directly opposing a gold inlay. Because both restorations are wet with saliva, an electrical circuit exists with a difference in potential between the dissimilar restorations (Fig. 3.10). When the two restorations are brought into contact, there is a sudden short-circuit through the two alloys. This can result in a sharp pain, called **galvanic shock**, which is well known in dentistry. An undetected piece of aluminum foil in a baked potato can produce the same effect.

When the teeth are not in contact, there is still an electrical circuit associated with the difference in potential or EMF between the two restorations. The saliva forms the electrolyte and the hard and soft tissues can constitute the external circuit, although the electrical resistance of the external circuit is considerable in comparison with that which exists when the two restorations are brought into contact. The current generated is inversely related to the electrical resistance of the metal of interest.

A current is present even in a single isolated metallic restoration, although it is less intense. In this situation, the electrochemical cell is generated as a result of the electrical potential differences created by the two electrolytes: saliva and tissue fluids. The term *tissue fluid* is used to denote the dentinal fluid, soft tissue fluid, and blood that provide the means for completing the external circuit. Because the chloride ion concentration is seven times higher than that of saliva, it is assumed that the interior surfaces of a dental restoration exposed to dentinal fluid will have a more active electrochemical potential. Possible current pathways are diagrammed in Figure 3.11.

Although the magnitude of these currents usually diminishes somewhat as the restoration ages, it remains indefinitely at the

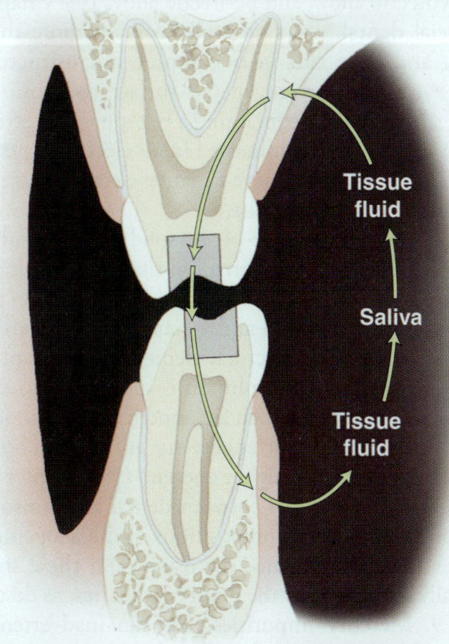

• **Fig. 3.10** Possible path of a galvanic current in the mouth.

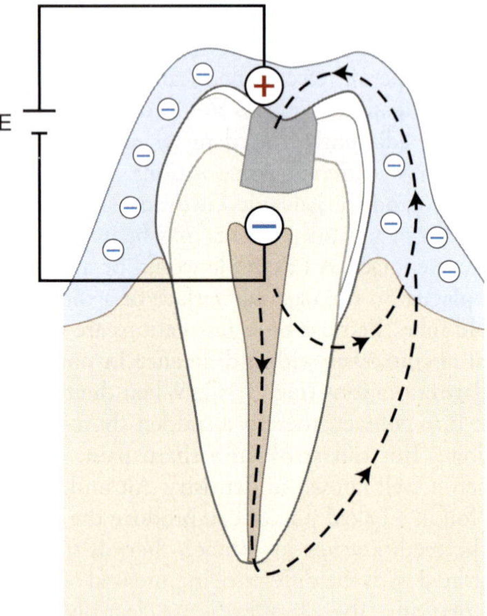

• **Fig. 3.11** Schematic illustration of a single metallic restoration showing two possible current pathways between an external surface exposed to saliva and an interior surface exposed to dentinal fluid. Because the dentinal fluid contains a higher Cl^- concentration than saliva, it is assumed that the electrode potential of the interior surface exposed to dentinal fluid is more active; it is therefore given a negative sign (−). The potential difference between the two surfaces is represented by E. (From *Metals Handbook*, 9th ed, Vol. 13. Metals Park, OH, American Society for Metals, 1978, p 1342.)

approximate value cited. The clinical significance of these currents, other than their influence on corrosion, will be discussed later in this chapter. Coating with a varnish helps to eliminate galvanic shock.

Heterogeneous Surface Composition

Another type of galvanic corrosion is associated with the heterogeneous composition of the surfaces of dental alloys; examples include the eutectic alloys and peritectic alloys (see Chapter 9).

- Commercial dental alloys generally contain more than three elements, and they can have complex microstructures that result in even more heterogeneous surface compositions. For example, when an alloy containing a two-phase eutectic microstructural constituent is immersed in an electrolyte, the lamellae of the phase with the more negative electrode potential are attacked, and corrosion results.
- In an alloy that is a single-phase solid solution, any cored structure is less resistant to corrosion than is the homogenized solid solution because of differences in electrode potential caused by microsegregation and variations in composition between individual microstructural elements (see Chapter 9).
- Even a homogenized solid solution is susceptible to corrosion at the grain boundaries, which are anodic to the cathodic grain interiors, because atomic arrangements at the grain boundaries are less regular and have higher energies (see Chapter 9).
- Solder joints (Chapter 16) between dental alloys also corrode because of differences in compositions of the alloy and solder.
- Impurities in alloys enhance corrosion, and these impurities are typically segregated at the grain boundaries, as described in Chapter 9. Mercury impurities that can inadvertently contaminate gold alloys during handling by dental personnel have electrode potentials different from those of the bulk grains of the gold alloys.
- Nominally pure metals, which do not contain significant quantities of impurities or secondary microstructural phases acting as miniature electrodes with different potentials, corrode at much slower rates than alloys do.

Stress Corrosion

Since the imposition of stress increases the internal energy of an alloy, the tendency to undergo corrosion will be increased. It is plausible that, for most metallic dental appliances, the deleterious effects of stress and corrosion, called **stress corrosion**, are most likely to occur during fatigue or cyclic loading in the oral environment. Small surface irregularities, such as notches or pits, act as sites of stress concentration so that ordinary fatigue failure (in the absence of corrosion) occurs at nominal stresses below the normal elastic limit of the alloy. Thus, any cold working of an alloy by bending, burnishing, or malleting causes localized permanent deformation in some parts of the appliance. Electrochemical cells consisting of the more deformed metal regions (anodic), saliva, and undeformed or less deformed metal regions (cathodic) are created, and the deformed regions will experience corrosion attack. This is one reason why excessive burnishing of the margins of metallic restorations is contraindicated.

Stress-corrosion occurs when a material exists in a relatively inert environment but corrodes due to an applied **stress**. The **stress** may be externally applied or residual.

CRITICAL QUESTION

How can a small pit in the surface of a metallic restoration or a gap between a metal restoration and a tooth become susceptible to and sustain aggressive, localized corrosive attack?

Concentration Cell Corrosion

An important type of electrochemical corrosion is called **concentration cell** corrosion, which occurs whenever there are variations in the electrolytes or in the composition of the given electrolyte within the system. For example, there are often accumulations of food debris in the interproximal areas between the teeth, particularly if oral hygiene is poor. This debris then produces an electrolyte in that area, which is different from the electrolyte that is produced by normal saliva at the occlusal surface. Electrochemical corrosion of the alloy surface underneath the layer of food debris will take place in this situation.

A similar type of attack may occur from differences in the oxygen concentration between parts of the same restoration, with the greatest attack at the areas containing the least oxygen (the anode). Irregularities such as pits, scratches, and cracks in restoration surfaces are important examples of this phenomenon. The region at the bottom of such a defect is oxygen-deprived and becomes the anode because it will typically be covered with food debris and mucin, while the alloy surface around the rim of a scratch or pit becomes the cathode, as diagrammed in Figure 3.12. Consequently, metal atoms at the base of the pit ionize and go into solution, causing the pit to deepen. The rate of such corrosion may be very rapid, since the area of the anodic region is much smaller than that of the cathodic region and there must be a balance of charge transport in both regions. Consequently, failure

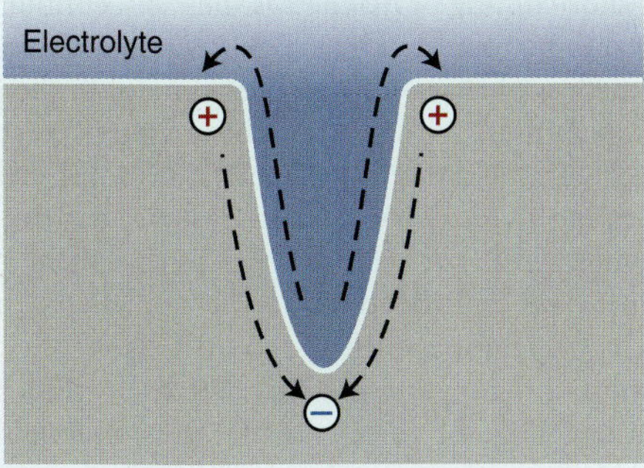

• **Fig. 3.12** A pit on a dental alloy as a corrosion cell. The region at the bottom of the pit is an anode, and the surface around the rim of the pit is the cathode. The ionic current flows through the electrolyte and the electronic current flows through the metal. (With permission from Richman, MH: *An Introduction to the Science of Metals*. Ginn Custom Publishers, 1974.)

may occur much more rapidly than would be expected from a uniform surface attack. Thus, to protect against such **pitting corrosion**, all metallic dental restorative materials should be polished. A closely related category of concentration cell corrosion is "**crevice corrosion**," in which preferential attack occurs at crevices and marginal gaps of crowns, bridges, and cavity restorations because of the presence of food debris and other deposits.

Protection Against Corrosion

Gold coating is employed to enhance the appearance of many commercial nondental products. However, this noble metal is soft, and when its surface becomes scratched or pitted to such a depth that the base metal is exposed, the base metal will be corroded at a very rapid rate because concentration cells have been created and two dissimilar metals are in direct contact. Attempts to use metallic and nonmetallic coatings to provide corrosion protection for dental gold alloys have generally been ineffective because such coatings: (1) were too thin, (2) were incomplete, (3) did not adhere to the underlying metal, (4) were readily scratched, or (5) were attacked by oral fluids.

However, in the case of two dissimilar metals in contact, paint or another nonconductive film can be used to advantage if it is applied to the more noble metal. The corrosion rate of the more active metal will be reduced because the surface area available for the reduction reaction has been decreased, and a scratch in the coating over the noble alloy will not lead to rapid attack of the active metal.

A highly effective protection utilizes certain metals that develop a thin, adherent, highly protective film by reaction with the environment; such a metal is said to be passive. A thin surface oxide forms on chromium, which is a good example of a passivating metal. The most common example is stainless steel, which contains sufficient amounts of chromium added to iron and its alloys to passivate the alloy, as described in Chapter 9. Iron, steel, and certain other metals that are subject to corrosion may also be electroplated with nickel followed by chromium for corrosion protection and esthetic reasons. However, it should be pointed out that tensile stress and certain ions, such as chloride ions, can disrupt the protective oxide film, leading to rapid corrosion. Chromium-passivated metals can be susceptible to stress corrosion and pitting corrosion; therefore, patients should be warned against using household bleaches for cleaning partial denture frameworks or removable orthodontic appliances that are alloyed with chromium. Titanium (Ti) also forms a passivating titanium oxide film, which is of interest, since both commercially pure Ti and alloys in which Ti is a major component are used for a variety of dental applications, such as cast restorations, orthodontic wires, endodontic instruments, and implants (see Chapters 9 and 12). Titanium and its alloys are widely used in dentistry because of their favorable combination of chemical, physical, and biological properties as well as their resistance to corrosion. Their consequent biocompatibility is among their major advantages. Nevertheless, corrosion can occur and the long-term accumulation of corrosion products can lead to fractures of the alloy–implant interface, implant abutment, or implant body. The combination of stress, corrosion, and bacteria contributes to implant failure.

Noble metals resist corrosion because their EMF is positive with regard to any of the common reduction reactions found in the oral environment. In order to corrode a noble metal under such conditions, an external current (overpotential) is required. A guideline that has been employed by the manufacturers of many dental alloys is that at least half the atoms should be noble metals (gold, platinum, and palladium) so as to ensure against corrosion. Palladium has been found to be effective in reducing the susceptibility to sulfide tarnishing for alloys containing silver. If noble metals are used to avoid corrosion, it is important that the more active constituents of the alloy be uniformly dispersed in a random solid solution, since the formation of a second phase that is enriched in an active metal will produce a galvanic corrosion cell.

Clinical Significance of Galvanic Currents

Small galvanic currents associated with electrogalvanism are known to be continually present in the mouth, promoting corrosion, as discussed earlier. As long as metallic restorative materials are employed, it is unlikely that these galvanic currents can be eliminated. Although postoperative pain caused by galvanic shock is not common, it can be a source of discomfort to an occasional patient. However, such postoperative pain usually occurs immediately after insertion of a new restoration and generally subsides and disappears in a few days. It is likely that the physiological condition of the tooth is the primary factor responsible for the pain resulting from this current flow. Once the tooth has recovered from the injury of preparing the cavity and has returned to a more normal physiological condition, the current flow produces no response. Currently, the most practical method for reducing or eliminating galvanic shock is a varnish coating on the surface of the metallic restoration. As long as the varnish remains, the restoration is insulated from saliva and no electrochemical cell is established. By the time the varnish has worn away, the pulp has usually healed sufficiently that no pain persists.

The balance of evidence shows that galvanic currents are deleterious only from the standpoint of patient discomfort, and even then only rarely. Nevertheless, dentists should avoid clinical procedures that exacerbate the condition, such as insertion of an amalgam restoration directly in contact with a gold crown. Mercury released from the corroding amalgam (the anode) may interact with the gold alloy (the cathode) and weaken it. A discoloration of both restorations may also occur, and often a metallic taste develops that can persist indefinitely.

Magnetic Materials

Magnetic materials are ubiquitous, being found in a wide range of everyday items, from magnetic bulletin boards to compasses to electrical generators. In dentistry, they are primarily used for retention of implant-borne prostheses and for orthodontic tooth movement. The force that magnets deliver is biologically safe and can be directed and exerted both within the mouth and through soft and hard tissues.

Magnetism occurs in nature in *magnetite*, a magnetic iron oxide, and in the synthetic alloys aluminum–nickel–cobalt (AlNiCo), platinum–cobalt (PtCo), samarium–cobalt (SmCo), and neodymium–iron–boron (NdFeB). Magnetism develops from circulating electrical currents. In magnetic materials, the circulation is caused by electrons orbiting within the atoms. In most materials, the magnetic effects among the electrons cancel out, but in iron and the alloys just mentioned, a net magnetic field is induced when the atoms are properly aligned. This alignment produces a magnetic field, which emerges from one pole (north pole) and returns to the other (south) pole. A magnetic field induces changes in the surrounding medium in proportion to flux density, the unit of which is Tesla (T), and the flux density is proportional to the size of the magnet. Attraction or repulsion between two magnets is dependent on their pole orientation and is inversely proportional to the square of the distance between them. These properties result in a dramatic reduction in attractive or repulsive force when magnets are not optimally aligned and not in close proximity.

A major shortcoming of magnets is their susceptibility to corrosion and need to be protected by a highly durable coating. Another problem is the loss of magnetic flux over time or in the presence of elevated temperatures. In dentistry, the magnetic materials used generate a constant field that is permanent at mouth temperatures. However, heating to relatively modest temperatures can cause irreversible magnetic loss. For example, this can occur in applications where magnets are embedded in acrylic appliances that, during curing, reach temperatures of 80°C to 90°C from the exothermic setting reaction of the methyl-methacrylate resin (see Chapter 11).

Within their range of current dental uses, magnets and static magnetic fields have been found to be biologically safe if the flux is less than 40 mT, according to the guidelines of the International Commission on Non-Ionizing Radiation Protection and the World Health Organization. According to these organizations, vertigo and nausea are experienced when the head moves rapidly in a field greater than 2 T, as might occur during medical magnetic resonance imaging. These symptoms derive from the disturbance of vestibular function by induced current in the central nervous system. There is little evidence of other effects, including carcinogenesis, although experimental data are still sparse. Magnetic fields developed near the gingiva by magnetic attachments for removable partial dentures have been reported to be well below 40 mT—in the 10- to 15-mT range.

Summary

- **Physical properties** are based on the laws of mechanics, acoustics, optics, thermodynamics, electricity, magnetism, radiation, atomic structure, and nuclear phenomena.
- **Mechanical properties**, a subset of physical properties based on the laws of mechanics.
- **Chemical properties** are based on the ways in which substances interact, combine, and change, as governed by their outer orbital electrons.
- **Rheology** is the study of the deformation and flow characteristics of matter, whether liquid or solid. Viscosity is the resistance of a fluid to flow.
- **Pseudoplastic, dilatant, and plastic behavior**
- The viscosity of many dental materials decreases with increasing strain rate until it reaches a nearly constant value. This is **pseudoplastic** viscosity.
- Liquids that show the opposite behavior are **dilatant** and become more rigid as the rate of deformation (shear strain rate) increases.
- Finally, some classes of materials behave like a rigid body until some minimum value of shear stress is reached.
- **Thixotropic behavior**

The viscosity of most fluids decreases rapidly with increasing temperature. Viscosity may also depend on previous deformation of the liquid. Such fluids become less viscous and more flowable upon repeated applications of pressure and are termed **thixotropic**.

- **Stress relaxation**

After a substance has been permanently deformed (plastic deformation), there are trapped internal stresses. The displaced atoms are not in equilibrium positions and are therefore unstable. Through a solid-state diffusion process driven by thermal energy, the atoms can slowly return to their equilibrium positions. The result is a change in the shape or contour of the solid as the atoms or molecules change positions. The material warps or distorts.

- **Creep and flow**
- **Creep** is defined as the time-dependent plastic strain of a material under a static load or constant stress.
- The related phenomenon of **sag** occurs in the permanent deformation of long-span metal bridge structures at porcelain-firing temperatures under the influence of the mass of the prosthesis.
- **Color and optical effects—nature of light and the role of human vision**
- Light is electromagnetic radiation that can be detected by the human eye. The eye is sensitive to wavelengths from approximately 400 nm (violet) to 700 nm (dark red).
- For an object to be visible, it must reflect or **transmit** light incident on it from an external source.
- **Nature of the object under view**
- Electromagnetic radiation in the visible region interacts with an object through:
  - **reflection** from its surface,
  - **absorption,**
  - **refraction**, or
  - **transmission** (i.e. by passing through unchanged).
- These phenomena determine the **opacity**, **translucency**, or **transparency** of an object. Light reflected from rough surfaces *scatters* in many directions because it is reflected at many angles by the uneven surface.
- A perfectly smooth surface gives a mirror-like finish termed **specular reflectance.**
- Whereas, a flat surface such as chalk gives a dull appearance termed **diffuse reflectance.**
- This influences the appearance of resin composite restorations, which should mimic the reflective pattern of surrounding natural tooth structure.
- **Three dimensions of color**
- **Hue**: The dominant color of an object, for example red, green, or blue. This refers to the dominant wavelengths present in the spectral distribution.
- **Value**: Value is also known as the gray scale. Value identifies the lightness or darkness of a color, which can be measured independently of the hue.

- **Chroma**: Chroma is the degree of saturation of a particular hue. For example, red can vary from scarlet to light pink, where scarlet has a high saturation and pink has a low saturation.
- **Color matching**

In dental practice, color matching is most often performed with the use of a shade guide. Shade guide tabs are used in much the same way as paint chips to match the color of house paint. The individual shade tabs are grouped according to hue:

- A = red-brown
- B = red-yellow
- C = gray
- D = red-gray

Recently, however, the trend is to arrange shade guides in decreasing order of value (lightest to darkest):

B1, A1, B2, D2, A2, C1, C2, D4, A3, D3, B3, A3.5, B4, C3, A4, C4

- **Effect of the light source**
- **Metamerism:** The phenomenon when objects that appear to be color-matched under one type of light may appear different under another type.
- **Fluorescence:** Natural sunlight, photoflash lamps, certain types of vapor lamps, and ultraviolet lights used in decorative lighting ("black lights") are sources containing substantial amounts of near-ultraviolet radiation. The energy that the tooth absorbs is converted into light with longer wavelengths, in which case the tooth actually becomes a light source. This phenomenon is called fluorescence.
- **Thermal properties**
- **Thermal conductivity** (κ) is the physical property that governs heat transfer through a material by conductive flow. The conduction of heat within a solid involves the transfer of thermal energy from one part of a material to another across a temperature gradient.
- **Thermal diffusivity** is a measure of the speed with which a temperature change will spread through an object when one surface is heated. A material with a high density and high specific heat will likely have a low thermal diffusivity.
- **Coefficient of thermal expansion**

It is defined as the change in length per unit of the original length of a material when its temperature is raised 1°C (1 K). A tooth restoration may expand or contract more than the tooth during a change in temperature; thus, there may be marginal microleakage adjacent to the restoration, or the restoration may debond from the tooth.

- **Electrochemical properties: tarnish and corrosion**
- **Tarnish** is a surface discoloration on a metal or a slight loss or alteration of the surface finish or luster. In the oral environment, tarnish often occurs from the formation of deposits on the surface of a restoration. Tarnish also arises from the formation of thin films, such as oxides, sulfides, or chlorides.
- **Corrosion** is an electrochemical process and is dependent on the ability to conduct electrical current, either by means of free electrons in metals or via ions in solution.

Corrosion is a process whereby deterioration of a metal is caused by reaction with its environment. In due course, corrosion can cause severe and catastrophic disintegration of metals.

- **Chemical corrosion** is the direct combination of metallic and nonmetallic elements to yield a chemical compound through oxidation reactions. A good example is the discoloration of silver by sulfur, where silver sulfide forms by chemical corrosion. It can also be a corrosion product of dental gold alloys that contain silver. This mode of corrosion is also referred to as dry corrosion, since it occurs in the absence of water or another fluid electrolyte.
- **Electrochemical mechanism of corrosion**

Electrochemical corrosion/galvanic corrosion. When a metal is in contact with a fluid electrolyte, the chemical potential causes enough ions to dissolve to form a saturated solution and produce an equal number of free electrons. The loss of electrons by a metal is known as oxidation and is the initial electrochemical event in the corrosion process.

- **Dissimilar metals**

An important type of electrochemical reaction occurs when combinations of dissimilar metals are in direct physical contact in a moist environment, which causes a sudden short-circuit through the two alloys. This can result in a sharp pain, called **galvanic shock**, which is well known in dentistry.

- **Heterogeneous surface composition**

Another type of galvanic corrosion is associated with the heterogeneous composition of the surfaces of dental alloys; examples include the eutectic alloys and peritectic alloys.

- **Stress corrosion**

It is plausible that, for most metallic dental appliances, the deleterious effects of stress and corrosion, called **stress corrosion**, are most likely to occur during fatigue or cyclic loading in the oral environment.

- **Concentration cell corrosion**

An important type of electrochemical corrosion is called **concentration cell** corrosion, which occurs whenever there are variations in the electrolytes or in the composition of the given electrolyte within the system.

- **Crevice corrosion** occurs at crevices and marginal gaps of crowns, bridges, and cavity restorations because of the presence of food debris and other deposits.
- **Magnetic materials:** In dentistry, they are primarily used for retention of implant-borne prostheses and for orthodontic tooth movement.

Review Questions

1. Discuss in detail tarnish and corrosion.
2. Discuss in detail optical properties influencing shade selection.
3. Discuss in detail tooth color. Add a note on shade selection.
4. What is the effect of light on tooth color? Add a note on metamerism.
5. Discuss in detail factors influencing corrosion of dental materials.
6. Discuss in detail physical and chemical properties influencing restorative materials.
7. Discuss in brief concentration cell corrosion.
8. Discuss in brief metamerism and fluorescence.
9. Discuss in brief hue, chroma, and value.
10. Discuss in brief shade selection.
11. Discuss in brief corrosion.
12. Discuss in brief thixotropic and pseudoplastic behavior.
13. Discuss in brief electrochemical corrosion.
14. Discuss in brief tarnish and its influence on the restoration.
15. Discuss in brief influence of light on the tooth and restorative material.

16. Discuss in brief coefficient of thermal expansion.
17. Discuss in brief thermal properties affecting restorative materials.
18. Discuss in detail optical and thermal properties of restorative materials.
19. Write a short note on galvanic corrosion.
20. Discuss in brief creep and flow.
21. Discuss in brief rheology of dental materials.
22. Write a short note on pseudoplastic materials.
23. Discuss in brief influence of coefficient of thermal expansion on microleakage restorative materials.
24. Discuss briefly pitting corrosion and stress corrosion.
25. Discuss in brief shade guides used in dentistry.

Selected Readings

Physical Properties

O'Brien WJ: Biomaterials Properties Database, University of Michigan, Ann Arbor, MI: http://www.lib.umich.edu/node/21860; An online database of dental materials properties compiled in a handbook format. Properties include: bond strengths between hard tissues and various dental materials, friction, hardness and other mechanical properties of dental tissues and dental materials, expansion and other thermal properties, optical properties including color range of natural teeth and dental shade guide colors, surface properties, density, and electrical properties.

Haidary A.; Leider J.S.; Silbergleit R. Unsuspected Swallowing of a Partial Denture. Am J Neuroradiol 28 1734–1735 (2007); A recent case report of a swallowed partial denture lodged in the hypopharynx and upper esophagus. The subtle imaging appearance and difficulty of detection and location of the swallowed denture is discussed.

McArthur D.R.; Taylor D.F. A determination of the minimum radiopacification necessary for radiographic detection of an aspired or swallowed object. Oral Surg 39 329–338 (1975).

Color and Optical Effects

American Dental Association: Dental product spotlight: Dental shade guides. J Am Dent Assoc 133 366–367 (2002).

American Dental Association. Esthetic dentistry: A new direction. J Am Dent Assoc (1987). (special issue); This is a series of papers covering the many facets of selecting materials and clinical procedures used in aesthetic dentistry. Depicted are the improved services available through bonding technology, with particular emphasis on the organization of color in the design and fabrication of restorative materials.

Antonson S.A.; Anusavice K.J. Contrast ratio of veneering and core ceramics as a function of thickness. Int J Prosthodont 14 316–320 (2001).

Barna G.J.; Taylor J.W.; King G.E.; et al. The influence of selected light intensities on color perception within the color range of natural teeth. J Prosthet Dent 46 450 (1981); Based on a study of the influence of light intensity on the ability to discriminate color differences within the color range of natural teeth. A significant number of the dentists in the study were found to be color-deficient. In such instances, the dentist should obtain assistance when matching tooth shades.

Calamia J.R.; Wolff M.S.; Simonsen R.J. Dental Clinics of North America: Successful Esthetic and Cosmetic Dentistry for the Modern Dental Practice. Elsevier Saunders Inc.; Presents the clinical steps needed to achieve predictable aesthetic color management.

Chu S.; Devigus A.; Mieleszko A. The Fundamentals of Color: Shade Matching and Communication in Esthetic Dentistry. Quintessence: Carol Steam, IL.

Cleland TM: The Munsell Color System. A Practical Description with Suggestions for Its Use. http://www.applepainter.com; An especially useful explanation of complementary colors is given in Chapter 5; http://www.applepainter.com/Chap05/

Goldstein R.E. Change Your Smile. ed 2 Quintessence: Chicago; Although this book is written for the patient, it is a useful reference for dentists to illustrate the possible aesthetic and reconstructive changes. The color illustrations before and after restorative treatment are evidence of the satisfactory end result when based on an understanding of parameters involved in color phenomena.

Goodacre C.J.; Paravina R.D.; Bergen S.F.; et al. A contemporary guide to color and shade selection for prosthodontists. American College of Prosthodontists (2009).

Haddad H.J.; Jakstat H.A.; Arnetzl G.; et al. Does gender and experience influence shade matching quality? J Dent 37 e40–4 (2009 Jan).

Johnston W.M.; Kao E.C. Assessment of appearance by visual observation and clinical colorimetry. J Dent Res 68 819–822 (1989).

Judd D.B.; Wyszecki G. Color in Business, Science, and Industry. John Wiley & Sons: New York; This book reviews the principles of color vision, color matching, color deficiencies, colorimetry, and the physics of colorant layers.

McLean J.W. The Science and Art of Dental Ceramics. The Nature of Dental Ceramics and Their Clinical Use. Vol. 1 Quintessence: Amador City, CA; Essential reading for those interested in an in-depth discussion of principles of color as related to dental ceramics. Basic fundamentals are clearly interwoven with clinical procedures.

Miller LL A. Scientific approach to shade matching. In: Proceedings of the Fourth International Symposium on Ceramics. Quintessence: Chicago, p. 193.

Paravina Rade D: Dental Color Matcher/an online education and training program for esthetic dentistry. http://scad.vpscustomer.com/Default.aspx; This online CE course presents a novel approach to practical shade matching and advanced aesthetics.

Parker R.M. Shade matching for indirect restorations in the esthetic zone. J Cosmet Dent 23 (4) 98–104 (2008).

Yuan J.C.-C.; Brewer J.D.; Monaco E.A.; et al. Defining a natural tooth color space based on a 3-dimensional shade system. J Prosthet Dent 98 (2) 110–119 (2007); doi:10.1016/S0022-3913(07)60044-4; Not all commercial shade guides cover all the areas of value, hue, and chroma present in human tooth structure. These articles analyze and present examples of this problem.

Electrochemical Properties

Berzins D.W.; Kawashima I.; Graves R.; et al. Electrochemical characteristics of high-Pd alloys in relation to Pd-allergy. Dent Mater 16 266–273 (2000); In vitro electrochemical evaluations of a variety of palladium-containing alloys provide insight into the mechanism of palladium allergy for some patients.

Chaturvedi T.P. An overview of the corrosion aspect of dental implants (titanium and its alloys). Indian J Dent Res 20 91–98 (2009); http://www.ijdr.in/text.asp?2009/20/1/91/49068.

Marek M. Interactions between dental amalgams and the oral environment. Adv Dent Res 6 100–109 (1992); http://adr.sagepub.com/content/6/1/100.full.pdf+html; A review of corrosion in dental amalgam and its physical, chemical, and biological consequences.

Meyer J.-M.; Reclaru L. Electrochemical determination of the corrosion resistance of noble casting alloys. J Mater Sci Mater Med 6 534–540 (1995); The in vitro corrosion resistance is compared for a large number of noble casting alloys.

Mueller H.J. Tarnish and corrosion of dental alloys. In: ASM Handbook. American Society for Metals Int: Metals Park, OH, pp. 1336–1366.

Sturdevant J.R.; Sturdevant C.M.; Taylor D.F.; et al. The 8-year clinical performance of 15 low-gold casting alloys. Dent Mater 3 347–352 (1987); Reports the tarnish and corrosion behavior of numerous gold casting alloys of known compositions over a prolonged period of time.

Upadhyay D.; Panchal M.A.; Dbey R.S.; et al. Corrosion of alloys used in dentistry: A review. Mater Sci Eng A 432 1–11 (2006); doi:10.1016/j.msea.2006.05.003. (1–2).

Walker R.S.; Wade A.G.; Iazzetti G.; et al. Galvanic interaction between gold and amalgam: effect of zinc, time and surface treatments. J Am Dent Assoc 134 (11) 1463–1467 (2003).

4

Mechanical Properties of Dental Materials

CHAPTER OUTLINE

KEY TERMS

Brittle—Relative inability of a material to deform plastically before it fractures.

Deformation—Change in dimension caused by force application. If the deformation recovers when the force is removed, it is called *elastic deformation.* If deformation does not recover completely when the force is removed, the amount of deformation that does not recover is called *permanent* or *plastic deformation.*

Ductility—The amount of plastic deformation a material can sustain under tension before fracture. This property is reported quantitatively as percent elongation.

Elastic limit—Magnitude of elastic stress above which plastic deformation occurs.

Elastic modulus (also modulus of elasticity and Young's modulus)—Resistance to elastic deformation of a material by force that is calculated as the ratio of elastic stress to elastic strain.

Fracture toughness—The critical stress-intensity factor at the point of rapid crack propagation in a solid containing a crack of known shape and size.

Hardness—Resistance of the surface of a material to plastic deformation, which is typically produced by forcing a pointed indenter on the surface.

Malleability—Ability to be hammered or compressed plastically into thin sheets without fracture.

Pressure—Force per unit area acting on the surface of a material. This is different from *stress*, which refers to the distribution of force within the material.

Proportional limit—Magnitude of elastic stress below which stress remains proportional to strain on a stress–strain curve.

Resilience—The amount of elastic energy per unit volume that is sustained on loading and released on unloading of a test specimen.

Strain—Change in dimension per unit initial dimension. In mechanical testing, the change in length is used. There are elastic strain and plastic strain.

Strain hardening (work hardening)—Increase in strength and hardness and decrease in ductility of a metal that result from plastic deformation.

Strength—(1) Stress at the point the material fractures; depending on method of loading, there are tensile, compressive, shear, torsional, flexural, and impact strengths. (2) Maximum stress that a structure can withstand without sustaining a specific amount of plastic strain; this is known as *yield strength* or *proof stress*.

Stress—Force per unit area within a structure subjected to a force; depending on the direction of force relative to the object, there are tensile, compressive, and shear stresses.

Stress concentration—Area or point of significantly higher stress that occurs because of a structural discontinuity such as a crack or pore or a marked change in dimension.

Stress intensity (stress intensity factor)—Relative increase in stress at the tip of a crack of given shape and size when the crack surfaces are displaced in the opening mode (also known as *fracture toughness*).

Toughness—Ability of a material to absorb elastic energy and deform plastically before fracturing; measured as the total area under a plot of tensile stress versus strain.

Tribology—The study and application of the principles of friction, wear, and lubrication.

True stress—Ratio of applied force to the actual (true) cross-sectional area; however, for convenience, stress is often calculated as the ratio of applied force to the initial cross-sectional area.

Yield strength—The stress at which a test specimen exhibits a specific amount of plastic strain.

The purpose of this chapter is to develop a conceptual foundation of the reasons for fracture of restorative materials and a basic framework of design features that will help you increase the fracture resistance of restorative materials in the oral environment. This knowledge will allow you to differentiate the potential causes of clinical failures that may be attributed to material deficiencies, design features, dentist errors, technician errors, or patient factors such as diet, biting force magnitude, and force orientation.

We learned in Chapter 1 that partially edentulous patients may receive removable partial dentures (RPDs) when the construction of a fixed bridge is not the best treatment option. You will learn later that RPDs are retained and supported by abutment teeth, to which they are attached by clasps, which are often made of alloys as the frameworks (Fig. 1.13). Figure 4.1 illustrates the stages of seating a clasp to an abutment tooth. The dotted patches represent the cross sections of the clasp as it is being seated. The greatest convexity or bulge, farthest from the axis of the tooth, is called the *height of contour* of the tooth. The area that is recessed relative to the height of the contour of the tooth or recessed relative to any part of the tooth surface is known as the *undercut.* The clasp that engages an undercut area on the abutment tooth for the purpose of retention is known as a *retentive arm.* The clasp opposite the retentive arm, which engages the surface area occlusal to the height of contour of the tooth, is known as the *reciprocal arm.* Greater than 180° encirclement of the abutment tooth allows for stabilization of the RPD.

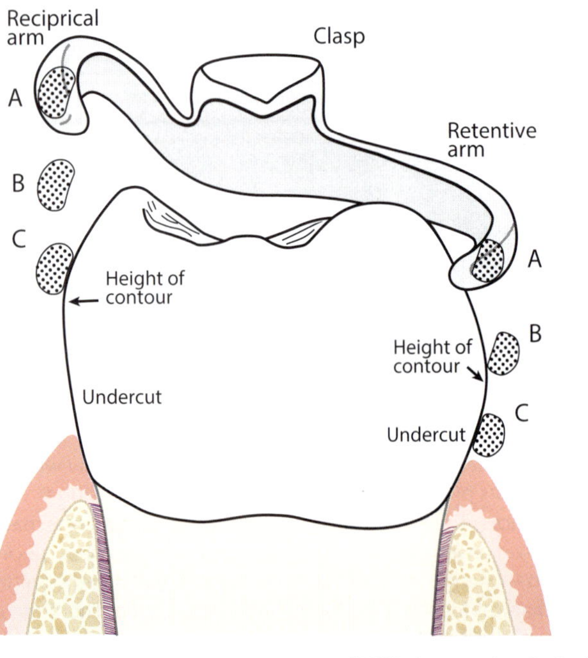

• **Fig. 4.1** Stages of removable partial denture (RPD) clasp seating. Dotted patches represent the cross sections of the clasp arms. The area recessed relative to the height of the contour is known as the undercut. **(A)** Before seating. **(B)** The retentive clasp passing the height of contour. **(C)** Seating completed.

During the insertion of the device, the patient positions the clasps above their respective abutment teeth (position *A* in Fig. 4.1) and forces the device to seat completely, which requires the clasp to traverse. This design means that the retentive clasp arm must flex open to slide past the height of contour of the tooth (position *B* in Fig. 4.1) and then flexes back to engage the undercut area (position *C* in Fig. 4.1). Meanwhile, the reciprocal arm will properly engage the tooth above the height of contour (position *C* in Fig. 4.1).

After wearing the device over some period of time, the patient begins to notice that the RPD is no longer retentive and moves up and down during chewing. The dentist will recognize that most likely, the retentive arm has lost adaptation to the tooth surface because of **deformation** resulting from repeated insertion and removal followed by chewing on the device. For metallic clasps, the dentist will use a pair of pliers to adjust the clasp to the original position by bending. The process can be repeated but there is a limit to the number of times the clasp can be bent. Eventually, the clasp breaks during adjustment.

This sequence of events illustrates how a material responds to applied force through changes of configuration. First, the clasp flexes slightly to slide over the height of contour and returns to the initial dimension to engage the undercut. A material is an elastic solid, or is said to behave elastically, when it exhibits the ability to deform (change in configuration) under an applied force and regain the original shape and size when the force is removed. When the clasps become loose because of permanent deformation after a period of service, they are adjusted to restore their original configuration. *Plasticity* is the ability of solids to change shape permanently when subjected to forces without rupture, whereas the quantity of permanent deformation the clasp can sustain before rupture is known as **ductility**. This sequence can also be demonstrated by flexing an orthodontic wire (elastic deformation), bending the wire further to make a 90° angle (plastic deformation), and bending back and forth several times at the same bend until the wire breaks.

The focus of this chapter is to describe the mechanical characteristics of these materials and discuss the basic principles behind these mechanical properties.

CRITICAL QUESTION

Why is strength not a true property of brittle dental materials?

What are Mechanical Properties?

Elastic solids may be stiff or flexible, hard or soft, brittle or ductile, and fragile or tough. However, these are qualitative mechanical properties that do not describe how similar or dissimilar dental materials of the same type may be. Mechanical properties are defined by the laws of mechanics—that is, the physical science dealing with forces that act on bodies and the resultant motion, deformation, or stresses that those bodies experience. This chapter focuses primarily on static bodies—those at rest—rather than on dynamic bodies, which are in motion. However, fatigue properties, determined from cyclic loading, are also important for brittle materials, as discussed later. Mechanical properties of importance to dentistry include **brittleness**, **compressive strength**, **ductility**, **elastic modulus**, fatigue limit, flexural modulus, **flexural strength**, **fracture toughness**, hardness, impact strength, **malleability**, **percent elongation**, Poisson's ratio, **proportional limit**, shear modulus, **shear strength**, **tensile strength**, torsional strength, **yield strength**, and Young's modulus.

All mechanical properties are measures of the resistance of a material to deformation, crack growth, or fracture under an applied force or pressure and the induced stress. An important factor in the design of a dental prosthesis is strength, a mechanical property of a material, which ensures that the prosthesis serves its intended functions effectively and safely over extended periods of time.

- In a general sense, strength is the ability of the prosthesis to resist induced stress without fracture or permanent deformation **(plastic strain)**.
- Plastic deformation occurs when the elastic **stress** limit (proportional limit) of the prosthetic material is exceeded.

Although **strength** is an important factor, it is not a reliable property for estimating the survival probabilities over time, (for example) of prostheses made of brittle material because strength increases with specimen size and stressing rate, decreases with the number of stress cycles, and is strongly affected by surface processing damage. Thus, strength is not a true property of a material compared with fracture toughness, which more accurately describes the resistance to crack propagation of brittle materials.

Why do dental restorations or prostheses fracture after a few years or many years of service?

The simplest answer is that the mastication force exerted by the patient during the final mastication cycle (loading and unloading) has induced a failure level of stress in the restoration. But why did the fracture not occur during the first month or year of clinical service? One can assume that the stress required to fracture a restoration must decrease somehow over time, possibly because of the very slow propagation of minute flaws to become microcracks through a cyclic fatigue process. The failure potential of prosthesis under applied forces is related to the mechanical properties and the microstructure of the prosthetic material. Mechanical properties are the measured responses, both elastic (reversible upon force reduction) and plastic (irreversible or nonelastic), of materials under an applied force, distribution of forces, or **pressure**. Mechanical properties are expressed most often in units of stress and/or **strain**. They represent measures of (1) elastic or reversible deformation (e.g., proportional limit, **resilience**, and modulus of elasticity); (2) plastic or irreversible deformation (e.g., percent elongation and hardness); or (3) a combination of elastic and plastic-deformation (e.g., toughness and yield strength). To discuss these properties, one must first understand the concepts of stress and strain and the differences between force, pressure, and stress.

CRITICAL QUESTION

How can two different compressive forces applied to the same ceramic crown produce different stresses within the crown surface?

Stresses and Strains

When a force or pressure is exerted on an elastic solid, the atoms or molecules respond in some way at and below the area of loading, but the applied force has an equal and opposite reaction at the area at some other point in the structure (e.g., an area that supports the solid and resists its movement).

The stress induced near the surface decreases with distance from the loading point and increases as the supporting surface is approached. This pattern is called a stress distribution or stress gradient.

The physical process by which atoms or molecules become displaced from their equilibrium positions under the application of an external force or pressure is related to yielding or plastic deformation on a broader scale. Stress is the force per unit area acting on millions of atoms or molecules in a given plane of a material. Except for certain flexural situations, such as four-point flexure, and certain nonuniform object shapes, stress typically decreases as a function of distance from the area of the applied force or applied pressure. Thus, stress distributions in an elastic solid are rarely uniform or constant. However, for purposes of determining mechanical properties, we assume that the stresses are uniformly distributed.

For dental applications, the most important stresses are

- Tensile stress,
- Shear stress, and
- Compressive stress.

The strength of a material is defined as the average level of stress at which it exhibits a certain degree of initial plastic deformation (yield strength) or at which fracture occurs (ultimate strength) in test specimens of the same shape and size.

Strength is dependent on several factors, including:

(1) Stressing rate
(2) Shape of the test specimen
(3) Size of the specimen
(4) Surface finish (which controls the relative size and number of surface flaws)
(5) Number of stressing cycles
(6) Environment in which the material is tested

However, the clinical strength of brittle materials (such as ceramics, amalgams, composites, and cements) is reduced when large flaws are present or if **stress concentration** areas exist because of improper design of a prosthetic component (such as a notch along a section of a clasp arm on a partial denture). Under these conditions a clinical prosthesis may fracture at a much lower applied force because the localized stress exceeds the strength of the material at the critical location of the flaw (stress concentration).

When one chews a hard food particle against a ceramic crown, the atomic structure of the crown is slightly deformed elastically by the force of mastication. If only elastic deformation occurs, the surface of the crown will recover completely when the force is eliminated. Elastic stresses in materials do not cause permanent (irreversible) deformation. On the other hand, stresses greater than the proportional limit cause permanent deformation and, if high enough, may cause fracture. For brittle materials that exhibit only elastic deformation and do not plastically deform, stresses at or slightly above the maximal elastic stress (proportional limit) result in fracture. These mechanical properties of brittle dental materials are important for the dentist to understand in designing a restoration or making adjustments to a prosthesis.

Based on Newton's third law of motion (i.e., for every action there is an equal and opposite reaction), when an external force acts on a solid, a reaction occurs to oppose this force which is equal in magnitude but opposite in direction to the external force. The stress produced within the solid material is equal to the applied force divided by the area over which it acts. A tensile force produces **tensile stress**, a compressive force produces compressive stress, and a shear force produces **shear stress**. A bending force can produce all three types of stresses, but in most cases fracture occurs because of the tensile stress component. In this situation, the tensile and compressive stresses are principal axial stresses, whereas the shear stress represents a combination of tensile and compressive components.

When stress is induced by an external force or pressure, deformation or strain occurs.

In the English or Imperial system of measurement, the stress is expressed in pounds per square inch. However, the megapascal unit is preferred because it is consistent with the SI system of units. SI stands for Systéme Internationale d'Unités (International System of Units). The pound-force (lbf) is not an SI unit of force or weight. It is equal to a mass of 1 pound multiplied by the standard acceleration of gravity on earth (9.80665 m/s^2). The newton (N) is the SI unit of force, named after Sir Isaac Newton. To illustrate the magnitude of 1 MPa, consider a McDonald's quarter-pound hamburger (0.25 lbf or 113 g before cooking) suspended from a 1.19 mm diameter monofilament fishing line. The stress per unit area within the line is 1 N/mm^2, or 1 MPa. If the line is 1.0 m long and if it stretches 0.001 m under the load, the strain (ϵ) is the change in length, Δl, per unit original length, l_o, or

$$\epsilon = \frac{\Delta l}{l_0} = \frac{0.001\ \text{m}}{1.0\ \text{m}} = 0.001 = 0.1\%$$

We can conclude that the line reaches a stress of 1 MPa at a tensile strain of 0.1%. Note that although strain is a dimensionless quantity, units such as meter per meter or centimeter per centimeter are often used to remind one of the system of units employed in the actual measurement. The accepted equivalent in the English system is inch per inch, foot per foot, and so forth.

CRITICAL QUESTION

Why is the maximum **elastic strain** of a cast alloy used for an inlay or crown an important factor in burnishing a margin? Use a sketch of a gap (e.g., Fig. 4.5) between a crown and the tooth margin or a stress–strain diagram (e.g., Fig. 4.4) to explain your answer.

Strain, or the change in length per unit length, is the relative deformation of an object subjected to a stress.

Strain may be either elastic, plastic, elastic and plastic, or viscoelastic. Elastic strain is reversible. The object fully recovers its original shape when the force is removed. Plastic strain represents a permanent deformation of the material; it does not decrease when the force is removed. When a prosthetic component such as a clasp arm on a partial denture is deformed past the elastic limit into the plastic deformation region, elastic plus plastic deformation has occurred, but only the elastic strain is recovered when the force is released. Thus, when an adjustment is made by bending an orthodontic wire, a margin of a metal crown, or a denture clasp, the plastic strain is permanent but the wire, margin, or clasp springs back a certain amount as elastic strain recovery occurs.

Viscoelastic materials deform by exhibiting both viscous and elastic characteristics. These materials exhibit both properties and a time-dependent strain behavior. **Elastic strain** (deformation) typically results from stretching but not rupturing of atomic or molecular bonds in an ordered solid, whereas the viscous component of viscoelastic strain results from the rearrangement of atoms or molecules within amorphous materials.

Stress is described by its magnitude and the type of deformation it produces. Three types of "simple" stresses can be classified: tensile, compressive, and shear. Complex stresses, such as those produced by applied forces that cause flexural or torsional deformation, are discussed in the section on **flexural stress**.

Tensile Stress

A **tensile stress** is always accompanied by tensile strain, but it is very difficult to generate pure tensile stress in a body—**that is, a stress caused by a load that tends to stretch or elongate a body**.

There are few pure tensile stress situations in dentistry. However, a tensile stress can be generated when structures are flexed. The deformation of a bridge and the diametral compression of a cylinder described later represent examples of these complex stress situations. In clinical practice we may encounter, a sticky candy or chikki may dislodge crowns by means of a tensile force when patients try to open their mouths after the candy has mechanically bonded to opposing teeth or crowns. However, tensile, compressive, and shear stresses can also be produced by a bending force, as shown in Figure 4.2 and as discussed in the following sections.

Compressive Stress

When a body is placed under a load that tends to compress or shorten it, the internal resistance to such a load is called a compressive stress. A compressive stress is associated with a compressive strain. To calculate compressive stress, the applied force is divided by the cross-sectional area perpendicular to the axis of the applied force.

CRITICAL QUESTION

Although the shear bond strength of dental adhesive systems is often reported in manufacturers' advertisements, most dental prostheses and restorations are not likely to fail by the development of pure shear stresses. Which two factors tend to prevent the occurrence of pure shear failure?

Shear Stress

This type of stress tends to resist the sliding or twisting of one portion of a body over another. Shear stress can also be produced by a twisting or torsional action on a material. For example, if a force is applied along the surface of tooth enamel by a sharp-edged instrument parallel to the interface between the enamel and an orthodontic bracket, the bracket may debond by shear stress failure of the resin luting agent. Shear stress is

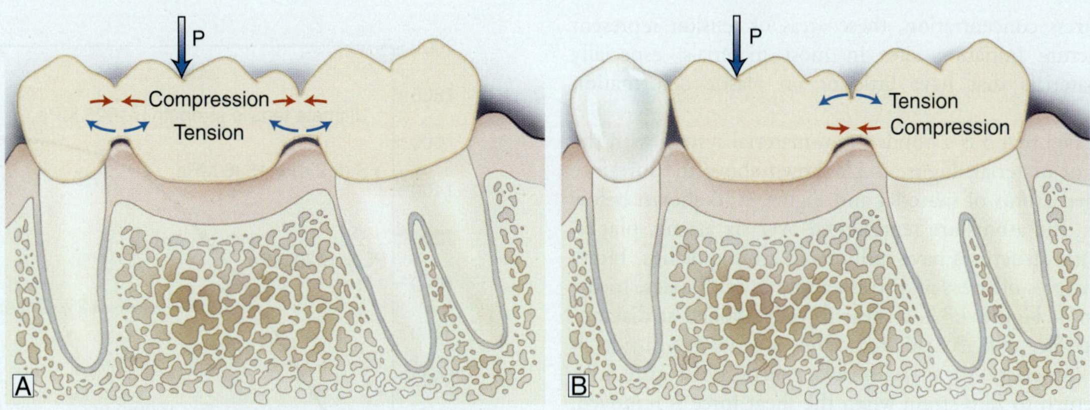

• **Fig. 4.2** **(A)** Stresses induced in a three-unit bridge by a flexural force (P). **(B)** Stresses induced in a two-unit cantilever bridge. Note that the tensile stress develops on the gingival side of the three-unit bridge and on the occlusal side of the cantilever bridge.

calculated by dividing the force by the area parallel to the force direction.

In the mouth, shear failure is unlikely to occur for at least four reasons:

(1) Many of the brittle materials in restored tooth surfaces generally have rough, curved surfaces.
(2) The presence of chamfers, bevels, or changes in curvature of a bonded tooth surface would also make shear failure of a bonded material highly unlikely.
(3) To produce shear failure, the applied force must be located immediately adjacent to the interface, as shown in Figure 4.3B. This is quite difficult to accomplish even under experimental conditions, where polished, flat interfaces are used. The farther away from the interface the load is applied, the more likely it is that tensile failure rather than shear failure will occur because the potential for bending stresses would increase.
(4) Because the tensile strength of brittle materials is usually well below their shear strength values, tensile failure is more likely to occur.

CRITICAL QUESTION

Why do brittle structures that are flexed usually fail on the surface that exhibits increasing convexity?

Flexural (Bending) Stress

Examples of flexural stresses produced in a three-unit fixed dental prosthesis (FDP) and a two-unit cantilever FDP are illustrated in Figure 4.2A and B, respectively. These stresses are produced by bending forces in dental appliances in one of two ways: (1) by subjecting a structure such as an FDP to three-point loading, whereby the endpoints are fixed and a force is applied between these endpoints, as in Figure 4.2A; and (2) by subjecting a cantilevered structure that is supported at only one end to a load along any part of the unsupported section, as in Figure 4.2B. Also, when a patient bites into an object, the anterior teeth receive forces that are at an angle to their long axes, thereby creating flexural stresses within the teeth.

As shown in Figure 4.2A, tensile stress develops on the tissue side of the FDP, and compressive stress develops on the occlusal side. Between these two areas is the neutral axis that represents a state with no tensile stress and no compressive stress. For a cantilevered FDP such as that shown in Figure 4.2B, the maximum tensile stress develops within the occlusal surface area since it is the surface that is becoming more convex (indicating a stretching action). If you can visualize this unit bending downward toward the tissue, the upper surface becomes more convex or stretched (tensile region) and the opposite surface becomes compressed. As explained in the

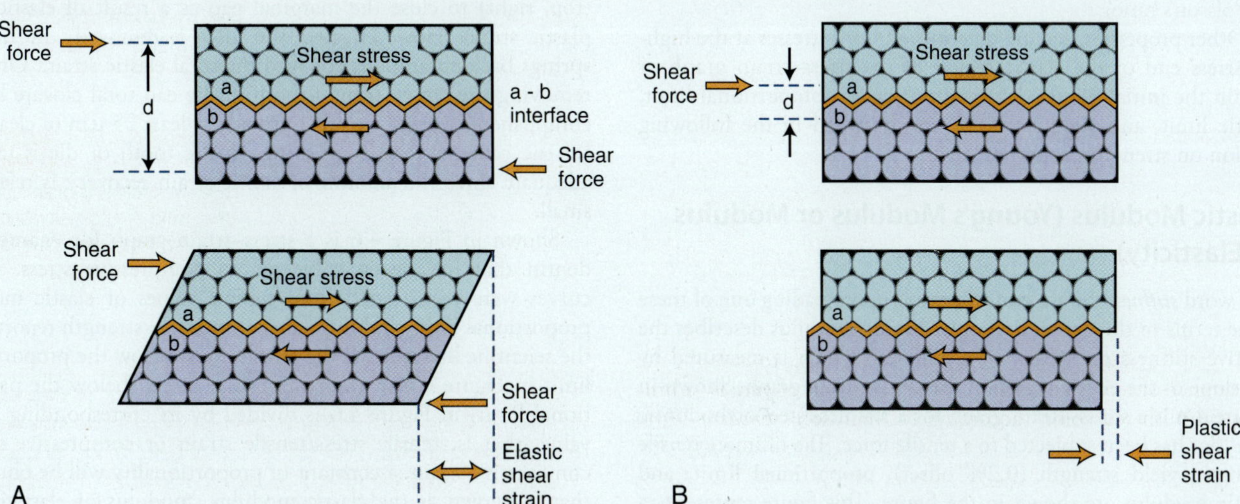

• **Fig. 4.3** Atomic model illustrating elastic shear deformation **(A)** and plastic shear deformation **(B)** for the unit length of a material structure.

section on stress concentration, these areas of tension represent potential fracture initiation sites in most materials, especially in brittle materials that have little or no plastic deformation potential.

Shown in Figure 4.3 is a bonded two-material system with the white atoms of material, Figure 4.3A shown above the interface and the shaded atoms of material and Figure 4.3B shown below the interface. The atoms are represented over six atomic planes, although dental structures have millions of atomic planes. However, the principles of stress and strain apply in both cases. In the upper section of Figure 4.3A, a shear force is applied at distance d/2 from interface a–b. As this force increases in magnitude, it first produces an elastic shear strain (lower section of Figure 4.3), which will return to zero strain when the shear force is removed. As shown in Figure 4.3B, if the shear force on the external surface is increased sufficiently, a permanent or plastic deformation will be produced.

For the case in Figure 4.3B, the force is applied along interface a–b and not at a distance away, as shown in Figure 4.3A. Because of this application of force along the interface, pure shear stress and shear strain develop only within the interfacial region. Because atoms have been displaced at near-neighbor locations, localized plastic deformation has also occurred. In the lower section of Figure 4.3B, the force has been released and a permanent strain of one atomic space has occurred. For Figure 4.3A, the stress induced is not pure shear since the force is applied at a distance from the interface. This is the reason why most shear bond tests do not actually measure shear strength but a tensile component of bending stress. These strength values are reported erroneously as shear strength rather than "apparent shear strength," which indicates that pure shear was unlikely.

Elastic Properties

Mechanical properties and parameters that are measures of the elastic strain or plastic strain behavior of dental materials include:

- **Elastic modulus** (also called **Young's modulus** or modulus of elasticity),
- Dynamic Young's modulus (determined by the measurement of ultrasonic wave velocity),
- Shear modulus,
- Flexibility,
- Resilience, and
- Poisson's ratio.

Other properties that are determined from stresses at the highest stress end of the elastic region of the stress–strain graph or within the initial plastic deformation region (proportional limit, elastic limit, and yield strength) are described in the following section on strength properties.

Elastic Modulus (Young's Modulus or Modulus of Elasticity)

The word *stiffness* should come to mind upon reading one of these three terms in the dental literature. Elastic modulus describes the relative stiffness or rigidity of a material, which is measured by the slope of the elastic region of the stress–strain graph. Shown in Figure 4.4 is a stress–strain graph for a stainless steel orthodontic wire that has been subjected to a tensile force. The ultimate tensile strength, yield strength (0.2% offset), proportional limit, and elastic modulus are shown in the figure. This figure represents a plot of true stress versus strain because the force has been divided by the changing cross-sectional area as the wire was being

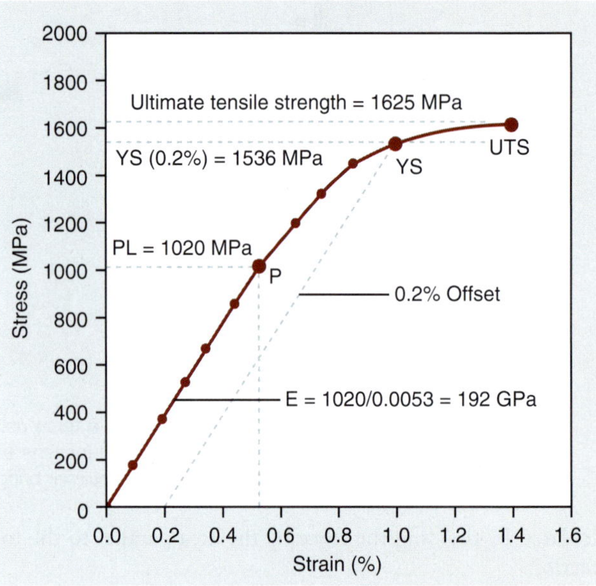

• **Fig. 4.4** Stress–strain plot for a stainless steel orthodontic wire that has been subjected to tension. The proportional limit (*PL*) is 1020 MPa. Although not shown, the elastic limit is approximately equal to this value. The yield strength (*YS*) at a 0.2% strain offset from the origin (*O*) is 1536 MPa and the ultimate tensile strength (*UTS*) is 1625 MPa. An elastic modulus value (*E*) of 192,000 MPa (192 GPa) was calculated from the slope of the elastic region.

stretched. The straight-line region represents reversible elastic deformation, because the stress remains below the proportional limit of 1020 MPa, and the curved region represents irreversible plastic deformation, which is not recovered when the wire fractures at a stress of 1625 MPa. However, the elastic strain (approximately 0.52%) is fully recovered when the force is released or after the wire fractures. We can see this easily by bending a wire in our hands a slight amount and then reducing the force. Assuming that the induced stress has not exceeded the proportional limit, it straightens back to its original shape as the force is decreased to zero.

This principle of elastic recovery is illustrated in Figure 4.5 for a burnishing procedure of an open metal margin (top, left), where a dental abrasive stone is shown rotating against the metal margin (top, right) to close the marginal gap as a result of elastic plus plastic strain. However, after the force is removed, the margin springs back an amount equal to the total elastic strain. Only by removing the crown from a tooth or die can total closure be accomplished. Because we must provide at least 25 μm of clearance for the cement, total burnishing on the tooth or die is usually adequate since the amount of elastic strain recovery is relatively small.

Shown in Figure 4.6 is a stress–strain graph for enamel and dentin that have been subjected to compressive stress. These curves were constructed from typical values of elastic moduli, proportional limit, and ultimate compressive strength reported in the scientific literature. If the tensile stress below the proportional limit in Figure 4.4 or the compressive stress (below the proportional limit) in Figure 4.6 is divided by its corresponding strain value, that is, tensile stress/tensile strain or compressive stress/compressive strain, a constant of proportionality will be obtained that is known as the elastic modulus, modulus of elasticity, or Young's modulus. These terms are designated by the letter E. The units of E are usually expressed as MPa for highly flexible materials

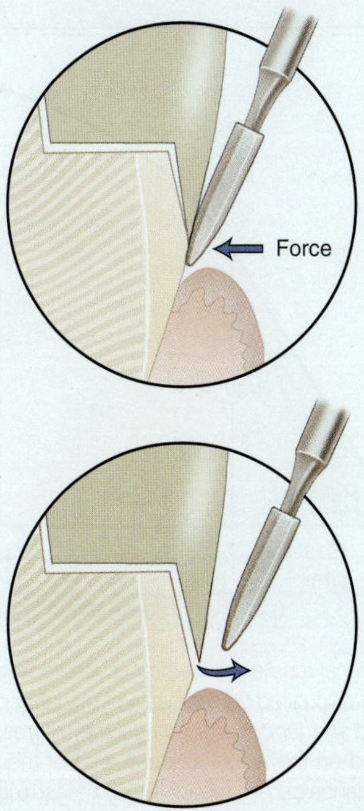

• **Fig. 4.5** Schematic illustration of a procedure to close an open margin of a metal crown by burnishing with a rotary instrument. Note that after the rotating stone is removed (*bottom*), the elastic strain has been recovered and a slight marginal discrepancy remains.

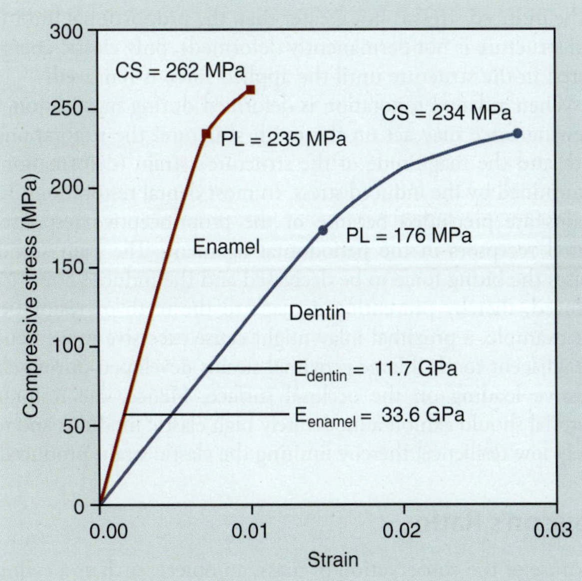

• **Fig. 4.6** Stress–strain plots for enamel and dentin that have been subjected to compression. The ultimate compressive strength (*CS*), proportional limit (*PL*), and elastic modulus (*E*) values are shown. (Data from Stanford JW, Weigel KV, Paffenbarger GD, and Sweeney WT: Compressive properties of hard tooth tissue. *J Am Dent Assoc* 60:746, 1960.)

or GPa for most of the stiffer restorative materials. The slope of the straight-line region (elastic range) of the stress–strain graph is a measure of the relative rigidity or stiffness of a material. Although the stiffness of a dental prosthesis can increase by increasing its thickness, the elastic modulus does not change. The elastic modulus has a constant value that describes a material's relative stiffness as determined from a stress–strain graph, which compensates for differences in cross-sectional area and length by plotting force per unit area by the relative change in dimension, usually length, relative to its initial value.

Variations in values of proportional limit, elastic modulus, and ultimate compressive strength have been reported for enamel and dentin relative to the area of the tooth from which the test specimens were obtained. Note that the proportional limit, ultimate compressive strength, and elastic modulus of enamel are greater than the corresponding values for dentin (Figure 4.6). In fact, the elastic modulus of enamel is about three times greater than that of dentin and, depending on the study considered, it can be as much as seven times higher. Dentin is capable of sustaining significant plastic deformation under compressive loading before it fractures. Thus, enamel is a stiffer and more brittle material than dentin and unsupported enamel is more susceptible to fracture. Conversely dentin is more flexible and tougher.

Because the elastic modulus of a material is a constant, it is unaffected by the amount of elastic or plastic stress induced in the material. It is independent of the ductility of a material, since it is measured in the linear region of the stress–strain plot. Thus, elastic modulus is not a measure of its plasticity or strength. Materials with a high elastic modulus can have either high or low strength values. Although a compressive test was selected to measure the properties of tooth structures in Figure 4.6, the elastic modulus can also be measured by means of a tensile test.

Because the elastic modulus represents the ratio of the elastic stress to the elastic strain, it follows that the lower the strain for a given stress, the greater the value of the modulus. For example, if one wire is much more difficult to bend than another of the same shape and size, considerably higher stress must be induced before a desired strain or deformation can be produced in the stiffer wire. Such a material would possess a comparatively high modulus of elasticity. A polyether impression material has a greater stiffness (elastic modulus) than all other elastomeric impression materials. Thus, a greater force is needed to remove an impression tray from undercut areas in the mouth. The modulus of elasticity of most dental biomaterials is given in units of giganewtons per square meter (GN/m^2), also referred to as gigapascals (GPa). This property is indirectly related to other mechanical properties. For example, two materials may have the same proportional limit but their elastic moduli may differ considerably.

The elastic modulus (E) of a tensile test specimen can be calculated as follows:

(3)

$$\text{Stress} = P/A = \sigma$$

(4)

$$\text{Stain} = \Delta l/l_0 = \epsilon$$

where P = the applied force or load
A = the cross-sectional area of the material under stress
Δl = the increase in length
l_0 = the original length.
Thus,

(5)

$$\Delta E = \frac{\text{Stress}}{\text{Strain}} = \frac{\sigma}{\epsilon} = \frac{P/A}{\Delta l/l_0}$$

Dynamic Young's Modulus

Elastic modulus can be measured by a dynamic method as well as the static techniques described in the previous section. Since the velocity at which sound travels through a solid can be readily measured by ultrasonic longitudinal and transverse wave transducers and appropriate receivers, the velocity of the sound wave and the density of the material can be used to calculate the elastic modulus and Poisson's ratio. This method of determining dynamic elastic moduli is less complicated than conventional tests of tensile or compressive strength, but the values are often found to be higher than those obtained by static measurements. For most purposes, however, these values are acceptable.

If a shear stress was induced instead of uniaxial tensile or compressive stress, the resulting shear strain could be used to define a shear modulus for the material. The shear modulus (G) can be calculated from the elastic modulus (E) and Poisson's ratio (ν) using Eq. (6):

(6)

$$G = \frac{E}{2\,(1+\upsilon)} = \frac{E}{2(1+.03)} = 0.38E$$

A value of 0.25–0.30 for Poisson's ratio is typical. Thus, the shear modulus is usually about 38% of the elastic modulus value.

Flexibility

For materials used to fabricate dental appliances and restorations, a high value for the elastic limit (the stress above which a material will not recover to its original state when the force is released) is a necessary requirement because the structure is expected to return to its original shape after it has been stressed and the force is removed (elastic recovery). Usually a moderately high modulus of elasticity is also desirable because only a small deformation will develop under a considerable stress, as in the case of an inlay or an impression material.

However, there are instances where a larger strain or deformation may be needed with a moderate or slight stress. For example, in an orthodontic appliance, a spring is often bent a considerable distance under the influence of a small stress. In such a case, the structure is said to be flexible and to possess the property of flexibility. *The maximum flexibility is defined as the flexural strain that occurs when the material is stressed to its proportional limit.*

Resilience

As interatomic spacing increases, internal energy increases. As long as the stress is not greater than the proportional limit, this energy is known as **resilience**. Popularly, the term *resilience* is associated with springiness, but it means precisely the amount of energy absorbed within a unit volume of a structure when it is stressed to its proportional limit. The resilience of two or more materials can be compared by observing the areas under the elastic region of their stress–strain plots assuming that they are plotted on the same scale. The material with the larger elastic area has the higher resilience.

Shown in Figure 4.7 is a stress–strain diagram illustrating the concepts of resilience and **toughness**. The area bounded by the elastic region is a measure of resilience and the total area under the stress–strain curve is a measure of toughness. This figure is explained further in the following section. Work is the product of the force times the distance through which the force acts. When work is performed on a body, energy is imparted to it. Consequently, when a dental restoration is deformed, it absorbs energy. If the induced stress is not greater than the proportional limit (the oral structure is not permanently deformed), only elastic energy is stored in the structure until the applied force is removed.

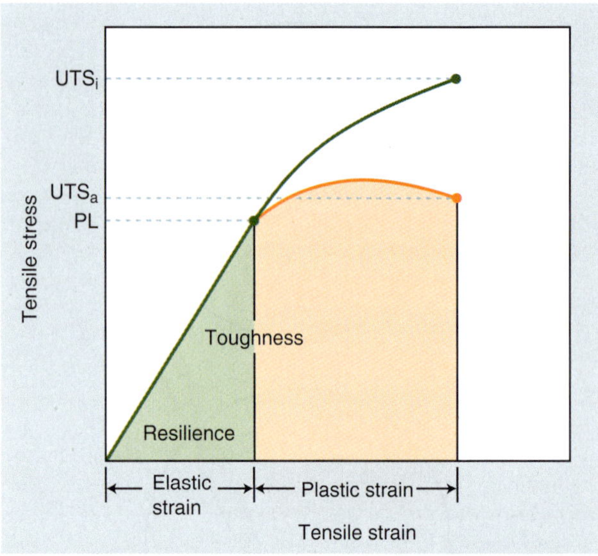

• **Fig. 4.7** Conventional tensile stress–strain curve (*orange line*) in the plastic deformation region calculated on the basis of the initial cross-sectional area of a rod. The solid line (*above the orange line*) represents the calculated stress values based on the actual reduced area of the rod as deformation increases. The resilience can be calculated by measuring the area within the elastic region. The toughness is related to the total area within the elastic and plastic regions. In this case, the proportional limit (PL) remains constant, but the toughness and ultimate strength (UTSi) are different.

When a dental restoration is deformed during mastication, the chewing force may act on the tooth structure, the restoration, or both and the magnitude of the structure's strain (deformation) is determined by the induced stress. In most dental restorations, large strains are precluded because of the proprioceptive response of neural receptors in the periodontal ligament. The pain stimulus causes the biting force to be decreased and the induced stress to be reduced, thereby preventing damage to the teeth or restorations. For example, a proximal inlay might cause excessive movement of the adjacent tooth if large proximal strains developed during compressive loading on the occlusal surface. Hence, the restorative material should exhibit a moderately high elastic modulus and relatively low resilience, thereby limiting the elastic strain produced.

Poisson's Ratio

Because of the conservation of mass, an object, such as a cylinder, becomes longer and thinner when a tensile force is applied to it. Conversely, a compressive force acts to make such an object shorter and thicker. An axial tensile stress, σ_z, along the z (long axis) of a mutually perpendicular xyz coordinate system produces an elastic tensile strain and an accompanying elastic contraction in the x and y directions (ϵ_x and ϵ_y, respectively). The ratio of ϵ_x/ϵ_z or ϵ_y/ϵ_z is an engineering property of the material called the Poisson's ratio (ν).

(7)

$$\upsilon = -\frac{\epsilon_x}{\epsilon_z} = -\frac{\epsilon_y}{\epsilon_z}$$

Poisson's ratio can be similarly determined in an experiment involving an axial compressive stress. Poisson's ratio is related to the nature and symmetry of the interatomic bonding forces described in Chapter 2. For an ideal isotropic material of constant volume, the ratio is 0.5. Most engineering materials have values between 0.25 and 0.30.

CRITICAL QUESTION

How can two identical forces produce two different stresses in an all-ceramic crown? Is it possible for a stiff material with a high modulus of elasticity to fail with no plastic deformation and at a lower strength than a more flexible material?

Strength Properties

How much strength do we need in materials for dental restorations to resist fracture for the lifetimes of our patients? An engineer would answer this question with another question. How large can the restorations be and still provide adequate aesthetics and masticatory function? Obviously for restorations to last forever without fracture, we would have to build excessively large structures for some materials, such as pure glass or unfilled acrylic resin. For other materials with great ductility and/or high fracture toughness and high flexural strength, the prostheses or restorations could be designed with approximately the same dimensions and anatomic form as existed for the original teeth. For the latter materials, we could assume the strength properties to be adequate if we followed some well-established engineering principles. **Strength** is equal to the degree of stress necessary to cause either fracture (ultimate strength) or a specified amount of plastic deformation (yield strength).

When we describe the strength of an object or a material, we are most often referring to the maximum stress that is required to cause fracture. Keep in mind, however, that strength values reported by manufacturers usually represent mean values, which means that 50% of the tested specimens have failed below this strength. Both types of deformational behavior can be described by strength properties, but we should use proper strength terms to differentiate between the stress causing permanent deformation and that required to produce fracture.

For specific dental materials, particularly metals, we are equally interested in the maximum stress that a structure can sustain before it becomes permanently or plastically deformed. This stress can be described either by the proportional limit or elastic limit. At stresses above these limits, plastic deformation occurs. The strength of a material can be described by one or more of the following properties:

(1) proportional limit, the stress above which stress is no longer proportional to strain;
(2) elastic limit, the maximum stress a material can withstand before it becomes plastically deformed;
(3) yield strength or proof stress, the stress required to produce a given amount of plastic strain; and
(4) ultimate tensile strength, shear strength, compressive strength, and flexural strength, each of which is a measure of stress required to fracture a material.

When a force is applied to a ceramic crown, the magnitude of stress that develops within the surface of the crown will depend on how the force was applied and on the orientation of the force. If the force is well distributed over an area, the stress that is induced in the crown will be reduced compared with a much more concentrated force of the same magnitude. Strength is not a measure of individual atom-to-atom attraction or repulsion but rather of the interatomic forces collectively over the entire wire, cylinder, implant, crown, pin, or whatever structure is stressed. Furthermore, the ultimate strength may not necessarily be equal to the actual instantaneous average stress at fracture, since the original cross-sectional area has changed in size.

CRITICAL QUESTION

How can the ultimate tensile stress (ultimate strength) sometimes be less than the maximum tensile stress?

Shown in Figure 4.7 is a stress–strain plot of a metal rod that has been subjected to a tensile test. The stress is calculated by dividing the applied force at any instant by the original cross-sectional area and is represented by the bold dashed line above the lightly shaded area. However, the diameter actually decreases as the metal is stretched.

The **true stress** is calculated as the force divided by the actual cross-sectional area at each measured strain value and is represented in Figure 4.7 by the bold line in the plastic deformation region above the dashed curve. It is evident that the cross-section of the wire decreases as it lengthens under tensile stress. Because of the reduction in area, the force required to increase deformation actually decreases. Thus, the stress calculated for testing purposes (force per unit initial area) decreases, and the ultimate tensile strength based on the initial area (lower UT'S value) as indicated in Figure 4.7 is less than the maximum tensile stress that occurs at the peak of the curve.

Although the true stress–strain curve represents the situation more accurately, the stress–strain curve as indicated by the dashed line in Figure 4.7 is commonly used. When we calculate the tensile strength of a certain wire, we wish to know the maximum stress it supports in tension without regard to the small changes that may occur in the cross-sectional area. Therefore, the ultimate tensile strength is defined as the **tensile stress** within a structure at the point of rupture.

Proportional Limit

When a wire is stretched steadily in tension, the wire eventually fractures. However, in dentistry we are interested also in the stress at which plastic deformation begins to develop. One method by which to determine this point is to plot a stress–strain diagram similar to that in Figures 4.4, 4.6, or 4.7. If the material obeys Hooke's law, the elastic stress will be proportional to elastic strain. For such a material, the stress–strain diagram shown in Figure 4.4 starts from the origin (O) as a straight line. Along this line the material behaves elastically, and it springs back to its initial shape and size at the instant the force is removed. When a certain stress value corresponding to point P is exceeded, the line becomes nonlinear and stress is no longer proportional to strain. When a straight edge is laid along the straight-line portion of the curve from O to P, the stress value at P, the point above which the curve deviates from a straight line, is known as the proportional limit.

For a material to satisfy Hooke's law, the elastic stress must be directly proportional to the elastic strain. The initial region of the stress–strain plot must be a straight line. Because direct proportionality between two quantities is graphically represented by a straight line, the linear portion of the graph in Figures 4.4, 4.6, and 4.7 satisfies this law. Because the proportional limit (stress corresponding to point P) is the greatest elastic stress possible in accordance with this law, it represents the maximum stress above which stress is no longer proportional to strain. For the stress–strain curve of dentin that is shown in Figure 4.6, the strain corresponding to the proportional limit is important because it represents the percent deformation that can be sustained in dentin before it becomes deformed permanently.

Elastic Limit

When a small tensile stress is induced in a wire, the wire will return to its original length when the load is removed. If the load is increased progressively in small increments and then released after each increase in stress, a stress value will be reached at which the wire does not return to its original length after it is unloaded. At this point the wire has been stressed beyond its elastic limit. The elastic limit of a material is defined as the greatest stress to which the material can be subjected such that it returns to its original dimensions when the force is released. Although tensile stress was used in the example, similar elastic limit measurements can be made for any type of stress, although different values of elastic limit are obtained in tension, compression, and shear.

CRITICAL QUESTION

Yield strength is a commonly reported property for metals and alloys but not for ceramics. Why is it not possible to measure the yield strength of ceramics or other purely brittle materials? Use a stress–strain plot to explain your answer.

Yield Strength (Proof Stress)

Yield strength often is a property that represents the stress value at which a small amount (0.1% or 0.2%) of plastic strain has occurred. A value of either 0.1% or 0.2% of the plastic strain is often selected and is referred to as the percent offset. The yield strength is the stress required to produce the particular offset strain (0.1% or 0.2%) that has been chosen. As in Figure 4.4, the yield strength for 0.2% offset is greater than that associated with an offset of 0.1%. If yield strength values for two materials tested under the same conditions are to be compared, identical offset values should be used. To determine the yield strength for a material at 0.2% offset, a line is drawn parallel to the straight-line region (Fig. 4.4), starting at a value of 0.002, or 0.2% of the plastic strain, along the strain axis and is extended until it intersects the stress–strain curve. The stress corresponding to this point is the yield strength. Although the term *strength* implies that the material has fractured, it is actually intact but has sustained a specific amount of plastic strain (deformation). For brittle materials such as dental ceramics, the stress–strain plot is a straight line with no plastic region. Thus, a determination of yield strength is not practical at either a 0.1% or 0.2% strain offset because there is no plastic strain. The material has actually fractured at a lower strain value.

Elastic limit, proportional limit, and yield strength are defined differently, but their values (of stress) are fairly close to each other in many cases. Elastic and proportional limits are usually assumed to be identical, although their experimental values may differ slightly. As shown in Figure 4.4, the yield strength (proof stress) is greater than the proportional limit. These values are important in the evaluation of dental materials because they represent the stress at which permanent deformation of the structure begins. If they are exceeded by mastication stresses, the restoration or appliance may no longer function as originally designed.

Permanent (Plastic) Deformation

As shown in Figure 4.4, the stress–strain graph is no longer a straight line above the proportional limit (PL); instead, it curves until the structure fractures. The stress–strain graph shown in Figure 4.4 is more typical of actual stress–strain curves for ductile materials. Unlike the linear portion of the graph at stresses below the proportional limit, it is not possible to extrapolate the shape of the curve above P because stress is no longer proportional to strain.

If the material is deformed by stress at a point above the proportional limit before fracture, removal of the applied force will reduce the stress to zero, but the plastic strain (deformation) remains. Thus the object does not return to its original dimension when the force is removed. It remains bent, stretched, compressed, or otherwise plastically deformed.

Cold Working (Strain Hardening or Work Hardening)

When most metal alloys have been stressed beyond their proportional limits, their hardness and strength increase at the area of deformation, but their ductility decreases. As dislocations move and pile up along grain boundaries, further plastic deformation in these areas becomes more difficult. As a result, repeated plastic deformation of the metal, as occurs during the bending of orthodontic wire or adjustment of a clasp arm on a removable dental prosthesis, can lead to embrittlement of the deformed area of the wire, and it may fracture when further permanent adjustment is attempted. Since the elastic modulus remains constant, the stress–strain curve of the deformed area would extend above the level of ultimate strength of the metal, but the plastic deformation part of the curve would be decreased progressively with each bend of a wire or clasp arm. The key to minimizing the risk of reduced plasticity (embrittlement) is to deform the metal in small increments so as not to plastically deform the metal excessively.

Diametral Tensile Strength

Tensile strength can generally be determined by subjecting a rod, wire, or dumbbell-shaped specimen to tensile loading (a uniaxial tension test). Since this test is quite difficult to perform for brittle materials because of alignment and gripping problems, another test can be used to determine this property for brittle dental materials. It is referred to as the diametral compression test, which is represented schematically in Figure 4.8. This test should be used only for materials that exhibit elastic deformation primarily and little or no plastic deformation. In this method, the compressive load is placed by a flat plate against the side of a short cylindrical specimen (disk), as illustrated in Figure 4.8. The vertical compressive force along the side of the disk produces a tensile stress that is perpendicular to the vertical plane passing through the center of the disk. Fracture occurs along this vertical plane (the dashed vertical line on the disk). In such a situation, the tensile stress is directly proportional to the compressive load applied. It is calculated by the following formula:

$$\text{Tensile Stress} = \frac{2F}{\pi D t} \tag{8}$$

where F = applied force
D = diameter
t = thickness

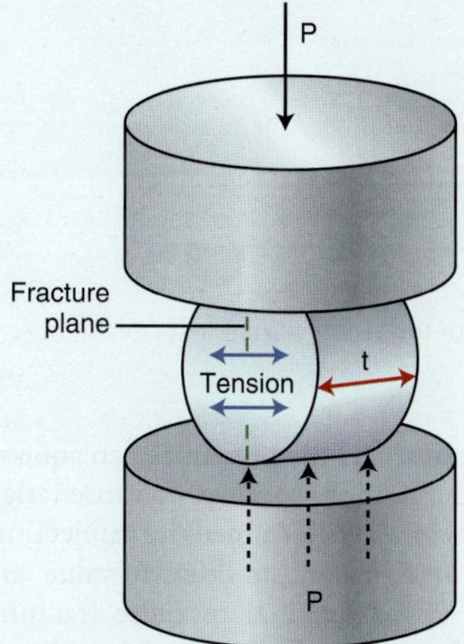

• **Fig. 4.8** Diametral compression test. Although a compressive force is applied along the side of the disk, a tensile fracture is produced. The tensile strength is calculated from the fracture load P, the disk diameter D, and the thickness t.

This test is simple to conduct and provides excellent reproducibility of results. However, use of this test on materials that exhibit appreciable plastic deformation before fracture results in erroneously high tensile strength values. Fracture of the specimen into several pieces rather than the ideal fragmentation into two segments suggests an unreliable test result.

Flexural Strength

Flexural strength, which is also called transverse strength and **modulus of rupture**, is essentially a strength test of a bar supported at each end or a thin disk supported along a lower support circle under a static load. For the disk specimen, the failure stress value is referred to as the biaxial flexural strength; the theory involved is beyond the scope of this textbook. For a bar with a rectangular cross-section subjected to three-point flexure (upper central loading in Fig. 4.9), the following equation may be used to calculate the flexural strength (maximum flexural stress at the lower midpoint surface):

(9)

$$\sigma = \frac{3PL}{2wt^2}$$

where σ = maximum flexural stress (MPa)
P = load at fracture (N)
L = distance between two supports (mm)
w = width of specimen (mm)
t = thickness or height of specimen (mm)

Typical specimen dimensions are a minimum span length of 20 mm, a width of 4 mm, and a thickness of 1.2–2.0 mm.

One of the limitations of the three-point flexural test is that if the bar specimen does not fracture at the midpoint directly under the applied force (F), a correction must be made to calculate the fracture stress at the actual point of fracture. If the fracture occurs in the middle of the lower span, Eq. (9) may be used.

The four-point flexural test shown in Figure 4.10 is preferred over the three-point test because the stress within the central loading span is constant. Therefore, no correction is required for specimens that fracture within the central loading span but that do not fracture precisely at the midpoint. The flexural stress within the midspan area can be calculated from Eq. (10) as follows:

(10)

$$\sigma = \frac{3PL}{4wt^2}$$

where σ = flexural strength
P = total applied load
L = distance between lower supports
w = width of specimen
t = thickness or height of specimen

The units of stress are force per unit area, most often given in the SI unit of megapascal (MPa). This test is, in a sense, a

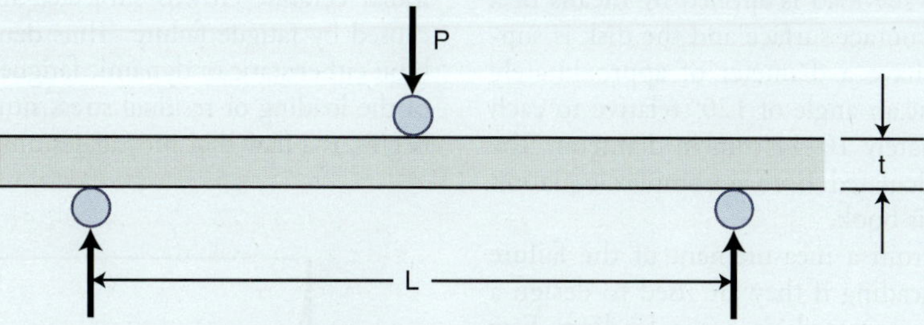

• **Fig. 4.9** Three-point flexure test design.

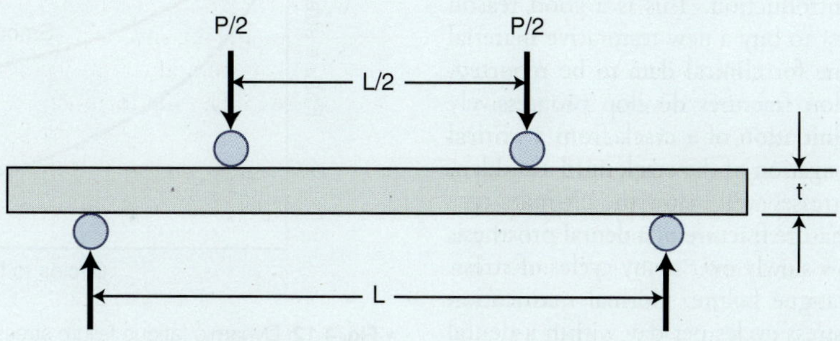

• **Fig. 4.10** Four-point flexure test design.

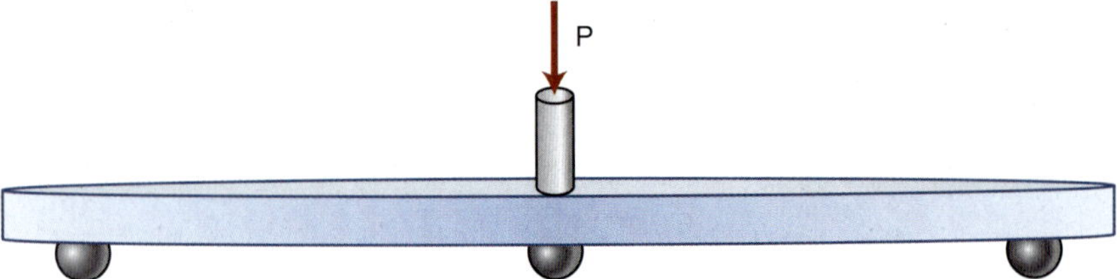

• **Fig. 4.11** Schematic illustration of the piston-on-three-ball test for the biaxial flexure test.

collective measurement of tensile, compressive, and shear stresses simultaneously. However, for sufficiently thin specimens, it is usually dominated by the tensile stress that develops along the lower surface. When the load is applied, the specimen bends. For a flat bar specimen, the resulting strain is represented by a decrease in the length of the top surface (compressive strain) of the specimen and an increase in the length of the lower surface (tensile strain). Consequently, the principal stresses on the upper surface are compressive whereas those on the lower surface are tensile. Obviously, the stresses change direction within the specimen between the top and bottom surfaces, with both stress and strain being zero at the region of change. This neutral surface does not change in dimension and is known as the neutral axis. Shear stress is also produced near the supported ends of the specimen, but it does not play a significant role in the fracture process. For brittle materials such as ceramics, flexural tests are preferred to the diametral compressive test because they more closely simulate the stress distributions in dental prostheses such as cantilevered bridges and multiple-unit fixed dental prostheses (FDPs or bridges) as well as the clasp arms of removable dental prostheses (RDPs).

Biaxial Flexural Test

This test is preferred by some scientists to avoid the problem of edge fractures, which can occur in flexural tests of bar specimens. For the typical biaxial flexural tests, disk-shaped specimens 12 mm in diameter and 1.2 mm in thickness are used. The biaxial flexure test based on the piston-on-three-ball design is shown schematically in Figure 4.11. The load is applied by means of a piston with a slightly curved contact surface and the disk is supported by steel balls, which have a diameter of approximately 3.2 mm. These are arranged at an angle of 120° relative to each other on a circle of approximately 10–12 mm in diameter. The biaxial flexural strength is calculated from a complex equation that is beyond the scope of this book.

Strength values obtained from a measurement of the failure load described earlier are misleading if they are used to design a structure that is subjected to repeated or cyclic loading. Few clinical fractures occur during a single-load application. If such fractures were common, these products would be withdrawn from the market soon after their introduction. This is a good reason why one should not be the first to buy a new restorative material but rather allow sufficient time for clinical data to be reported. Most prosthesis and restoration fractures develop progressively over many stress cycles after initiation of a crack from a critical flaw and subsequently by propagation of the crack until a sudden, unexpected fracture occurs. Stresses well below the ultimate tensile strength can produce premature fracture of a dental prosthesis because microscopic flaws grow slowly over many cycles of stress. This phenomenon is called fatigue failure. Normal mastication induces several thousands of stress cycles per day within a dental restoration. For glasses and certain glass-containing ceramics, the induced tensile stress and the presence of an aqueous environment further reduce the number of cycles to cause fatigue failure.

Fatigue behavior is determined by subjecting a material to a cyclic stress of a maximum known value and determining the number of cycles required to cause fracture. As shown in Figure 4.12, a plot of the failure stress versus the number of cycles to failure enables calculation of a maximum service stress or an endurance limit—the maximum stress that can be maintained without failure over an infinite number of cycles. For brittle materials with rough surfaces, the endurance limit is lower than it would be if the surfaces were more highly polished (Fig. 4.12). For a given applied stress, the rougher material would fail in fewer cycles of stress.

Some materials or prosthetic appliances exhibit static fatigue, a phenomenon attributed to the interaction of a constant tensile stress with structural flaws over time. The influence of flaw size on the stress to cause failure is shown in Figure 4.13. Note that for a given flaw size, less stress is required to produce failure if the stress is cycled between high and low values. Furthermore, aqueous solutions are known to corrosively degrade dental ceramics by converting surface flaws to one or more cracks over time in the presence of tensile stress. This environmental factor further reduces the magnitude of tensile stress that can be sustained by ceramics over time.

Ceramic orthodontic brackets and activated wires within the brackets represent a clinical system that can exhibit static fatigue failure in which a sustained stress in the presence of water causes cracks to develop and progress over time. The delayed fracture of molar ceramic crowns subjected to periodic cyclic forces may be caused by fatigue failure. Thus dental restorative materials can exhibit either static or dynamic fatigue failure depending on the nature of the loading or residual stress situation. In either case, the failure begins as a flaw that propagates until catastrophic fracture occurs.

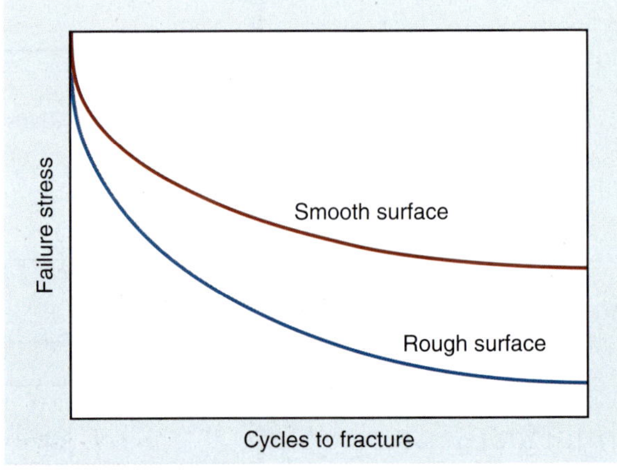

• **Fig. 4.12** Dynamic fatigue failure stress for a brittle material as a function of surface roughness and number of stress cycles.

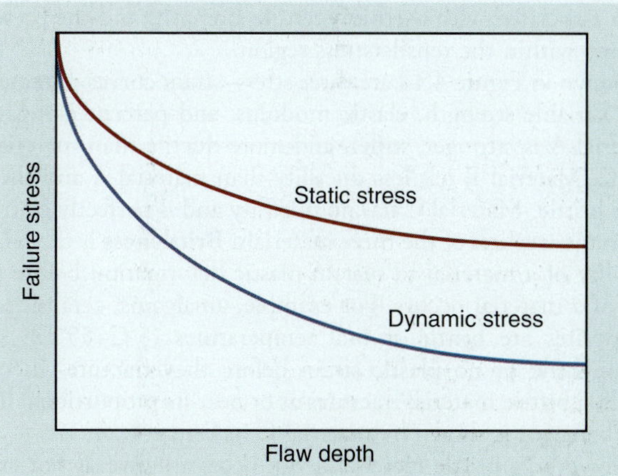

• **Fig. 4.13** Dynamic and static fatigue failure stress for a brittle material as a function of flaw depth.

Impact Strength

This property may be defined as the energy required to fracture a material under an impact force. The term *impact* is used to describe the reaction of a stationary object to a collision with a moving object. A Charpy-type impact tester is usually used to measure impact strength. A pendulum is released that swings down to fracture the center of a bar specimen supported at both ends. The energy lost by the pendulum during the fracture of the specimen can be determined by a comparison of the length of its swing after the impact with that of its free swing when no impact occurs. The energy units are joules, foot-pounds, inch-pounds, and so forth. Unlike the case in most mechanical tests, the dimensions, shape, and design of the specimen to be tested should be identical for uniform results.

With appropriate values for the velocities and masses involved, a blow by a fist or other object to the lower jaw can be considered an impact situation. In the impact process, the external forces and resulting stresses change rapidly, and a static property such as the proportional limit is not useful in predicting the resulting deformations. However, a moving object possesses a known amount of kinetic energy. If the struck object is not permanently deformed, it stores the energy of the collision in an elastic manner. This ability is reflected by the resilience of a material, which is measured by the area under the elastic region of the stress–strain diagram. Thus a material with a low elastic modulus and a high tensile strength is more resistant to impact forces. A low elastic modulus and a low tensile strength suggest low-impact resistance. For dental materials of low-impact resistance, the elastic moduli and tensile strengths, respectively, are as follows:

- Resin-based composite: 17 GPa and 30−90 MPa
- Dental porcelain: 40 GPa and 50−100 MPa
- Poly (methylmethacrylate): 3.5 GPa and 60 MPa
- Amalgam: 21 GPa and 27−55 MPa
- Alumina ceramic: 350−418 GPa and 120 MPa

Thus, if one simply calculates the area under the stress versus strain graph, the greatest resilience is associated with the composite, followed in decreasing order by the porcelain, PMMA, amalgam, and alumina.

Weibull Statistics

When a manufacturer reports the strength of a restorative material, one might assume that a restoration made with that material would have the reported strength. Unfortunately, such a restoration could have a strength lying in the lowest 5% of test values. In some cases, such extreme values are called outliers. The reported strength typically represents the mean value of a range of strengths determined from a specific test such as a tensile test, a compression test, a shear test, a flexure test, or an impact test. Thus it would be more useful if we knew the 95% stress level—that is, the stress level below which 95% of specimens of identical shape, size, and processing conditions would survive a given fracture test. However, it would be even more useful if we knew the 95% stress level for cyclic fatigue test conditions, which would more closely simulate clinical conditions. Nevertheless, for brittle materials such as some dental restorative materials (e.g., resin-based composites and ceramics), the distribution of strength values tends to be non-normal or non-Gaussian. If the strength distribution does not exhibit a normal or symmetrical distribution with values clustered uniformly around a mean value, the distribution may be better described by the use of Weibull statistics, which is based on the concept of the weakest link.

Ceramic strength data are typically asymmetrical. Thus, they are better described using the Weibull distribution than the Gaussian distribution function. Weibull plots of log fracture probability as a function of fracture stress can be used as a factor in the design of dental restorations that are produced from brittle biomedical materials. A Weibull plot can be used to determine the cumulative probability that a sample will fail under a given load or induced stress. These plots are based on data obtained on a representative population (ideally 30 or more) of specimens tested in a manner similar to that which the materials will experience during clinical service. If a dental practice specifies that less than one ceramic restoration in 100 should fracture during use, the Weibull distribution data can be analyzed to estimate the stress that would cause this 1% level of failure. With knowledge of this 99% survival stress, the design of restorations can be optimized by changing dimensions or restricting use conditions such that no location within the restoration sustains stresses above the failure stress.

Another important Weibull parameter is the Weibull modulus (designated by m), which represents the distribution of flaws in brittle materials or the distribution of strength determined from a plot of log fracture probability versus failure stress. The failure strengths of brittle materials are statistically distributed as a function of the homogeneity of the material. The Weibull distribution is described by Eq. (11):

$$Pf = 1 - \exp\left[-\left(\sigma/\sigma_o\right)^m\right] \quad (11)$$

where Pf = fracture probability defined by the relation Pf = i/(N + 1)

i = rank in strength

N = total number of specimens in the sample

m = shape parameter or Weibull modulus

σ = fracture stress

σ_o = scale parameter or characteristic strength (63.2% failure level)

A low Weibull modulus reflects a high variation in measured strength values and an increase in the probability that flaws will interact to weaken a brittle material. A low Weibull modulus suggests that products with strength that is substantially lower than the mean will exhibit a greater inconsistency in strength. The use of these products for prostheses will result in a greater variation in fracture force and decreased reliability. Higher values of Weibull modulus correspond to a higher level of homogeneity of the material and greater reliability as a structural material. Most ceramics exhibit m values in the range of 5–15, and metals, which are ductile, have m values above 20.

Other Important Properties

Toughness

Toughness is defined as the amount of elastic and plastic deformation energy required to fracture a material. Fracture toughness is a measure of the energy required to propagate critical flaws in the structure. Toughness is measured as the total area under the stress–strain graph (such as shown in Fig. 4.7) from zero stress to the fracture stress. Toughness increases with increases in strength and ductility. Greater the strength and higher the ductility (total plastic strain), greater the toughness. Thus, it can be concluded that a tough material is generally strong, although a strong material is not necessarily tough. In comparison, the modulus of resilience is the energy required to stress a structure to its proportional limit. It can be measured as the area under the linear elastic portion of the stress–strain curve.

Fracture Toughness

The strength of ductile materials such as gold alloys and certain resin-based composites is useful for determining the maximum stress that restorations of these materials can withstand before a certain amount of plastic deformation or fracture occurs. For brittle materials such as dental ceramics, strength is of only limited value in the design of ceramic prostheses. Small defects (porosity and microcracks) are randomly distributed in location and size throughout a ceramic, causing large strength variations in otherwise identical ceramic specimens. Furthermore, surface flaws caused by grinding—as from coarse-, medium-, or fine-grit diamond particles—can greatly weaken an otherwise strong ceramic, especially in the presence of tensile stress in the area of the flaws. Strength is inversely proportional to the square root of the flaw depth within the surface.

Fracture toughness, or the critical **stress intensity**, is a mechanical property that describes the resistance of brittle materials to the catastrophic propagation of flaws under an applied stress. Fracture toughness is given by the symbol K_{Ic} in units of stress times the square root of crack length; that is, $MPa{\bullet}m^{1/2}$ or the equivalent form, $MN{\bullet}m{-}^{3/2}$. Thus, the fracture resistance of a porcelain veneer with a K_{Ic} of 0.75 $MPa{\bullet}m^{1/2}$ is much lower than that of the tougher supporting core ceramics used for all-ceramic prostheses, such as alumina and yttrium-stabilized zirconia with K_{Ic} values of 3.4 and 7.9 $MPa{\bullet}m^{1/2}$, respectively.

CRITICAL QUESTION

Is a stiff material (high elastic modulus) stronger than a more flexible material?

Brittleness

Materials that are very brittle have a tensile strength markedly lower than their corresponding compressive strength because of their inability to plastically deform and reduce the tensile stress at flaw tips. This is true of all brittle dental materials, such as amalgams, composites, cements, ceramics, and some base metal alloys. The failure of these materials in clinical usage is most often associated with their low tensile strengths and the presence of flaws within the tensile stress region.

Shown in Figure 4.14 are three stress–strain curves of materials with variable strength, elastic modulus, and percent elongation. Material A is stronger, stiffer, and more ductile than materials B and C. Material B has less ductility than material A and thus, is more brittle. Material C has no ductility and is perfectly brittle; it is also the weakest of the three materials. **Brittleness** is the relative inability of a material to sustain plastic deformation before fracture of a material occurs. For example, amalgams, ceramics, and composites are brittle at oral temperatures (5°C–55°C). They sustain little or no plastic strain before they fracture. In other words, a brittle material fractures at or near its proportional limit. This behavior is shown by material C in Figure 4.14.

However, a brittle material is not necessarily weak. For example, a cobalt-chromium partial denture alloy may have a percent elongation of less than 1.5% but an ultimate tensile strength of 870 MPa. The tensile strength of a glass-infiltrated alumina core ceramic (In-Ceram Alumina) is moderately high (450 MPa), but it has 0% elongation.

If a glass is drawn into a fiber with very smooth surfaces and insignificant internal flaws, its tensile strength may be as high as 2800 MPa (400,000 psi), but it will have no ductility (0% elongation). Thus, dental materials with low or zero percent elongation—including amalgams, composites, ceramics, and nonresin luting agents—will have little or no burnishability because they have no plastic deformation potential.

CRITICAL QUESTION

What is the difference in appearance between a stress–strain graph for a material that has high strength, high stiffness, and high ductility and one for a material that is weak, flexible, and more brittle?

Ductility and Malleability

When a cast dental alloy is stressed beyond its proportional limit, it becomes permanently deformed. If it sustains tensile stress and

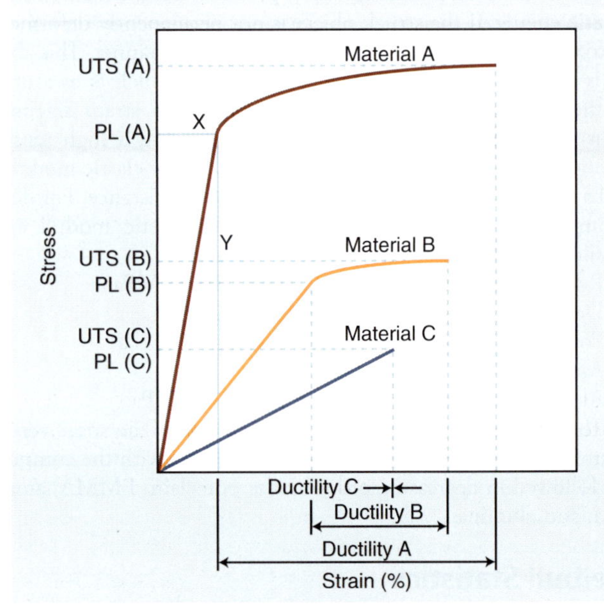

• **Fig. 4.14** Stress–strain plots of materials that exhibit different mechanical properties. UTS, ultimate tensile stress; PL, proportional limit.

considerable permanent deformation without rupture, it is classified as a ductile alloy. **Ductility represents the ability of a material to sustain a large permanent deformation under a tensile load up to the point of fracture**. For example, a metal that can be drawn readily into a long thin wire is considered to be ductile.

Examples of three materials with different degrees of ductility (percent elongation) are shown in Figure 4.14. Material A is the most ductile as shown by the longest plastic strain range (curved region). Material C is typical of brittle materials because no plastic deformation is possible and fracture occurs at the proportional limit.

Malleability is the ability of a material to sustain considerable permanent deformation without rupture under compression, as in hammering or rolling into a sheet. Gold is the most ductile and malleable pure metal, and silver is second. Of the metals of interest to the dentist, platinum ranks third in ductility, and copper ranks third in malleability.

Ductility is the relative ability of a material to be stretched plastically at room temperature without fracturing. Its magnitude can be assessed by the amount of permanent deformation indicated by the stress–strain curve. For example, the plastic strain indicated in Figure 4.14 is a relative measure of the ductility of the solid material. After fracture, the mechanical stress decreases instantly to zero, and the residual strain represents the amount of permanent deformation that has been produced in the object.

Which Tests Are Used to Determine Ductility?

Three common methods are used to determine ductility: (1) the percent elongation after fracture, (2) the reduction in area of tensile test specimens, and (3) the maximum number of bends performed in a cold bend test. Probably the simplest and most commonly used method is to compare the increase in length of a wire or rod after fracture in tension to its length before fracture. Two marks are placed on the wire or rod at a specified distance apart and this distance is designated as the gauge length. For dental materials, the standard gauge length is usually 51 mm. The wire or rod is then pulled apart under a tensile load. The fractured ends are fitted together and the gauge length is again measured. The ratio of the increase in length after fracture to the original gauge length, expressed in percent, is called the percent elongation and represents the quantitative value of ductility.

CRITICAL QUESTION

Hardness is a property used to predict the wear resistance of a material and its ability to abrade opposing dental structures. What other factors may be responsible for excessive wear of natural tooth enamel or prosthetic surfaces by a hard material?

Hardness

Except for comparing one material with another, this term is difficult to define. In mineralogy the relative hardness of a substance is based on its ability to resist scratching. In metallurgy and most other disciplines, the concept that is most generally accepted is that of "resistance to indentation." It is on the basis of this process that most modern hardness tests are designed.

An indentation produced on the surface of a material from the applied force of a sharp point or abrasive particle results from the interaction of numerous properties. Among the properties that are related to the hardness of a material are compressive strength, proportional limit, and ductility.

Hardness data for dental materials are useful to the dentist and materials scientist. Hardness tests are included in numerous specifications for dental materials developed by the American Dental Association (ADA) and standards promoted by the International Organization for Standardization (ISO). There are several types of surface hardness tests. Most are based on the ability of the surface of a material to resist penetration by a diamond point or steel ball under a specified load. The tests most frequently used in determining the hardness of dental materials are known by the names Barcol, Brinell, Rockwell, Shore, Vickers, and Knoop. Selection of the test should be determined on the basis of the material being measured.

The *Brinell hardness test* has been used extensively for determining the hardness of metals and metallic materials used in dentistry. The Brinell hardness number is related to the proportional limit and the ultimate tensile strength of dental gold alloys. Because the test is a relatively simple one, it may often be conveniently used as an index of properties that involve more complex test methods. The Brinell hardness test is one of the oldest tests employed for determining the hardness of metals. In this test, a hardened steel ball is pressed under a specified load into the polished surface of a material, as shown in Figure 4.15. The load is divided by the area of the projected surface of the indentation, and the quotient is referred to as the Brinell hardness number, usually abbreviated as HB or BHN, or more recently, HBW. Thus, for a given load, the smaller the indentation, the larger is the number and the harder the material.

The *Rockwell hardness test* is somewhat similar to the Brinell test in that a steel ball or a conical diamond point is used, as diagrammed in Figure 4.15. Instead of measuring the diameter of the impression, the depth of penetration is measured directly by a dial gauge on the instrument. A number of indenting points of different sizes are available for testing a variety of different materials. The Rockwell hardness number (abbreviated as RHN) is designated according to the particular indenter and load employed. The convenience of the Rockwell test, with direct reading of the depth of the indentation, has led to its wide usage in industry. However, neither the Brinell test nor the Rockwell test is suitable for brittle materials.

The *Vickers hardness test* employs the same principle of hardness testing that is used in the Brinell test. However, instead of a steel ball, a square-based pyramid is used (Fig. 4.15). Although the impression is square instead of round, the method for calculating the Vickers hardness number (usually abbreviated as HV or VHN) is the same as that for the BHN in that the load is divided by the projected area of indentation. The lengths of the diagonals of the indentation are measured and averaged. The Vickers test is employed in the standard testing of dental casting gold alloys. The test is suitable for determining the hardness of brittle materials; therefore, it has also been used for measuring the hardness of other cast dental alloys as well as of tooth structure.

The *Knoop hardness test* employs a diamond-tipped tool that is cut in the geometric configuration shown in Figure 4.15. The impression is rhombic in outline, and the length of the largest diagonal is measured. The load is divided by the projected area to give the Knoop hardness number (usually abbreviated as HK or KHN). When the indentation is made and the indenter is subsequently removed, the shape of the Knoop indenter causes elastic recovery of the projected impression to occur primarily along the shorter diagonal. The stresses are distributed in such a manner that only the dimensions of the minor axis are subject to change by relaxation. Thus, the hardness is virtually independent of the ductility of the tested material. The hardness of tooth enamel can

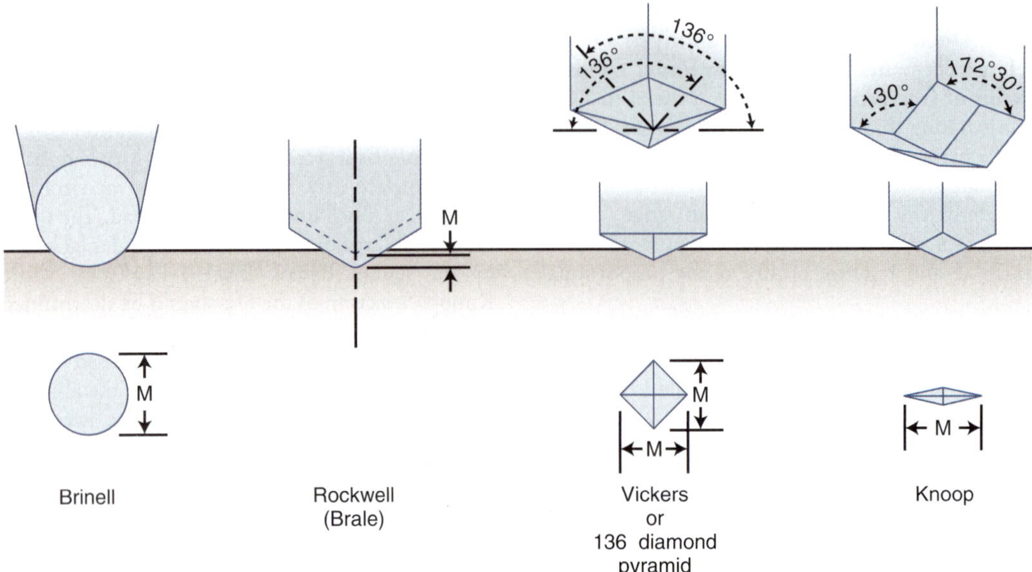

• **Fig. 4.15** Shapes of hardness indenter points (*upper row*) and the indentation depressions left in material surfaces (*lower row*). The measured dimension M that is shown for each test is used to calculate hardness. The following tests are shown: Brinell test—a steel ball is used, and the diameter of the indentation is measured after removal of the indenter. Rockwell test—a conical indenter is impressed into the surface under a minor load (*dashed line*) and a major load (*solid line*), and M is the difference between the two penetration depths. In the Vickers or 136° diamond pyramid test, a pyramidal point is used, and the diagonal length of the indentation is measured. In the Knoop test, a rhombohedral pyramid diamond tip is used and the long axis of the indentation is measured.

be compared with that of gold, porcelain, resin, and other restorative materials. Also, the load may be varied over a wide range, from 0.1 kgf to more than 1 kgf, so that values for both exceedingly hard and very soft materials can be obtained by this test.

The Knoop and Vickers tests are classified as microhardness tests in comparison with the Brinell and Rockwell macrohardness tests. Both Knoop and Vickers tests employ load less than 9.8 N. The resulting indentations are small and limited to depths of less than 19 μm. Hence, they are capable of measuring the hardness in small regions of thin objects. The Rockwell and Brinell tests give average hardness values over much larger areas.

Friction and Wear (Tribology)

When we write on a blackboard with a piece of chalk, we feel there is a resistance between the chalk and the blackboard. The resistance felt during writing is called friction. The friction effects are those that arise from the tangential forces transmitted across the interface of contact when solid surfaces are pressed together by our hands. The wear phenomena consist of the removal of material from the surfaces of one of the contacting bodies as a result of interaction with the other contacting body. Adhesion is the ability of contacting bodies to withstand tensile force after being pressed together. A layer of oil on the board surface keeps the chalk from contacting the blackboard, which effectively eliminates wear of the chalk. In engineering terms, this process is called lubrication. In dental material manipulation, this behavior has been used to keep materials from sticking together. For example, a separating medium is used to keep denture resin from adhering to the gypsum mold in denture processing (Chapter 11).

Tribology is the term referring to the study and application of the principles of friction, wear, and lubrication. The following segment focuses on friction and wear as they occur during clinical service.

Friction

Friction is the force that opposes the relative motion that exists when a solid object is moved tangentially with respect to the surface of another that this object touches or when an attempt is made to produce such motion. Although friction is an obstacle to motion, the presence of friction makes the completion of certain tasks possible. We fight against friction as we walk or drive to a destination; however, we need the friction to stop the motion when we reach the destination. In the dental office, operators holding various instruments in their hands, such as a tool for condensing amalgam or scaling teeth, cannot carry out their work if the friction between the operator's hand and the instrument is too low. When this occurs, we call that condition "slippery." Take the RPD as an example, the friction between the retentive clasp and the abutment tooth plays an important role in keeping the RPD stable.

Mechanism of Friction

Macroscopically, a surface may look shiny as light is reflected well from the surface. The same surface in submicron scale could look like a mountain terrain filled with peaks called asperities (Fig. 4.16). Consider two solid materials stacked upon each other; there are points of contact called asperity junctions (Fig. 4.16A), and the sum of the areas of all the junctions constitute the real area of contact, Ar. The interfacial area between the two surfaces is known as the apparent surface area as observed by our eyes.

Because the real area of contact is only a small fraction of the apparent surface area, the stress at each junction could be one or several magnitudes higher than that calculated using the apparent surface area. One or both materials may be plastically deformed. The harder asperity will dent the softer one, as shown in Figure 4.16B, when additional load is applied. Recall the discussion in Chapter 2 that attractions between atoms and molecules occur at a very short range, on the order of magnitude of only a few Angstroms. If both surfaces are free of contaminants, the

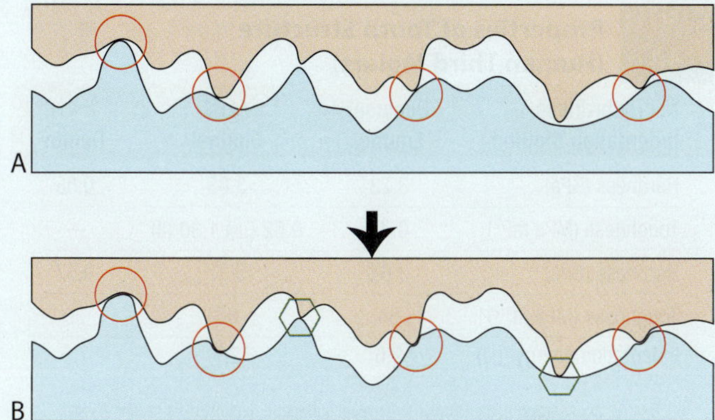

• **Fig. 4.16** Microscopical aspect of the interface between two objects. **(A)** The weight of the top object is supported by the bottom object at the points of contact. **(B)** Additional pressure causing plastic deformation of the bottom object and additional contacts. This illustration indicates that the top object is harder than the bottom one. If one is to slide the top object horizontally to the right, it needs to overcome the obstacles of bottom object at the areas of contact. The force needed to break through is the friction, and fracture of asperities of either object at the contact could occur. The residue of fracture asperities is the wear debris.

stress at the asperity/asperity interface can be high enough to cause bonding at the atomic or molecular level, forming asperity junctions. To begin sliding between opposing surfaces, these junctions need to be broken. As the sliding continues, asperities of opposing surfaces collide, which can result in fracture of the weaker asperities or harder asperities plowing through the softer surface. The combined effort to make the object move is reflected in the frictional force.

The friction is expressed in quantitative terms as a force. The initial force needed to start sliding is called static friction, and the force needed to continue sliding is called kinetic friction. The force required to begin sliding is greater than the force needed to keep the object sliding.

Laws of Sliding Friction

The following are the laws of friction expressing the magnitude of the friction force as a function of macroscopically observable variables: the applied load, the size of the region of contact, and the sliding velocity:

1. The friction force F is proportional to the normal force P: $F = \mu P$. This relationship enables us to calculate the coefficients of static friction, μs, and kinetic friction, μk.
2. The friction force is independent of the apparent area of contact, Aa. Thus large and small objects have the same coefficients of friction. Keep in mind that the interaction that occurs at the real areas of contact is what contributes to friction. Additional load increases the real area of contact but not the apparent area of contact (Fig. 4.16B).
3. The kinetic friction force is independent of the sliding velocity. This implies that the force needed to maintain sliding is the same at any specified velocity.

Friction plays important roles in various dental appliances and instruments. For example, we can consider static friction as a mechanism for preventing a restoration from falling off its intended location.

Wear

Wear may be defined as the removal of material from solid surfaces as a result of mechanical action. The wear process is generally thought of as destructive because it often leads to failure of prostheses or appliances. In fact, there are a considerable number of practical uses for the wear process. Here are some examples where controlled wear is needed to accomplish the work. In the making of a composite restoration, there is a need to shape the restoration and finish to a pleasing appearance. Finishing involves a sequence of abrasive processes. Among these are the use of burs, abrasive paper, and finally, loose abrasive grains to achieve a very smooth surface. In cutting operations as part of cavity preparation, having a sharp edge for the cutting tool is essential. If during the operation, the edge becomes blunted, cutting no longer occurs; the process must be stopped, and the edge must be re-formed.

Types of Wear

Research has established that there are four main forms of wear: (1) adhesive, (2) abrasive, (3) corrosive, and (4) surface-fatigue wear. Each wear process obeys its own laws; however, on many occasions, one of the modes of wear acts in such a way as to affect the others

Adhesive wear results from the strong bonding that occurs whenever atoms or molecules come into intimate contact under pressure. The asperity junctions are broken near the interface within one of the materials during sliding. In consequence, a transferred fragment will be formed. That fragment might be broken off when this fragment collides with another asperity from the opposing material. The repeated process of asperity-junction formation, fracture near the junction, and detachment of transferred fragments yields debris of adhesive wear.

Abrasive wear arises when a hard, rough surface slides against a softer surface, digs into this surface, and plows a series of grooves. The material originally in the grooves is normally removed in the form of loose fragments, or else the material forms a pair of mounds along each groove. A harder surface is less likely to wear than a softer surface because the harder surface resists denting, but the softer surface does not. This is known as two-body abrasive wear. Abrasive wear can also arise in a somewhat different situation, when hard, abrasive particles are introduced between sliding surfaces and abrade material from each surface. The mechanism of this form of abrasive wear seems to be that an abrasive grain adheres temporarily to one of the sliding surfaces or is embedded in the material and plows out a groove in the other. **This is known as three-body abrasive wear.**

Corrosive wear occurs in situations where the environment surrounding a sliding surface interacts chemically with the surface. If the products of reaction are worn off the surface, corrosive wear has occurred. The first stage of corrosive wear is corrosive attack of the surface, which is identical with ordinary corrosion. Some corrosion processes can result in a protective layer that slows down the corrosion process, such as with aluminum, titanium, and alloys with sufficient chromium. The second step of the corrosive wear process consists of wearing away the reaction product film, as a result of sliding, and exposing a fresh surface for corrosive attack.

Surface-fatigue wear is closely related to the general phenomenon of fatigue of materials in that there is a characteristic interrelation between the stresses in the contacting materials and the number of cycles required to produce fracture. As stressing and unstressing of the material of occluding continue, a subsurface crack propagates. For a long time, the material appears to be quite unaffected by this stress cycling, but suddenly, perhaps after a few hundred thousand hours of loading, a particle spalls off the surface, and thereafter, deterioration of the surface and flaking of fragments become rapid.

There are a few marginal processes that are often classified as forms of wear that include actions of fretting, erosion, cavitation, and impact. Each type describes a different way in which the load and sliding action are introduced. Briefly, fretting wear arises when contacting surfaces undergo oscillatory tangential displacement of small amplitude. Erosion wear is a process in which a particle carried in a fluid medium hits a solid surface and removes material from this surface. Cavitation-erosion wear occurs as a result of the cavitation of a liquid. The liquid is put through a cycle of compression, then tension, and then compression again, and so on. Impact wear is a short sliding motion, such as grit-blasting, where two solid bodies interact for an exceptionally short time interval.

Factors Influencing Abrasive Wear

The amount of abrasive wear in volume loss (V) is found to be proportional to the size of the actual contact area. This actual contact area is proportional to the pressure applied (P) and inversely proportional to the hardness of the surface (H). In addition, the wear increases as the distance of travel by one surface increases. In dentistry, the distance is often in the form of the chewing cycle (N). Mathematically, the relationship is expressed as $V \propto (N \cdot P/H)$. This equation does not necessarily hold true in all cases but clearly points out the influence of three major factors on wear. In reality, many other factors may be involved in the wear process, such as surface roughness, temperature, and environment (e.g., moisture). Roughness increases the actual contact area and the wear. Polishing to attain a smooth surface is highly advisable to reduce wear. The thermal properties of the surface become important when sliding takes place at high speeds, such as grinding and polishing. The oral environment provides natural lubrication that reduces wear. Soft foods reduce wear because they serve to cushion and lubricate during mastication. The resulting wear debris may be washed away by saliva or may be trapped between the two opposing surfaces, creating the so-called three-body abrasive wear. This phenomenon occurs when the diet is impregnated with fine, solid particles and during brushing of the teeth with an abrasive.

CRITICAL QUESTION

Why do prostheses sometimes fail under a very small force even though the strength of the prosthetic material is relatively great?

Strength of Tooth Structure

The relatively wide variation in mechanical properties of human tooth structure is attributed to the technical problems associated with preparing and testing such small specimens, which in some instances are less than 1 mm in length. The results reported in one study are shown in Table 4.1. This study investigated the effect of enamel–rod orientation by propagating cracks in the occlusal surface and in axial sections in directions parallel and perpendicular to the occlusal surface. The cracks in the axial enamel section were longer in the direction perpendicular to the occlusal surface rather than parallel to the surface. The cracks that propagated toward the dentinoenamel junction (DEJ) were arrested and did not penetrate the DEJ into dentin. The fracture toughness of dentin varied by a factor of 3 as a function of enamel–rod orientation. The elastic modulus of enamel also varied between the occlusal surface and the axial section. The results of this study demonstrate that the mechanical properties of tooth structure are a function of

TABLE 4.1 Properties of Tooth Structure (Human Third Molars)

Microhardness Indentation Method	Occlusal Enamel	Axial Enamel	Dentin
Hardness (GPa)	3.23	3.03	0.58
Toughness (MPa·m$^{1/2}$)	0.77	0.52 (⊥) 1.30 (II)	—
Hardness (GPa)	3.62	3.37	0.57
Toughness (MPa·m$^{1/2}$)	94	80	20
Indentation energy (μJ)	2.6	2.7	7.5

⊥Enamel axial section perpendicular to occlusal surface; II, enamel axial section parallel to occlusal surface.
From Xu HHK, Smith DT, Jahanmir S, Romberg E, Kelly JR, Thompson VP, Rekow ED: Indentation damage and mechanical properties of human enamel and dentin. *J Dent Res* 77:472–480, 1998.

microstructural orientation. Indentation energy is a recently introduced property that is used to predict the machinability and wear behavior of ceramics. Research data suggest that during indentation or cutting, brittle enamel may be removed by microfracture, whereas dentin may be removed by forming ductile chips.

Although the data in Table 4.1 indicate a variation in the properties of enamel and dentin from one type of tooth to another, the difference is more likely the result of variations within individual teeth than between teeth. The properties of enamel vary somewhat with the position on the tooth; that is, occlusal enamel is stronger than enamel on other surfaces of the tooth. Also, the properties of enamel vary according to the microscopic structure. For example, enamel is stronger under longitudinal compression than when subjected to lateral compression. On the other hand, the properties of dentin appear to be independent of structure, regardless of the direction of compressive stress.

The tensile properties of tooth structure have also been measured. Dentin is considerably stronger in tension (50 MPa) than enamel (10 MPa). Although the compressive strengths of enamel and dentin are comparable, the proportional limit and modulus of elasticity of enamel are greater than the corresponding values for dentin. The higher modulus of elasticity of enamel results in less resilience compared with dentin.

Typically, the energy of a biting or chewing event is absorbed by the food bolus during mastication and by the teeth, periodontal ligament, and bone. Also, the design of the tooth enables the tooth to absorb significant static and dynamic (impact) energies. The modulus of resilience of dentin is greater than that of enamel and is better able to absorb impact energy. Enamel is a brittle substance with a comparatively high modulus of elasticity, a low proportional limit in tension, and a low modulus of resilience.

CRITICAL QUESTION

Why do prostheses sometimes fail under a very small force even though the strength of the prosthetic material is relatively great?

Stress Concentration Effects

Unexpected fractures of dental prostheses and restorations occur occasionally even when high-quality materials have been used.

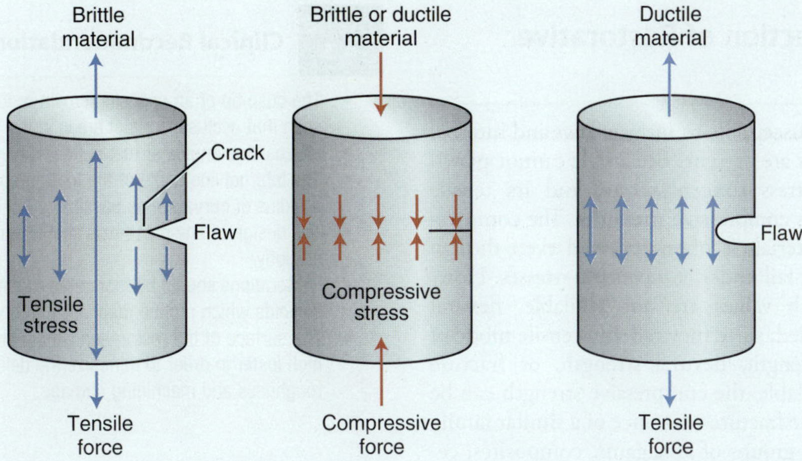

• **Fig. 4.17** Influence of tensile and compressive stresses on flaws in brittle and ductile materials.

These failures result from locally high stresses in specific areas even though the average stress in the structure is low. The cause of this strength reduction is the presence of small microscopic flaws or microstructural defects on the surface or within the internal structure. These flaws are especially critical in brittle materials in areas of tensile stress because tensile stress tends to open cracks; therefore, the stress at the tips of these flaws is greatly increased and may lead to crack initiation and broken bonds. Shown in Figure 4.17 is a theoretical tensile stress distribution in brittle and ductile materials. Although the tensile stress has increased at the flaw tip in each case, it has increased by a smaller amount in the ductile material (right-side illustration of Fig. 4.17), in which plastic deformation has occurred with subsequent widening of the flaw tip, thereby reducing the magnitude of localized tensile stress. As shown on the left side of Figure 4.17, the tensile stress in a brittle material cannot be relieved by plastic deformation at the flaw tip and a crack develops as the stress increases to a critical level. Note the increased level of tensile stress at the tip of the flaw. However, the stress at areas far away from these flaws will be much lower if flaws are absent in these areas.

The flaw does not play a significant role when the material is subjected to an external compressive force, as shown in the center of Figure 4.17. In this case, the compressive stress that develops in the material tends to close the crack, and this stress distribution is more uniform. There are two important aspects of these flaws: (1) the stress intensity increases with the length of the flaw, especially when it is oriented perpendicular to the direction of tensile stress, and (2) flaws on the surface are associated with higher stresses than are flaws of the same size in interior regions. Thus, surface finishing of brittle materials—such as ceramics, amalgams, and composites—is extremely important in areas subjected to tensile stress.

Reduced strength of a brittle restorative material may be caused by localized areas of stress enhancement can also result from factors other than the inherent microscopic flaws on the surface of a material. Areas of high stress concentration are caused by one or more of the following factors:

1. Surface defects, such as porosity, grinding roughness, and machining damage, can be reduced by polishing the surface to reduce the depth of the defects.
2. Interior flaws, such as voids or inclusions, which are difficult to minimize but we can ensure the highest quality of the structure or to increase the size of the object.
3. Marked changes in contour, such as the point of attachment of a clasp arm to a partial denture framework or a sharp internal angle at the pulpal–axial line angle of a tooth preparation for an amalgam or composite restoration. The design of any prosthesis should vary gradually rather than abruptly. Smooth internal line angles reduce the risk of cusp fracture.
4. A large difference in elastic moduli or thermal expansion coefficient across a bonded interface. The elastic moduli of the two materials should be more closely matched. The materials must be closely matched in their coefficients of expansion or contraction. If a thermal mismatch cannot be avoided, the weaker, more brittle material should have a slightly lower expansion or contraction coefficient so that a protective compressive stress is sustained in its structure next to the interface.
5. A Hertzian load (or point contact). The cusp tip of an opposing crown or tooth should be well rounded such that occlusal contact areas in the brittle material are large. In addition, the internal line angle of the tooth preparation should have as large a radius of curvature as possible (Table 4.2).

TABLE 4.2 Clinical Implications

- Choice of restorative materials should be based on type of restoration, size, and location.
- Materials which exhibit superiority in some areas may be lacking in other properties. The choice of restorative material may be dictated by the physical requirements for a given situation and prosthesis.
- Test results reported by manufacturers represent a mean value and may not accurately represent the performance of a material under actual clinical conditions.
- From an ultraconservative viewpoint, the lowest 5%–10% of a strength distribution, not mean values, should be used to design a prosthesis intended to resist fracture at a high level of confidence
- Patients who exhibit evidence of extreme bruxism represent a higher risk population for the fracture of brittle restorative materials.
- The best test of a successful restorative material is the test of time under actual clinical conditions. Laboratory data should always be correlated with clinical data.

Criteria for the Selection of Restorative Materials

A brittle material is highly susceptible to surface flaws and internal defects when tensile stresses are present. Because it cannot plastically deform to reduce stress concentrations, and its tensile strength is far lower than its compressive strengths. The compressive strength of brittle materials is often reported even though most brittle materials rarely fail under compressive stresses. However, when tensile strength values are not available, flexural strength values should be used, since they reflect a tensile mode of fracture. When tensile strength, flexural strength, or fracture toughness data are not available, the compressive strength can be useful for comparisons of the fracture resistance of a similar family of brittle materials, such as groups of amalgams, composites, ceramics, or cements.

The physical properties described earlier have been obtained using specimen shapes and sizes that are quite different from those of tooth restorations. Thus, material products must be selected intuitively on the basis of property comparisons. Engineers employ similar criteria for the selection of materials to be used for the construction of large structures. Engineers have an advantage over dentists in this respect because they know beforehand the maximum "average" stresses that structures are expected to sustain before fracture occurs. Furthermore, these expected stresses are multiplied by a "safety factor" to ensure that the structure will be able to withstand a certain amount of excess stress. However, the tensile strength values reported for restorative materials represent the mean stress values below which 50% of the test specimens have fractured and above which only 50% had survived. Because this is an unacceptable failure rate for restorative dentistry, the range of measured values should be known. *From an ultraconservative viewpoint, the lowest 5–10% of a strength distribution, not mean values, should be used to design a prosthesis intended to resist fracture at a high level of confidence. We can also use the 95% survival stress as determined from Weibull analyzes of the data.*

It is unfortunate that the magnitudes of mastication forces are not known for individual patients to the extent that the dentist can predict the stresses that will be induced in dental restorations. However, patients who exhibit evidence of extreme bruxism represent a higher risk population for the fracture of brittle restorative materials. The knowledge of the relationships between the properties of restorative materials known to exhibit excellent long-term survival performance is reinforced by clinical experience. As is true for the field of engineering, the dental profession is aware that the best test of a successful restorative material is the test of time under actual clinical conditions (Table 4.3).

TABLE 4.3 Clinical Recommendations

- The cusp tip of an opposing crown or tooth should be well rounded such that occlusal contact areas in the brittle material are large.
- Internal line angles of restorations should be rounded.
- The internal line angle of the tooth preparation should have as large a radius of curvature as possible.
- The design of any prosthesis should vary gradually rather than abruptly.
- Restorations should be fabricated to minimize internal flaws such as voids which reduce mechanical properties.
- The surface of the restoration should always be polished to a high luster in order to minimize the deleterious effects of grinding roughness and machining damage.

Summary

- **Mechanical properties**—the physical science dealing with forces that act on bodies and the resultant motion, deformation, or stresses that those bodies experience.
- Stress is the force per unit area acting on millions of atoms or molecules in a given plane of a material.
- Types of stresses are **tensile stress, shear stress, and compressive stress.**
- Elastic stresses in materials do not cause permanent (irreversible) deformation. On the other hand, stresses greater than the proportional limit cause permanent deformation and, if high enough, may cause fracture.
- **Brittle materials** exhibit only elastic deformation and do not plastically deform.
- A bending force can produce all three types of stresses, but in most cases fracture occurs because of the tensile stress component.
- **Strain,** or the change in length per unit length, is the relative deformation of an object subjected to a stress.
- **Tensile stress** is a stress caused by a load that tends to stretch or elongate a body.
- When a body is placed under a load that tends to compress or shorten, it results in compressive stress.
- The type of stress that tends to resist the sliding or twisting of one portion of a body over another is called shear stress.
- Elastic modulus describes the relative stiffness or rigidity of a material.
- If the tensile/compressive stress below the proportional limit is divided by its corresponding strain value, a constant of proportionality will be obtained that is known as the **elastic modulus, modulus of elasticity, or Young's modulus.**
- Enamel is stiffer and brittle whereas dentin is more flexible and tougher.
- The maximum flexibility is defined as the flexural strain that occurs when the material is stressed to its proportional limit.
- When a larger strain or deformation happens with a moderate or slight stress, it is termed as **flexibility.**
- Resilience is associated with springiness, i.e., the amount of energy absorbed within a unit volume of a structure when it is stressed to its proportional limit.
- Toughness is defined as the quantity of elastic and plastic deformation energy required to fracture a material. The total area under the **stress–strain curve** is a measure of toughness.
- Strength is equal to the degree of stress necessary to cause either fracture (ultimate strength) or a specified amount of plastic deformation (yield strength).
- Strength is not a measure of individual atom-to-atom attraction or repulsion but rather of the interatomic forces collectively exerted over the entire wire, cylinder, implant, crown, pin, or whatever structure that is stressed.
- The ultimate **tensile strength** is defined as the tensile stress within a structure at the point of rupture.

- The point in the stress–strain curve above which the curve deviates from a straight line or above which plastic deformation occurs on stress application is called as **proportional limit.**
- For a material to satisfy Hooke's law, the elastic stress must be directly proportional to the elastic strain.
- The elastic limit of a material is defined as the greatest stress to which the material can be subjected such that it returns to its original dimensions when the force is released.
- **Yield strength** is used in cases where the proportional limit cannot be determined with sufficient accuracy.
- Yield strength often is a property that represents the stress value at which a small amount (0.1% or 0.2%) of plastic strain has occurred.
- For brittle materials such as dental ceramics, the stress–strain plot is a straight line with no plastic region.
- When most metal alloys have been stressed beyond their proportional limits, their hardness and strength increase at the area of deformation, but their ductility decreases.
- Dimetral tensile strength test should be used only for materials that exhibit elastic deformation primarily and little or no plastic deformation for determining the tensile strength.
- **Flexural strength**, which is also called transverse strength and modulus of rupture, is done by three point and four point bending test.
- **Impact strength** may be defined as the energy required to fracture a material under an impact force. The term impact is used to describe the reaction of a stationary object to a collision with a moving object. A Charpy-type impact tester is usually used to measure impact strength.
- **Fracture toughness,** or the **critical stress intensity**, is a mechanical property that describes the resistance of brittle materials to the catastrophic propagation of flaws under an applied stress.
- **Ductility** represents the ability of a material to sustain a large permanent deformation under a tensile load up to the point of fracture when, a metal is drawn readily into a long thin wire.
- **Malleability** is the ability of a material to sustain considerable permanent deformation without rupture under compression, as in hammering or rolling into a sheet. Gold is the most ductile and malleable pure metal, and silver is second.
- The relative hardness of a substance is based on its ability to resist scratching or resistance to indentation.
- Properties that are related to the hardness of a material are compressive strength, proportional limit, and ductility.
- The **Brinell hardness** test has been used extensively for determining the hardness of metals and metallic materials and is related to the proportional limit and the ultimate tensile strength of dental gold alloys.
- **Stress concentration** develops in areas of small microscopic flaws or microstructural defects on the surface or within the internal structure. These flaws are especially critical in brittle materials in areas of tensile stress because tensile stress tends to open cracks.
- Cuspal enamel is stronger than enamel on other surfaces of the tooth. Enamel is stronger under longitudinal compression than when subjected to lateral compression. The properties of dentin appear to be independent of structure regardless of the direction of compressive stress.
- The **tensile properties** of tooth structure have also been measured. Dentin is considerably stronger in tension (50 MPa) than enamel (10 MPa).
- The proportional limit and modulus of elasticity of enamel are greater than the corresponding values for dentin. The higher modulus of elasticity of enamel results in less resilience compared with dentin.
- Friction is the force that opposes the relative motion that exists when a solid object is moved tangentially with respect to the surface of another, that this object touches or when an attempt is made to produce such motion.
- **Wear may be defined as the removal of material from solid surfaces as a result of mechanical action.**
- There are four main forms of wear: (1) adhesive, (2) abrasive, (3) corrosive, and (4) surface-fatigue wear.

Review Questions

Define the following:

1. Hardness. Also describe various tests for hardness
2. Proportional limit
3. Stress–strain curve
4. Poisson's ratio
5. Types of stress
6. Proportional limit, elastic limit, and yield strength
7. Resilience
8. Diametral tensile strength
9. Biaxial flexural test
10. Ductility and malleability
11. Stress concentration effects and how to minimize stress concentration
12. Fatigue strength.
13. Discuss friction and wear in dentistry
14. Write a short note on wear

Selected Readings

Callister W.D.; Rethwisch D.G. Materials Science and Engineering: An Introduction. John Wiley & Sons: Hoboken, NJ.

Frechette V.D. Failure Analysis of Brittle Materials. The American Ceramic Society: Westerville, OH; This classic textbook on fracture surface analysis provides an excellent overview of fractographic techniques. Since many dental materials are brittle in nature, the identification of fracture patterns and the crack origin are useful to identify the principal sites of crack initiation.

Gibbs C.H.; Mahan P.E.; Mauderli A.; et al. Limits of human bite strength. J Prosthet Dent 56 (2) 226–229 (1986); The maximum biting force (4337 N) measured in this study was listed in the *Guinness Book of Records* as the greatest bite force ever recorded for humans.

Gibbs C.H.; Anusavice K.J.; Young H.M.; et al. Maximum clenching force of patients with moderate loss of posterior tooth support: a pilot study. J Prosthet Dent 88 (5) 498–502 (2002); The ability to sustain a maximum clenching force for a period of 2 s was reported in this study.

Griffith A.A. The phenomena of rupture and flow in solids, Philosophical Transactions of the Royal Society of London. A 221 163–198 (1921); Griffith proposed that minute cracks in a general glass act as a stress raiser that reduces the theoretical strength of glass to 1% of that predicted for its theoretical strength. He also concluded that the magnitude of the fracture stress and the square root of the critical flaw depth was a constant.

Irwin G. Analysis of stresses and strains near the end of a crack traversing a plate. J Apple Mech 24 361–364 (1957); Based on the shortcomings of Griffith's theory for ductile materials, Irwin modified Griffith's equations by accounting for inelastic behavior at the crack tips.

Handbook Metals. Desk Edition. ASM International: Metals Park, OH; This handbook provides a comprehensive overview of metals and metal technology including properties and selection criteria, processing information, and testing and inspection guidelines on failure analysis, mechanical testing, nondestructive testing, metallography, fractography, and quality control.

O'Brien W.J. Biomaterials Properties Database. University of Michigan: Ann Arbor, MIhttp://www.lib.umich.edu/taubman-health-sciences-library/biomaterials-properties-toc; This database provides an electronic reference to the following properties of dental materials: bond strength between restorative materials and tooth structures, Brinell hardness number, coefficient of friction, coefficient of thermal expansion, color range of natural teeth, colors of dental shade guides, contact angle, creep of amalgam, critical surface tension, density, dynamic modulus, elastic modulus, flow, heat of fusion, heat of reaction, Izod impact strength, index of refraction, Knoop hardness number, melting temperatures and ranges, Mohs' hardness, penetration coefficient, percent elongation, permanent deformation, Poisson's ratio, proportional limit, shear strength, Shore A hardness, solubility and disintegration in water, specific heat, strain in compression, surface free energy, surface tension, tear energy, tear strength, thermal conductivity, thermal diffusivity, transverse strength, ultimate compressive strength, ultimate tensile strength, vapor pressure, Vickers hardness, water sorption, yield strength, and zeta potential.

Stanford J.W.; Weigel K.V.; Paffenbarger G.D.; et al. Compressive properties of hard tooth tissue. J Am Dent Assoc 60 746 (1960); Although this study was published in 1960, it remains one of the most authoritative references on the mechanical properties of tooth structure.

Van Vlack L.H. Elements of Materials Science and Engineering. ed 6 Addison-Wesley: Reading, MA; This reference book presents an overview of the structure of matter, the properties of materials, and engineering.

PART II

Direct Restorative Materials

5

Resin-Based Composites

CHAPTER OUTLINE

KEY TERMS

Activation—Process by which sufficient energy is provided to induce an initiator to generate free radicals and cause polymerization to begin.

Activator—Source of energy used to activate an initiator and produce free radicals; the source of energy can be an electron-donating chemical, light, and/or heat.

C-factor—Configuration factor. This represents the ratio between the bonded surface area of a resin-based composite restoration and the nonbonded or free surface area. The greater the C-factor, the greater the stress that develops at the restoration margin, which can lead to gap formation, marginal breakdown and leakage, and other problems (e.g., secondary caries).

Chemical-activated/self-cured/resin/composite—Composite system consisting of two pastes—one containing an initiator and the other an activator—which, when mixed together, release free radicals that initiate polymerization. Many terms have been used throughout the development of this material; we will use either *chemical-activated* or *self-cured* in this book.

Coupling agent—A compound that provides chemical bonds between two dissimilar classes of materials. For example, organosilane compounds are applied to the surfaces of silicate-based fillers to ensure that they are chemically bonded to the resin matrix of a dental composite.

Degree of conversion (DC)—Percentage of carbon–carbon double bonds (–C=C–) converted to single bonds (–C–C–) during curing to form a polymeric resin. Also known as *degree of cure* and *degree of monomer-to-polymer conversion*.

Dental composite—Highly crosslinked polymeric materials reinforced by a dispersion of amorphous silica, glass, crystalline, mineral, or organic resin filler particles and/or short fibers bonded to the matrix by a coupling agent. In dentistry, it is often called just "composite."

Depth of cure—Depth or thickness of a light-cured resin that has attained adequate mechanical strength from polymerization when exposed to a light source under a specific set of conditions.

Dual-cured resin—Dental composite that contains both chemical-activated and light-activated components to initiate polymerization and potentially overcome the limitations of either the chemical- or light-cured system when used alone.

Filler—Inorganic, glass, and/or organic-resin particles that are dispersed in a resin matrix to increase rigidity, strength, and wear resistance and to decrease thermal expansion, water sorption, and polymerization shrinkage. Radiopaque fillers can also be added to impart radiopacity to dental composites. Aluminofluorosilicate fillers can be added to release fluoride from dental composites.

Flowable composite—Hybrid composite with reduced filler level and a narrower particle-size distribution to increase flow and promote intimate adaptation to prepared tooth surfaces. Flowable composites are often used as the first layer of a cavity filling to improve filling adaptation to the cavity.

Free radical—An atom or group of atoms (R) with an unpaired electron (•). R•-producing reactions initiate and propagate polymerization and eventually lead to a final set.

Gel point/gelation—The point in the polymerization reaction where sufficient crosslinks have formed to produce a rigid, glassy state in which internal flow among the developing polymer chains has stopped. All but localized molecular motion has stopped. After the gel point, stresses cannot be relieved but instead continue to increase and concentrate near the bonded interfaces. Thus, reducing the polymerization rate provides more time for adjacent polymer chain segments to slip among themselves to lower energy configurations and relieve developing stresses before the polymerization reaches gel point.

Inhibitor—A chemical added to resin systems to minimize spontaneous polymerization to extend the storage life of the resin through free radical–scavenging mechanisms. It also increases the working time of self-cured resin composites.

Initiator—A free radical–forming chemical used to start the polymerization reaction. It enters into the chemical reaction and becomes part of the final polymer compound; thus, it is not a catalyst, although it is often incorrectly labeled as such.

Light-cured/light-activated resin/composite—Resin or particle-filled resin consisting of a single component that becomes polymerized through the use of a photosensitive initiator system (typically camphorquinone and an amine) and a light-source activator (typically visible blue light). *Photocured* and *photoinitiated* are also used in the literature; we will use either *light-activated* or *light-cured* in this book.

Matrix—A plastic resin material that forms a continuous phase upon curing and binds the reinforcing filler particles.

Oxygen-inhibited layer—The thin surface region of a polymerized resin containing unreacted methacrylate groups arising from dissolved oxygen, which acts to inhibit the free radical polymerization curing reaction; also known as the *air-inhibited layer.*

Resin—Blend of monomers and/or macromolecules with other components that form a material with a set of useful properties.

Dental resin-based composites are structures composed of three major components: a highly cross-linked polymeric ***matrix*** reinforced by a dispersion of glass, mineral, or resin ***filler*** particles and/or short fibers bound to the matrix by ***coupling* agents**. Such resins are used to restore and replace dental tissue lost through disease or trauma and to **lute** and cement crowns and veneers and other indirectly made or prefabricated dental devices.

The gold standard of reference for these materials is amalgam. However, amalgam has its own disadvantages, such as (1) poor esthetics, (2) unfounded concerns about health hazards from the leakage of mercury, and (3) waste disposal concerns. Because resin-based composites can be made to match the natural appearance of teeth, they have become the most popular of the esthetic or tooth-colored filling materials and are widely used for a variety of dental applications.

Another key advantage of resin materials is that they can be made in a range of consistencies, from highly fluid to rigid pastes, which allows them to be conveniently manipulated and molded, to a custom-made form and then converted through a polymerization *curing* reaction to a hard, strong, attractive, and durable solid.

History

There have been remarkable developments in filler, bonding, and curing technologies in esthetic restorative materials over the past 55 years, as shown in Figure 5.1. During the first half of the twentieth century, silicates were the tooth-colored material of choice for cavity restoration. Silicates release fluoride and are excellent for preventing caries, but they are currently used almost exclusively for deciduous teeth because they become severely eroded within a few years (see Chapter 7). Acrylic resins, similar to the materials used to make dentures and custom impression trays (polymethylmethacrylate [PMMA]; see Chapter 11), soon replaced silicates because of their tooth-like appearance, insolubility in oral fluids, ease of manipulation, and low cost. Unfortunately, these acrylic resins had relatively poor wear resistance and tended to shrink severely during curing, which caused them to pull away from the cavity walls, thereby producing crevices or gaps that facilitate leakage within these gaps. Excessive thermal expansion and contraction caused further stresses to develop at the cavity margins when hot or cold beverages and foods were consumed.

These problems were reduced somewhat by the addition of quartz powder particles to form a composite structure. The filler occupies space, but it does not take part in the setting reaction. In addition, commonly used fillers have an extremely low coefficient of thermal expansion, approaching that of tooth structure, thus greatly reducing thermal expansion and contraction. However, these early PMMA-based composites were not very successful, in part because the filler particles simply reduced the volume of polymer resin without being bonded (coupled) to the resin. Thus, defects developed between the particles and the surrounding resin, which led to leakage, staining, and poor wear resistance.

In 1962, Bowen developed a new type of composite material that largely overcame these problems. Bowen's main innovations were bisphenol-A glycidyl dimethacrylate (*bis*-GMA), a monomer that forms a cross-linked matrix that is highly durable (see Chapter 6), and a surface treatment utilizing an organic silane compound called a *coupling agent* to bond the filler particles to the resin matrix. Current tooth–colored restorative materials continue to use this technology, but many further innovations have been introduced since 1962.

Many of these advances have occurred through developments in the filler component. The filler has evolved to ever-smaller sizes, mainly in order to improve appearance and polishability. Barium and other specialty glass and inorganic mineral fillers have been developed to impart radiopacity, enhance manipulation and handling, offset curing shrinkage, and improve mechanical properties. In the 1970s, a category now known as traditional composites (also known as conventional or macrofilled composites) was developed; this contained very large particles of ground amorphous silica and quartz (Fig. 5.2), which imparted significant improvements in mechanical properties, water sorption,

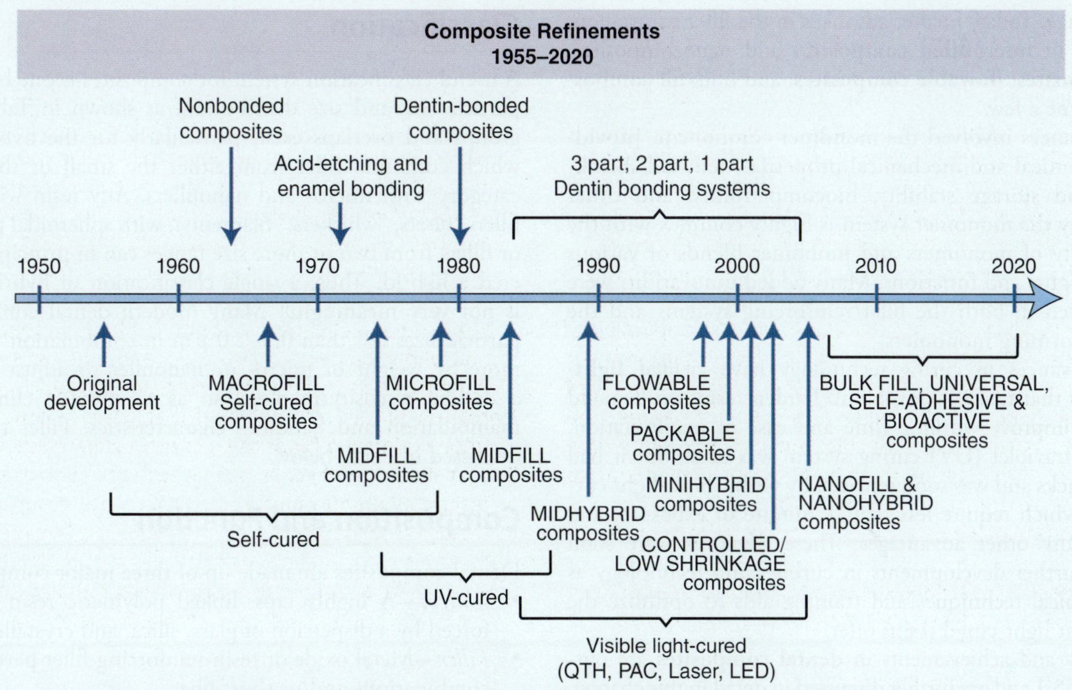

• **Fig. 5.1** Chronology of dental composite developments in monomer, filler, bonding, and curing technologies. (Adapted from Bayne SC: Dental biomaterials: where are we and where are we going? *J Dent Educ* 69:571–585, 2005.)

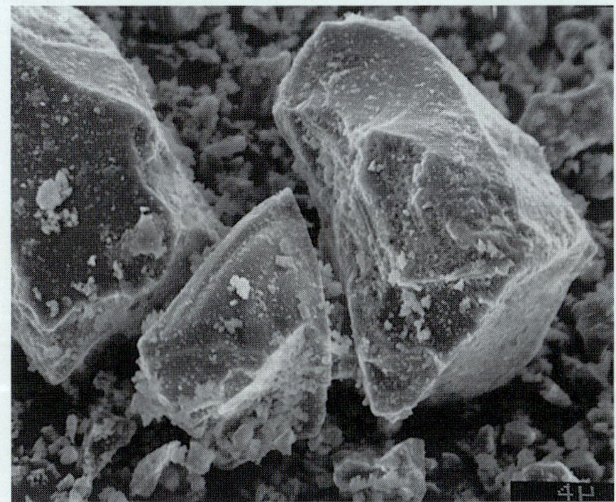

• **Fig. 5.2** Ground quartz filler particles with diameters of about 1–30 μm. Such relatively large fillers were used in early formulations of traditional composites. The smaller particles seen in the background contribute to a broad particle size distribution. (Courtesy of K-J M Söderholm.)

polymerization shrinkage, and thermal expansion compared with unfilled acrylic. However, these composites suffered from roughening of the surface as a result of the selective abrasion of the softer resin matrix surrounding the harder filler particles. To improve surface smoothness and retain or improve the physical and mechanical properties of traditional composites, small-particle-filled composites were developed, using inorganic fillers ground to a size range of about 0.5–3 μm but with a broad size distribution (Fig. 5.3), allowing a higher filler loading (80–90% by weight and 65–77% by volume). This resulted in not only smoother surfaces but also greater wear resistance and some decrease in

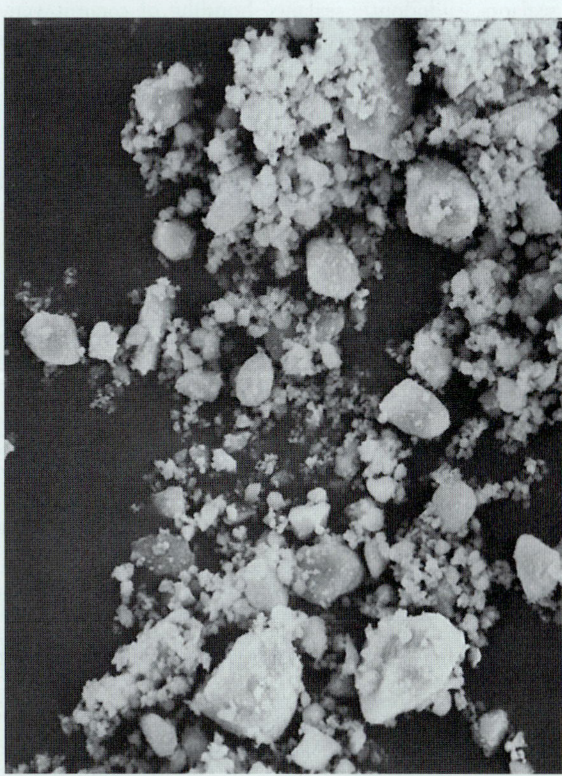

• **Fig. 5.3** Typical particles of a small-particle-filled composite, with sizes in the range of 0.1–10 μm. (Courtesy of EA Glasspoole and RL Erickson.)

curing shrinkage. Today, further advances in the filler component have resulted in **microfilled composites** and nanocomposites, **hybrid composites**, **flowable composites**, and bulk fill composites just to name a few.

Other advances involved the monomer component, providing better chemical and mechanical properties, reduced shrinkage, color and storage stability, biocompatibility, and other features. Today the monomer system is highly complex with the use of a variety of monomers and monomer blends of various molecular weights and functions. Many added innovations were later introduced in both the filler/reinforcing systems and the resin matrix-forming monomers.

Finally, advances in curing technology have yielded **light-cured** systems that make it possible to harden resins on demand as well as to improve working time and ease of manipulation. Initially an ultraviolet (UV) curing system was used, but it had several drawbacks and was soon replaced by visible blue–light curing systems, which require less than 1 minute of exposure, and they have many other advantages. These advances were soon followed by further developments in curing-lamp technology as well as in clinical techniques and training aids to optimize the advantages that light-cured resins offer.

The history and achievements in **dental composites** are outlined in Figure 5.1 and are further discussed in detail in this chapter.

Applications

Dental applications for resin-based composites include cavity and crown restoration materials, adhesive bonding agents, pit and fissure sealants, endodontic sealants, bonding of ceramic veneers, and cementation for crowns, bridges, and other fixed prostheses.

Classification

A useful classification system for composites is one based on filler particle size and size distribution, as shown in Table 5.1. Subgroups and overlaps exist, particularly for the hybrid category, which combines filler from either the small or the traditional category with micro- and nanofillers. Any resin with elongated fillers (fibers, "whiskers," filaments), with spheroidal particle fillers or fillers from two or more size ranges can in principle be considered a hybrid. Thus, a single classification of hybrid composite is not very meaningful. Many modern dental composites have particle sizes less than 0.5–1.0 μm in combination with 10% or more by weight of micro- or nanofiller to adjust the paste to a desired viscosity/rheology so as to provide clinically useful manipulation and handling characteristics. Filler technology is discussed in detail below.

Composition and Function

Dental composites are made up of three major components:

- *Matrix*—A highly cross-linked polymeric resin matrix reinforced by a dispersion of glass, silica, and crystalline.
- *Filler*—Metal oxide or resin-reinforcing filler particles or their combinations and/or short fibers.
- *Coupling agents*—Bonded to the matrix by silane coupling agents.

In addition, dental composites contain a number of other components, including an **activator-initiator** system that is required to convert the resin paste from a soft, moldable filling material to a hard, durable restoration. Pigments help to match the color of tooth structure. Ultraviolet (UV) absorbers and other

TABLE 5.1 Classification of Resin-Based Composites and Indications for Use

Class of Composite	Particle Size	Clinical Use
Traditional (large particle)	1–50 μm glass or silica	High-stress areas
Hybrid (large particle)	(1) 1–20 μm glass (2) 40 nm silica	High-stress areas requiring improved polishability (Classes I, II, III, IV)
Hybrid (midfilled)	(1) 0.1–10 μm glass (2) 40 nm silica	High-stress areas requiring improved polishability (Classes III, IV)
Hybrid (minifilled/SPF[a])	(1) 0.1–2 μm glass (2) 40 nm silica	Moderate-stress areas requiring optimal polishability (Classes III, IV)
Nanohybrid	(1) 0.1–2 μm glass or resin microparticles (2) ≤100 nm nanoparticles	Moderate-stress areas requiring optimal polishability (Classes III, IV)
Packable hybrid	Midfilled/minifilled hybrid, but with lower filler fraction	Situations where improved condensability is needed (Classes I, II)
Flowable hybrid	Midfilled hybrid with finer particle size distribution	Situations where improved flow is needed and/or where access is difficult (Class II)
Homogeneous microfilled	40 nm silica	Low-stress and subgingival areas that require a high luster and polish
Heterogeneous microfilled	(1) 40 nm silica (2) Prepolymerized resin particles containing 40 nm silica	Low-stress and subgingival areas where reduced shrinkage is essential
Nanofilled composites	<100 nm silica or zirconia Homogeneous independent nanoparticles or nanoclusters	Anterior and noncontact posterior areas

[a]SPF, small particle–filled.

additives improve color stability, and polymerization **inhibitors** extend storage life and provide increased working time for **chemically activated resins**. Other components may be included to enhance performance, appearance, and durability.

CRITICAL QUESTION

What are the three essential components of resin composite materials?

What are the potential uses of composites in dentistry?

What roles do coupling agents, fillers, *bis*-GMA, and other high-molecular-weight dimethacrylate monomers play in the function and performance of dental resins?

Matrix

The resin matrix in most dental composites is based on a blend of aromatic and/or aliphatic *dimethacrylate* monomers such as *bis*-GMA (Fig. 5.4) and urethane dimethacrylate (UDMA, Fig. 5.4) to form highly cross-linked, strong, rigid, and durable polymer structures (see Figs 6.3 and 13.16). This matrix forms a continuous phase in which the reinforcing filler is dispersed. Because of the large molecular volume of these monomers, polymerization shrinkage can be as low as 0.9% (average of 1.5% compared with a range of 2%–3% for most composites) when combined with inorganic particulate fillers at levels of up to 88% by weight. However, UDMA and *bis*-GMA are highly viscous (800,000 centipoise, similar to honey on a cold day) and are difficult to blend and manipulate. Thus, it is necessary to use varying proportions of lower molecular-weight highly fluid monomers such as triethylene glycol dimethacrylate (TEGDMA, 5–30 centipoise; Fig. 5.4) and other lower molecular-weight dimethacrylates to blend with and dilute the viscous components to attain resin pastes sufficiently fluid for clinical manipulation and for incorporating enough filler to reinforce the cured resin. Unfortunately, these smaller, diluent monomers undergo greater polymerization shrinkage, partially offsetting the advantage of using large monomers such as *bis*-GMA. Generally the greater the proportion of these "diluting" monomers, the greater the polymerization shrinkage and the greater the risk of eventual leakage in marginal gaps and the problems that may result.

Various dimethacrylate resin combinations have been explored through the years in attempts to reduce viscosity and increase the DC. The UDMAs have shown particular promise. UDMA resins are any monomer containing one or more urethane groups (–NH–CO–O–) and two methacrylate end groups (Fig. 5.4).

Because of the large molecular volume of these monomers, polymerization shrinkage can be as low as 0.9% (average of 1.5% compared with a range of 2% to 3% for most composites) when combined with inorganic particulate fillers at levels of up to 88% by weight. UDMA (about 20 Pa•s) and *bis*-GMA (about 800 Pa•s, similar to honey on a cold day) are highly viscous and are difficult to blend and manipulate. Thus, varying proportions of lower molecular-weight highly fluid monomers such as triethylene glycol dimethacrylate (TEGDMA; 0.005–0.05 Pa•s; Fig. 5.4) and other lower molecular-weight dimethacrylates to blend with and dilute the viscous components to attain resin pastes sufficiently fluid for clinical manipulation and for incorporating enough filler to reinforce the cured resin are necessary. For example, a blend of 75% *bis*-GMA and 25% TEGDMA by weight has a viscosity of about 4.3 Pa•s, whereas the viscosity of a 50% *bis*-GMA/50% TEGDMA blend is about 0.2 Pa•s (similar to thin syrup). Unfortunately, these smaller, diluent monomers undergo greater polymerization shrinkage that generates more shrinkage stress, which may cause the formation of marginal gaps and increase the risk of eventual leakage and the problems that may result, partially offsetting the advantage of using large monomers such as *bis*-GMA.

CRITICAL QUESTION

What are the problems that result from shrinkage and cure-induced stress during the polymerization of restorative resins?

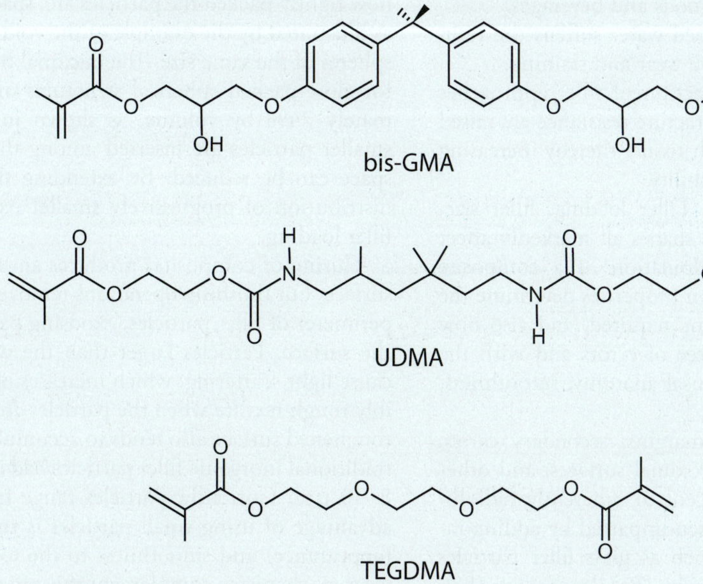

bis-GMA

UDMA

TEGDMA

• **Fig. 5.4** Chemical structure of bisphenol A glycidyl dimethacrylate (bis-GMA), urethane dimethacrylate (UDMA), and triethylene glycol dimethacrylate (TEGDMA).

Filler

Various transparent mineral fillers are employed to strengthen and reinforce composites as well as to reduce curing shrinkage and thermal expansion (generally between 30% and 70% by volume or 50% and 85% by weight of a composite). These include the so-called "soft glass" and borosilicate "hard glass", fused quartz, aluminum silicate, lithium aluminum silicate (beta-eucryptite, which has a negative coefficient of thermal expansion), ytterbium fluoride, and barium (Ba), strontium (Sr), zirconium (Zr), and zinc glasses. The latter five types of fillers impart radiopacity because of their heavy metal atoms.

Quartz had been used extensively as a filler in the early versions of dental composites. It has the advantage of being chemically inert but it is also very hard, making it abrasive to opposing teeth or restorations as well as difficult to grind into very fine particles; thus, it is also difficult to polish. The so-called amorphous silica has the same composition and refractive index as quartz; however, it is not crystalline and not as hard, thus, greatly reducing the abrasiveness of the composite surface structure and improving its polishability.

For acceptable esthetics, the translucency of a composite restoration must be similar to that of tooth structure. Thus, the index of refraction of the filler must closely match that of the resin. For *bis*-GMA and TEGDMA, the refractive indices are approximately 1.55 and 1.46, respectively, and a mixture of the two components in equal proportions by weight yields a refractive index of approximately 1.50. Most of the glasses and quartz used for fillers have refractive indices of approximately 1.50, which is adequate for sufficient translucency.

Function of Fillers

Fillers can provide the following benefits:

- **Reduction of polymerization shrinkage/contraction.** Although shrinkage varies from one commercial composite to another, it typically ranges from slightly less than 1% up to about 4% by volume.
- **Reduction in thermal expansion and contraction.** As the overall expansion coefficient decreases with filler loading and approaches that of tooth tissue, less interfacial stress is produced because of differential volumetric changes while an individual consumes hot and cold foods and beverages.
- **Decreased water sorption.** Absorbed water softens the resin and makes it more prone to abrasive wear and staining.
- **Reinforcement.** As the volume fraction of filler approaches approximately 70%, abrasion and fracture resistance are raised to levels approaching those of tooth tissue, thereby increasing both clinical performance and durability.
- **Control of workability/viscosity.** Filler loading, filler size, and the range of particle sizes and shapes all markedly affect the consistency and clinical manipulation of a composite paste. Consistency and manipulation properties determine the ease of operation, the skill and time required, and also how reliably a cavity can be restored free of errors and with the proper interproximal contact, occlusal anatomy, smoothness, and appearance.
- **Imparting radiopacity.** Leaking margins, secondary caries, poor proximal contacts, wear of proximal surfaces, and other problems cannot be detected adjacent to inherently radiolucent resins. Radiopacity is most often imparted by adding radiopaque inorganic compounds such as glass filler particles with heavy-metal atoms, such as barium (Ba), lanthanum (La), strontium (Sr), ytterbium (Yb), zinc (Zn), or zirconium (Zr). For optimal diagnostic contrast, the restoration should have a radiopacity approximately equal to that of enamel, which is about twice that of dentin. Exceeding the radiopacity of enamel by a large degree will have the effect of obscuring radiolucent areas caused by gap formation or secondary caries.
- **Fluoride release.** Ytterbium fluoride (YbF_3) and aluminofluorosilicate glass (traditionally used in glass ionomers) are able to release fluoride from dental composites.

CRITICAL QUESTION

Why is there a tradeoff among workability, durability, and esthetics when fillers are incorporated in resins?

Characteristic of Fillers

The most commonly used glass filler is barium (Ba) glass. Although glass fillers containing metals of a high atomic number provide radiopacity, they are not as inert as quartz and amorphous silica and are slowly leached and weakened in acidic liquids such as citrus juices, high pH solutions, and other oral fluids. The glass filler is also attacked over time by caries-protective acidulated phosphate fluoride solutions or gels. Because of differences in the composition of saliva among patients, it is difficult to predict the clinical effects of exposure to saliva. However, the implication is that glass-filled composites will gradually become more susceptible to abrasive wear and hence they will have a shorter functional lifetime compared with silica-reinforced resins.

For acceptable esthetics, the translucency of a composite restoration must be similar to that of tooth structure. Thus, the refractive index of the filler must closely match that of the resin. For *bis*-GMA and TEGDMA, the refractive indices are approximately 1.55 and 1.46, respectively, and a mixture of the two components in equal proportions by weight yields a refractive index of approximately 1.50. Most of the glasses and quartz used for fillers have refractive indices of approximately 1.50, which is adequate for sufficient translucency.

Most important properties are improved by increased filler loading. A *distribution* of particle sizes is used to maximize loading (volume fraction of filler). If particle size is uniform, no matter how tightly packed the particles are, spaces will exist among them, as illustrated by the example of the void spaces in a box filled with spheres of the same size. The maximal theoretical packing fraction for close-packed spherical structures of uniform-size is approximately 74% by volume, as shown in Figure 5.5. However, if smaller particles are inserted among the larger spheres, the void space can be reduced. By extending this process, a continuous distribution of progressively smaller particles can yield maximal filler loading.

Curing of composites produces an initially smooth, resin-rich surface, but finishing operations remove the resin matrix from the perimeter of filler particles, exposing particles that protrude from the surface. Particles larger than the wavelength of visible light cause light scattering, which increases opacity and produces a visibly rough texture when the particles are exposed at the surface. A roughened surface also tends to accumulate stains and plaque. The traditional inorganic filler particles had average diameters of about 8–40 μm. Currently, particles range from 5 nm to 2 μm. The advantage of using small particles is that they improve esthetics (appearance) and smoothness to the tongue (polishability). Oral wear mechanisms complement this process, such that the ultimate smoothness that can be maintained is highly dependent on particle size.

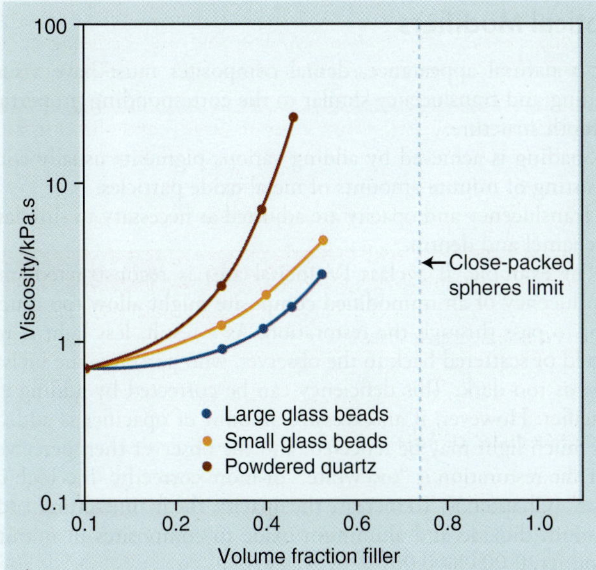

• **Fig. 5.5** The effect of filler-specific surface area on the viscosity (log scale) of the uncured resin matrix. The smaller the particle, the larger is the surface area and the greater the viscosity buildup. (Adapted from Darvell BW: *Materials Science for Dentistry*, ed 9, Woodhead Publishing Ltd, Cambridge, UK, 2009.)

However, the smaller the filler particle size, the higher the surface-to-volume ratio available to form polar or hydrogen bonds with monomer molecules to inhibit their flow and increase viscosity (resistance to mixing and manipulation) thus, the less filler that can be added. The proportion of filler is limited to about 80% by volume. Therefore, there is always a tradeoff among the requirements for workability, durability, and esthetics. The clinician's challenge is to make an informed judgment concerning the claims for the many products offered and to select one that is well suited to a particular clinical application.

Types of Fillers

Various transparent mineral fillers are employed in formulating composite resins. These include the so-called "soft glass" and borosilicate "hard glass;" fused quartz; aluminum silicate; lithium aluminum silicate (beta-eucryptite, which has a negative coefficient of thermal expansion); ytterbium fluoride; and barium, strontium, zirconium, and zinc glasses. More discussion on the particle size and fabrication of related fillers is provided later in the section on the classification of composites by filler particle size.

In the quest for improved aesthetics and, hence, smaller particle sizes, two filler systems, ormocer and polyhedral oligomeric silsesquioxane (POSS), in which a portion of the reinforcing component operates at molecular scale, have been introduced.

Ormocer

Ormocer is an acronym for *organically modified ceramics.* They are considered to be molecule-sized hybrid structures consisting of inorganic–organic copolymers. These molecular hybrids consist of, for example, methacrylate-terminated chains grafted onto a central cyclic polysiloxane 2- to 3-nm particle. These nanoparticles are dispersed on a molecular scale, and high-molecular-weight, flexible, relatively low-viscosity, crosslinkable molecules ("oligomers") result. The large spacing between crosslinks resulting from curing produces a low level of polymerization shrinkage, and the inorganic network provides abrasion resistance through the glasslike structure and low water sorption resulting from hydrophobicity.

Ormocers are used in the formulation of several commercial composites (e.g., Definite and Admira, Voco GmbH, Cuxhaven, Germany; Ceram-X, Dentsply International, York, PA). While the molecule-sized silicate particles provide some reinforcement, ground glass and/or other fillers are typically required for sufficient reinforcement. Therefore, ormocer is often considered as part of the matrix of the composite. Advantages of ormocer-based dental materials include limited cure shrinkage, very high biocompatibility, good manipulation properties, and excellent esthetics.

POSS

POSS is an acronym for *polyhedral oligomeric silsesquioxane.* The molecules are 12-sided silicate cages produced from silane and functionalized to copolymerize with other monomers. Silsesquioxane is a chemical structure with the composition $R_nSi_nO_{1.5n}$; for example, $(CH_3)_8Si_8O_{12}$. For the POSS materials used in dental applications, the R-group is typically a methacrylate (Fig. 5.6).

POSS is a molecule-sized hybrid organic–inorganic oligomeric compound that can disperse homogeneously in compatible monomers and become covalently incorporated into crosslinked networks upon curing. Like the ormocer-type materials, the silicate cage structures provide a reinforcing function, but filler particles must also be included to achieve the balance of mechanical and other properties required for adequate performance as dental composites. Depending on the dispersed filler, POSS-based resins are characterized as being highly polishable and having excellent polish retention, mechanical properties, and wear resistance. Current commercial products based on silsesquioxane technology include Artiste Nano-Hybrid Composite (Pentron Clinical, Wallingford, CT).

CRITICAL QUESTION

What roles do the coupling agents play in the function and performance of dental resins?

Coupling Agent

As stated previously, it is essential that filler particles be bonded to the resin matrix. This allows the more flexible polymer matrix to

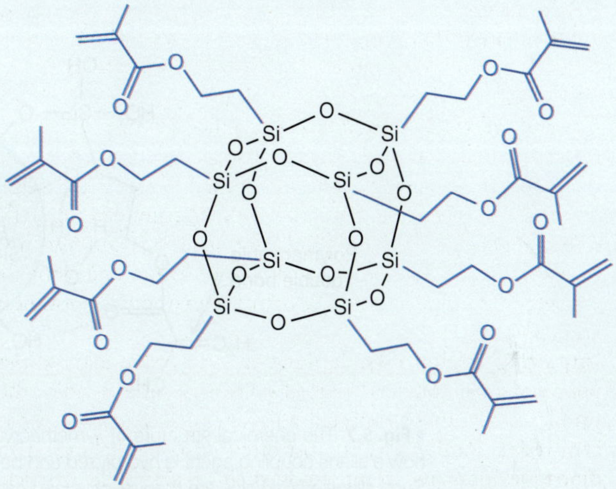

• **Fig. 5.6** Methacryl polyhedral oligomeric silsesquioxane, a 12-sided silicate cage structure having polymerizable methacrylate pendant groups. (Courtesy of Hybrid Plastics, Inc. Hattiesburg, MS.)

transfer stresses to the higher modulus (more rigid and stiffer) filler particles. The chemical bond between the two phases of the composite is formed by a coupling agent, a difunctional surface-active compound that adheres to filler particle surfaces and also co-reacts with the monomer forming the resin matrix. A properly applied coupling agent can impart improved physical and mechanical properties and inhibit leaching by preventing water from penetrating along the filler–resin interface.

Although titanates and zirconates can be used as coupling agents, organosilanes—such as γ-methacryloxypropyl trimethoxysilane—are used most commonly (Fig. 5.7). In the presence of water, the methoxy groups ($-OCH_3$) are hydrolyzed to silanol (–Si–OH) groups, which can bond with other silanols on the filler surfaces by forming siloxane bonds (–Si–O–Si–). The organosilane methacrylate groups form covalent bonds with the resin when the resin is polymerized, thereby completing the coupling process. Proper coupling by means of organosilanes is extremely important to the clinical performance of resin-based composite restorative materials.

Inhibitors

Inhibitors are added to resin systems to minimize or prevent spontaneous or accidental polymerization of monomers. Inhibitors have a strong reactivity potential with free radicals. If a free radical is formed, for example, by brief exposure to room lighting when the material is dispensed, the inhibitor reacts with the free radical faster than the free radical can react with the monomer. This prevents the initiation of monomers and subsequent chain propagation. After all of the inhibitor is consumed, chain propagation can begin. A typical inhibitor is butylated hydroxytoluene, which is used in concentrations on the order of 0.01% by weight. Thus, inhibitors have two functions: to extend the resin's storage life and to ensure sufficient working time.

Optical Modifiers

For a natural appearance, dental composites must have visual shading and translucency similar to the corresponding properties of tooth structure.

- Shading is achieved by adding various pigments usually consisting of minute amounts of metal oxide particles.
- Translucency and opacity are adjusted as necessary to simulate enamel and dentin.

For example, if a class IV incisal area is reconstructed, the translucency of an unmodified composite might allow too much light to pass through the restoration. As a result, less light is reflected or scattered back to the observer, who perceives the incisal edge as too dark. This deficiency can be corrected by adding an opacifier. However, if an excessive amount of opacifier is added, too much light may be reflected, and the observer then perceives that the restoration is "too white," or more correctly, "too high in value" (Chapter 3). To increase the opacity, the manufacturer adds titanium dioxide and aluminum oxide to composites in minute amounts (0.001%–0.007% by weight).

- All optical modifiers affect light transmission through a composite.
- Darker shades and greater opacities have a decreased depth of light-curing ability and require either an increased exposure time or a thinner layer when cured.
- Studies have shown that for optimal polymerization, resins with darker shades and opacifiers should be placed in thinner layers. This consideration has added importance when a bonding agent covered by a composite layer is being cured.

Classification of Dental Composites

As the variety of dental composites increases in response to new innovations and needs, there are also several ways of classifying

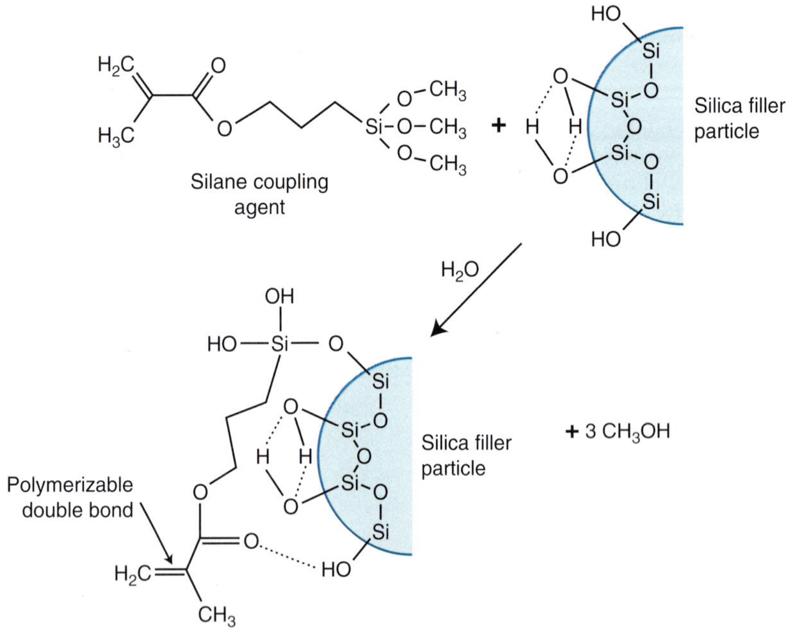

• **Fig. 5.7** The chemical structure of γ-methacryl-oxypropyltrimethoxy silane and an idealized diagram of how a silane coupling agent is hydrolyzed and becomes attached to silica and glass filler particle surfaces. Such silanized particles are then reactive and can "couple" the particles to the resin matrix by copolymerization with the double bond in the silane propylmethacrylate group ($CH_2{=}C(CH_3)COO{-}C_3H_6{-}Si{-}$). (Data taken from Söderholm K-J M and Shang S-W: Molecular orientation of silane at the surface of colloidal silica. *J Dent Res* 72:1050−1054, 1993.)

dental composites, depending on various aspects of the composites. A useful classification system for composites is one based on filler particle size and size distribution, as shown in Table 5.1.

Dental composites can also be classified based on

- Classification by filler particle size,
- Curing method,
- Manipulation characteristics,
- Application,
- Unique characteristics, and
- Any combination of these.

Classification by Filler Particle Size

The classification of fillers by particle size is shown in Table 5.2. In conjunction with the chronology of dental composite developments shown in Figure 5.1, it can be seen that the distribution and average size of filler particles played a major role in the advancement of dental composites. As such, a classification of dental composites based on the filler particle size can be used (Table 5.1).

Traditional/Large-Particle/Macrofill Composites

These are the traditional composites with glass or silica macrofiller particles in the size range of between 8 and 40 μm (Fig. 5.2). Because of their large particle size, these composites have lower relative viscosity and are easier to fill at higher loadings than microfills and nanofills. As such, they tend to be stronger and can be used in high-stress areas. However, the visibly rough texture after polishing, caused by the exposure of larger particles, has made this category of dental composite obsolete.

TABLE 5.2 Classification of Reinforcing Filler Particles by Size Range

Class of Filler	Particle Size
Macrofillers	10–100 μm
Small/fine fillers	0.1–10 μm
Midfillers	1–10 μm
Minifillers	0.1–1 μm
Microfillers	0.01–0.1 μm (agglomerated)
Nanofillers	0.005–0.1 μm[a]

[a]5–100 nm, nonagglomerated.

Homogeneous Microfill Composites

The solution to rough surfaces and an opaque appearance was the homogeneous microfill composites, which used filler particles with a mean diameter much smaller than the wavelength of visible light. Such fillers are made by a pyrolytic precipitation process where a silicon compound such as $SiCl_4$ is burned in an oxygen/hydrogen atmosphere to form macromolecular chains of colloidal silica (see Fig. 5.8), resulting in *amorphous silica* with an average size of 40 nm.

However, these particles, because of their extremely small size, have extremely large surface areas ranging from 50 to 400 m^2/g. In addition, the pyrolytic process results in particle "agglomeration" into long, molecular-scale chains (Figs 5.9 and 5.10). These nondiscrete, 3-D, chainlike networks drastically increase monomer viscosity and make clinical manipulation difficult. Thus, filler incorporation at high enough loading to adequately reinforce the resin is difficult. In fact, when incorporated directly in "homogeneous" microfill composites, only about 2% by weight produces a stiff paste that is much too viscous for clinical manipulation (Fig. 5.5). They are often just called *microfill composite.*

CRITICAL QUESTION

Why is the polymerization shrinkage of microfilled (heterogeneous microfill) composites not higher than that of conventional composites even though the inorganic filler loading in microfill is substantially lower?

Microfilled (Heterogeneous Microfill) Composites

To increase the inorganic filler loading of microfill composites, a resin-based filler loaded with 10- to 100-nm inorganic colloidal silica is used instead. These resin-based, heterogeneous fillers are made by incorporating about 50 vol% of silane-treated colloidal silica microfiller into the monomer at a slightly elevated temperature to lower the viscosity and by using large industrial machines capable of mixing high-viscosity blends. The mixture is cured and then pulverized to make a filled resin powder consisting of 5- to 50-μm particles. These amorphous colloidal silica-containing particles are then used as an "organic" filler, which is incorporated into the monomer with additional silane-treated colloidal silica to form a workable paste. In this way, the overall *inorganic* filler content of the final, cured composite is increased to about 50% by weight. However, if the composite particles are counted as filler particles, the filler content is closer to 80% by weight (approximately 60% by volume). A diagram representing the preparation of the filler in microfilled resins of this type is shown in Figure 5.11. This class of material is called *heterogeneous microfill* or *microfilled composite.*

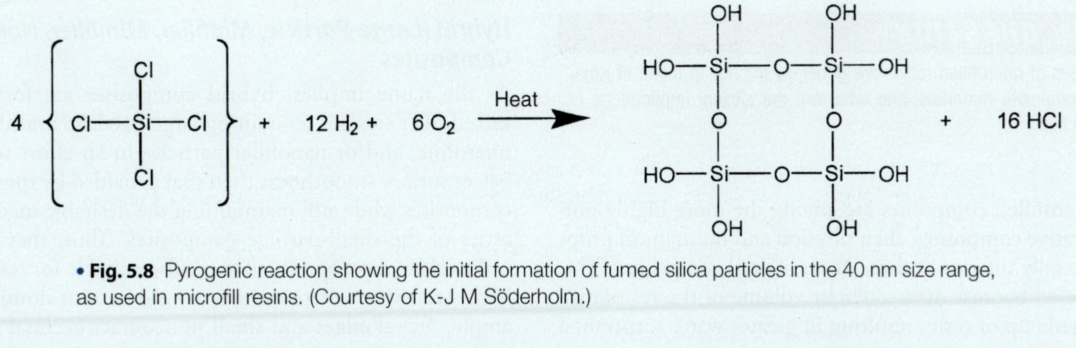

$$4\left\{\begin{array}{c} Cl \\ | \\ Cl{-}Si{-}Cl \\ | \\ Cl \end{array}\right\} + 12\,H_2 + 6\,O_2 \xrightarrow{\text{Heat}} \begin{array}{c} OH \qquad\quad OH \\ | \qquad\qquad | \\ HO{-}Si{-}O{-}Si{-}OH \\ | \qquad\qquad | \\ O \qquad\qquad O \\ | \qquad\qquad | \\ HO{-}Si{-}O{-}Si{-}OH \\ | \qquad\qquad | \\ OH \qquad\quad OH \end{array} + 16\,HCl$$

• **Fig. 5.8** Pyrogenic reaction showing the initial formation of fumed silica particles in the 40 nm size range, as used in microfill resins. (Courtesy of K-J M Söderholm.)

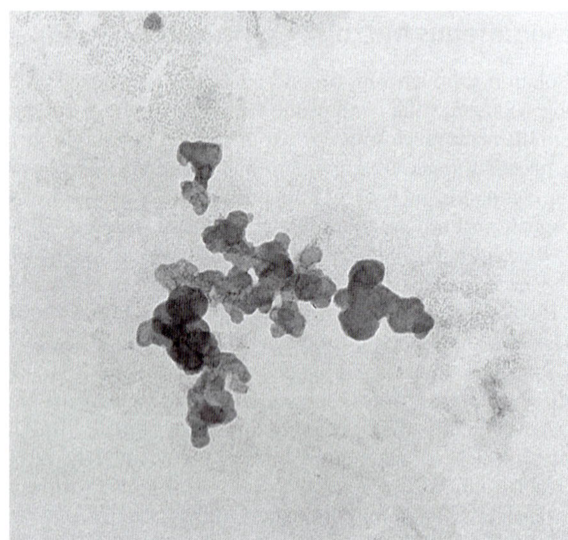

• **Fig. 5.9** Transmission electron microscopic image of fumed silica particles produced by the pyrogenic reaction shown in Figure 5.8. The particle diameters average approximately 0.04 μm or 40 nm. (Courtesy of K-J M Söderholm.)

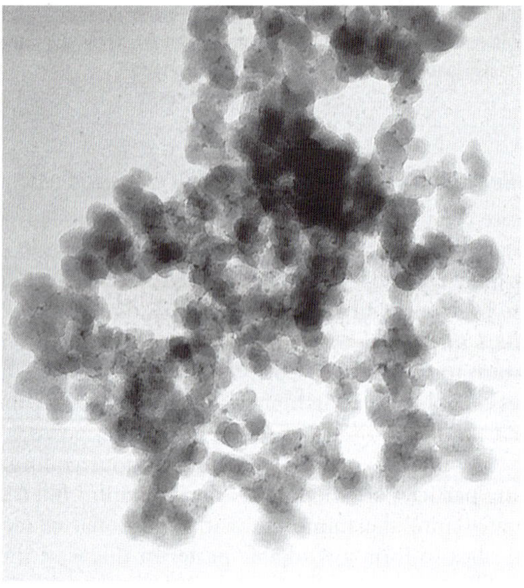

• **Fig. 5.10** The pyrogenic silica used in microfilled composites has a very large total surface area because of its extremely small average particle size of about 0.04 μm/40 nm. These particles agglomerate and form long chains, as seen in this transmission electron micrograph. The chains of silica particles act similarly to resin polymer chains, as described in Chapter 6, and dramatically increase the viscosity of the monomer. (Courtesy of K-J M Söderholm.)

CRITICAL QUESTION

Which properties of microfilled resins are generally inferior to those of other resin-based composite materials, and what are the clinical implications of these deficiencies?

While microfilled composites are among the more highly polishable restorative composites, their physical and mechanical properties are generally inferior to those of traditional composites. This is to be expected because 40%–80% by volume of the restorative material is made up of resin, resulting in greater water sorption, a

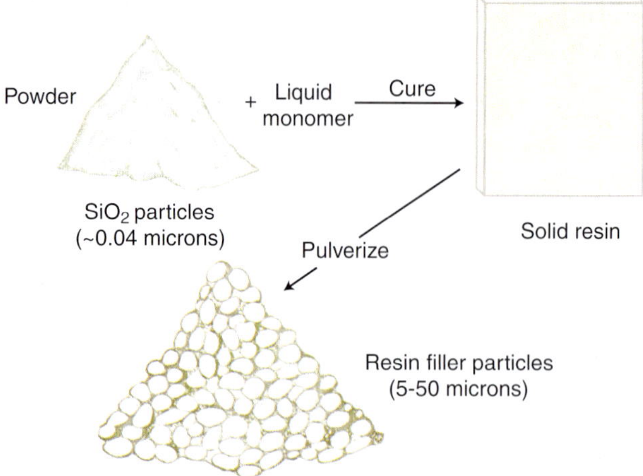

• **Fig. 5.11** Preparation of resin filler particles for use in microfilled composites. The filler particles in a microfilled composite consist of pulverized "composite filler particles" dispersed in a cured resin matrix. Pyrogenic colloidal silica particles of about 0.04 μm (about 40 nm) are incorporated into both the precured resin filler particles and the curable monomer, with the precured resin containing a substantially higher concentration. (Modified from P Lambrechts: *Basic Properties of Dental Composites and Their Impact on Clinical Performance*. Thesis. Leuven, Belgium, Katholieke University, 1983.)

higher coefficient of thermal expansion, and decreased elastic modulus. In addition, the weak bond of the prepolymerized particles to the clinically cured resin matrix results in decreased tensile strength, similar to that of composites with nonsilanized filler particles. Table 5.3 shows various properties of different types of composites for reference.

CRITICAL QUESTION

What features of microfilled resins make them the material of choice for certain types of restorations?

Which types of restorations are produced ideally from microfilled composites?

In the longer term, if microfilled composites are placed in wear-prone areas, they eventually break down and wear at a rate too fast for acceptable clinical performance. If placed in areas of proximal contact, anterior tooth "drifting" may occur. The wear process has also been related to fracture propagation around the poorly bonded "organic" filler particles (Fig. 5.12). Thus, diamond burs, rather than fluted tungsten-carbide burs, are recommended for trimming microfilled composites so as to minimize the risk of chipping. Microfilled composites are the resins of choice for restoring teeth with carious lesions in smooth surfaces (classes III and V) but not in stress-bearing situations (classes II and IV).

Hybrid (Large-Particle, Midfiller, Minifiller, Nanohybrid) Composites

As the name implies, hybrid composites are formulated with mixed filler systems containing large-particle, midfiller, minifiller, microfine, and/or nanofiller particles in an effort to obtain even better surface smoothness than that provided by the small-particle composites while still maintaining the desirable mechanical properties of the small-particle composites. Thus, they are a general utility class of composite that are also suitable for restoring certain high-stress sites where esthetic considerations dominate—for example, incisal edges and small noncontact occlusal cavities. They

TABLE 5.3 Properties of Composite Restorative Materials

Characteristic/Property	Unfilled Acrylic	Traditional	Hybrid (Small-Particle)	Hybrid (All-Purpose)	Microfilled	Flowable Hybrid	Packable Hybrid	Enamel	Dentin
Size (μm)	—	8–12	0.5–3	0.4–1.0	0.04–0.4	0.6–1.0	Fibrous	—	—
Inorganic filler (vol%)	0	60–70	65–77	60–65	20–59	30–55	48–67		
Inorganic filler (wt%)	0	70–80	80–90	75–80	35–67	40–60	65–81	—	—
Compressive strength (MPa)	70	250–300	350–400	300–350	250–350	—	—	384	297
Tensile strength (MPa)	24	50–65	75–90	40–50	30–50	—	40–45	10	52
Elastic modulus (GPa)	2.4	8–15	15–20	11–15	3–6	4–8	3–13	84	18
Thermal expansion coefficient (ppm/°C)	92.8	25–35	19–26	30–40	50–60	—	—	—	—
Water sorption (mg/cm²)	1.7	0.5–0.7	0.5–0.6	0.5–0.7	1.4–1.7	—	—	—	—
Knoop hardness (KHN)	15	55	50–60	50–60	25–35	—	—	350–430	68
Curing shrinkage (vol%)	8–10	—	2–3	2–3	2–3	3–5	2–3	—	—
Radiopacity (mm Al)	0.1	2–3	2–3	2–4	0.5–2	1–4	2–3	2	1

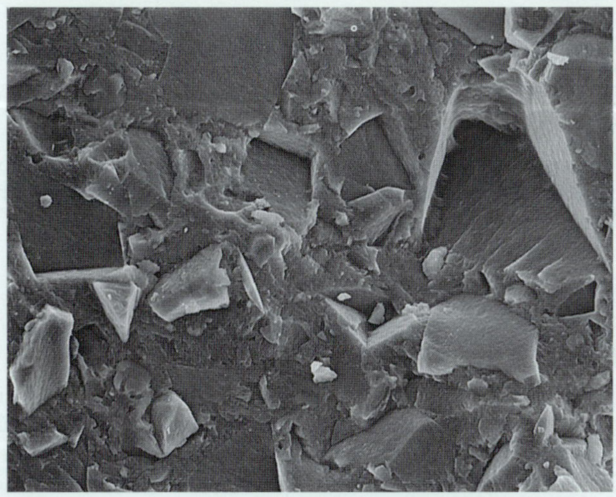

• **Fig. 5.12** Fractured microfilled composite. The fractured surface shows that the organic filler (composite filler) particles have been plucked out of the matrix resin, suggesting adhesive failure due to a weak interface between the precured microfill particles and the clinically cured resin. (Courtesy of K-J M Söderholm.)

are widely used for anterior restorations, including class IV sites (Fig. 5.13). Most commercial hybrid composites are marketed as nanohybrids because they are supposed to contain discrete nanofillers, but whether that is true or not, any hybrid could be marketed as a nanohybrid because hybrids contain nanoparticles. Thus, checking whether the nanoparticles are discrete, in aggregates, or in clusters is important.

- Most modern hybrid fillers consist of colloidal silica and ground particles of glasses containing heavy metals constituting a filler content of approximately 75%–80% by weight.
- The glasses have an average particle size of about 0.4–1.0 μm, with a trend to steadily reduce this size range as improvements are made.
- In a typical size distribution, 75% of the ground particles are smaller than 1.0 μm, and colloidal silica represents 10%–20% by weight of the total filler content.

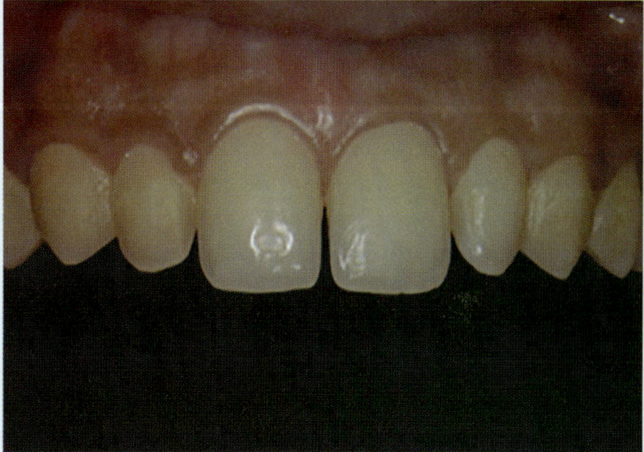

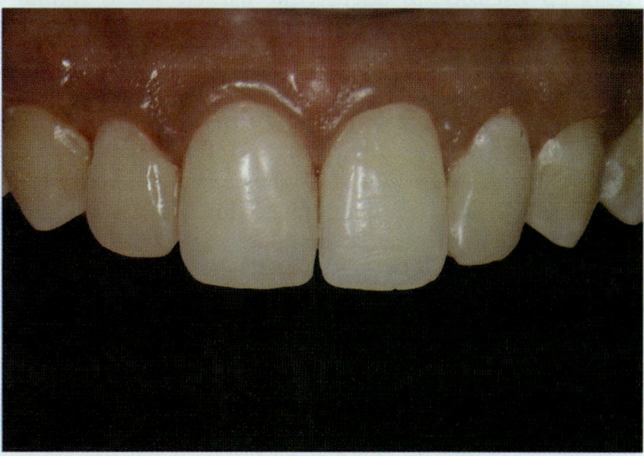

• **Fig. 5.13** Diastema closure of multiple anteriors using a hybrid composite. These restorations of the teeth produced a highly esthetic result. (Courtesy of Arvind Shenoy.)

- The smaller microfiller sizes increase the surface area, which generally increases the viscosity and requires a decrease in overall filler loading compared with small-particle composites. A polished surface is shown in Figure 5.14.

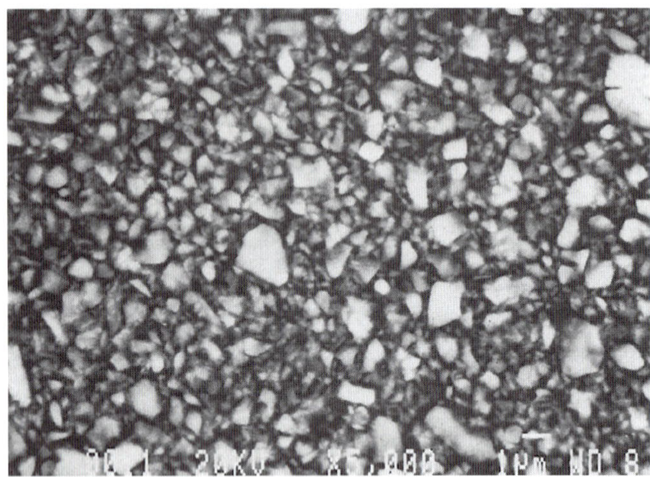

• **Fig. 5.14** Polished surface of a hybrid composite similar to that shown in Figure 5.13. Particle sizes range from about 0.1 to 3 μm (SEM magnification ×5000). (Courtesy of Robert L Erickson.)

CRITICAL QUESTION

How can the particle size and size distribution of resin-based composites be used to select clinical materials for various restorative situations?

Compared with amalgam, what disadvantages are associated with the use of resin composites as esthetic posterior resins?

Nanofilled Composites/Nanocomposites/Nanohybrid Composites

More recently, nanoparticles (1–100 nm) have been fabricated by a different method from the pyrolytic precipitation process used for colloidal silica. This allows the individual, primary particles to be surface-coated (with γ-methacryloxypropyltrimethoxysilane, for example) *prior* to becoming incorporated into three-dimensional macromolecule chains, thereby preventing or limiting particle agglomeration into large networks and driving up viscosity. In essence, the particle size is similar to that in microfilled composites, but the difference is that the particles in microfilled composites are in three-dimensional agglomerates or networks that increase viscosity whereas those in nanofilled composites are mostly discrete and have a minimal effect on viscosity. Thus, these composites have optical properties and superior polishability like those of microfilled composites, but the surface treatment reduces the increase in viscosity when incorporated into the monomer, which allows an increased filler loading of upwards of 60% by volume and 78% by weight. Filler loading in this range is expected to lead to the necessary mechanical properties for use in posterior, stress-bearing restorations, but these properties have not yet been confirmed.

One of the reasons that increased mechanical properties are not observed is that no commercial products have as yet been reported to contain only isolated, discrete, homogeneously dispersed nanoparticles as the sole filler component. In fact, few if any dental resins currently designated as nanocomposites meet the strict requirement of having essentially all filler less than 100 nm. This is because some of the nanoparticles exist as loosely bound "clusters" (loose agglomerates, such as in Filtek Supreme, 3M ESPE) of primary nanoparticles, which are sometimes reported to extend into the micron size range (e.g., 60 nm to 1.4 μm). Above 100 nm, clusters, like any particles, begin to scatter visible light and thereby reduce the translucency and the **depth of cure** of the composite. In addition, these clusters are not chemically bound to each other and act to decrease mechanical properties. Thus, while these nanocomposites with clusters have increased filler loading and hence better mechanical properties than a true homogeneous nanocomposite, they are not as strong as a hybrid composite or a microfilled composite.

To combat this deficiency, larger particles of either finely ground glass or precured nanoparticle-filled resin organic filler particles (essentially the same as those found in the microfilled composites) are combined with the monomer-dispersed nanoparticles. Thus, most, if not all, of these products are more accurately designated as "hybrid" nanocomposites or nanohybrids consisting of a blend of two or more size ranges of filler particles, one or more of which is in the nanoparticle range (see Table 5.1).

CRITICAL QUESTION

What are the relationships and tradeoffs among particle size, composition, and percentage of filler relative to their effect on manipulation consistency, polishability, radiopacity, durability, and appearance of resin-based composite materials?

Classification of Composites by Manipulation Characteristics

There are three distinct classes of composite materials based on the flow characteristics of the composite materials during the placement:

- Flowable
- Condensable
- Bulk fill

Flowable Composites

A modification of the small-particle composite and hybrid composite results in the so-called flowable composites, which have become popular since 1995. These resins typically have a lower viscosity through a reduced filler loading, which enables the resin to flow readily, spread uniformly, intimately adapt to a cavity form, and produce the desired dental anatomy. This improves the clinician's ability to form a well-adapted cavity base or liner, especially in class II posterior preparations and other situations in which access is difficult. However, while these materials tend to be less sticky during handling than microfills and hybrids, they are inherently inferior in mechanical properties owing to the lower filler loading and higher susceptibility to wear and other forms of attrition. Because of their greater ease of adaptation and flexibility as a cured material, flowable composites are also useful in class I restorations in gingival areas. They may also be applied in a manner similar to the use of fissure sealants as minimal class I restorations to prevent caries.

Condensable (Packable) Composites

Compared with amalgam, the technique of composite placement is far more time-consuming and demanding. Because of their highly plastic, paste-like consistency in the precured state, composites cannot be packed vertically into a cavity in such a way that the material flows laterally as well as vertically to ensure intimate contact with the cavity walls. In particular, the restoration of a tooth in which a proximal contact with the adjacent tooth is required, the paste consistency of most composites dictates that a matrix band be carefully contoured and wedged to obtain an acceptable proximal contact. These are tedious, time-consuming procedures and can produce variable results without a high level of skill. Packable composites, also known as condensable composites, were developed by adjusting their filler distribution to increase the strength and stiffness of the uncured material. They have consistency and handling characteristics similar to lathe-cut amalgam.

Specifically the packable/condensable characteristics are derived from the inclusion of elongated, fibrous filler particles of about 100 μm in length and/or rough-textured surfaces or branched geometries that tend to interlock and resist flow. This causes the uncured resin to be stiff and resistant to slumping yet moldable under the force of amalgam condensers. Rough surfaces and blends of fibrous and particulate fillers produce a packable consistency and enable other properties to be optimized for clinical performance. In certain products, larger than average filler particles (15–80 μm) are used, and the resin matrix is modified chemically to allow a slight increase in filler content over hybrids. Some have the same filler particles as their companion hybrids from the same manufacturer; and the only difference is that the resin matrix is adjusted to allow approximately 1%–2% of additional filler loading. However, many of the limitations of resin composites still prevail, and approximately twice the time required for amalgam placement is needed. At present, these materials have not demonstrated any advantageous properties or characteristics over the hybrid resins other than being somewhat similar to amalgam in their placement technique. Despite manufacturers' claims to the contrary, packable composites have not yet proven to be an answer to the general need for highly wear-resistant, easily placed posterior resins with low curing shrinkage and a depth of cure greater than 2 mm.

Bulk Fill Composites

In the recent past a new variety of composite resins have been launched which claim to provide ease of use with large increments.

Two types of bulk-filled composites are available:

- Low-viscosity materials like Venus Bulk Fill (Heraus Kulzer; Hanau, Germany), Filtek Bulk Fill (3M ESPE), and SureFil SDR (Dentsply Caulk) are placed in 4-mm increments. Low-viscosity composites are generally used as dentin replacement layers or are recommended for small occlusal restorations. They have lower filler rates, and most wear more than highly filled composites.
- High-viscosity bulk placement materials such as Tetric EvoCeram Bulk Fill (Ivoclar Vivadent; Amherst, NY) handle like highly filled composite resins. They can be used to restore large preparations, and have 4 mm depths of cure depending upon the shade and curing light used. Adding new photo-initiators like Ivocerin (Ivoclar Vivadent) increase the depth of cure for Tetric EvoCeram Bulk Fill, while combining this with a photo-inhibitor creates adequate working time.

Bulk fill composites should ideally satisfy the following requirements:

- They must have low polymerization shrinkage stress to decrease microleakage and counter polymerization shrinkage, reducing stress by exhibiting some elasticity.
- Should demonstrate an improved depth of cure, at least 4 mm, which is accomplished by being translucent and highly conducive to light transmission.
- They should be more flowable to allow for easy cavity adaptation, including in cervical margins and existing boxes.
- Should have good compressive strength and wear resistance.

Bulk-fill composites typically have good mechanical properties within the range of universal composites (transverse strength ~120 to 160 MPa and elastic modulus ~10 GPa) with very low shrinkage (<2% volumetrically). One study reported that despite being placed in a 4-mm layer, SDR Flow (Dentsply) performed just as well clinically as a nanohybrid placed in 2-mm layers after 5 years.

Because of the use of an amine-based activator, dual-cured bulk-fill composites are expected to have poorer initial color and color stability. Also, some studies have shown that only a few bulk-fill composites had volumetric shrinkages <2% and that shrinkages may be more in the range between 1.7% and 3.5%. Finally, volumetric shrinkages are not well correlated to the production of shrinkage stress because shrinkage stress is not a material property, and various factors, such as rate of polymerization and composite modulus, affect shrinkage stress. In fact, the method of shrinkage-stress measurement strongly affects the measured stress values and sometimes, even sample ranking. Thus, although shrinkage stress may be more important than volumetric shrinkage in predicting composite longevity, using this parameter to compare products is more difficult, and relative rankings would need to be used instead.

Bulk-fill composites may be too translucent to be esthetic. To address this concern, monomers that change in refractive index as they polymerize have been used so that this will match with the filler's refractive index before curing to allow deep light penetration. However, as the cure progresses, the composite will become opaquer and achieve a better match with the surrounding tooth structure. Examples include 3M Filtek One Bulk Fill Smart Contrast Ratio Management system and Ivoclar Tetric EvoCeram Bulk Fill Aessencio Technology.

The most recent advancement in bulk-fill composites is the introduction of bulk-fill flowable composites. Most of these products are recommended as the first layer of a restoration like conventional flowable composites, except this time, the first layer could be 4 mm (e.g., 3M Bulk Fill Flowable and Ivoclar Vivadent EvoFlow Bulk Fill). Thus, only a second top esthetic layer is needed to complete the restoration, and often the corresponding bulk-fill composites from the same company are recommended with these bulk-fill flowables. The methods in making these bulk-curable are similar to those in regular bulk-fill composites, except the filler loading tends to be significantly lower to decrease viscosity (64–73 wt% vs 77–87 wt% in conventional bulk-fill composites), and thixotropic properties are used to make these composites injectable. Despite that, transverse strengths are still in the range of regular bulk-fill composites (120–173 MPa), but the elastic modulus is lower, with some products having a deliberately lower modulus to reduce polymerization shrinkage stress (1.1–2.1 MPa) despite having higher volumetric shrinkage (2.5%–3.5%). Examples include 3M Bulk Fill Flowable and Shofu Beautifil Bulk Flowable. A lower elastic modulus means the material is not as stiff, and hence, some polymerization stress is relieved.

CRITICAL QUESTION

What are the similarities and differences in the mechanisms involved in chemical-activated and light-activated dental resins?

Classification by Curing Method

Methacrylate-functionalized monomers polymerize by the addition polymerization mechanism (also known as *chain-growth polymerization*) initiated by free radicals. Free radicals can be generated by chemical activation or by external energy activation (heat, light, or microwave). Because dental composites for direct placement use chemical activation, light activation, or a combination of the two, only these systems are discussed here.

Chemical-Activated (Self-cured) Resins

Chemical-activated resins are supplied as two pastes, one of which contains the benzoyl peroxide initiator, and the other contains monomers and an aromatic tertiary amine activator (e.g., N, N-dimethyl-p-toluidine). When the two pastes are mixed together, the amine activates the benzoyl peroxide to form free radicals, and addition polymerization is initiated. There are inherent limitations with chemical activation. First, air is incorporated during mixing, leading to the formation of pores that weaken the structure and trap oxygen, which inhibits polymerization on the inner surfaces of the pores.

Second, the operator has no control over the working time after the two components have been mixed. Therefore, both insertion and contouring must be completed quickly once the resin components are mixed. Thus, today they are mainly used for restorations and large foundation structures (buildups) that are not readily cured with a light source.

Third, the reactivity of oxygen to a radical is much higher than that of a monomer inhibiting polymerization on the surface. During the inhibition period, this oxygen diffuses into the resin and is consumed by the radicals formed. This reaction forms an oxygen-inhibited layer. The thickness of the oxygen-inhibited layer is dependent on the viscosity of the resin, the solubility of oxygen in the monomer, and the initiating system used.

Fourth, self-cured resins tend to have higher initial color and lower color stability as a result of the aromatic amine. This is another reason self-cured resins are not used as direct restorations.

Table 5.4 lists the advantages and disadvantages of chemical-activated resins.

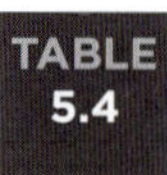

TABLE 5.4 Advantages and Disadvantages of Chemically Activated (Self-cure) Resins

Advantages	Disadvantages
Convenience and simplicity: no equipment needed, hazard-free Long-term storage stability	Mixing causes air entrapment, leading to porosity that weakens the material and increases susceptibility to staining. This has been reduced by the use of mixing syringes
Manipulation of working/setting time by varying proportions	Aromatic amine accelerators oxidize and turn yellow with time—i.e., color instability
Degree of cure equal throughout material if mixed properly	Difficult to mix evenly, causing unequal degree of cure and consequent poor mechanical properties
Marginal stress buildup during curing is much lower than for photocured resins owing to relatively slower rates of cross-link formation	

Light-Activated (Light-Cured) Resins

To overcome the problems associated with chemical activation, systems using a photosensitive initiator system and a light source for activation were developed. The first light-activated systems were formulated for UV light, which has been replaced by visible blue-light–activated systems, with great improvements in the quality of the cured composites (Box 5.2). Light-curable dental composites are supplied as a single paste contained in a light-proof syringe or capsule because there is no chemical activator in the material. The free radical–initiating system, consisting of a photosensitizer and an amine co-initiator, is contained in this paste. As long as these two components are not exposed to light, they do not interact. However, exposure to light in the blue region (wavelength of about 468 nm) produces an excited state of the photosensitizer, which then interacts with the amine to form free radicals that initiate addition polymerization (Fig. 5.15). Camphorquinone (CQ) is a commonly used photosensitizer that absorbs blue light with wavelengths between 400 and 500 nm. Only small quantities of CQ are required (0.2% by weight or less in the paste). A number of amine initiators are suitable for interaction with CQ, such as dimethylaminoethyl methacrylate (DMAEMA), which is also present at low levels of about 0.15% by weight.

In addition to avoiding the porosity of chemical-activated resins, light-activated materials allow the operator to complete insertion and contouring before curing is initiated. Furthermore, once curing is initiated, an exposure time of 40 s or less is required to light-cure a 2-mm-thick layer, compared with several minutes for self-cured materials. Finally, light-cured systems are not as sensitive to oxygen inhibition as are the self-cured systems. Because of these advantages, visible light–activated composites are more widely used than chemical-activated materials.

However, light-cured composites have inherent limitations. For example, they must be placed incrementally when the bulk exceeds approximately 2–3 mm because of the limited depth of light penetration. Thus, light-cured composites can actually require more time when making large restorations (e.g., in class II cavity preparations). The depth of cure has been raised to at least 4 mm with the development of bulk-fill composites (see Bulk-Fill Composites section). Other issues are related to the light-curing unit and are discussed in three areas: the curing lamps, the depth of cure, and the safety precautions for using lamps.

Table 5.5 lists the advantages and disadvantages of light-activated resins. Box 5.1 and 5.2 provide clinical recommendations for placement of light activated composite resins.

CRITICAL QUESTION

What are the tradeoffs among the several types of light sources used to photoactivate dental restorative resins?

Curing Lamps

The two main types of lamps currently used for photoinitiation of the polymerization process are quartz–tungsten–halogen (QTH) lamps and LED lamps, with LED lamps quickly overtaking QTH lamps in popularity.

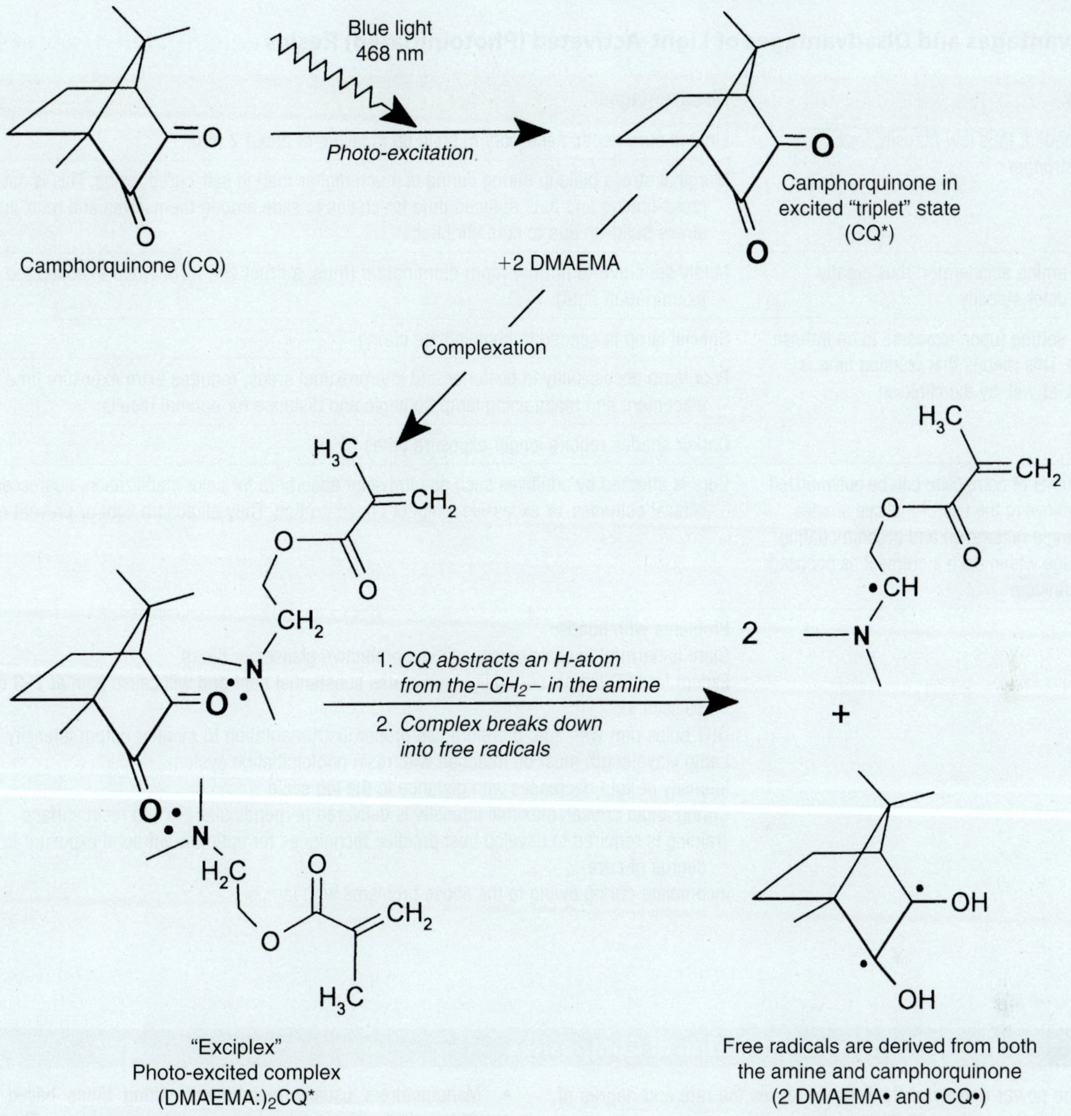

Blue light
468 nm
Photo-excitation
Camphorquinone (CQ)
Camphorquinone in excited "triplet" state (CQ*)
+2 DMAEMA
Complexation
"Exciplex"
Photo-excited complex
(DMAEMA:)$_2$CQ*
1. CQ abstracts an H-atom from the–CH_2– in the amine
2. Complex breaks down into free radicals
Free radicals are derived from both the amine and camphorquinone
(2 DMAEMA• and •CQ•)

• **Fig. 5.15** The light-cured process is activated when a diketone photosensitizer such as camphorquinone (CQ) absorbs a quantum of blue light and forms an excited-state complex (exciplex) with an electron donor such as an amine (e.g., dimethylaminoethyl methacrylate [DMAEMA]). In the figure, "••" denotes the unshared pair of electrons "donated" by the amines to the > C = O (ketone) groups in CQ. While in this activated complex, CQ extracts a hydrogen atom from the α-carbon adjacent to the amine group, and the complex decomposes into amine and CQ free radicals. The CQ free radical is readily inactivated. Thus, in photoinitiation, only the amine-free radicals act to initiate the addition polymerization reaction (see Fig. 6.8).

QTH or halogen lamps have a quartz bulb with a tungsten filament that irradiates both UV and white light, which must be filtered to remove heat and all wavelengths except those in the violet-blue range (about 400–500 nm) to match the photoabsorption range of CQ. The irradiance of the bulb (200–400 mW/cm^2) diminishes with use, so a calibration meter is required to measure the irradiance.

LED lamps use a solid-state electronic process to emit radiation only in the blue part of the visible spectrum, between 440 and 480 nm, and do not require filters. LEDs require low wattage, can be battery-powered and cordless, generate very little heat, and are quiet because no cooling fan is needed. Initially, they produced similar irradiance as QTH lamps (200–400 mW/cm^2), but the latest versions are more intense and use two or more LED units to both increase irradiance (>1000 mW/m^2) and extend the wavelength range. As such, significantly less time is needed to cure the composite using LED lamps. Their light bulbs are also cheaper to replace (up to a third of the price of QTH light bulbs) and more reliable.

CRITICAL QUESTION

What are the benefits and drawbacks of increasing the irradiance of curing lamps?

TABLE 5.5 Advantages and Disadvantages of Light-Activated (Photoinitiated) Resins

Advantages	Disadvantages
No mixing needed: thus low porosity, less staining, stronger	Limited cure depth: necessary to build up in layers of about 2 mm
	Marginal stress buildup during curing is much higher than in self-cured resins. This is due to faster cross-linking and thus reduced time for chains to slide among themselves and relax interfacial stress build-up due to cure shrinkage
No aromatic amine accelerator: thus greatly improved color stability	Mildly sensitive to normal room illumination (thus, a crust will form when exposed too long to an examination light)
"Command" setting (upon exposure to an intense blue light). This means that working time is controlled, at will, by the clinician	Special lamp is needed to photoinitiate curing
	Poor lamp accessibility in posterior and interproximal areas; requires extra exposure time and care in placement and maintaining lamp tip angle and distance for optimal results
	Darker shades require longer exposure times
Small increments of composite can be polymerized at a time allowing the use of multiple shades within a single restoration and accommodating for shrinkage within each increment as opposed to bulk shrinkage	Cure is affected by additives such as ultraviolet absorbers for color stabilization, fluorescent dyes for clinical esthetics, or excessive inhibitor concentration. They all absorb light or prevent reaction.
	Problems with lamps: Glare is harmful to clinic personnel; use protective glasses or filters Except for LED lamps, curing light generates substantial heat and will cause pain at 2–3 mm in about 20 seconds QHT bulbs dim with age; therefore use proper instrumentation to monitor output intensity Lamp wavelength must be matched with resin photoinitiation system Intensity of light decreases with distance to the log scale Curing angle critical; maximal intensity is delivered perpendicular (90°) to resin surface Training is required to develop best practice techniques for optimum intraoral exposure to maximize degree of cure Incomplete curing owing to the above problems with lamps

• BOX 5.1 Factors Influencing Light Curing of Composites

- Increasing the power density of the lamp increases the rate and degree of cure. However, faster curing with higher intensity light sources can increase shrinkage stress
- Increased intensity will allow either shorter curing times for a given depth of cure or increased depth of cure for a given exposure time. The practical consequence is that curing depth is limited to 2–3 mm unless excessively long exposure times are used, regardless of lamp intensity
- Manufacturers usually recommend curing times based on a particular curing device for each shade and type of resin. *These recommended times are typically the absolute minimum required*
- Darker shades and greater opacities have a decreased depth of light-curing ability and require either an increased exposure time or a thinner layer when cured

• BOX 5.2 Clinical Recommendations for Placement of Composite Resins

- The adhesive preparation design requires maximum preservation of remaining tooth structure, and there is no extension for prevention. Healthy tooth structure should only be removed when the occlusal outline requires extension to a point within or beyond the functional stops
- The preparation is limited to what is needed for access to the lesion or defect, since composite requires less volume to resist clinical fracture than does amalgam
- To allow for a better resin adaptation, all internal line angles should be rounded and cavity walls should be smooth
- The occlusal cavosurface margin should not be beveled; this increases the width of the preparation and may infringe on the centric holding area, increasing the wear rate of the restoration
- When one is replacing old G V Black style amalgam or composite restorations, which invariably have high C, factor shrinkage some technique modifications are indicated:
- Option 1: Use RMGIC as a liner to replace missing dentin
- Option 2: Use strategic and incremental layering of flowable composite or bulk fill composite to rebuild the dentin
- Subsequently build up cusps incrementally, with hybrid or nanocomposites following which the cusps can be cross-linked. Do not fill the cavity horizontally
- Opposing enamel walls should not be contacted by the same increment; this will minimize the wall-to-wall shrinkage and thus reduce intercuspal stress

Polymerization is initiated when a critical concentration of free radicals is formed. This requires that a particular number of photons be absorbed by the initiator system, which is directly related to the wavelength, irradiance, and time of exposure. For maximum curing, a radiant energy influx of approximately 16 J/cm^2 is required for a 2-mm-thick layer of resin. This can be delivered by a 40-s exposure to a lamp emitting 400 mW/cm^2 (40 s $\times$ 400 mW/cm^2 = 16,000 mJ/cm^2 or 16 J/cm^2). By the law of reciprocity, the same result can be produced by a 20-s exposure at 800 mW/cm^2 or an exposure of about 13 s with a 1200-mW/cm^2 lamp. Thus, increasing the irradiance of the lamp increases the rate and degree of cure. However, research studies have shown that a longer-than-calculated time might be needed when higher irradiance light is used. In addition, faster curing with higher irradiance light sources can increase shrinkage stress, as discussed in the following section.

CRITICAL QUESTION

How does lamp irradiance affect the depth of cure?

What are the most important factors that affect the depth of cure for a lamp with a given irradiance?

Depth of Cure and Exposure Time

LED lamps with substantially increased irradiances (>1000 mW/cm^2) have opened the possibility of reduced exposure times with a greater depth of cure. However, with conventional composites, light absorption and scattering in resin composites reduces the irradiance and DC exponentially with the depth of penetration. Irradiance can be reduced by a factor of 10–100 in a 2-mm-thick layer of composite. This reduces monomer conversion to an unacceptable level at depths greater than 2–3 mm. Thus, the surface must be irradiated for a longer time to deliver sufficient energy well below the surface. Given the limits imposed by the light scattering and absorption inherent in current restorative resins, the tradeoffs are such that increased irradiance will allow either shorter curing times for a given depth of cure or an increased depth of cure for a given exposure time, but there is little advantage in attempting to achieve both simultaneously. The practical consequence is that the curing depth is limited to 2–3 mm unless excessively long exposure times are used, regardless of lamp irradiance.

Light attenuation can also vary considerably from one type of composite to another, depending, for example, on the opacity, filler size, filler concentration, and pigment shade (i.e., darker shades and/or more opaque resins require longer curing times). For these reasons, manufacturers usually recommend curing times based on a particular curing device for each shade and type of resin. These recommended times are typically the absolute minimum required. To maximize both the degree of polymerization and the long-term clinical durability, the clinician should adjust the exposure time and curing technique to the irradiance of the light source used. Light is also absorbed and scattered as it passes through tooth structure, especially dentin, thereby causing incomplete curing in such critical areas as proximal boxes. Therefore, when one attempts to polymerize the resin through tooth structure, the exposure time should be increased by a factor of 2–3 to compensate for the reduction in light irradiance.

CRITICAL QUESTION

What are the critical exposure techniques and lamp-maintenance practices required for optimal curing and ensuring maximal longevity of resin-based composite restorations?

For the halogen (QHT) lamps, light irradiance is particularly susceptible to aging of the light source. For all types, faulty orientation of the light tip and too great of a distance between the light tip and restoration will reduce light output. Several surveys have shown that the curing units in many dental offices worldwide do not deliver an adequate light output. The bulbs, LEDs, reflectors, and internal filters in dental light-curing units of all types have been shown to degrade with use. In addition, autoclaving, the use of disinfectant chemicals, or restorative material adhering to the light tip can dramatically reduce light output.

Consequently, the lamp's output irradiance should be checked regularly, and the operator should always place the light tip as close as possible perpendicular to the restorative material and maintain this distance and orientation throughout the exposure time. Studies reported in 2010 and 2011 by Price and colleagues concluded that specialized training in these technique-related details substantially improves the intraoral degree of monomer-to-polymer conversion that is obtained.

Safety Precautions for Using Curing Lamps

The light emitted by curing units can cause retinal damage if a person looks directly at the beam. Thus, never look directly into the light tip and minimize observation of the reflected light for longer periods. Protective eyeglasses and various types of shields that filter the light are available for increased protection for both clinical personnel and patients.

Dual-Cured Resins

One way to overcome the limits on curing depth and some of the other problems associated with light curing is to combine chemical-curing and light-curing components in the same resin. Dual-cured resins consist of two light-curable pastes, one containing benzoyl peroxide and the other containing an aromatic tertiary amine accelerator. They are formulated to cure very slowly when mixed for the self-cured mechanism. The curing process is then accelerated on "command" via light curing. The chief advantage of this system is assurance of completion of cure throughout, even if light curing is inadequate. The major disadvantage is the porosity caused by the required mixing, but this has been greatly alleviated by the use of mixing syringes. There is also less color stability than with the light-cured resins as a result of the aromatic amine accelerators, but this is still better than the self-cured systems because the concentration of the accelerators is reduced compared with self-cured resins. Finally, as with the self-cured resins, oxygen inhibition and porosity are problems with dual-cured resins. Dual-cured materials are intended for any situation that does not allow sufficient light penetration to produce adequate monomer conversion—for example, cementation of bulky ceramic inlays. This technology has been incorporated into direct composites to develop bulk-fill composites with unlimited depth of cure. Examples include Parkell HyperFil, Apex Injectafil DC, and Coltene Fill-Up!.

Classification of Composites by Unique Properties

As composites have become the dominant materials in restorative dentistry, they have also been formulated to address additional demands from the material. The unique properties discussed in this section include low-shrinkage composites, self-adhesive flowable composites, and bioactive composites.

Low-Shrinkage Composites

With polymerization shrinkage being a major deficiency with dental composites, there have been many advancements to develop low-shrinkage composites. These advancements can be separated into advancements that maximize filler loading and those in low-shrinkage monomers.

Maximizing Filler Loading

The role of fillers in reducing polymerization shrinkage has been discussed earlier. The first dental composite marketed as a low-shrinkage composite was the Bisco Aelite LS with optimized filler loading as high as 89% by weight and 75% by volume, which is still the highest filler loading by volume reported. The Aelite LS has a filler particle size range of 0.04 to 3.5 μm and a volumetric shrinkage of 1.5%, but because of the larger particles, this material is only recommended for posterior class I, II, and VI restorations and not for aesthetic applications.

CRITICAL QUESTION

What are the key strategies used in the new monomers to make composites low shrinkage?

The Shofu Beautifil Bulk Restorative similarly has a filler loading as high as 87% by weight and 75% by volume and a volumetric shrinkage of 1.7%. This material is also only indicated for posterior, nonaesthetic class I and II applications. Interestingly, the Shofu Beautifil II LS has lower filler loading at 83% by weight but lower volumetric shrinkage at 0.85%, yet higher shrinkage stress than the Beautifil Bulk Restorative (2.72 MPa vs 1.06 MPa, respectively). This surprising difference in shrinkage stress is caused by Beautifil Bulk Restorative having a lower elastic modulus.

Low-Shrinkage Monomers

The influence of monomers on polymerization shrinkage has also been discussed earlier. In this section, we will discuss four monomers that have been used to formulate low-shrinkage composites.

Kalore, also known as *DX-511* (GC America) (Fig. 5.16), has a high molecular weight and a long rigid central section with flexible methacrylate end groups; these provide rod-like shapes that facilitate self-assembly into compact molecular structures. This, together with dilution of the number of polymerizable end groups as a result of the high molecular weight (895 vs 512 for *bis*-GMA), reduces polymerization shrinkage, and the flexible end groups promote reactivity and enhance monomer–polymer conversion.

N'Durance (Septodont USA) is a dimer dicarbamate dimethacrylate (DDCDMA) product that also contains a bulky central group, somewhat analogous to TDC-urethane dimethacrylate. The bulky center is made up of a six-carbon aliphatic ring with two long hydrocarbon side chains derived from a linoleic acid dimer (Fig. 5.17). The center section is connected to two methacrylate end groups via urethane groups (−NH−CO−O−, also referred to as *carbamate* groups). The chain length between reactive ends is very long (having a molecular weight of 843), similar to that of DX-511 (see Fig. 5.15), which provides double-bond dilution and hence reduced shrinkage; the bulky center section allows greater conversion during copolymerization and greater stress relaxation prior to the gel point. A further advantage is the hydrophobic nature of the center group, which restricts water absorption and solubility with the other dimethacrylates in the formulation. This leads to the formation of two separate phases during polymerization and produces a small expansion that partially offsets the polymerization shrinkage.

Venus Diamond (Kulzer) is a resin product based on 4,8-di(methacryloxy methylene)-tricyclodecane (TCDDMA), a bulky, space-filling dimethacrylate monomer (Fig. 5.18). The bulky three-ring central group provides steric hindrance, which holds the monomers apart and thus slows the rate of polymerization. This lengthens the time needed for the crosslinking reaction to reach the gel point and provides time for adjacent polymer chain segments to slip among themselves, rearrange to lower energy configurations, and relieve developing stresses before the gel

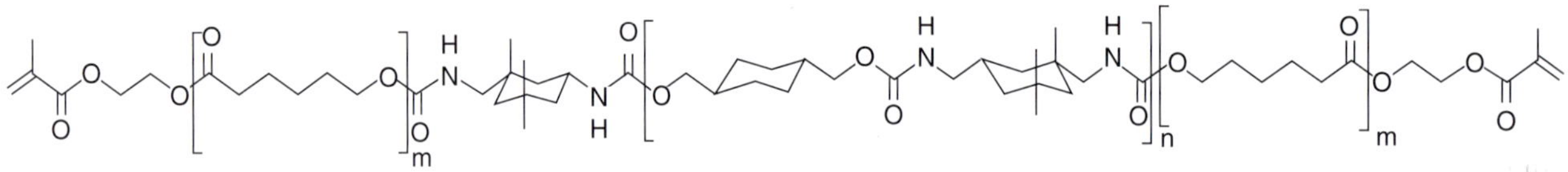

• **Fig. 5.16** A high-molecular-weight polyurethane dimethacrylate monomer, DX-511, that contains a long, rigid central section between flexible methacrylate end groups ("Kalore," GC America, Alsip, IL). Like UDMA, DX-511 has urethane (-NH-CO-O-) groups that connect a central segment between two ethyl-methacrylate end groups. It also contains 2m +1 cyclohexane rings. (Courtesy of Barry K Norling.)

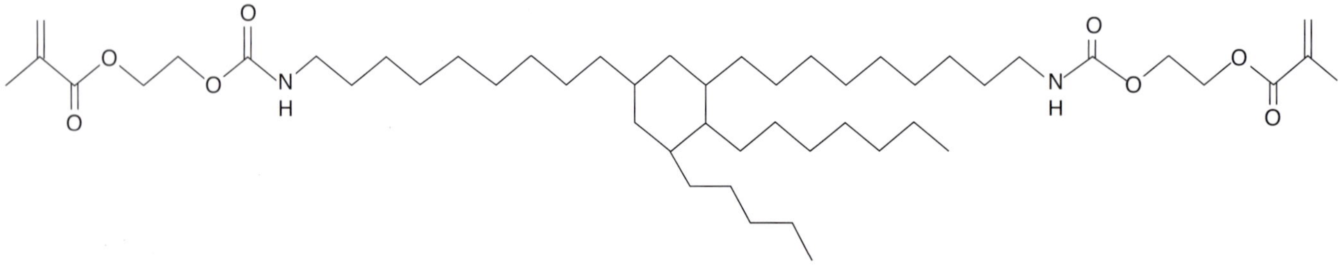

• **Fig. 5.17** Dimer dicarbamate dimethacrylate (DDCDMA), a phase-separating cycloaliphatic urethane dimethacrylate with a bulky center, is composed of a six-carbon aliphatic ring with two long hydrocarbon side chains derived from a linoleic acid dimer. (Courtesy of Barry K Norling.)

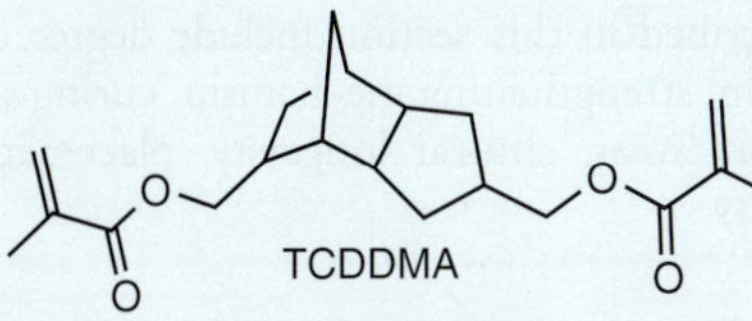

TCDDMA

• **Fig. 5.18** 4,8-Di(methacryloxymethylene)-tricyclodecane (TDC, TCDDMA), a bulky, space-filling urethane dimethacrylate monomer.

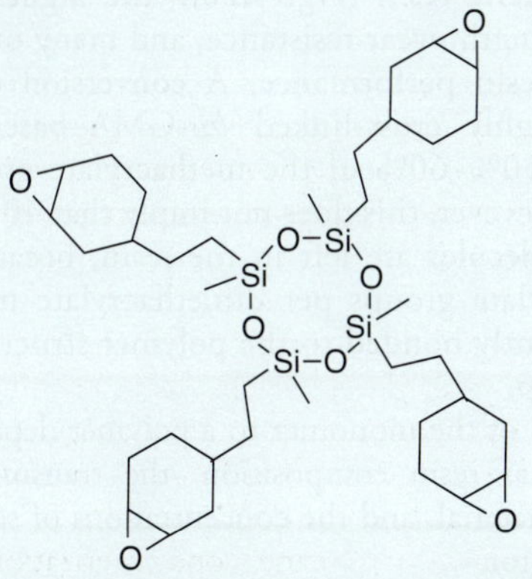

• **Fig. 5.19** Tetrafunctional silorane monomer polymerizes via a cationic-initiated, epoxy ring-opening, cross-linking mechanism. When the rings open, the chains lengthen and occupy more space and partially offset the polymerization shrinkage. (From Weinmann, et al: Siloranes in dental composites. *Dent Mater* 21[1]: 2005.)

point is reached, resulting in one of the lower curing-stress resins currently reported among commercial products.

Filtek LS (3M ESPE) involves an entirely different chemistry based on epoxy, rather than acrylic functionality. This product is no longer available on the market but is included here in case future products contain epoxy chemistry. These tetra-functional "silorane" monomers (Fig. 5.19) use ring-opening polymerization. Silorane chemistry uses a combination of epoxy functionality (three-unit ring with two carbons and one oxygen) combined with siloxane units (–O–Si–O–) that can be cured with low shrinkage via a cationic crosslinking mechanism by means of ring-opening polymerization. When the rings open, they lengthen and occupy more space; the resulting expansion offsets a substantial proportion of the polymerization shrinkage. Previously, epoxy systems were not used for dental applications because a nontoxic curing initiator with hydrolytic stability could not be found.

CRITICAL QUESTION

What technology is employed to make composites self-adhesive?

Self-adhesive Flowable Composites

The process of bonding composites to the tooth is complicated. As such, the development of dentin bonding agents has gone from "three step" to "one step" with one bottle of liquid. Self-adhesive flowable composites, which contain self-etching and adhesive monomers for bonding to hydroxyapatite, may practically eliminate the bottles and the use of a separate bonding agent. These composites would be used like conventional flowable composites in small class I cavities, as a first or base layer under fillings, and as pit and fissure sealants, but without the need for a bonding agent.

Currently, three commercial self-adhesive flowable composites exist, each containing a monomer that etches and adheres to tooth structure. DMG Constic contains 10-methacryloyloxydecyl dihydrogen phosphate (MDP) monomer, which was found to form stable bonds with hydroxyapatite with the formation of 10-MDP-Ca salts. Kerr Vertise Flow contains glycerol phosphate dimethacrylate (GPDM) monomers, which have a strong etching effect but form a weaker chemical bond with hydroxyapatite compared with other self-adhesive monomers. Pentron Fusio Liquid Dentin uses 4-methacryloxyethyl trimetellitic acid (4-META) to etch and bond via its carboxylate groups to the calcium in hydroxyapatite.

Product brochures show dentin shear bond strengths of 24, 20, and 15 MPa for Constic, Vertise Flow, and Fusio Liquid Dentin, respectively. However, Peterson et al. reported that after thermocycling for 5000 cycles at temperatures of 5°C to 55°C, dentin bond strengths deteriorated to 0.3, 0.7, and 2.4 MPa, and enamel bond strengths deteriorated to 3.9, 1.4, and 2.5 MPa for Constic, Vertise Flow, and Fusio Liquid Dentin, respectively. The results are suspected to be caused by the low filler loading of these flowables and the hydrophilic nature of the self-etching and adhesive monomers, which may increase water imbibition and subsequent polymer degradation.

CRITICAL QUESTION

What is the main characteristic of a bioactive composite?
Which released ions are responsible for hydroxyapatite formation?

Bioactive Composites

The definition of a *bioactive material* in biomedical science is a material that is not just biocompatible or bioinert but one that produces a favorable biological response, such as repair or regeneration of tissue. In dental materials, bioactive materials have traditionally included those that release fluoride ions, such as glass ionomers (see Chapter 7), resin-modified glass ionomers (RMGIs), and compomers. Released F^- ions can induce remineralization and bind with apatite to form stronger fluorapatite to protect the tooth from acid demineralization. However, glass ionomers and RMGIs are not very aesthetic and have poor mechanical properties. As such, they are mainly used as class V restorations and as cements.

New and improved bioactive composites include DMG's Ecosite Bulk Fill composite, Parkell's Predicta Bioactive composites (Bulk, Core-Stackable, and Core-Flowable), Shofu's Beautifil composites (II LS, Bulk Flowable, Flow Plus, and Flow Plus X), and Pulpdent's ACTIVA BioACTIVE restorative. Interestingly, DMG's Ecosite Bulk Fill composite is not marketed as a bioactive composite, despite claims that this product release F^- ions. Parkell's Predicta Bioactive composites simply release Ca^{2+}, $PO_4^{=}$, and F^- to trigger apatite formation. However, there is currently not much information available for how Predicta Bioactive composites release these ions.

Shofu's Beautifil composites are "hybrid" composites called *Giomer* that are like RMGIs and compomers with modified filler. The aim is to combine the fluoride-releasing and recharging ability of glass ionomers with the mechanical properties of nanohybrid composites. The advancement here is that instead of using alumino-silicate glass particles to release F^- ions, Giomers use fluoro-boro-alumino-silicate glass particles with a surface coating of a glass ionomer trapped in a polyacid matrix to also release

Na^+, Sr^{2+}, Al^{3+}, $SiO_4^{=}$, and $BO_3^{\equiv}$. The $SiO_4^{=}$ and F^- ions are used to promote remineralization, and the F^- and Sr^{2+} ions are used for converting hydroxyapatite to the stronger fluoroapatite and strontium-apatite. The ion exchange from Giomer fillers is also supposed to neutralize acid that leads to tooth demineralization.

Pulpdent's ACTIVA BioACTIVE restorative is a dual-cured RMGI/compomer, which is based on urethane dimethacrylate that increases composite toughness and reduces wear compared with RMGIs and compomers. This composite releases and recharges with Ca^{2+}, $PO_4^{=}$, and F^- to stimulate apatite formation and teeth remineralization and releases more $PO_4^{=}$ under acidic conditions to claim its "smart" material status. This product is also self-adhesive as a result of the polyacrylic acid in the glass ionomer component and phosphate-based monomers in the ionic resin (Chapter 7). The system is a dual-cured material that uses an automix syringe that will entail some of the disadvantages inherent in dual-cured composites. Its transverse strength is toward the lower end of universal composites (120 MPa). However, a 2019 randomized controlled study by van Dijken et al. suggested that ACTIVA BioACTIVE, as used in posterior restorations, may not bond to dentin or prevent secondary caries. The article cited a significantly higher failure rate compared with a nonbioactive nanofill composite as soon as 1 year (24.1% vs 2.5%, respectively) as a result of lost restorations, postoperative symptoms, and secondary caries.

Properties of Resin-Based Composites

Table 5.3 presents a compilation of selected physical and mechanical properties of various types of composites. Additional properties described in this section include degree of cure, resin matrix constrain, strengthening mechanism, curing shrinkage and shrinkage stress, wear, clinical longevity, placement time, and biocompatibility.

Degree of Conversion (DC)

The DC is a measure of the percentage of carbon-carbon double bonds that have been converted to single bonds to form a polymeric resin (Fig. 5.20). The higher the DC, the better the strength, wear resistance, and many other properties essential to resin performance. A conversion of 50%–60%, typical of highly cross-linked *bis*-GMA–based composites, implies that 50%–60% of the methacrylate groups have polymerized. However, this does not imply that 40%–50% of the monomer molecules are left in the resin, because one of the two methacrylate groups per dimethacrylate molecule could still be covalently bonded to the polymer structure, forming a pendant group.

Conversion of the monomer to a polymer depends on several factors, such as resin composition, the transmission of light through the material, and the concentrations of sensitizer, initiator, and inhibitor.

The total DC within resins does not differ between chemically activated and light-activated composites containing the same monomer formulations as long as adequate light curing is employed. Conversion values of 50%–70% are achieved at room temperature for both curing systems. Likewise, polymerization shrinkage of comparable light-activated and chemically activated resins is not significantly different. However, in light-cured materials, curing shrinkage leads to substantially greater stress buildup

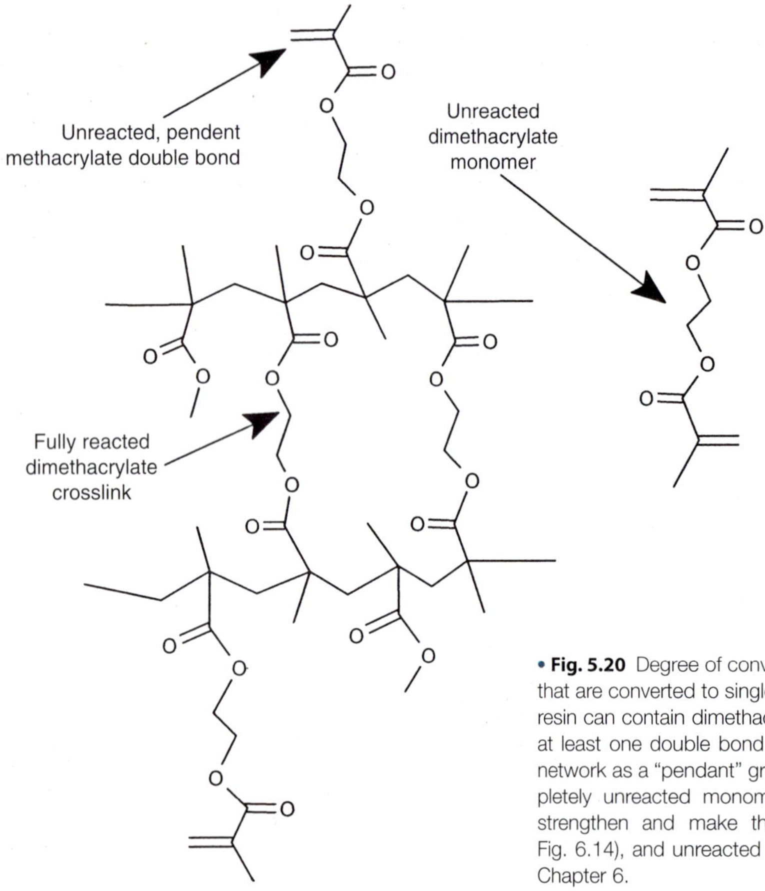

• **Fig. 5.20** Degree of conversion (DC) reflects the percentage of methacrylate double bonds that are converted to single bonds during the curing reaction. This figure shows that a cured resin can contain dimethacrylates groups with zero, one, or two unreacted double bonds. If at least one double bond has reacted, the dimethacrylate group is bound to the polymer network as a "pendant" group with one double bond available for further reaction. Any completely unreacted monomers can migrate out of the cured resin. Cross-linked groups strengthen and make the resin rigid while pendant groups plasticize the resin (see Fig. 6.14), and unreacted monomer softens and swells the resin structure, as explained in Chapter 6.

and leakage at the resin margins, in turn leading to staining, sensitivity, and secondary caries.

Matrix Constraint

As mentioned above, the presence of filler particles bonded to the matrix via coupling agents reduces thermal expansion and contraction of the composite. When thermal stresses arise, the interfacial bond and the presence of a filler with a lower coefficient of thermal expansion (nearly zero in some cases) prevents or reduces the contraction or expansion of the matrix. Thus, during expansion, while the space occupied by the filler tries to increase, the filler with lower coefficient of expansion does not—and since the filler is chemically bonded to the matrix, it prevents the space from getting larger and hence prevents or reduces the expansion. Conversely, during cooling, the matrix contracts and decreases the space occupied by the filler, but since the filler occupies that space, contraction is prevented or reduced. Thus, the filler particles lower thermal expansion and contraction by occupying space that polymers, which are susceptible to thermal expansion, would otherwise have occupied, and they also constrain the interfacial bond from expanding thermally.

This constraint does have its limits. During expansion, the composite can fracture within the matrix because of the added tension caused by the nonexpansion of the filler particle, within the filler particle, or at the interfacial bond, depending on whether the interfacial bond is stronger than the fracture toughness of the filler or the matrix. In contraction, the composite can fracture within the matrix or within the filler particle, depending on which is weaker.

Toughness

The strength of composites is highly dependent on the ability of the coupling agent to transfer stresses from the weak matrix to the strong filler particles. Without the coupling agent, the filler particles cannot absorb stresses in the matrix and act as if they were voids, thereby weakening instead of strengthening the matrix. Thus, a crack traveling through the matrix simply bypasses the particles. In a true composite, the matrix and filler are chemically bonded. As the crack propagates to a bonded filler particle, the crack must pass around the particle, since it is stronger than the matrix and the interfacial bond. Thus, the path the crack must take and the total new surface area that the crack must form is increased; therefore the energy needed for the crack to propagate is increased. This makes the composite tougher.

If the interfacial bond is weaker than the matrix, a process of crack blunting occurs (Fig. 5.21). As the crack propagates to the weak interface, a void or tear opens up in front of the advancing crack because of the stresses that the weak bond experiences. However, this void is perpendicular to the propagating crack; thus, when the crack arrives, the tip of the crack has been blunted and significantly more stress is required to propagate the crack.

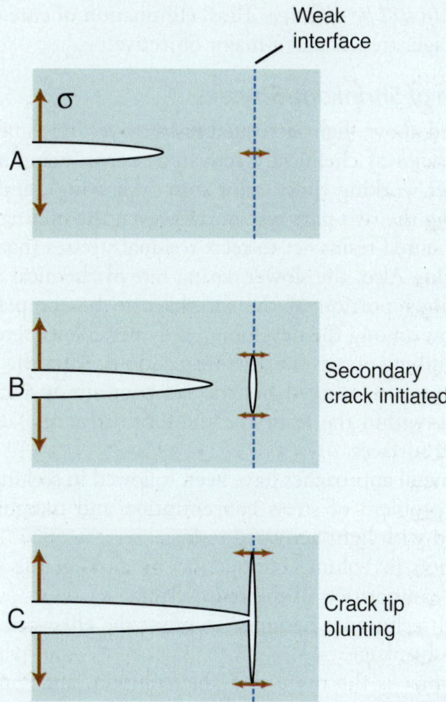

• **Fig. 5.21** A crack propagates through the resin matrix under the influence of a tensile stress toward a weak interface **(A)**, and initiates a secondary crack when the stress induced at the weak interface is greater than the interfacial bond strength **(B)**. When the main crack reaches the extended secondary crack, its propagation is impeded by a process called crack blunting **(C)**. (Adapted from Darvell BW: *Materials Science for Dentistry*, ed 9, Woodhead Publishing Ltd, Cambridge, UK, 2009.)

CRITICAL QUESTION

What are the problems that result from shrinkage and curing-induced marginal stress during the polymerization of restorative resins?

How are polymerization stresses affected by the presence of reinforcing fillers in dental composites?

Curing Shrinkage and Shrinkage Stress

Curing shrinkage arises as the monomer is converted to polymer and the free space it occupies reduces (approximately 20% less than that among unreacted monomers). In turn, this polymerization shrinkage produces unrelieved stresses in the resin after it reaches the "**gelation**" point and begins to harden. The polymerization shrinkage and resultant stress can be affected by the following:

1. Total volume of the composite material
2. Type of composite
3. Polymerization speed
4. Ratio of bonded/nonbonded *surfaces* or the configuration of the tooth preparation (**C-factor**)

These stresses tend to develop at the tissue/composite interface, weakening the bond, and eventually producing a gap at the restoration margins. Consequently, the risk for marginal leakage and the ensuing problems of marginal staining and secondary caries are exacerbated. Undoubtedly this is one of the greatest problems of composites used for class II and class V restorations.

Traditionally this problem has been combated in two ways. First, larger monomers used to "dilute" the number of double bonds that need to be reacted. *Bis*-GMA and UDMA have five times or more the molecular weight of methyl methacrylate (MMA), so the density of methacrylate double-bond groups is approximately two-fifths as high in MMA. This reduces polymerization shrinkage proportionately.

Another method has been the addition of inorganic fillers that do not enter into the polymerization process, although they do bond to the polymer. Thus, because a percentage of the volume does not enter into the reaction, the amount of monomer necessary and the cure shrinkage are both reduced. When prepared correctly, commercial composites have done quite well, *but this shrinkage can still be excessive*. Thus, elimination of cure shrinkage and shrinkage stress is still a major objective.

Reduction of Shrinkage Stresses

As discussed above, light-activated resins have overcome many of the deficiencies of chemically activated resins, including lack of control over working time, color shift (yellowing), and porosity from mixing the two-part system. However, the internal pores in chemically cured resins act to relax residual stresses that build up during curing Also, the slower curing rate of chemical activation allows a larger portion of the shrinkage to be compensated by internal flow among the developing polymer chains before extensive cross-linking occurs (i.e., before gelation). After the gel point, stresses cannot be relieved but instead continue to increase and concentrate within the resin and the tooth structure adjacent to the bonded surfaces.

Two general approaches have been followed in seeking to overcome the problem of stress concentration and marginal failure experienced with light-activated resins:

(1) Reduction in volume contraction by altering the chemistry and/or composition of the resin system.

(2) Clinical techniques designed to offset the effects of polymerization shrinkage.

The former is the more desirable solution, and intensive research and development efforts are currently in progress to develop resins with low shrinkage and low thermal expansion. In the meantime, a variety of techniques have been investigated that can immediately be put into practice by the clinician. These techniques are associated with incremental buildup and control of the curing rate.

CRITICAL QUESTION

How can the composite clinical manipulation technique be used to improve the integrity of the marginal seal in a composite restoration?

Incremental Buildup and Cavity Configuration

One technique attempts to reduce the C-factor, which is related to the geometry of the cavity preparation and represented by the ratio of bonded to nonbonded surface areas. Residual polymerization stress increases directly with this ratio. During curing, shrinkage leaves the bonded cavity surfaces in a state of stress; the nonbonded, free surfaces (i.e., those that reproduce the original external tooth anatomy) relax some of the stress by contracting inward toward the bulk of the material. A layering technique (Fig. 5.22) in which the restoration is built up in increments, curing one layer at a time, effectively reduces polymerization stress by minimizing the C-factor. That is, thinner layers reduce bonded surface area and maximize nonbonded surface area, thus minimizing the associated C-factor. In any case, as discussed previously, limitations on the depth of cure of photoinitiated resins dictate the use of incremental buildup of the composite. Thus, an incremental technique overcomes both limited depth of cure and residual stress concentration but adds to the time and difficulty of placing a restoration.

Soft-Start, Ramped Curing, and Delayed Curing

- Soft-Start—In the soft-start technique, curing begins at low light irradiance and finishes with high irradiance. This approach allows for a slow initial rate of polymerization and a high initial level of stress relaxation during the early stages and ends at the maximum irradiance once the gel point has been reached. This drives the curing reaction to the highest possible conversion only after much of the stress has been relieved. A number of studies have demonstrated that varying levels of stress reduction in tooth-cavity walls can be achieved in this way while not increasing the total exposure time or sacrificing either degree of cure or depth of cure.
- Ramped Curing—In ramping, the irradiance is gradually increased or "ramped up" during the exposure. Such ramping employs stepwise, linear, or exponential modes.
- Delayed Curing—In delayed curing, the restoration is initially incompletely cured at low irradiance. The clinician then sculpts and contours the resin to the correct occlusion and later applies a second exposure of light for the final cure. This delay allows substantial stress relaxation to take place. The longer the time that is available for relaxation, the lower is the residual stress that is expressed.
- Delayed curing and exponential ramp curing appear to provide greater reductions in curing stress but do require more time.

In response to this situation, care should be taken when high-irradiance lamps are used. Increased lamp irradiance allows for shorter exposure times for a given depth of cure in a particular shade and type of resin. Thus, these high-irradiance lamps should, in principle, provide substantial savings in chair time. However, a

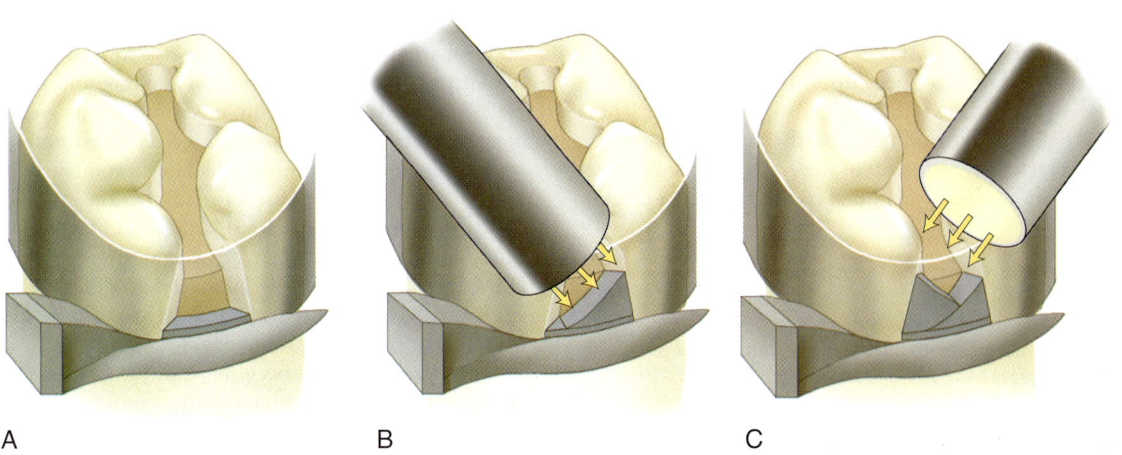

• **Fig. 5.22** **(A)** First incremental layer of resin composite (gray area) has been placed and cured. **(B)** Second increment being cured with a light source. **(C)** Third composite increment during curing.

high-irradiance, short-exposure time causes an accelerated rate of curing, which inevitably leads to substantial residual stress buildup because of the inherently less time for stress-relaxation mechanisms to take place. *Because of these tradeoffs, there appears to be little advantage to ramped, delayed, or soft-start curing techniques.* Numerous laboratory studies and some clinical evidence support this conclusion. Thus, the clinician should carefully consider the tradeoffs before investing in these more expensive types of curing lamps.

Wear (Volume Loss by Abrasion and Other Mechanisms)

In addition to polymerization shrinkage, other frequent clinical problems have been occlusal (Fig. 5.23 and interproximal wear, especially in the case of posterior composites. The mechanism of occlusal wear is a complex problem that has been the subject of much research. Unfortunately, before clinical use, abrasion and wear resistance can be measured only by a laboratory test that simulates simplified environmental conditions. As yet, no single test method has been agreed upon as a valid predictor of clinical performance. Controlled clinical evaluations are the only reliable means of evaluating the durability and useful lifetime of restorative materials. However, based on such studies, the best composites designed for posterior restorations still wear more than natural enamel under identical conditions. Although wear rate differences of 10–20 μm/year may seem small for posterior composites, this wear rate still amounts to 0.1–0.2 mm more than enamel over 10 years. Thus, it is important to be cautious in selecting the clinical cases to be treated with posterior composites.

Two principal mechanisms of composite wear have been proposed:

- The first mode is two-body wear, based on direct contact of the restoration with an opposing cusp or with adjacent proximal surfaces to mimic the high stresses developed in the small area of contact. This is related to the higher force levels exerted by the opposing cusp or forces transferred to proximal surfaces.
- The second mode is three-body wear, which simulates loss of material in noncontacting areas, most probably owing to contact with food as it is forced across the occlusal surfaces. This type of wear is affected in a complex way by a number of composite properties such as toughness, porosity, stability of the silane coupling agent, degree of monomer conversion, filler loading, and the size and types of filler particles.

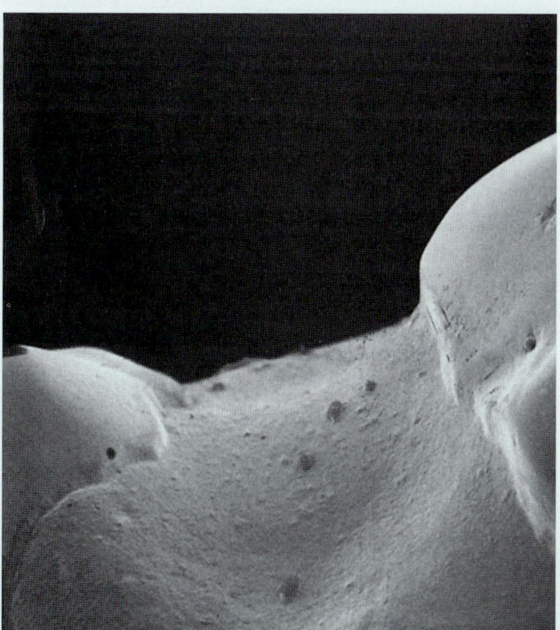

• **Fig. 5.23** Scanning electron micrograph of a 9-year-old small-particle-filled composite, illustrating generalized, three-body wear. (Courtesy of Robert L Erickson.)

Clinically, although direct tooth to restoration contact occurs infrequently during mastication, the loss of material caused by direct wear in areas of tooth-to-tooth contact appears to be greater than that of three-body abrasion by food in noncontact areas. Composites in which the filler particles are small (1 μm or less), high in concentration, and well bonded to the matrix are the most resistant to wear. Large restorations tend to wear more than do smaller ones, as do restorations in molars compared with those in premolars.

Variations among patients—such as differences in chewing habits, force levels, and variations in oral environments—also play a significant role in the wear process. A typical wear pattern for a composite is shown in Figure 5.23 for a 9-year-old, chemically activated, small-particle-filled composite restoration. Although the loss of material shown in this figure is more severe than that for current restorative materials, it illustrates the wear phenomenon. Notice the smoother anatomical contours and the exposed cavity walls where the composite has been worn away by abrasion.

The major indications for composites for class II restorations place emphasis on the demand for esthetics. A conservative preparation is preferred so that the tooth, rather than the composite, absorbs more of the stress. The dentist must also be familiar with the rigorous placement procedures essential for success, as described in textbooks on operative dentistry (Box 5.2). However, there are obvious contraindications. A composite class II restoration is doomed to failure in the mouth of a patient who bruxes because of the greater potential for wear. Use of posterior composites in a caries-active mouth is also questionable because few current restorative materials have the ability to provide an anticariogenic effect or to resist leakage. If composites are used for such situations, the application of a hydrophilic sealing resin along the margins may be beneficial. Nonetheless, with the greater demand for esthetics and continual improvements in composite formulations, the use of these materials in stress-bearing situations continues to increase. In response, academic and industry research can be expected to continue to improve the clinical durability of composite materials.

Ongoing advances in composite technology have considerably reduced the problem of wear in posterior resin applications. Nevertheless difficulties still exist in high-stress situations related to inherent problems with both the mechanical and chemical degradation of composites.

Indirect Posterior Composites

Indirect composites for fabrication of onlays and inlays are polymerized externally and then luted to the tooth with a compatible resin cement. Indirect composite inlays or onlays reduce wear and leakage and overcome some of the limitations of resin composites. Several different approaches to resin inlay construction have been proposed:

- The use of both direct and indirect fabrication methods.
- The application of light, heat, pressure, or a combination of these curing systems.
- The combined use of hybrid and microfilled composites.

The fabrication process for direct composite inlays first requires the application of a separating medium (e.g., agar solution or glycerin) to the prepared tooth. The restorative resin pattern is then formed, light-cured, and removed from the preparation. The rough inlay is then exposed to additional light for approximately 4–6 minutes or heat-activated at approximately 100°C for 7 minutes, after which the preparation is etched, the inlay cemented into place with (typically) a dual-cure resin, and the inlay is then polished.

Composite systems are also available as indirect products. Indirect inlay resins require an impression and a dental laboratory technician to fabricate the inlay. In addition to conventional light- and heat-curing, laboratory processing may employ heat (e.g., 140°C) and pressure (e.g., 0.6 MPa for 10 minutes). Other techniques have also been recommended. The first consists of substituting the normal atmospheric conditions in the curing chamber to one without oxygen. This is accomplished by evacuating the oxygen-containing atmosphere and carefully substituting a nitrogen atmosphere. The second method consists of curing at a slow rate (soft-start polymerization). The third and final method for improving wear resistance consists of introducing light and heat simultaneously to the curing chamber. All of these methods, for various reasons, enhance the conversion level of double carbon bonds to single carbon bonds, thereby increasing the degree of polymerization.

The potential advantage of these materials is that a significantly higher degree of polymerization is attained, which improves physical properties and resistance to wear. The polymerization shrinkage does not occur in the prepared teeth, so induced stresses and bond failures are reduced, which reduces the potential for leakage. Furthermore, these resins are repairable in the mouth and are not as abrasive to opposing tooth structure as ceramic inlays.

Laboratory studies support these expected advantages: for example, a recent review revealed that the annual clinical failure rates in class I and II posterior stress-bearing cavities are the same for composite inlays as for amalgam restorations (1.9%), somewhat superior to those for direct composites (3.6%), and only slightly (but not significantly) inferior to cast gold inlays and onlays (1.4%) (Manhart et al., 2004). However, technique sensitivity for indirect resin restoration systems remains high and their appropriateness as a substitute for amalgam or cast restorations in *all* posterior applications is not clear, even though the esthetics are appealing.

Longevity of Composites

The most commonly cited reasons for the failure of composites in clinical studies are secondary caries, fracture, marginal deficiencies, and wear. However, these reasons vary greatly depending on the type of study (randomized clinical trial versus private practice setting), type of composite used, period of observation, and other aspects of study design. Nonetheless, properly placed, composites can last many years even in posterior regions, where wear and bite forces are greatest.

The clinical performance of dental restorations is best judged on the basis of long-term clinical trials, preferably those based on randomized controlled designs. However, very few studies of this type exist in the dental literature.

A critical review of clinical data over 10 years by Chadwick et al. shows that the survival rates of composites are significantly lower than those of amalgam. Amalgam also demonstrated less variability in survival rates (Fig. 5.24). The comparative survival rates for amalgam versus composite restorations in permanent teeth at 3, 4, 5, and 7 years are summarized in Table 5.6. Similar comparative data for restorations in primary teeth after 3 and 4 years are also listed in this table. The overall survival rate for composites in permanent teeth after 7 years was 67.4%, compared with 94.5% for amalgam restorations. More than 90% of amalgam restorations in permanent teeth survived longer than 9 years. In comparison, only 64% of glass ionomer restorations

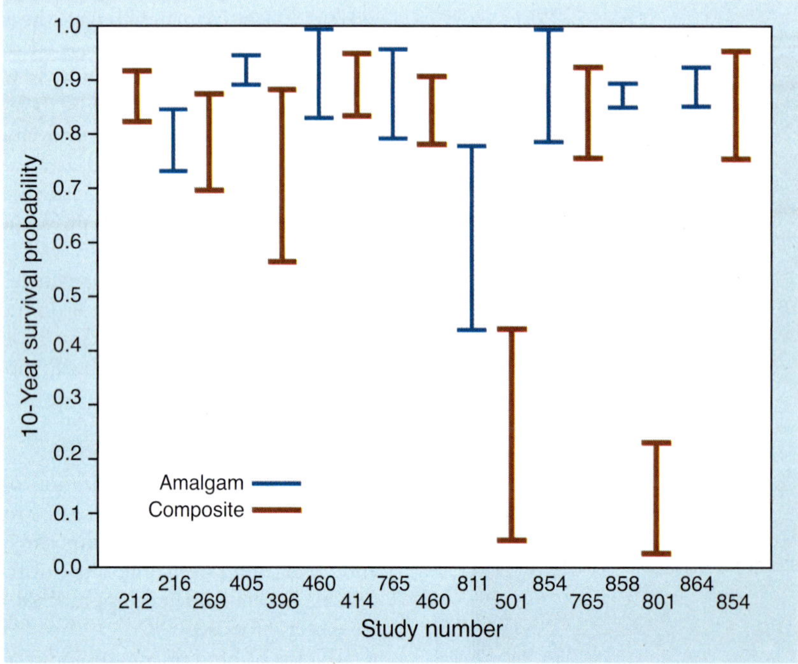

• **Fig. 5.24** Ten-year survival probability for posterior composite and amalgam restorations. (Data from Chadwick BL, Dummer PMH, Dunstan F, et al: *The Longevity of Dental Restorations: A Systematic Review.* National Health Service Centre for Reviews and Dissemination, University of York, 2001.)

TABLE 5.6 Comparison of Survival Probabilities for Various Types of Restorations After 3, 4, 5, and 7 Years

Restoration	3 YEARS PRIMARY PERMANENT		4 YEARS PRIMARY PERMANENT		5 YEARS PRIMARY PERMANENT		7 YEARS PRIMARY PERMANENT	
Type	Teeth	Teeth	Teeth	Teeth	Teeth	Teeth	Teeth	Teeth
Amalgam	95.3	97.2	95.1	96.6	90.8	95.4	—	94.5
Composite	82.4	90.0	67.2	85.6	—	78.2	—	67.4
Glass Ionomer	51.5	73.8	51.5	73.8	31.2	64.9	—	—
DBA and Composite	—	83.7	—	47.7	—	41.5	—	—
Ceramic or Composite Inlay	—	93.3	—	90.1	—	85.3	—	

DBA, dentin bonding agent.
Modified from Chadwick BL, Dummer PMH, Dunstan F, et al: *The Longevity of Dental Restorations: A Systematic Review.* National Health Service Centre for Reviews and Dissemination, University of York, Heslington York, YO10 5DD, United Kingdom, 2001.

survived after 5 years. Only 41% of class V composites placed with dentin bonding agents survived longer than 5 years. The study concluded that the class II glass ionomer/composite restorations should be avoided because of a high percentage of failures at the gingival margin of the proximal box.

In a retrospective study on the longevity of 1955 posterior composites placed between 1990 and 1997 in a private-practice setting, Opdam et al. reported a survival rate for composite resin of 91.7% at 5 years and 82.2% at 10 years. There was a significant effect of the size of restored surfaces on the survival of the restorations—that is, the more conservative the restoration, the longer these restorations survived.

In a 22-year follow-up of 362 restorations placed between 1986 and 1990, da Rosa Rodolpho et al. reported survival rates of midfill hybrid composites at 74% and minifill hybrid composites at 64%, respectively. The study also reported that the annual failure rate in the second part of the observation period had become constant for midfill composite, whereas minifill composite had shown an increase, suggesting that the physical properties of the composite might have some impact on restoration longevity.

One systematic review by Alvanforoush and colleagues compared composite failure between the two decades of 1995–2005 and 2006–2016 using studies that were at least 24 months long. Twelve studies that were used for the systematic review had observation periods of posterior composites of longer than 6 years. Five were published between 1995 and 2005 and observed posterior composites for 10 years. Seven were published between 2006 and 2016 that ranged from 6 to 22 years. Interestingly, overall, they found that composite survival rates actually decreased from 89.4% in the studies from 1995 to 2005 to 86.9% in the studies from 2006 to 2016. However, the incidence of failure from secondary caries decreased from 29.5% to 25.7%, and additionally, the incidence of composite fracture increased from 28.8% to 39.1%. The authors note that these findings may be attributable to the increased use of composites for larger restorations. Table 5.5 summarizes long-term survival rates for the different types of composites in this review.

Opdam (2014) in a meta-analysis of 12 clinical studies based on raw data found that caries risk and number of restored surfaces play a significant role in restoration survival, and that, on average, posterior resin composite restorations show a good survival, with annual failure rates of 1.8% at 5 years and 2.4% after 10 years of service.

Hientze (2015) evaluated the clinical effectiveness of anterior composites and found that Class IV restorations showed more fractures than Class III restorations. Class IV restorations with hybrid composites showed less fractures than microfilled composites and that the overall performance of hybrid composites was better than that of microfilled composites.

CRITICAL QUESTION

How does the extent to which monomer is converted to polymer affect the longevity of composite restorations?

What factors related to the curing process affect the integrity of the seal between a photocured resin composite and the margins of a cavity preparation?

Placement Time of Composites

Although the performance of posterior composites has greatly improved during the past decade relative to amalgams, the placement time is significantly higher for composites, as shown in Figure 5.25. The placement time of ceramic and composite inlays is significantly higher than that for either amalgam or composite restorations. Obviously the cost of restorations for the patient is also proportionately higher for the inlay prostheses. In fact, the relative cost per tooth per year over a 5-year period for amalgam, composite, and ceramic or composite inlay restorations, in terms of multiples, is 1, 1.62, and 6.35, respectively. The relative cost per tooth per year of amalgam restorations is significantly less than that of composites after 10 years (1 versus 3.36, respectively). A comparative analysis of the placement times is summarized in Table 5.7 for class I, class II (two-surface), class II (three-surface, mesial-occlusal-distal), and pin-retained cusp replacement restorations.

Biocompatibility of Composites

Concerns about the biocompatibility of restorative materials usually relate to the effects on the pulp from two aspects: (1) the inherent chemical toxicity of the material and (2) the marginal leakage of oral fluids.

A chemical insult to the pulp from composites is possible if components leach out or diffuse from the material and

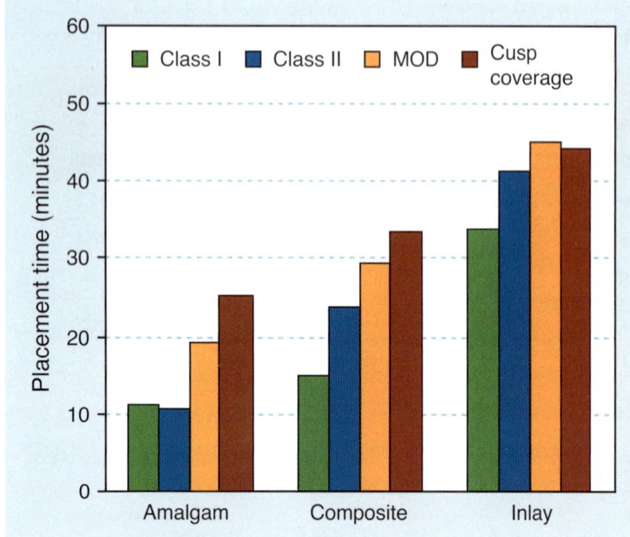

• **Fig. 5.25** Placement time required for posterior amalgam, composite, and ceramic and composite inlay restorations. (Data from Chadwick BL, Dummer PMH, Dunstan F, et al: *The Longevity of Dental Restorations: A Systematic Review.* National Health Service Centre for Reviews and Dissemination, University of York, 2001.)

subsequently reach the pulp. Inadequately cured composite materials at the floor of a cavity can serve as a reservoir of diffusible components that can induce long-term pulp inflammation. This situation is of particular concern for light-activated materials. If a clinician attempts to polymerize too thick a layer of resin or if the exposure time to the light is inadequate (as discussed previously), the uncured or poorly cured material can release leachable constituents adjacent to the pulp. Nonetheless, adequately polymerized composites are relatively biocompatible because they exhibit minimal solubility, and unreacted species are leached in very small quantities. From a toxicological point of view, these amounts should be too small to cause toxic reactions. However, from an immunological point of view, under extremely rare conditions, some patients and dental personnel can develop allergic responses to these materials.

The second concern is associated with polymerization shrinkage of the composite and the subsequent marginal leakage. The marginal leakage might allow bacterial ingrowth, and these microorganisms may cause secondary caries or pulp reactions. Therefore, the restorative procedure must be designed to minimize polymerization shrinkage and marginal leakage. A comprehensive review of biocompatibility is presented in Chapter 17.

Bisphenol A Toxicity

Bisphenol A (BPA), a precursor of *bis*-GMA, has been shown to be a xenoestrogen, a synthetic compound that mimics the effects of estrogen by having an affinity for estrogen receptors. BPA and other endocrine-disrupting chemicals (EDCs) have been shown to cause reproductive anomalies, especially in the developmental stages of fetal wildlife. Although the effects on humans are still unclear, testicular cancer, decreased sperm count, and hypospadias (displacement of the urethral meatus) have been seen as the result of exposure to EDCs.

BPA has recently also been shown to exhibit antiandrogenic activities, which may prove to be detrimental in organ development. Studies have shown that the **estrogenicity** of resin compounds is mainly associated with BPA and BPA dimethacrylate (*BPA-DM*), monomers found in the base paste of some dental sealants. *In vitro* reports have confirmed that BPA and BPA-DM applied to cancer cells significantly increase cell proliferation and DNA synthesis, similar to the effect of estrogen. *In vitro* studies with mammals have revealed numerous effects, such as delayed and sustained hyperprolactinemic changes in estrogen receptors in the hypothalamus and pituitary glands.

Controversy surrounds this issue because it is unclear how much BPA or BPA-DM is released to the oral cavity and what dosage is enough to affect human health. A clinical study (Olea et al., 1996) revealed that BPA was collected in saliva after 1 hour of sealant placement, leading the authors to conclude that sealant application led to xenoestrogen exposure in children. This led to a deluge of follow-up examinations to determine the validity of the results. More recent studies have shown that BPA-DM should be restricted to use in resin-based composites because of its very potent estrogenic effect and because of high levels found in the body; however, the effect of BPA is negligible. Further research should be conducted *in vivo* to show the chemical activity of these compounds and their effects on human development. Additional information on the biocompatibility of restorative materials is presented in Chapter 17.

Finishing of Composites

The term *finishing* usually refers to the process of adapting the restorative material to the tooth (e.g., removing overhangs and

TABLE 5.7 Comparison of Average Time (minutes) Required for Initial (I) and Replacement (R) Restorations

	AMALGAM		COMPOSITE		COMPOSITE AND CERAMIC INLAY	
Restoration Type	I	R	I	R	I	R
Class I	11	11	15	16	34	34
Class II	15	13	24	24	41	40
MOD: mesio-occlusal-distal	19	19	29	31	45	45
Cusp replacement with pins	25	26	33	34	44	44

I: Initial restoration; R: replacement restoration.
Adapted from Chadwick BL, Dummer PMH, Dunstan F, et al: *The Longevity of Dental Restorations: A Systematic Review.* National Health Service Centre for Reviews and Dissemination, University of York, Heslington York, YO10 5DD, United Kingdom, 2001.

shaping occlusal surfaces), whereas *polishing* refers to removing surface irregularities to achieve the smoothest possible surface. Optimal finishing and polishing of resin-based composites is a very important step in the completion of a restoration. Residual surface roughness can encourage bacterial growth, which can lead to a myriad of problems including secondary caries, gingival inflammation, and surface staining. Several methods for the finishing and polishing of resin-based composites have been advocated. The best possible finish is produced by not polishing surfaces at all, at least surfaces that have polymerized next to a smooth matrix strip. This minimizes porosities as well as the oxygen-inhibited layer. However, it is often difficult to achieve proper contours and margin adaptation without some amount of finishing because the plastic strip is often difficult to adapt to the convex and concave surfaces of the tooth. Therefore, different finishing and polishing systems are being marketed to achieve the best possible surface.

Research has been conducted to examine the effect of several significant factors on the finish and polish of a composite restoration: (1) environment, (2) delayed versus immediate finish, (3) the types of materials, and (4) surface coating and sealing.

Environment

Environment involves whether the process of finishing and polishing should be performed in a wet or dry field in the mouth. Some advocates say that finishing in a dry field with the finishing equipment mounted on a slow-speed handpiece allows for better visualization of the restoration margins. However, studies have shown that a dry polishing technique results in an increase in marginal leakage, possibly because of heat production, which can disturb the marginal sealing ability of the adhesive resins. Other studies have shown that structural and chemical changes occur on the surfaces of restorations as a result of a dry environment. However, still other research has confirmed that the dry polishing technique has no effect on the hardness or surface structure. As with many dental procedures, grinding and finishing are best accomplished in moderation. The clinician should finish the restoration in an environment where the margins are clearly discernible and where minimal heat is generated. Excessive heat results in smearing of the surface and depolymerization. Water-cooling during grinding and finishing should ensure a standard surface quality.

Elapsed Time Between Curing of the Composite and Finishing and Polishing

Elapsed time may also have an effect on surface characteristics and resistance to leakage that develops. Some advocate delaying the finishing of composite restorations for up to 24 hours because polymerization is incomplete at placement, although composite manufacturers recommend that finishing be accomplished shortly after placement. Studies have shown that delayed finishing can actually increase marginal leakage and has no effect on surface characteristics compared with immediate finishing. Also, delayed finishing has a minimal effect on hardness. Thus, for all practical purposes, almost all composite restorations should be finished and polished shortly after placement during the same appointment, although the finishing should be delayed for approximately 15 minutes after curing.

Types of Materials and Devices

A variety of materials and devices can be used to finish and polish composite restorations. Use of a scalpel blade or any thin, sharp-edged instrument to remove flash on the proximal areas is recommended. However, this is a very risky procedure, especially if the trimming procedure involves shearing in a direction toward the composite and away from the gingival margin, which can lead to localized debonding and leakage. Trimming forces should be applied either parallel to the margin or toward the gingival tissue. Coarse to ultrafine aluminum oxide discs can be applied to areas with difficult access around the proximal surfaces or in embrasures (see Chapter 16). Tungsten carbide burs or fine diamond tips can be used to adjust occlusal surfaces and blend the composite to the surfaces of the teeth. Several studies in the literature have rated many of these systems as to their effect on surface smoothness and microleakage. Currently, aluminum oxide disks produce the best surface while also inducing minimal trauma. Other systems include resin-finishing devices that use fine and extrafine polishing pastes, silicone-based systems, and silicone carbide–impregnated polishing brushes and points. Recent studies suggest that while the use of successively finer disks is still very effective, recently developed two- and one-step systems may be slightly better at producing the highest gloss for most types of dental composite. Though the high initial shine may be important to the patient, especially for the anterior teeth, the main concern of the dentist is the surface quality after months and years of service. Although high stresses may be associated with surface grinding and polishing, a recent study has shown that the type of polishing system used does not significantly affect the development of microleakage.

Surface Coating and Sealing

An important step in finishing and polishing is the application of a bonding agent or a surface sealer. It has been widely documented that the finishing (and possibly polishing) process is detrimental to composite surfaces in that surface microcracks are introduced and the highly polymerized outer surface of the resin composite material is removed. Application of a penetrating surface sealer or a low-viscosity resin with little or no filler ensures that surface porosities are filled and microcracks sealed. Studies have shown that this "rebonding" technique also significantly decreases microleakage by improving the marginal seal of restorations.

Repair of Composites

Composites can be repaired by replacing lost material. This is a useful procedure for correcting defects or altering contours on existing restorations. The procedures for adding new material differ depending on whether the restoration is freshly polymerized or an older restoration.

When a restoration has just been placed and polymerized, it may still have an oxygen-inhibited layer of resin on the surface. Additions of new composite can be made directly to this layer because this represents, in essence, an excellent bonding substrate. Even after the restoration has been polished, adding more material can still repair a defect. A restoration that has just been cured and polished may still have more than 50% of unreacted methacrylate groups to copolymerize with the newly added material.

As the restoration ages, fewer and fewer unreacted methacrylate groups remain and greater cross-linking reduces the ability of fresh monomer to penetrate the matrix. The strength of the bond between the original material and the new resin decreases in direct proportion to the time that has elapsed between polymerization and addition of the new resin. Furthermore, polished surfaces

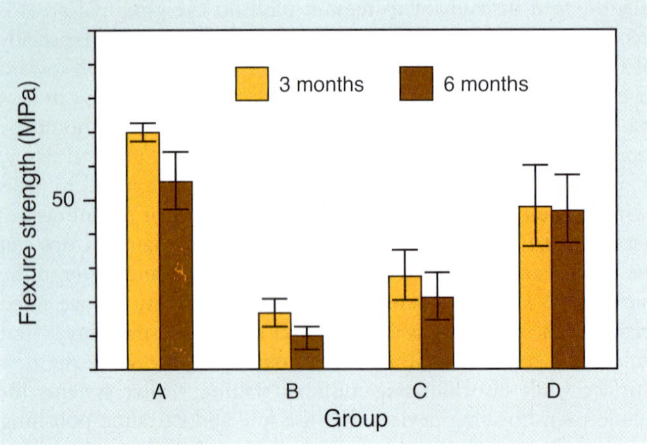

• **Fig. 5.26** The influence of the method of composite repair on strength under in vitro conditions. Flexural strength after storage in distilled water at 37°C for 3 and 6 months. **(A)** Original, unbroken samples serving as a control. **(B)** Repair without first acid-etching. **(C)** Repair after acid-etching and the application of an unfilled resin. **(D)** Repair after toluene/silane treatment to soften the broken surfaces and facilitate permeation by new monomer. (Data from K-J M Söderholm: Flexure strength of repaired dental composites. *European J Dent Oral Science* 94:364–369, 1986.)

expose filler surfaces that are free from silane. Thus, the filler surface area does not chemically bond to the new composite layer. Even ideally—that is, with the addition of a silane-bonding agent to the surface before the addition of new composite—the strength of repaired composite is less than half the strength of the original material (Fig. 5.26).

Even though repair is essential to the overall longevity of composite restorations, there are very few reports of formal investigations or long-term trials concerning composite repair. Recently, however, 2- to 3-year clinical results have been reported showing good outcomes for repairs or the resealing of marginal defects, and a recent 7-year recall reinforced the use of a conservative repair strategy. A survey of general practitioners found that half always repair defective composite margins adjacent to enamel but most replace a restoration if the defective margin is adjacent to dentin. Thus, it would appear that the repair of composite restorations with defective margins adjacent to enamel is becoming the standard of care.

Mechanical bonding can be achieved by roughening the intraoral surface through air abrasion followed by phosphoric acid application to clean the surface of debris and etch any available enamel. The repair can then be completed using a bonding agent and resin composite of choice. Recent studies also suggest that air abrasion combined with silica coating (and possibly silane) is a very effective preparation method for composite repair.

Acid Etching

As described in Chapter 6, acid etching is used to aid and enhance the formation of a resin bond to the teeth. For example, when aqueous 30%–50% phosphoric acid is applied to enamel, the enamel rods are attacked and dissolved to depths of 10–100 μm. The differential etching of the rods and interprismatic material results in etch pits about 4 μm in diameter. When a composite is applied, resin can readily wet the etched surfaces and flow into the pits, thus forming microscale mechanical bonds (micromechanical interlocking) and anchoring the resin to the enamel. Thus, etching increases surface area, increases surface energy to enhance wetting, and creates porous enamel-rod ends for resin penetration.

Because some conventional restorative cavity walls are roughly parallel to the enamel rods, it may be necessary to overextend the restoration onto uncut enamel, or (better) to add chamfers or bevels to the enamel of the cavity preparation periphery to obtain bonding. More restorative tags are produced if an unfilled "bonding agent" resin is applied prior to application of the composite.

Use of Composites for Resin Veneers

Originally resin veneering materials were heat-polymerized polymethylmethacrylate, which were improved subsequently by the addition of fillers and cross-linking agents. Microfilled materials that use *bis*-GMA, UDMA, or other high-molecular-weight dimethacrylates—such as 4, 8-dimethacryloxymethylene-tricyclodecane (Fig. 5.18)—as resin matrices have created renewed interest in resin-veneered metal restorations. These resins are polymerized using visible light or a combination of heat and pressure. In general, these new microfilled resins have physical properties superior to those of the original unfilled resin.

The first resin veneers were mechanically bonded to metal substrates using wire loops or retention beads. Recent improvements in bonding mechanisms have included micromechanical retention created by acid etching the base metal alloy and the use of chemical bonding systems such as 4-META, phosphorylated methacrylate, epoxy resin, or silicone dioxide flame-sprayed to the metal surface followed by the application of a silane coupling agent (silicoating).

Prosthetic resin-veneering materials have several advantages and disadvantages compared with ceramics. The advantages include ease of fabrication, predictable intraoral reparability, and less wear of opposing teeth or restorations. The drawbacks include low proportional limit and pronounced plastic deformation, which contribute to distortion on occlusal loading. Therefore, the resin should be protected with metal occlusal surfaces whenever feasible. Leakage of oral fluids and staining below the veneers, particularly those attached mechanically, are caused by dimensional changes from water sorption, heating, and cooling. Surface staining and intrinsic discoloration tend to occur with these resins.

Resins are also susceptible to wear during toothbrushing. Thus, it is necessary to instruct the patient on proper cleaning procedures using a soft toothbrush and mild abrasive toothpastes. Resin-veneered metal restorations are not suitable for use as removable partial denture abutment retainers where the clasp arm engages an undercut on the veneered surface because the resin is not as wear-resistant as porcelain.

Resin composites can also be used as a conservative alternative to conventional prosthodontic restorations, such as veneers for masking tooth discoloration or malformation. The resins are used as preformed laminate veneers, in which resin shells are adjusted by grinding and the contoured facing is bonded to tooth structure using the acid-etching technique with either chemically activated, visible light–activated, or dual-cure luting resin cements. Resins used to cement indirect restorations, veneers, and prosthetic devices are similar to flowable restorative resins but are adjusted to match the needs of luting applications. This type of resin material is discussed further in Chapter 11.

Selection Criteria for Posterior Composites

Not all patients should be considered as candidates for these posterior restorations. The primary indication for using direct posterior composites in place of amalgam is esthetics. Unless the patient's esthetic demands are high, there are minimal advantages to using resin restorations in posterior regions. Often the disadvantages coupled with the difficulty in manipulation far outweigh the benefits. Selection criteria for composite resins are described in Box 5.3.

The Academy of Operative Dentistry–European Section (Lynch 2014) considers the placement of resin composites to be appropriate in the following clinical scenarios in posterior teeth:

- Treatment of primary lesions of caries.
- Replacement of existing defective direct restorations.
- Replacement of most inlays.
- Repair of existing restorations, both direct and indirect.
- Restoration of endodontically treated teeth which do not
- require the protection afforded by an extracoronal restoration.
- Restoration of fractured and cracked teeth.
- Restoration of teeth affected by tooth wear or erosion.

Other indications might include the need for conservative preparations along with conservation of tooth structure. Because composite restorations do not depend on mechanical undercuts for retention, the concepts of resistance form and retention form do not really apply to resin preparations. However, because of their inferior physical properties

- Composites should not be used for cuspal coverage or for large restorations exceeding one-third the buccolingual width of the tooth.
- If possible, occlusal load should always be borne by sound tooth structure and never by resin.
- Because wear is also an issue, posterior composites should not be placed in patients experiencing parafunctional habits.

Photocuring Training, Evaluation, and Process Management

In order to reach a high degree of cure, light-cured resins must receive sufficient energy at the appropriate wavelengths. The light energy delivered to the composite is dictated by the operator technique of focusing light on the restoration, the type of curing light, and the location of the restoration, and the energy needed for proper curing depends on the type of resin used. Clinicians may have dental radiometers to measure the irradiance at the emitting tip of a curing light but might not be certain if sufficient energy has been delivered to the restoration to reach an adequate cure level and depth of cure.

The "MARC" (an acronym for "managing accurate resin curing," BlueLight Analytics Inc., Halifax, NS) device and training system shifts the paradigm away from measuring the average irradiance of a curing light and only including the wavelengths and energy actually received by the resin being polymerized. The MARC device combines precise laboratory spectral technology with clinically relevant measuring conditions within prepared dentoform teeth in a mannequin head. Spectrum-corrected sensors inside the dentoform teeth are attached to a laboratory-grade spectroradiometer embedded within the manikin's head to record the light received from curing units. Output from the spectrometer is fed into a laptop computer, where custom software provides real-time and accumulated comparison data: spectral irradiance, total energy delivered over a given exposure duration, and the estimated exposure duration needed to deliver a specified energy dosage.

In addition to providing real-time feedback to judge when adequate photoenergy has been delivered, the MARC device can also be used as a training aid for performing optimal photocuring in clinics (Box 5.4). The effect of minor alterations in tip distance and angle and movement during exposure is displayed in real time, and the ultimate consequence in terms of altered energy delivered is determined. The device can also be used to determine the ability of various lamps to deliver adequate energy levels between different tooth locations.

• BOX 5.3 Selection of Composite Resins

- Microfilled composites are the resins of choice for restoring teeth with carious lesions in smooth surfaces (Classes III and V) but not in stress-bearing situations (Classes II and IV)
- Small (fine) particle composites have an excellent balance among polishability, appearance, and durability, making this category suitable for general anterior use
- Hybrid composites are a general utility class of composites that are also suitable for restoring certain high-stress sites where esthetic considerations dominate
- Nanocomposites with clusters have increased filler loading and hence better mechanical properties than a true homogeneous nanocomposite
- Despite manufacturers' claims to the contrary, packable composites have not yet proven to be an answer to the general need for highly wear-resistant, easily placed posterior resins with low curing shrinkage and a depth of cure greater than 2 mm

• BOX 5.4 Clinical recommendations for improving performance of curing light

1. Monitor the performance of the curing light and keep a logbook of the output from the light from the date of purchase. Repair or replace the light when necessary.
2. Maximize the output from the curing light by routinely examining the light tip for damage and remove remnants of previously cured resin. Clean or replace the tip as necessary.
3. Place the central axis of the tip of the curing light directly over the resin surface; the emitting end should be parallel to the resin surface being exposed.
4. Where undercuts are present that cause shadows, move the light tip around and increase the exposure time. Use supplementary buccolingual interproximal curing (but beware of overheating).
5. Beware of damaging the pulp or oral mucosa when using a powerful curing light. Use a lower power setting when curing the bonding system in deep cavities. Protect the oral mucosa from the light with gauze and either air cool or wait several seconds between each light curing cycle when using a curing light that might produce a damaging temperature increase.

Acknowledgments

The authors would like to acknowledge Dr Josephine Esquivel-Upshaw and Dr Barry K Norling for their contribution to the previous edition of this chapter.

Summary

- **Terminology**
  Dental resin-based composites are structures composed of three major components:
  - A highly cross-linked polymeric resin matrix reinforced by a dispersion of glass, silica, crystalline,
  - Metal oxide or resin-reinforcing filler particles or their combinations and/or short fibers, which are bonded to the matrix by
  - Silane *coupling agents*
- **Classification**
  - Traditional (large particle): Particle size 1–50 μm glass or silica
  - Hybrid (large particle): Particle size 1–20 μm glass or 40 nm silica
  - Hybrid (midfilled): Particle size 0.1–10 μm glass or 40 nm silica
  - Hybrid (minifilled/SPF): Particle size 0.1–2 μm glass or 40 nm silica
  - Nanohybrid: Particle size 0.1–2 μm glass or resin microparticles or ≤100 nm nanoparticles
  - Nanofilled composite: Particle size <100 nm silica or zirconia homogeneous independent nanoparticles or nanoclusters.
- **Classifications of filled resins**
  Two general classifications are used to categorize resin based composites:
  - One **based on the size and combination of sizes of the reinforcing filler particles.**
  - **Ano**ther is based on the manipulation characteristics of the filled monomer paste.
- **Classification based on size**
  - **Small (fine) particle composites:** Small-particle composites have mean particle diameters between 0.1 and 10 mm (minifiller and midfiller).
  - **Microfilled composites:** Microfilled composites are agglomerates of 0.01–0.1 mm inorganic colloidal silica particles embedded in 5–50 mm resin filler particles.
  - **Hybrid composites: nanofilled composites/nanocomposites/nanohybrid composites.**
- **Classification of composites by manipulation characteristics**
- ***Flowable composites***
  A modification of the small-particle composite and hybrid composite, results in the so-called flowable composites. These resins typically have a lower viscosity through reduced filler loading, which enables the resin to flow readily, spread uniformly, intimately adapt to a cavity form, and produce the desired dental anatomy.
- ***Condensable (packable) composites***
  Packable composites, also known as condensable composites were developed by adjusting their filler distribution to increase the strength and stiffness of the uncured material. They have consistency and handling characteristics similar to lathe-cut amalgam.
- **Bulk fill composites**
  In the recent past a new variety of composite resins have been launched which claim to provide ease of use with large increments of 4 mm. Two types of bulk filled composites are available.
  - Low-viscosity materials.
  - High-viscosity bulk placement materials.
- **Composition**
- **Matrix:** The resin matrix in most dental composites is based on a blend of aromatic and/or aliphatic *dimethacrylate* monomers such as *bis*-GMA and urethane dimethacrylate (UDMA) to form highly cross-linked, strong, rigid, and durable polymer structures which forms a continuous phase in which the reinforcing filler is dispersed.
- **Filler:** Various transparent mineral fillers are employed to strengthen and reinforce composites as well as to reduce curing shrinkage and thermal expansion (generally between 30% and 70% by volume or 50% and 85% by weight of a composite). Fillers can provide the following benefits:
  - Reinforcement
  - Reduction of polymerization shrinkage/contraction
  - Reduction in thermal expansion and contraction
  - Control of workability/viscosity
  - Decreased water sorption
  - Imparting radiopacity.
- **Coupling agent**
  The two phases of the composite are chemically bound together by a coupling agent; this is a difunctional surface active compound that adheres to filler particle surfaces and also coreacts with the monomer forming the resin matrix.
- **Activation/initiation system**
- **Chemically activated (self-cure) resins**
- **Photochemically activated (light-cure) resins**
- ***Curing lamps***
  - Light-emitting diode (LED) lamps
  - Quartz-tungsten-halogen (QTH) lamps
  - Plasma arc curing (PAC) lamps
  - Argon laser lamps.
- **Dual-cured resins**
- **Curing shrinkage and shrinkage stress**
- **Reduction of shrinkage stresses**

Review Questions

1. Discuss in brief configuration factor (C factor).
2. Discuss in brief polymerization shrinkage.
3. Discuss in detail composition of composites.
4. Discuss in brief light curing units.
5. Techniques to overcome polymerization shrinkage.
6. Classify composites.
7. Discuss in brief dual cured composites.
8. Discuss in brief hybrid composites.
9. Discuss in brief flowable composites.
10. Discuss in brief bulk fill composites.
11. Discuss in brief fillers in composites.
12. Recent advances in composites.
13. Discuss in brief low shrink composites.
14. Discuss in detail composite placement techniques.
15. Describe the composition and classification of composite restorative resins.
16. Classify composite resins. Give its composition and describe the role of fillers in composite resins.

17. Classify composite resins. Give its composition and describe the role of fillers in composite resins add a note on visible light-activated composite resins.
18. Name 3 structural components in composite resin. Give two examples for each component. Give two advantages and disadvantages of light-cured composite.
19. Classify composite resins. What are bonding and coupling agents?
20. Classify composite resins. Discuss in detail each ingredient in composite, with strong emphasis on matrix, filler, and coupling agent.
21. Discuss pit and fissure sealants.
22. Discuss in brief curing systems for composites.
23. Discuss in detail factors influencing optical properties of composite resins.
24. Discuss in detail the physical properties of composite resins and factors affecting the same.
25. Discuss in detail properties of composite resins.
26. Discuss in brief sandwich technique.
27. Discuss in brief preventive resin restorations.
28. Compare the various curing systems for composites.
29. Discuss in detail curing lights and technique of ramp curing.
30. Discuss in brief soft start polymerization.

Selected Readings

Publications and Patents

Academy of Dental Materials. International Congress on Dental Materials, Transactions. Academy of Dental Materials, Baylor College of Dentistry: Houston, TX; A host of review papers are presented on many aspects of dental composite chemistry, systems usage, dentin bonding agents, and microleakage.

Albers H. Tooth-Colored Restoratives: Principles and Techniques. ed 9 BC Decker: Hamilton, Ontario, Canada; The author discusses a complete array of composite systems, with emphasis on clinical applications. The book combines the science of dental polymers with discussions of clinical applications.

Boaro L.C.C.; Goncalves F.; Guimarães T.C.; et al. Polymerization stress, shrinkage and elastic modulus of current low-shrinkage restorative composites. Dent Mater 26 (12) 1144–1150 (2010); This investigation found that not all composites that claimed "low-shrinkage" exhibited reduced polymerization shrinkage. It was also concluded that in order to effectively reduce polymerization stress (not just shrinkage), a low post-gel shrinkage must be accompanied by a relatively low elastic modulus.

Bowen R.L. Dental filling material comprising vinyl-silane treated fused silica and a binder consisting of the reaction product of bisphenol A and glycidyl methacrylate. US Patent 3,006,112 US Patent and Trademark Office: Washington, DC; This patent marks a milestone in dentistry. It resulted in superior resin-based materials and was issued a few years after Buonocore's discovery that resins could be bonded to acid-etched enamel. With Bowen's invention and Buonocore's discovery, it became possible to restore class IV cavities in a conservative and predictable way, which had been impossible previously.

Chadwick B.L.; Dummer P.M.H.; Dunstan F.; et al. The Longevity of Dental Restorations: A Systematic Review. National Health Service Centre for Reviews and Dissemination, University of York: York, UK; A comprehensive evidence-based review of dental restorations.

Chen M.-H. Update on dental nanocomposites. J Dent Res 89 549–560 (2010); This article reviews recent studies of the development of dental nanocomposites and their clinical applications, as of 2010.

da Rosa Rodolpho P.A.; Cenci M.S.; Donassollo T.A.; et al. A clinical evaluation of posterior composite restorations: 17-year findings. J Dent 34 427–435 (2006).

Darvell B.W. Materials Science for Dentistry. ed 9 Woodhead Publishing Ltd: Cambridge, UK; A comprehensive dental materials science textbook that connects clinical performance properties to first principles and underlying mechanism in much greater detail than is typically presented to dental students. An excellent reference for researchers, materials scientists, and those in academic dentistry as well as students at all levels.

Darvell B.W. Glossary of Terms for Dental Materials Science. ed 11 Kuwait Publishing Ltd: Cambridge, UK.

Drummond J.L. Degradation, fatigue, and failure of resin dental composite materials. J Dent Res 87 710–719 (2008).

Ferracane, J. L., et al. (2017). "Academy of Dental Materials guidance-Resin composites: Part II-Technique sensitivity (handling, polymerization, dimensional changes)." Dent Mater **33**(11): 1171-1191. OBJECTIVE: The objective of this work, commissioned by the Academy of Dental Materials, was to review and critically appraise test methods to characterize properties related to critical issues for dental resin composites, including technique sensitivity and handling, polymerization, and dimensional stability, in order to provide specific guidance to investigators planning studies of these properties. RESULTS: The properties for evaluating resin composites were ranked in the priority of measurement as follows: (1) porosity, radiopacity, sensitivity to ambient light, degree of conversion, polymerization kinetics, depth of cure, polymerization shrinkage and rate, polymerization stress, and hygroscopic expansion; (2) stickiness, slump resistance, and viscosity; and (3) thermal expansion.

Ferracane J.L. Resin composite—state of the art. Dent Mater 27 (1) 29–38 (2011); This review concludes that in 2010 the commercial materials available to the dental profession were of high quality and when used appropriately have proven to deliver excellent clinical outcomes of adequate longevity.

Gallegos L.L.; Nicholls J.I. In vitro two-body wear of three veneering resins. J Prosthet Dent 60 172 (1988); Three veneering resins were tested for wear. A significant difference in wear against porcelain was found among the three resins, but no difference in wear was found against enamel.

Heintze, S. D., et al. (2015). "Clinical effectiveness of direct anterior restorations—a meta-analysis." Dent Mater 31(5): 481-495.

This is the first meta-analysis on the efficacy of composite resin restorations in anterior teeth. The objective of the present meta-analysis was to verify whether specific material classes, tooth conditioning methods and operational procedures influence the result for Class III and Class IV restorations. Of the 84 clinical trials, 21 studies met the inclusion criteria, 14 of them for Class III restorations, 6 for Class IV restorations and 1 for closure of diastemata; the latter was included in the Class IV group. Twelve of the 21 studies started before 1991 and 18 before 2001. The estimated median overall success rate (without replacement) after 10 years for Class III composite resin restorations was 95% and for Class IV restorations 90%. The main reason for the replacement of Class IV restorations was bulk fractures, which occurred significantly more frequently with microfilled composites than with hybrid and macrofilled composites.

Ilie, N., et al. (2017). "Academy of Dental Materials guidance-Resin composites: Part I-Mechanical properties." Dent Mater 33(8): 880-894.

OBJECTIVE: The objective of this project, which was initiated from the Academy of Dental Materials, was to review and critically appraise methods to determine fracture, deformation and wear resistance of dental resin composites, in an attempt to provide guidance for investigators endeavoring to study these properties for these materials. RESULTS: The properties for evaluating resin composites were ranked in the priority of measurement as following: (1) Strength, Elastic Modulus, Fracture toughness, Fatigue, Indentation Hardness,

Wear-abrasion (third body) and Wear-attrition (contact/two body), (2) Toughness, Edge strength (chipping) and (3) Wear determined by toothbrush.

Joniot S.B.; Gregoire G.L.; Auther A.M.; et al. Three dimensional optical profilometry analysis of surface states obtained after finishing sequences for three resin-based composites. Oper Dent 25 311–315 (2000).

Khurana S.; Rammal S.; Ben-Jonathan N. Exposure of newborn male and female rats to environmental estrogens: Delayed and sustained hyperprolactinemia and alterations in estrogen receptor expression. Endocrinology 141 4512–4517 (2000).

Lambrechts P.; Braem M.; Vanherle G. Evaluation of clinical performance for posterior resin-based composites and dentin adhesives. J Oper Dent 12 53 (1987); These authors have been leaders in the clinical evaluation of resin systems. This paper is a superb treatment of the subject and emphasizes the limitations of current adhesives and composites.

Lutz F.; Phillips R.W. A classification and evaluation of composite resin systems. J. Prosthet Dent 50 480 (1983); This article presents a structure-based classification scheme for composites, one that has been almost universally accepted since its publication. Knowledge of the structure makes it possible to make decisions as to the inherent properties and selection for specific situations. (See also Willems et al. [1992], below).

Lynch, C. D., et al. (2014). "Guidance on posterior resin composites: Academy of Operative Dentistry - European Section." J Dent 42(4): 377-383.

This paper presents the position of the Academy of Operative Dentistry European Section (AODES) in relation to posterior resin composites. The AODES considers adhesively bonded resin composites of suitable composition and properties to be the "material of choice" for use in direct minimal intervention approaches to the restoration of posterior teeth. In so doing, the AODES emphasises the importance of the practice of evidence-based minimal intervention dentistry, including the use of refurbishment and repair techniques to extend the longevity of restorations. Guidance, based on best available evidence, has been made in relation to certain aspects of resin composite placement techniques in posterior teeth.

Malhotra N.; Mala K. Light-curing considerations for resin-based composite materials: a review. Part I. Compend Contin Educ Dent 31 (7) 498–505 (2010). ibid, Part II, 31(8):584–591, 2010; These articles provide an excellent overview of the performance and limitations of four types of curing lights for resin-based composites: LED, QTH, PAC, and laser curing. The type of curing light and curing mode impact the polymerization kinetics of resin-based composite (RBC) materials. They also affect the polymerization shrinkage and associated stresses, microhardness, depth of cure, degree of conversion, and color change of RBCs. These factors can also influence the microleakage in an RBC restoration. Apart from the type of unit and mode used, the polymerization of RBCs is also affected by how a light-curing unit is used and handled, as well as the aspects associated with RBCs and the environment. Part II discusses the various clinical issues that should be considered while curing RBC restorations in order to achieve the best possible outcome.

Manhart J.; Chen H.V.; Hickel R. The suitability of packable resin-based composites for posterior restorations. J Am Dent Assoc 132 (5) 639–645 (2001).

Manhart J.; Chen H.Y.; Hamm G.; et al. Review of the clinical survival of direct and indirect restorations in posterior teeth of the permanent dentition. Oper Dent 29 481–508 (2004); These reviewers surveyed the literature from about 1990 to 2004 to assess the longevity of restorations in stress-bearing posterior cavities, and possible reasons for clinical failure. Indirect resin restorations were found to have lower annual failure rates than direct restorations ($P = 0.0031$). Principal reasons for failure were secondary caries, fracture, marginal deficiencies, wear, and postoperative sensitivity.

Manhart J.; Kunzelmann K.-H.; Chen H.Y.; et al. Mechanical properties of new composite restorative materials. J Biomed Mater Res (A) 53 353–361 (2000); An evaluation of the new class of hybrid composites known as "packable" or "condensable." These authors demonstrate that although the handling character of these materials is analogous to that of lathe-cut amalgams, they do not offer any other advantage compared with other hybrid composites as restorative resins.

Naciff J.M.; Jump M.L.; Torontalli S.M.; et al. Gene expression profile induced by 17 alpha-ethynyl estradiol, bisphenol A and genistein in the developing female reproductive system of the rat. Toxicol Sci 68 184–199 (2002).

Olea N.; Pulgar R.; Perez P.; et al. Estrogenicity of resin-based composites and sealants used in dentistry. Environ Health Perspect 104 298–305 (1996).

Opdam, N. J., et al. (2014). "Longevity of posterior composite restorations: a systematic review and meta-analysis." J Dent Res 93(10): 943-949.

The aim of this meta-analysis, based on individual participant data from several studies, was to investigate the influence of patient-, materials-, and tooth-related variables on the survival of posterior resin composite restorations. Following Preferred Reporting Items for Systematic Reviews and Meta-Analyses (PRISMA) guidelines, we conducted a search resulting in 12 longitudinal studies of direct posterior resin composite restorations with at least 5 years' follow-up. Of all restorations, 2,816 (2,585 Class II and 231 Class I) were included in the analysis, of which 569 failed during the observation period. Main reasons for failure were caries and fracture. The regression analyses showed a significantly higher risk of failure for restorations in high-caries-risk individuals and those with a higher number of restored surfaces.

Opdam N.J.M.; Bronkhorst E.M.; Roeters J.M.; et al. A retrospective clinical study on longevity of posterior composite and amalgam restorations. Dent Mater 23 (1) 2–8 (2007).

Paris F.; Balaguer P.; Terouanne B.; et al. Phenylphenols, biphenols, bisphenol-A and 4-tert-octylphenol exhibit alpha and beta estrogen activities and antiandrogen activity in reporter cell lines. Mol Cell Endocrinol 193 43–49 (2002); This article concludes that the environmental chemicals studied may have a negative impact on androgen action during fetal and postnatal life.

Ramos R.P.; Chinelatti M.A.; Chimello D.T.; et al. Assessing microleakage in resin composite restorations rebounded with a surface sealant and three low-viscosity resin systems. Quintessence Int 33 450–456 (2002).

Price R.B.; Felix C.M.; Whalen J.M. Factors affecting the energy delivered to simulated class I and class V preparations. J Can Dent Assoc 76 A94 (2010)http://www.jcda.ca/article/a94.

Price R.B.; Labrie D.; Whalen J.M.; et al. Effect of distance on irradiance and beam homogeneity from four light-emitting diode curing units. J Can Dent Assoc 77 B9 (2011)http://www.jcda.ca/article/B9; These two articles by Price et al. present an analysis of both technical variations among curing lamps and human operator variables on clinical outcomes and implications for best practice techniques.

Ravasini, F., et al. (2018). "Treatment Outcome of Posterior Composite Indirect Restorations: A Retrospective 20-Year Analysis of 525 Cases with a Mean Follow-up of 87 Months." Int J Periodontics Restorative Dent 38(5): 655-663.

The purpose of this study was to evaluate the survival of 525 composite indirect restorations in premolars and molars after a follow-up of 20 years. For each patient, the following variables were recorded and analyzed: age, sex, smoking status, presence of plaque according to O'Leary index, and presence of bruxism. The results of this study demonstrate the efficacy of indirect composite restorations, confirming their reliability as a posterior prosthetic clinical option.

Roulet J.-F.J.F. Degradation of Dental Polymers. Karger: Basel and New York; A thorough discussion is presented of the chemistry and composition of modern dental restorative resins. Emphasis is placed on how composition and clinical usage influence the longevity of a restorative material in vivo.

Roulet J.-F.J.F. The problems associated with substituting resin-based composites for amalgam: a status report on posterior composites. J Dent 16 101 (1988); A comprehensive review is presented of the factors to be considered in the use of posterior composites as an alternative to dental amalgam. The author concludes that the indications for posterior composites are very limited.

Rueggeberg F.A. An Expert's Buying Guide for Curing Lights. ADA Professional Product Review. Vol. 4 American Dental Association: Chicago, IL.

Schafer T.E.; Lapp C.A.; Hanes C.M.; et al. Estrogenicity of bisphenol A and bisphenol A dimethacrylate in vitro. J Biomed Mater Res 45 192–197 (1999).

Setcos J.C.; Tarim B.; Suzuki S. Surface finish produced on resin composites by new polishing systems. Quintessence Int 30 169–173 (1999).

Stansbury J.W. J Polymer science: Part A. Polym Chem 44 3921–3929 (2006); Article on N'Durance, a high-molecular-weight, phase-separating dicarbamate with composite resin having hydrophobic side chains.

Summitt J.B.; Robbins W.J.; Hilton T.J.; et al. Fundamentals of Operative Dentistry: A Contemporary Approach. ed 3 Quintessence: Chicago; The technical procedures used in the placement of resin-based composites in various types of restorations are discussed and illustrated. Many clinical illustrations are included that show the variety of applications for dental composites.

Tsujimoto, A., et al. (2018). "Wear of resin composites: Current insights into underlying mechanisms, evaluation methods and influential factors." Jpn Dent Sci Rev 54(2): 76-87.

Van Ende, A., et al. (2017). "Bulk-Fill Composites: A Review of the Current Literature." J Adhes Dent 19(2): 95-109.

Wendt S.L. Jr.; Leinfelder K.F. The clinical evaluation of heat-treated composite resin inlays. J Am Dent Assoc 120 177 (1990); One of a few papers available that report the clinical performance of heat-polymerized composite inlays. Although marginal integrity was superior, no difference was detected in wear resistance as compared with light-cured inlays.

Weinmann W.; Thalacker C.; Guggenberger R. Siloranes in dental composites. Dent Mater 21 (1) 68–74 (2005).

Wilder A.D. Jr.; May K.N. Jr.; Bayne S.C.; et al. Seventeen-year clinical study of ultraviolet-cured posterior composite class I and II restorations. J Esthet Dent 11 135–142 (1999).

Willems G.; Lambrechts P.; Braem M.; et al. A classification of dental composites according to morphological and mechanical characteristics. Dent Mater 81 310–319 (1992); A classification scheme for composites, based on structure, that revises and updates the earlier one of Lutz and Phillips (1983; see above).

Wolter H.; Storch W.; Ott H. New inorganic/organic copolymers (ORMOCERS) for dental applications. Mat Res Soc Symp Proc 346 143–149 (1994).

Wu J.; Mather R.T. POSS polymers: Physical properties and biomaterials applications. J Macromol Sci R, Part C: Polymer Rev 49 25–63 (2009).

Yap A.U.J.; Sau C.W.; Lye K.W. Effects of finishing/polishing time on surface characteristics of tooth-colored restoratives. J Oral Rehab 25 456–461 (1998).

Yap A.U.J.; Wong M.L.; Lim A.C. The effect of polishing systems on microleakage of tooth-coloured restoratives. Part 2: Composite and polyacid-modified resin-based composites. J Oral Rehabil 27 205–210 (2000).

Useful Websites

Biomaterials Properties Database: http://www.lib.umich.edu/node/21860

The Biomaterials Network: http://www.biomat.net/

Dentistry Today, Advanced Resin Technologies: http://www.dentistrytoday.com/dental-materials/972

Dental products newsletters: http://www.dentaladvisor.com/, http://www.cliniciansreport.org/page/additonal-studies-archive, http://adeptinstitute.com/members/000_source/membership/list.php

Managing Accurate Resin Curing (MARC): http://curingresin.com/dental_clinicians.html

Ormocer technology: http://www.ormocer.de/EN/herstellungsver fahren/index.jsp

Polyhedral oligomeric silsesquioxane (POSS) technology, Hybrid Plastics: http://www.hybridplastics.com/docs/

Polymer Learning Center, acrylic polymers: http://www.pslc.ws/mactest/level3.htm

Virtual Textbook of Polymer Science: http://plc.case.edu/tutorial/enhanced/files/textbook.htm

6

Bonding Mechanism and Bonding Agents

CHAPTER OUTLINE

KEY TERMS

Acid-etching/Acid-etch technique—The process of cleaning and roughening a solid surface by exposing it to an acid and thoroughly rinsing the residue to promote micromechanical bonding of an adhesive to the surface.

Adhesion—A molecular or atomic attraction between two contacting surfaces promoted by the interfacial force of attraction between the molecules or atoms of two different materials. Adhesion may occur as chemical adhesion (formation of covalent bonds, hydrogen bonds, or polar bonds via van der Waals attraction [Chapter 2]), mechanical adhesion (structural interlocking), or a combination of both types.

Cement/Cementing—Substance that hardens from a viscous state to a solid union between two surfaces. For dental applications, cements act as a base, liner, restorative filling material, or adhesive to bond devices and prostheses to tooth structure or to each other. See also *Luting agent*.

Contact angle—Angle of intersection between a liquid and a surface of a solid that is measured from the solid surface through the liquid to the liquid–vapor tangent line originating at the terminus of the liquid–solid interface; used as a measure of wettability, whereby absolutely no wetting occurs at a contact angle of 180 degrees and complete wetting occurs at an angle of 0 degrees.

Dentin-bonding agent—A thin layer of resin between conditioned dentin and the resin matrix of a resin-based composite restorative material.

Dentin conditioner—An acidic agent that dissolves the inorganic structure in dentin, resulting in a collagen mesh that allows infiltration of an adhesive resin.

Hybrid layer—An intermediate layer of resin, collagen, and dentin that is produced by acid etching of dentin and infiltration of resin into the conditioned dentin.

Luting agent—A viscous, cement-like material that also fills a gap between the bonded materials. It originally referred to nonadhesive agents only but now also includes adhesive agents.

Microleakage—The flow of oral fluid and bacteria into the microscopic gap between a prepared tooth surface and a restorative material.

Obturation—In endodontic dentistry, filling of a root canal completely and densely with a nonirritating hermetic sealing agent to prevent leakage.

Primer—A hydrophilic, low-viscosity resin that promotes bonding to a moist substrate, such as dentin.

Resin tag—Extension of resin that has penetrated into etched enamel or dentin. Resin tags form micromechanical interlocks analogous to screw threads.

Smear layer—Poorly adherent layer of ground dentin produced by cutting a dentin surface; also, a tenacious deposit of microscopic debris that covers enamel and dentin surfaces that have been prepared for a restoration.

Bonding and **adhesion** comprise a complex set of physical, chemical, and mechanical mechanisms that allow the attachment and binding of one substance to another. A dental-bonding system performs three essential functions:

1. Provides resistance to separation of an **adherend** substrate (i.e., enamel, dentin, metal, composite, ceramic) from a restorative or **cementing** material.
2. Distributes stress along bonded interfaces.
3. Seals the interface via adhesive bonding between dentin and/or enamel and the bonded material, thus increasing resistance to **microleakage** and decreasing the risk for postoperative sensitivity, marginal staining, and secondary caries.

Historical Background

Prior to the middle of the twentieth century, dental bonding consisted of various methods of mechanical retention, such as forming undercuts in cavity preparations for amalgam restorations (see Chapter 8). **Luting**, using zinc phosphate and other nonadhesive dental cements, also falls into this category of bonding (see Chapter 7). In the late 1940s, Oskar Hagger, at the De Trey division of Amalgamated Dental, developed the first bonding agent, Sevriton Cavity Seal. This system was based on glycerophosphoric acid dimethacrylate (see Fig. 6.5 on page 136) as a self-adhesive or self-etching component for both enamel and **dentin bonding**. However, this product had very limited clinical durability because of the large interfacial stresses that developed because of the high polymerization shrinkage and high thermal expansion of the unfilled methacrylate-based resins used at that time. Shortly after, Michael Buonocore investigated stronger acids and discovered that phosphoric acid provides superior enamel etching, and it is still in use today.

As shown in Figure 6.1, these discoveries of **acid etching** led to our ability to produce clean, high-energy, roughened enamel surfaces capable of establishing a durable micromechanical retentive interface with resin-based cementing and restorative materials, which launched the current era of **adhesive** dentistry. These events soon led to a burgeoning growth in the development of adhesive materials and bonding techniques, into the beginning of the twenty-first century. This progress is summarized in Figure 6.1 and is discussed in detail in several of the later sections of this chapter. Presently, **adhesive bonding** can only be relied on for long-term retention in very select circumstances using highly specialized materials and clinical techniques, many of which are discussed in detail below. Nevertheless, dentistry is now well into the era of adhesive bonding and its associated field of esthetic dentistry. In order for bonding to be completely predictable and reliable, the following criteria would need to be satisfied:

1. The procedure must be safe and biologically acceptable.
2. The bond strength should be clinically significant to avoid discoloration at the margins and secondary caries.
3. The bond strength must be achieved easily with minimal technique sensitivity.
4. High early bond strengths should be achieved to facilitate immediate finishing of restorations.
5. The bond must be stable in vivo for a clinically significant period of time.

Applications for Bonding

It has always been the endeavor of the dental fraternity to create long-lasting restorations, with minimal removal of tooth structure. To that end, research has focused on adhesive technology as the most efficient way to bond dissimilar materials. Today, acid etching is one of the most predictable ways to promote restoration retention and to ensure a sealed interfacial joint at restoration margins. This procedure has markedly expanded the use of resin-based restorative materials because it provides a strong, durable bond between resin and tooth structure and has formed the basis for many innovative dental procedures as diverse as orthodontic bracket bonding and porcelain laminate veneer bonding. Additional applications include pit and fissure sealants; amalgam bonding, ceramic bonding; both enamel and dentin bonding; adhesive cements, including glass ionomer restorative materials; and endodontic sealers. Many of these applications are discussed in this chapter; however, other bonding applications are also discussed in greater detail throughout the book but with particular emphasis in Chapters 2, 5, 7, 10 and 11.

CRITICAL QUESTION

Why is good wetting of tooth structure by a dental adhesive not adequate for long-term adhesive bonding of a restorative material?

Mechanisms of Adhesion

True adhesion has been the "holy grail" of dental restorative materials for many decades. If true adhesion of restorative materials to tooth structure is to be achieved, three conditions must be satisfied:

1. Sound tooth structure must be conserved.
2. Optimal retention must be achieved.
3. Microleakage must be prevented.

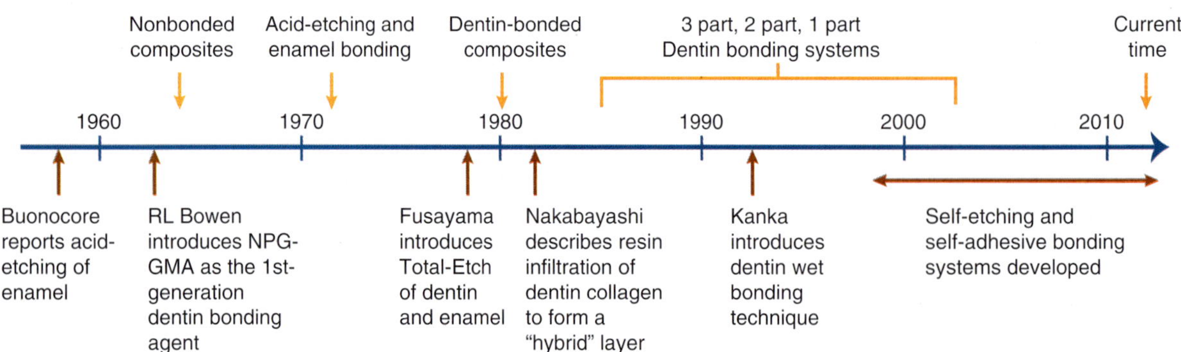

• **Fig. 6.1** Major turning points and events in dental bonding technologies.

The science of adhesion has been covered in Chapter 2. In this chapter, only those principles of adhesion needed for an understanding of dental bonding will be discussed.

Oral hard tissues and their environment are complex. However, the fundamental mechanism of adhesion to tooth structure can be regarded simply as an exchange by which inorganic tooth material (hydroxyapatite) is replaced by synthetic resins. This process involves two parts:

1. Removing hydroxyapatite to create micropores.
2. Infiltration of resin monomers into the micropores and subsequent polymerization.

As a result, **resin tags** are formed that micromechanically interlock or interpenetrate with the hard tissue. There may also be chemical interactions with the tooth substrate if monomers having acidic or chelating functional groups are present. In general, the following factors can play major or minor roles in achieving adhesive bonds:

1. Surface energy and wetting,
2. Interpenetration (formation of a hybrid zone),
3. Micromechanical interlocking,
4. Chemical bonding.

Wetting is the essential first step for the success of all adhesion mechanisms. An adhesive cannot form micromechanical interlocks, chemical bonds, or interpenetrating networks with a surface unless it can form intimate contact with the surface, spread over it, and penetrate by capillary attraction into any microscopic and submicroscopic irregularities. These conditions are, by definition, achieved if the adhesive wets the surface.

As explained in Chapter 2, **wettability** of a liquid on a solid can be characterized by the **contact angle** that forms between a liquid and solid, as measured within the liquid. Categories of wettability include "mostly nonwetting" (>90 degrees), "absolutely no wetting" (180 degrees), "mostly wetting" (<90 degrees), and absolute wetting (0 degrees). See Figure 2.40 for a schematic illustration of wetting situations.

Generally, wettability can be enhanced by increasing the **surface energy** of the substrates (e.g., dentin, enamel, and synthetic materials). Since a clean, microroughened tooth surface has higher surface energy than unprepared tooth surfaces, organic adhesives are inherently able to wet and spread over such a surface unless a low **surface tension** material contaminates it before the adhesive can be applied. The **acid-etch technique**, by which contaminants are removed and microporosities are created, is widely used to generate high-energy tooth surfaces and promote wetting by adhesive monomers.

Although wetting is an essential requirement for intraoral adhesion, it is not sufficient to ensure durable bonding. As explained below, to achieve strong bonding through the micromechanical interlocking mechanism, wetting monomers must intimately adapt to enamel and fill enamel surface irregularities and/or infiltrate into a demineralized collagen network in dentin. Some acid monomers with a phosphate (e.g., phenyl-P) or carboxyl group (e.g., 4-MET) have the additional potential of forming chemical bonds with calcium in the residual tooth tissue. The chemical structures of these acidic monomers are shown in Figs 6.4 and 6.6.

A key requirement for achieving lasting intraoral bonds is hydrolytic stability (resistance to chemical degradation by water). Enamel and dentin are hydrated, hydrophilic, and permeable to water. Even if an enamel or dentin surface is initially dried before applying an adhesive, inadvertent contamination and diffusion can easily result in water becoming strongly bound to both the hard tissue and the adhesive. Thus, for an adhesive monomer to wet hard tooth tissue as well as form a durable bond in the moist environment of the mouth, it must be both hydrophilic for water compatibility and hydrolytically stable to ensure longevity.

Smear Layer

Whenever both enamel and dentin tissues are mechanically cut, especially with a rotary instrument, a layer of adherent grinding debris and organic film known as a **smear layer** is left on their surfaces and prevents strong bonding. Different quantities and qualities of smear layer are produced during restorative and endodontic cavity preparation. The thickness would depend to a large degree on the types of instruments used and the instrumentation technique. In dentin, the smear layer becomes burnished into the underlying dentinal tubules and lowers dentin permeability, which is a protective effect. However, it is also weakly cohesive to the underlying dentin with a bond strength of 5–10 MPa, which interferes with strong bonding. It is essential, therefore, to employ various cleaning or treatment agents and procedures to either remove the smear layer or enhance its **cohesive strength** and other properties.

To achieve predictable bonding, it is essential to either remove the smear layer completely by using an acid or to modify it, and use adhesive monomers to penetrate the smear layer and bond to underlying intact dentin structures below.

The term "hybrid layer" is one of the key factors in the bonding of resins to etched dentin. *Without a hybrid layer, a strong and stable bond will not be formed to the dentin.* Therefore, it is essential to modify the dentin surface through conditioning, so a mechanical interlocking of resin around dentinal collagen can occur. The hybrid layer has also been referred to as the "resin dentin interdiffusion zone."

Acid-Etch Technique

Whenever both enamel and dentin tissues are mechanically cut, especially with a rotary instrument, a layer of loosely held debris and organic film known as a smear layer is left on their surfaces and prevents strong bonding. Different quantities and qualities of smear layer are produced by various cutting and instrumentation techniques, which play an important role in both restorative and endodontic treatments, as explained further in Chapter 9 (Cements). In dentin, the smear layer becomes burnished into the underlying dentinal tubules and lowers dentin permeability, which is a protective effect. However, it is also a very weakly cohesive material and thus detaches easily, consequently interfering with strong bonding. Thus, various cleaning or treatment agents and procedures must be employed to remove the smear layer and expose the intact substrate for bonding. As explained in greater detail in the discussion that follows, acid etching is used to remove the smear layer from both enamel and dentin. Alternatively, in dentin, the smear layer can be left partially in place and modified such that adhesive resins penetrate through it and bond to the intact dentin structures below.

Enamel Etching

The first meaningful demonstration of intraoral adhesion was reported by Michael Buonocore (1955). Buonocore etched enamel surfaces with various acids, placed an acrylic restorative material on the micromechanically roughened surfaces, and found a great increase in the resin–enamel bond strength (~20 megapascals [MPa]). One of the surface conditioning agents he used, phosphoric acid, is still the most widely used etchant today for bonding to both enamel and dentin. Depending on the concentration,

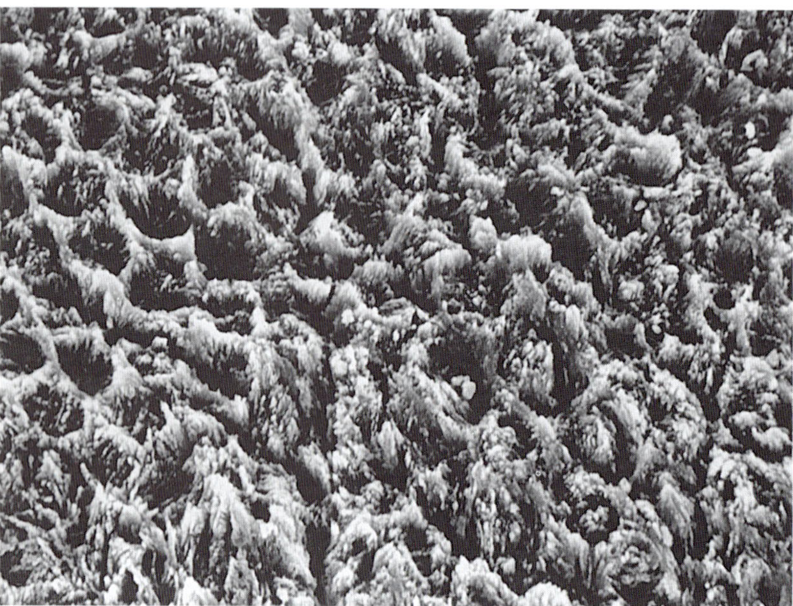

• **Fig. 6.2** Surface of etched enamel in which the centers of enamel rods have been preferentially dissolved by phosphoric acid. (Courtesy of K-J Söderholm.)

phosphoric acid removes the smear layer and about 10 microns of enamel to expose prisms of enamel rods to create a honeycomb-like, high-energy retentive surface (Fig. 6.2). The higher surface energy ensures that resin monomers will readily wet the surface, infiltrate into the micropores, and polymerize to form resin tags. The pattern of etching enamel may vary from selective dissolution of either the enamel rod centers (type I etching) as shown in Figure 6.2, or the peripheral areas (type II etching) as indicated by the resin tags in Figure 6.3. In either case, the resin tags are approximately 6 μm in diameter and 10–20 μm in length and lead to micromechanical interlocking.

Prior to the introduction of enamel acid etching and the use of enamel bonding agents, restorative materials were placed directly on the smear layer of the prepared tooth. It is evident that the apparent bond strength is the cohesive strength (5–10 MPa) of the smear layer, which is not sufficient to withstand the daily mechanical forces experienced in the mouth. As a result, debonding and leakage of oral fluids within the microscopic space between prepared teeth and restorative materials was an ongoing problem.

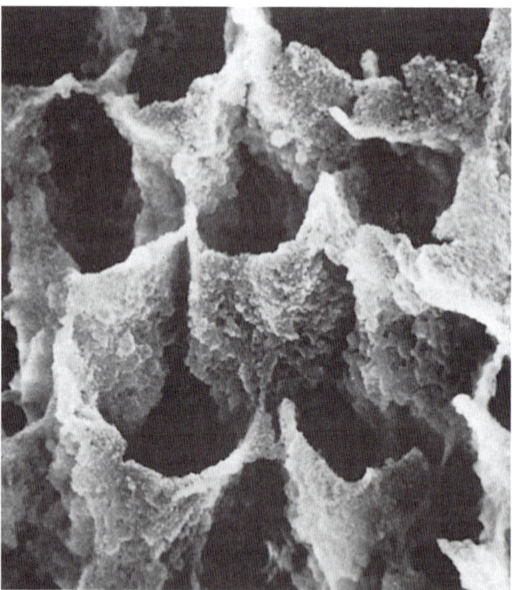

• **Fig. 6.3** Scanning electron microscopy image of tags formed by the penetration of resin into etched areas of enamel. The resin was applied to the etched enamel, and enamel was then dissolved by acid to reveal the tags (×5000). (Courtesy of K-J Söderholm.)

In earlier generations of restorative materials like amalgam, the microleakage was countered to a large extent by the deposition of corrosion products such as tin oxide. Resin-based composites also cause problems because of the shrinkage stress (~15 MPa) generated during polymerization, exacerbating fracture of the tooth-restorative interface. Stronger and longer lasting bonds result if the smear layer is removed, because resins can then directly bond to the intact hard tissue.

Dentin Etching

As illustrated in Figure 6.1, dentin etching did not gain wide acceptance until Fusayama introduced the total-etch concept in 1979. For this method, both dentin and enamel are etched simultaneously, typically using 37% phosphoric acid. His study demonstrated that not only was restoration retention substantially increased but also pulp damage did not occur as had been generally assumed. A subsequent study by Nakabayashi et al (1984) revealed that hydrophilic resins can infiltrate the surface layer of acid-demineralized collagen fibers that are produced in etched dentin and it can form a layer of resin-infiltrated dentin with high cohesive strength. Such a **hybrid layer** structure forms very strong resin bonds through the development of an interpenetrating network of polymer and dentinal collagen, together with numerous micromechanical interlocks at the resin–hybrid layer interface. Since the total-etch technique usually involves etching with an acid followed by rinsing to remove the acid, this technique is also known as the *etch-and-rinse technique* (Box 6.1).

Dentin etching is more technique-sensitive than enamel etching because of the complexity of the dentin structure. Unlike enamel, dentin is a living tissue, consisting of 50 vol% (volume percentage) of calcium phosphate mineral (hydroxyapatite), 30 vol% of organic material (mainly type I collagen), and 20 vol%

• BOX 6.1 Clinical Tips for Etch-and-Rinse Technique

- Acid gel is preferable to liquid: application is easier to control
- Concentration 35%; time minimum: 15–30 seconds
- Rinsing time: 5–10 seconds
- Complete removal of etchant through rinsing is crucial for success. This ensures removal of etchant as well as dissolved calcium phosphates
- Complete isolation of etched surface with no saliva contamination crucial to ensure longevity of bond
- Despite careful handling, the composition of the primer solution may change after the bottle has been opened and closed several times due to quick evaporation of solvent
- *Many clinicians, however, still dry the tooth preparation after rinsing away the etching gel to check for the classic etched enamel appearance. Because it is clinically impossible to dry enamel without simultaneously drying dentin, the dentin collagen collapses easily upon air drying*
- Rewetting the dried etched dentin with water or with aqueous rewetting agents has been demonstrated to restore bond strength values and to raise the collapsed collagen network to a level similar to a "wet bonding" technique

fluid. Acid etching removes hydroxyapatite almost completely from several microns of sound dentin, exposing a microporous network of collagen suspended in water. In order to achieve predictable bonds in dentin, it is essential to penetrate and integrate these collagen fibers into the hybrid layer. To achieve this, it is essential that the collagen fibers remain distended in a moist environment. A ***priming*** step, which involves using a hydrophilic monomer with a solvent, is used to achieve resin infiltration into conditioned dentin. The solvent helps remove the water while the hydrophilic resin penetrates the spaces between the collagen fibers, thus achieving interdiffusion. The amount of water left in etched dentin is critical. If insufficient water is present, the collagen network will collapse and produce a relatively impermeable layer that prevents resin infiltration and subsequent hybridization. If too much water remains, resin infiltration cannot fully replace the water in the collagen network and, consequently, sets the condition for later leakage into those locations.

Process and Procedural Factors

Several aspects of the total-etch, etch-and-rinse, and related techniques are critical to the success or failure of bonding systems, as discussed below.

Etching Time

The optimal application time for the etchant may vary somewhat, depending on previous exposure of the tooth surface to fluoride and other factors. For example, a permanent tooth with a high fluoride content may require a somewhat longer etching time, as do primary teeth. In the latter, increased surface conditioning time is needed to enhance the etching pattern on primary tooth enamel that is more aprismatic than permanent tooth enamel. Currently, the etching time for most etching gels is approximately 15 seconds. The advantage of such short etching times is that they yield acceptable bond strength in most instances, while conserving enamel and reducing treatment time.

Rinsing and Drying Stage

Once the tooth is etched, the acid should be rinsed away thoroughly with a stream of water for about 20 seconds, and the rinsed water must be removed. In clinical scenarios like diastema closure or orthodontic bracket placement where enamel alone is etched and is to be bonded with a hydrophobic resin (e.g., bisphenol A glycidyl methacrylate [bis-GMA]–based resin; see Chapter 5), it must be dried completely with warm air until it takes on a white, frosted appearance. Dentin, in contrast, cannot withstand such aggressive drying, which would cause bond failure because of the formation of impermeable, collapsed collagen fibers. In the total-etch technique, a **dentin bonding agent** and **primer** must be used that are compatible with both moist dentin and moist enamel.

Cleanness of the Bonding Surfaces

The etched surfaces must be kept clean (free of contaminants) and sufficiently dry until the resin is placed to form a sound mechanical bond. Although etching raises the surface energy, contamination can readily reduce the energy level of the etched surface. Reducing the surface energy, in turn, makes it more difficult to wet the surface with a bonding resin that may have too high a surface tension to wet the contaminated surface. Thus, even momentary contact with saliva or blood can prevent effective resin tag formation and severely reduce the bond strength. Another potential contaminant is oil that is released from the air compressor and transported along the airlines to the air–water syringe. *If contamination occurs, the contaminant should be removed, and the surface should be etched again for 10 seconds.*

Other Factors

The acid-etch technique was not widely used in the years immediately following its introduction (Fig. 6.1). The principal reason was the inferior properties of the unfilled acrylic restorative materials used at that time. With those resins, high polymerization shrinkage (>6 vol%) and coefficients of thermal expansion in excess of 100 ppm/°C generated interfacial stresses sufficient to rupture the bond to etched enamel. After highly filled resin-based composites were marketed beginning in the mid-1960s, the acid-etch technique was "rediscovered." Therefore, the choice of restorative materials also plays an important factor in the success of bonding.

CRITICAL QUESTION

What types of bond formations result from the use of a dentin bonding agent?

Dentin-Bonding Agents

Dental bonding agents are designed to provide a sufficiently strong interface between restorative composites and tooth structure to withstand mechanical forces and shrinkage stress. The success of adhesives is dependent on two types of bonding:

1. Micromechanical interlocking, chemical bonding with enamel and dentin, or both.
2. Copolymerization with the resin matrix of composite materials.

Before the total-etch technique was adopted, predominately hydrophobic enamel bonding agents were used only to enhance the wetting and adaptation of resin to conditioned enamel surfaces. Generally, enamel bonding agents are made by combining different dimethacrylates from resins of composite materials (e.g., bis-GMA) with diluting monomers (e.g., triethylene glycol dimethacrylate [TEGDMA], Fig. 6.4) to control viscosity and to

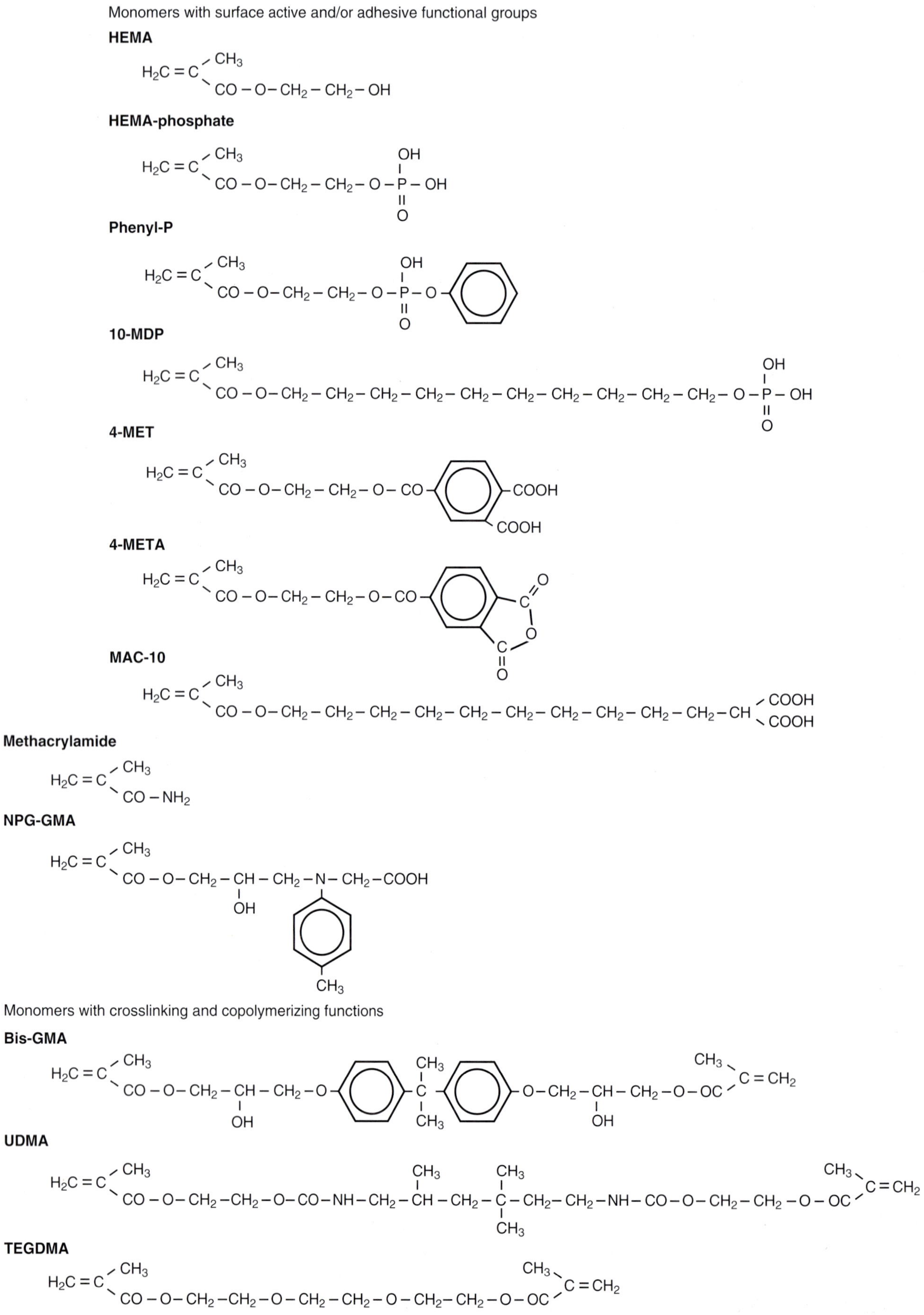

Monomers with surface active and/or adhesive functional groups

HEMA

$H_2C=C(CH_3)-CO-O-CH_2-CH_2-OH$

HEMA-phosphate

$H_2C=C(CH_3)-CO-O-CH_2-CH_2-O-P(=O)(OH)-OH$

Phenyl-P

$H_2C=C(CH_3)-CO-O-CH_2-CH_2-O-P(=O)(OH)-O-C_6H_5$

10-MDP

$H_2C=C(CH_3)-CO-O-CH_2-CH_2-CH_2-CH_2-CH_2-CH_2-CH_2-CH_2-CH_2-CH_2-O-P(=O)(OH)-OH$

4-MET

$H_2C=C(CH_3)-CO-O-CH_2-CH_2-O-CO-C_6H_3(COOH)_2$

4-META

$H_2C=C(CH_3)-CO-O-CH_2-CH_2-O-CO-C_6H_3(CO-O-CO)$

MAC-10

$H_2C=C(CH_3)-CO-O-CH_2-CH_2-CH_2-CH_2-CH_2-CH_2-CH_2-CH_2-CH_2-CH_2-CH(COOH)_2$

Methacrylamide

$H_2C=C(CH_3)-CO-NH_2$

NPG-GMA

$H_2C=C(CH_3)-CO-O-CH_2-CH(OH)-CH_2-N(C_6H_4CH_3)-CH_2-COOH$

Monomers with crosslinking and copolymerizing functions

Bis-GMA

$H_2C=C(CH_3)-CO-O-CH_2-CH(OH)-CH_2-O-C_6H_4-C(CH_3)_2-C_6H_4-O-CH_2-CH(OH)-CH_2-O-OC-C(CH_3)=CH_2$

UDMA

$H_2C=C(CH_3)-CO-O-CH_2-CH_2-O-CO-NH-CH_2-CH(CH_3)-CH_2-C(CH_3)_2-CH_2-CH_2-NH-CO-O-CH_2-CH_2-O-OC-C(CH_3)=CH_2$

TEGDMA

$H_2C=C(CH_3)-CO-O-CH_2-CH_2-O-CH_2-CH_2-O-CH_2-CH_2-O-OC-C(CH_3)=CH_2$

• **Fig. 6.4** Structures of representative monomers used in enamel and dentin bonding agents.

enhance wetting. These agents have no potential for adhesion, but they improve **micromechanical bonding** by optimal formation of resins tags within the enamel. Because enamel can be kept fairly dry, these rather hydrophobic resins work well as long as they are restricted to enamel.

During the past few years, these bonding agents have been replaced by the same systems that are used on dentin. This transition occurred because of the benefit of simultaneously bonding resin to both enamel and dentin, not because of any substantial improvement in bond strength.

A wide variety of chemistries have been explored and marketed in the search for species that can produce strong, permanent bonds to dentin. As discussed in the earlier section on adhesion mechanisms, a successful dentin-bonding system must meet several requirements:

1. Adequate removal or dissolution of the smear layer from enamel and dentin,
2. Maintenance or reconstitution of the dentin collagen matrix,
3. Good wetting,
4. Efficient monomer diffusion and penetration,
5. Polymerization within tooth structure,
6. Copolymerization with the resin composite matrix.

Irrespective of the number of bottles or components (see Fig. 6.7 and Table 6.1), a typical dentin-bonding system includes etchants, resin monomers, solvents, initiators and inhibitors, fillers, and sometimes other functional ingredients such as antimicrobial agents. Some of the newer multi mode (Universal) adhesives also contain silane to promote bonding to ceramics and 10-MDP to promote bonding to metallic substrates.

Design of Dentin-Bonding Systems

All bonding systems consist of three key components:

1. Conditioning (cleaning),
2. Priming (wetting, adapting),
3. Bonding (mechanical adhesion, curing).

Composition

Etchants

Etchants are relatively strong acids (pH = 1–2) used to remove smear layers and to dissolve the mineral phase to allow formation of micromechanical interlocking in enamel and in dentin. A number of acidic agents have been used to produce the required microporosity. However, phosphoric acid at a concentration between 30% and 50%, typically 37%, is the preferred etching agent to produce consistent etching patterns while not damaging the pulp. Concentrations greater than 50% result in the deposition of an adherent layer of monocalcium phosphate monohydrate on the etched surface, which inhibits further dissolution. Generally, the etchant is supplied as an aqueous gel to allow precise placement over a specific area. These gels are often made by adding colloidal silica (the same fine particles used in microfilled composites) or polymer beads to the acid. Brushes are used to place the acidic gel, or the acid may be supplied in a disposable syringe from which it can be expressed onto enamel and dentin. *During placement, it is important to be aware of the risk for air bubbles that may be introduced at the interface. Regions with air pockets will not be etched.*

TABLE 6.1 Classification of Dental-Bonding Systems and Representative Examples of Commercial Products Currently Available for Clinical Use

ETCH-AND-RINSE		SELF-ETCH	
Three-Step (Fourth Generation)	**Two-Step (Fifth Generation)**	**Two-Step (Sixth Generation)**	**One-Step (Seventh Generation)**
1. Etch Apply for 15 seconds, rinse 15 seconds gently air-dry, while keeping dentin moist	1. Etch Apply for 15 seconds, rinse 15 seconds, gently air-dry while keeping dentin moist	1. Etch and Prime One application without rinsing, gently air-dry	1. Etch, Prime, and Bond Apply 1–5 layers without rinsing, gently air-dry, light-cure
2. Prime Apply 1–5 layers, gently air-dry	2. Prime and Bond Apply 1–5 layers, gently air-dry, light-cure	2. Bond Apply one layer, gently air-dry, light-cure	
3. Bond Apply one layer, gently air-dry, light-cure			
Representative Products Currently Marketed for Clinical Use			
Adper Scotchbond Multi-Purpose (3M ESPE)	DenTASTIC UNO (Pulpdent)	Adper Prompt (3M SPE)	AdheSE One (Ivoclar Vivadent)
All Bond 3 (Bisco)	Excite (Vivadent)	AdheSE (Ivoclar Vivadent)	Adper Easy Bond Self Etch (3M ESPE)
DenTASTIC All-Purpose (Pulpdent)	Gluma Comfort Bond (Heraeus Kulzer)	All-Bond SE (Bisco)	Adper Prompt L-Pop (3M ESPE)
Gluma Solid Bond (Heraeus Kulzer)	One-Step Plus (Bisco)	Clearfil Protect Bond (Kuraray)	Clearfil S3 Bond (Kuraray)
Optibond FL (Kerr)	PQI (Ultradent)	Nano-Bond (Pentron)	Futurabond DC (VOCO)
Syntac (Ivoclar Vivadent)	Prime & Bond NT (Dentsply)	One-Step P/TYRIAN (Bisco)	G-Bond (GC), XENO V (Dentsply)
	Single Bond (3M ESPE)	Peak (Ultradent)	I-Bond (Heraeus Kulzer)

Primers

As discussed earlier, dentin etching is highly technique-sensitive because the demineralized collagen network readily collapses when dried. Therefore, priming is necessary to maintain an expanded collagen network while removing residual water to allow for the infiltration of the hydrophobic adhesive monomer. Primers are solutions containing hydrophilic monomers dissolved in a solvent such as acetone, ethanol, or water. Such monomers exhibit hydrophilic properties through phosphate, carboxylic acid, alcohol, or ester functional groups. HEMA (2-hydroxyethyl methacrylate; shown in Fig. 6.4) is a widely used primer monomer because of its high hydrophilicity and solvent-like nature.

Primer mixtures have a wide pH range because of variations in the functional groups of the corresponding monomers. The rank of functional groups in their acidity is as follows: sulfonic acid > phosphonic > phosphoric > carboxylic > alcohol. If the concentration of acidic monomers is increased in a HEMA base, a primer formulation may reach a pH low enough (e.g., 1–2) to remove smear layers and etch underlying dentin. If a primer has the ability to both etch and prime, it is categorized as a self-etching primer. For this purpose, acidic monomers are frequently used to formulate self-etching primers. Representative of these are:

- HEMA-phosphate, phenyl-P (2-[methacryloyloxyethyl]phenyl hydrogen phosphate),
- 10-MDP (10-methacryloyloxydecyl dihydrogen phosphate),
- 4-MET (4-methacryloyloxyethyl trimellitic acid),
- 4-META (4-methacryloyloxyethyl trimellitic anhydride),
- MAC-10 (11-methacryloyloxy-1,1′-undecanedicarboxylic acid).

The chemical structures of these primer components and other representative bonding system monomers are illustrated in Figure 6.4.

Early dentin-bonding agents were based on the successful model of silane coupling agents as used to bond the inorganic filler to the matrix resin in composites (see Chapter 5), to bond porcelain laminate veneers through resin cements to acid-etched enamel, and to repair fractured porcelain with composites (see Chapter 10). As shown in Figure 6.5 (*left*), generically, a silane coupling agent may be represented as M–R–X.

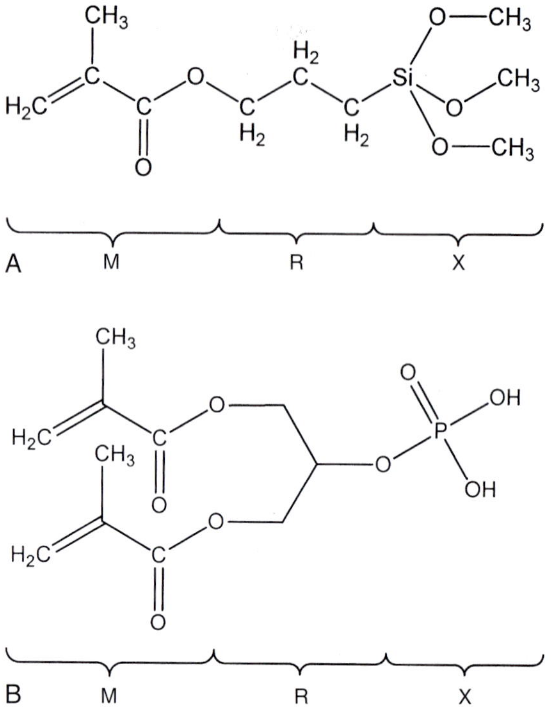

M–R–X Concept

- M represents an unsaturated methacrylate group or groups capable of copolymerizing with the other monomers of a resin cement or composite.
- X represents a group capable of chemically reacting with siliceous materials such as glass and silicate filler particles in composites, and porcelain crowns and veneers, and/or the calcium ions (Ca^{++}) in dental hard tissues.
- R is a spacer group that provides flexibility and mobility, and thus enhanced reactivity, for the M group after the X group has been immobilized by reaction at a surface. Similarly, the adhesive phosphate monomer in Figure 6.5 (*right*) also has the M–R–X structure. This adhesive phosphate compound was the self-etching monomer used in the first dentin-bonding system, Sevriton (DeTrey division of Amalgamated Dental, now Dentsply DeTrey, Konstanz, Germany), which was introduced in the 1950s. The silane monomer shown, γ-methacryloxypropyl trimethoxysilane, is currently used in all dental applications of coupling agents (Fig. 6.6).
- Analogous to silane coupling agents, it was believed that dentin bonding could be achieved by forming chemical bonds between a resin system and either the inorganic or the organic components of dentin, in particular, the Ca^{++} within the hydroxyapatite mineral phases of dentin. Phosphate and carboxylic groups form chelation bonds with Ca^{++} and, therefore, are expected to form such bonds during dentin priming, as has been found with polycarboxylate cements. Then, during polymerization, the methacrylate group of the M–R–X molecule can react with the resin matrix of the composite material and thereby form a chemical bond between composite and dentin. Several compounds that were believed to possess these properties are shown in Figure 6.4: NPG-GMA (a condensation product of *N*-phenyl glycine and glycidyl methacrylate, and the first dentin-bonding agent), polymerizable phosphates (e.g., phenyl-P and 10-MDP), and carboxylate compounds (e.g., 4-MET, MAC-10, and 4-META). Also in this category are poly(alkenoic) acids as used in carboxylate and glass ionomer cements (GICs). However, in spite of theoretical evidence that chemical bonding to tooth structure is possible, no convincing experimental evidence has yet been validated to prove that *significant* chemical bonding occurs between dentin adhesives and tooth structure under intraoral conditions. Rather, the adhesive functional groups facilitate surface cleaning and etching, and development of micromechanical interlocking and monomer penetration of dentin to form a hybrid layer of molecular entanglements between collagen and polymer.

• **Fig. 6.5** M-R-X structures of γ-methacryloxypropyl trimethoxysilane (*A*) and glycerophosphoric acid dimethacrylate (*B*). The surface interaction or bonding mechanism of the silane is shown in Figure 5.7. The chemical adhesion or bonding mechanism of phosphoric acid is shown in Figure 6.6.

Solvents

The addition of solvents to resins is indispensable to the composition of adhesives that need to bond to dentin. Primers and/or adhesive resins tend to have a low viscosity, which is partly due to the dissolution of the monomers in a solvent, which improves

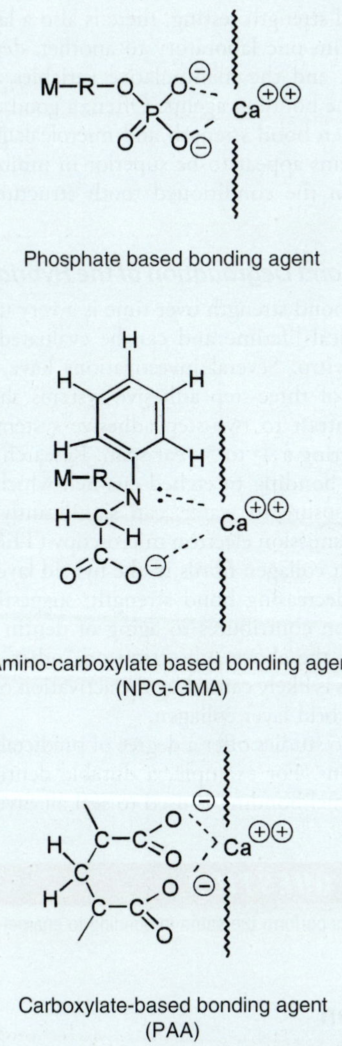

• **Fig. 6.6** Chemical bonding mechanisms to hard tooth tissues through calcium salt formation with monomers having adhesive functional groups. (Courtesy of K-J Söderholm.)

their diffusion ability in the microretentive tooth surface. The most commonly used solvents are water, ethanol, and acetone. In addition to the enhancement of wetting of hydrophilic dentin, each solvent has a specific contribution to improve bond adhesion. Water can ionize acidic monomers as well as re-expand the collapsed collagen network.

Usually ethanol is used in conjunction with water as co-solvent. Moreover, water–alcohol mixtures are known to be "azeotropic." This implies the formation of hydrogen bonds between water and ethanol molecules, resulting in a better evaporation of these water–ethanol aggregates than pure water. Acetone has a high vapor pressure, about four times as high as that of ethanol, which is a main advantage. However, its high volatility may also lead to reduce shelf-life of acetone-containing adhesives, by rapid evaporation of the solvent.

Ethanol and acetone have better miscibility with relatively hydrophobic monomers, and their "water-chasing" ability facilitates water removal.

Adhesives

For dentin bonding, the primary purpose of adhesives is to fill the interfibrillar space of the collagen network, creating a hybrid layer and resin tags to provide micromechanical retention upon polymerization. In addition, adhesive layers also should prevent fluid leakage along the restorative material's margin, since they make up the major part of the intermediate layer between dentin and/or enamel and restorative composites.

It is evident that adhesives need to be hydrophobic so that fluid will not be allowed to permeate through the intermediate layer. At the same time, adhesives require a certain hydrophilicity to diffuse into the hydrophilic, primer-wetted dentin. Generally, adhesive resins are composed mainly of hydrophobic dimethacrylates such as bis-GMA, TEGDMA, and urethane dimethacrylates (UDMA), and a small amount of a hydrophilic monomer such as HEMA. Although dimethacrylate adhesives yield strong bond strengths, the polar ester bond inevitably absorbs water and gradually hydrolyzes. Since carbamides are more hydrolytically stable than ester groups, methacrylamides have recently been adopted to replace methacrylates in several commercial products (e.g., AdheSE One F, Ivoclar Vivadent, Amherst, NY). These monomers are also shown in Figure 6.4.

Initiators

Similar initiator systems are used in both adhesives and restorative composites. Polymerization can be initiated either through a photoinitiator system consisting of a photosensitizer (e.g., camphorquinone) and an initiator (e.g., tertiary amine), through a self-cure system that includes a chemical initiator (e.g., benzoyl peroxide [BPO]), or through a dual-cure initiator system. (See Chapter 5 for details concerning initiator systems.)

Filler Particles

Nanometer-sized silica particles have been added to some adhesives to reinforce the adhesive and thereby produce higher bond strengths. However, the strengthening effect of the fillers in adhesives is uncertain because it is not clear whether these fillers can actually penetrate into the demineralized collagen networks, since the interfibrillar space of the collagen networks is within the range of 20 nanometers (nm) while the filler particles have a size of approximately 40 nm. The other reason for the addition of fillers is to effectively modify adhesive viscosity to a thicker, pastier consistency. When such an adhesive is applied to an etched dental surface, it yields a thicker bonding layer that can promote increased bond strength by preventing oxygen inhibition. Moreover, a thick adhesive layer can reduce shrinkage stress because it is more compliant compared with restorative composites.

Other Ingredients

Some manufacturers sometimes add specific ingredients, which purportedly improve bonding efficiency. The adhesives manufactured by 3M ESPE (Adper Prompt, Single Bond, Scotchbond Multipurpose) often contain a specific polyalkenoic copolymer. The rationale for the use of this polymer is to provide better moisture stability.

It is unclear whether this compound actually influences the bond strength. Moreover, some studies have suggested that this monomer does not dissolve in the adhesive's solution, leading to a separate phase producing many globules within the polymer of the adhesive layer.

Sometimes additional ingredients are used with dentin bonding agents for a variety of specific purposes. A few examples include the following:

Glutaraldehyde (Probond, Dentsply, York, PA) is added as a desensitizer. The monomer 12-methacryloyloxydodecylpyridinium bromide, MDPB (Clearfil Protect Bond, Kuraray America,

New York, NY) and parabene (Adper Prompt-L-Pop, 3M ESPE, St. Paul, MN) are used as antimicrobials. Fluoride (Prime and Bond NT, Dentsply, York, PA) is added to prevent secondary caries. Benzalkonium chloride (e.g., Etch 37, Bisco, Schamburg, IL) and chlorhexidine (e.g., Peak LC Bond Resin, Ultradent Products, South Jordon, UT) are used to prevent collagen degradation. The latter products have recently been shown in laboratory studies to prevent protease enzymes (matrix metalloproteinase enzymes or proteins [MMPs]) from being activated and subsequently denaturing the hybrid layer collagen. Unfortunately, only the early stages of long-term clinical trial results are available at this time to show whether such additives are ultimately effective.

CRITICAL QUESTION

Why are dentin bond strength values so variable?

Properties

Measurement of Bond Strength

Evaluation of the efficacy of dentin adhesives is generally based on measurement of bond strength as determined by loading bonded test specimens in shear or in tension until fracture occurs. Such tests offer only indirect evidence of how the adhesive is likely to perform in vivo. Data published on bond strengths for a given material often varies widely, and the standard deviation of the mean value for a given bond test is usually high. This wide variance in data, that is better described by the coefficient of variation (standard deviation/mean), may be attributed to the variables inherent at the dentin surface, such as water content, the presence or absence of a smear layer, dentin permeability, orientation of the tubules relative to the surface, and differences in the in vitro test design and stress distribution adjacent to the interface. Furthermore, although no universal agreement on the minimal bond strength necessary to provide successful bonding has been established, a value of 20 MPa or higher has been proposed as a reasonable goal.

Recently, a number of studies have adopted the microtensile test methodology. By using very small specimens (approximately 1 mm^2 in cross-section), one can prepare multiple specimens from a single tooth. Even with very high indicated strengths, for example, 30 MPa or higher, failure occurs at the adhesive interface rather than within dentin. This interfacial failure has led some proponents of the method to suggest that it is the only valid measure of bond strength because significant fractions of specimens rarely fail along the tooth–resin interface using traditional test specimen geometries, such as shear-test designs.

Regardless of the numerical differences generated by different laboratory test methods, it is clear that current dentin bonding agents are capable of yielding higher bond strength values that can shift the site of clinical failure from the interface to within dentin adjacent to the restoration or, in some cases, within the restoration adjacent to the interface. Regardless of the bond test selected, it is clear that the inherent bond strength is no longer the limitation in the effectiveness of bonded restorations. The limiting factor now appears to be, at least for large restorations, induced stresses generated during curing shrinkage within the resin-based composite itself.

Studies have shown bond strength in specimens without enamel borders was significantly lower than in specimens with enamel borders, especially in peripheral dentin.

Measurement of Microleakage

The degree of microleakage at the restoration–tooth interface can be monitored by the penetration of tracers and staining agents. As is true for bond strength testing, there is also a large variation in leakage data from one laboratory to another, depending on the technique used and the manipulative variables adopted during placement of the bonding agents. Often, a good correlation does not exist between bond strength and microleakage. Nonetheless, the newer systems appear to be superior in inhibiting interfacial leakage between the conditioned tooth structure and adhesive resin.

Aging Effects and Degradation of the Hybrid Layer

The change of bond strength over time is a very useful indication of relative clinical lifetime and can be evaluated by accelerated aging tests in vitro. Several investigations have found that the bond strength of three-step adhesive systems show little or no decrease in contrast to two-step adhesive systems that decrease significantly during a 4- to 5-year span. Research has also shown that peripheral bonding to etched enamel, which seals the resin bond from exposure to water, can significantly increase bond durability. Transmission electron microscopy (TEM) observations have shown that collagen fibrils in the hybrid layer degrade coincidently with decreasing bond strength, suggesting that hybrid layer degradation contributes to aging of dentin bond integrity. As indicated in the above subsection on "other" bonding agent ingredients, this is likely caused by the activation of MMPs, which denature the hybrid layer collagen.

Some in vitro studies offer a degree of predictability for certain clinical situations. For example, a durable dentin bond can be expected if enamel bonding is used to seal all cavity margins.

CRITICAL QUESTION

Do bonding agents perform the same in bonding to enamel and dentin?

Classification

When discussing dentin-bonding agents, it has become customary to describe the generations (first generation, second generation, etc.) of bonding agents that have led sequentially from the earliest, relatively ineffective materials to the current materials, which provide reliable functional bonds. This organization into generations of bonding agents is a somewhat artificial device, which only marks advances in materials and techniques along a developmental pathway and does not necessarily indicate improvement in performance. A stepwise evolution of bonding agents is described in Box 6.2. Therefore, this chapter uses a more logical and straightforward classification for contemporary adhesive systems based rather on their mechanism of adhesion and the number of clinical steps involved. This classification was developed by van Meerbeek et al. (2003). As shown in Figure 6.7 and Table 6.1, it is based on two general approaches to etching, priming, and applying the bonding resin to dentin and enamel surfaces, and further subdivided into the number of steps in the process. Thus, the major categories of bonding systems are known as "etch-and-rinse" and "self-etch" systems, with two subcategories, each according to the number of clinical steps involved.

Etch-and-Rinse Adhesives

- *Three-step (fourth generation):* At this time, the most established, most reliable adhesion method in this category consists of three steps: (1) an acid etchant application, (2) application of the primer, and (3) application of the actual bonding agent or bonding resin. The primer contains hydrophilic functional

• BOX 6.2 Classification of Bonding Systems by Generations

- First-generation adhesives contained GPDM as active ingredient. GPDM has ionic bonding potential to hydroxyapatite (HAp) via its phosphate functional group. These early adhesives, however, presented unstable, very low 2–3 MPa bond strengths to dentin.
- Second-generation adhesives were categorized into calcium- and collagen-bonding types. These incorporated functional monomers, all designed to chemically interact with either inorganic (HAp) or organic (collagen) dentinal components. Some additional bond strength was gained, but it seldom exceeded 5–6 MPa.
- The basis for the third-generation adhesives was laid when the earlier Japanese concept of etching dentin to remove the smear layer was introduced by Fusayama in 1979. Phosphoric-acid etching was followed by the application of a two-component chemically curing bonding agent that already contained the functional monomer 10-MDP.
- Fourth-generation adhesives make use of the "TOTAL-ETCH" technique; these total-etch adhesives evolved towards multi-step systems that included the separate use of a CONDITIONER and PRIMER prior to the application of the actual ADHESIVE RESIN in a typical three-step application procedure. The fourth-generation adhesives are today called three-step etch&rinse adhesives (3E&Ras), as they involve the successive application of a conditioner, primer, and adhesive resin in three application steps.
- Fifth-generation adhesives are 2-STEP ETCH&RINSE ADHESIVES (2-E&Ras) that combine the primer and bonding agent in "one-bottle" adhesives. While being popular in routine clinical practice, a significant price is paid for EASE-OF-USE, as 2-E&Ras generally presents lower laboratory and clinical performance.
- Sixth-generation adhesives are today called 2-STEP SELF-ETCH ADHESIVES (2-SEas) that provide an acidic self-etch primer, basically combining the acid etchant with a primer, followed by the application of a classic adhesive resin.
- Seventh-generation adhesives are the true 1-STEP SELFETCH ADHESIVES or "all-in-one" adhesives that combine all three etching, priming, and bonding functions in one single application step without a water rinse phase.
- The newest eighth-generation adhesives are the so-called UNIVERSAL ADHESIVES (UAs) that can be applied according to the dentist's personal choice in both full E&R or SE bonding modes, or the combined mode involving selective enamel E&R with a 1-SE bonding mode.

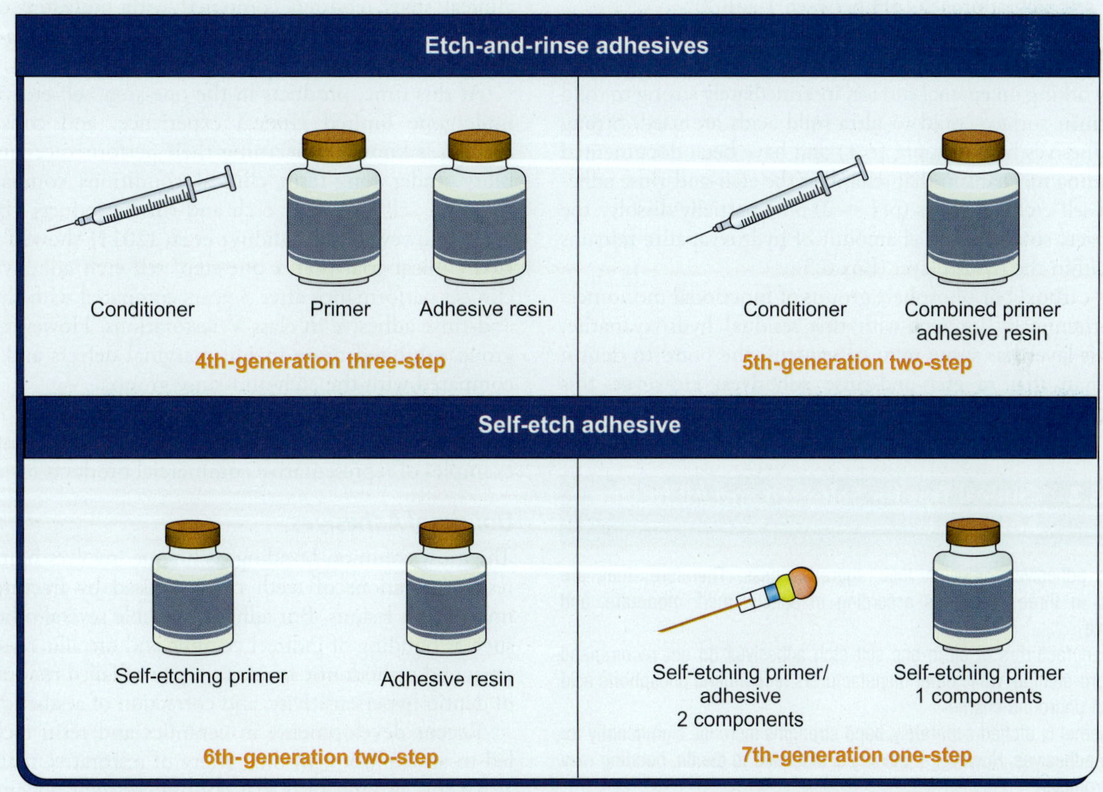

• **Fig. 6.7** Classification of current adhesive systems according to van Meerbeek et al. (2003). (Figure adapted with permission from Cardoso MV, de Almeida Neves A, Mine A, et al: Current aspects on bonding effectiveness and stability in adhesive dentistry. *Aust Dent J* 56(S1):31–44, 2011.)

monomers dissolved in an organic solvent such as acetone, ethanol, or water. The third step is the application of a hydrophobic resin, as mentioned earlier in the chapter.

- *Two-step (fifth generation):* A simplified method in this category combines the primer and adhesive resin into one application. This etch-and-rinse strategy is the most effective to achieve efficient and stable bonding to enamel. Etching, usually with a 30%–40% phosphoric gel that is rinsed away, promotes the dissolution of enamel rods, creating porosities that are filled by bonding agents through capillary action and then followed by polymerization of resin.

However, when dealing with a dentinal substrate, bonding is more difficult and less predictable than in enamel because of the organic characteristics of dentin. In this case, phosphoric acid treatment exposes a collagen network that is nearly devoid of hydroxyapatite. Bonding occurs by diffusion and infiltration of the resin within the collagen mesh, forming a hybrid layer. After in situ polymerization, this hybrid layer provides micromechanical retention to the restoration. True chemical-adhesive bonding is unlikely to contribute significantly to bond strength, as the monomer functional groups have only very weak affinities for collagen. Further, in the two-step category, hydrophilic and ionic monomers are combined, with the result that the bonded interface does not develop a hydrophobic resin layer and, thus, leaves the bond susceptible to water penetration and subsequent degradation, which greatly reduces bond durability.

Self-Etch Adhesives

With the self-etch adhesives, acidic monomers (self-etching primer) that simultaneously demineralize and prime tooth surfaces are applied and dried on the tooth surface. Depending on their interaction depth, these are sub-classified as follows:

- A few hundreds of nanometers following an "ultra-mild" self-etch approach (pH > 2.5), which sometimes is being referred to as "nano-interaction."
- An interaction depth of around 1 m for a "mild" self-etch approach (pH ≈ 2).
- An interaction depth between 1 and 2 m for an "intermediately strong" self-etch approach (pH between 1 and 2).
- Interaction of several micrometers deep for a "strong" self-etch approach (pH ≤ 1) (van Meerbeek et al., 2003).

When working on enamel surface, intermediately strong to mild and for dentin surfaces mild to ultra-mild acids are used. Strong self-etch adhesives have low pH (<1) and have been documented with a bonding mechanism that resembles the etch-and-rinse adhesives. Mild self-etch adhesives (pH $= 2$) only partially dissolve the dentin surface, so a substantial amount of hydroxyapatite remains available within the hybrid layer (Box 6.3).

Specific carboxyl or phosphate groups of functional monomers can then chemically interact with this residual hydroxyapatite. Because this layer has some mineral content, the bond to dentin is better than that of etch-and-rinse adhesives. However, this interfacial zone can be more prone to hydrolytic degradation because the structure is more hydrophilic. The dentin bond durability of mild self-etch primer systems seems to be adequate.

- *Two-step (sixth generation):* This approach does not involve a separate etching step. In this case, an acidic monomer, which is not rinsed, is used to condition and prime the tooth at the same time. Then, a bonding agent from a separate bottle is used.
- *One-step (seventh generation):* The simplified method in this category combines conditioner, primer, and bonding resin into a single step. Most one-step or "all-in-one" systems are delivered by a bottle, vial, or single-unit dose applicator, which are formulated as a single component. However, Adper Promp L-Pop (3M ESPE, St. Paul, MN) is a variation on this theme, in which two liquid components are packaged in separate "blister" compartments in a single dispenser. Bursting one blister causes the two components to blend and form a single component, which is then applied immediately using a brush that forms the handle of the blister pack. This version of one-step, two-component, self-etching primer–adhesive is illustrated in Figure 6.7.

One-step, self-etch adhesives are an attractive approach for clinicians because of the reduced and less complex number of clinical steps required compared with multistep etch-and-rinse adhesives. There is no need for rinsing or drying of the tooth structure because of the lack of an etch step.

At this time, products in the one-step, self-etch category have undergone limited clinical experience, and consequently not enough is known concerning their performance and bond durability under long-term clinical conditions compared with the two-step self-etch and etch-and-rinse products (Box 6.2). Recently, however, van Landuyt et al. (2011) showed in a randomized clinical trial that a one-step, self-etch adhesive had similar clinical performance after 3 years compared with that of an etch-and-rinse adhesive in class V restorations. However, the one-step group exhibited more incisal marginal defects and discoloration compared with the etch-and-rinse group.

These four categories are described further in Table 6.1 and Box 6.3, which also provide typical application instructions and examples of representative commercial products for each category.

• BOX 6.3 Clinical Tips for Self-Etch and All-in-One Adhesives

- Self-etch adhesives differ in their aggressiveness. Therefore, they are classified in three categories according to acidity: mild, moderate, and aggressive
- Some manufacturers of all-in-one self-etch adhesives do not recommend enamel pre-etching, while other manufacturers recommend phosphoric acid etching of unground enamel
- When enamel is etched separately, bond strengths increase significantly for self-etch adhesives. However, if etching is extended to dentin, bonding may be compromised
- If using a single-bottle adhesive, the amount required should be dispensed immediately prior to use in order to reduce the risk of solvent loss, which could potentially result in phase separation of monomer and water
- Apply the self-etch adhesive to the enamel first, followed by application to the dentin. Some products recommend agitation of the adhesive to enhance its penetration
- If using a one-step self-etch adhesive, apply multiple applications to help ensure adequate coating and penetration
- Thoroughly dry the adhesive (with a gentle stream of air) once it has been placed, to ensure removal of any volatile solvent and prevent interference with polymerization
- Storage criteria should be scrupulously adhered to. Most self-etch adhesives need to be refrigerated

Universal Adhesives

The most common bonding technique involves bonding to direct resin restorations of teeth compromised by fractures, carious or non-carious lesions. But adhesives enable several other procedures, such as bonding of indirect ceramic and metallic restorations, fiber posts and orthodontic brackets, repair of failed restorations, control of dentin hypersensitivity, and correction of aesthetic impairments.

Recent developments in ceramics and resin technology have led to an explosion in the variety of restorative material options. What this also means is that bonding systems now need to be able to bond reliably to all these substrates preferably chemically. Clinically, there is a challenge to ensure that the correct protocol is followed to ensure predictable bonding.

Manufacturers are constantly trying to provide us a one-step solution and Universal adhesives are supposed to enable one to bond multiple substrates. This new family of dental adhesives is known as "universal" or "multi-mode" and represents the latest generation of adhesives on the market. They are designed under the "all-in-one" concept of the already existing one-step self-etch adhesives but also incorporate the versatility of being adaptable to the clinical situation. An adhesive that can be applied both ways enables the practitioner to decide on a specific adhesive protocol that is most suited for the cavity being prepared.

• BOX 6.4 Comparative Clinical Capabilities of Commercially Available Universal Adhesives

	Scotchbond Universal	All-Bond Universal	Xeno Select	Peak Universal Bond	Adhese Universal	Clearfil Universal Bond	Futurabond U	Optibond XTR	iBond Universal	G-Premio BOND
Total etch	Yes	Yes	Yes	Yes	Yes	Yes	Yes	No	Yes	Yes
Selective etch	Yes	Yes	Yes	Yes	Yes	Yes	Yes	Yes	Yes	Yes
Self-etch	Yes	Yes	Yes	Yes	Yes	Yes	Yes	Yes	Yes	Yes
Dual-cure without separate activator	No	Yes	No	No	Yes	No[a]	Yes	Yes	Yes	No
Bonds to ceramics without separate primer	Yes	Yes	No	No	No	Yes[b]	Yes	Yes	No	No
Bonds to Zirconia and metal without separate primer	Yes	Yes	No	No	No	Yes	Yes	Yes	Yes	Yes

[a]*Except when used with own cement.*
[b]*But recommended for optimal performance.*

Thus, manipulation has been simplified by reducing the number of steps to a one-step system, with all components (etchant, primer, and bonding resin) incorporated into a single dental material.

What are Universal Adhesives?

According to Gary Alex (2015), universal adhesives have been described by some manufacturers and opinion leaders as ideally a single-bottle, no-mix, adhesive system that can be used in total-etch, self-etch, or selective-etch mode depending on the specific clinical situation and personal preferences of the operator. The term "UNIVERSAL" refers to their application options, enabling them to be used either following an E&R or SE bonding mode, while offering application versatility with (claimed) bonding potential to glass-rich (via silane) and glass-poor zirconia (via 10-MDP) ceramics for indirect tooth-restoration indications. Additionally, manufacturers typically state that universal adhesives can be used for the placement of both direct and indirect restorations and are compatible with self-cure, light-cure, and dual-cure resin-based cements. In principle, this would enable bonding to these surfaces without the need for dedicated and separately placed primers such as silane and various products marketed as metal and zirconia primers.

Although universal adhesives have a composition similar to that of traditional one-step SE adhesives, most universal adhesives also contain specific carboxylate and/or phosphate monomers that bond ionically to calcium in hydroxyapatite

Scotchbond Universal Adhesive (3M ESPE; Seefeld, Germany) was the first "universal" single-bottle adhesive. Subsequently, most manufacturers have developed and launched products in this category. They vary widely based on their composition and capabilities. Some are capable of bonding to glass ceramics, since they contain silane, while others need a separate primer to be used. In a sense, the term "Universal" can be quite confusing since there is nothing universal about these systems. A brief summary of the capabilities of these systems is available in Box 6.4

One can see that they vary widely both in their capabilities as well as their clinical applications.

Universal adhesives can be applied using a total-etch, self-etch, or selective-etch technique. By and large, the selective enamel etching (SEE) technique would be the most preferred technique for use with universal adhesives.

Selective Etch

The selective-etch procedure is a concept in which the enamel is etched with phosphoric acid and rinsed, followed by applying the self-etching adhesive to the enamel and dentin. The main purpose is to improve the bond strength to enamel and provide an effective peripheral enamel seal. A typical example of use with selective etch technique is described in Box 6.5.

Universal adhesives have a higher pH than traditional adhesives (Table 6.2) and consequently most bond to etched enamel better than unetched enamel.

Unfortunately, self-etching adhesives produce lower bond strengths to phosphoric acid–etched dentin. The universal systems claim that they are less technique-sensitive and not affected by partial etching of the dentin in the selective etch technique. However, when a self-etching adhesive is applied to cut dentin, etched intentionally or unintentionally, bond strengths to the etched dentin are reduced. Two "universal" adhesives (Scotchbond Universal

• BOX 6.5 Selective Etch Protocol for Bonding

The preferred bonding protocol combines selective enamel E&R with 2-step SE in three application steps:

1. Selectively etch enamel with 30–40% phosphoric acid, avoiding etching adjacent dentin. If dentin is not touched, enamel etching can even be extended beyond 15 s. Thoroughly water rinse and air-dry as described above for the recommended full 3-E&R route.
2. As the most important adhesive step, actively rub the 10-MDP-based mild self-etch primer for at least 15 s. Self-etch priming cannot be done long enough; continuously supply "fresh" primer onto the dentin substrate. Priming is ended with gentle air drying to promote solvent evaporation.
3. As for the full E&R route, apply in the final step a solvent—poor/free adhesive resin in a visibly thick layer with stress-absorbing potential. After gently air blowing to uniformly spread the adhesive resin, the adhesive resin should ALWAYS be separately and immediately light-cured on dentin.

Considering being the most intimate contact achievable between atoms and molecules, chemical bonding should always be strived for to attain durable bonding to dentin. Therefore, the latter 3-step combined selective enamel E&R followed by 2-step SE bonding route should be considered as today's PREFERRED bonding protocol.

TABLE 6.2 Comparing Universal Adhesives

	Scotchbond Universal	Prime and Bond Elect	All-Bond Universal
Film thickness	5–7 μ	3–5 μ	<10 μ
Compatibility with chemical cured composites	Needs dual-cure activator	Needs dual-cure activator	No dual-cure activator needed
pH	2.7	2.5	3.2
Solvent	Ethanol	Acetone	Ethanol

and All-Bond Universal) contain a phosphate monomer (MDP phosphate monomer) that allows them to bond to multiple substrates. As mentioned earlier MDP is mainly used as an etching monomer, due to the dihydrogen phosphate group, which can dissociate in water to form two protons. This monomer is quite hydrophobic and, as a consequence, ethanol and acetone are most suitable solvents for this monomer. 10-MDP will be relatively hydrolysis stable, as water will be kept at a distance.

This monomer is capable of forming strong ionic bonds with calcium due to the low dissolution rate of the resulting Ca-salt in its own solution.

Scotchbond Universal contains silane to bond to ceramic without a separate silane application, and it also bonds directly to zirconia and alumina oxide abraded metal.

All-Bond Universal will bond to zirconia but requires a separate application of Z-Prime (Bisco), a phosphate-containing monomer.

Two of the currently marketed "universal" adhesives (Scotchbond Universal and Prime and Bond Elect) can efficiently bond to chemical or dual-cured cements, core materials, or composites using a dual-cured activator.

Universal Adhesives are often marketed to clinicians as user-friendly simplified adhesives, which offer ease of use and quick application. Despite this aggressive marketing, ultra-simplified 1-step self-etch adhesives, which combine dentin-enamel conditioner, primer and bonding adhesive resin in one bottle without requiring mixing, have resulted in low dentin bond strengths, deficient bonding to intact enamel, incompatibility with self-curing resins, and poor clinical outcomes in non-carious cervical lesions and posterior composite restorations. Ideal adhesion and sealing of enamel are only feasible with adhesives that rely on enamel phosphoric acid etching.

Though there is limited data available on the overall bonding, durability of these adhesives Nagarkar (2019) based on literature analysis recommended the following:

- Use of SEE strategy for permanent teeth and ER strategy for primary teeth.
- For glass-matrix ceramic restorations, such as lithium disilicate, an additional silane application step is necessary even if the UA contains a silane in its composition.
- For zirconia restorations, relying solely on bonding for retention should be avoided even though laboratory studies suggest the use of air-abrasion with aluminum oxide or silica-coated aluminum oxide particles (tribochemical silica coating) or ceramic coating for acceptable bonding using an MDP-based UA.
- For repair of direct composite resins and pre-polymerized composite resins for indirect restorations, the use of air-abrasion with aluminum oxide and UA application is recommended.

BOX 6.6 Clinical Recommendations for Use of Bonding Agents in Specific Situations

- For bonding composite cores, three-step, etch-and-rinse (fourth-generation) systems are usually recommended.
- For bonding anterior and posterior composites and cementation of veneers with resin cements, two-step etch-and-rinse (fifth-generation) systems provide the best performance.
- For bonding posterior composites, self-etch, two-step (sixth-generation) systems are the better choice.
- Self-etch two-step bonding systems are also the material of choice for the immediate dentin sealing (IDS) technique. The IDS technique is characterized by the sealing of the exposed dentin immediately after tooth preparation and before taking the impression.
- Self-adhesive resin cements are dual-cured materials and can be used for cementation of indirect restorations in most clinical situations. The exception would be cementation of veneers, in which case a light-cured cement would be preferred.

- Clinical studies recommend ER or SEE strategy for improving survival rates of composite restorations in non carious cervical lesions (NCCLs); and SEE strategy for Class II composite restorations.

The sheer variety of bonding systems available in the market necessitates the use of different materials and techniques in specific clinical scenarios. Recommendations for selecting an appropriate system in different clinical scenarios are provided in Box 6.6.

Bonding to Root Dentine

Advancements in endodontic techniques and armamentarium have led to a large number of teeth needing post endodontic restorations. Bonding to endodontically treated teeth can be challenging, especially when one needs to bond fiber posts to root dentine. The most common reason for clinical failure of fiber posts is the debonding of these posts from dentin. There have been conflicting results regarding the bond strength of different resin-luting agents to posts and intraradicular dentin.

Attaining clean dentin surfaces after mechanical post space preparation is an essential step for optimal post retention and bonding. Acidic monomers presented in self-etching dentin adhesives or the self-etching resin cements are less predictable to modify the thick smear layer and to form the hybrid layer along the walls of the post space. Acid etching of root dentin with phosphoric acid followed by copious water rinsing with an endodontic needle is helpful to remove the smear layer created after post space preparation. However, the effectiveness of acid etching is questionable at the apical level, because intricate narrow and deep canals cannot be completely cleaned and free from the smear layer.

Phark (2012) recommended the following to improve boning efficiency to root dentine:

- A composite core buildup must be incrementally made to reduce polymerization shrinkage and microleakage.
- Chlorhexidine is indicated for final irrigation (at the end of endodontic treatment) and after post space preparation.
- Cleaning of the post with ethanol is indicated after post manipulation to ensure adequate bonding to the resin cement.
- Dual-cured resin cements/adhesives and self-adhesive resin cements are recommended for post adhesive cementation.
- A waiting period of 24–48 hours before final tooth preparation must be respected to ensure maximum polymerization and post retention.

• BOX 6.7 Recommended Protocol for Cementing Posts to Root Dentin

- After making the intra-radicular preparation, clinical and radiographic assessments and sectioning the fiberglass post to appropriate length, secure absolute isolation of the area.
- Moisture must be controlled when using adhesive techniques to guarantee the success and longevity of adhesion.
- Create roughness throughout the prepared area with a diamond bur. Afterwards, rinse thoroughly with water and dry with an endodontic suction. Diamond burs produce a smear layer that is easier to dissolve than that resulting from the use of carbide drills.
- Apply 37% phosphoric acid to all root walls of the preparation. Activate the acid with a disposable brush or paper cone/point for 15 seconds.
- Wash for an equal amount of time and use clean paper cones to dry the preparation.
- Apply the universal adhesive inside the preparation with a disposable brush and remove the excess with light air jets and paper cones. Afterwards, rub the adhesive vigorously over the surface for 15 seconds and remove the excess in the same way as described above.
- Try the post to check its adaptation. Afterwards, remove the post and polymerize the adhesive for 20 seconds, using a photopolymerization unit.
- Apply the adhesive resin cement inside the intraradicular preparation with a cementation tip.
- Seat the post until it reaches the bottom of the preparation. Remove excess cement with a brush and photopolymerize for at least 40 seconds.

A clinical recommendation for adhesive cementation of fiber posts is provided in Box 6.7.

CRITICAL QUESTION

Can a single luting agent be used for cementation of indirect restorations in all clinical scenarios?

Luting Agents and Resin Cements

For many years, retention of indirect restorations could only be attained by the use of favorable tooth preparations and by micromechanical interlocking of the **luting agent** into irregularities present on the surface of the restoration and the tooth. Adhesive bonding completely changed the use of direct and indirect restorations. A number of materials are available for cementation, including zinc phosphate cements, polycarboxylate cements, GICs, RMGI cements, and resin cements that are described in more detail below and in Chapter 7. This section will concentrate on their bonding mechanism and new developments, especially regarding resin cements.

Resin cements must bond to different substrates, including tooth structure, resin composites, gold, metal alloys, titanium, and porcelain, and other ceramics. Most resin cements require pretreatment of the dental substrate to promote bonding to the dental tissues. The bonding of resin cements can be facilitated through a separate bonding step or they could have self-etch bonding components incorporated within them. The former can be considered either as an etch-and-rinse adhesive resin cement or as a self-etch adhesive resin cement, according to its bonding agent system. Self-adhesive resin cements, for which no extra clinical step is necessary for bonding, such as RelyX Unicem (3M ESPE, St. Paul, MN), were developed in the past decade. In vitro studies have reported better enamel bonding performance for non–self-adhesive resin cements compared with self-adhesive cements. Despite the initial low pH ($pH < 2.0$), the enamel and dentin demineralization is only superficial. An increase in pH (up to 7.0) is observed as a consequence of the reaction between the phosphate groups and alkaline fillers and the hydroxyapatite from enamel and dentin, neutralizing the resin's inherent acidity. The bonding mechanism of these newly developed resins relies more on chemical bonding than on micromechanical retention. The acid groups chelate the calcium ions of the hydroxyapatite, promoting chemical adhesion. In addition, carboxylic groups of polyalkenoic acid (found in RelyX Unicem, 3M ESPE) form ionic bonds with calcium present in the hydroxyapatite, positively influencing the chemical bonding. With regard to biocompatibility, these cements showed no adverse pulp response according to one study (Pedro et al., 2006).

Zinc phosphate cement shows low bond strength to dentin because of the lack of adhesion and absence of chemical bond formation with tooth structure. Bonding in this case occurs primarily by mechanical interlocking at the interfaces. However, GIC can chemically bond by ionic interaction of the carboxyl groups of the polyalkenoic acid with the calcium of the hydroxyapatite that remained attached to the collagen fibrils. However, GIC and zinc phosphate cement show similar clinical results.

Most resin cements show superior mechanical properties and higher bond strengths of restorative materials to tooth structure than that of conventional luting agents. Some studies have shown that even when bonding to zirconia that has high polycrystalline content and lack of glass matrix, higher values can be achieved. Preparation of the tooth structure for cementation remains the same regardless of the indirect restoration material used. However, the preparation of an all-ceramic restoration can include, but is not limited to, sandblasting, application of hydrofluoric acid for etching, silanization, or application of a ceramic primer to improve bond strength. For cementation of all-ceramic restorations, resin cement is the material of choice. Depending on the polymerization process, resin cements can be chemically cured, light-cured, or dual-cured. Self-adhesive resin cements are dual-cured materials and can be used for cementation of indirect restorations in most clinical situations. The exception would be cementation of veneers, in which case a light-cured cement would be preferred.

For cementation of indirect restorations where most of the tooth structure is dentin, resin cements have shown better mechanical properties compared with conventional cements. Long-term clinical data are needed to corroborate in vitro studies.

CRITICAL QUESTION

Why are self-adhesive cements currently not used to bond orthodontic brackets?

Orthodontic Bracket Bonding Resins

Orthodontic treatment with fixed appliances involves the use of attachments such as brackets and bands. Bands are metal rings that go around teeth and are usually used on molars. Brackets can be welded to bands but are most commonly used today bonded to enamel. The development of bonding has contributed to a decrease in banding even in posterior teeth. A variety of luting agents have been used in orthodontics such as polycarboxylate cement, GIC, and resin-modified glass ionomer (RMGI) cements. Contemporary bonding process to enamel involves the following:

1. Prophylaxis of bonding surface
2. Etching with phosphoric acid gel or aqueous solutions

3. Rinsing with water
4. Drying with air
5. Application of sealant or primer
6. Bonding of brackets with resin cement
7. Light-curing the dual-cured or light-cured cement

Self-adhesive cements are not recommended by manufacturers as luting agents for orthodontic fixed appliances. Self-adhesive cements exhibit a lower bond strength to intact enamel in comparison with conventional orthodontic resin cements that require phosphoric acid etching. However, self-etching systems have shown acceptable results for bonding orthodontic brackets.

In orthodontic treatment, bonding most likely involves mainly enamel as the substrate. However, adults are increasingly undergoing tooth alignment. This population has larger amalgam restorations, porcelain fused to metal (PFM) crowns, and all-ceramic crowns. Therefore, bonding of brackets to those surfaces also plays an important role in orthodontic treatment. It is important that the bonding of brackets be reliable, since replacing loose brackets is inefficient, time-consuming, and costly.

Several types of surface treatments can be used with restorative materials to increase bond strength. For example, roughening with a diamond bur, and sandblasting enhance bonding, especially in the case of metals. These treatments create irregularities and increase surface area, promoting both micromechanical retention and chemical adhesion in the case of resins such as those containing 4-META, 10-MDP, and others as shown in Figure 6.4. Bond strength of brackets bonded to amalgam is lower than that to etched enamel. In addition to forming a reliable bond, the ability of a resin to reduce or prevent demineralization ("white spot" caries) in the difficult-to-clean areas around orthodontic brackets and bands and to reduce damage to enamel during the treatment period are also important properties in this clinical scenario.

CRITICAL QUESTION

What are the materials and techniques needed to overcome the root canal system environment and create a hermetic seal with endodontic obturation systems?

Root Canal Sealers

Endodontic sealers are used in conjunction with a solid or semisolid core material to fill voids and to seal root canals during **obturation**. These sealers, sometimes called *cements*, should fill and promote a close seal between the core and the dentinal walls of the canal, preventing or minimizing leakage, entombing residual microorganisms, and possibly filling inaccessible areas of the root canal system. Sealer selection may influence the outcome of endodontic treatment. However, low levels of evidence are available in the literature, with no randomized clinical trials to corroborate this statement. Traditionally, gutta-percha has been used as the solid core material in combination with a zinc oxide and eugenol or calcium hydroxide cement, or an epoxy-based sealer. Clinical studies have shown predictable results with these conventional root canal sealers. GICs and resin-modified GICs are also used as root canal sealers. These can chemically bond to root canal dentin, but no bond is obtained to gutta-percha.

Recently, new materials have been introduced on the market to improve the seal of the root canal system. These include different types of core materials, the development of low-viscosity methacrylate resin-based sealers, and the incorporation of dentin bonding agents. One system uses conventional cones that are coated with a proprietary resin coating (EndoRez, Ultradent, South Jordan, UT) in combination with a methacrylate-based, dual-cured resin sealer and no dentin-bonding agent. In this case, the endodontic seal is dependent on the penetration of the hydrophilic sealer into the dentinal tubules and lateral canals following removal of the smear layer. Another system, called Resilon (SybronEndo Corporation, Orange, CA) is a thermoplastic composite polycaprolactone-based core material that contains dimethacrylate resin, radiopaque fillers, and glass-ionomer particles. Resilon cones are applied in combination with a methacrylate-based sealer to root dentin treated with self-etching primers. At the present time, obturation systems also include the use of self-etch cementing sealers.

Because of the highly complex environment of the root canal system, it is very difficult to promote adequate bond strength and low microleakage through the formation of a hybrid layer in root canal dentin, even with the latest bonding technologies. The configuration of the cavity or "C-factor" (ratio of bonded to unbonded walls as described in Chapter 5) is an especially important factor. The greater the C-factor, the greater the stress that can develop at any particular biomaterial interface. In turn, this stress can lead to interface breakdown, gap formation, microleakage, and ultimately to such problems as apical infection and caries. In the case of root canals, C-factors can be extremely high, over 1000. Thus, a resin endodontic sealer is subjected to severe polymerization shrinkage stresses during setting, which may cause debonding and gap formation along the periphery of the root canal obturation and adhesive interfaces. Gaps can form between the sealer and dentin wall or in between the solid core material (e.g., gutta-percha) and the sealer. Therefore, root canal obturation inherently requires a number of different materials and involves multiple interfaces, thereby creating a greater challenge than most other applications of adhesive dentistry.

In a long, narrow space such as the root canal, the application of self-etching adhesives or any other bonding system becomes challenging and might not be uniform throughout the entire interface. Therefore, if resin infiltration into demineralized dentin and hybrid formation is not adequate to prevent movement of fluids inward through dentin, over time, the bond will be compromised and the seal will fail. In addition, in bonding systems that contain volatile solvents, evaporation might be hindered. The canal anatomy is not only problematic to adhesive root canal obturation but also for the bonding of prefabricated posts. A further problem is that some irrigating solutions (e.g., sodium hypochlorite) and intracanal medicaments can also have adverse effects on root canal dentin collagen and, consequently, to the longevity of endodontic bonding. Different endodontic treatment protocols are currently under investigation to optimize bonding quality in root canal obturation.

CRITICAL QUESTION

Why are glass ionomer cements (GICs) not used routinely as pit and fissure sealants?

Glass Ionomer Restoratives

GICs are described in some detail in the discussion of dental cements (see Chapter 7). However, they are also pertinent to this chapter, since they represent a class of materials that exhibit chemical bonding to tooth structure. They consist of a powder, an acid-soluble aluminosilicate glass, and an aqueous solution of polyacrylic acid or an analogous polyacid. Ca^{2+} and aluminum (Al^{3+}) ions released from the powder react with the carboxylic acid (–COOH) groups to form divalent salts, which cross-link and cure the polymeric acid. The same carboxylate groups also interact strongly with surface Ca^{2+} ions in enamel or dentin to affect chemical adhesion to tooth structure.

This occurs through ionic bond formation between the carboxyl groups of the polyalkenoic acid with calcium of hydroxyapatite. Thus, the chelation of carboxyl groups that are derived from polyalkenoic acid with the calcium in apatite can be obtained as represented below:

$$\text{Polyalkenoic acid R} - \text{COO} - H_3O^+ + \text{Hydroxyapatite } (OH^-) \rightarrow Ca^{+2} + PO4^{3-}$$

This chemical adhesion may also be beneficial in terms of resistance to hydrolytic degradation. A short polyalkenoic acid pretreatment can be used to clean the tooth surface and to remove the smear layer, exposing collagen fibrils to a depth of about 0.5–1 micron.

Micromechanical bonding of the glass ionomer components occur by interdiffusion. Most of the current glass ionomer restorative materials also contain resin and are referred to as RMGI. They contain a light-curable acrylic resin that provides for rapid polymerization at and near the surface, together with the same bonding mechanisms as are produced with traditional glass ionomers.

Because of their fluorine-releasing capability, glass ionomer restoratives are especially useful for patients who are at a high risk for carious lesions. For teeth requiring class II restorations, a **sandwich technique** is sometimes used. This technique consists of placing a type II GIC in the cervical area of a proximal box or the floor of other tooth preparations and building the remainder of the restoration with a resin-based composite because of its greater strength and durability in occlusal sites. Long-term clinical studies have shown that this technique might not be advantageous for class II restorations in comparison with directly bonding composite resins in posterior restorations.

GICs can be used as esthetic alternatives to amalgam restorations in class V erosion lesions, as shown schematically in Figure 6.8. Although shear bond strengths measured in the laboratory are only approximately 3 MPa, clinical retention is excellent. Until recently, glass ionomers were the only materials that yielded 100% retention rates in class V lesions without mechanical retention or enamel etching, based on certain clinical studies of 3 years or more in duration.

Clinical longevity depends not just on bond strength but also on dislodging forces. Composite restoratives undergo significant polymerization shrinkage, which creates stresses adjacent to the resin–dentin interface that can rupture dentinal bonds in all but the smallest restorations. Because glass ionomers generate low stresses on setting, they are well retained even with their low bond strengths in areas such as class V sites, where occlusal forces and other external forces induce relatively little stress. However, they have also been used with somewhat limited success as pit and fissure sealants. Because of the higher stresses induced by intraoral forces in occlusal areas, a greater degree of dislodgment and fracture occur in these sites. GIC may be used as an interim preventive agent when a resin-based sealant is indicated, but concerns about moisture control may compromise such placement.

CRITICAL QUESTION

How does amalgam bonding to dentin differ from composite bonding to dentin?

Amalgam Bonding

Although mechanical retention and resistance forms were the hallmark of traditional amalgam preparation design, modern conservative philosophy has stimulated a search for improved methods for retaining and sealing amalgam restorations. Amalgam bonding or bonded amalgam restorations combine the reliability of this traditional material with a dentin-bonding system, potentially reducing microleakage and increasing fracture resistance. Mechanical adjuncts, including threaded pins or retentive grooves placed in dentin, have served well for years toward these ends. More recently, bonding agents employing M–R–X-type adhesive monomers have achieved some clinical success. One system uses 4-META (see Fig. 6.4). However, the mechanism responsible for bonding amalgam to resin is predominantly mechanical in nature. It is produced during condensation of the amalgam mass into the viscous plastic adhesive layer, thereby producing macroretentive areas that will interlock after polymerization. The results of controlled clinical trials have been mixed, but it is safe to say that amalgam bonding has a place as an adjunct to conventional retentive means if employed so as to maximize sealing and minimize dislodging stresses. In this regard, thicker adhesive layers or interfaces have been shown to promote greater retention under certain conditions. One example is Amalgambond Plus with HPA (high performance additive) powder (Parkell Inc., Edgewood, NY), which contains polymethylmethacrylate fibers to form a thick, viscous layer when mixed with the Amalgambond Plus base and catalyst liquids. Studies such as that of Overton (2005) have shown that amalgam bonding bond strengths range from 6 to 15 MPa.

CRITICAL QUESTION

Can sealants prevent secondary caries progression when placed over underlying carious enamel or dentin?

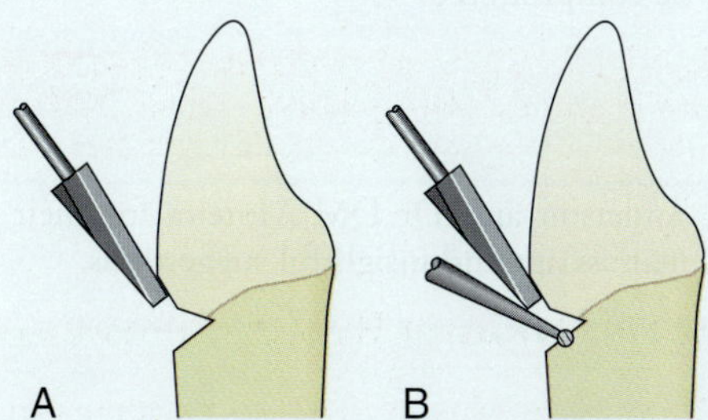

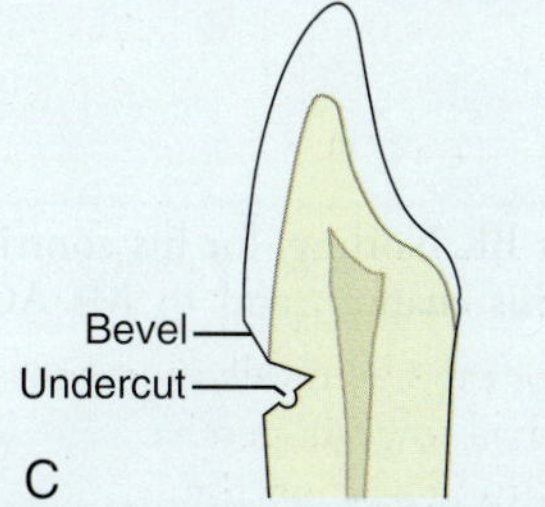

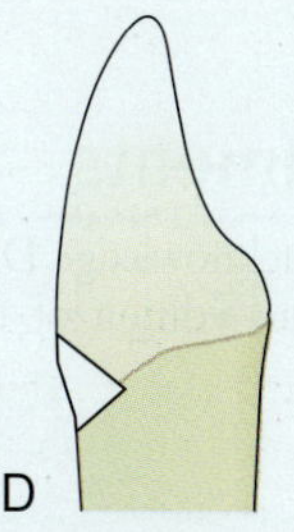

• **Fig. 6.8** Glass ionomer restoration of enamel class V lesion. Because of the low curing shrinkage and thermal and mechanical stresses experienced by this material in a relatively sheltered location, clinical retention is vertically 100% despite low bond strengths of about 3 MPa. The use of an undercut for retention may not be necessary in most cases.

Pit and Fissure Sealants

Various materials and techniques have been advocated for preventing caries in the susceptible pit and fissure areas of posterior teeth, particularly in the pediatric patient or for the patient at a high caries risk in general. The most popular sealant techniques make use of resin systems that can be applied to the occlusal surfaces of teeth. The objective of sealant use is for the resin to penetrate into the pits and fissures and to seal these areas against oral bacteria and debris. A cross-section of a tooth to which a pit and fissure sealant has been applied is shown in Figure 6.9.

Several types of resins, both filled and unfilled, have been employed as pit and fissure sealants. These resin systems include those based on cyanoacrylates, UDMA, and bis-GMA. The commercially available products are based on either the UDMA or bis-GMA monomers (see Fig. 6.4) that may be polymerized either by the amine-benzoyl peroxide chemical activation-initiation system or by light activation, as discussed in Chapter 5. The unfilled resins are available as colorless or tinted transparent materials. The filled resins are opaque and available either as tooth-colored or white materials.

The success of the sealant technique is highly dependent on obtaining and maintaining an intimate adaptation of the sealant to the tooth surface. Therefore, the sealants must be of relatively low viscosity so that they will wet the tooth and flow readily into the depths of the pits and fissures. To enhance wetting and mechanical retention of the sealant, the tooth surface is first conditioned by etching with acid, as described earlier. The physical properties of the sealants are closer to those of unfilled direct resins than to those of resin-based composites.

The reduction in occlusal caries resulting from the careful use of pit and fissure sealants has been impressive. Consequently, the American Dental Association, the American Academy of Pediatric Dentistry, the American Society of Dentistry for Children, and the American Association of Public Health Dentistry have all endorsed the use of sealants as an effective therapy. Clinical studies have shown that the failure frequency of sealants is approximately 5% per year after one single application of the sealant. In one report, at the end of 10 years, 78% of first permanent molars were free of caries when a single application of sealant had been placed compared with only 31% of caries-free teeth in the unsealed matched pairs. Mertz-Fairhurst et al. (1998) reported even more dramatic results in a study of sealed class I composite restorations where carious dentin was not removed. They showed that the lesions did not progress over a period of 10 years as long as the sealants remained intact.

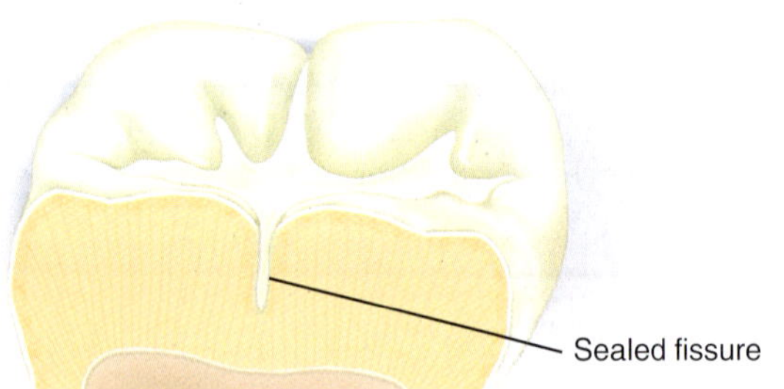

• **Fig. 6.9** Schematic of a tooth cross-section, illustrating penetration of a sealant into an occlusal fissure.

If doubt exists about whether the pit or fissure is free from caries or not, it is still justified to place a sealant. Clinical trials in which sealants were intentionally placed in pits and fissures that were diagnosed as having caries have shown that as long as a sealant is well retained, no caries progression will occur. If a dentist feels uncomfortable about sealing in a potential carious lesion and believes that a visual inspection of the potential lesion is required, another conservative approach can be taken that consists of a minimal cavity preparation and the placement of an enamel–dentin-bonded composite restoration combined with a sealant application. With such an approach, most of the occlusal surface is sealed. This restoration is called a **preventive-resin restoration (PRR)**. The PRR treatment has exhibited a success rate of 75% after 9 years, a remarkably high success rate, compared with traditional amalgam treatment.

There is indirect evidence that use of the four-handed technique when placing resin-based sealants is associated with improved retention rates. Sealant retention can be improved if the clinician uses an etch-and-rinse technique with a primer and bonding agent.

Presently available self-etching bonding agents provide comparable or less retention than do bonding agents that involve a separate acid etching step.

Evidence suggests that sealant effectiveness on cavitated lesions into dentin is limited. Losing sealant does not increase caries risk compared to never sealed teeth in children and teeth at similar risk.

Future Developments

Hybrid layer degradation, whether from within the adhesive layer or the dentin, remains a matter of concern for long-term stability of the bond. No matter where biodegradation starts, research should focus on the use of non-hydrolyzing polymers and inhibition of enzymatic activity in dentin. Dentin in NCCLs is still the most challenging and unpredictable coronal substrate for adhesion. In vitro results cannot be directly extrapolated to clinical practice.

While it is desirable that technique-sensitive adhesive systems should be simplified in terms of application steps, it is essential to ensure that the requisite bond strength and its stability should not be compromised.

Acknowledgments

The authors wish to acknowledge Dr BK Norling, for his contribution to the previous edition of this chapter; and to Ms AC Anderson and Dr DM Moreira for their critical review of the manuscript and insightful suggestions.

Summary

- **Bonding** and **adhesion** comprise a complex set of physical, chemical, and mechanical mechanisms that allow the attachment and binding of one substance to another.
- **Mechanisms of adhesion**
- The fundamental mechanism of adhesion to tooth structure can be regarded simply as an exchange by which inorganic tooth material (hydroxyapatite) is replaced by synthetic resins. This process involves two parts:

- Removing hydroxyapatite to create micropores.
- Infiltration of resin monomers into the micropores and subsequent polymerization.
  The following factors can play major or minor roles in achieving adhesive bonds:
  - Surface energy and wetting
  - Interpenetration (formation of a hybrid zone)
  - Micromechanical interlocking
  - Chemical bonding.
- **Smear layer**
- Whenever both enamel and dentin tissues are mechanically cut, especially with a rotary instrument, a layer of adherent grinding debris and organic film known as a **smear layer** is left on their surfaces and prevents strong bonding.
- It is also weakly cohesive to the underlying dentin with a bond strength of 5–10 MPa, which interferes with strong bonding.
- To achieve predictable bonding, it is essential to either remove the smear layer completely by using an acid or to modify it, and use adhesive monomers to penetrate the smear layer and bond to underlying intact dentin structures below.
- The **hybrid layer** is the primary bond mechanism for dentin. There is an interdiffusion or **micromechanical interlocking** of resin with demineralized collagen of intertubular dentin. Resin tags are also formed, but are an insignificant bonding mechanism. *Without a hybrid layer a strong and stable bond will not be formed to the dentin.* The hybrid layer has also been referred to as the 'resin dentin interdiffusion zone'.
- **Acid-etch technique**
- **Enamel etching**
- Phosphoric acid removes the smear layer and about 10 microns of enamel to expose prisms of enamel rods to create a honeycomb-like, high energy retentive surface.
- **Dentin bonding agents**
- Dental bonding agents are designed to provide a sufficiently strong interface between restorative composites and tooth structure to withstand mechanical forces and shrinkage stress. The success of adhesives is dependent on two types of bonding:
  - Micromechanical interlocking, chemical bonding with enamel and dentin, or both.
  - Copolymerization with the resin matrix of composite materials.
- A successful dentin-bonding system must meet several requirements:
  - Adequate removal or dissolution of the smear layer from enamel and dentin
  - Maintenance or reconstitution of the dentin collagen matrix
  - Good wetting
  - Efficient monomer diffusion and penetration
  - Polymerization within tooth structure
  - Copolymerization with the resin composite matrix
- **Design of dentin-bonding systems**
  All bonding systems consist of three key components:
  - Conditioning (cleaning)
  - Priming (wetting, adapting)
  - Bonding (mechanical adhesion, curing).
- **Classification**
- **Etch-and-rinse adhesives**
  - *Three-step (fourth generation):* At this time, the most established, most reliable adhesion method in this category consists of three steps: (1) an acid etchant application, (2) application of the primer, and (3) application of the actual bonding agent or bonding resin.
  - *Two-step (fifth generation):* A simplified method in this category combines the primer and adhesive resin into one application. This etch-and-rinse strategy is the most effective to achieve efficient and stable bonding to enamel. Etching, usually with a 30%–40% phosphoric gel that is rinsed away promotes the dissolution of enamel rods, creating porosities that are filled by bonding agents through capillary action and then followed by polymerization of resin.
- **Self-etch adhesives**
  With the self-etch adhesives, acidic monomers (self-etching primer) that simultaneously demineralize and prime tooth surfaces are applied and dried on the tooth surface.
  - *Two-step (sixth generation):* In this case an acidic monomer, which is not rinsed, is used to condition and prime the tooth at the same time. Then, a bonding agent from a separate bottle is used.
  - *One-step (seventh generation):* The simplified method in this category combines conditioner, primer, and bonding resin into a single step. Most one-step or "all-in-one" systems are delivered by a bottle, vial, or single-unit dose applicator, which are formulated as a single component.
- **Universal adhesives**
  Universal adhesives are ideally a single-bottle, no-mix, adhesive system that can be used in total-etch, self-etch, or selective-etch mode depending on the specific clinical situation and personal preferences of the operator.
  The term "UNIVERSAL" refers to their application options, enabling them to be used either following an E&R or SE bonding mode, while offering application versatility with (claimed) bonding potential to glass-rich (via silane) and glass-poor zirconia (via 10-MDP) ceramics for indirect tooth-restoration indications.
  - Universal adhesives can be applied using a total-etch, self-etch, or selective-etch technique.
- **Glass ionomer restoratives**
  Bonding occurs through ionic bond formation between the carboxyl groups of the polyalkenoic acid with calcium of hydroxyapatite. Thus, the chelation of carboxyl groups that are derived from polyalkenoic acid with the calcium in apatite can be obtained as represented below:
- **Pit and fissure sealants**
- The objective of sealant use is for the resin to penetrate into the pits and fissures and to seal these areas against oral bacteria and debris.
- Another conservative approach can be taken that consists of a minimal cavity preparation and the placement of an enamel–dentin-bonded composite restoration combined with a sealant application. With such an approach, most of the occlusal surface is sealed. This restoration is called a **PRR.**

Review Questions

1. Discuss in detail enamel and dentin-bonding agents.
2. Discuss in detail principles of dentin bonding.
3. Discuss in brief conditioner or dentin conditioner.
4. Discuss in detail composition of dentin-bonding systems.
5. Discuss in detail difference between bonding to enamel and dentin.
6. Discuss in brief enamel bonding.
7. Discuss in brief acid etching and its effect on enamel and dentin.
8. Discuss in detail patterns of etching seen in enamel.
9. Discuss in brief classification of dentin-bonding systems.
10. Discuss in brief self-etch bonding systems.
11. Discuss in brief etch-and-rinse bonding systems.
12. Discus in brief mechanism of bonding of glass ionomer cements.
13. Write a short note on amalgam bonding.
14. Discuss in brief preventive resin restorations.
15. Discuss in brief ideal requirements of bonding agents.
16. Discuss in brief challenges in bonding to dentin.
17. Discuss in brief acid etching.
18. Discuss in brief self-etching primers.
19. Discuss in brief role of primers in bonding.
20. Discuss in brief hybrid layer.
21. Write a short note on universal adhesives.
22. Discuss in brief selective enamel etching.

Selected Readings

Asmussen E.; Munksgaard E.C. Bonding of restorative resins to dentine: Status of dentine adhesives and impact on cavity design and filling techniques. Int Dent J 38 97 (1988); The chemistry of dentin bonding agents is described, and bond strength data are presented. Also, factors involved in clinical usage that influence retention are cited.

Beauchamp J.; Caufield P.W.; Crall J.J.; Donly K.; Feigal R.; Gooch B.; Ismail A.; Kohn W.; Siegal M.; Simonsen R. American Dental Association Council on Scientific Affairs. Evidence-based clinical recommendations for the use of pit-and-fissure sealants: a report of the American Dental Association Council on Scientific Affairs. J Am Dent Assoc 139 (3) 257–268 (2008 Mar); This article presents a systematic review and clinical recommendations for the use of pit and fissure sealants.

Bedran-Russo A, Leme-Kraus AA, Vidal CMP, Teixeira EC. An Overview of Dental Adhesive Systems and the Dynamic Tooth-Adhesive Interface. Dent Clin North Am. 2017;61(4):713-31.

Bowen R.L.; Eichmiller F.C.; Marjenhoff W.A.; et al. Adhesive bonding of composites. J Am Coll Dent 56 10 (1989); This article discusses the merits of several of the popular dentin and enamel bonding systems, noting differences in chemical components and instructions for use.

Buonocore M.G. A simple method of increasing the adhesion of acrylic filling materials to enamel surfaces. J Dent Res 34 849 (1955); In this paper, published approximately 50 years ago, Buonocore suggested that etching enamel would improve mechanical bonding of an unfilled resin (composites were nonexistent at that time). The technique is now an essential step in the use of all modern composites.

Buonocore M.G. The use of adhesives in dentistry. Charles C Thomas: Springfield, IL; In this book, Buonocore, the developer of the acid-etch technique, identified potential problems associated with the use of adhesives in dentistry that are still germane to current systems, for example, dentin bonding agents.

Cardoso M.V.; de Almeida Neves A.; et al. Current aspects on bonding effectiveness and stability in adhesive dentistry. Australian Dental Journal 56 (S1) 31–44 (2011).

De Munck J.; van Landuyt K.L.; Peumans M.; et al. A critical review of the durability of adhesion to tooth tissue: Methods and results. J Den Res 84 (2) 118–132 (2005); This review examines the fundamental processes that cause the adhesion of biomaterials to enamel and dentin to degrade over time. This paper critically appraises methodologies that focus on chemical degradation patterns of hydrolysis and elution of interface components, as well as mechanically oriented test setups, such as those designed for fatigue and fracture toughness measurements.

Douglas W.H. Clinical status of dentine bonding agents. J Dent 17 209 (1989); An excellent review and update of the evolution of earlier dentin bonding agents, the problems associated with adhesion, and the clinical criteria involved in phenomena such as microleakage and tooth strengthening. This reference is essential for individuals interested in this highly controversial area.

Fusayama T.; Nakamura M.; Kurosaki M.; et al. Nonpressure adhesion of a new adhesive restorative resin. J Dent Res 58 1364 (1979); A breakthrough in dentin bonding was demonstrated when acid etching of dentin was reported to increase retention of restorations, but with no increase in pulpal trauma.

Gary Alex, D. (2015). "Universal Adhesives: The Next Evolution in Adhesive Dentistry?" Compend Contin Educ Dent **36**(1). This article provides a comprehensive overview of Universal adhesives.

Glantz P. On wettability and adhesiveness. Odont Rev 20 1 (Suppl 17) 1 (1969); The first in a series of publications by this author suggesting that the use of topical fluorides provides an additional mechanism involved in reduction of dental caries, that is, lowering of the surface energy of tooth structure, thereby reducing plaque accumulation over a given interval.

Haller B. Which self-etch bonding systems are suitable for which clinical indications? Quintessence Int 44 (9) 645–661 (2013 Oct); This article assesses self-etch bonding systems, which comprise a great variety of different types of products, each with specific strengths and weaknesses. It gives clinical recommendations for use of bonding systems in specific clinical situations.

Houpt M.; Fuks A.; Eidelman E. The preventive resin (composite resin/sealant) restoration: Nine-year results. Quintessence Int 25 155 (1994); Nine-year data presented to show the efficiency of using preventive resin restorations (PRRs) to treat pits and fissures with carious lesions.

Ikemura K.; Endo T. A review of our development of dental adhesives—Effects of radical polymerization initiators and adhesive monomers on adhesion. Dent Mater J 29 (2) 109–121 (2010); The authors present a thorough review of their development of monomers for self-etching and self-adhesive bonding systems, the role of initiators, and chemical structure–property relationships. A rare look behind the scenes of the tremendous scientific and technical effort required for the development of dental materials.

Imazato S. Antibacterial properties of resin composites and dentin bonding systems. Dent Mater 19 (6) 449–457 (2003); This paper reviews the research conducted on the evaluation of antibacterial properties of commercial composites and adhesive systems, in addition to the discussion of many attempts to achieve antibacterial composites or adhesives.

Liu Y.; Tjäderhane L.; Breschi L.; et al. Limitations in bonding to dentin and experimental strategies to prevent bond degradation. J Dent Res 90 (8) 953–968 (2011).

Marshall S.J.; Bayne S.C.; Baier R.; et al. A review of adhesion science. Dent Mater 26 11–16 (2010).

Mertz-Fairhurst E.J. Current status of sealant retention and caries prevention. National Institutes of Health Consensus Development Conference. Dental sealants in the prevention of tooth decay. J Dent Res

48 18 (1984); Ten-year data presented to show a substantial reduction in caries following the placement of sealant as compared with untreated control surfaces.

Mertz-Fairhurst E.J.; Curtis J.W.; Ergle J.W.; et al. Ultraconservative and cariostatic sealed restorations: Results at year 10. J Am Dent Assoc 129 55 (1998); A classic 10-year study that demonstrates the efficacy of sealed composites in preventing caries progression even when the carious dentin was not removed.

Nagarkar, S., et al. (2019). "Universal dental adhesives: Current status, laboratory testing, and clinical performance." J Biomed Mater Res B Appl Biomater **107**(6): 2121-2131.

The aim of this review was to synthesize the literature regarding the current status of UAs, their adhesion potential to various substrates and their performance in different restorative situations.

Nakabayashi N.; Kojima K.; Masuhara E. Sealants consensus development conference statement on dental sealants and the prevention of tooth decay. J Am Dent Assoc 108 233 (1984); Recommendations are made from a consensus conference on the state of the art of sealant therapy. The data presented were strongly supportive of sealant use.

Overton J.D.; Vance R.I. Effect of adhesive volume on the bond strength of bonded complex amalgam restorations. Am J Dent 18 (6) 320–322 (2005).

Özcan M, Volpato CAM. Current perspectives on dental adhesion: (3) Adhesion to intraradicular dentin: Concepts and applications. Japanese Dental Science Review. 2020;56(1):216-23.

Pashley D.H.; Carvalho R.M.; Sano H.; et al. The microtensile bond test: A review. J Adhes Dent 1 (4) 299 (1999); A review of the microtensile bond test, which permits true interfacial bond strength measurement in modern bonded systems for which conventional shear bond tests yield cohesive dentin failure.

Pashley D.H.; Tay F.R.; Carvalho R.M.; et al. From dry bonding to water-wet bonding to ethanol-wet bonding. A review of the interactions between dentin matrix and solvated resins using a macromodel of the hybrid layer. Am J Dent 20 (1) 7–20 (2007).

Pedro P.C.; Souza A.M.F.; Aranha J.H.; et al. Dental Materials 22 (9) 838–844 (2006); In vitro cytotoxicity and in vivo biocompatibility of contemporary resin-modified glass-ionomer cements.

Perdigão, J. (2020). "Current perspectives on dental adhesion: (1) Dentin adhesion – not there yet." Japanese Dental Science Review **56**(1): 190-207.

Perdigão J.; Lopes M. Dentin bonding—questions for the new millennium. J Adhes Dent 1 (3) 19 (1999); An update on the state of dentin bonding with a discussion of unanswered questions.

Perdigão J. Dentin bonding—variables related to the clinical situation and the substrate treatment. Dent Mater 26 (2) 24–37 (2010).

Peutzfeldt A.; Sahafi A.; Flury S. Bonding of restorative materials to dentin with various luting agents. Oper Dent 36 (3) 266–273 (2011).

In: (editors: Phillips R.W.; Ryge G.) Proceedings on adhesive restorative dental materials. Owen Litho Service: Spencer, IN; These historical transactions resulted from the first workshop on the problems of, and potential solutions to, the development of adhesive dental materials. The recommendations for critically important areas of research have provided an impetus for investigations in this area.

Perdigão J. Current perspectives on dental adhesion: (1) Dentin adhesion – not there yet. Japanese Dental Science Review. 2020;56(1):190-207.

Jin-Ho Phark, N. S., Luana Oliveira, and J. Sillas Duarte (2012). "Biomaterials Update- A Comprehensive Guide for Post and Core Restorations." Quintessence of Dental technology

Powers J.M.; O'Keefe K.L. Update on seventh-generation bonding agents. Inside Dentistry 5 (2) 52–56 (2009).

Simonsen R.J. Retention and effectiveness of dental sealant after 15 years. J Am Dent Assoc 122 34–42 (1991); This paper represents a long-term evaluation of sealants based on a single application.

Simonsen R.J.; Neal R.J. A review of the clinical application and performance of pit and fissure sealants. Aust Dent J 56 (Suppl 1) 45–58 (2011); This paper focuses on the clinical aspects of pit and fissure sealant application and the most recent publications that support an evidence-based clinical application technique.

Schwartz R.S.; Fransman R. Adhesive dentistry and endodontics: Materials, clinical strategies and procedures for restoration of access cavities: A review. J Endod 31 151–165 (2005).

van Landuyt K.L.; Snauwaert J.; De Munck J.; et al. Systematic review of the chemical composition of contemporary dental adhesives. Biomaterials 28 (26) 3757–3785 (2007); This article systematically reviews the ingredients commonly used in current dental adhesives as well as the properties of these ingredients. It also includes an extensive table with the chemical formulation of contemporary dental adhesives.

van Landuyt K.L.; Peumans M.; De Munck J.; et al. Three-year clinical performance of a HEMA-free one-step self-etch adhesive in non-carious cervical lesions. Eur J Oral Sci 119 511–516 (2011).

Van Meerbeek, B., et al. (2020). "From Buonocore's Pioneering Acid-Etch Technique to Self-Adhering Restoratives. A Status Perspective of Rapidly Advancing Dental Adhesive Technology." J Adhes Dent **22**(1): 7-34.

This literature-based OPINION PAPER reflects in an introductory historical perspective on the rapid advancement of dental adhesive technology. Past and current techniques to bond to tooth tissue, in particular to dentin as the most challenging bonding substrate, are critically appraised.

Van Meerbeek B. Adhesion to enamel and dentin: current status and future challenges. Oper Dent 28 (3) 215–235 (2003).

van Meerbeek B.; Van Landuyt K.L.; De Munck J.; et al. Technique-sensitivity of contemporary adhesives. Dent Mater J 24 (1) 1–13 (2005).

van Meerbeek B.; Peumans M.; Poitevin A.; et al. Relationship between bond-strength tests and clinical outcomes. Dent Mater 26 (2) 100–121 (2010).

van Meerbeek B.; Yoshihara K.; Yoshida Y.; et al. State of the art of self-etch adhesives. Dent Mater 27 17–28 (2011); An excellent overview of the types of adhesive systems and application strategies in current use as of 2011.

Vaught R.L. Mechanical versus chemical retention for restoring complex restorations: What is the evidence? J Dent Educ 71 (10) 1356–1362 (2007).

Zisman W.A. Influence of constitution on adhesion. Ind Eng Chem 55 19 (1963); One of the pioneers in surface phenomena discusses parameters that influence wetting. Zisman was a leader in the use of contact angle measurements to screen the potential wetting of adhesives to selected adherends.

Useful Websites

Biomaterials Properties Database: http://www.lib.umich.edu/node/21860

The Biomaterials Network: http://www.biomat.net/

Dentistry Today, Advanced Resin Technologies: http://www.dentistrytoday.com/dental-materials/972

http://www.faqs.org/abstracts/Health/Clinical-guidelines-for-photocuring-restorative-resins-Assessing-the-effect-of-extraneous-light-on-p.html

http://adeptinstitute.com/members/000_source/membership/list.php?view=3&title=Bonding+%28Direct+Resin%29

http://www.dentalcompare.com/

http://www.afms.af.mil/

7 Dental Cements

CHAPTER OUTLINE

KEY TERMS

Acid–base reaction—Chemical reaction between a compound containing replaceable hydrogen ions (acid) and a substance containing replaceable hydroxide ions (base) that yields salt and water; for aqueous liquid and powder cements, the liquid is the acid, and the powder is the base.

Atraumatic restorative treatment (ART)—Clinical procedure performed without dental burs, air/water spray, or anesthesia that consists of manual excavation of cavitated carious tissues and restoration of the tooth cavity with a fluoride-releasing cement.

Bioactivity—Reactive potential of a material to form a layer of hydroxyapatite-like material on their surface in vivo.

Calcium phosphate cements—Cement that is used for bone regeneration that consists of powder (dicalcium, tricalcium, or tetracalcium phosphates) that is mixed with an aqueous solution from which hydroxyapatite precipitates.

Cavity liner—Material to coat the bottom of a cavity preparation to protect the pulp; a liner is applied in a thin layer.

Cement—Substance that hardens from a viscous state to a solid union between two surfaces; for dental applications, cements act as a base, liner, filling material, root canal sealer, or adhesive to bind devices and prostheses to tooth structure or to each other.

Cement base—Material used to protect the pulp in a cavity preparation by providing thermal insulation and sometimes a medicament, usually thicker and more distant from the pulp than a cavity liner.

Cement thickness—Distance between an abutment tooth and cemented prosthesis, influenced by the design of the prosthesis and the viscosity of the cement during seating.

Compomer—A term derived from the terms *composite* and *ionomer*; a resin-based composite consisting of a silicate glass filler phase and a methacrylate-based matrix with carboxylic groups; also known as *polyacid-modified glass ionomer cement.*

Endodontic sealer—Material to prevent any transmittance of fluid or bacteria from the coronal to the apical region, used in conjunction with an obturation material such as gutta-percha.

Film thickness—Thickness in micrometer of a cement 7 minutes after 150 N has been applied, which is the International Organization for Standardization (ISO) and American Dental Association (ADA) method for determining the ability of a cement to spread under pressure.

Glass ionomer cement (GIC)—Cement that hardens following an acid–base reaction between fluoroaluminosilicate glass powders and an aqueous-based polyacrylic solution; also known as *polyalkenoate cement.*

Hydraulic cement—Cement that requires water to cause the material to set.

Luting agent—A viscous cement-like material that fills a gap between two surfaces to prevent dislodgment. The term *luting agent* originally referred to nonadhesive agents only but now also includes adhesive agents.

Maturation—Process of aqueous cement strengthening after setting.

Mineral trioxide aggregate (MTA)—A tricalcium and dicalcium silicate-based cement used for vital pulp therapy and other endodontic indications.

Pulp capping—A procedure to treat pulp that has been exposed through caries removal or trauma, by the application of a medicament; *indirect pulp capping* is the term used when the pulpal exposure is incipient, such as when dentinal tubules are visible in the cavity.

Resin cement—A resin-based composite material used for attaching fixed prostheses or orthodontic brackets; these cements are less viscous than resin composite restorative materials.

Resin-modified glass ionomer cement (hybrid ionomer cement)—Cement that combines a glass powder and an aqueous solution of polymerizable groups attached to the polyacrylic acid.

Varnish—Material applied to the floor of a cavity; a solution of natural gum, synthetic resins, or resins dissolved in volatile solvent, such as acetone, ether, or chloroform; material applied superficially to a tooth to release fluoride.

Zinc oxide–eugenol (ZOE) cement—Cement based on the reaction between zinc oxide and eugenol.

Zinc phosphate cement—Substance formed by the reaction between zinc oxide powder and phosphoric acid liquid that can be used either as a base or as a luting agent.

Dental **cements** are materials that set intraorally and are commonly used to join a tooth and a prosthesis. They are classified according to their major chemical reacting components, as shown in Table 7.1. Every cement must be assessed for its biocompatibility, safety, and effectiveness. Ideally a cement does not cause damage to a tooth, has suitable physical properties for its intended use, and provides passive or active (bioactive) properties. Ultimately, the body should not recognize the cement as foreign, so that healing of affected tissues can begin as soon as possible.

History of Dental Cements

In the 1800s, zinc oxide (ZnO) powder of good purity was found to react with eugenol at room temperature to form a functional cement. The ZnO–eugenol (ZOE) material was used as an impression material and temporary restoration and was eventually found to be obtundent with the pulp and suitable as a root canal sealer. ZnO was observed to react with phosphoric acid to yield a material stronger than ZOE, capable of securing gold alloy restorations to tooth preparations. The high acidity of the ZnO–phosphate cement was unsuitable for pulpal contact but a good insulator for use as a base. In the mid-20th century, ZnO was also used with carboxylic acid to produce a cement that was lower in acidity and capable of bonding to tooth structure.

When the ZnO in zinc phosphate cement was replaced with a glass powder, a semitranslucent esthetic filling called *silicate cement* was created. The longevity of the silicate cement restorations was unimpressive (<4 years) because the silicate cements have high solubility. Gradually, the silicate cements lost anatomical contour and degraded at the margins. Despite the deficiency, the occurrence of recurrent caries adjacent to these cements was rare. Laboratory studies showed that fluoride was released from the glass in the silicate cements. The impressive anticariogenic potential of the silicate cements highlighted the ability of fluoride ions (F^-) to inhibit demineralization.

The lessons learned from silicate cement and zinc carboxylate cement led to the development of glass ionomer cements (GICs), which contained a modified glass for the powder and polyacrylic acid for the liquid. Incorporating the polymerization technology of methacrylate resin into the liquid created dual-cured materials: acid–base and polymerization reactions. From this combination, resin-modified glass ionomer cement (RMGI) evolved. Replacing the liquid component of RMGI with a water-free acidic polymerizable monomer created a light-curable single-component material called compomer, a term derived from the terms *composite* and *ionomer*. The goal of these two hybrid materials was to combine the strength of composite with the fluoride release and self-adhesion of glass ionomer into one material.

Around the mid-20th century, new attributes for dental cements were needed for use with gutta-percha points in endodontic therapy. These cements are denoted as endodontic sealers, which must cure in the moist root canal dentin. Furthermore, endodontic materials must ensure that oral bacteria cannot percolate through the root to the periapical bone; otherwise, serious infection persists or occurs. Esthetics are less important for endodontic cements than for supragingival indications. Several dental materials were adapted for endodontic use: ZOE, polyvinyl siloxane, epoxy resins, and hydraulic ceramics (tricalcium/dicalcium silicate). In the 1990s, the bioactivity and sealing ability of tricalcium/dicalcium silicate cements became recognized and appreciated in dentistry. This ceramic dental cement is now widely indicated for pulpal and periradicular contact, including endodontic indications.

Varnish has been used for pulpal protection, especially with amalgam in a cavity preparation. The use of varnish has declined with decreased amalgam use. However, surficial varnishes are

TABLE 7.1 Overview of Dental Cements

Powder/Liquid Systems

Materials	Powder	Liquid	Reaction Type	Indications
Zinc phosphate	Zinc oxide and magnesium oxide	Phosphoric acid, water	Acid–base reaction	Cementing metallic fixed prostheses
Zinc oxide–eugenol	Zinc oxide	Eugenol	Acid–base reaction	Pulp protection, temporary cement
Zinc oxide–eugenol (EBA modified)	Zinc oxide	Eugenol, EBA	Acid–base reaction	Pulp protection, temporary cement
Zinc polycarboxylate	Zinc oxide and magnesium oxide	Polyacrylic acid, water	Acid–base reaction	Metallic fixed prostheses short spans or crowns
Glass ionomer	Fluoroaluminosilicate glass	Polyacrylic acid, polybasic carboxylic acid, water	Acid–base reaction	Cementing crowns (alumina, zirconia metal), metal posts, and core restoration
Resin-modified glass ionomer (hybrid ionomer)	Fluoroaluminosilicate glass, chemical- and/or light-activated initiator(s)	Polyacrylic acid, water-soluble methacrylate monomer, water, activator	Light- or chemical-activated polymerization and acid–base reaction	Metal, lithium disilicate, alumina or zirconia prostheses,[a] metal posts/core
	Fluoroaluminosilicate glass, metallic oxides, sodium fluoride, chemical- and/or light-activated initiator(s)	Dimethacrylate/carboxylic monomers, multiple functional acrylate monomers, water, activator for chemical activation	Polymerization by light and chemical activation, and acid–base reaction	
	Fluoroaluminosilicate glass, nonreactive filler, reactive monomers	Nonreactive filler, methacrylate-modified polyalkanoic acid, water-soluble methacrylate monomer, water	Light-activated polymerization and acid–base reaction	
Epoxy	Methenamine, titania, silver	Bisphenol A, epichlorohydrin resin	Chemical crosslinking polymerization of epoxide	Root canal sealing
Tricalcium/dicalcium silicate	Tricalcium/dicalcium silicate and radiopaque powder	Water-based liquid	Hydration with liquid	Pulpal protection, periradicular contact, endodontic sealing

Two-Paste Systems

Materials	Base Paste	Catalyst Paste	Reaction Type	Indications
Compomer	Fluoroaluminosilicate glass, metallic oxides, sodium fluoride, chemical- and/or light-activated initiator(s)	Dimethacrylate/carboxylic monomers, multiple functional acrylate monomers water, activator (for chemical cure)	Light or chemical activation of polymerization and acid–base reaction	Cavities in deciduous teeth, cervical cavities in adults, anterior proximal restorations in adults, small load-bearing restorations in adults, temporary
Resin cement	Methacrylate monomers, fillers, light-activated initiator(s)	Methacrylate monomers, fillers, activator (for chemical cure)	Polymerization by light and chemical activation, or chemical activation only	Ceramic veneers, Maryland bridges, lithium disilicate, alumina, zirconia, cores, and posts
	Polymethyl methacrylate polymer beads	Liquid 1: Methacrylate monomers Liquid 2: Catalyst	Chemical-activated polymerization	
Disalicylate	Butyl ethylene glycol salicylate resin, bismuth oxide	Resimpol natural resin, 13% "MTA" (tricalcium/dicalcium silicate and tricalcium aluminate?), titania, and silica	Chemical-activated polymerization	Endodontic sealing
Disalicylate	Glycol disalicylate, titanium dioxide and barium sulfate, titania, zinc oxide	Ethyl toluene sulfonamide, calcium hydroxide, zinc oxide, zinc stearate	Chemical-activated polymerization	Pulp capping
Epoxy	Bisphenol-A epoxy resin, bisphenol-F epoxy resin, calcium tungstate, zirconium oxide, silica, iron-oxide pigments	Dibenzydiamine, aminoadamantane, tricyclodecane-diamine, calcium tungstate, zirconium oxide, silica, silicone oil	Chemical-activated polymerization	Endodontic sealing

Continued

TABLE 7.1 Overview of Dental Cements—cont'd

Materials	Paste or Liquid	Reaction Type	Indications
Single Component			
Compomer	Methacrylate monomer, acidic monomer, fluoroaluminosilicate glass, initiator	Light-activated polymerization	Cavities in deciduous teeth, cervical cavities in adults, anterior proximal restorations in adults, small load-bearing restorations in adults, temporary
Varnish	Resins, organic solvent (acetone); chloroform ether may include silver, fluoride, or calcium compounds	Evaporation of solvent	Pulp protection, surficial ion release for caries prevention or remineralization
Inert	Methacrylate monomers, initiator, ceramic fillers	Light-activated polymerization	Cementing ceramic restorations or orthodontic brackets
Tricalcium/dicalcium silicate	Methacrylate monomers, initiators, tricalcium/dicalcium silicate, barium zirconate	Light-activated polymerization	Pulp-capping, pulpotomies
Tricalcium/dicalcium silicate	Organic liquid, tricalcium/dicalcium silicate, radiopaque powder	Hydration in vivo	Pulpotomies, endodontic sealing
Calcium hydroxide	Iodoform, silicone, calcium hydroxide	Nonsetting	Primary tooth pulpectomy
Tricalcium/dicalcium silicate	Tricalcium silicate, salicylate resin, titanium oxide, calcium tungstate	Nonsetting	Primary tooth pulpectomy

EBA, ethoxybenzoic acid.
[a]Do not use for anterior because of opacity.

popular, especially among pediatric dentists. These varnishes are placed on enamel to release fluoride to provide protection against caries and promote remineralization from acids in the oral cavity with calcium ions. Sealants based on resins are also used superficially on teeth to provide protection against caries.

In the 20th century, varnishes included silver ions, silver nitrate, and silver diamine fluoride solutions for arresting caries and reducing sensitivity. The hazard with silver compounds is imparting a black color to the caries, as discussed later.

Most current cements include polymers and ceramic powders. The remainder of this chapter is organized by general indications: pulp protection and enamel protection, fixed prosthodontic device cementation, endodontic restoratives, and sealing.

CRITICAL QUESTION

Dental cements are not as strong as composites or amalgams. Why do we use cement for restorations in certain situations?

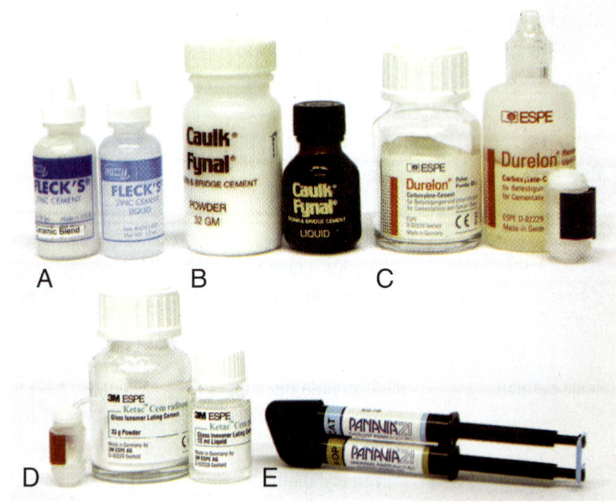

• **Fig. 7.1** Dental cements as luting agents. **(A)** Zinc phosphate. **(B)** Reinforced zinc oxide–eugenol. **(C)** Polycarboxylate with capsule. **(D)** Glass ionomer with capsule. **(E)** Resin cement. Each material system consists of two components: **(A)** to **(D)** are powder–liquid systems and **(E)** is a paste–paste system.

Many types of dental cements are supplied as a powder and a liquid or as two pastes (Fig. 7.1), so that mixing starts a chemical reaction. The liquids are usually acids (proton donors), and the powders are basic (alkaline) in nature, commonly composed of **glass** or metal oxides. The reaction between the powder and liquid is usually an **acid–base reaction**, although mineral trioxide aggregate (MTA) undergoes a hydration reaction. **Resin cements** do not rely on an acid–base reaction but set through polymerization activated by light or a chemical. When mixed, cement hardens (or sets) within a reasonable time. Set cements are strong enough to be used as a **base** for pulp protection, as a restorative material for temporary or **permanent restorations,** or as a **luting agent.**

Many viscosities of cements are available in dentistry, ranging from a paste-like consistency to a highly flowable form. For cementing an **appliance,** a luting agent must exhibit a sufficiently low viscosity to flow readily along the interfaces between hard tissue and a fixed prosthesis, and they must be capable of wetting both surfaces to retain the prosthesis in place. For a pulp that may have been irritated or damaged from the caries process or prepared cavity, a protective layer may be needed, such as a cavity **varnish,** liner, or base material that flows and sets within the prepared cavity. For fixing a post in a root canal, a more viscous cement is needed. For a root-tip filling, a viscous paste that does not dissolve out of the root apex is necessary. In orthodontics, the cement must be adhesive and possess a viscosity that is low enough to seat a band and high enough to keep brackets from drifting before the cement is cured. This chapter is organized so that cements for luting are described first, followed by pulp protection and restorative cements, including some endodontic specialty applications.

Cements may have mechanical or chemical adhesion or a combination of the two, as discussed in the following.

Classification of dental cements is as follows:

- Cements for luting
- Cements for pulp protection
- Cements for restoratives

The first ZnO-based cement for cementing fixed prostheses was not adhesive to the tooth or metal prostheses. The cement functioned by filling the microscopic space between the device and the tooth and hardening to a high cohesive mass, which prevented dislodgment (Fig. 7.2). The mechanical retention is obtained by the combination of the microscopically rough tooth and prosthesis surfaces along with the rigid cement that fills the gaps. This mechanical retention is referred to as *luting,* where zinc phosphate is the dominating cement. The degree of cement retentiveness for a given restoration relies on many factors: prepared tooth form, height, number of abutments, accuracy of superstructure fit, distribution of the cement, and occlusion.

Dental prostheses that are mechanically retained include the following:

(1) fixed prosthodontics made of metal, ceramic-veneered metal, or ceramic;
(2) temporary restorations;
(3) pins and posts used for retention of restorations; and
(4) implant superstructures.

As discussed in Chapter 6, *luting* traditionally refers to the use of nonadhesive materials for retaining prostheses, and *bonding* refers to the use of adhesive bonding materials. The distinction has faded in the literature; the use of adhesive bonding medium is also referred to as *luting.*

When a device is seated without a luting agent, point contacts are made between the tooth and the appliance (Fig. 7.3A and B).

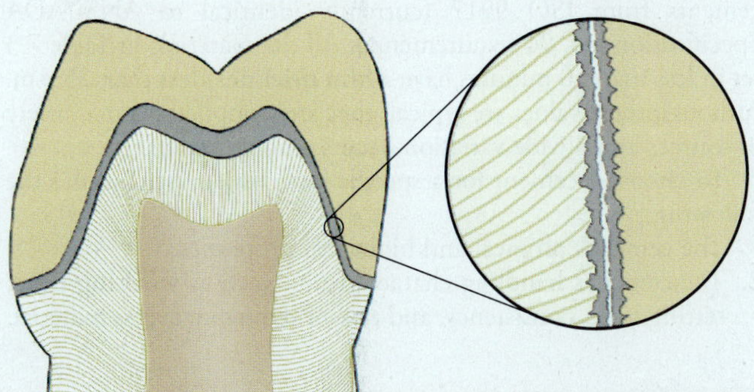

• **Fig. 7.2** Diagram of the suggested mechanism through which a dental cement provides mechanical retention of a gold crown. The cement penetrates irregularities in the tooth structure and the casting. Upon hardening, these retentive sites aid in retaining the cast crown in place. The enlargement shows a fracture through the cement, resulting in dislodgment of the crown.

The cement is used to fill the areas that are not in contact. The cement prevents oral fluid from flowing between the surfaces, thereby preventing bacterial invasion. Luting of a device to a tooth requires a cement of low viscosity and low contact angle to the tooth and the appliance to form a continuous film (Fig. 7.3C), without the formation of voids at interface (Fig. 7.3D). Voids impair the cement's ability to support and retain a prosthesis.

Porosity in powder–liquid cements is created from incorporating air while mixing powder into liquid. One study with luting agents showed that the method of mixing had no influence on the formation of small pores, but hand mixing yielded more large pores than triturator mixing. Porosity measurement of hand-mixed powder-to-liquid cements showed that polycarboxylate cement had the highest porosity, followed by zinc phosphate and GICs. Higher viscosity generally leads to more pores during mixing. If air bubbles are entrapped, masticatory forces may fracture weak appliances such as veneers. When a void-free layer is formed and hardens, one surface is wedged against another to resist the shearing stresses that might dislodge the appliance.

To choose a cement for attaching a fixed prosthesis, the key characteristics are the working time, setting time, consistency, ease of removal of excess material, and adhesion. Any cement for attachment must flow under pressure and wet (spread over) the tooth and prosthetic surfaces. The internationally accepted requirements for luting cements are shown in Table 7.2A and B. Luting cements are required to have a film thickness less of than 25 μm when tested according to American National Standards Institute (ANSI)/American Dental Association (ADA) Specification No. 96 and ISO 9917-1 or 9917-2. For endodontic sealers, which are discussed later, the maximum film thickness is 50 μm per ISO 6876. The film thickness essentially reflects the consistency of the cement mixture and is affected by the size of particles and the P/L ratio. The ISO film-thickness test method requires freshly mixed cement to be placed between two optically flat surfaces, and a 150-N vertical load is applied. Seven minutes later, the thickness of the film is measured. Such samples should appear to create continuous films.

The intaglio of a crown must be cleaned before the application of luting cement. The interior surface should be carefully abraded with a stone or sandblasted with alumina abrasive. Prolonged sandblasting can deform metal margins or erode ceramic margins and should be avoided. Crowns should be thoroughly rinsed to remove debris and dried. Cementing a prosthesis to a tooth occurs in three steps after the cement is mixed, if mixing is required: cement placement, seating, and excess-cement removal.

After mixing, a luting cement should be as free of bubbles as possible and then placed in the intaglio of a crown or bridge (Fig. 7.4A and B). The cement should coat the entire intaglio surface but fill only a portion of the intaglio. Filling the entire intaglio increases the risk for bubble entrapment, the time and pressure needed for seating, and the time and effort required to remove excess cement. A fixed prosthesis should be fully seated with moderate finger pressure, displacing excess cement.

Microscopically the tooth and prosthesis surfaces are rough and the cement fills the irregular crevices between both surfaces to form a void-free continuum that microscopically locks one surface against another to resist shear stresses that might dislodge the appliance Figure 7. 2. Mechanical retention may be insufficient. Chemical adhesion of the cement, tooth, and device improves retention.

Glass ionomer cements (GICs), based on polyacrylic acids, bond to teeth by chelating acrylic acids to both organic and inorganic tooth components, and continue to cure after the defined **setting time**. If glass ionomers are allowed to mature in an

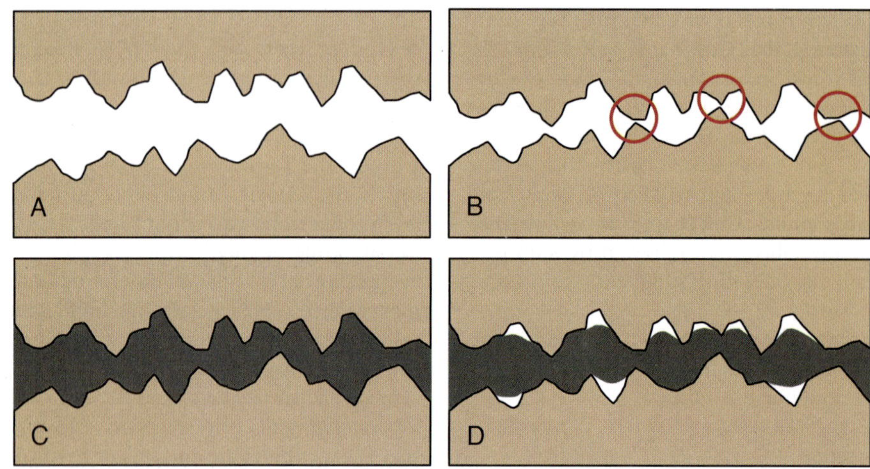

• **Fig. 7.3** Schematic illustration of the abutment–prosthesis interfaces. **(A)** Irregular surface morphology of the two surfaces to be bonded. **(B)** Two surfaces pressed against each other without an intermediate layer. Note the small number of points of contact illustrated by the circles. **(C)** Continuous interface when a third material, either cement or adhesive, is used as the intermediate layer. **(D)** Voids generated as a result of the inability of the intermediate layer to wet the surfaces completely.

TABLE 7.2A ISO 9917-1 Requirements

	ZINC PHOSPHATE		ZINC POLYCARBOXYLATE		GLASS IONOMER	
Cement Type→	**Luting**	**Liner or Base**	**Luting**	**Liner or Base**	**Luting**	**Liner or Base**
Maximum mixing time (min)	2.5	2	2.5	2	1.5	1.5
Final setting time (min)	8	6	8	6	8	6
Maximum film thickness (μm)	25	nr	25	nr	25	nr
Minimum compressive strength (MPa)	50					
Maximum acid erosion (mm)	0.3		0.4		0.17	

nr, no requirement.

TABLE 7.2B ISO 9917-2 Requirements

Cement Use→	Luting	Liner or Base	Restorative
Minimum working time (min)	1.5	1.5	1.5
Minimum setting time (min)	8	6	6
Maximum film thickness (μm)	25	No requirement	
Minimum flexural strength (MPa)	10	10	25

isolated environment (i.e. free of contamination from surrounding moisture and protected from loss of water through evaporation), the cements increase in strength and become more resistant to dissolution. Varnish coats applied at the margins of fresh GICs facilitate **maturation**; details are discussed later in this chapter.

Hydrophilic dentin bonding agents penetrate pores in dentin created by acid etching; these also have high bond strength through micromechanical retention. Resin cements based on NPG-GMA, polymerizable phosphates, and methacryloxyethyl trimellitic anhydride (4-META) bond to calcium within dentin.

Table 7.3 represents a compilation of the physical properties of various luting agents and the requirements for water-based dental cements from ISO 9917 (currently identical to ANSI/ADA Specification No. 96 requirements). All the materials in Table 7.3 set in less than 10 minutes have a **film thickness** less than 25 μm. Although these values are typical, they are compiled from a variety of sources and a wide variation occurs among brands.

To choose a cement for a specific task, one must consider the following:

1. The cement's physical and biological properties.
2. The cement's handling characteristics, such as **working time**, setting time, consistency, and ease of removing excess material.

CRITICAL QUESTION

During the initial try-in of a three-unit fixed dental prosthesis (bridge), the prosthesis fits the prepared teeth perfectly and appears to be retained on the teeth so tenaciously that removal requires a great deal of force. Why is cement required for retention in this situation?

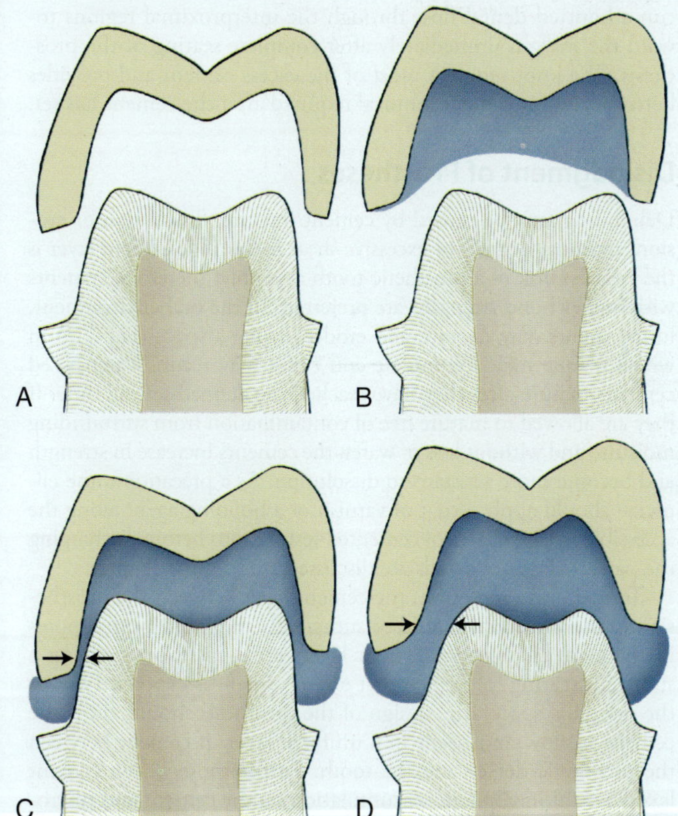

• **Fig. 7.4** Mechanics of cementing a prosthesis. **(A)** Assembly of a fixed prosthesis and respective tooth preparation. **(B)** Luting agent placed in the prosthesis should cover the entire surface. **(C)** Space for expelling excess cement decreases as the prosthesis reaches its final position. Arrows show the thickness of space for expelling excess cement. **(D)** Higher degree of the abutment taper provides a greater space for expelling excess cement.

Luting Interface

Luting cements are designed to fill the microscopic gaps between a prosthesis and a prepared tooth. As shown in Fig. 7.3A, each surface is microscopically rough, having peaks and valleys, and only point contacts are made by the peaks (Fig. 7.3B). The areas that are not in contact must be filled by the cement to prevent oral fluid flow and bacterial invasion. One can seal the space by placing a soft adhesive between the two surfaces, which can conform under pressure to the roughened surface features.

The first dental luting cements were not adhesive to the tooth or prostheses, but they filled the microscopic space and created a strong physical attraction to both substrates that prevented dislodgment. The current approach for cementing prostheses or appliances involves the use of an adhesive technique that forms a solid sealing layer within a few minutes (Fig. 7.3C) to improve retention of the prosthesis. The cement should flow under pressure and wet the surfaces. A luting agent must form a continuous film without forming voids (Fig. 7.3D), which are detrimental to retention and support of the prosthesis.

Procedure for Luting a Single Crown

Luting of a single crown is described as an example (Fig. 7.4A) in three steps: cement placement, seating of the crown, and excess cement removal.

Cement Placement

The cement should coat the entire inner surface of the crown and extend slightly over the margin to ensure that the space between the crown and tooth will be completely sealed. Cement should fill about half of the inner cavity volume of the crown (Fig. 7.4B) and must be free of bubbles. Air entrapment must be avoided in the critical occlusal region; otherwise masticatory forces may fracture any ceramic prosthesis. Do not fill the entire crown cavity because

TABLE 7.3 Typical Properties of Dental Cements Used for Luting Applications

Cement	Setting Time (min)	Film Thickness (μm)	24-h Compressive Strength (MPa)	24-h Diametral Tensile Strength (MPa)	Elastic Modulus (GPa)	Solubility in Water (wt%)	Pulp Response
Zinc phosphate	5.5	20	104	5.5	13.5	0.06	Moderate
ZOE[a]	4.0–10	25	6–28	–	–	0.04	Mild
Zinc polycarboxylate	6.0	21	55	6.2	5.1	0.06	Mild
Glass ionomer	7.0	24	86	6.2	7.3	1.25	Mild to moderate
Resin-modified glass ionomer	4.25	11–22	85–185	18–26	2.5–7.8	1.00	Mild to moderate
Compomer	4.0	36	165	–	3.6	0.69	Moderate
Resin	2.0–4.0	<25	70–172	40–77	2.1–3.1	0–0.01	Moderate
ISO 9917	2.5–8	25 (max)	50	N/A	N/A	0.20 (max)	See note[b]

[a]ZOE, zinc oxide–eugenol.
[b]Note: Response compared with the severe irritation of silicate cement.

this increases the risk for bubble entrapment, the time and pressure required for seating, and the time and effort to remove excess cement.

Seating

Use moderate finger pressure to displace excess cement and seat the crown on the prepared tooth. Tapping or vibration of the crown or using an ultrasonic device may also help to achieve complete seating of the crown. Evaluate three points on the margin with an explorer to ensure that seating is adequate, and ask the patient to bite on a soft substance such as wood or a cotton roll to ensure complete seating; this will also expel excess cement (Fig. 7.4C). Complete seating is essential. Re-evaluate at least three points of the margin and the occlusion before the cement has set.

Three characteristics make seating a crown easier: (1) lower-viscosity cements, (2) more taper of the prepared tooth (Fig. 7.4D), and (3) decreased height of the prepared tooth. Note that higher taper and lower tooth height compromise the retention.

CRITICAL QUESTION

Why does the technique of removing excess cement differ among types of cements?

Removal of Excess Cement

Excess cement should be present at the margin of a crown just after seating, but its removal depends on the properties of the cement used. Zinc phosphate and **ZOE** cements do not adhere to the surrounding surfaces, the tooth, or the prosthesis, so the cement should set completely before the excess cement is removed. Glass ionomer, polycarboxylate, and resin cements adhere chemically and physically to the surrounding surfaces and should be removed as soon as the seating is completed to prevent adhesion to the exterior of the prostheses or to the surrounding teeth. A separating medium, such as petroleum jelly, can be applied carefully to external and surrounding surfaces to inhibit cement adherence, making cement removal easier when these cements are allowed to set completely.

Some GICs and dual-cure resin cements can be removed easily in about 1.5–3 minutes after mixing begins but before setting by an acid–base reaction or light curing is finished. At this point the cement has acquired some strength but is not strong enough to resist separation from the margin, which allows removal of larger pieces of the excess cement.

Zinc polycarboxylate cement transforms to a rubbery state before setting. At this stage, the cement is so thick that any attempt to remove the excess may inadvertently pull the cement away from the marginal area, or it may remove some of the cement from within the cemented prosthesis.

The technique of removing excess cement is usually described in the instructions for use provided by the manufacturer. Regardless of which cement the dentist may use, it is always advisable to run a knotted dental floss through the interproximal regions toward the margin immediately after complete seating of the prosthesis. The knot removes most of the excess cement and provides better access for cement removal required after the cement has set.

Dislodgment of Prostheses

Debonding may be caused by cement fracture, dissolution or erosion, secondary caries, or excessive shear forces. The cement layer is the weakest link of a prosthetic tooth assembly; therefore, cements with higher bond strengths are preferred. In the oral environment, luting agents may dissolve and erode; leaving a space (Fig. 7.5) in which plaque may accumulate and caries may recur. Water-based cements mature after they have reached the defined setting time. If they are allowed to mature free of contamination from surrounding moisture and without loss of water, the cements increase in strength and become more resistant to dissolution. As a precaution, the clinician should apply a coat of varnish or a bonding agent along the accessible marginal area of cemented restorations before discharging the patient. Further details are discussed later in this chapter.

To maximize retention, the cement layer between the prosthesis and the abutment should be sufficiently thin to minimize pores in the cement. Thinner cement layers are created by applying a sufficient seating force such that excess cement is expressed out of the marginal space. The design of the prosthesis should allow the cement to flow and result in a uniform layer of cement between the prosthetic device and the tooth. Furthermore, when cement layers are thinner, plaque accumulation on the cement and microleakage are less likely. Cements should be insoluble in water and should not absorb water. Preferably the coefficient of thermal expansion between the tooth, the prosthesis, and the cement should be similar over the range of temperature associated with consumed foods and beverages. Cements having high compressive, shear, and flexural strengths are preferred. Dislodgment is minimized for cements with high shear bond strength (chemically bonded cements). When chemical bonding occurs, failure may occur cohesively through the cement (Fig. 7.6A). With a thin

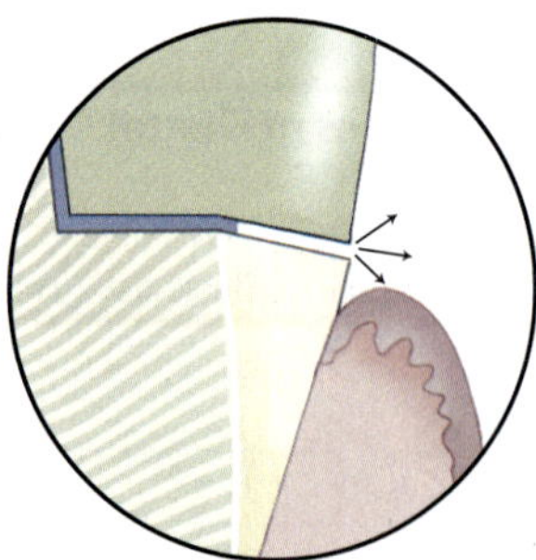

• **Fig. 7.5** Loss of cement at the marginal area resulting from exposure to oral fluid.

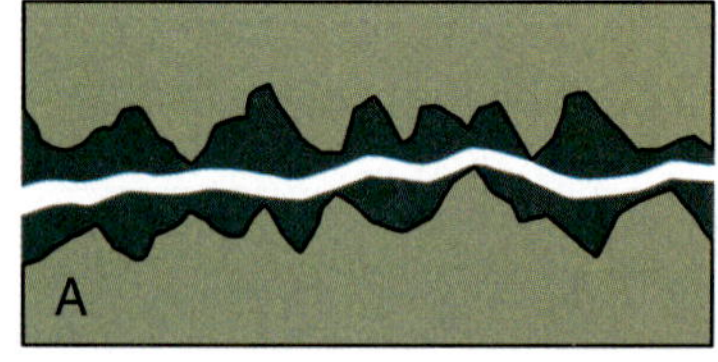

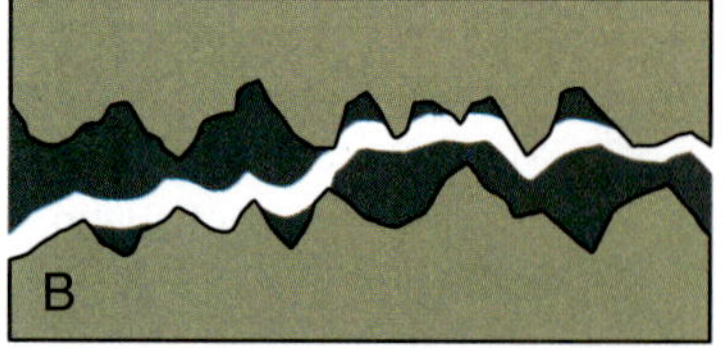

• **Fig. 7.6** Failure modes of the interface. **(A)** Cleavage through the cement layer. This is unlikely because of the small thickness of the cement involved. **(B)** The most likely failure occurs at the luting agent/prosthesis interface. Remnants of the luting agent often remain on the opposing surface.

chemically bonded cement, the prosthesis may become dislodged when the luting cement fractures or dissolves. When a cement produces only mechanical retention, failure begins at the interfaces (Fig. 7.6B). A low setting contraction is preferred to minimize interfacial stresses.

CRITICAL QUESTION

The terms *film thickness* and *cement thickness* are used to describe the properties of dental cements. What is the difference between these terms and what is the clinical significance of these terms?

Film Thickness

This property is often confused with **cement thickness**. *Film thickness* refers to the thickness of a continuous cement after setting under pressure, according to ANSI/ADA Specification No. 96 (ISO 9917-1). To determine film thickness, freshly mixed cement is placed between two optically flat surfaces and a 150-N vertical load is applied 10 seconds before the end of the measured working time. After 10 minutes have elapsed since application of the load, the thickness of the film between the two flat surfaces is measured as the film thickness. The cement film should be continuous and no voids should exist in the film. Thus, film thickness is an indication of the viscosity of the cement during seating. A lower film thickness implies lower viscosity. For luting applications, the maximum allowable film thickness is 25 μm for the ADA specification or ISO standard indicated earlier; a low film thickness is preferred, so that excess cement can be expressed more easily. The size of particles and the **P/L ratio** significantly affect the film thickness. For temporary and final restorations, the maximal acceptable film thickness is larger. However, there is no film thickness specification for base and liner and restorative applications. For root canal sealers, the maximal film thickness is 50 μm. For comparison, the diameter of flaxen human hair ranges between 17 and 50 μm.

Cement thickness refers to the thickness of the cement between the tooth structure and a cemented cast crown, inlay, onlay, or veneer. It plays a significant role in the retention of prostheses and varies with:

1. The amount of force applied during seating of the prosthesis.
2. The direction in which the force is applied to the prosthesis during seating.
3. The design of the prosthesis relative to its potential to inhibit or facilitate the flow of cement.
4. The fit of the prosthesis on the prepared tooth.
5. The inherent film thickness of the cement.

An acceptable cement thickness in the literature ranges from 25 to 120 μm. However, cement thickness associated with resin cements can exceed 150 μm.

Cements for Pulp Protection

Specialized materials are used in prepared cavity to protect the pulp from thermal or chemical irritation. For instance, metallic restorations are excellent thermal conductors, but they promote thermal sensitivity when hot and cold foods or beverages are consumed. Cements containing phosphoric acid, direct filling resins, and some GICs cause a chemical irritation. Generally, the inflammation caused by chemically irritating cements increases in the order of polycarboxylate cement, **zinc phosphate cement**, and GIC. The setting contraction of amalgam or composite can lead to marginal leakage as well as pulpal irritation.

Cavity varnishes, liners, and base materials have been used as adjuncts to restorative materials to protect the pulp from such injuries. Some of these agents may also provide caries prevention benefits, as described in the following. Most of materials used for this application are cements, although some are not. For example, copal varnish and calcium hydroxide are not cements, but they are discussed here because of the pulp protection they offer.

CRITICAL QUESTION

What is the purpose of using cavity varnishes and why is copal varnish no longer used as often as it was between 1960 and 1990?

Cavity Varnishes

Varnishes are composed of natural gums—such as copal, rosins, or synthetic resins—dissolved in an organic solvent (acetone, chloroform, or ether). The varnish forms a thin coating on the tooth as the solvent evaporates. Varnishes have a high solvent content and at least two thin layers should be applied to produce a continuous coating; otherwise small pinholes may occur. A brush, or a small pledget of cotton may be used as an applicator, but it should be discarded after each application to the tooth to avoid introducing microorganisms into the varnish bottle.

In vitro studies suggest that varnish reduces the infiltration of irritating fluids through marginal crevices and lessens pulpal irritation. Clinical observations based on tooth sensitivity, as reported by patients, have yet to confirm these benefits in vivo. Varnish is also claimed to prevent the penetration of corrosion products of amalgams into the dentinal tubules, thereby reducing the unsightly tooth discoloration often associated with amalgam restorations. However, high-copper amalgam products, which are more corrosion resistant than their predecessors, have diminished the need for varnish.

A varnish is not indicated when adhesive materials such as GICs or bonding agents for resin-based composite are used. Dentin bonding agents serve the same purpose as varnish.

Cavity Liners

Calcium hydroxide is the chief ingredient in many cavity liners and cement base materials because calcium hydroxide is antimicrobial, has an elevated pH (basic, alkaline), and stimulates the formation of secondary dentin over an injured pulp to protect it over the long term. As a **cavity liner**, the calcium hydroxide powder is suspended in a solvent carrier with a thickening agent. When it is placed on the pulpal floor, the solvent evaporates and leaves a thin film of calcium hydroxide. The liner does not possess significant mechanical strength or thermal insulation capability but it can neutralize acids that migrate toward the pulp and, in the process, it can induce the formation of secondary dentin. Eventually, the calcium hydroxide forms calcium carbonate and becomes inactive. Calcium hydroxide is soluble in water and must not be left on the margin of the prepared cavity or the margin will not be properly sealed.

Many formulas that are available for cavity lining materials are based on adding calcium hydroxide to low-viscosity ZOE, GI, or resin cements. Some of these liners adhere to the tooth-restoration interface; therefore, the function of liners has been expanded to include the sealing of dentin from the potential influx of microorganisms and irritants from restorative procedures.

Calcium hydroxide liners are commonly used for direct and indirect **pulp capping** and as a dressing after vital pulpotomy procedures on primary teeth. MTA is a newer cavity liner material that forms calcium hydroxide as it sets. Both MTA and calcium hydroxide undergo a transformation of hydroxide to calcium carbonate from exposure to carbon dioxide in the blood and oral fluids, causing their antimicrobial effectiveness to diminish. Newer cements containing calcium silicate are also very promising in terms of pulp protection. A detailed discussion on cements used for pulp protection is provided later in the chapter.

CRITICAL QUESTION

Why does the strength requirement of the cement base material depend on the type of restorative material to be placed?

Cement Bases

In contrast to liners, cement bases are applied in thicker layers (greater than 0.75 mm) beneath restorative materials to protect the pulp against thermal injury, galvanic shock, and chemical irritation. Clinical experience has shown that temperature changes have a more acute effect on the pulp when a base does not insulate teeth containing large amalgam fillings. Zinc phosphate and ZOE cements are commonly used, as well as some polycarboxylate and fast-setting GICs. Table 7.4 shows that zinc phosphate and ZOE cements are better insulators (having lower thermal conductivity) than metals, although they have less insulating ability than Portland cement, corkboard, or glass. The insulating abilities of polycarboxylate, glass ionomer, and calcium hydroxide materials also fall within this range. Their actual heat transfer is more complex and depends on the material's heat capacity, thickness, and density.

The choice of base will very often be dictated by the depth of the cavity. Zinc phosphate cement is an effective base for thermal insulation, but its low pH (acidity) may require a cavity liner under the cement to protect the pulp. However, the risk of low pH in contact with the pulp is minimized if the zinc phosphate cement is mixed to a thick, nontacky, putty-like consistency, which does not have excess acid. Calcium hydroxide, ZOE, polycarboxylate, and **glass ionomer cement** are effective barriers against the penetration of irritating constituents from restorative materials. When glass ionomer is used as a base in very deep cavities, a calcium hydroxide liner should be applied first to protect the deep areas where pulp exposure is more likely to occur.

Cement bases should be strong enough to withstand forces during the placement of fillings and mastication forces during service. Restorative materials should be placed after the initial set of the base cement has occurred. Table 7.5 shows the compressive strength of representative dental cements over time. Their strength increases rapidly over the first 30 minutes and continues to increase over 24 hours.

The minimal strength required to resist masticatory forces has not been determined because of their complexity and the influence of the design of the prepared tooth cavity. A base cement should be selected after considering:

- The design of the cavity
- The direct restorative material
- The proximity of the pulp chamber relative to the cavity floor or wall

For amalgam restorations, calcium hydroxide and ZOE materials are effective base cements. For direct filling gold restorations, which are relatively ductile, a stronger base cement—such as zinc phosphate, polycarboxylate, or GIC—is indicated. In those cases where a liner of calcium hydroxide or ZOE cement on the cavity floor is desired the liner should be overlaid with a strong base cement.

Neither microleakage nor acid penetration is prevented by using a base cement in conjunction with amalgam or direct filling gold foil. When a cavity varnish or dentin bonding agent is indicated to seal a restoration, the base often governs the order of material application.

- If a zinc phosphate cement base is used, a sealing (varnish) material should be applied to the cavity walls before placement of the base.
- For the more biocompatible cement base materials (e.g. calcium hydroxide, ZOE, polycarboxylate, and GIC), the base cement is placed, followed by the cavity varnish after the base has hardened.
- For resin-based composites, calcium hydroxide and GIC are satisfactory base cements.

MTA is also used as a base because it is insulating, antimicrobial, and nonacidic. However, currently available products have slow setting characteristics. Thus, MTA is primarily a specialty material.

TABLE 7.4 Thermal Conductivity of Cement Base Materials and Other Common Materials

Material	Thermal Conductivity (W/m•K)
Zinc phosphate cement (dry)	1.26
Zinc phosphate cement (wet)	1.63
Zinc oxide–eugenol	1.67
Corkboard	0.04
Gypsum plaster board	0.17
Portland cement	0.29
Glass	1.01
Zirconia ceramic	1.7
Ice	2.18
Stainless steel	15.9
Alumina	30
Pure gold	297

TABLE 7.5 Compressive Strength (MPa) of Cement Base Materials after Setting

Material	7 min	30 min	24 h
Zinc oxide–eugenol	2.8	3.5	5.2
	6.2	6.9	12.4
	15.9	20.7	24.1
Calcium hydroxide	3.8	4.8	10.3
	7.6	6.2	8.3
Zinc phosphate	6.9	86.9	119.3
MTA	–	–	28.0

Cements for Restoratives

Cements can be employed for temporary or short-term periods (days to weeks), intermediate-term periods (weeks to months), or long-term periods (years) in the restoration of anterior teeth. The general procedure for using cements as restoratives is essentially the same as for the use of resin-based composites. In the early 1900s, ZOE, zinc phosphate, and **silicate cement** were the major material systems used for restoratives. Silicate cement, based on silicate glass particles and phosphoric acid, was a translucent restorative material and it was the primary esthetic material before resin composites were introduced. The mean survival time of silicate cement restorations was unimpressive—about 4 years—because of their high solubility rate, loss of anatomical contour, and margin degradation. In 1972, GICs, based on new silicate glass formulas and polyacrylic acid, were introduced. The use of silicate cement diminished markedly with the advent of resin composite, and silicate cement is rarely used today.

Zinc Oxide Eugenol and Noneugenol Cements

ZOE cements have been formulated as powder–liquid and two-paste systems. The powder–liquid combination contains zinc oxide powder and eugenol liquid. The two-paste system includes a base paste containing zinc oxide powder, and the eugenol is in the accelerator (or catalyst). The ZOE setting reaction starts with water present in the tooth or the eugenol solution hydrolyzing the zinc oxide to form zinc hydroxide. The zinc hydroxide and eugenol chelate and solidify. The reaction proceeds more rapidly in a warm, humid environment, such as inside a tooth. When zinc acetate dihydrate is included in the powder, the reaction is faster; zinc acetate is more soluble than zinc oxide or hydroxide. Acetic acid in the eugenol solution also accelerates the dissolution of zinc oxide. The setting reaction is slower for the other zinc oxide cements. A wide variety of ZOE cements are available, with compressive strengths ranging from 3 to 55 MPa. Finer powders increase the strength of the resulting cement.

The versatility of ZOE is reflected in ISO 3107:2011 (ANSI/ADA Standard No. 30), which lists four clinical types of ZOE cement:

(I) temporary cementation,
(II) long-term cementation of fixed prostheses,
(III) temporary fillings and thermal insulating bases, and
(IV) intermediate restorations. ZOE cements are also used as root canal sealers and periodontal dressings.

Temporary ZOE restorations are expected to last a few weeks. The antimicrobial attribute of ZOE is a benefit compared with GICs or resin composites. However, ZOE cements can cause pulpal necrosis; therefore, ZOE should not be used directly on pulp. Indirectly used, ZOE has a sedative effect by sealing the dentinal tubules against the ingress of oral fluids until a more permanent restoration can be fabricated and cemented.

Intermediate-duration ZOE cements serve as a restorative material for about 1 year. To achieve the properties necessary for this use, a stiff, putty-like restorative consistency must be used (high P/L ratio). The higher the P/L ratio, the faster the material sets. A cool glass mixing slab slows the setting, which should be above the dew point to avoid moisture condensation and dilution of the cement.

An excellent application for these ZOE cements is for temporary or provisional (short-term or intermediate-term) luting of provisional fixed prosthodontics. Long-term ZOE luting cements are somewhat difficult to manipulate because their film thicknesses are high, and excess cement is difficult to remove; therefore long-term ZOE luting cements should never be used for temporary cementation. ZOE cement is used for implant superstructure cementation, where more retentive cements could lead to damage of the supporting implant if retrieval is required. The consequence of the less adhesive cement is potential loosening of the implant prosthesis.

To improve the strength of ZOE cements, part of the eugenol liquid has been replaced by orthoethoxybenzoic acid and alumina added to the powder. Another system, called *polymer-reinforced ZOE,* incorporates a powder containing 20 to 40 wt% fine polymer particles and zinc oxide particles treated with carboxylic acid. Residual eugenol is thought to interfere with the proper polymerization of resin-based composites or cements; therefore some carboxylic acids have been used to replace eugenol and produce a ZOE-like material. Such products are called *zinc oxide–noneugenol cements.* The compressive strength of these improved ZOE cements is acceptable, but their strength values are inferior to those of glass ionomer and resin cements (Table 7.5).

Zinc Phosphate Cement

Zinc phosphate cement first appeared in the literature in 1879, and the chemistry of the modern-day cement was established in 1902. It is the oldest luting cement and its long clinical record of success serves as a standard by which newer cements are compared.

Chemistry and Setting

Zinc phosphate cement consists of a powder and liquid which are mixed just before use. The powder contains more than 75% of zinc oxide and up to 13% of magnesium oxide; these powders are sintered above 1000°C, then ground into a fine powder, and blended with radiopaque powders. The liquid contains phosphoric acid (38%–59%), water (30%–55%), aluminum phosphate (2%–3%), and in some cases zinc phosphate (up to 10%). The liquid controls the pH and the rate of the liquid–powder (acid–base) reaction. Also, the finer the particle size, the faster the cement sets.

When mixed, phosphoric acid dissolves the zinc oxide, which reacts with the aluminum phosphate and forms zinc aluminophosphate gel on the remaining undissolved zinc oxide particles. The set cement contains unreacted zinc oxide particles encased in an amorphous matrix of zinc aluminophosphate. Loss of water from the liquid lengthens the setting reaction, while incorporation of additional water during mixing accelerates the reaction.

CRITICAL QUESTION

Why does an extended spatulation prolong the setting time of zinc phosphate cement whereas it shortens the setting time of gypsum products?

Clinical Manipulation

The reaction between zinc oxide and phosphoric acid is exothermic and requires a careful mixing procedure to minimize the effect of heat generation. The zinc oxide cement powder should be dispensed on a glass slab and divided into several portions (Fig. 7.7A). The manufacturer's instructions should describe the amount of powder by including a measuring device, the number of liquid drops, the method for dividing powder increments, the mixing time for each increment, and the total mixing time. The

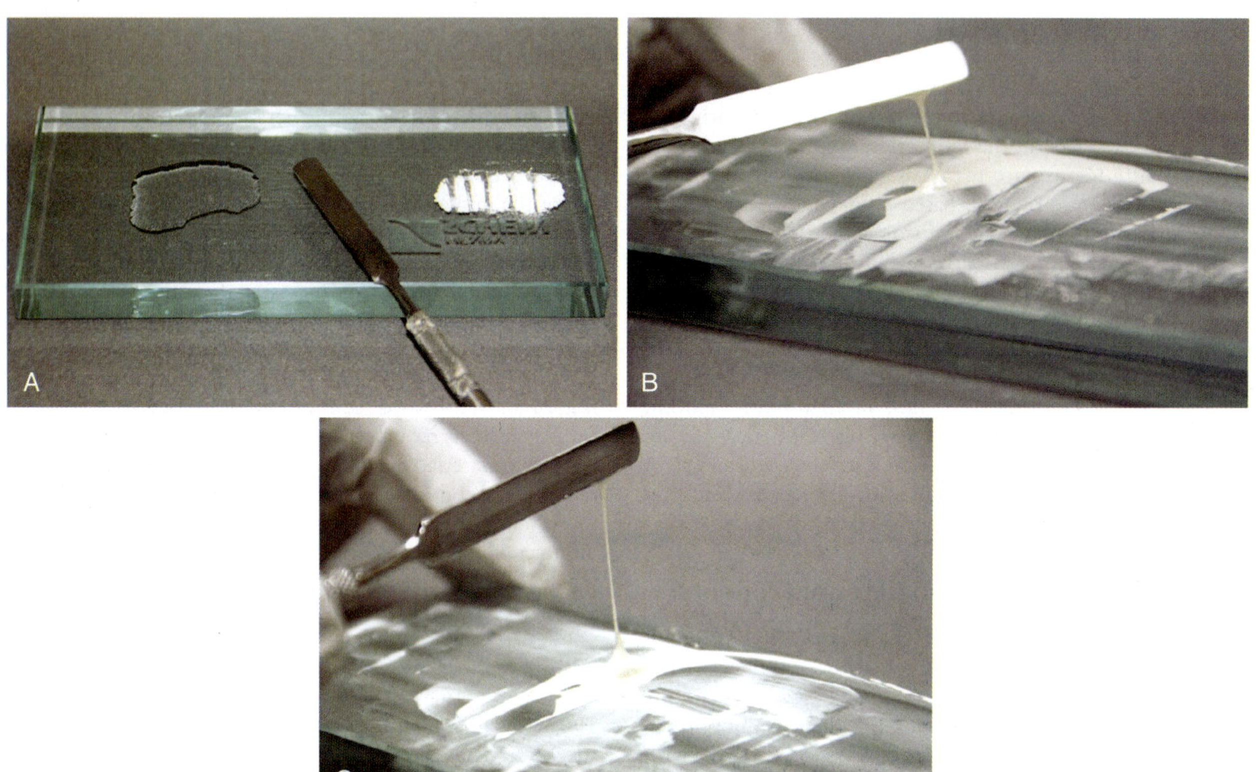

• **Fig. 7.7** Manipulation of zinc phosphate cement. **(A)** Powder and liquid dispensed on mixing slab; powder is divided into six increments: 1/16, 1/16, 1/8, 1/4, 1/4, and 1/4. **(B)** Proper consistency for cementation; the mixture is strung up about 1/2–3/4 inch (~12–19 mm) at separation. **(C)** The mixture is strung up more than 3/4 inch without separation; this indicates that the cement has become too thick for cementation.

liquid should not be dispensed onto the slab until the powder is dispensed and divided, and the cement is ready for use because the water from the liquid will evaporate, as shown in Fig. 7.8.

Mixing of Zinc Phosphate Cement

Mixing of this cement should be initiated by incorporating the smallest portion of powder using a thin spatula and brisk spatulation. Most of the area of the mixing slab should be used to dissipate heat. A good rule to follow is to spatulate each increment of powder for 15–20 seconds before adding another increment, and all mixing should be completed within 1.5–2 minutes (see Table 7.6). After the powder is completely incorporated and a creamy mixture has been created, the cement is drawn across the slab and the flat blade of the mixing spatula contacts the mixture and is slowly drawn away. If a string of cement can be lifted from 12 (1/2 inch) to 19 mm (~3/4 inch) before separating from the spatula (Fig. 7.7B), the cement is considered fluid enough for cementing a prosthesis. If the string exceeds 19 mm, the cement is too viscous for proper seating of prostheses (Fig. 7.7C) and another mixture should be made. After the prosthesis is coated with the cement and is seated, it should be held under pressure until the cement sets. The field of operation should be kept dry during the entire seating procedure.

Removal of Excess Zinc Phosphate Cement

Excess cement must be removed from the interproximal area immediately with a knotted dental floss after complete seating and remaining excess cement should be allowed to set before removal. A layer of varnish or other impermeable coating should be applied to the margin after removal of excess cement to allow the cement more time to mature and to develop an increased resistance to dissolution in oral fluid.

Control of Working Time

The length of working time may be varied to some degree to fit the clinical situation. For example, a fixed dental prosthesis with multiple crowns requires more working time for cementation. Four techniques can extend the working time of zinc phosphate cement.

- First, the P/L ratio can be reduced to produce a thinner mixture. However, this change will result in a lower initial pH of the cement and it will adversely affect the mechanical properties of the cement (Fig. 7.8).
- Second, smaller portions of powder should be mixed for the first few increments. Initial small increments of powder dissolve in the liquid, which reduces the acidity of the liquid and retards the reaction rate with subsequent increments. Meanwhile, the heat generated from the reaction will be dissipated sufficiently during spatulation. If a large portion of powder is used initially, the quantity of heat generated cannot be dissipated fast enough to prevent it from accelerating the reaction.
- Third, the operator can prolong the spatulation of the last increment of powder. The spatulation effectively destroys the matrix as it forms, which means that extra time is needed to rebuild the bulk of the matrix. This is not a preferred method for extending the working time.

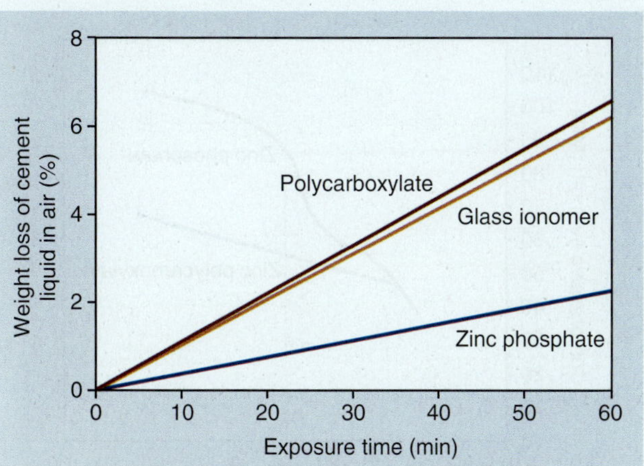

• **Fig. 7.8** Loss of water from cement liquids when they are exposed to air.

- Fourth, a colder mixing temperature will retard the chemical reaction between the powder and the liquid, thereby delaying formation of the matrix. However, the temperature of the slab should be above the **dew point**; otherwise, water condenses, dilutes the liquid, and reduces the compressive and tensile strength of the zinc phosphate cement. The use of a cool slab for mixing is the most viable method of extending the working time of zinc phosphate cement, and this should apply whenever multiple-unit prostheses are being cemented. This procedure yields lower cement viscosity at the completion of mixing, as indicated by a much lower height of the cement at separation when lifted by the spatula. The lower viscosity cement facilitates the seating of multiple-unit cast restorations.

Retention

Zinc phosphate does not chemically bond to teeth or prostheses; its bond is simply mechanical. A cavity liner applied on the tooth surface for pulp protection before application of zinc phosphate cement will reduce retention by creating a smoother surface with less interlocking.

Mechanical and Biological Properties

Zinc phosphate luting cements have a compressive strength as high as 104 MPa, a diametral tensile strength of 5.5 MPa, and an elastic modulus of 13 GPa (Table 7.3), making it relatively strong and stiff compared with other cements. Generally zinc phosphate cements have a relatively low solubility in water; however, in vivo disintegration occurs in the presence of lactic, acetic, and citric acids.

The phosphoric acid in the liquid makes the mixture quite acidic and therefore cytotoxic when a prosthesis is luted with this cement on a prepared tooth (Table 7.7). As setting occurs, the acidity is partially neutralized, but the cement remains acidic after 24 hours, with the pH rising from 3 to 6. For thin layers of dentin, a cavity liner (i.e. $Ca[OH]_2$) is recommended to prevent an adverse pulpal response from the pressure of luting, which forces acid into the pulp tissue. Younger patients are especially susceptible because they have a more open dentin tubule area, whereas older patients with sclerotic dentin will have a more tortuous path that restricts the penetration of acid toward the pulp.

Zinc Polycarboxylate Cement

Zinc polycarboxylate cement was the first dental cement to exhibit chemical bonding to teeth, marking an improvement over the mechanical bonding of zinc phosphate cement. Zinc polycarboxylate cement is not used for restorative purposes because the cement is opaque.

Chemistry and Setting

The polycarboxylate cements are powder–liquid systems that set by an acid–base reaction.

TABLE 7.6 Manipulation and Clinical Issues Related to Cements

	Mixing Technique	Clinical Issues
Zinc phosphate	Glass slab/steel spatula Small increments Mix over wide surface area, 20 s per increment Total mixing time 1.5–2 min	High initial pH Protection with varnish prior to cement application recommended
Zinc polycarboxylate cement	Glass slab/steel spatula Liquid should not be refrigerated Powder should be rapidly incorporated into the liquid	Bottle should be capped immediately or else water in liquid evaporates rapidly Cement must be used before it loses its glossy appearance Excess cement should not be removed while the cement is rubbery
Glass ionomer cement (GIC)	Paper pad/flexible spatula preferred Powder divided into two increments Half of the powder is mixed into the liquid for 5–15 s Remaining half then added rapidly. Total mixing time 45 s	Glossy appearance indicates the presence of unreacted polyacid, which is critical for bonding to the tooth Setting cement should be protected from moisture for about 5 min Finishing procedures should be delayed Care should be taken to prevent dehydration and cement should be protected with varnish/bonding agent
Resin cement	Paper pad/flexible spatula Usually two pastes Mix thoroughly Very easy to not mix adequately	For dual-cured and light-cured cements tack cure for 5 s and remove all excess Protect margins with gel to prevent oxygen inhibition during setting Light cure for 20 s from all surfaces with an LED light

TABLE 7.7 pH of Cements for Luting Applications

Time (minutes)	Zinc Phosphate	Polycarboxylate	GLASS IONOMER Polyacid Liquid	GLASS IONOMER Water-Settable
2	2.1	3.4	2.3	1.8
5	2.6	3.9	3.0	2.0
10	3.1	4.4	3.8	3.4
15	3.3	4.8	3.9	3.9
20	3.6	4.9	4.0	4.2
30	3.7	5.0	4.2	4.5
60	4.3	5.1	4.6	4.8
1440	5.5	5.9	5.7	6.0

Composition

The liquid is a water solution of polyacrylic acid or a copolymer of acrylic acid with other carboxylic acids, such as itaconic acid. The molecular weight of the polyacids ranges from 30,000 to 50,000 and the acid concentration varies from 32% to 42% by weight. The powder contains mainly zinc oxide with some magnesia, tin oxide, bismuth oxide, and/or alumina. Small amounts of stannous fluoride are used in some brands to adjust the setting time, increase the strength, and enhance the manipulative properties. The amount of fluoride released from such cements is minor, that is, only 15%–20% of that released from GICs.

Setting Reaction

The reaction of zinc polycarboxylate cement is similar to that of zinc phosphate cement. Setting begins by dissolution of powder particles by the acid, which releases zinc, magnesium, and tin ions; these bind and cross-link the carboxyl groups. The result is a cross-linked polycarboxylate matrix phase encapsulating the unreacted portion of the particles. The hardened zinc polycarboxylate cement is an amorphous gel matrix in which unreacted powder particles are dispersed, as occurs also with zinc phosphate cement. The pH of the cement liquid is initially slightly less acidic than that of zinc phosphate cements but it is still very low (about 1.7). The pH of the mix rises rapidly from 3 to 6 as the setting reaction proceeds (Table 7.7). The setting time ranges from 6 to 9 minutes, which is an acceptable range for luting cements.

Mechanism of Adhesion

The outstanding characteristic of zinc polycarboxylate cement is its chemical bond to tooth structure. The polyacrylic acid bonds to calcium ions on the surface of enamel or dentin. The bond to enamel is greater than that to dentin, because the enamel has a higher concentration of calcium. See Fig. 7.9 for a comparison of its tensile bond strength with that of zinc phosphate cement. Thermal cycling of the cement reduces the bond strength of zinc phosphate cements to dentin or enamel to zero, unlike that of polycarboxylate cements.

Clinical Manipulation of Polycarboxylate Cement

Despite the adhesion of the cement to tooth structure, polycarboxylate cements are not superior to zinc phosphate cement in the retention of cast noble metal prostheses. The likely cause is their surface contamination of the prostheses. The inner surface of a crown must be cleaned to improve wettability and the mechanical bond at the cement–metal interface. The surface can be carefully abraded with a stone or sandblasted with alumina abrasive. Note that long sandblasting times or excessive air pressure can deform metal margins and such procedures should be avoided. Crowns should be thoroughly rinsed to remove debris and dried. The outer surface of the prosthesis should be coated carefully with a separating medium, such as petroleum jelly, to prevent excess polycarboxylate cement from adhering to its surface.

A meticulously clean tooth surface is necessary to achieve adhesion and ensure intimate contact between the polycarboxylate cement and the tooth. A 10% polyacrylic or maleic acid solution should precede cement application and be applied to the tooth for 10–15 seconds, followed by rinsing with water. After cleansing, the prepared tooth should be isolated to prevent contamination by oral fluids and blotted dry. Drying with an air syringe is acceptable, although the patient may experience discomfort if a vital tooth is not anesthetized.

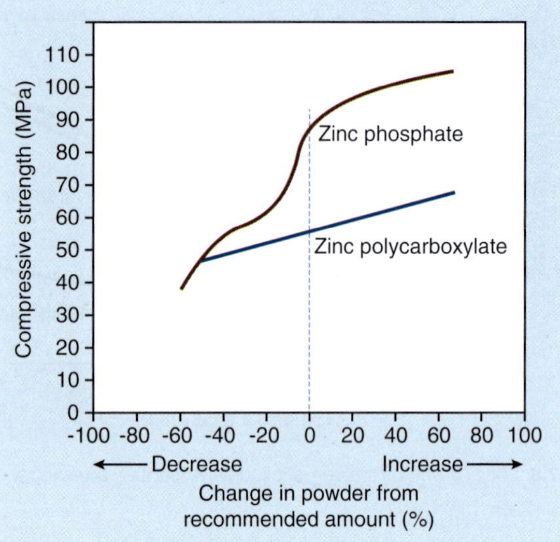

• **Fig. 7.9** Effect of powder/liquid ratio on the strength of two cements. Cement specimens were prepared with greater and lesser amounts of powder (higher and lower powder/liquid ratio) than recommended by the manufacturers (represented by a 0% change).

CRITICAL QUESTION

Why should zinc polycarboxylate cement be applied on the prepared tooth before the cement loses its glossy appearance?

Mixing of Cement

The P/L ratio of polycarboxylate cements varies from product to product, but is about 1.5 by weight. This cement should be mixed on a nonabsorbent surface, such as a glass slab. The liquid component of polycarboxylate cement is viscous and should not be refrigerated. The liquid's viscosity depends on its molecular weight and the concentration of the polyacrylic acid in each brand. The liquid should be dispensed just before use because the water in the liquid evaporates quickly (Fig. 7.10), which raises its viscosity. The powder should be rapidly incorporated into the liquid. A long mixing time can yield a cement that is too viscous

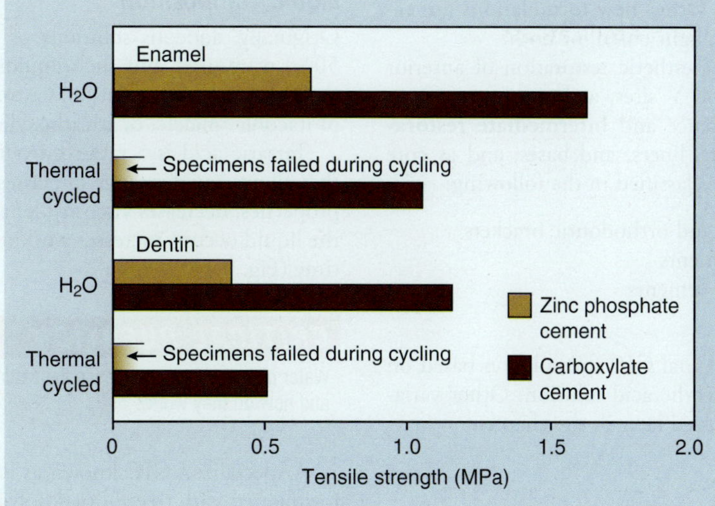

• **Fig. 7.10** The tensile strength required to separate enamel and dentin surfaces luted with a polycarboxylate cement after storage in water for 1 week. Thermally stressed specimens were subjected to 2500 cycles between water baths maintained at 10°C and 50°C.

for its intended application (Table 7.6). The cement must be used before it loses its glossy appearance because the glossy surface indicates free carboxylic acid groups are still present for good bonding to the tooth. A dull-looking mixture means insufficient carboxyl groups are present for bonding to the calcium in the tooth.

Removal of Excess Cement

During setting, the polycarboxylate cement passes through a rubbery stage. Excess cement should not be removed while the cement is rubbery because some of the cement may be pulled out from beneath the margins, leaving a void. Excess cement can be removed as soon as the cementing process is completed, or when the cement becomes hard, provided that the outer surface of the prosthesis is coated with a separating medium.

Control of Working Time

The working time for polycarboxylate cement is much shorter than that for zinc phosphate cement, approximately 2.5–5 minutes. Figure 7.11 shows the relative viscosities and working times of zinc phosphate, polycarboxylate, and GICs as they set. A cool slab lengthens the working time for zinc carboxylate cement, although it causes the polyacrylic acid to thicken, which hinders mixing. Refrigerating the powder is useful because it retards the reaction without raising the viscosity of the liquid.

Polycarboxylate cements are more viscous than a comparable mix of GIC; however, the polycarboxylate mix undergoes thinning at an increased shear rate. Clinically, this means that rapid spatulation and fast seating will reduce the viscosity of the polycarboxylate cement to ensure complete seating.

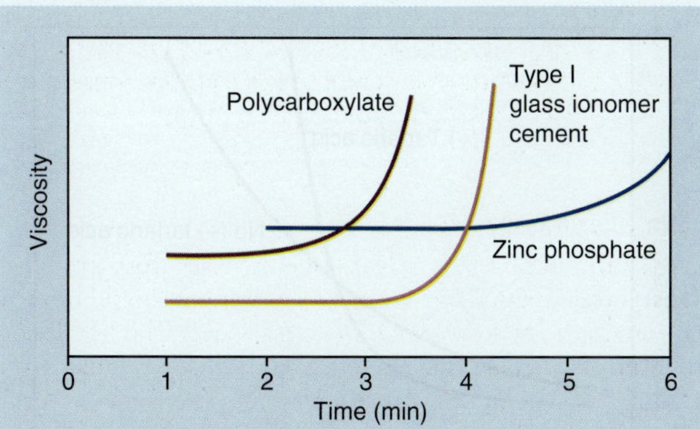

• **Fig. 7.11** Viscosity of freshly mixed cements. The viscosity is related to the relative ability to allow complete seating of the prosthesis. Zinc phosphate cement is more viscous initially but provides a longer working time for seating compared with either polycarboxylate or GICs.

Mechanical and Biological Properties

The compressive strength of polycarboxylate cement is approximately 55 MPa, which is lower than that of zinc phosphate cement. Zinc polycarboxylate cement is more elastic than zinc phosphate cement (Table 7.3), which makes it more difficult to remove excess polycarboxylate cement after setting. As with zinc phosphate cement, acids dissolve this cement, and lower P/L ratio increase solubility.

Polycarboxylate cements produce minimal irritation to the pulp. The larger size of the polyacrylic acid molecules compared with those of phosphoric acid limits acid penetration into the dentinal tubules, contributing to the excellent biocompatibility and lack of postoperative sensitivity of polycarboxylate cement.

Glass Ionomer Cement (GIC)

GIC is the generic name for materials based on the reaction of glass powder and polyacrylic acid. The cements were developed in the 1970s to improve clinical performance compared with silicate cements and to reduce the risk of pulp damage.

The use of polyacrylic acid makes GIC capable of bonding to tooth structure. GIC is considered superior to many types of cements because it is adherent and translucent. Various formulas are available depending on the intended clinical application. Water-soluble polymers and polymerizable monomers have been replacing part of the liquid content. Particles of metal, metal-ceramic, and ceramic have been added to some products to enhance mechanical properties. Other new formulations are capable of being chemically cured, light cured, or both.

GICs have been used for the esthetic restoration of anterior teeth, for example, Class III and V sites, as luting cements; as adhesives for orthodontic appliance and **intermediate restorations**; as pit and fissure sealants, liners, and bases; and as core buildup materials. The GICs are classified in the following:

Type I: Luting crowns, bridges, and orthodontic brackets
Type IIa: Esthetic restorative cements
Type IIb: Reinforced restorative cements
Type III: Lining cements, base

This section describes the original GIC formulation based on silicate glass particles and polyacrylic acid solution. Other variations of glass ionomers are discussed later in the chapter.

Chemistry and Setting

The chemistry of GICs is essentially the same for all three types, with variations in powder composition and particle size to achieve the desired function. The consistency of the mixed GIC varies widely among manufacturers, from low to very high viscosity as influenced, by their use of various particle size distributions and the P/L ratio. Larger particles (about 50 μm) are used for various restorative indications, and finer glass particles (about 15 μm) are used for cementing.

Glass Composition

The glass composition in GIC varies among manufacturers, but it always contains silica, calcia, alumina, and fluoride, as shown in Table 7.8. The ratio of alumina to silica is the key to their reactivity with polyacrylic acid. Barium, strontium, or other higher atomic number metal oxides are added to the glass to increase the radiopacity. The silica glass is melted at temperatures between 1100°C and 1500°C, depending on the raw materials and the overall composition. The glass is ground into a powder with particles ranging from less than 15 to about 50 μm, depending on the indication.

TABLE 7.8 Composition of Three Glass Ionomer Cement Powders (weight percent)

Component	Composition A	Composition B	Composition C
SiO_2	41.9	35.2	20–30
Al_2O_3	28.6	20.1	10–20
AlF_3	1.6	2.4	–
CaF_2	15.7	20.1	–
NaF	9.3	3.6	–
$AlPO_4$	3.8	12.0	–
F	–	–	10–15
Na_2O	–	–	1–5
BaO	–	–	10–20
CaO	–	–	10–20
P_2O_5	–	–	1–5

Liquid Composition

Originally, aqueous solutions of polyacrylic acid (about 40%–50%) were used, but such liquids were viscous and had a short shelf life because of gelation. Currently, the liquids are copolymers of itaconic, maleic, or tricarboxylic acids (Fig. 7.12).

Tartaric acid is a rate-controlling additive in the GIC liquid that allows a wider range of glasses to be used, improves handling properties, decreases viscosity, lengthens shelf life before gelling of the liquid occurs, increases working time, and shortens the setting time (Fig. 7.13).

CRITICAL QUESTION

Water plays two critical roles in the setting of conventional GIC. What are they and how do they work?

A specialized GIC known as a water-settable glass ionomer is formulated with freeze-dried polyacrylic acid solid and glass powder, which is mixed with water or an aqueous solution containing tartaric acid. This type of GIC has an extended working time because additional time is needed to dissolve the dried polyacrylic acid in water and start the acid–base reaction.

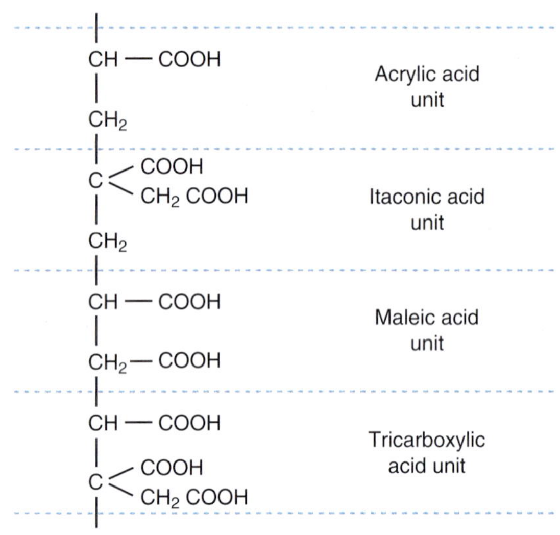

• **Fig. 7.12** Structure of various types of alkenoic acids that make up polyacids of GICs.

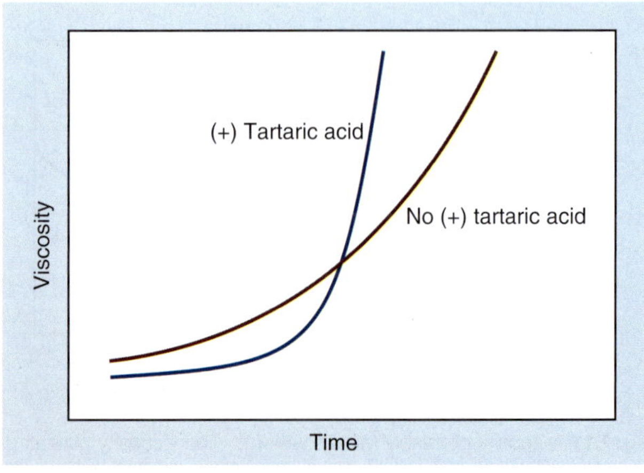

• **Fig. 7.13** Effect of tartaric acid on the viscosity–time relationship for a GIC during setting.

Setting Reaction

When the powder and liquid are mixed for a GIC, the acid starts to dissolve the glass, releasing calcium, aluminum, sodium, and fluorine ions. Water serves as a reaction medium. The polyacrylic acid chains are then cross-linked by the calcium ions; however, over the next 24 hours, the calcium ions are replaced by aluminum ions. Sodium and fluorine ions from the glass do not participate in the cross-linking of the cement. Some of the sodium ions may replace the hydrogen ions of carboxylic groups, and fluorine ions are dispersed within the cross-linked (matrix) phase of the set cement. The cross-linked phase becomes hydrated over time as it matures. A silica-rich gel that is formed on the surface of the glass particles sheaths the undissolved portion of glass particles. Thus, the set cement consists of undissolved glass particles with a silica gel coating embedded in an amorphous matrix of hydrated calcium and aluminum polysalts containing fluoride. Fig. 7.14 illustrates the structure of set GIC restoration, and Fig. 7.15 is a photomicrograph of set GIC.

Mechanism of Adhesion

Glass ionomers bond to tooth structure by chelation of the carboxyl groups of the polyacrylic acids with the calcium in the apatite of the enamel and dentin (see Fig. 7.14), in a manner similar to polycarboxylate cement.

CRITICAL QUESTION

Under what condition might zinc phosphate cement be preferred over GIC for luting of ceramic crowns?

Clinical Manipulation

The following conditions for GIC must be satisfied for cementing fixed prostheses: (1) the surface of the prepared tooth must be clean and blotted dry, (2) the entire intaglio of the prosthesis must be coated with luting cement and seated completely, and (3) excess cement must be removed at the appropriate time. For restorative indications, the GIC surface must be protected to prevent dehydration or premature exposure to saliva. Surface finishing of GIC restorations must be carried out without excessive drying to ensure their survival.

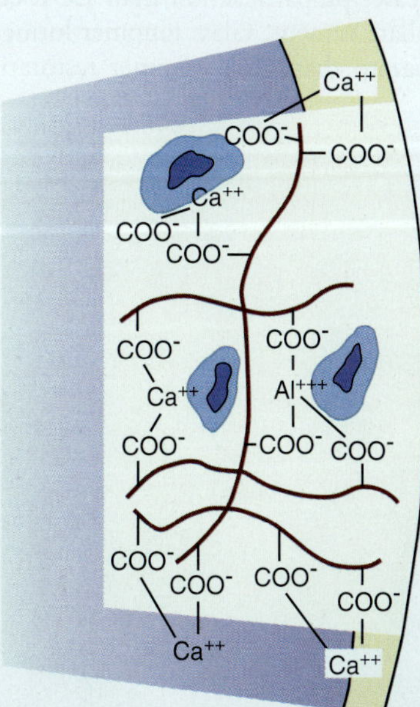

• **Fig. 7.14** Diagram depicting the structure of GIC. The solid blue particles represent unreacted glass particles surrounded by the gel (*light blue-shaded structure*) that form when Al^{3+} and Ca^{2+} ions are leached from the glass as a result of attack by the polyacrylic acid. The Ca^{2+} and Al^{3+} ions form polysalts with the COO− groups of the polyacrylic acid to form a cross-linked structure. The carboxyl groups react with the calcium in enamel and dentin.

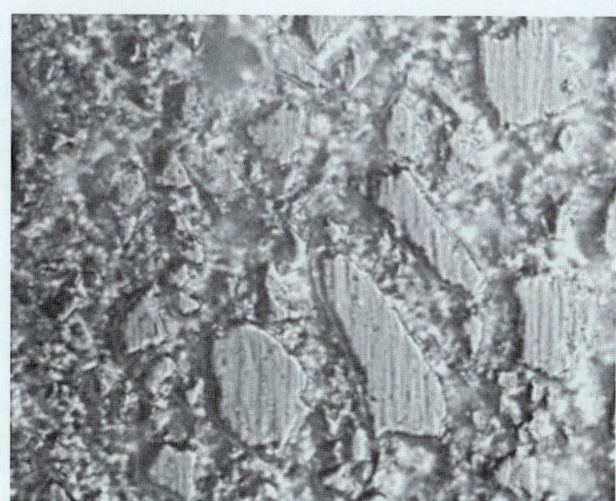

• **Fig. 7.15** Photomicrograph of a set GIC showing unreacted particles surrounded by the continuous matrix.

Surface Preparation

Clean tooth surfaces are essential for sustained adhesion. A pumice slurry can be used to remove the smear layer produced by prepared cavity. Alternatively, the tooth may be etched (conditioned) with an organic acid-like polyacrylic acid (10%–20%) for 10–20 seconds, followed by a 20–30-second water rinse. Fig. 7.16

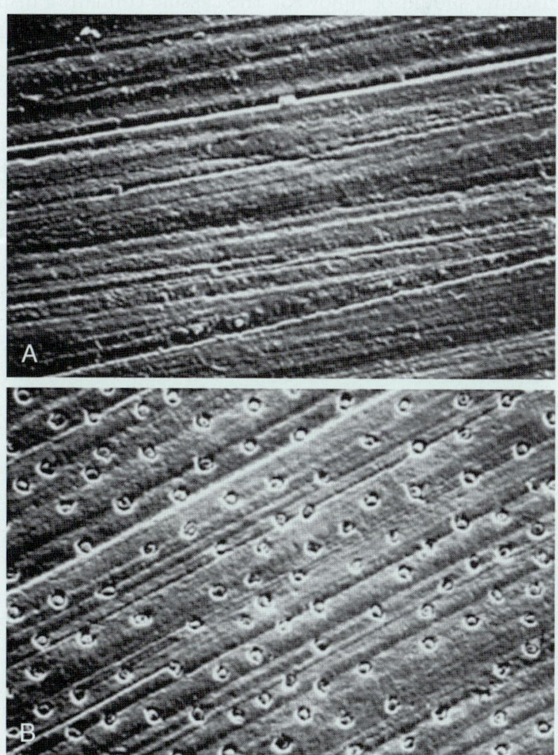

• **Fig. 7.16** **(A)** Prepared dentin surface showing the presence of the smear layer. **(B)** After cleansing with polyacrylic acid, the smear layer is removed yet the tubules remain plugged.

shows the desired etching and smear layer removal on dentin after a 10-second swabbing action with a 10% polyacrylic acid solution. After conditioning and rinsing the preparation, the surface should be dried but not desiccated and it must remain uncontaminated by saliva or blood. For cases where the residual dentin thickness from the pulp is less than 0.5 mm, a calcium hydroxide liner is recommended.

Material Preparation

The P/L ratio recommended by the manufacturer should be followed. A paper pad or a cool, dry glass slab may be used for mixing. The latter serves to retard the reaction and extend the working time. The slab should not be colder than the dew point. The powder and liquid should be dispensed just before mixing is begun; otherwise evaporation of water increases the acid/water ratio of the liquid. The powder should be incorporated rapidly into the liquid using a stiff spatula for restorative applications or a flexible metal or plastic spatula for luting applications. Normally half of the powder is mixed into the liquid for 5–15 seconds; the rest of the powder is then quickly added and mixed by folding the cement on itself until a uniform, glossy appearance is achieved. The mixing time should not exceed 45 seconds but may be less for certain products (see Table 7.6).

- A glossy appearance indicates the presence of unreacted polyacid, which is critical for bonding to the tooth.
- A dull appearance indicates that the acid has reacted too much with the glass particles for good bonding.

Glass ionomers are supplied in two bottles or capsules containing preproportioned powder and liquid (Fig. 7.17). The capsules are convenient and offer a consistent P/L ratio with less variation than that for hand spatulation. A triturator is used to mix the powder and liquid after the seal between the powder and liquid has been broken. The trituration time and speed given by the manufacturer should be followed. The capsule contains a dispensation tip that facilitates direct injection of the mix into the prepared tooth cavity or onto a fixed prosthesis for bonding.

Placement of Material

A tooth cavity should be slightly overfilled with GIC restorative. A freshly prepared glass ionomer mixture is hygroscopic, which means that it absorbs water from the surrounding environment. After placement, the GIC surface should be covered with a plastic matrix for about 5 minutes to protect the material from gaining or losing water during the initial set. Water dilutes the matrix-forming cations and anions, destroying the ability to form the hydrated matrix. When the matrix is removed, the surface must immediately be protected with the varnish supplied with the GIC or with petrolatum while the excess GIC is removed from the margins. Finishing is improved if the cement sets while protected, which lowers the risk of dehydration and the tendency to **craze** the surface, which would make the restoration more opaque. Before the patient is dismissed, a type II GIC restoration should be coated with varnish, since the exposed cement is still vulnerable to dehydration until it has fully matured over a period of a few weeks. If these recommended procedures are not followed, the surface will inevitably become chalky or crazed (Fig. 7.18).

For luting applications, the GIC is applied by a plastic instrument to the prosthetic device. The excess cement can be removed immediately upon seating or after a length of time as prescribed in the manufacturer's instructions. No matrix protection is needed during the initial setting. Coating of the margin of the cemented prosthesis with a varnish after complete removal of the excess will allow proper maturation of the GIC cement.

Release of Fluoride

After setting, glass ionomers release fluoride in amounts comparable to those released initially from silicate cement (Table 7.9). Whereas in vitro studies have shown the ability of the glass ionomer restorations to inhibit enamel and dentin **demineralization** produced by acidic gels or demineralizing buffer solutions, not all clinical studies confirm the ability of GIC to prevent secondary caries or the effectiveness of GIC over other nonfluoridated materials like composites. More information on fluoride release is presented later.

Biological and Mechanical Properties

GICs elicit a greater pulpal reaction than ZOE cement but less than zinc phosphate cement. Glass ionomer luting agents pose a greater pulpal hazard than glass ionomer restorations when the

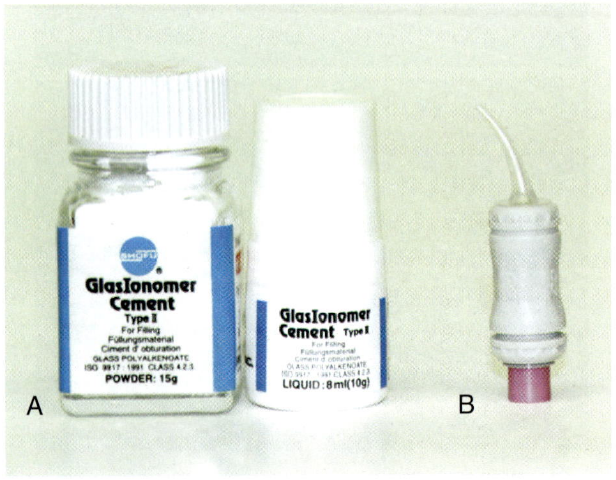

• **Fig. 7.17** Two powder–liquid type II restorative GICs. **(A)** Two-bottle system for hand mixing. **(B)** Capsule for trituration (GC Fuji Triage capsule).

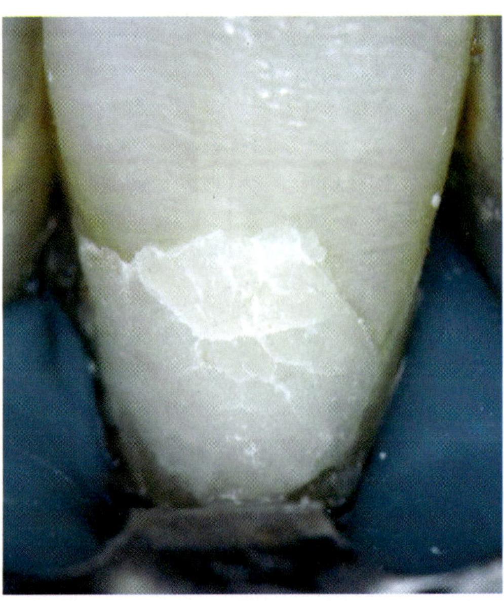

• **Fig. 7.18** Crazed surface on glass ionomer restorations resulted from inadequate protection of the material during maturation. (Courtesy of Dr S Geradeli)

TABLE 7.9 Cumulative Fluoride Release From Various Glass Ionomer Products

Material	FLUORIDE RELEASED (μG) 14 Days	30 Days
Type II	440	650
Cermet	200	300
Silver alloy admix	3350	4040
Type I	470	700
Liner (conventional)	1000	1300
Liner (hybrid)	1200	1600

GIC is mixed with a low P/L ratio because the pH remains acidic longer. With any GIC, a protective liner such as $Ca(OH)_2$ should be used if the preparation is closer than 0.5 mm to the pulp chamber.

Table 7.10 lists the properties of several restorative glass ionomers showing their compressive and tensile strengths. The compressive strength is similar to that of zinc phosphate, and its diametral tensile strength is slightly higher. The modulus of elasticity is only about half that of zinc phosphate cement (Table 7.3). Thus, the GIC is less stiff and more susceptible to elastic deformation.

GIC restoratives are more vulnerable to wear than are composites when subjected to in vitro toothbrush abrasion tests and simulated occlusal wear tests. Fracture toughness (Table 7.11), which is a measure of the energy required to cause crack propagation leading to fracture, is another property pertinent to restorative materials. Restorative GICs are less tough than resin-based composites.

Metal-Reinforced Glass Ionomer Cements

Metallic fillers have been incorporated in GICs to improve their fracture toughness and stress-bearing capacity. The metallic fillers are derived from silver alloy powder or particles of silver sintered to glass that make the cement grayish and more radiopaque; these **metal-reinforced glass ionomer cements** are called alloy admixture and **cermet**, respectively. All of the concerns and procedures that apply to conventional GICs apply to metal-reinforced GICs.

TABLE 7.10 Properties of Restorative Glass Ionomer Cements

Materials	Compressive Strength (MPa)	Diametral Tensile Strength (MPa)	Hardness (KHN)
Type II	196–251	18–26	87–177
Cermet	176–212	19–22	30–45
High-viscosity	301	24	108
Hybrid	202–306	20–48	64–85

Data from Xie D, Brantley WA, Culbertson BM, Wang G: Mechanical properties and microstructures of glass-ionomer cements. *Dent Mater* 16:129, 2000.

These cement systems release appreciable amounts of fluoride, but the release rate decreases over time (Table 7.9). Less fluoride is released from the cermet cements because a portion of the glass particles is metal coated. For the alloy admixed cement, the metal filler particles are not bonded to the glass; thus, the entire surface of the glass is available for fluoride leaching.

The adhesion and fluoride release from the metal-reinforced GICs are very useful for core buildups of teeth to be restored with cast crowns and for restoratives on occlusal surfaces of primary molars. However, metal-reinforced GICs are of limited in use as an alternative to amalgam or composite for posterior restorations. Studies show that these cements fall short of expectations. For example, in vitro studies have shown that metal-reinforced GICs are weaker than resin-based composite cores; therefore, they should not be used if the cement represents greater than 40% of the total core buildup. The auxiliary use of pins or other retention forms is advisable in such cases. In addition, metallic fillers do not improve mechanical properties, including fracture toughness, compared with other restorative glass ionomers (Tables 7.10 and 7.11). Compared with conventional glass ionomers, the metal-reinforced GICs exhibit no improvement in clinical performance and life expectancy for Class II restorations in deciduous teeth. However, these cements harden rapidly, so they can be finished in a relatively short time, which is useful for pedodontic cases.

CRITICAL QUESTION

For the atraumatic restorative treatment technique, why is a high-viscosity GIC the most appropriate material?

TABLE 7.11 Fracture Toughness of Glass Ionomer Materials and Selected Other Materials

Type of Material	Fracture Toughness (MPa•$m^{1/2}$)
Amalgam[a]	0.97–1.60
Hybrid composite[b]	1.75–1.92
Conventional GIC (luting)[c]	0.27–0.37
Conventional GIC (restoration)[d]	0.72
Metal-reinforced GIC (cermet)[e]	0.51
Metal-reinforced GIC (admixture)[e]	0.30
High-viscosity GIC[f]	0.45–0.72
Hybrid GIC (luting)[c]	0.79–1.08
Hybrid GIC (restoration)[e]	1.37
Compomer (restoration)[b]	0.97–1.23
Resin cement[c]	1.30

[a]Data from Lloyd CH, Adamson M: The fracture toughness (K_{IC}) of amalgam. *J Oral Rehab* 12:59–68, 1985.
[b]Data from Yap AU, Chung SM, Chow WS, et al: Fracture resistance of compomer and composite restoratives. *Oper Dent* 29:29–34, 2004.
[c]Data from Mitchell CA, Douglas WH, Cheng YS: Fracture toughness of conventional, resin-modified glass–ionomer and composite luting cements. *Dent Mater* 15:7–13, 1999.
[d]Data from Bonilla ED, Mardirossian G, Caputo AA: Fracture toughness of various core build-up materials. *J Prosthodont* 9:14, 2000.
[e]Data from Kovarik RE, Muncy MV. Fracture toughness of resin-modified glass ionomers. *Am J Dent* 8:145–148, 1995.
[f]Data from Yamazaki T, Schricker SR, Brantley WA, et al: Viscoelastic behavior and fracture toughness of six glass-ionomer cements. *J Prosthet Dent* 96:266–272, 2006.

High-Viscosity Glass Ionomer Cement

Atraumatic restorative treatment (ART) is a preventive and restorative caries management concept developed for dentistry in regions of the world that do not have an infrastructure with electricity or piped water systems. ART relies on hand instruments for opening tooth cavities, removing carious dentin, and mixing the material. GIC, which releases fluoride and bonds chemically to tooth structure, is the natural choice of material for these situations. GIC may be superior to nonfluoridated materials, especially when the complete removal of carious tissue cannot be accomplished because of inadequate dental treatment facilities.

Initial results of using conventional GIC have proven the feasibility for ART, which has led to the development of **high viscosity glass ionomer cements** for general dental practices. These GICs contain smaller glass particle sizes and use a higher P/L ratio, yielding greater compressive strength (Table 7.10). They exhibit excellent packability for better handling characteristics. The high-viscosity GICs are also used for core buildups, primary tooth fillings, nonstress-bearing restorations, and intermediate restorations in general practices. Encapsulated packaging of the high-viscosity GICs (Fig. 7.19) is convenient and increases their acceptance in developed countries.

Clinical Manipulation

The clinical steps in the ART procedure with high-viscosity GICs are as follows:

1. Isolating the tooth with cotton rolls.
2. Accessing the carious lesion with a hand instrument.
3. Removing the soft tissue with an excavator.
4. Using a weak acid to prepare the tooth and enhance chemical bonding.
5. Placing the high-viscosity GIC using finger pressure.

Results of a study using the ART showed that the survival rate of partially and fully retained single-surface restorations on permanent teeth was 99% after 1 year and 88% after 3 years. The same study showed that the partial and full retention of sealants in the permanent dentition was 90% after 1 year and 71% after 3 years. A recent study followed two groups of children: one group received high-viscosity GIC by the ART procedure and one group received amalgam restorations. The cumulative survival rates after 6.3 years for ART and amalgam restorations were 66.1% and 57.0%, respectively.

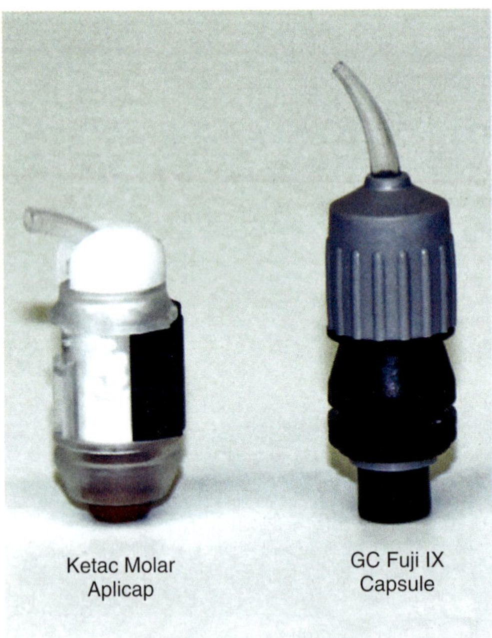

• **Fig. 7.19** Two high-viscosity GICs. Ketac Molar Aplicap (*left*), GC Fuji IX Capsule (*right*).

In a general practice office, where electricity and water lines are available, the same procedures can be used, augmented by rotary instruments. Short-term clinical studies confirm that high-viscosity GICs are suitable alternatives to amalgam for Class I and II restorations in primary teeth. A 2-year study that compared the survival of high-viscosity GICs revealed no statistically significant differences between the ART procedure and the conventional procedure of preparing prepared cavities cavity using rotary instruments for Class I preparations. However, the use of conventional preparation techniques leads to a higher survival rate for Class II preparations. A retrospective clinical study of Class II restorations made of a high-viscosity GIC showed 100%, 93%, and 60% survival rates after 1.5, 3.5, and 6 years, respectively, based on conventional techniques.

CRITICAL QUESTION

What are the advantages of incorporating polymerizing resin in GICs?

Resin-Modified Glass Ionomer Cement (Hybrid Ionomer)

Water-soluble methacrylate-based monomers have been used to replace part of liquid component of conventional GIC results in a group of materials called **resin-modified glass ionomer cements** (Fig. 7.20), also known as **hybrid ionomer** cement. The monomers can be polymerized by a chemical or light activation or both, and the GIC acid–base reaction will occur along with polymerization. Some hybrid ionomer cements also contain nonreactive filler particles, which lengthen the working time, improve early strength, and make the cement less sensitive to moisture during setting.

Chemistry and Setting

The liquid component of hybrid ionomer cements usually contains a water solution of polyacrylic acid, hydroxyethyl metharylate (**HEMA**), and polyacrylic acid modified with methacrylate. The powder component contains fluoroaluminosilicate glass particles of a conventional GIC plus initiators, such as camphorquinone, for light curing and/or chemical curing. The acid–base reaction begins upon mixing and continues after polymerization at a much slower rate than for conventional GICs because less water is present and the reaction is much slower in the solid phase than in the liquid phase.

Some hybrid ionomers are designed for restorative purposes and contain nonreactive fillers normally found in the resin composite, replacing some silicate glass; the quantity of carboxylic acid groups is also decreased. These changes do not affect the setting mechanism but impart changes in the characteristics of the material, such as bonding and strength.

Mechanism of Bonding

The bonding mechanism for hybrid ionomer cements to tooth structure is the same as that for conventional GICs. However, the use of polymerizable monomers in hybrid ionomers leads one to

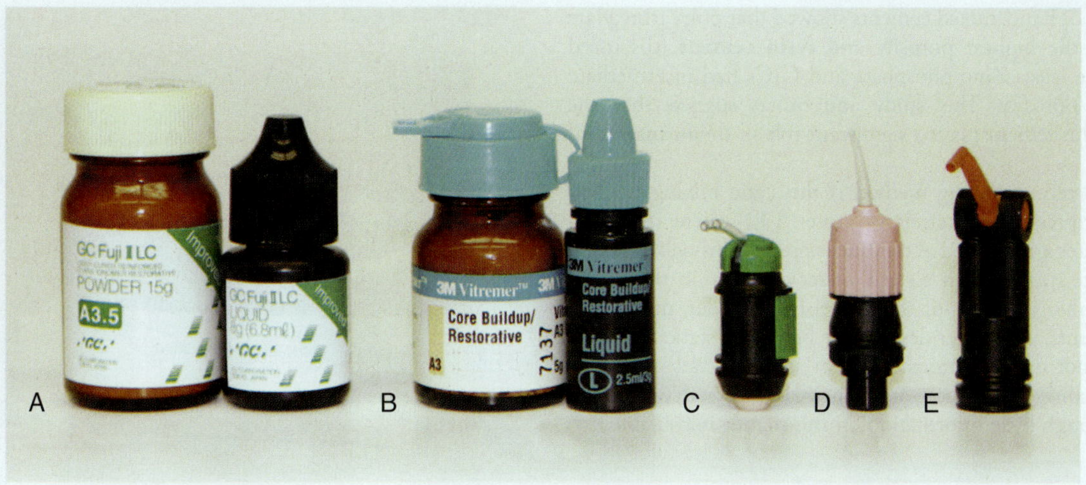

• **Fig. 7.20** Representative resin-modified GICs. **(A)** and **(B)** Two-bottle powder–liquid system. **(C)** Photac Fil Quick Aplicap. **(D)** GC Fuji Plus Capsule. **(E)** Ketac Nano; a paste–paste system using static mixing.

speculate that the bonding mechanism should also include the "hybrid layer" of the cement that infiltrates the tubules. Currently no conclusive evidence exists of hybrid layer formation with hybrid ionomer cements. Studies have reported the presence of an "indistinct" or "structureless" layer at the ionomer–dentin interface, although other studies show no evidence of resin infiltration into the etched dentin. Higher bond strengths to teeth and resin-based composites have been reported for hybrid ionomer cements than for conventional glass ionomers, which are probably associated with enhanced micromechanical interlocking to the roughened tooth surface.

Unfortunately, the methacrylate polymerization of resin-based composites causes more shrinkage of hybrid ionomers during setting as compared with a conventional GIC. The lower water and carboxylic acid contents also reduce the ability of the cement to wet tooth substrates, causing more microleakage than with conventional glass ionomers.

Clinical Manipulation

Clinical applications of hybrid ionomers include liners, fissure sealants, base materials, core buildups, restoratives, adhesives for orthodontic brackets, repair materials for damaged amalgam cores or cusps, and retrograde root filling materials. For any indication, surface conditioning of the tooth structure with a mild acid is essential for bond formation. For the hybrid ionomer containing nonreactive filler particles, less carboxylic acid is available for bonding to tooth structure and a dentin bonding system is needed.

Fissure Sealant

Low-viscosity hybrid ionomers or conventional GICs may be used for fissure/sealant indications. One clinical study shows that the retention rate of glass ionomer sealant is poor after 1 year, but patches of GIC are retained within the fissures and no signs of carious lesions are observed.

Liner and Base

As a liner or base material, hybrid ionomer serves as an intermediate bonding material between the teeth and composite restorations. Hybrid ionomer is not indicated for direct pulp capping. If the situation warrants a direct pulp capping procedure, a calcium hydroxide liner should be used prior to the application of a hybrid ionomer. The adhesion of GIC to dentin reduces the probability of gap formation at gingival margins located in dentin or cementum, compensating for the polymerization shrinkage of the overlying resin-based composite restoration on the hybrid ionomer base. Furthermore, a hybrid ionomer base or liner reduces the technique sensitivity of resin bonding agents and provides the **anticariogenic** effect from fluoride (Table 7.9). This procedure is often referred to as the sandwich technique, which combines the desirable qualities of the glass ionomer and the esthetics of the composite restoration. This **sandwich technique** is recommended for Class II and V composite restorations when individual patients are at a moderate-to-high risk for caries.

Restorations

The monomers in hybrid GICs make the cements more translucent. Fluoride release is unchanged from that of conventional GICs, and the diametral tensile strengths of hybrid glass ionomers are higher than those of GICs (Table 7.10). This increase in tensile strength (but not compressive strength) is attributed to their lower elastic modulus and the greater amount of plastic deformation that can be sustained before fracture occurs.

Water Uptake

The presence of HEMA in hybrid ionomers increases water absorption and causes expansion of up to about 8% by volume. This expansion has been linked to the fracture of all-ceramic crown restorations when used for core buildups or as luting cements. However, recent in vitro studies show that all-ceramic crowns cemented on natural teeth or titanium abutments with hybrid ionomer luting agents did not crack after 12 months of storage in water.

Delivery System

Porosity in cement is the result of air incorporation during mixing of powder and liquid. One study of luting agents showed that the method of mixing had no influence on the formation of small pores but that hand mixing yielded more large pores than triturator mixing of capsules. A later study showed that hand mixing yielded significantly greater compressive strength with the luting cement whereas capsule mixing resulted in a stronger restorative cement, although the difference was small. Porosity measurements in four types of hand-mixed cements showed that polycarboxylate cement had the highest porosity and **resin cement** (discussed later) had the least. Zinc phosphate and GICs had intermediate amounts of porosity. This study and others suggest that the viscosity of the cement plays a significant role in the formation of porosity.

The most recent mixing method is the static mixing used in preparing impression materials (Chapter 13), where dual cartridges of pastes are blended as they are expressed through a mixing tip. Complete mixing with a static mixer depends on the paste's properties, inner diameter of the dispensing cylinder, number of mixing elements, and mixer design. The benefit of static mixing is that it does not mix air into the cement and it takes less time to complete mixing. A low-porosity cement is expected with static mixing, although little information on this matter is available.

CRITICAL QUESTION

What is the setting mechanism of calcium aluminate GIC?

Calcium Aluminate Glass Ionomer Cements

A hybrid product with a composition between that of calcium aluminate and GIC, designed for luting fixed prostheses, is a new addition to the family of GICs. The calcium aluminate component is made by sintering a mixture of high-purity Al_2O_3 and CaO (approximately 1:1 molar ratio) to create monocalcium aluminate. The material is crushed and milled to a specified particle size distribution. When mixed with water, the calcium aluminate powder starts to dissolve Ca^{2+}, $Al(OH)_4-$, and $OH-$ ions and a weak acid–base reaction begins. The powder acts as the base and water as the weak acid. At low water-to-cement volume ratio, the reaction is followed by an immediate precipitation of hydrates, caused by saturation of the solution, which grows and hardens over time. This type of cement is also known as a hydraulic cement and has been advocated as a restorative material. This reaction has been paired with glass ionomer ingredients to create the hybrid calcium aluminate GIC.

The main ingredients in the powder of this hybrid cement are calcium aluminate, polyacrylic acid, tartaric acid, strontium-fluoro-alumino glass, and strontium fluoride. The liquid component contains 99.6% water and 0.4% additives for controlling setting. The glass ionomer components of the cement are responsible for the early properties (i.e. viscosity, setting time, and strength). The calcium aluminate contributes to a basic pH during curing, reduction in microleakage, excellent biocompatibility, and long-term stability and strength. The polyacrylic acid has a dual function in this hybrid material. As in a conventional GIC, the polyacrylic acid is cross-linked by $Ca^{2}+$ ions leached from both the soluble glass and the calcium aluminate. The polyacrylic acid also acts as a dispersing agent for the calcium aluminate. The resulting material is a composite of hydrated ceramic material and a cross-linked polyacrylate polymer. The cement is packaged in capsules for mechanical mixing (Fig. 7.21).

In vitro retention and shear bond test strength are excellent, as is compressive strength for the hybrid calcium aluminate cement. The working and setting times are reported to be 2 and 5 minutes, respectively. The film thickness is 15 ± 4 μm. Setting expansion of 0.4% in vitro has been reported. A study of cement set inside glass tubes showed no fracture of the glass; therefore, this amount of expansion was considered acceptable. A microstructure study showed formation of hydroxyapatite in a phosphate buffer solution on the surface of the luting cement. Results of a 2-year clinical study revealed a favorable performance of this cement.

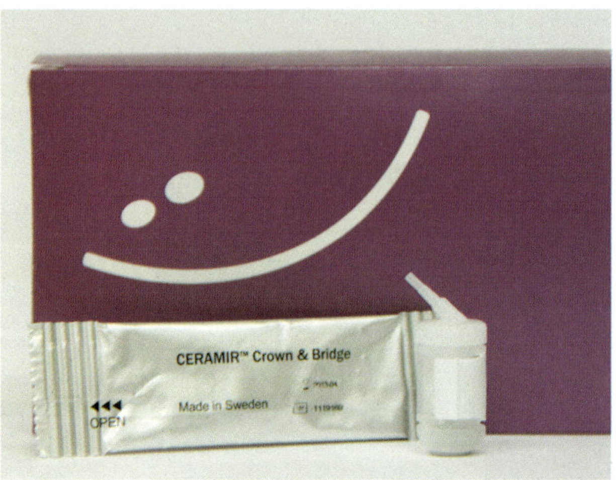

• **Fig. 7.21** A calcium aluminate GIC.

CRITICAL QUESTION

How does *compomer* differ from resin-based composite?

Compomer

Compomer is a polyacid-modified composite made by incorporating glass particles of GIC in water-free polyacid liquid monomer with appropriate initiator. The rationale for using this material is the integration of the fluoride-releasing capability of glass ionomers with the durability of resin composites. Compomers possess properties distinctly different from those of resin composites and glass ionomers.

Chemistry and Setting

Compomers are usually a one-paste, light-cure materials for restorative applications, although powder–liquid systems for luting applications are available (Fig. 7.22). These water-free materials

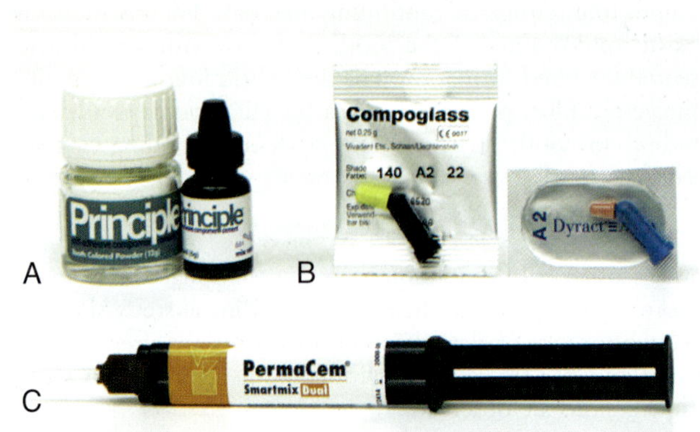

• **Fig. 7.22** Typical compomer materials. **(A)** A powder–liquid system. **(B)** Two single-component systems. **(C)** A paste–paste dual cartridge using static mixing. All systems are light curable.

contain nonreactive inorganic filler particles, reactive silicate glass particles, sodium fluoride, and polyacid-modified monomers, such as a diester of 2-hydroxyl methacrylate with butane carboxylic acid and photoactivators. Setting of these one-component compomers is initiated by photopolymerization of the acidic monomer. Compomer cements are sensitive to moisture and are packaged to protect against moisture absorption, even though their acid–base reaction is slow. Like resin composites, compomers are functionally hydrophobic but to a lesser extent, and intraorally they absorb water from the saliva that begins the slow acid–base reaction of GIC between the acidic functional groups and silicate glass particles, which lead to fluoride release.

For the powder–liquid compomer products, the powder contains strontia-alumina-fluorosilicate glass, metallic oxides, and initiators. The liquid contains polymerizable methacrylate/carboxylic monomers, multifunctional acrylate monomers, and water. Depending on the initiators, the material can be chemically cured, light cured, or dual cured to augment the slower acid–base reaction.

Bonding Mechanism

Compomer restorative materials require a dentin-bonding agent prior to their placement because they do not contain water, which could make them **self-adhesive,** like conventional GIC or hybrid ionomer. Bond strength of one-paste compomers to tooth structure using a dentin-bonding agent is similar to or higher than that of hybrid ionomers. The powder–liquid compomer cements for luting are self-adhesive, because water in the liquid makes the mixture acidic, like hybrid ionomers.

Clinical Manipulation

The restorative compomer materials are mainly used in low-stress-bearing areas such as Class III and V prepared cavity, or as an alternative to glass ionomer restoratives or resin-based composites. The tooth structure should be etched prior to application of the dentin bonding agent and the compomer. Compomers are finished just like resin composites.

Compomer luting systems are indicated for cementing prostheses with a metallic substrate. The cement mixture is placed only on the prosthesis, which is seated with finger pressure. The margin should be light cured immediately to stabilize the prosthesis. The chemical-cure compomers complete their setting reaction in approximately 3 minutes in the oral environment, although they may take 10 minutes or more to set on the bench top. Ninety seconds from the end of mixing, the material will reach a gel state, at which point the excess cement may be removed.

Water Uptake

Water absorption by restorative compomers, which is as high as 3.5% by weight, is a desired process to complete the acid–base reaction and subsequent fluoride release. As expected, restorative compomer releases less fluoride than that from conventional GICs and hybrid ionomers. Studies have shown that the compressive strength and flexural strength of compomers decrease on storage in saline solution, a phenomenon not observed in resin composites. The decrease in strength is associated with the water uptake and the acid–base reaction. However, the surface hardness and microtensile strength appear to be unchanged. When manufacturers treat the reactive glass with silane, water uptake is reduced and strengths are higher.

Clinical Performance

Not all compomers exhibit acceptable clinical performance in Class V restorations, and the color stability of compomer cements is a problem. The change in refractive index on the surface by water absorption and staining by food are the likely causes. A 24-month clinical study shows that, except for marginal integrity, they perform as well as resin-based composite sealants when used to seal fissures. Compomers perform as well as resin composites for Class I and II restorations and acceptably as luting agents for orthodontic bands.

Resin Cements

Resin cements are low-viscosity versions of resin-based composites. These cements have a matrix of methacrylate monomers with dispersed fillers. Silane coating is required on the filler particle surfaces to bond them to the monomers during polymerization for a durable, wear-resistant material. Polymerization of the resin cement can be by self-, light- or dual-cured mechanisms. Most resin cements for adhering devices are dual-cured materials. Dual- or self-cured cements are used for prostheses made with medium- or high-opacity materials. For dual-cured cements, blue light initiates the curing at the margins, and the self-cure progresses over time. The light-cured resin cements are indicated for cementing ceramic veneers and direct bonding of ceramic or polymeric orthodontic brackets. Because of light attenuation by the translucent prostheses, longer light exposure is often required than with direct composites. However, the duration of light exposure should be minimized to avoid heating the pulp. Many brands are available worldwide, which vary widely in physical properties (Fig. 7.23).

Chemistry and Setting

Resin cements, like resin-based composite, require the same bonding systems as resin-based composites for adhesion to teeth. Many bonding systems are available, which vary in the steps needed. The one-, two-, and three-component systems were discussed in Chapter 6. The one-component system combines etching and priming. Bonding systems, like the resin cements, may be self-, dual-, or light-cured materials, but all incorporate at least

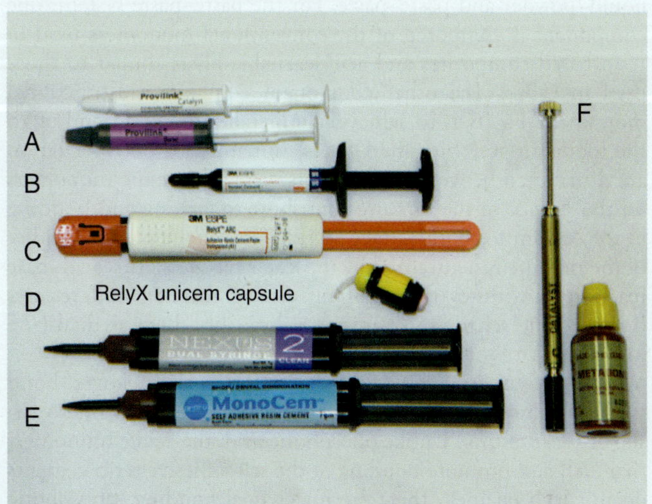

• **Fig. 7.23** Commercial resin cements. **(A)** A hand-mixing paste–paste dual-cure system for temporary prostheses. **(B)** A single-component light-cure system for porcelain veneers. **(C)** A paste–paste dual-cartridge dispensing system that requires hand mixing. **(D)** A powder–liquid capsule system that is triturated. **(E)** Two paste–paste dual-cartridge systems that require static mixing; the top one requires a bonding agent and the bottom one is self-adhesive. **(F)** A liquid–liquid system.

one hydrophilic monomer. Thirty hydrophilic monomers have been used, each with a methacrylate functionality, to infiltrate the dentinal collagen and establish a micromechanical bond. Typically, these monomers are acidic or amide formulas in a water-miscible solution. Examples are HEMA, 4-META, carboxylic acids, and an organophosphate (e.g. 10-methacryloyloxydecamethylene phosphoric acid [MDP]). For systems that require a bonding agent, the resin primers partially infiltrate the collagen fibrils that have been demineralized by acid etching. The resin tags fill the space to reduce adverse pulpal responses from the osteoblastic processes in the tubules.

Self-cured and dual-cured resin cements contain two components (base and catalyst) that require mixing. Chemical activation is slower than with light curing and provides extended working time. In dual-cured cements, setting starts when the cement is exposed to a curing light. Components are mixed on a paper pad for 20–30 seconds, or two pastes can be mixed when dispensed through a dual-chambered syringe through a static mixing tip. The most esthetic resin cements are light cured only, and their color stability over time is better than the dual-cured resins.

Some bonding agents are called "universal" bonding agents by the manufacturer. Most universal bonding agents can be used with total, self-, and selective etching before placement of dual- or self-curing cements. Some universal adhesives release fluoride, and some are two-part liquids that require mixing. The adhesive agent may also be used as a primer on metal and ceramic-based restoratives.

Not all resin cement systems require a bonding agent. One system based on 4-META uses liquid monomers and catalysts without any traditional inorganic fillers and relies on mixing with various amounts of polymer beads to adjust the viscosity of the cement for intended applications. This cement eliminates the steps of etching, priming, and bonding and allows the clinician to bond prostheses directly to clean abutments. These cement systems rely on modified dimethacrylate monomers with acid-containing side chains, such as phosphoric acid, attached as pendant groups. Upon contact with the tooth surface, the acidic group binds with calcium in the hydroxyapatite to bond to the tooth.

The current self-adhesive resin cements are two-part systems: liquid–powder and paste–paste. For the paste–paste system, one component is composed of the conventional monomers used in resin-based composites and acid-leachable fillers similar to those used in GICs. The other component contains acid-functional monomers (Fig. 6.4) to achieve demineralization and bonding to the tooth surface, with inert fillers. Initiators for polymerization are distributed between components. Only the acidic monomers on the surface of the mixture contribute to etching and bonding of the cement to tooth surface, as in GICs. The remaining acidity of the mixture is neutralized by the leachable glass. This acid–base reaction constitutes the recurrent setting reaction and releases fluoride. The setting mechanisms also qualify them as dual-cure materials.

The self-adhesive resin cements usually show lower bond strength values than nonself-adhesive resin cements in microtensile or shear testing. Unlike phosphoric acid, the acidic monomers that etch and promote bonding of the self-adhesive resin cements do not etch enamel. Therefore for enamel bonding, phosphoric acid etching is needed.

Clinical Manipulation and Evaluation

Liquid–powder formulations are often packaged in capsule form and mixed by trituration (Fig. 7.23D). Two-paste resin systems are often sold with a static mixer tube to use on the end of a two-barrel syringe; the static mixer dispenses a mixed cement (Fig. 7.23E). Static mixing or trituration of capsules has largely replaced hand mixing. Static mixing is convenient and does not mix air into the cement, unlike hand mixing. The mechanism of static mixing is discussed in Chapter 13 with mixing of impression materials.

For bonding inlays or crowns, a separate phosphoric acid etching of the enamel margins improves marginal sealing and adaptation. However, phosphoric acid decreases bond strength to dentin because the viscous cements cannot penetrate a demineralized collagenous matrix created by phosphoric acid. However, the self-adhesive resin cements have fairly strong bonds to dentin, despite the lack of formation of the classical hybrid layer shown for enamel bonding.

The chemical and physical properties of self-adhesive resin cements reported in the literature show that self-adhesive resin cements may be expected to perform as well as other resin-based and nonresin-based dental cements; however, few long-term studies are available. Nonetheless, the handling properties of these materials appear to be excellent, and their acceptance by the profession is increasing.

The monomers in uncured resin cements are irritating to the pulp. To prevent the infiltration of irritants, pulp protection with a liner is important when the thickness of the remaining dentin is less than 0.5 mm. The procedure for preparing the tooth remains the same for each resin system, but the treatment of the prosthesis differs depending on the prosthesis material, as described next.

Polymerization of the resin cement occurs by chemical-, light-, or dual-cure mechanisms. The majority of resin cements today are of the dual-cure variety. Light-cured resin cement is less common because of the potential for incomplete polymerization of the cement under a prosthesis; it is used for cementing porcelain veneers.

Classification: Based on Adhesive Scheme

- Etch-and-rinse resin cements
- Self-etch resin cements
- Self-adhesive resin cements.

Etch-and-Rinse Resin Cements

Etch-and-rinse resin cements combine an etch-and-rinse dentin adhesive system with methacrylate-based resin cement. Most manufacturers of resin cements recommend the use of two-step etch-and-rinse adhesives or "one-bottle" adhesive systems, which combine the primer and adhesive resin into one solution, theoretically making it more user friendly than multibottle etch-and-rinse adhesives.

Phosphoric acid is generally used to etch the enamel and dentine. Etch-and-rinse adhesives must be used with a wet bonding technique to avoid the collapse of the collagen network exposed after etching. This is followed by application of the primer and bonding agent. Multiple coatings may be required to achieve sufficient micromechanical interlocking. Following adhesive application the solvent should be completely evaporated to decrease permeability and improve bond strength.

Subsequently, the adhesive system is polymerized to yield adequate mechanical and physical properties. The use of a self- or dual-cured adhesive may be considered especially for indirect restorations, when effective light polymerization is uncertain. Some etch-and-rinse resin cements include chemical coinitiators or activators to convert the light-polymerized adhesive into a self- or dual-cured adhesive. However, the use of an activator is not always helpful in improving the bond between dual-cured adhesives and self- or dual-cured composites. In addition, the degree of conversion is significantly lower in the self-polymerizing mode than when the same adhesive is used in dual-cure mode. Therefore, dentin adhesives used in conjunction with resin cements must be light polymerized, irrespective of the activation mode. Extended curing times are also helpful in ensuring complete polymerization.

Self-Etch Resin Cements

The intrinsic technique sensitivity of the etch-and-rinse resin cements led to the development of resin cements which were compatible with self-etch adhesives.

Self-etch systems apply a self-etching primer to prepare the tooth surface, and mixed cement is applied over the primer. Bonds to tooth structure using this category of cements are almost as high as those of the total-etch cements. Two-step self-etch adhesives comprise a self-etching primer and a hydrophobic adhesive resin, whereas one-step self-etch adhesives combine etchant, primer, and bonding in a single solution. Self-etch adhesives simultaneously demineralize and infiltrate the dental substrate. The etching characteristics are dependent on the pH of the acidic solutions. Self-etch adhesives do not require rinsing and drying, the smear layer is not removed but impregnated by the acidic monomers. Micromechanical interlocking is still the main source of bonding for self-etch adhesives.

Caution is advised when bonding one-step self-etch adhesive to dual-cured resin cements because of the adverse chemical interaction between the acidic adhesive and resin cement.

Self-Adhesive Resin Cements

A number of resin cements have recently been introduced as one-component "universal adhesive cements." These claim to have good bond strengths to dentin, enamel, and porcelains without the need for separate bonding agents.

These cements contain phosphoric acid, which is grafted into the resin. After mixing, the phosphoric acid methacrylate is able to demineralize the hard tissues. The phosphoric acid reacts with filler particles and dentin in the presence of water, forming a bond. The resin is polymerized into a cross-linked polymer, as is the case with composite resin bonding.

Self-adhesive resin cements can bond to dental hard tissues without conditioning procedures or the use of bonding adhesive. Most cements have an initial low pH (pH <2.0). An increase in pH (up to 7.0) is observed as a consequence of the reaction between the phosphate groups and alkaline fillers and the hydroxyapatite from enamel and dentin, neutralizing the resin's inherent acidity.

Self-adhesive resin cements rely more on chemical bonding than on micromechanical retention. The acid groups chelate the calcium ions of the hydroxyapatite, promoting chemical adhesion. In some cases, the addition of polyalkenoic acid (found in RelyX Unicem, 3M ESPE) provides carboxylic groups, which form ionic bonds with calcium present in the hydroxyapatite, positively influencing the chemical bonding.

Self-adhesive resin cements are able to partially dissolve the smear layer without removing the smear plug within the dentinal tubules. The type of instrument used for tooth preparation would determine the thickness of the smear layer, which in turn could influence the bond strength.

Pretreatment of enamel with strong acid, such as 35% phosphoric acid, is highly recommended. Most self-adhesive resin cements yield bond strengths lower than etch-and-rinse resin cements or 10-MDP self-etch resin cements. With the exception of RelyX Unicem, most self-adhesive resin cements maintain low pH for a long time after setting, which can adversely influence the bonding.

A recent clinical trial revealed good performance of a self-adhesive cement (RelyX Unicem) over 38 months for luting alloy–based restorations.

At present there is no long-term clinical data to fully recommend self-adhesive resin cements as substitutes for etch-and-rinse resin cements.

Classification: Based on Polymerization Mechanism

1. Light-cure resin cements
2. Dual-cure resin cements
3. Chemical-cure resin cements.

Newer resin cements such as Rely X Ultimate (3M) offer greater flexibility in terms of usage. These can be used with compatible Universal bonding systems in either selective etch, total etch or self-etch mode. Other manufacturers are also now offering resin cements which can be used in the self-adhesive mode, but should one need greater flexibility it is possible to use them in conjunction with compatible bonding systems. These cement/bonding combos offer a wider variety of options in bonding to various substrates.

CRITICAL QUESTION

Why are different types of surface treatment protocols used in the treatment of prosthesis surfaces?

The procedure for preparing tooth surfaces remains the same for each system, but the treatment of the prosthesis differs depending on the composition of the prosthesis, as described in Box 7.1.

Metallic Prostheses

The bondable surface of base metal prostheses should be roughened by electrochemical etching or by grit blasting with 30–50 μm

• BOX 7.1 Surface Treatment for Restorations

Glass-Ceramic Restorations

1. Surface treatment of porcelain 5%–9.5% hydrofluoric acid. Hydrofluoric acid is used to selectively dissolve the glass matrix, creating microporosities around the leucite crystals
2. Conditioned with silane
3. Sandblasting contraindicated

Glass-Infiltrated Alumina-Based Ceramics

Surface treatment

- Acid etchants – do not adequately roughen
- Tribochemical silica coating process (Rocatec)
- Cleaning the surface with 110 μm high-purity Al_2O_3
- Conditioned with silane

Pretreatment Techniques for Zirconia-Based Ceramics

Pretreatment techniques for promoting bonding to zirconia-based ceramics include:

- Air-particle abrasion
- Tribochemical silica coating (Rocatec)
- 10-MDP containing ceramic primer

alumina particles at an air pressure of 0.4–0.7 MPa. Some bonding systems include a metal primer containing an adhesion promoter. Oxide formation on the base metal surfaces contributes to the bond strength when resin cement containing MDP or a 4-META-based resin is used. To enhance bonding to noble alloys, which lack a stable oxide at room temperature, one can electrochemically deposit a thin (about 0.5 μm) layer of tin on noble metal and heat it to an appropriate temperature to form a tin oxide surface. Silica deposition on noble and base alloy surfaces can be achieved by blasting silica-coated Al_2O_3 particles on these surfaces. Subsequent silanization improves metal surface bonding to resin cements, although the bond strength is similar to that measured for grit blasting and electrochemical etching.

Polymeric Prostheses

Resin-based veneers, inlays, onlays, crowns, and fixed dental prostheses are cemented with resin cements. The polymer's surface should be grit blasted to increase the roughness for mechanical adhesion. Some polymer prosthesis systems have a special adhesive based on the same monomer that is used to fabricate the prosthesis. Sufficient time, as much as 30 minutes, must be allowed for adequate penetration and diffusion of the adhesive into the cross-linked polymer prosthesis to occur before curing.

Ceramic Prostheses

Some dental ceramic restorations are translucent and the shade of the luting cement can affect the esthetics of the ceramic restoration. Resin cements are the luting agents of choice for all-ceramic inlays, crowns, and bridges because of their ability to reduce fracture of the ceramic structures and the range of shades available to produce an optimal esthetic appearance.

- If the ceramic prostheses are silica based, like feldspathic porcelain, the inner surfaces of the prostheses are etched with hydrofluoric acid, and a silane coating is applied prior to cementation, either by the dental laboratory or chairside.
- Etching and silanization are not effective with ceramics that do not contain silica, such as alumina- and zirconia-based ceramics.
- Zirconia-based systems need to be sandblasted and benefit from an additional coat of 10 MDP containing ceramic primer.
- Zirconia-based restorations should never be etched with phosphoric acid, since doing so will prevent the zirconia from bonding effectively with bonding agents and resin cements.
- After try in zirconia-based restorations should be cleaned with either Ivoclean (Ivoclar Vivadent) or sodium hypochlorite to provide a clean surface for bonding.

Clinical technique for cementation of monolithic zirconia crowns is presented in Box 7.2.

Light-cure resin cements are indicated for the cementation of thin ceramic prostheses such as veneers, resin-based prostheses, and direct bonding of ceramic or plastic orthodontic brackets (Box 7.3). Seat the prosthesis with light pressure to expel excess cement, secure the prosthesis in place by spot curing part of the prosthesis without irradiating the excess cement, clean the excess cement from the margin and then light cure the remaining area for the specific duration recommended by the manufacturer.

To match the resin cement with the ceramic prosthesis, some systems provide water-soluble try-in materials with the same shades as the cements. The try-in gels are applied in the same way as a cement, and the prosthesis is seated and examined in situ for its esthetic appearance. This process can be repeated with various try-in gel shades until the clinician is satisfied with the esthetic appearance. After the proper cement shade has been selected, the residual try-in paste must be rinsed off the tooth and the prosthesis is thoroughly rinsed with a water spray. The cementation process is then completed using a cement of the same shade as the selected try-in gel.

• BOX 7.2 Clinical Technique for Cementation of Monolithic Zirconia Crowns

- Try in the restorations
- Adjust the contacts, and if needed occlusion
- Polish with the appropriate zirconia polishers
- Microetch the internal surface with 30-μm alumina oxide and clean the internal surface with a surface treatment of Ivoclean (Ivoclar Vivadent)
- Rinse and dry
- Coat the internal surface with and MDP containing zirconia primer that supports chemical adhesion of cements to the zirconia restorations
- Use a dual-cured resin cement or a resin-modified glass ionomer luting cement
- If using a dual-cure cement tack cure for 5 s with the LED curing light to help set the material that is expressed on the crown margins then let set for 3 min to auto cure
- Remove excess cement
- Use of phosphoric acid for etching the intaglio surface of the crown is contraindicated

• BOX 7.3 Bonding Procedure for Ceramic Veneers

1. Etch the veneer with hydrofluoric acid and wash off etchant thoroughly. Clean the surface of the restoration prior to bonding. Place the restoration in acetone to remove all organic debris from the internal surface of the restoration. Dry the restoration.
2. Apply bonding agent and luting material to the veneer. Use the micro applicator tip to apply the bonding agent to the etched surface of the veneer. Lightly dry the bonding agent with gentle stream of compressed air to evaporate the solvent in the bonding agent. Place a thin layer of light-activated resin veneer cement to cover the inner surface of the veneer. Put the veneer aside where it is not exposed to light to prevent premature polymerization of the luting composite.
3. Acid etch the tooth preparation. Use a Mylar matrix band to protect the adjacent teeth during the etching procedure. Apply a 37% phosphoric acid gel for 20 s on the enamel surfaces and slightly beyond the margins. Wash thoroughly and dry.
4. Application of bonding agent. Use a Mylar matrix band to protect the adjacent teeth during the placement of the bonding agent. Use the micro applicator tip to apply the bonding agent to the prepared tooth. Lightly dry the bonding agent with gentle stream of compressed air to evaporate the solvent in the bonding agent.
5. Insertion of the restoration. Place the restoration onto the preparation and apply gentle finger pressure until the restoration is completely seated. The pressure should be gentle to prevent breaking the restoration. Use continuous pressure in an incisal to gingival direction to allow the composite to flow until the restoration appears to be seated.
6. Removal of excess luting material. Use the micro applicator tips to remove excess luting material from the margins. A small brush can also be used to remove the excess material from the gingival embrasures. Use an explorer to remove additional excess from the embrasures as required. Tack cure for 3 s and remove excess cement with explorer and floss.
7. Polymerize the bonding material. Light cure from the gingival, facial, incisal, and lingual for 40 s in each area. Keep the light as close to the restoration as possible to maximize its effectiveness.

Orthodontic Brackets

Orthodontic bonding is a specialized use of cement that must be strong enough to withstand the forces exerted on the device for about 2 years, but then the bond must be broken for removal with minimal effect on the tooth. The bonding of orthodontic brackets requires proper isolation and etching of the enamel surface to secure the bond between the tooth and the bracket. The tooth-facing side of the bracket requires some means of mechanical retention, such as the metal mesh of a metal bracket or retentive dimples or ridges on ceramic or polymer brackets. Ceramic bracket bases are commonly precoated with an organosilane, like that used to bond the inorganic fillers to the resin matrix of resin-based composites. Polycarbonate brackets are primed with a solvent containing methylmethacrylate monomer.

Mechanical and chemical adhesion to the bracket and tooth are important for the prevention of premature debonding. Because of the cement exposure to the oral cavity, the bond strength decreases over the course of treatment and bracket removal can be uneventful. Debonding of brackets at the tooth/cement interface, or less preferably at the cement/bracket interface, is desirable, but not within the tooth enamel.

Orthodontic bands are commonly cemented with GIC. Their removal is facilitated by using air to desiccate and weaken the cement.

CRITICAL QUESTION

What is the benefit of calcium hydroxide in contact with pulpal tissue?

Pulp Protection

Tooth enamel is a translucent crystalline bioceramic but is vulnerable to acids and the repeated stress of a lifetime of chewing. The underlying dentin may be exposed to the oral cavity when the enamel is worn, chemically eroded by acidic foods or cariogenic bacteria, mechanically abraded by food or opposing teeth, fractured, or prepared for restoration. Depending on the remaining dentin thickness, the exposed dentinal tubules provide a communication path to the pulp for acids and microbiological insults. The dentin must be covered to minimize further damage. When metallic material is used to restore the tooth, discomfort may arise from hot or cold nutrition or galvanic contact with metal restoratives on opposing dentition. During restorative procedures, the acidic components of some dental cements may irritate the pulp before setting. Therefore pulp protectants are required when little protective dentin is left after a cavity preparation.

Pulp protectants for cavity preparations approximating the pulp are denoted as *pulp-capping materials, varnishes, cavity liners,* or *base materials.* Pulp-capping materials are in direct contact with the pulp, and their biocompatibility is crucial to the pulp's healing. Varnishes as very thin resin layers used to plug and block the dentinal tubules exposed in a cavity preparation. Cavity liners are thin layers and are used for indirect pulp capping when the remaining dentin is less than 1 mm and are more protective than varnishes. Base materials are placed in thicker layers than liners and are commonly placed farther from the pulp. The base material is needed for insulation from the thermal, chemical, or galvanic irritations that may occur with restorative materials.

Pulp-Capping Materials

Pulp-capping agents are used when the pulp has been exposed and bleeding is frank. The best pulp-capping and cavity-liner materials are bioactive and antimicrobial. *Bioactivity,* as defined in ISO 22317, is the spontaneous formation of a thin layer rich in Ca and P, similar to hydroxyapatite, on the surface of a material in vivo or synthetic body fluid. Bioactivity occurs by the release of calcium and hydroxide ions that create a high pH (alkaline), thus causing the precipitation of calcium phosphate from the supersaturated body fluids in the vicinity of their surface. Bone morphogenic protein (BMP) and transforming growth factor-beta one (TGF-β1) may be solubilized from the bone or dentine by the high pH and released to stimulate repair. The pulp can heal by forming pulpal odontoblasts on the calcium phosphate layer of the bioactive materials, forming reparative dentin. Such a histological result is shown in Fig. 7.24. Bioactive pulp-capping agents include calcium hydroxide powder and tricalcium/dicalcium silicate materials.

Calcium Hydroxide

Calcium hydroxide medicaments are available as powder, one-paste, or two-paste products with radiopaque fillers. Calcium hydroxide powder may simply be mixed with water and placed, or some products disperse the powder in a carrier such as polyethylene glycol liquid, such as UltraCal (Ultradent Inc.). Other products may include calcium hydroxide in a resin formula that sets chemically or with light, such as Dycal (Caulk Dentsply Sirona). Calcium hydroxide is sparingly soluble in water and does not set into a hardened cement during the procedure but gradually converts to calcium carbonate by carbon dioxide in the blood and oral fluids over time. Such products must not be left on the margins of the cavity preparation; otherwise, the margin will not be properly sealed. Calcium hydroxide is beneficial because of a high pH, which makes this material antimicrobial. However, calcium hydroxide alone does not set or provide much thermal insulation but is bioinert. Histologically, calcium hydroxide stimulates reparative dentin when placed on the pulp, although the reparative dentin may have tunnel defects.

CRITICAL QUESTION

Why is MTA cement biocompatible and considered bioactive?

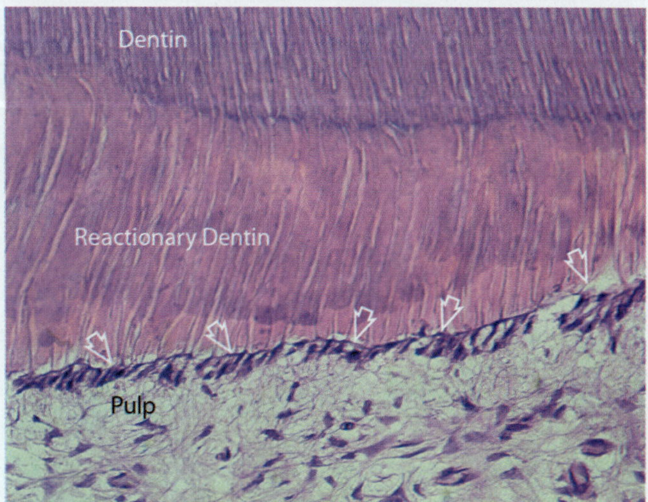

• **Fig. 7.24** Reactionary dentin. Histological section of a human tooth submitted to a slight pathological stimulus from a deep cavity filled with light-cured glass ionomer cement and then extracted 30 days after the procedure. The remaining dentin thickness is 287 µm at the thinnest region. Note that the pulp tissue subjacent to the continuous odontoblast layer *(hollow arrows)* does not show inflammation. (Courtesy of Dr Carlos Alberto de Souza Costa)

Tricalcium/Dicalcium Silicate

Tricalcium/dicalcium silicate (tricalcium silicate, for short) products are also known by the names MTA, *calcium silicate, biosilicates,* or *bioceramics.* Chemically, the predominant compounds in these cements are tricalcium silicate and dicalcium silicate powders with inert radiopaque ceramic powders. The tricalcium silicate powders are unique ceramic compounds because they set with water and form calcium hydroxide as a reaction product within a hard matrix of hydrated tricalcium and dicalcium silicate. The calcium hydroxide reaction product renders bioactivity and imparts antimicrobial properties. Furthermore, because the calcium hydroxide is within a matrix, the alkalinity is sustained longer than in calcium hydroxide alone. This type of cement is thermally insulating and seals very well, without shrinkage.

For pulpotomies, hemorrhage should be controlled with a cotton pellet moistened with saline, a dilute solution of sodium hypochlorite (0.5%–1.0%) before placement, to avoid blood seeping into the cement and ensure removal of enough affected pulp. The consistency of the tricalcium silicate can be fluid or putty-like for pulpal placement. After placement, any restorative material, including ZOE, GIC, hybrid ionomer liner, or flowable compomer or composite, can be placed immediately over the tricalcium silicate without waiting for a full set of tricalcium silicates. Bonding agents do not adhere to tricalcium silicates, and etching should not be performed directly on tricalcium silicates. The precipitation of hydroxyapatite at interfaces with the tissue should prevent the tricalcium silicates from being dislodged. After pulpotomy treatment, the pulp should be periodically assessed for vitality, as an indication of a dentinal barrier forming beneath the tricalcium silicate cement. Tricalcium silicates have been added to the resin matrix as pulp protectant, such as TheraCal and TheraCal PT (Bisco). These products set by light curing or dual curing of the resin, but their bioactivity is lessened by the resin encapsulation of the bioactive component.

The properties and applications of tricalcium/dicalcium silicate will be discussed in more detail later in the chapter.

Formocresol and Ferric Sulfate

Formocresol and ferric sulfate have been used as protective medicaments for partial or complete pulpotomy procedures, among other techniques, including electrosurgery and laser cautery. Ferric sulfate and formocresol staunch the bleeding pulp, but neither material is bioactive. By far, formocresol has been the most popular among pediatric dentists. Ferric sulfate–treated pulpotomies have led to the unfortunate consequence of root resorption. Calcium hydroxide has not been popular in pediatric dentistry because this material has been less successful with pulpal inflammation and tooth resorption in small, thin primary teeth. The bioactive tricalcium silicate–based products are superseding the use of formocresol or ferric sulfate medicaments for pediatric pulpotomies, with a better success rate for retention before exfoliation.

Pediatric pulpotomies may fail or may not be suitable because of deeper infection of the pulp. For these cases, the pulp is extirpated, and the canal is filled with a nonsetting medicament. The filling material is nonsetting to avoid interference with the primary tooth's exfoliation. These materials should be radiopaque. Two such materials contain calcium hydroxide in silicone oil or tricalcium silicate powder in salicylate resin.

CRITICAL QUESTION

Why is MTA cement biocompatible and considered bioactive?

Tricalcium/Dicalcium Silicate Cement

Dental cements based on tricalcium and dicalcium silicates (*tricalcium silicate,* for short) are beneficial because of their sealing ability, biocompatibility, and bioactivity. These cements are less cytotoxic than GICs or polymeric materials. These hydraulic cements need water to set, which is ever present in the oral cavity. The first tricalcium/dicalcium silicate product was called *mineral trioxide aggregate* (MTA) and later, *bioceramic.* These names are widely used in dentistry to denote the tricalcium/dicalcium silicates products (Fig. 7.25).

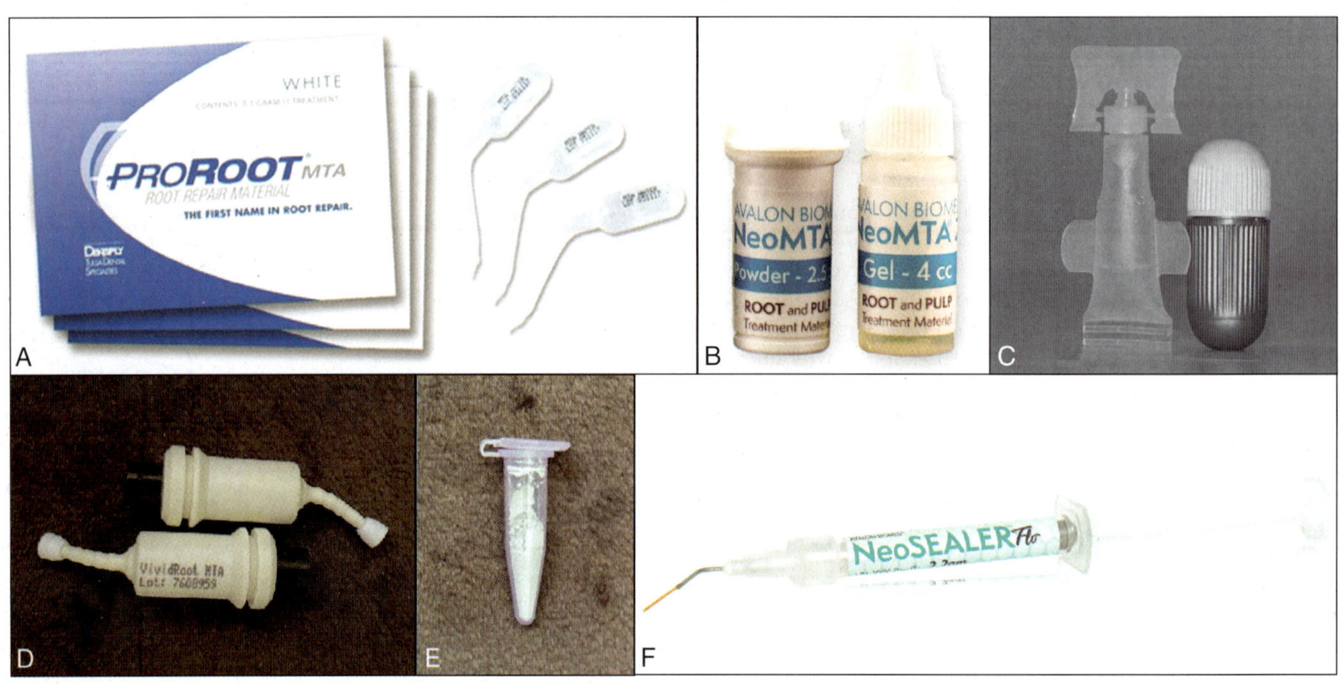

• **Fig. 7.25** An assortment of tricalcium silicate products with various packaging for the bioactive powder. **(A)** Schets. **(B)** Bottles. **(C)** Amalgam-type cartridges. **(D)** Ampoules. **(E)** Vials. **(F)** Paste.

TABLE 7.12 Phases in Tricalcium Silicate Cement Before Hydration

Ceramic Phases	Wt%
Tricalcium silicate $3(CaO)\bullet SiO_2$	45–75
Dicalcium silicate $2(CaO)\bullet SiO_2$	7–32
Radiopaque filler (Bi_2O_3, ZrO_2, $CaWO_4$, Ta_2O_5)	20–55
Minor phases, optional	
Tricalcium aluminate $3(CaO)\bullet Al_2O_3$	0–13
Tetracalcium aluminoferrite $4(CaO)\bullet Al_2O_3\bullet Fe_2O_3$	0–18
Gypsum $CaSO_4\bullet 2H_2O$	2–10
Calcium carbonate ($CaCO_3$)	<10

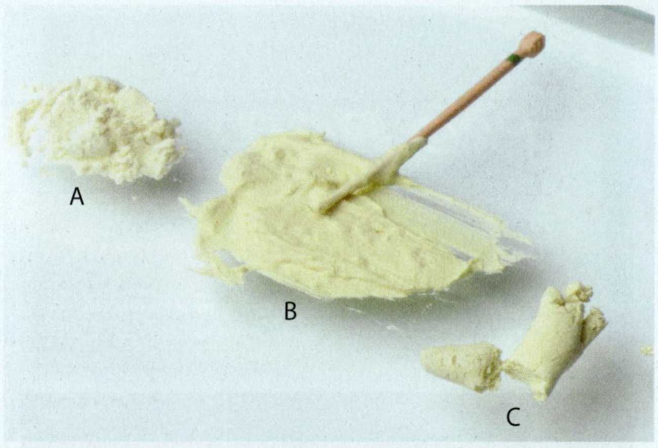

• **Fig. 7.26** Mixing of mineral trioxide aggregate. **(A)** Dispense powder and liquid. **(B)** Bring the powder to liquid and spatulate until a putty-like consistency. **(C)** Roll to the desire shape for usage.

The essential components of these bioactive cements are tricalcium silicate and dicalcium silicate ceramic powders blended with inert radiopaque powders, usually bismuth oxide, zirconia, calcium tungstate, barium zirconate, or tantalum oxide. Minor phases of tricalcium aluminate, calcium sulfate (Table 7.12), calcium carbonate, and tetracalcium aluminoferrite are sometimes present, depending on the brand. The ferrite compound makes the cement gray.

Tricalcium silicate cement sets by reaction with water to form a rigid matrix of calcium silicate hydrates with embedded calcium hydroxide. The hydration starts on the surface of the tricalcium silicate particles and gradually penetrates inward, although never completely. Setting times for these products vary from a few minutes to 2 hours for the original ProRoot MTA. The long setting time, washout, and high price were major drawbacks of early products. Improved products are now available with shorter setting times based on finer particle sizes and modified water-based liquids containing calcium chloride, polycarboxylate, or various water-soluble organic materials.

Products are available for a range of indications, from pulpal to periradicular contact. The primary indications are for pulp and periradicular tissue contact. The tricalcium/dicalcium silicate cements are vulnerable to acid dissolution; therefore periodontal and coronal usage is only temporary. The cement sets over a wide range of P/L ratios, roughly between 4:1 and 2:1. The P/L ratio can be varied to suit the case and the clinician's preference. The powder should be dispensed onto a glass slab (Fig. 7.26A), with a drop of the liquid next to the powder. A medium-stiffness metal spatula should be used to bring powder to liquid and spatulate until a putty-like consistency is reached (Fig. 7.26B). The mixture can be formed into a "roll" with gloved fingers (Fig. 7.26C), and then the spatula can be used to cut off small sections for insertion into a pulpotomy preparation, a root-end filling of a perforation site, a cavity preparation, or a pulp exposure such as a pulpotomy. A plastic filling instrument or a small amalgam carrier is commonly used to transport the cement into the surgical location, and the cement is then gently compacted. If the mixed cement is not used immediately, a moist gauze "tent" can be placed over the material to prevent dehydration. If the mixture appears dry, usually more liquid can be added to prolong the working time.

The pH of MTA rises rapidly after contact with water by releasing calcium hydroxide as a reaction product. The calcium hydroxide in the set tricalcium silicate makes this material antibacterial, antifungal, and bioactive. That is, the high pH on the surface causes the precipitation of hydroxyapatite crystals on the surface in vitro or in vivo. MTA should not be allowed to stay in contact with the mucosa because the high pH can cause a superficial lesion. Excess material should be washed out of the oral cavity. The surficial layer of hydroxyapatite that forms in vivo causes a chain of healing reactions to the bone-like surface, which does not appear as a foreign body to the cells. Reparative dentin forms in apposition to the tricalcium/dicalcium silicates in pulpal indications. Cementum-like layers form over the tricalcium silicate used to fill perforations, resorption defects, or root ends. When the tricalcium/dicalcium silicate materials set, the dimensional change is <0.1% expansion, which is highly desirable for sealing, unlike polymers that shrink.

New bioactive, hydraulic paste products have been introduced. For these, the tricalcium/dicalcium silicate cement and radiopaque powders are suspended in organic liquids. When used in vivo, the organic liquid diffuses away from the powder, and water diffuses inward to cause setting. Such one-component paste products are being used for pulpal and periradicular containing cements, including endodontic sealing with gutta-percha.

Other hydraulic cements are likely to be developed that incorporate calcium monoaluminate to make a more acid-resistant cement suitable for infected (acidic) sights. Also, the reaction of silica hydrate (silicic acid) with calcium hydroxide (pozzolan reaction) will be used for new products to create a hydrated silica cement.

Mineral Trioxide Aggregate Cements

A new category of cement, based on some of same compounds found in Portland cement, has gained popularity for endodontic applications (Fig. 7.27A). This material is beneficial because of its sealing ability and biocompatibility. In 1878, Witte published a case report in Germany on using Portland cement to fill root canals; however, Portland cement–type materials were not used in common practice until the 1990s. The first product, called **mineral trioxide aggregate (MTA)**, is made of a hydraulically active powder that combines calcium oxide (calcia, CaO), aluminum oxide (alumina, Al_2O_3), and silicone dioxide (silica, SiO_2) into hydraulically active ceramic compound.

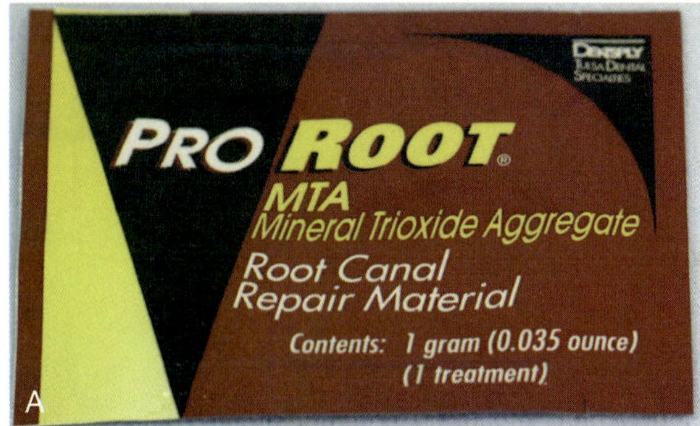

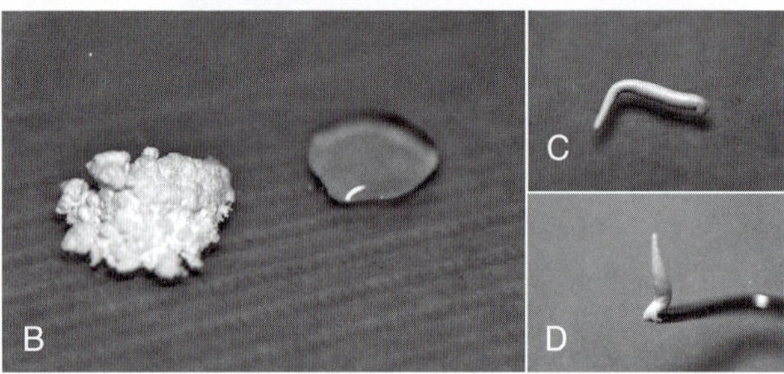

• **Fig. 7.27** Manipulation of MTA. **(A)** A package of MTA powder. **(B)** Powder and water on a glass slab ready for hand mixing. **(C)** The mixture should exhibit a putty-like consistency as it is rolled into a log. **(D)** The log can be cut into suitable pieces for placement.

Chemistry and Setting

The essential phases of MTA cement powder are tricalcium silicate, dicalcium silicate, and radiopaque filler. Usually minor phases of tricalcium aluminate and calcium sulfate (Table 7.13) are present. Some MTA-type products contain calcium carbonate or tetracalcium aluminoferrite. MTA has been denigrated in the literature as expensive Portland cement because the same phases are present in both materials; however, MTA-type products contain a radiopaque agent—usually bismuth oxide, zirconia, or tantalum oxide—without which MTA would not be distinguishable on a radiograph. The term *MTA* is used here to denote all of the tricalcium and dicalcium silicate products.

MTA sets by reaction with water (Fig. 7.27B) and forms a highly alkaline (pH about 12) cement composed of a rigid matrix of calcium silicate hydrate and calcium hydroxide. These hydrates form on the surface of the original calcium silicate particles and hydration gradually progresses inward. The setting time for MTA is lengthy, about 165 minutes for the initial set and less than 6 hours for the final set, which is a major drawback to using this cement. When MTA sets, it expands less than 0.1%, which helps to create a barrier that is especially important for endodontics.

After mixing with water, the pH of MTA cement rises rapidly by the release of calcium hydroxide. The remarkable success of MTA as a biocompatible material has been attributed to the calcium hydroxide in the set MTA, which makes the material antibacterial and antifungal. For example, MTA cement is less cytotoxic than GIC, and hydroxyapatite crystals form on the surface of MTA in vitro with a phosphate-buffered saline, making this cement uniquely bioactive. Cementum-like layers have formed over root ends where MTA has been used for endodontic surgeries.

New formulations are being introduced that include polymers, salts (especially calcium chloride), and water-reducing agents to improve handling and to shorten the setting time for MTA products. Such products will expand the indications and utility of these calcium silicate powders.

TABLE 7.13 Phases in MTA-Type Powders Before Hydration

Ceramic Phases	Wt%
Tricalcium silicate: $(CaO)_3 \bullet SiO_2$	45–75
Dicalcium silicate: $(CaO)_2 \bullet SiO_2$	7–32
Radiopaque filler: Bi_2O_3 or Ta_2O_5	20–35
Tricalcium aluminate: $(CaO)_3 \bullet Al_2O_3$	0–13
Tetracalcium aluminoferrite: $(CaO)_4 \bullet Al_2O_3 \bullet Fe_2O_3$	0–18
Gypsum: $CaSO_4 \bullet 2H_2O$	2–10

Clinical Manipulation

MTA was first used for root apex filling in endodontic surgeries, but its indications have expanded to include procedures for **vital pulp therapy** (pulp capping and pulpotomy dressing) and procedures that contact the periradicular tissues, such as root-end filling, apexification, perforation repair, root resorption repair, obturation, and root canal sealing. Because it is caustic, MTA should not be allowed to stay in contact with the mucosa because the high pH can cause a superficial lesion. Excess material should be removed from the oral cavity.

MTA will set over a wide range of P/L ratio, roughly between 4:1 and 2:1, although most products employ a P/L ratio of 3:1. To mix MTA, the powder should be dispensed onto a glass slab, with a drop of the liquid from the kit next to the powder. A stiff metal spatula should be used to incorporate the powder gradually into the liquid until a putty-like consistency is reached (Fig. 7.27C). Thorough mixing and repeated spatulation should be performed. The mixed material can be formed and rolled into a "log" with gloved fingers (Fig. 7.27D); then the spatula can be used to cut off small sections for insertion in a root-end filling or a perforation site. A spatula, a small amalgam carrier, or a condenser is commonly used to transport the MTA delicately into the surgical location. If mixed MTA is not used immediately, a moist gauze "tent" can be placed over the material to prevent dehydration. If drying occurs, the material can be reconstituted with water within the first hour because its setting time is so long. If hemorrhage is not controlled before placement, MTA may be discolored by blood seeping into the MTA material via capillary action as it gradually sets. Inhomogeneity of the radiopaque phases has been noted in some MTA products, and other MTA products have coarse powders. The products are evolving in the marketplace and improving.

Thorough flushing of root canal irrigants should be performed before placing an MTA mixture. Common canal irrigants and debridement preparations often contain ethylenediaminetetraacetic acid (EDTA) or other organic acids that partially dissolve and impair the seal of MTA by the chelation of EDTA to the calcium in MTA.

Endodontic Applications

MTA cement is starting to replace the use of calcium hydroxide for certain indications in endodontics. For long calcium hydroxide powder has been used as a disinfectant material for apexification when the tooth necrosed before the root was completely formed. In these cases, the dressing is used to allow the tooth to remain in place and encourage normal root development. The apexification procedure removes the pulp, cleans and shapes the root canal, removes the smear layer, disinfects the canal, and concludes by placing calcium hydroxide to promote osteocementum at the apex. The calcium hydroxide powder can plug the tubules and neutralize acid, minimize adverse pulpal responses, help dissolve residual tissue after debridement, and induce a calcified apical tissue barrier that allows a deciduous tooth to remain in place and the apex to finish development. MTA has been used for apexification of immature roots instead of $Ca(OH)_2$ because it facilitates development of normal periradicular architecture by inducing hard tissue barriers.

Calcium hydroxide is also used as a dressing after vital pulpotomy procedures in primary teeth and as a temporary intracanal medicament during root canal therapy. MTA and tricalcium phosphate (TCP) slurries have also been used for these indications.

Pulp Capping

For treating pulp exposures, the consistency of MTA can be more fluid. Hemorrhage should be controlled by pressure on the exposure site with a cotton pellet moistened with saline, a dilute solution of sodium hypochlorite (0.5%–1.0%), or a commercially available mild hemostatic agent. The material can be applied with a Dycal instrument or other similar instrument to access the area. A hybrid ionomer liner or flowable compomer may be placed and light cured over MTA and the immediately surrounding dentin. The remaining preparation can be acid etched, followed by placing an adhesive and a resin-based composite. Resin-based composite or an interim glass ionomer can be placed directly over MTA; however, etchant should not be applied on the MTA because acid destroys the integrity of the material and prevents MTA from setting. The pulp should be periodically assessed for its responsiveness, as indicated by a dentinal barrier forming adjacent to the MTA cement.

Compatibility with Restorative Materials

Research has shown that GIC placed over the setting MTA does not affect the setting of the MTA even though a calcium salt formed at the interface. No change was observed in the setting time, susceptibility to crazing of the GIC, or the shear bond strength between glass ionomer and MTA. A study of the bonding of resin-based composite and compomer to MTA, which had set for 48 hours in a moist condition, shows that the use of total-etch single-bottle bonding agent yields a higher bond strength. The results may differ from one brand of material to another; more studies are needed to confirm these effects.

Mechanical Properties

The hydration reactions of MTA continue for about 28 days, while the strength increases over this period to about 50 MPa. Its 24-hour compressive strength is significantly less than that of amalgam, ZOE intermediate-type restorations, and ZOE-ethoxybenzoic acid materials. However, after 3 weeks, no significant differences were measured in compressive strength between ZOE, calcium hydroxide, and MTA cements. Flexural strength is not usually measured for such ceramic materials and is low for MTA compared with metals or resin composites. The bond strength of MTA to endodontic post materials is not high and MTA should not be used for post retention. Set MTA is quite insoluble and has low setting expansion, a property required by ISO 6876 for root canal sealers (<3% solubility and <0.01% expansion after 30 days).

Biodentine

Biodentine is a calcium silicate-based material which is touted as a dentine substitute which is bioactive and favorable for pulpal heath and healing. The powder consists of tricalcium silicate, dicalcium silicate, calcium carbonate and oxide filler, iron oxide shade, and zirconium oxide. Tricalcium silicate and dicalcium silicate are the core materials and zirconium oxide serves as a radiopacifier. The liquid, contains calcium chloride as an accelerator and a hydrosoluble polymer that serves as a water reducing agent. It has a fast setting time, due to the increase in particle size, adding calcium chloride to the liquid component, and decreasing the liquid content. The setting period of the material is as short as 9–12 minutes.

Setting Reaction

Just after mixing, the calcium silicate particles of Biodentine react with water to from a high pH solution containing Ca^{2+}, OH^-, and silicate ions. The hydration of the tricalcium silicate leads to the formation of a hydrated calcium silicate gel on the cement particles and calcium hydroxide nucleates. With the passage of time, calcium silicate hydrated gel polymerizes to form a solid network and the alkalinity of the surrounding medium increases due to the release of calcium hydroxide ions. Further the hydrated calcium silicate gel surrounds the unreacted tricalcium silicate particles and due to its relatively impermeable nature to water, it helps in slow down the effects of further reactions. The complete reaction can be summarized as:

$$2(3CaO.SiO2) + 6H2O \rightarrow 3CaO.2SiO2.3H2O + 3Ca\ (OH)2$$

An interesting clinical and histological study performed on molars to be extracted for orthodontic reasons showed that Biodentine had a similar efficacy to MTA in clinical setting and may well be regarded as an alternative for pulp capping procedures. Biodentine showed complete dentinal bridge formation and no inflammatory response (Nowicka, 2013).

Relatively easier manipulation, low cost, and faster setting are the major advantages of this material when compared to MTA. Studies have also proved that its compressive and flexural strength are superior to that of MTA. High biocompatibility and excellent bioactivity further go in favor of this dental replacement material.

Calcium Phosphate Cements

Calcium phosphate cements are combinations of dicalcium phosphate dihydrate, dicalcium phosphate anhydrous, TCP, and tetracalcium phosphate that are mixed with an aqueous solution saturated with calcium phosphate, an organic acid, or a solution of polymers. An example is Sankin Apatite Root Canal Sealer (Dentsply Sankin, Tokyo, Japan).

The cement pastes gradually set and form hydroxyapatite. The calcium phosphate phases dissolve in the liquid and precipitate a less soluble calcium phosphate, which "sets" at 37°C, with some poorly crystalline hydroxyapatite being formed. The cements are suitable bone-substitute materials because they are gradually resorbed. They can sometimes be used in place of granular hydroxyapatite. However, their washout and low strength are problematic.

Experimental formulas of calcium phosphate base and liner products have been made that include polymerizable resins and additives in the liquid phase. The resins allow water diffusion that facilitates the conversion of calcium phosphate to hydroxyapatite. Clinical studies show that the caries-affected dentin underneath this cement had significantly more calcium and phosphorus content to a depth of 30 μm, and the mineral content was in the range of healthy dentin after 3 months. Research continues to investigate such biocompatible materials for pulpal protection and endodontic indications.

Endodontic Sealers

Endodontic sealers are specialized versions of dental cement (Fig. 7.28) that are used during **obturation** with gutta-percha to fill voids and promote a close seal between the core and the dentinal walls of the canal, preventing or minimizing leakage, entombing residual microorganisms, and preferably filling areas of the root canal system that are inaccessible by instrumentation. The requirements for the ideal root canal sealer are listed in Box 7.4, and the ISO 6876 requirements are shown in Table 7.14. Several dental cements have been adapted for this specialized use; the most popular are ZOE-based sealers. ZOE sealers are inexpensive, are slow setting, and have a long history of acceptable clinical use. However, the newer epoxy-based sealers are radiopaque and more biocompatible than ZOE. Polyvinylsiloxane (PVS) sealers are also available as powder–liquid and two-paste systems. GIC and resin-modified GICs have also been used. A filled biodegradable thermoplastic polymer, Resilon (Resilon Research LLC, Madison, CT), along with a resin-based sealer, Epiphany (Pentron Clinical Technologies, Wallingford, CT), was introduced in the 1990s. This system claimed to have less leakage than the traditional gutta-percha with sealer but performed poorly over time as a result of degradation of the polymer matrix. Another system uses gutta-percha cones that are coated with a proprietary resin coating (EndoRez, Ultradent, South Jordan, UT) for use in combination with a methacrylate-based, dual-cured resin sealer and no dentin-bonding agent. In this case the endodontic seal is dependent on the penetration of the hydrophilic sealer into the dentinal tubules and lateral canals following removal of the smear layer.

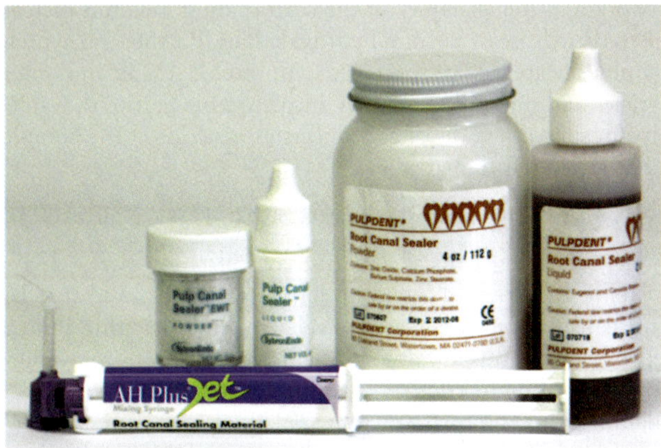

• **Fig. 7.28** Root canal sealers. The two materials in the back are powder–liquid systems. The dual cartridge syringe in the foreground is a paste–paste system with static mixing tip.

TABLE 7.14 ISO 6876 and ADA 57 Requirements for Endodontic Sealers

Property	Requirement
Flow (mm)	>17
Working time	To be stated by manufacturer in minutes or hours
Setting time	To be stated by manufacturer in minutes or hours
Maximum film thickness (μm)	50
Solubility (%)	<3
Radiopacity (mm of equivalent Al)	>3
Dimensional stability (ADA 57 only)	less than 0.1% expansion, less than 1% shrinkage

• BOX 7.4 Endodontic Sealer Criteria

Endodontic sealers should have the following characteristics:

- Make a hermetic seal
- Be tacky when mixed to provide good adhesion with the canal wall when set
- Contain particles of powder that are very fine so that they can mix easily with liquid, where appropriate
- Be radiopaque for visualization on a radiograph
- Not shrink upon setting
- Not discolor tooth structure
- Be bacteriostatic or at least not encourage bacterial growth
- Set slowly
- Be insoluble in tissue fluids
- Be well tolerated by the periapical tissue (and also not provoke an immune response, be mutagenic, or carcinogenic)
- Be soluble in common solvents, if necessary, to remove the root canal filling

In the long, narrow space of the root canal, the application of any bonding system to form a uniform interface is challenging. For example, in bonding systems that contain volatile solvents, evaporation might be hindered. The canal anatomy is not only problematic to adhesive root canal obturation but also for the bonding of prefabricated posts. A further problem is that some irrigating solutions (e.g. sodium hypochlorite) and intracanal medicaments have adverse effects on root canal dentin collagen and the longevity of endodontic bonding. Unlike other cements, endodontic sealers are not light cured because of the inability to complete the curing in the depths of a root canal (~2 cm), the complex anatomy of intercommunicating canals, and the inaccessible locations often in the posterior.

The configuration of the root canal also presents a high "C-factor" (Chapter 5) because a nonbonded area of the cement layer exists within the bonded canal. Thus a resin endodontic sealer is subjected to severe stresses induced by the sealer's polymerization shrinkage during setting. Debonding and gaps may occur between the sealer and dentin wall or in between the solid core material and the sealer along the periphery of the root canal obturation.

The newest category of endodontic sealers incorporates bioactive cements, such as Total Fill, Edge Endo, iRoot ES, and Endosequence BC Sealer. These materials are a single paste of tricalcium/dicalcium silicate powders suspended in organic liquids. Such sealers have a low setting expansion of 0.2% as a result of hydration-forming hydroxyapatite. Many sealers have shrinkage of 6% or higher, which leads to interface separation, whereas even a small expansion promotes hermetic interface sealing.

Resin-based sealers with bioactive fillers dispersed in the resin may not have the same bioactive effect as the single-paste sealer. The resins coat the bioactive particles and interfere with the release of calcium and hydroxide ions.

Fluoride-Releasing Materials

The anticariogenic potential of silicate cement confirms the ability of F^- to inhibit demineralization, leading to the development of several fluoride-containing restorative materials and cements: conventional glass ionomers, RMGI, polyacid-modified composites (compomers), composites, and even amalgams. For the fluorosilicate glass−based materials, fluoride is first released to the matrix from the glass during the acid–base reaction and then to the oral cavity over time. For composite and amalgam, the fillers—such as inorganic salts, leachable glasses, and organic fluoride compounds—incorporated in the material dissolve partially upon contact with water and diffuse into the material to provide the fluoride for release. The rate of fluoride release depends on the cement matrix, porosity, and nature of the fluoridated filler (i.e. type, amount, particle size, and silane treatment). Fig. 7.29 illustrates the typical behavior of fluoride release from dental materials.

Factors Affecting Fluoride Release In Vitro

Fluoride release studies are usually conducted in vitro, where the experimental conditions can be controlled and the fluoride is easier to measure. Also, intrinsic characteristics of the material—such as formulas, filler compositions, ratio of component mixing, mixing procedure, and curing time—can be studied more easily. For such in vitro tests the protocols have varied in terms of the composition and pH of storage media, frequency of the storage solution change, and plaque and pellicle formation.

The kinetics of fluoride release are similar among all materials, although composite and amalgam have much lower release levels than those from glass ionomer−based materials. When the demineralization–**remineralization** cycle was used, a higher fluoride release in an acidic medium was observed. Ion-enriched (ions other than F^-) storage media, such as artificial saliva, reduced the release. The presence of esterase or hydrolases in the storage media or on the surface of the material can increase the release further. Removal of the outer layer of compomers by air polishing or finishing was found to restore fluoride release near their initial release rates resulting from exposure of new surfaces. However, simulated toothbrushing with nonfluoridated dentifrice showed no changes in fluoride release, indicating insignificant change of the surface by toothbrushing.

Fluoride Recharging

In vitro data have shown that fluoride release from glass ionomer remains detectable for years, although the rate of release is reduced by a factor of 10 within the first few months (see Fig. 7.29A). To boost fluoride release from existing restoratives, recharging with fluoride has been suggested. The most common recharging method is to expose the restorative to a concentrated fluoride agent in the range of 0.02% for a NaF solution (90 ppm) to 1.23% acidulated phosphate fluoride (APF, 12,300 ppm) for 4–5 minutes. The ability of a restorative material to be recharged and serve as a fluoride reservoir depends on the type and permeability of the material, the frequency of fluoride exposure, and the concentration of the fluoridating agent. For example, recharging

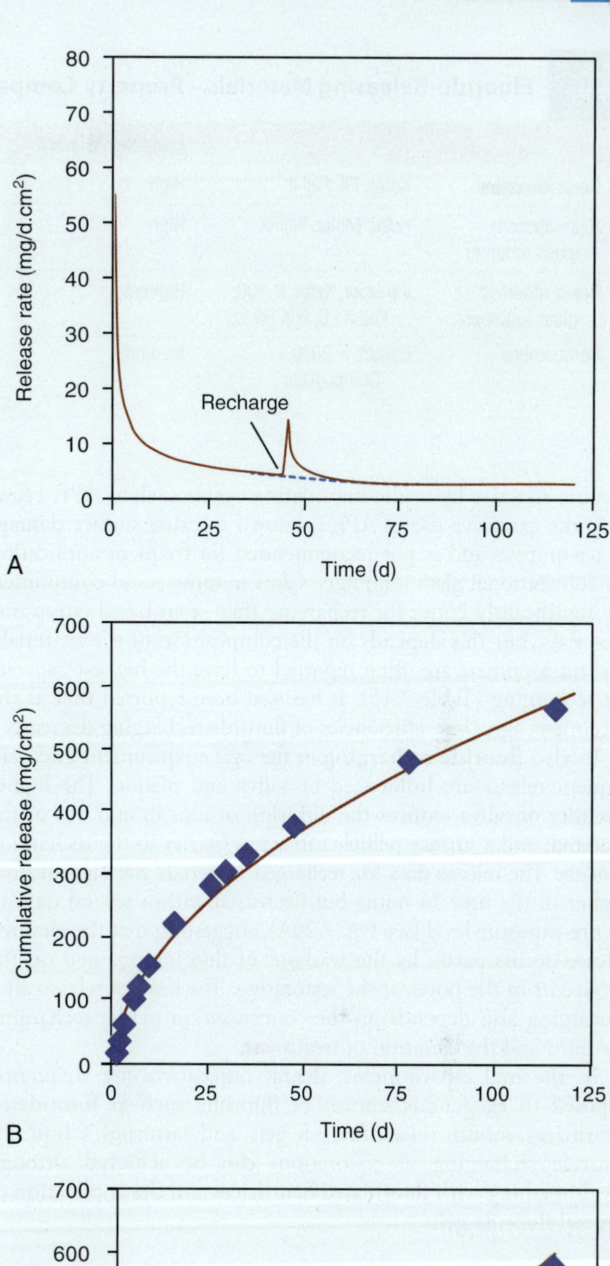

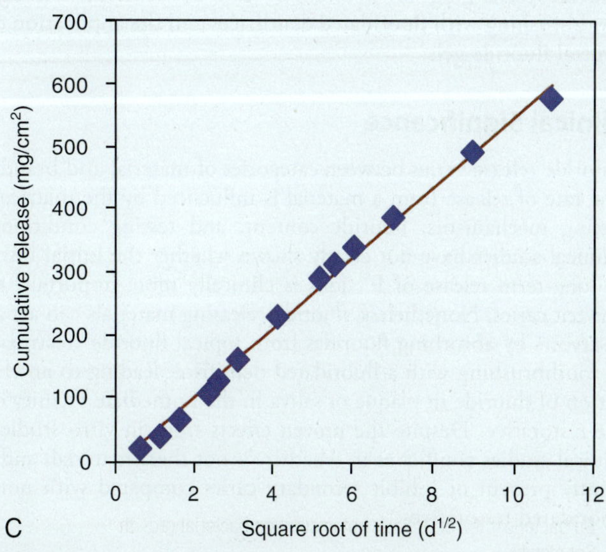

• **Fig. 7.29** Typical fluoride-release profiles. **(A)** Release rate versus time; the spike reflects fluoride recharging and the blue dotted line represents the fluoride release where no recharging has occurred. **(B)** Cumulative release over time; the diamonds are experimental data of **(A)** without recharging, and the curve is the best-fit curve of Y (total release) = a + b•(time)$^{1/2}$. **(C)** The same data in **(B)** plotted against square root of time; it reveals a linear relationship. The effect of recharging is not shown in **(B)** or **(C)**.

TABLE 7.15 **Fluoride-Releasing Materials – Property Comparisons**

		Fluoride Release	Bond Strength	Strength	Wear Resistance	Fluoride Recharge
Glass ionomers	Ketac-Fil, Fuji II	High	Low	Low	Low	Medium
High-viscosity glass ionomer	Ketac Molar, Fuji IX	High	Medium	Medium	Medium	Medium
Resin-modified glass ionomers	Vitremer, Ketac N 100, Fuji II LC, Fuji Fill LC	Highest	Medium	Low	Low–medium	Highest
Compomers	Dyract, F-2000, Compoglass	Medium	High	Medium	Medium	Medium

is more effective by acidic fluoridating agents such as APF. However, the extensive use of APF is known to cause surface damage of restoratives and is not recommended for frequent application on conventional glass ionomers. Glass ionomers and compomers are significantly better for recharging than resin-based composite materials, but this depends on the composition of the materials. Hybrid ionomers are often reported to have the highest capacity for recharging (Table 7.15). It has also been reported that as the specimens age, their efficiencies of fluoride recharging decrease.

In vivo **fluoride recharging** in the oral environment and subsequent release are influenced by saliva and plaque. The higher viscosity of saliva reduces the diffusion of ions in and out of the material, and a surface pellicle can act as barrier to the recharging process. The release data for recharged materials was significantly higher in the first 24 hours but decreased within several days to its pre-exposure level (see Fig. 7.29A), suggesting that the elevated release occurs partly by the washout of fluoride retained on the surface or in the pores of the restorative. The level of release after recharging also depends on the concentration of the recharging medium and the duration of treatment.

In the oral environment, dental restoratives are frequently exposed to exogenous sources of fluoride, such as fluoridated dentifrices, mouth rinses, fluoride gels, and varnishes. Clinically, fluoride recharging of restorations can be achieved through toothbrushing with fluoridated dentifrices and the application of neutral fluoride gels.

Clinical Significance

Fluoride release varies between categories of material and brands. The rate of release from a material is influenced by the matrices, setting mechanisms, fluoride content, and testing conditions. Clinical studies have not clearly shown whether the initial burst or long-term release of F^- ions is clinically more important to prevent caries. Nonetheless, fluoride-releasing materials can act as reservoirs by absorbing fluorides from topical fluoride treatment or toothbrushing with a fluoridated dentifrice, leading to an elevation of fluoride in plaque or saliva in the immediate vicinity of the restorative. Despite the proven effects from in vitro studies, clinical studies conflict as to whether or not these materials sufficiently prevent or inhibit secondary caries compared with nonfluoridated restoratives.

Solubility and Disintegration of Cements

Cements in the oral environment are continually exposed to a variety of acids produced by microorganisms or consumed in foods and drinks. A number of procedures have been used to assess the relative resistance of various cements to degradation in the mouth. ANSI/ADA Specification No. 96 (ISO 9917-1) describes the use of 0.1 M lactic acid/sodium lactate (pH 2.74) to test the erosion rate of glass ionomer, zinc polycarboxylate, and zinc phosphate cements. The depth at the center of each sample after 24 hours of immersion is measured and the value of eroded depth in millimeters per hour is calculated. The procedure described in ISO 4049 measures the weight (mg) and volume (mm^3) of the specimen before immersion in water and the weight of the specimen after 5 days of immersion and desiccation. The solubility is calculated by dividing the weight changes by the volume. A third method used in ANSI/ADA Specification No. 30 and No. 57 (ISO 6876) specifies measurement of specimen weight before 24 hours of immersion in water and weight of the residue after the water in the eluted solution has evaporated. The weight percentage is then reported.

To make the solubility results clinically relevant, various testing conditions—such as varying the pH of storage media between 3 and 10, the concentration of electrolytes of the storage media, the powder–liquid ratio of the material, and extended observation period 30 days or longer—have been used and each condition is found to have a statistically significant influence on solubility. Because of water sorption, some specimens have shown a negative solubility (weight gain) within the duration of the test. Several studies have reported that there is no correlation between solubility data from acidic erosion and weight loss. The vast amount of in vitro data shows that cement solubility differs among categories of materials and may be product specific. Therefore, the clinical relevance of in vitro solubility data is not clear.

Calcium hydroxide, ZOE, and early formulations of glass ionomer−based endodontic sealer often exhibited solubility near the maximum specified in the standards. However, despite their high solubility in laboratory tests, ZOE-based root canal sealers have been used successfully for decades in endodontics. Other sealers based on epoxy, PVS, new GIC, and polyketone all show significantly lower solubility than ZOE. A resin-based, calcium-hydroxide-containing cavity liner was found to be less soluble than its conventional counterparts. These results show that the cement's matrix phases derived from acid–base reactions exhibited higher solubility than those resulting from resin polymerization.

For the aqueous-based cements, the solubility increases in order as follows: conventional GIC, zinc phosphate cement, and polycarboxylate cement, although some studies reported no difference between zinc phosphate and polycarboxylate cements. The presence of polymerizing monomers reduces the solubility of hybrid glass ionomer relative to that of conventional GIC. Fully set RMGI cements have higher strength and lower early solubility than those of conventional glass ionomer. Acid impingement studies showed that erosion after 24 hours in 0.1 M lactic acid decreased in the following order: zinc phosphate, conventional GIC, and hybrid GIC to compomer.

Resin cements are the least soluble of all dental cements. It appears that the solubility is inversely proportional to the resin content, especially for hydrophobic resins. As for glass ionomer, the tooth preparation should be well isolated and saliva must not contact the cement for 7–10 minutes to minimize the loss by solubility of the cement at the margins.

In addition to the in vitro tests described earlier, the durability of cementing agents has been obtained in situ by placing small specimens of the cements in intraoral appliances that can be removed from the mouth to measure the loss of material. In one study cements were inserted in tiny wells placed in the proximal surfaces of cast crown restorations. These crowns were cemented with temporary ZOE cement. After 1 year, the crowns were removed and the cement loss was measured. GIC exhibited the least degradation, followed by zinc polycarboxylate cement, zinc phosphate cement, and zinc polycarboxylate cement mixed in a lower P/L ratio. The relative disintegration rates of the cements apparently bear no relationship to the solubility data presented in Table 7.3. The solubility of zinc polycarboxylate cement mixed at the recommended P/L ratio and zinc phosphate cement was not significantly different. However, a reduction of powder in the zinc polycarboxylate mixture produced a cement that disintegrated rapidly.

No single cement is applicable for all indications in dentistry. Prudent dentists have several types of cements in their armamentarium. Manufacturers' formulas and processes dictate most cement characteristics, but the clinician has some control over the handling, setting, and to some degree, the biocompatibility through the mixing ratios or technique.

The historic zinc phosphate cement has fallen out of use, but ZOE cements are used for luting, for temporary restorations, and for retaining fixed prostheses on implant-supported abutments, which facilitate retrievability of the prostheses. Zinc polycarboxylate cements are noninjurious to the pulp and adhesive to tooth structure, but they are not commonly used because of their short working time and viscous nature.

GICs work well for orthodontic bands and cementing of metal crowns on primary teeth. The fluoride-releasing capability makes GIC the material of choice for the replacement of restorations that have failed because of recurrent caries and for patients living in areas where fluoridated drinking water is not available. A primary disadvantage of GICs is the slow maturing process that is required to develop their highest strength.

Resin cements are insoluble in oral fluids, and their fracture toughness is higher than that of other cements. Resin cements can be used for all types of cementation, most notably for prostheses with poor retention, and for all-ceramic prostheses where the esthetic demand is very high. Resin cements require bonding agents to be effective. Etching may be required to obtain a strong attachment to enamel with bonding agents. Self-etching and self-adhesive resin cements are now available.

Hybrid ionomer cements are used as a liner, fissure sealant, and base material and in core buildups and orthodontic band cementation. Compomers are used for cementing metallic prostheses and some restorative indications. The durability of compomers is inferior to that of resin-based composites; thus, they should only be used for low-stress areas.

Glass-ionomer, polycarboxylate, and resin cements adhere chemically and physically to the surrounding surfaces. Excess cement should be removed as soon as the seating is completed to prevent adhesion to the exterior of the prostheses or surrounding teeth. A separating medium, such as petroleum jelly, spread on external and surrounding surfaces inhibits cement adherence, making cement removal easier when these cements fully set.

The important properties of cements for adhering devices are summarized in Table 7.16. A high elastic modulus was important for gold alloy restorations, and a lower elastic modulus is needed under ceramic restorations.

Pulp capping and cavity liners/base materials are important for pulpal health and protection from acidic cements. GICs elicit a greater pulpal reaction than ZOE cement but less than zinc phosphate cement. Calcium hydroxide and tricalcium silicate products are important for direct or indirect pulpal protection. These bioactive materials initiate subgingival or pulpal tissue healing, although the tricalcium silicates are superseding calcium hydroxide products, especially for pulpotomies.

Calcium aluminate GIC relies on the GIC to establish the early strength and the hydration of calcium aluminate for final properties and bioactivity. New formulas of cements are anticipated, based on calcium aluminates and pozzolanic cements. The latter cement is based on silicic acid reacting with calcium hydroxide, often called *Roman cement.*

Specialty areas of dentistry, such as orthodontics and endodontics, use variations of the cements discussed to achieve the unique needs for their procedures. Endodontic cement formulas include ZOE, epoxy, polyvinyl siloxane, and now the tricalcium silicates. The tricalcium silicates are used surgically and nonsurgically, depending on the viscosity of the cement used.

TABLE 7.16 Properties of Cements for Affixing Devices

Cement Type	Setting Time (min)	Film Thickness (μm)	24-h Compressive Strength (MPa)	24-h Diametral Tensile Strength (MPa)	Elastic Modulus (GPa)	Solubility in Water (wt%)
Zinc phosphate	5.5	20	104	5.5	13.5	0.06
ZOE (type I)	4.0–10	25	6–28	—	—	0.04
ZOE–EBA (type II)	9.5	25	55	4.1	5.0	0.05
ZOE + polymer (type II)	6.0–10	32	48	4.1	2.5	0.08
Zinc polycarboxylate	6.0	21	55	6.2	5.1	0.06
Glass ionomer	7.0	24	86	6.2	7.3	1.25
Resin	2.0–4.0	<25	70–172	—	2.1–3.1	0–0.01

EBA, ethoxybenzoic acid; ZOE, zinc oxide–eugenol.

Cements for dentistry continue to evolve and improve in their insolubility, sealing, esthetics, bonding, and durability. Filler particles, usually glass, continue to move to smaller sizes. *Nanoparticles* is now a commonly used term, which usually means silica particles are included, but the material may include other fillers that have some portion of particles finer than 0.1 μm (100 nm). New adhesive polymers and refinement of the fillers will continue to help dentists minimize tissue destruction and maximize preservation.

Acknowledgment

We thank Dr Jesper Lööf for reviewing and providing valuable information for the section on calcium aluminate glass ionomer cement.

Summary

- **Dental cements** are materials that set intraorally and are commonly used to join a tooth and a prosthesis, to protect the pulp or to restore a cavity.
- **Classification based on usage**
  - **Luting cements**
  - **Cements for pulp protection**
  - **Restorative cements**
- **Cements for luting**
- **Cavity varnishes**
- **Cavity liners**
  - **Calcium hydroxide** is the chief ingredient in many cavity liners and cement base materials because calcium hydroxide is antimicrobial, has an elevated pH (basic, alkaline), and stimulates the formation of secondary dentin over an injured pulp to protect it over the long term.
  - As a **cavity liner**, the calcium hydroxide powder is suspended in a solvent carrier with a thickening agent. When it is placed on the pulpal floor, the solvent evaporates and leaves a thin film of calcium hydroxide.
- **Cement bases**
- **Cements for restoratives**
  - **Zinc phosphate cement**
- **Zinc polycarboxylate cement**
  - The polycarboxylate cements are powder–liquid systems that set by an acid–base reaction.
  - The liquid is a water solution of polyacrylic acid or a copolymer of acrylic acid with other carboxylic acids, such as itaconic acid.
  - The powder contains mainly zinc oxide with some magnesia, tin oxide, bismuth oxide, and/or alumina.
  - The outstanding characteristic of zinc polycarboxylate cement is its chemical bond to tooth structure.
  - Polycarboxylate cements produce minimal irritation to the pulp.
- **Glass ionomer cement (GIC)**
  - GIC is the generic name for materials based on the reaction of glass powder and polyacrylic acid.
  - The use of polyacrylic acid makes GIC capable of bonding to tooth structure.
  - The glass composition in GIC varies among manufacturers, but it always contains silica, calcia, alumina, and fluoride.
  - The liquids are copolymers of itaconic, maleic, or tricarboxylic acids.
- Tricalcium silicate cement sets by reaction with water to form a rigid matrix of calcium silicate hydrates with embedded calcium hydroxide.
- **Mineral trioxide aggregate cements**
  - The essential phases of MTA cement powder are tricalcium silicate, dicalcium silicate, and radiopaque filler.
  - MTA sets by reaction with water and forms a highly alkaline (pH about 12) cement composed of a rigid matrix of calcium silicate hydrate and calcium hydroxide.
  - MTA cement is starting to replace the use of calcium hydroxide for certain indications in endodontics.
- The GICs are classified as:
  - Type I: Luting crowns, bridges, and orthodontic brackets
  - Type IIa: Esthetic restorative cements
  - Type IIb: Reinforced restorative cements
  - Type III: Lining cements, base.
- **Resin-modified glass ionomer cement (hybrid ionomer)**
- **Calcium aluminate glass ionomer cements**
  - A hybrid product with a composition between that of calcium aluminate and GIC, designed for luting fixed prostheses, is a new addition to the family of GICs.
  - The main ingredients in the powder of this hybrid cement are calcium aluminate, polyacrylic acid, tartaric acid, strontium-fluoro-alumino glass, and strontium fluoride.
  - The liquid component contains 99.6% water and 0.4% additives for controlling setting.
- **Compomer**
- **Resin cements**
- **Classification: based on adhesive scheme**
  - Etch-and-rinse resin cements
  - Self-etch resin cements
  - Self-adhesive resin cements
- **Classification: based on polymerization mechanism**
  - Light-cure resin cements
  - Dual-cure resin cements
  - Chemical-cure resin cements
- **Zinc oxide**–eugenol cement
  - ZOE cement is commonly used for luting and intermediate restorations because of its medicament quality and neutral pH.
  - The powder contains zinc oxide particles and the liquid is eugenol. For the two-paste system, the base paste contains zinc oxide powder and the eugenol is contained in the accelerator (or catalyst).
  - Tricalcium/dicalcium silicate cement: Dental cements based on tricalcium and dicalcium silicates (*tricalcium silicate,* for short) are beneficial because of their sealing ability, biocompatibility, and bioactivity.
  - These hydraulic cements need water to set, which is ever present in the oral cavity.
  - The essential components of these bioactive cements are tricalcium silicate and dicalcium silicate ceramic powders blended with inert radiopaque powders, usually bismuth oxide, zirconia, calcium tungstate, barium zirconate, or tantalum oxide.

Review Questions

1. Classify dental cements. Give the composition, setting action, and properties of zinc oxide–eugenol cement.
2. Classify dental cements. Discuss composition, properties, and uses of zinc phosphate cement.
3. Enumerate various cements used in dentistry mentioning their special uses. Discuss the composition and setting reaction of zinc phosphate cement.
4. Classify dental cements. Discuss composition, properties, and advantages of zinc polycarboxylate cement.
5. Describe the composition, setting and bonding reactions, properties and uses of zinc polycarboxylate cement.
6. Classify dental cements. Discuss in detail glass ionomer cements.
7. Enumerate various cements used in dentistry mentioning their special uses. Discuss composition and properties of GI cement.
8. Discuss in detail the composition, setting reaction, and bonding of tooth enamel and dentin of GIC. Add a note on modified GICs.
9. Classify dental cements. Discuss composition and properties and advantages of GI cement.
10. Compare the physical properties of ZnOE, $ZnPO_4$, and GIC cements.
11. Discuss agents of pulp protection under metallic restorations.
12. Classify restorative materials and mention their ideal requirements.
13. Ideal requirements of luting agents.
14. Modified zinc oxide–eugenol cements.
15. Intermediate restorations.
16. What are anhydrous or water settable GICs?
17. ASPA cement.
18. Anticariogenic properties of GIC.
19. Resin-modified GICs.
20. Enumerate different materials which can be used as base materials.
21. Cavity liners and bases.
22. Root canal sealers.
23. Describe the composition, advantages, and disadvantages of calcium hydroxide base.
24. Discuss in brief recent advances in glass ionomer cements.
25. Sandwich technique.
26. Discuss in brief calcium silicate cements.

Selected Readings

Ambard A.J.; Mueninghoff L. Calcium phosphate cement: Review of mechanical and biological properties. J Prosthodont 15 321–328 (2006); This article offers a review of the literature on the use of calcium phosphate up to 2003.

Balderamos L.P.; O'Keefe K.L.; Powers J.M. Color accuracy of resin cements and try-in paste. Int J Prosthodont 10 111–115 (1997); Color readings by instrument showed there were significant differences in color between resin cements and their corresponding try-in pastes.

Behr M.; Rosentritt M.; Wimmer J.; et al. Self-adhesive resin cement versus zinc phosphate luting material: A prospective clinical trial begun 2003. Dent Mater 25 601–604 (2009); This study evaluates the performance of self-adhesive cements and shows that these cements have performed well over a period of 3 years.

Berekally T.L.; Makinson O.F.; Pietrobon R.A. A microscopic examination of bond surfaces in failed electrolytically etched cast metal fixed prostheses. Aust Dent J 38 229–237 (1993); The study shows that clinical failure of debonded electrolytically etched (Maryland) bridge retainers occurred mostly by resin failure within the cement layer close to the enamel-resin interface.

Chaar M.S.; Att W.; Strub J.R. Prosthetic outcome of cement-retained implant-supported fixed dental restorations: A systematic review. J Oral Rehab 38 697–711 (2011); This article concludes that cement-retained implant-supported fixed restorations are a reliable and effective option for single crowns and short-span FDPs but did not provide accurate information about the ideal type of cement for stability and retrievability.

Costa C.A.S.; Mesas A.N.; Hebling J. Pulp response to direct capping with an adhesive system. Am J Dent 13 81–87 (2000); This paper reports the effect of direct pulp capping with an adhesive system and a zinc oxide–eugenol cement (ZOE) in rat molar teeth. Both materials allowed pulp repair.

Crisp S.; Kent B.E.; Lewis B.G.; et al. Glass ionomer cement formulations. II. The synthesis of novel polycarboxylic acids. J Dent Res 59 1055–1063 (1980); The synthesis of many polycarboxylic acids is reported. A copolymer of acrylic and itaconic acids was found to combine several favorable characteristics.

In: (editors: Davidson C.L.; Mjör I.A.) Advances in Glass Ionomer Cements. Quintessence: Chicago; This book comprises 14 chapters covering such topics as chemistry, physical properties, bonding, fluoride release, and clinical applications.

Darvell BW: *Materials Science for Dentistry,* 10th ed, Woodhead Publishing, Duxford UK, 2018. An excellent resource on chemistry of dental materials.

Davidson CL, Mjör IA (editors): *Advances in Glass Ionomer Cements.* Chicago, Quintessence, 1999. Fourteen chapters covering such topics as chemistry, physical properties, bonding, fluoride release, and clinical applications.

Dickens-Venz S.H.; Takagi S.; Chow L.C.; et al. Dickens B: Physical and chemical properties of resin-reinforced calcium phosphate cements. Dent Mater 10 100–106 (1994); This article describes the formulation of a resin-modified calcium phosphate cement and the evaluation of its properties.

Duarte S. Jr/N; Sartori A.; Sadan J.-H.; Phark. Adhesive Resin Cements for Bonding Esthetic Restorations: A Review. Quintessence of Dental Technology Vol 34 (2011); This article reviews all the developments in resin cements and provides compositional details of most commercial formulations.

Forsten L. Fluoride release from a glass ionomer cement. Eur J Oral Sci 85 503–504 (1977); The author measured release of fluoride from a glass ionomer cement and a silicate cement. The fluoride release during the first 2 weeks was more than that during the subsequent 5 weeks. Slightly more fluoride was released from the glass ionomer cement than from the silicate.

Frencken J.E.; Taifour D.; van't Hof M.A. Survival of ART and amalgam restorations in permanent teeth of children after 6.3 years. J Dent Res 85 622–626 (2006); This study followed a total of 1117 single- and multiple-surface restorations made of amalgam and ART GIC. They concluded that the restorations produced with the ART approach survived longer than those produced with amalgam.

Goldman M. Fracture properties of composite and glass ionomer dental restorative materials. J Biomed Mater Res 19 771–783 (1985); This investigator found that metal-reinforced GIC exhibited a lower fracture toughness than that of composite resins, a reflection of materialist brittleness.

Hermansson L.; Faris A.; Gomez-Ortega G.; et al. Calcium-aluminate based dental luting cement with improved sealing properties: An overview. In: (editors: Narayan R.; Colombo P.; Mathur S.; Ohji T.)

Frencken J.E.; Taifour D.; van't Hof M.A. Survival of ART and amalgam restorations in permanent teeth of children after 6.3 years. J Dent Res 85 622–626 (2006); This study followed a total of 1117 single- and multiple-surface restorations made of amalgam and ART GIC. They concluded that the restorations produced with the ART approach survived longer than those produced with amalgam.

Goldman M. Fracture properties of composite and glass ionomer dental restorative materials. J Biomed Mater Res 19 771–783 (1985); This investigator found that metal-reinforced GIC exhibited a lower fracture toughness than that of composite resins, a reflection of materialist brittleness.

Hermansson L.; Faris A.; Gomez-Ortega G.; et al. Calcium-aluminate based dental luting cement with improved sealing properties: An overview. In: (editors: Narayan R.; Colombo P.; Mathur S.; Ohji T.) Advances in Bioceramics and Porous Ceramics III. 31, pp. 27–38; This paper discusses a Ca-aluminate-based bioceramic as a luting agent for the fixation of crowns and bridges and presents data on biocompatibility, sealing and integration mechanisms, leakage, compressive strength, and shear bond strength values.

Jefferies SR: Bioactive and biomimetic restorative materials: A comprehensive review, Part I. *J Esthet Restor Dent* 26:14-26, 2014. An informative paper on use of calcium aluminate cement for crowns.

Jefferies S.R.; Pameijer C.H.; Appleby D.C.; et al. Prospective observation of a new bioactive luting cement: 2-year follow-up. J Prosthodont 21 33–41 (2012); After periodic recalls up to 2 years, the new bioactive cement tested thus far has performed favorably as a luting agent for permanent cementation.

Kaur, M. (2017). "MTA versus Biodentine: Review of Literature with a Comparative Analysis." *Journal of Clinical and Diagnostic Research*.

Knibbs P.J.; Walls A.W.G. A laboratory and clinical evaluation of three dental luting cements. J Oral Rehabil 16 467–473 (1989); A number of studies such as this one have reported a poor correlation between in vitro and in vivo disintegration of different luting agents. The possible explanations are discussed.

Malkondu, O., et al. (2014). "A review on biodentine, a contemporary dentine replacement and repair material." *Biomed Res Int 1-10*

McKinney J.E.; Antonucci J.M.; Rupp N.W. Wear and microhardness of a silver-sintered glass ionomer cement. J Dent Res 67 831–835 (1988); This investigation showed reduced wear with a cermet ionomer as compared with an unfilled cement by test procedures designed to replicate masticatory wear patterns. It also suggests that silver might have provided a lubrication effect.

McLean J.W. Limitations of posterior composite resins and extending their use with glass ionomer cements. Quintessence Int 18 517–529 (1987); The advantages and disadvantages of composite resins versus glass ionomer cements in posterior situations are reviewed.

Mennemeyer V.A.; Neuman P.; Powers J.M. Bonding of hybrid ionomers and, resin cements to modified orthodontic band materials. Am J Orthod Dentofac Orthop 115 143–147 (1999); Air abrasion of band materials provides highly increased bond strength of hybrid ionomer and resin cements to metal except for the conventional glass ionomer.

Mitchell C.A.; Douglas W.H.; Cheng Y.S. Fracture toughness of conventional, resin-modified glass-ionomer and composite luting cements. Dent Mater 15 7–13 (1999); This study found that differences existed between the fracture toughness of the three types of luting cements and it describes the effect of mixing method.

Mount G.J. An Atlas of Glass Ionomer Cements—A Clinician's Guide. ed 3 Martin Dunitz: London; This book is an excellent step-by-step presentation of the clinical usage of the various GIC formulations.

Nicholson J.W. Polyacid-modified composite resins ("compomers") and their use in clinical dentistry. Dent Mater 23 615–622 (2007); This paper describes the chemistry and properties of compomers designed for use in clinical dentistry and reviews the literature in this area.

Pameijer C.H.; Nilner K. Long term clinical evaluation of three luting materials. Swed Dent J 18 59–67 (1994); Clinical evaluations up to 4 years show the three luting cements performed satisfactorily. The choice of a final luting agent should be based on anticipated postoperative pulpal reactions rather than exclusive reliance on physical properties.

Peters M.C.; Bresciani E.; Barata T.J.; et al. In vivo dentin remineralization by calcium-phosphate cement. J Dent Res 89 286–291 (2010); This clinical study reveals the capacity of a Ca-P base to promote remineralization of caries-affected dentin.

Phillips R.W.; Crim G.; Swartz M.L.; et al. Resistance of calcium hydroxide preparations to solubility in phosphoric acid. J Prosthet Dent 52 358–360 (1984); Newer "hard-setting" calcium hydroxide-based materials are less soluble in acid than earlier versions.

Phillips R.W.; Swartz M.L.; Lund M.S.; et al. In vivo disintegration of luting agents. J Am Dent Assoc 114 489–492 (1987); The in vivo solubility of a GIC was superior to either zinc phosphate or carboxylic cement.

Powis D.R.; Folleras T.; Merson S.A.; et al. Improved adhesion of a glass ionomer cement to dentin and enamel. J Dent Res 61 1416–1422 (1982); The first of many studies showing improvement in the bond strength of a glass ionomer cement to tooth structure when the smear layer is removed with polyacrylic acid.

Primus CM, Tay FR, Niu L-N: Bioactive tri/dicalcium silicate cements for treatment of pulpal and periapical tissues. *Acta Biomater* 96:35–54, 2019. A thorough review of the tricalcium silicate cements.

Sidhu S.K.; Watson T.F. Resin-modified glass ionomer materials: A status report for the *American Journal of Dentistry*. Am J Dent 8 59–67 (1995); This report describes the difference between conventional and early version of hybrid ionomers.

Smith D.C. Development of glass-ionomer cement systems. Biomaterials 19 467–478 (1998); This article reviews bonding of polyacrylic acid to backgrounds that led to the development of glass ionomer cement.

Smith D.C.; Ruse N.D. Acidity of glass ionomer cements during setting and its relation to pulp sensitivity. J Am Dent Assoc 112 654–657 (1986); The data indicate that the glass ionomer luting cements show lower pH values for longer times than zinc phosphate and polycarboxylic cements.

Swartz M.L.; Phillips R.W.; Clark H.E. Long-term F release from glass ionomer cements. J Dent Res 63 158–160 (1984); Fluoride release from luting and filling GIC and silicate cement is similar over a 12-month period. The silicophosphate cement released somewhat less fluoride, while the release from a fluoride containing polycarboxylate was negligible after the first few days.

Ten Cate J.W.; Featherstone J.D. Mechanistic aspect of the interactions between fluoride and dental enamel. Crit Rev Oral Biol Med 2 283–296 (1991); This article critically reviews the information about tooth-fluoride interactions, both from laboratory and clinical studies.

Trairatvorakul C.; Itsaraviriyakul S.; Wiboonchan W. Effect of glass-ionomer cement on the progression of proximal caries. J Dent Res 90 99–103 (2011); This split-mouth study showed that lesions treated with GIC were more likely to remain in or regress to the outer half of enamel.

Tyas M.J. Milestones in adhesion: Glass-ionomer cements. J Adhes Dent 5 259–266 (2003); This article offers an excellent review of the conventional and hybrid glass ionomer cements.

Weiner R. Liners and bases in general dentistry. Aust Dent J 56 (Suppl 1) 11–22 (2011); This review article discusses the use of liners and bases and the types of materials that are available to the restorative dentist.

Welbury R.R.; McCabe J.F.; Murray J.J.; et al. Factors affecting the bond strength of composite resin to etched glass ionomer cement. J Dent 16 188–193 (1988); Omission of the etching process did not produce a significantly inferior bond but the results were less dependable.

Wiegand A.; Buchalla W.; Attin T. Review on fluoride-releasing restorative materials—fluoride release and uptake characteristics, antibacterial activity and influence on caries formation. Dent Mater 23 343–362 (2007); A review article covering the fluoride release and recharge capabilities and antibacterial properties of fluoride-releasing dental restoratives. It also discusses the status concerning the prevention or inhibition of caries development and progression.

Wilson A.D.; McLean J.W. Glass Ionomer Cements. Quintessence: Chicago; This book provides an in-depth discussion of the evolution and chemistry of different GIC formulations.

8 Dental Amalgams

CHAPTER OUTLINE

KEY TERMS

Amalgam—An alloy containing mercury.

Amalgamation—The process of mixing liquid mercury with one or more metals or alloys to form an amalgam.

Condensation—The process of pressing dental amalgam by force to remove excess mercury and ensure continuity of the matrix phase.

Creep—The time-dependent strain or deformation that is produced by a stress. The creep process can cause an amalgam restoration to extend out of the restoration site, thereby increasing its susceptibility to marginal breakdown.

Delayed expansion—The gradual expansion of a zinc-containing amalgam over a period of weeks to months. This expansion is associated with the development of hydrogen gas, which is caused by the incorporation of moisture in the plastic mass during its manipulation in a cavity preparation.

Dental amalgam—An alloy that is formed by reacting mercury with silver, copper, and tin and that may also contain palladium, zinc, and other elements to improve handling characteristics and clinical performance.

Dental amalgam alloy (alloy for dental amalgam)—An alloy of silver, copper, tin, and other elements that is processed in the form of powder particles or as a compressed pellet.

Marginal breakdown—The gradual fracture of the perimeter or margin of a dental amalgam filling, which leads to the formation of gaps between the amalgam and the tooth.

Trituration—The mixing of amalgam alloy particles with mercury in a device called a *triturator*; the term is also used to describe the reduction of a solid to fine particles by grinding or friction.

When metal particles are mixed with mercury in certain proportion at room temperature, the mixture appears plastic initially. At that consistency, the mixture can be adapted to any shape with a light pressure. Meanwhile the outer portion of the particle in the mixture dissolves into mercury that slowly hardens the mixture. When the solubility of the metal in mercury is exceeded, crystals of mercury-containing compounds start to precipitate within the mercury. The process increases the firmness of the mixture, which enables sculpting of the mixture to the desirable anatomical form with instruments. The reaction continues at a slower rate as the mixture transforms into a solid with sufficient strength to resist fracture. The reaction process is called amalgamation, and the metallic solid containing mercury is called amalgam.

CRITICAL QUESTION

After reacting with liquid mercury, how do the original powder particles become structural components of the set dental amalgams?

Dental Amalgam

The amalgams used today are largely based on the formulation published by G. V. Black in 1895. The major modifications to that formulation were raising the copper content and making of spherical particles during the early 1960s. Despite amalgam's long history of success as a restorative material, there have been periodic concerns regarding the potential adverse health effects arising from exposure to mercury in dental amalgam. Because of advances in resin-based composites and adhesive technology in dentistry, the use of amalgam has declined substantially. Dental amalgam use will be limited in the future and may eventually be phased out of the clinician's armamentarium.

There are billions of amalgam restorations remaining in patients' mouths. Many of these restorations will require attention, such as for replacement, repair, or refurbishing procedures.

By definition, an amalgam is an alloy that contains mercury. Mercury, a liquid at room temperature, can dissolve and react to form an alloy with numerous metals. When metal particles are mixed with mercury, the outer portion of the particles dissolves into mercury. At the same time, mercury diffuses into the metal particles. When the solubility of the metal in mercury is exceeded, crystals of mercury-containing compounds start to precipitate within the mercury. During this period of reaction the metal particles coexist with the liquid mercury, giving the mix a plastic consistency. This means that the mixture can be adapted to any shape with a light pressure. As the content of liquid mercury in the mixture decreases by the formation of precipitates, the mixture hardens. This process is called **amalgamation** and the material has been used for restoring tooth structure. The first use of amalgam for tooth filling was recorded in the Chinese medical literature in CE 659. In this chapter the term restoration refers to the amalgam filling and the adjacent tooth structure.

Despite its long history of success as a restorative material, there have been periodic concerns regarding the potential adverse health effects arising from exposure to mercury released from dental amalgam. Because of advances in resin-based composites and adhesive technology in dentistry, the use of amalgam has declined substantially. Its use may be limited in the near future and it may eventually disappear from the clinician's armamentarium.

In this chapter, amalgam structure, properties, and manipulation characteristics are discussed.

Amalgam Alloys

Before these alloys are reacted with mercury, they are known as **dental amalgam alloys** or alloys for dental amalgam. They are usually provided as:

1. Irregularly shaped particles (Fig. 8.1) produced by milling or lathe-cutting a cast ingot of the amalgam alloy,
2. As spherical particles (Fig. 8.2) produced by atomizing the liquid alloy in a chamber filled with inert gas, or
3. As a mixture of both lathe-cut and spherical particles (Fig. 8.3).

Originally, the dentist dispensed alloy powder and mercury in a mortar and mixed them together with a pestle by hand. The process of mixing is called **trituration**. Later, the powder was compacted in the form of pellets, which were dispensed along with mercury in a reusable capsule with a pestle (Fig. 8.4A) and triturated by a power-driven triturator or amalgamator (Fig. 8.5). Today, disposable amalgam capsules are widely available (Fig. 8.4B and C). Each capsule contains a predetermined amount of alloy powder and mercury in a sealed pouch, and the capsule is sealed to prevent evaporation of the mercury.

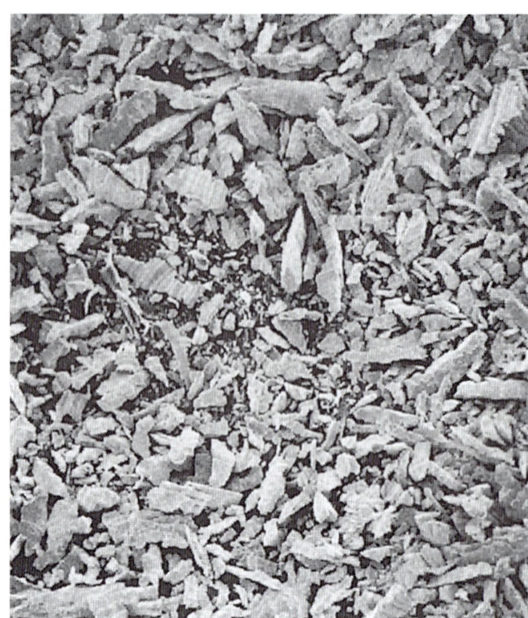

• **Fig. 8.1** Particles of conventional lathe-cut alloy for dental amalgam (×100).

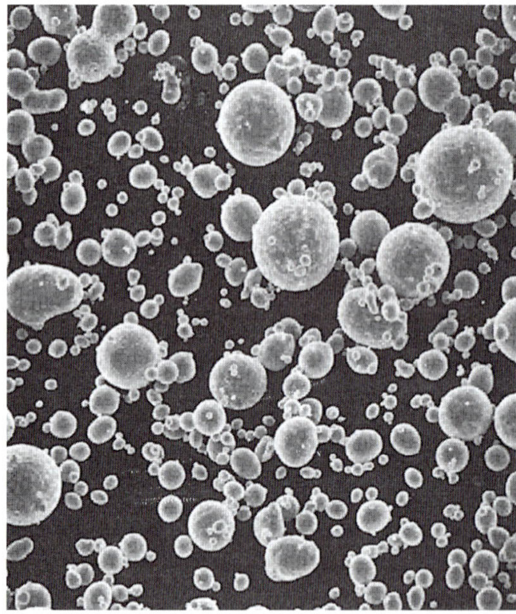

• **Fig. 8.2** Particles of spherical alloy for dental amalgam (×500).

Composition

The introduction of a higher copper content in amalgam alloys marked a significant change in the properties of amalgams. It is now customary to classify amalgam alloys as either low-copper (conventional) or high-copper alloys (Table 8.1). In both types, the major components of the alloys are silver and tin.

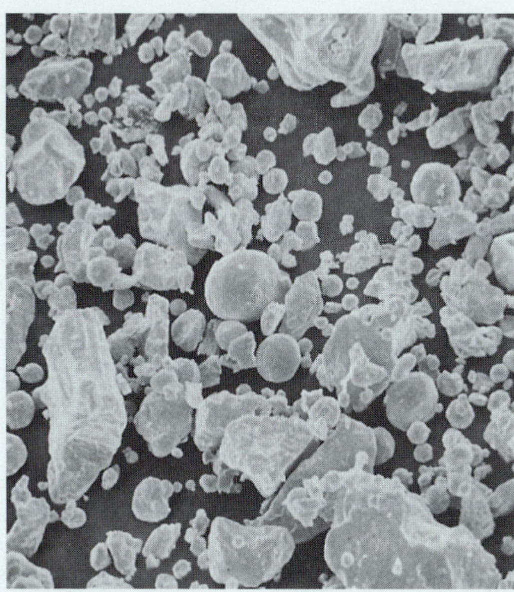

• **Fig. 8.3** Typical admix high-copper alloy powder showing the lathe-cut silver–tin particles and silver–copper spherical particles (×500).

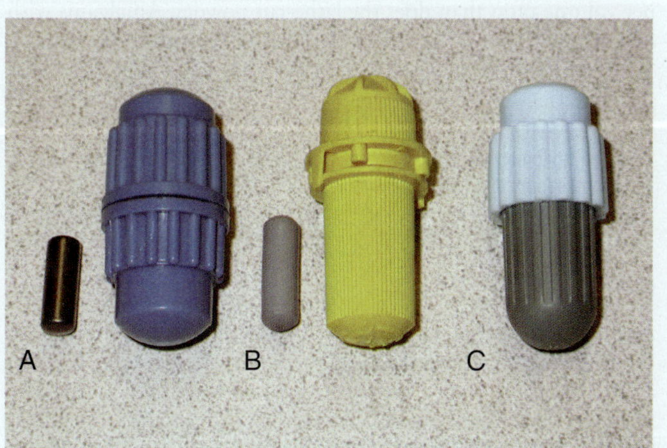

• **Fig. 8.4** Types of capsules. **(A)** Reusable capsules with pestle. **(B)** Preproportioned capsule with pestle. **(C)** Preproportioned capsule without pestle.

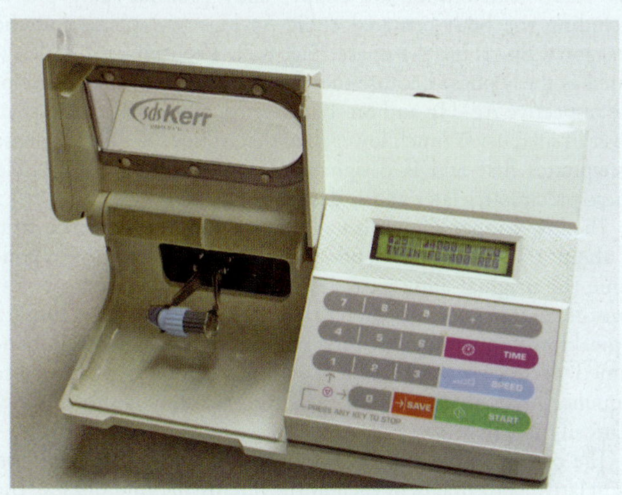

• **Fig. 8.5** A programmable triturator.

TABLE 8.1 Composition of Some Typical Commercial Amalgam Alloys

	COMPOSITION (MASS %)			
Amalgam	**Ag**	**Sn**	**Cu**	**Zn**
Low copper (lathe-cut)	70.3	25.9	2.8	0.9
Low copper (spherical)	72.0	25.0	3.0	-
High copper (admix)	69.5	17.7	11.8	1.0
High copper (spherical)	61.0	26.0	13.0	-

Silver–Tin System

Fig. 8.6 is an equilibrium-phase diagram of the silver–tin alloy system. Conventionally, starting from the left of the phase diagram, each phase is designated with a Greek letter in alphabetical order from 0% to 100% Sn. The ratio of silver to tin in Table 8.1 shows that amalgam alloys have a narrow range of compositions, falling within the $\beta + \gamma$ and the γ phases of the diagram shown in Fig. 8.6.

CRITICAL QUESTION

How can zinc be a beneficial additive to alloy for dental amalgam but also a component that can potentially cause significant postoperative discomfort to the patient?

Low-Copper Alloys

Silver–tin alloys are quite brittle and difficult to blend uniformly unless a small amount of copper is substituted for silver. Within the limited range of copper solubility, an increased copper content hardens and strengthens the silver–tin alloy. The chief function of

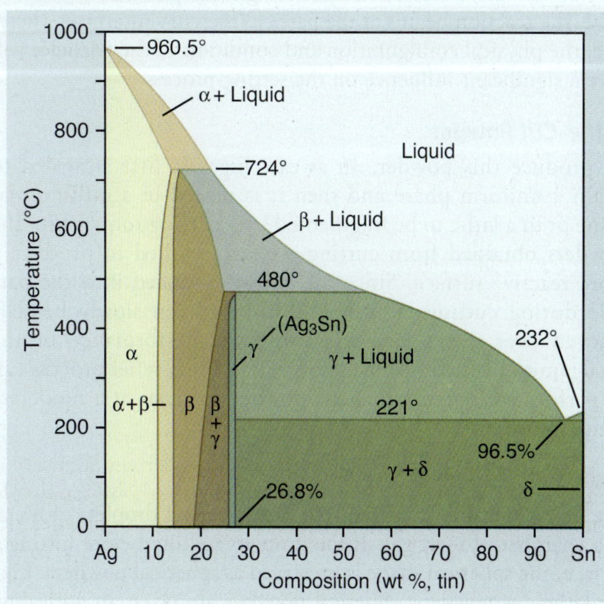

• **Fig. 8.6** Equilibrium-phase diagram of silver–tin system.

zinc in an amalgam alloy is to act as a deoxidizer, which is an oxygen scavenger that minimizes the formation of oxides of other elements in the amalgam alloys during melting. Alloys without zinc are more brittle, and their amalgams tend to be less plastic during condensation and carving. The American Dental Association (ADA) Specification No. 1 for amalgam alloys allows some mercury in the alloy powder.

The ranges of conventional alloy composition by weight in the early 1980s were 66.7%–71.5% silver, 24.3%–27.6% tin, 1.2%–5.5% copper, 0%–1.5% zinc, and 0%–4.7% mercury. The structure of these conventional alloys was dominated by Ag_3Sn (γ phase) with some Cu_3Sn (ϵ phase).

High-Copper Alloys

The first high-copper alloy was formulated by mixing one part of silver–copper, spherical eutectic (Ag–Cu; 71.9% silver and 28.1% copper by weight) particles to two parts of Ag_3Sn, provided as lathe-cut particles. This modification raises the copper content to 11.8% by weight. This is often called "dispersed-phase alloy" or "admixed high-copper alloy."

A second type of high-copper alloy was made by melting all components of the dispersed phase alloy. This process yields a single composition system. The presence of the higher copper content makes mechanical cutting of ingots into particles difficult. Thus, they are often provided in a spherical form that is produced by an atomization process. The copper content of this group of alloys can be as high as 30% by weight. Various amounts of indium or palladium have been included in some commercial systems.

Gallium-Based Alloys

In an attempt to eliminate mercury from direct metallic restorative materials, gallium, which is also a liquid when alloyed with indium and tin at room temperature, has been considered as a substitute. Like mercury, this metal element can be triturated with alloys for high-copper amalgam.

Powder Configuration

Dental amalgams are made by mixing alloy powders with mercury. The reaction begins at the particle/mercury interface. Therefore, the physical configuration and condition of the particles will have a significant influence on the setting process.

Lathe-Cut Powder

To produce this powder, an as-cast ingot is first annealed to retain a uniform phase and then it is placed in a milling machine or in a lathe to be fragmented by a cutting tool or bit. The powders obtained from cutting are acid washed to produce a more reactive surface. Since the stresses induced into the particle during cutting are not uniform and can slowly be self-relieved over time, they will cause the performance of the amalgam to be inconsistent. However, a stress-relief process can be performed by annealing the powder particles at a moderate temperature.

Atomized Powder

The liquid metal is atomized into fine spherical droplets of metal in a chamber of inert gas. If the droplets solidify before hitting a surface, the spherical shape is preserved as spherical powders. Like the lathe-cut powders, spherical powders are given an annealing heat treatment and surface washing.

Particle Size

The average particle sizes of modern powders range between 15 and 35 μm. Smaller particles greatly increase the surface area per unit volume of the powder. A powder containing tiny particles requires a greater amount of mercury to form an acceptable amalgam. It is critical to maintain an optimal particle size and size distribution.

The particle size distribution can affect the character of the finished surface. When the amalgam has partially hardened, the tooth anatomy is carved in the amalgam with a sharp instrument. During carving, the larger particles may be pulled out of the matrix, producing a rough surface. Such a surface is probably more susceptible to corrosion than a smooth surface. A smaller average particle size tends to produce a more rapid hardening of the amalgam with greater early strength.

Lathe-Cut Powder Versus Spherical Powder

Amalgams made from lathe-cut powders or admixed powders tend to resist condensation better than amalgams made entirely from spherical powders. Since freshly triturated amalgams from spherical powders are very plastic, one cannot rely on the pressure of condensation to establish a proximal contour for a class II restoration. Spherical alloys require less mercury than typical lathe-cut alloys because spherical alloy powder has a smaller surface area per volume ratio than does the lathe-cut powder. Amalgams with low mercury content generally have better properties.

CRITICAL QUESTION

Through what mechanism does the addition of 65% or more of copper by weight prevent the formation of the undesirable γ_2 phase?

Amalgamation

As discussed earlier, modern dental amalgam alloys are based on the intermetallic compound Ag_3Sn; therefore, the main reaction after trituration occurs between Ag_3Sn and mercury. Other elements in the alloy, especially copper, also play a significant role in the final microstructure of set amalgams.

Low-Copper Alloys

The main reactions of low-copper alloy produce alloy phases including the body-centered cubic Ag_2Hg_3 (γ_1) phase and the hexagonal $Sn_{7-8}Hg$ (γ_2) phase (Fig. 8.7). Both phases are designated as the γ phase because they happen to be the third phase of the respective Ag–Hg and Sn–Hg systems. Since the solubility of silver in mercury is much lower than that of tin, the Ag_2Hg_3 phase precipitates first and is designated as γ_1, whereas the $Sn_{7-8}Hg$ phase precipitates later and is designated as γ_2.

The low-copper alloy is usually mixed with mercury in a ratio of about 1:1. This is an insufficient amount of mercury to consume the original alloy particles completely; consequently, unconsumed particles are present in the set amalgam. Thus, a typical low-copper amalgam is a composite in which the unconsumed particles are embedded within γ_1 and γ_2 phases. The sequence of amalgamation of the silver–tin alloy is shown schematically in Fig. 8.8.

The physical properties of the hardened amalgam depend on the relative percentages of each of the microstructural phases. The greater the number of unconsumed Ag–Sn particles retained in

Low-copper alloy

$Ag_3Sn + Hg \longrightarrow Ag_2Hg_3 + Sn_{7\text{-}8}Hg$ + unreacted Ag_3Sn

High-copper admix alloy

Ag_3Sn + Ag-Cu + Hg $\longrightarrow Ag_2Hg_3$ + [$Sn_{7\text{-}8}Hg$ + unreacted Ag-Cu] + unreacted Ag_3Sn

Secondary solid-state reaction $\longrightarrow Cu_6Sn_5 + Ag_2Hg_3$ + unreacted Ag-Cu

High-copper spherical alloy

$[Ag_3Sn + Cu_3Sn] + Hg \longrightarrow Ag_2Hg_3 + Cu_6Sn_5$ + unreacted $[Ag_3Sn + Cu_3Sn]$

Symbols and stoichiometry of phases	
Phase Symbols	Composition
γ	Ag_3Sn
γ_1	Ag_2Hg_3
γ_2	$Sn_{7\text{-}8}Hg$
ϵ	Cu_3Sn
η (η')	Cu_6Sn_5

• **Fig. 8.7** Reactions of low-copper and high-copper amalgams, and symbols of phases involved in the setting of dental amalgams.

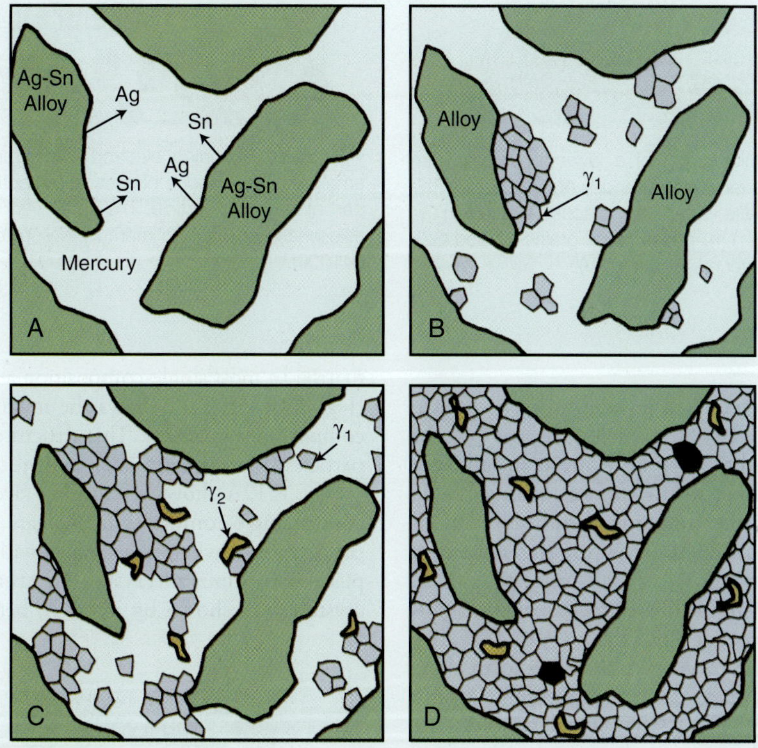

• **Fig. 8.8** Schematics that illustrate the development sequence of the amalgam microstructure when lathe-cut low-copper alloy particles are mixed with mercury. **(A)** Dissolution of silver and tin into mercury. **(B)** Precipitation of γ_1 crystals in the mercury. **(C)** Consumption of the remaining mercury by growth of γ_1 and γ_2 grains. **(D)** The final set amalgam.

the final structure, the stronger the amalgam will be. The γ_2 phase is the weakest and least stable in a corrosive environment and may suffer corrosion attack especially in crevices of the restorations.

A reaction between Cu_3Sn (ϵ phase) and γ_2 also occurs and yields Cu_6Sn_5 (η' phase). Because of the low copper content, a majority of γ_2 remains. Fig. 8.9 illustrates the features found in a typical microstructure of amalgam made from a lathe-cut, low-copper alloy. As described later, the addition of more than 6% of copper by weight can reduce or eliminate the γ_2 phase by formation of the Cu–Sn phase.

According to the phase diagram of Cu–Sn, the Cu_6Sn_5 phase exhibits a solid state transformation at 186–189°C. The new phase is different structurally from the previous phase with no change in composition. The high-temperature phase is designated as η and the lower temperature phase is η'. Since the formation of the Cu_6Sn_5 phase in amalgam occurs at room temperature, η' is used throughout the following discussion.

CRITICAL QUESTION

Compared with amalgams made from admixed high-copper alloys, what are the benefits and risks of the amalgams made from high-copper single-composition spherical particles?

High-Copper Alloys

Two different types of high-copper alloy powders are available. The first is a two-phase admixed powder and the second is a single-composition single-phase powder. Both types contain more than 6% of copper by weight.

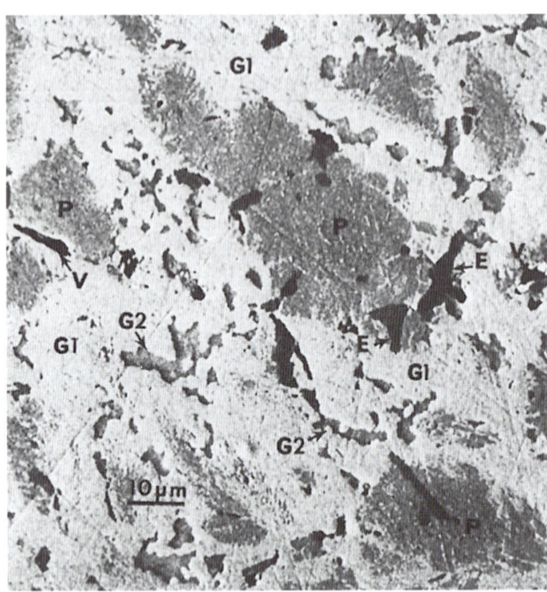

• **Fig. 8.9** A scanning electron micrograph of a low-copper amalgam (×1000). The micrograph features remaining β and γ Ag-Sn phases (the large dark areas labeled P), ϵ phase (small dark patches labeled E), γ_1 phase (light background labeled G1), γ_2 phase (small grains labeled G2), and voids (left center and right center areas labeled V).

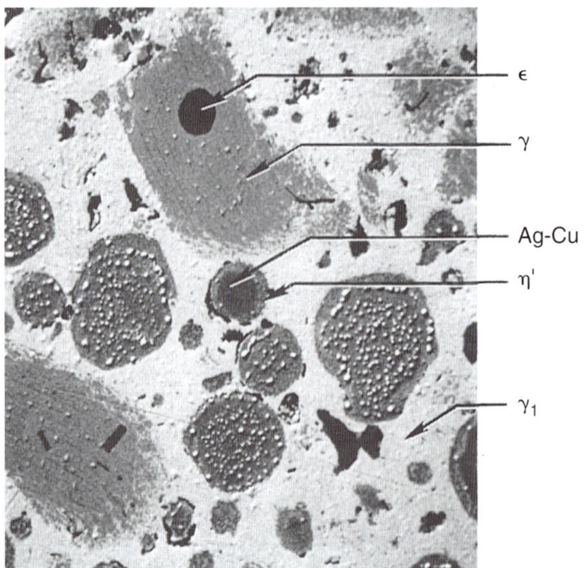

• **Fig. 8.10** Scanning electron micrograph of an admixed high-copper amalgam. The various phases and reaction layer are labeled. ϵ Phase is part of lathe-cut particle. The small, very light drop-shaped areas on particle phase are high in mercury owing to the freshly polished specimen (×1000).

Admixed Alloys

When mercury reacts with an admixed powder, silver in Ag–Cu spheres and silver and tin from Ag–Sn particles dissolve into the mercury. Whereas both γ_1 and γ_2 crystals form, as in lathe-cut alloys, the tin in mercury diffuses to the surfaces of the Ag–Cu alloy particles and reacts with the copper to form a layer of η′ phase crystals on the surface. The η′ layer on the surface of Ag–Cu alloy particles also contains γ_1 crystals, since γ_1 and η′ phases form simultaneously. As in the low-copper amalgams, γ_1 is the matrix phase (i.e., the phase that binds the unconsumed alloy particles together). In this reaction, the γ_2 phase does form along with the η′ phase but later reacts with copper from Ag–Cu particles, yielding additional η′ phase (the secondary solid-state reaction in Fig. 8.7). The γ_2 phase can be eliminated with at least 11.8% of copper by weight in the alloy powder.

Fig. 8.10 illustrates the microstructure of an admixed amalgam. Included in this structure are the γ phase particles, Ag–Cu particles, ϵ particles, the γ_1 matrix, and η′ reaction layers. In some admixed amalgams, a small number of the η′ crystals are also found amid the γ_1 matrix.

Single-Composition Alloys

The major components of single-composition particles are usually silver, copper, and tin. The copper content of various single-composition alloys ranges from 13% to 30% by weight. In addition, small amounts of indium or palladium are included in some of the single-composition alloys. A number of phases are found in each single-composition alloy particle, including the β phase (Ag–Sn), γ phase (Ag_3Sn), and ϵ phase (Cu_3Sn). Some of the alloys may also contain some η′ phase.

When triturated with mercury, silver and tin from the Ag–Sn phases dissolve in mercury. Very little copper dissolves in mercury. The γ_1 crystals grow, forming a matrix that binds together the partially dissolved alloy particles. The η′ crystals are found as meshes of rod-like crystals at the surfaces of alloy particles, dispersed in the matrix. In most single-composition amalgams, little or no γ_2 forms (Fig. 8.7). Fig. 8.11 shows the microstructure of a typical single-composition amalgam. This structure includes unconsumed alloy particles (P), γ_1 grains (G1), and η′ crystals (H).

Fig. 8.12A shows a scanning electron micrograph of a high-copper single-composition amalgam fractured a few minutes after condensation when the amalgamation reaction was still taking place. Two kinds of crystals are seen on the surface: polyhedral crystals (γ_1), shown by arrow A, between the unconsumed alloy

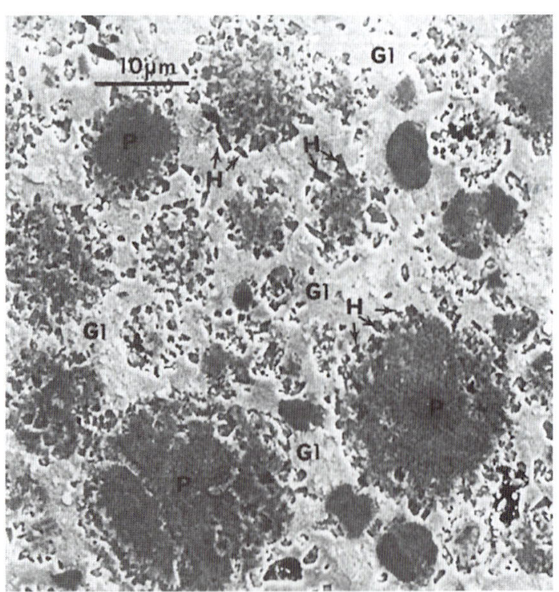

• **Fig. 8.11** A scanning electron micrograph of a high-copper single-composition amalgam (×560). The micrograph features unconsumed alloy particles (labeled P), γ_1 matrix phase (labeled G1), and η′ crystals (labeled H).

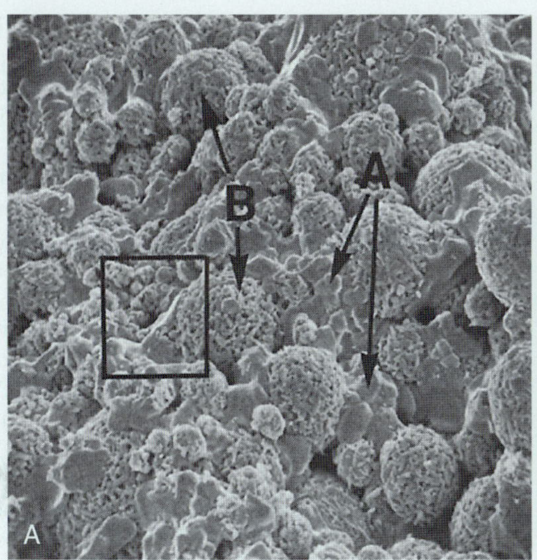

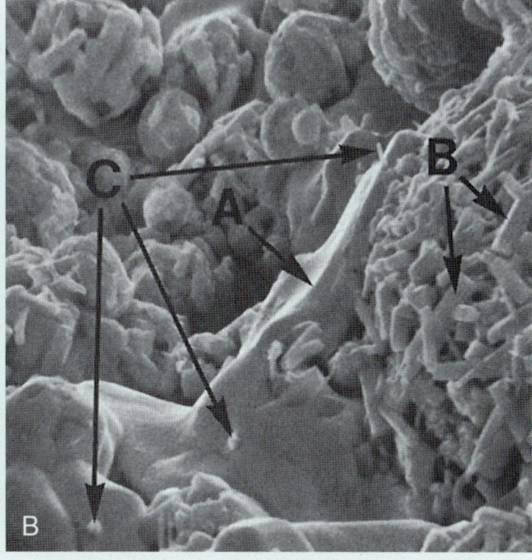

• **Fig. 8.12 (A)** Scanning electron micrograph of a high-copper single-composition amalgam fractured shortly after condensation, showing reaction products being formed: γ_1 (*arrow A*), and mesh of η' phase (*arrow B*) covering unreacted spherical particles. **(B)** Higher magnification of marked area in (A). η' Rods (*arrow C*) embedded in γ_1 crystals (*arrow A*) can be identified (×5000).

particles, and meshes of η' rod crystals, shown by arrow *B*, for the unconsumed alloy particles.

Fig. 8.12B shows details of the marked areas in Fig. 8.11A. In addition to a mesh of η' crystals (*arrow B*), which formed on an unconsumed particle, η' rods (*arrow C*) are seen embedded in a γ_1 crystal (A). Meshed η' crystals on unconsumed alloy particles may strengthen bonding between the alloy particles and γ_1 grains, and η' crystals dispersed between γ_1 grains may interlock γ_1 grains. This interlocking is believed to improve the amalgam's resistance to deformation.

CRITICAL QUESTION

What is the ideal mercury/alloy ratio for an admixed amalgam and a spherical particle amalgam? What are the consequences of insufficient and excess amounts of mercury for amalgam restorations?

Clinical Manipulation of Amalgam for Restorations

A good modern dental amalgam alloy can be manipulated so that the restoration lasts, on average, 15 years. The cavity preparation must be designed correctly and the amalgam must be manipulated properly so that the set amalgam restoration is not placed under excessive tensile stress.

Obviously the selection of one type of amalgam over others should be based on the clinical performance; lacking such information, it should be based on the physical and mechanical properties. However, the initial analysis of properties should be compared with clinical performance as such data become available. Another criterion is that the alloy should meet the requirements of the ADA's Specification No. 1 or ISO 1559. However, it is the operator who controls the performance of a restoration. Thus, it is essential that the alloy selected be one with which the dentist and the assistant feel comfortable. Use of alloys and techniques that are technique insensitive relative to the manipulation and placement of the amalgam will enhance the quality and durability of the restoration.

Mercury/Alloy Ratio

The amount of alloy and mercury to be used can be described as the mercury/alloy ratio, which signifies the number of parts by weight of mercury divided by the number of parts of alloy to be used for the particular technique. Sufficient mercury must be present in the original mix to provide a coherent and plastic mass after trituration, but it must be low enough that the mercury content of the restoration is at an acceptable level without the need to remove an appreciable amount of mercury during condensation. The mercury content of the lathe-cut alloy is about 50% by weight and that for spherical alloys is 42% by weight.

When mortar and pestle were used for mixing amalgam, it was necessary to use an excess amount of mercury to achieve a smooth and plastic amalgam. Removal of excess mercury was accomplished by squeezing or wringing the mixed amalgam in a squeeze cloth prior to insertion of the increments into the prepared cavity. However, the amount of mercury removed by the squeeze cloth process and during condensation varied. Thus, there was a considerable chance for error.

Proportioning of Mercury and Alloy

A wide variety of mercury and alloy dispensers are available. The most common is the dispenser based on volumetric proportioning. Preweighed pellets or tablets are first placed in a capsule. In mechanical mixing, the capsule serves as a mortar. As a liquid, mercury can be measured by volume without appreciable loss of accuracy. The dispenser should be held vertically to ensure consistent dispensing of mercury. The dispenser should be at least half full when it is used. If it is not, the weight of mercury dispensed may be erratic. Probably the most common cause of inaccurate delivery of mercury is the entrapment of contaminants in the reservoir and orifice of the device. This variable could decrease the amount of mercury by 3% or 4% and this may lead to an unusable mix. Regardless of the alloy or triturator used, no more than two pellets of alloy should be mixed in a capsule at one time.

Disposable capsules containing preproportioned aliquots of mercury and alloy are now widely used. To prevent any amalgamation from occurring during storage, the mercury and alloy are physically separated from each other. The older types of preproportioned capsules require activation before trituration to allow the mercury to enter the compartment with the alloy. Some alloys are now available in *self-activating capsules*, which bring the alloy and mercury together automatically during the first few oscillations of the triturator. Although the preproportioned material is more expensive, it is more convenient, it eliminates the chance of mercury spills during proportioning, and it should result in a reliable mercury/alloy ratio. However, these capsules do not provide an opportunity to make minor adjustments in the mercury/alloy ratio to accommodate personal preferences.

Regardless of the method used, the proper amount of mercury and alloy always must be proportioned before the start of trituration. The addition of mercury after trituration is contraindicated.

CRITICAL QUESTION

How should the optimal trituration time be determined for a given dental amalgam product?

Mechanical Trituration

The objective of trituration is to provide proper amalgamation of the mercury and alloy. There is always an oxide layer of the alloy surface that hinders diffusion of mercury into the alloy. This film must be disrupted so that a clean surface of alloy can make intimate contact with the mercury. The oxide layer is removed by abrasion when the alloy particles and mercury are triturated.

Triturators

The main mixing mechanism of a mechanical triturator is a reciprocating arm that holds the capsule under a protective hood. The purpose of the hood is to confine mercury that might escape into the room or to prevent a capsule from being accidentally ejected from the triturator during trituration. A commonly used older model is a single-speed device with an automatic timer for controlling the length of the mixing time. Later models have multiple speed settings. A modern triturator is often microprocessor controlled (Fig. 8.5) and contains preset trituration programs for a number of materials. It can also be programmed by the operator to include other materials. A cylindrical metal or plastic piston of smaller diameter than the capsule is inserted into the capsule, and this serves as the pestle (Fig. 8.4A and B). Spherical alloys often do not need a pestle (Fig. 8.4C).

A triturator should be used at the speed recommended by the alloy manufacturer. Older triturators do not operate at a sufficient rate of speed to amalgamate high-copper alloys properly with minimal mercury. Self-activating capsules are usually very sensitive to trituration speed.

Dentists and assistants can adjust the amalgamation time required to attain a mix of correct consistency. For a given alloy and mercury/alloy ratio, increased trituration time and/or speed shorten the working and setting times. In addition, alloys differ in their sensitivity to trituration time (Fig. 8.13).

A reusable capsule should be clean and free of previously mixed, hardened alloy. At the end of each trituration procedure, one should quickly remove the pestle from the capsule, replace the lid, reinsert the capsule in the triturator, turn it on for a second or two, and then remove the amalgam. This mulling process generally causes the mix to cohere so that it can be readily removed from the capsule with minimal residue in the capsule. It minimizes the need of scraping out partially hardened alloy, which usually produces scratches in the capsule.

Consistency of the Mix

The proper time of mixing can be determined by observing the consistency of the mix. For example, the very grainy mix (Fig. 8.14A) indicates undertrituration. Not only will the amalgam restoration made from this mix be weak, but also the rough surface left after carving of the granular amalgam will increase its susceptibility to tarnish. If the trituration has produced an amalgam of the general appearance shown in Fig. 8.14B, the strength will be optimal and the smooth carved surface will retain its luster long after polishing. Because of the friction between particles during trituration, such an amalgam mix should be warm (not hot) when it is removed from the capsule. This will have no effect on the physical properties of the amalgam other than to shorten the working time somewhat. Overtrituration that results from a higher speed or a longer mixing time results in a softer (mushy) mixture that often sticks to the wall of the capsule. Compared

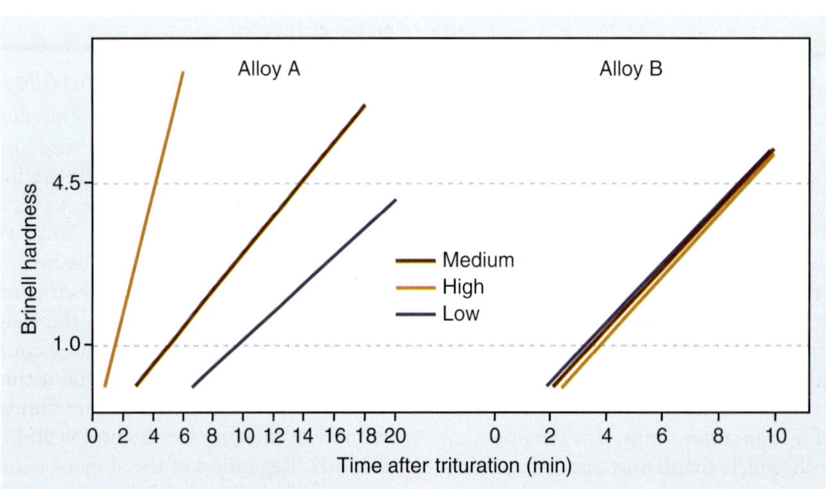

• **Fig. 8.13** Hardening data for two alloys mixed at low, medium, and high settings of trituration speed. Broken lines at 1.0 and 4.5 represent desirable working and carving consistencies, respectively.

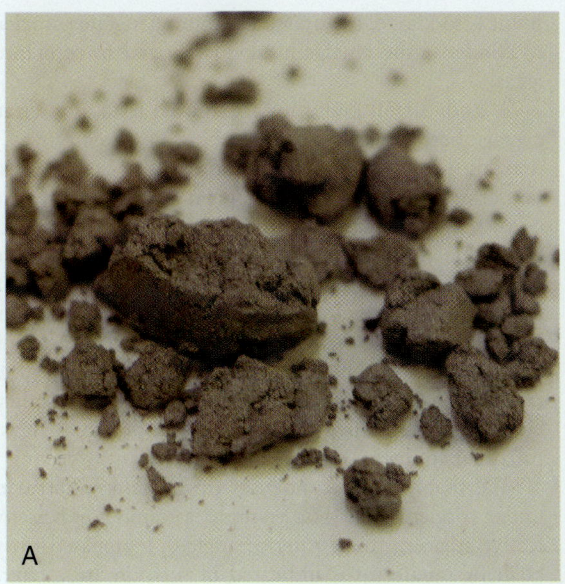

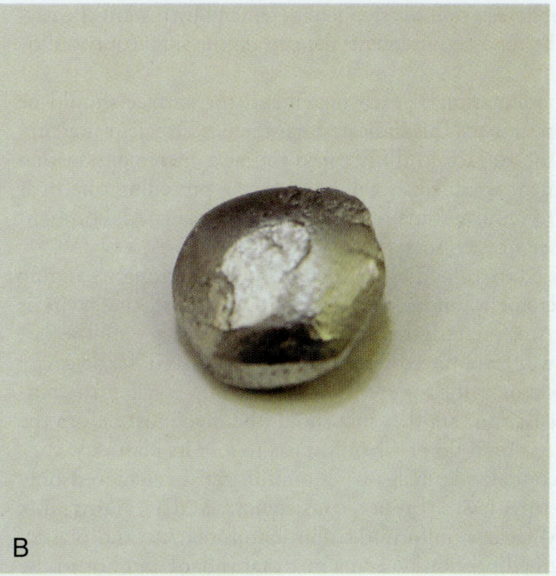

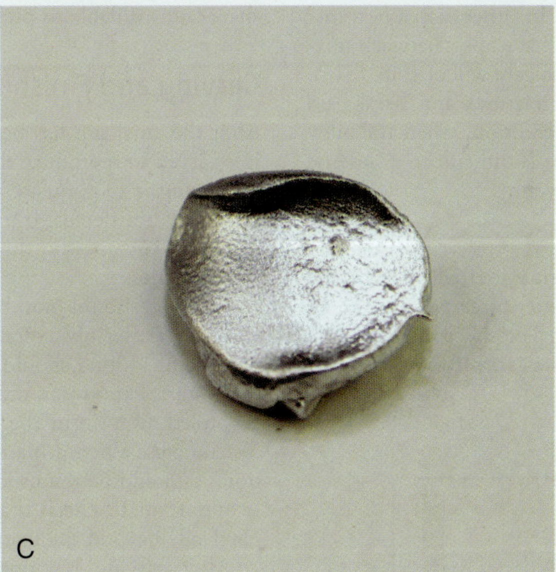

• **Fig. 8.14** Appearance of freshly triturated amalgam mixture. **(A)** A grainy undertriturated mixture; restoration made of such a mixture has low strength and poor resistance to corrosion. The mixture may appear in solid mass, but the surface remains without luster as shown. **(B)** A properly triturated amalgam that appears rounded with a smooth shiny surface. **(C)** An overtriturated amalgam mixture, which is shinier than that of the properly triturated one, and because of more fluid consistency the mass appears flattened by the force of trituration.

with the properly mixed amalgam, the surface of overtriturated amalgam is shinier, the shape of the mass is flatter (Fig. 8.14C), and the working time is shorter with a slightly higher setting contraction.

CRITICAL QUESTION

During the condensation of an amalgam, at what point in time should the triturated mixture be discarded and replaced by a new mixture?

Condensation

The goal of condensation is to compact the alloy into the prepared cavity so that the greatest possible density is attained, with sufficient mercury present to ensure continuity of the matrix phase (Ag_2Hg_3) between the remaining alloy particles. This results from a reduction of excess mercury and porosity within the set amalgam.

After the mixture is made, the increments of alloy should be carried to, and inserted in, the prepared cavity by means of instruments such as small forceps or an amalgam carrier designed for this purpose. Condensation of the amalgam should then be promptly initiated. The field of operation must be kept absolutely dry during condensation. Because of the nature of the operation, condensation is usually accomplished within four walls and a floor. One or more walls may be a thin sheet of stainless steel, called a *matrix*. Sufficient pressure should be used to remove voids and to adapt the material to the walls.

Condensation Procedure

The condenser tip, or face, is forced into the amalgam mass under hand pressure. Condensation is usually started at the center, and then the condenser point is stepped incrementally toward the cavity walls. The force requirements depend on the shape of the alloy particle.

After condensation of each increment, the surface should be shiny in appearance. This indicates that there is sufficient mercury present at the surface to diffuse into the next increment so that each increment is added, it will bond to the preceding one. It is important to remove some of the soft or mushy material brought to the surface of each increment.

The procedure of adding an increment, condensing it, adding another increment, and so forth is continued until the cavity is overfilled. Any mercury-rich material at the surface of the last increment will be removed when the filling is carved. If the cavity is a large one or if for some reason undue time is taken to complete condensation, another mix should be made just before the original one is used up or when it starts to lose its plasticity.

A well-condensed amalgam restoration can be achieved only if the mixture has a proper consistency. A dry, grainy mix (Fig. 8.14A) lacks a uniform distribution of mercury and plasticity, as described previously, and a mix that is hard and hot to the touch has probably been mixed too long. In either case, a new mix should be prepared. The longer the time that elapses between mixing and condensation, the weaker the amalgam will be (Fig. 8.15). Condensation of partially set material fractures and breaks up the matrix that has already formed. In addition, when the alloy has lost a certain amount of plasticity, it is difficult to condense without producing internal voids and layering.

Condensation Pressure

The area of the condenser tip and the force exerted on it by the operator govern the condensation pressure (force per unit area). When a given force is applied, the smaller the condenser, the greater is the pressure exerted on the amalgam. If the condenser point is too large, the operator cannot generate sufficient pressure to condense the amalgam adequately and force it into retentive areas.

A study of 30 practitioners showed that condensation forces average between 13.3 and 17.8 N (3–4 lb) employed. To ensure maximum density and adaptation to the cavity walls, the condensation force should be as great as the alloy will allow, and consistent with patient comfort. Many of the spherical alloys have little "body" and offer only minimal resistance to the condensation force. Therefore, the strength properties of spherical amalgam alloys tend to be less sensitive to condensation pressure. In many instances, condensation becomes a matter of attaining good adaptation. The potential disadvantages of a spherical alloy compared with an admixed alloy (lathe-cut and spherical particles) are the tendency for overhangs in proximal areas and weak proximal contacts.

The shape of the condenser tips should conform to the area under condensation. For example, a round condenser tip is ineffective adjacent to a corner or angle of a prepared cavity; a triangular or square tip is indicated in such an area. Tips of various shapes are available to provide effective condensation.

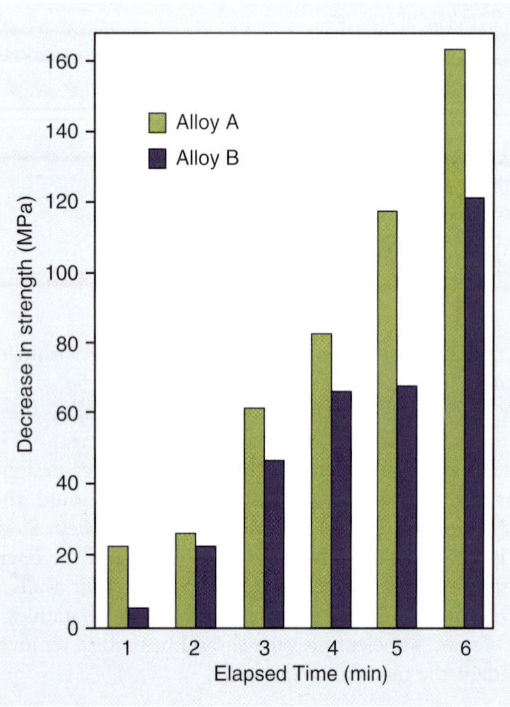

• **Fig. 8.15** Effect of elapsed time between trituration and condensation on the strength of the hardened amalgam. The greater the elapsed time, the lower is the strength.

Carving and Finishing

After the amalgam has been condensed into the prepared cavity, it is carved to reproduce the proper tooth anatomy. The objective of carving is to simulate the anatomy rather than to reproduce extremely fine details. If the carving is too deep, the bulk of amalgam may become too thin and it may fracture under direct occlusal loading.

Carving should not be started until the amalgam is hard enough to offer resistance to the carving instrument. A scraping or "ringing" sound should be heard when it is carved. If the carving is started too soon, the amalgam may be so plastic that it may be pulled away from the margins, even by the sharpest carving instrument. When a matrix band is used to facilitate condensation, it should be removed during the final carving procedure. It is important to check that excess amalgam has not been forced gingivally beyond the matrix during condensation.

After carving is completed, the surface of the restoration should be smoothed. This may be accomplished by judiciously burnishing the surface and margins of the restoration. Burnishing of the occlusal anatomy can be accomplished with a ball burnisher. Alternatively, a rigid flat-bladed instrument is best used on smooth surfaces. Smoothing can be concluded by gently rubbing the surface with a moist cotton pellet or by lightly smoothing the surface with a rubber polishing cup and an extremely fine polishing or prophylaxis paste. Clinical data on performance of restorations support the desirability of burnishing the fast setting, high-copper systems. Burnishing slow-setting alloys can damage the margins of the restoration. Undue pressure should not be exerted in burnishing, and heat generation should be avoided. Temperatures above 60°C (140°F) cause a significant release of mercury. The mercury-rich condition created at the margins results in accelerated corrosion, fracture, or both.

Regardless of alloy, trituration method, or condensation technique, the carved surface of the filling is rough, as demonstrated by the dull surface of the restorations in Fig. 8.16A. The surfaces are covered with scratches, pits, and irregularities, which can result in concentration cell corrosion over time. The smooth surface on the restorations shown in Fig. 8.16B, is produced by the final finishing procedure. The final finishing of the restoration should be delayed until the amalgam develops sufficient strength to resist

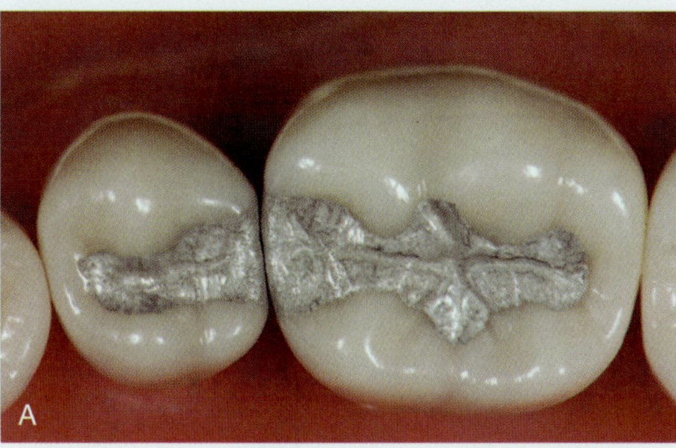

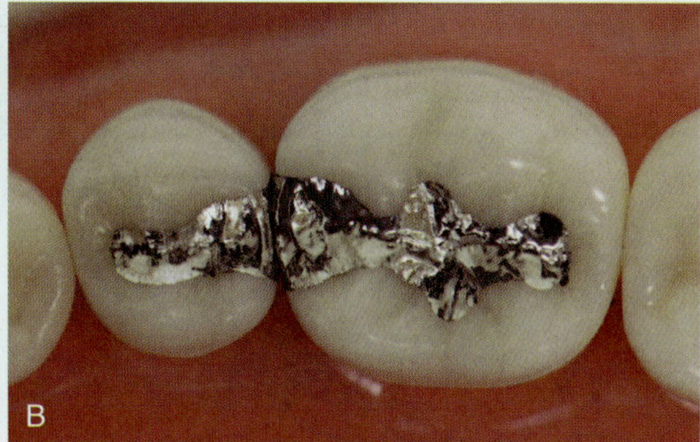

• **Fig. 8.16** **(A)** Amalgam restorations as they appear after carving. **(B)** The same restorations after final finishing. (Courtesy of S Geraldeli.)

the pressure of polishing. Generally, the recommendation is to wait for at least 24 hours or until the next appointment. However, the trend has been to forego the previously recommended final finishing procedure after 24 hours. The need for extremely high luster is questionable, but the metal surface should be smooth and uniform. The use of dry polishing powders and disks can easily raise the surface temperature to cause vaporization of mercury. Thus, a wet abrasive powder in a paste form is necessary.

Properties of Amalgam

ADA Specification No. 1 (ISO 1559) for amalgam alloys lists dimensional change, compressive strength, and creep as the measures of amalgam quality. The controlling variables and significance of these properties are described later.

CRITICAL QUESTION

How does the mercury content and condensation method affect the expansion or contraction that may occur during setting of an amalgam filling?

Dimensional Stability

Amalgam can expand or contract, depending on its manipulation. Severe contraction can lead to microleakage, plaque accumulation, and secondary caries. Excessive expansion can produce pressure on the pulp and postoperative sensitivity. Protrusion of a filling can also result from excessive expansion. ADA Specification No. 1 requires that the dimensional change of amalgam be in the range of 15–20 μm/cm measured at 37°C between 5 minutes and 24 hours after the beginning of trituration.

Mechanism of Dimensional Change

When the alloy and mercury are mixed, contraction results as the particles dissolve (and hence become smaller). Since the final volume of the γ_1 phase is less than the sum of the silver and liquid mercury volume needed to produce the γ_1 phase, contraction continues as long as the γ_1 phase keeps growing. As γ_1 crystals grow, they will impinge against one another. When there is sufficient liquid mercury present to provide a plastic matrix, expansion will occur when γ_1 crystals impinge on each other. After a rigid γ_1 matrix has formed, growth of γ_1 crystals cannot force the matrix to expand further. The reaction continues with γ_1 crystals growing into interstices containing mercury.

This model implies that expansion will occur if sufficient mercury is present in the mix when the dimensional change begins. Therefore, manipulation with less mercury in the mix, as occurs for lower mercury/alloy ratio and higher condensation pressures, will favor contraction. In addition, manipulative procedures that accelerate setting and consumption of mercury also favor contraction, including longer trituration times and use of smaller alloy particles.

Many modern amalgams exhibit a net contraction on setting, whereas in the past, measurements invariably indicated that an expansion occurred (Fig. 8.17). Two reasons for the difference are that older amalgams contained larger alloy particles and are mixed at higher mercury/alloy ratio than present-day amalgams. Likewise, hand trituration was used to prepare the specimens. Now high-speed mechanical triturators are employed.

Effect of Moisture Contamination

When a zinc-containing, low-copper or high-copper amalgam is contaminated by moisture during trituration or condensation, a large expansion, such as that shown in Fig. 8.18, can take place. This expansion usually starts 3–5 days after placement and may continue for months, reaching values greater than 400 μm/cm (4%). This type of expansion is known as **delayed expansion** or secondary expansion. The effect is caused by the hydrogen produced by electrolytic action involving zinc and water. The hydrogen does not combine with the amalgam but, rather, collects within the filling, increasing the internal pressure to levels high enough to cause the amalgam to creep, thus producing the observed expansion. The main source of contamination is saliva from poor isolation of the operative field. It should be noted that water must be incorporated into the bulk of amalgam during trituration or condensation to cause delayed expansion.

CRITICAL QUESTION

What is the mechanism of marginal breakdown? What are the steps that can be taken to reduce the risk or extent of this process?

Strength

A lack of adequate strength to resist masticatory forces is one of the inherent weaknesses of amalgam restorations. In properly designed restorations, such failures are relatively rare. More common are defects at the margins of amalgams.

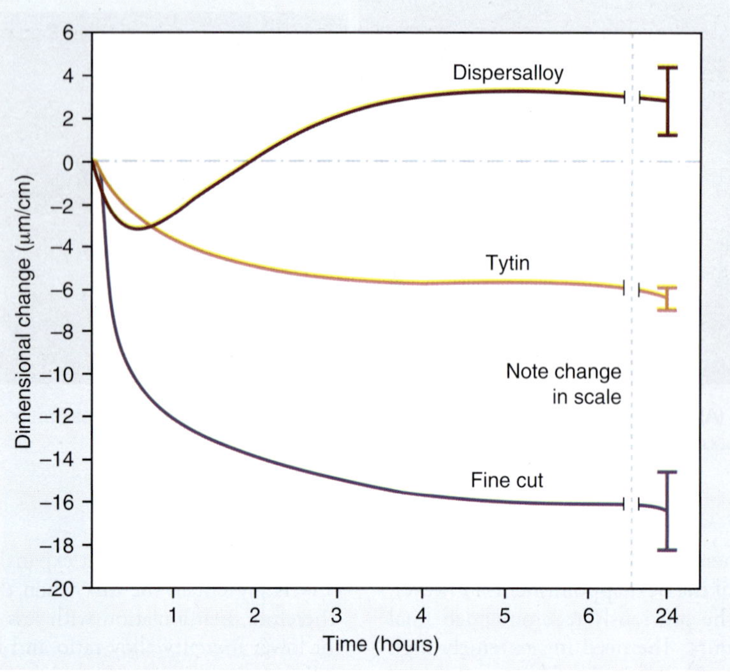

• **Fig. 8.17** Dimensional change of three amalgam products over a 24-h period. **(A)** A high-copper admixed amalgam (Dispersalloy). **(B)** A high-copper single-composition amalgam (Tytin). **(C)** A lathe-cut low-copper amalgam (Fine Cut).

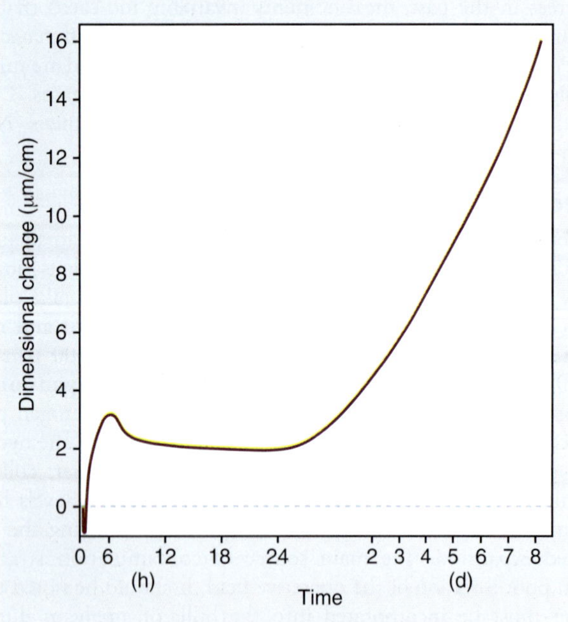

• **Fig. 8.18** Delayed expansion of an amalgam.

Traditionally, the strength of dental amalgam has been measured under compressive stress using specimens of dimensions comparable to the volume of typical amalgam fillings. When strength is measured in this manner, the compressive strength of a satisfactory amalgam probably should be at least 310 MPa. Table 8.2 shows typical compressive and tensile strengths at 1 hour and 7 days after preparation for a low-copper amalgam and two high-copper amalgams.

The significance of the 7-day compressive strength to clinical performance has been questioned. The strength of amalgam is more than adequate under compressive loads. However, amalgam is much weaker in tension than in compression (Table 8.2). For example, a compressive stress on a restored cusp introduces complex stresses that result in tensile stresses in the area. Since dentin has a relatively low elastic modulus, as much tooth structure as possible should be preserved to prevent the dentin from bending, which allows amalgam to bend and for tensile stresses to develop. Since amalgam cannot withstand high tensile or bending strength, the design of the restoration should include a stiff supporting structure whenever there is danger that it will be flexed in tension.

Effect of Trituration

The effect of trituration depends on the type of amalgam alloy, the trituration time, and the speed of the triturator. Either undertrituration or overtrituration will decrease the strength for both conventional and high-copper amalgams.

Effect of Mercury Content

The strength of an amalgam is a function of the volume fractions of unconsumed alloy particles and mercury-containing phases, and the inherent flaw density and depth of flaws. Insufficient mercury between particles yields a dry, granular mix. Such a mix results in a rough, pitted surface that promotes corrosion. Increasing the final mercury content increases the volume fraction of the matrix phases at the expense of the alloy particles. A higher mercury content promotes the formation of γ_2 phase, even in a high-copper amalgam. As a result the higher the mercury content, the incidence and severity of fracture increase as the amalgam restorations age. The effect of the mercury content upon the compressive strength of amalgam is shown in Fig. 8.19.

Mercury analysis of a large number of restorations reveals that the mercury content of the marginal areas averages between 2% and 3% higher than the bulk of the restoration. This is true regardless of the condensation method or the "dryness" of the increments used to build the restoration.

TABLE 8.2 Compressive Strength, Creep, and Tensile Strength of Low-Copper and High-Copper Amalgams

	COMPRESSIVE STRENGTH (MPA)			
	1 h	7 Days	Creep (%)	Tensile Strength at 24 h (MPa)
Low copper[a]	145	343	2.0	60
Admix (high copper)[b]	137	431	0.4	48
Single composition (high copper)[c]	262	510	0.13	64

[a]Fine Cut.
[b]Dispersalloy.
[c]Tytin.

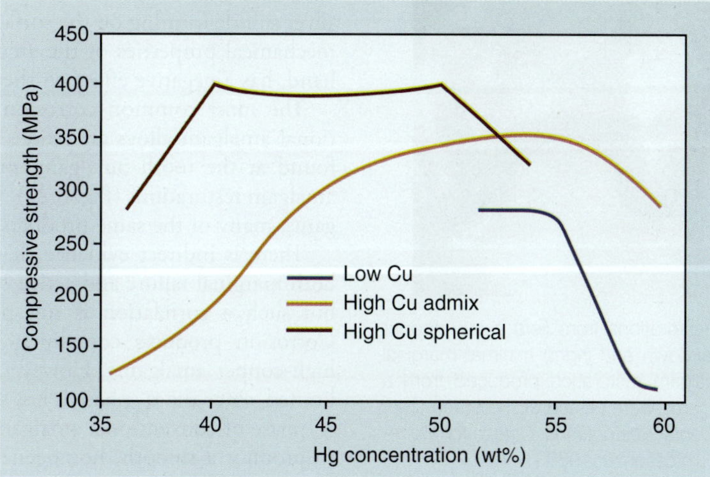

• **Fig. 8.19** Effect of mercury content (percent by weight) on the compressive strength of amalgam prepared with representative low-copper, high-copper admix, and high-copper single-composition spherical alloys.

Effect of Condensation

Good condensation techniques will express mercury and result in a smaller volume fraction of matrix phase. Higher condensation pressures are required to minimize porosity and express mercury from lathe-cut amalgams. On the other hand, spherical amalgams condensed with lighter pressures produce adequate strength. Greater condenser pressure will simply punch through the amalgam.

Effect of Porosity

Voids and porosity are factors that may reduce the compressive strength of set amalgams. The lack of plasticity of amalgam mixes caused by delayed condensation or undertrituration leads to porosity in set amalgams. Insufficient condensation pressure on lathe-cut alloys results in more porosity.

Effect of Amalgam Hardening Rate

Since a patient may be dismissed from the dental chair within 20 minutes after trituration of the amalgam, a vital question is whether the amalgam has gained sufficient strength to prevent fracture caused by a prematurely high occlusal force imposed by the patient. Amalgams do not gain strength as rapidly as might be desired. When the patient is dismissed, the compressive strength of the amalgam may be only 6% of the 1-week strength. Thus, it is likely that a high percentage of fractures in amalgam restorations occur within the first few hours after insertion.

ADA Specification No. 1 requires a minimal compressive strength of 80 MPa at 1 hour. The 1-hour compressive strength of high-copper single-composition amalgams is exceptionally high (Table 8.2). This strength will make fracture less probable if the patient accidentally bites on the restoration soon after leaving the dental office. In addition, these amalgams may be strong enough shortly after placement to permit amalgam buildups to be prepared for crowns and allow earlier impressions of crown preparations to be made. Nonetheless, patients should be warned not to subject the restoration to high biting stresses for at least 8 hours after placement. By that time a typical amalgam will have reached at least 70% of its strength.

Creep

Creep occurs when a solid material slowly deforms plastically under the influence of stresses. Creep of amalgam is determined by placing a cylinder of set amalgam (4 mm in diameter and 6 mm long) under a 36 MPa compressive stress. The specimen is prepared and stored at 37°C for 7 days before testing. The change of length between 1 and 4 hours as a percentage of the original length is the creep value reported in Table 8.2.

Creep rate has been found to correlate with marginal breakdown of conventional low-copper amalgams; that is, the higher the amount of creep, the greater is the degree of marginal deterioration. Creep causes the amalgam to flow over time such that unsupported amalgam protrudes at the margin of the restoration. Because of low tensile strength and the onset of corrosion, the protruded segment of amalgam fractures and leaves a ditch around the margin (left restoration in Fig. 8.20). Fig. 8.20 shows marginal breakdown in a class II amalgam (left side) filling that was produced with a high-creep amalgam.

When an amalgam creeps, it is the γ_1 phase that deforms plastically. Higher creep rates should be expected for low-copper amalgam with higher γ_1 volume fractions and vice versa. The presence of the γ_2 phase increases the creep rate. In addition to the absence of the γ_2 phase, the very low creep rates in single-composition high-copper amalgams may be associated with η' phase rods, which act as barriers to deformation of the γ_1 phase. Therefore, the manipulative factors discussed previously that maximize strength also minimize creep for any given type of amalgam.

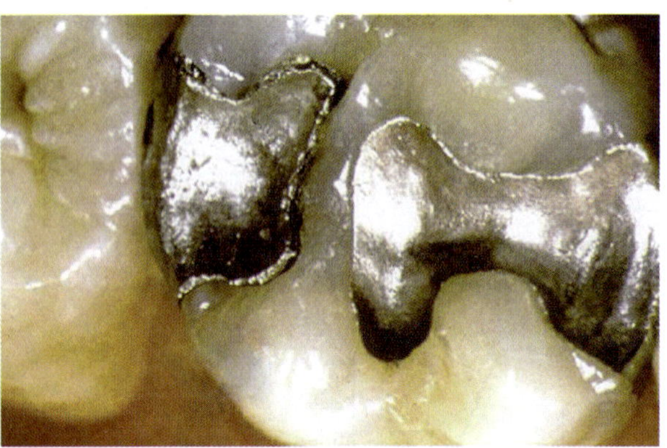

• **Fig. 8.20** Two-surface amalgam restorations from (*left*) a low-copper amalgam with severe marginal breakdown and (*right*) minimal marginal discrepancy of a higher-quality amalgam restoration produced from a high-copper admix alloy. Both amalgams were placed at the same time. (Adapted from *Quality Evaluation of Dental Restorations: Criteria for Placement and Replacement.* Chicago, Quintessence, 1989.)

CRITICAL QUESTION

How can corrosion of an amalgam restoration lead to both positive and negative outcomes?

Tarnish and Corrosion Resistance

Amalgam restorations often tarnish and corrode in the oral environment. A tendency toward tarnish, which is the result of silver sulfide forming on the surface, does not affect or change the mechanical properties of the amalgam. Corrosion, on the other hand, has a negative effect on the properties.

The most common corrosion products found with conventional amalgam alloys are oxides and chlorides of tin. These are found at the tooth–amalgam interface and within the bulk of amalgam restorations (Fig. 8.21). In the case of high-copper amalgams, many of the same products are found (Fig. 8.22).

There is indirect evidence that the γ_2 phase is implicated in both marginal failure and active corrosion in conventional alloys, but such a correlation is not possible for high-copper alloys. Corrosion products containing copper can also be found in high-copper amalgams. However, the corrosion process is more limited, since the η' phase is less susceptible to corrosion than the γ_2 phase of conventional amalgams. Every effort should be made to produce a smooth, homogeneous surface on a restoration in

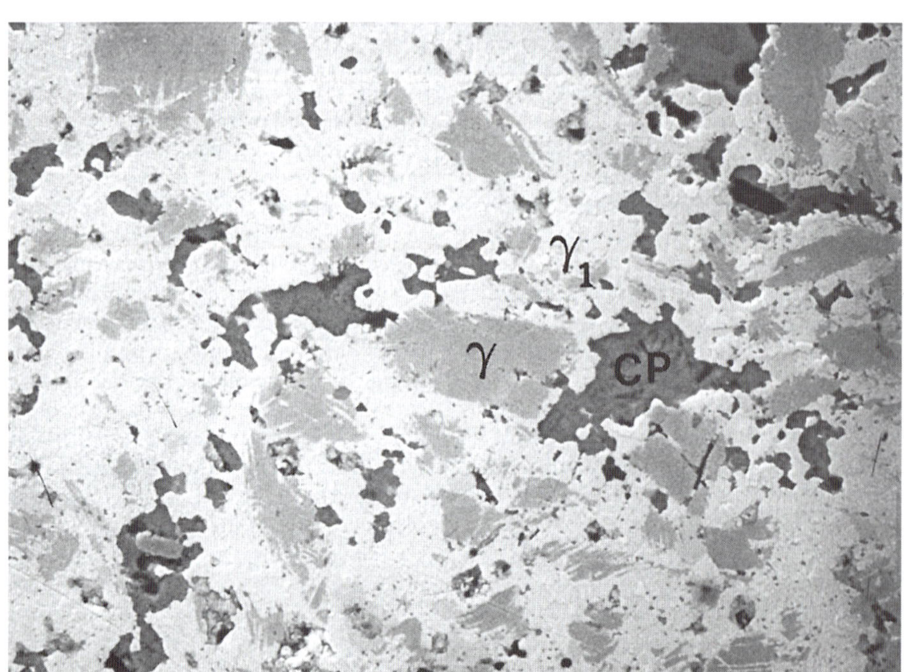

• **Fig. 8.21** Microstructure of 7-year-old conventional amalgam alloy filling. The various phases are marked. Note extensive porosity and that the γ_2 area has been replaced by a Sn-Cl corrosion product (CP). (Courtesy of GW and SJ Marshall.)

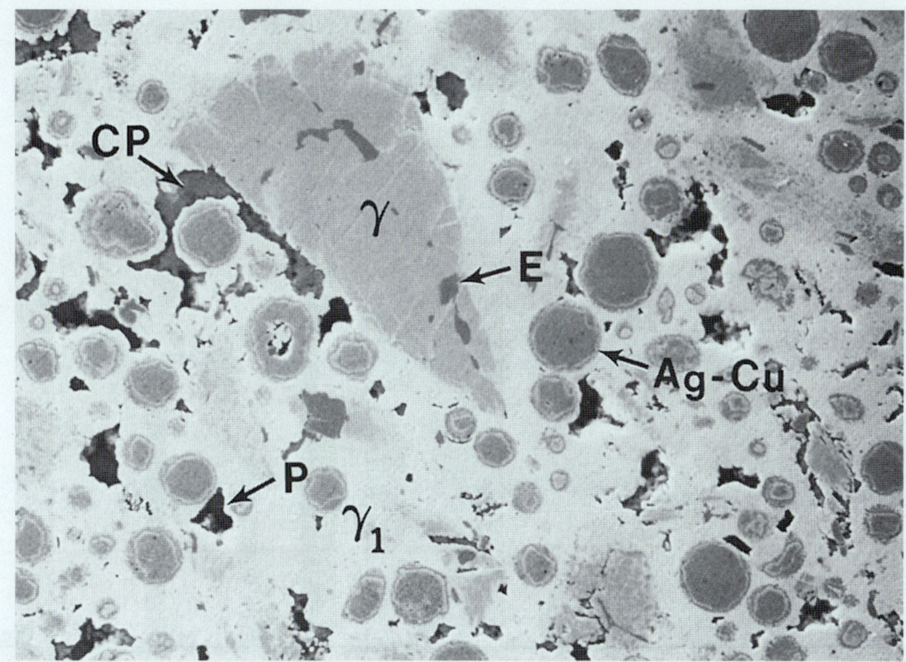

• **Fig. 8.22** Microstructure of an 8-year-old high-copper amalgam restoration. The gamma and gamma 1 phases are labeled. Although some porosity (P) is seen, it is less than that in the microstructure the conventional alloy restoration seen in Figure 8.21. The high-copper amalgam shown here also has less corrosion product (CP). (Courtesy of GW and SJ Marshall.)

order to minimize tarnish and corrosion, regardless of the alloy system used.

Whenever a gold restoration is placed in contact with an amalgam, corrosion of the amalgam can be expected as a result of the large differences in electromotive force (EMF) of the two materials. The corrosion process can liberate free mercury, which can contaminate and weaken the gold restoration. Biological effects such as galvanism can also result.

Clinical Performance of Amalgam Restorations

Amalgam does not adhere to the tooth structure. At best it affords only a reasonably close adaptation to the walls of the prepared cavity. For this reason cavity varnishes are used to reduce the gross leakage that occurs around a new filling. The use of dentin bonding agents with amalgam is another relatively new method to reduce microleakage. Clinical trials using the bonded amalgam technique continue to show promise. Results after 2–5 years appear to be equivalent to those from conventional amalgams. The long-term promise of this method is that it may allow more conservative cavity preparations with reduced mechanical retentive features.

If the amalgam is properly inserted, leakage decreases as the restoration ages in the mouth. This may be caused by corrosion products that form in the interface between the tooth and the filling, sealing the interface, thereby preventing leakage. The presence of calcium and phosphorus and the demineralization of tooth structures adjacent to the amalgam filling also strongly suggest a possible biological interaction in this corrosion process. The ability to seal against microleakage is exhibited by both the older low-copper amalgams and the newer high-copper amalgams. However, the accumulation of corrosion products is slower for the high-copper alloys.

After the amalgam is placed, a variety of changes occur at both the microstructural and the visual levels. At the visual level, many amalgam restorations must be replaced because of problems, including secondary caries, gross fracture of the amalgam, "ditched" or fractured margins, excessive tarnish and corrosion, and a variety of other factors. At the microstructural level, changes occur as a result of corrosion and stresses associated with mastication forces. All of these factors are probably interrelated, and the precise contribution of each to a specific case of failure is uncertain.

The ultimate lifetime of an amalgam restoration is determined by a number of factors: (1) the material, (2) the dentist and the assistant, and (3) the patient's environment. The first two parameters are the dominant factors controlling the amalgam performance during the early life of the restoration. Changes in the amalgam structure during clinical use and survival of amalgam restorations of various types are discussed in the following.

Clinical Significance of Dimensional Change

There are several causes for excessive expansion of amalgam. One is insufficient trituration and condensation; the other is delayed expansion brought about by the contamination of the Zn-containing amalgam with moisture during trituration or condensation. At 20 weeks, amalgam specimens prepared from both types of alloys (alloy A, low copper, and alloy B, high copper) when contaminated by moisture, expanded far more than the same uncontaminated amalgams (Fig. 8.23). The expansion of the alloys at 20 weeks was also accompanied by a substantial reduction in compressive strength (Fig. 8.24).

Delayed expansion of amalgam often causes intense pain. It is presumed that when an expansion of this magnitude occurs, the

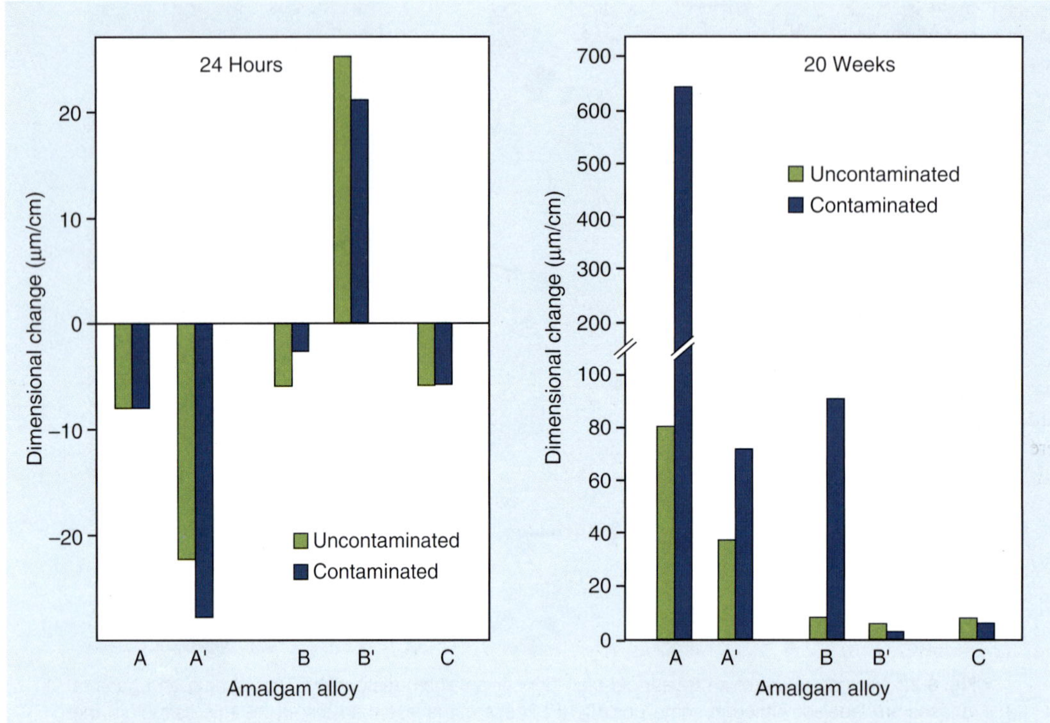

• **Fig. 8.23** Effect of moisture contamination on the dimensional change of various types of amalgam alloys. **(A)** Zinc-containing low-copper lathe-cut alloy. **(A')** Zinc-free low-copper lathe-cut alloy. **(B)** Zinc-containing high-copper lathe-cut alloy. **(B')** Zinc-free high-copper lathe-cut alloy. **(C)** Zinc-free high-copper spherical alloy.

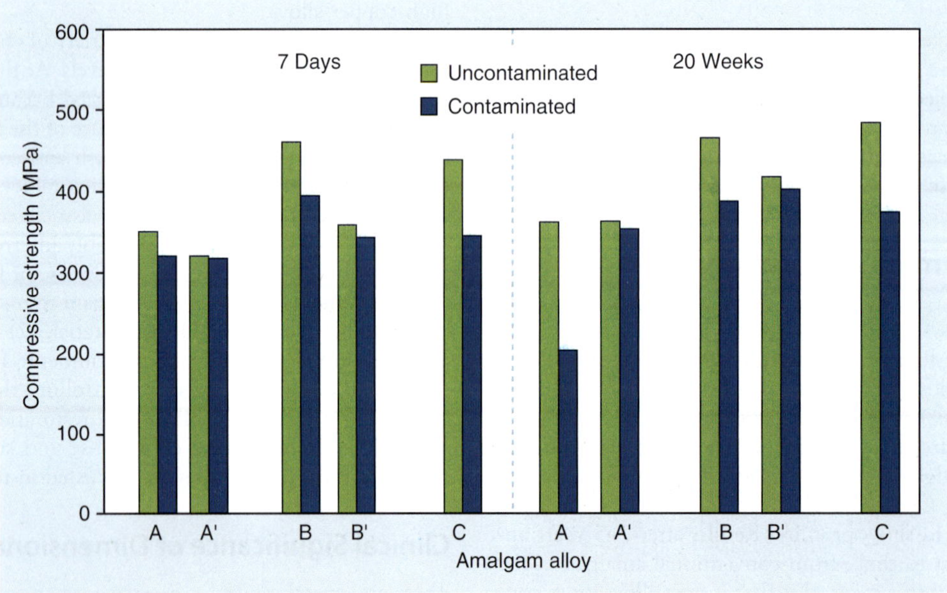

• **Fig. 8.24** Effect of moisture contamination on the compressive strength of various types of amalgam alloys. **(A)** Zinc-containing low-copper lathe-cut alloy. **(A')** Zinc-free low-copper lathe-cut alloy. **(B)** Zinc-containing high-copper lathe-cut alloy. **(B')** Zinc-free high-copper lathe-cut alloy. **(C)** Zinc-free high-copper spherical alloy.

filling may become wedged so tightly against the cavity walls that pressure develops in the pulp chamber. Such pain may be experienced 10–12 days after the amalgam is inserted. If it is not removed, a contaminated amalgam continues to expand, and the final result may be a protruding filling. Because the brittle amalgam margins are unsupported, they are susceptible to fracture, and marginal defects result. Leakage at the amalgam/enamel interface can produce marginal discoloration, with further corrosion and pitting by the concentration cells (Chapter 3). Pitting and corrosion, regardless of the cause, reduce the strength of amalgam restorations.

CRITICAL QUESTION

Which variables affect the marginal breakdown of amalgam restorations? Which of these factors are under the control of the dentist?

Marginal Breakdown

Although the ditching of a margin (Fig. 8.25) may not have progressed to the point where secondary caries may have developed, the restoration is unsightly and further deterioration may be anticipated. Examination of clinical restorations has associated secondary caries with marginal discrepancies that exceed 400 μm. Many such restorations are replaced as a preventive measure. Recent studies have shown that for a population with good oral hygiene, the incidence of secondary caries is quite low even in the presence of severe marginal deterioration. Thus, a more conservative approach, such as repair or recontouring, has been suggested.

Improper Cavity Preparation or Finishing

If unsupported enamel is left at the marginal areas of the cavity preparation, the tooth structure may fracture over time. Thus, the ditched amalgam may involve fracture of adjacent enamel as well as the amalgam.

Improper carving and finishing of the filling and/or failure to remove a mercury-rich surface layer may leave a thin, weak ledge of amalgam extending over the enamel that will eventually fracture, leaving a ditched margin (Fig. 8.26). Such thin extensions beyond the finish line of the tooth preparation are often difficult to detect and remove. One method is to finish the margins lightly with a soft, unribbed, prophylactic polishing cup and a fine, slightly moist prophylaxis paste. However, the cup should be tilted such that the edge rotates from amalgam to tooth, as shown in Fig. 8.27.

Creep

There appears to be little correlation between creep and marginal breakdown with alloys having creep values below 1%. However, when creep values are above this level, restorations made from higher-creep alloys generally experience greater marginal breakdown than do restorations of lower-creep alloys.

The absence of the corrosion-susceptible γ_2 phase in the microstructure of high-copper amalgams is assumed to be the principal factor responsible for the superior resistance of these alloys to marginal breakdown. If this assumption is correct, the property of creep is not an important property for the prediction of marginal breakdown in high-copper amalgams. Expansion of the amalgam from moisture contamination of a zinc-containing alloy can also cause this type of failure.

Thus, several mechanisms, separately or working synergistically, may be responsible for marginal breakdown. The precise mechanism of marginal breakdown and these specific properties are not completely understood. However, it is advisable to select alloys that inherently have low creep and possess excellent resistance to corrosion.

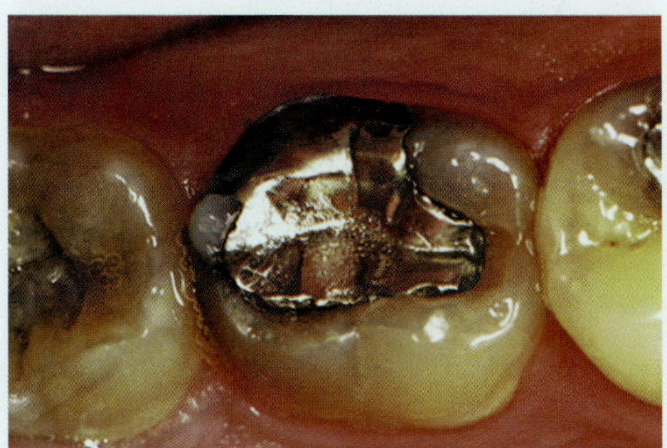

• **Fig. 8.25** A "ditched" amalgam restoration with severe marginal breakdown. (Courtesy of S Geraldeli.)

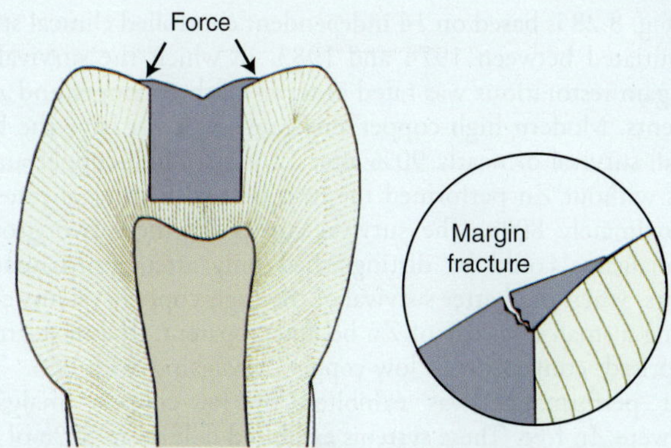

• **Fig. 8.26** Marginal ditching of an amalgam restoration. If a feather edge of the amalgam is left overlapping the enamel at the margin or if a mercury-rich surface layer is not properly removed, the marginal extension may fracture under masticatory stress.

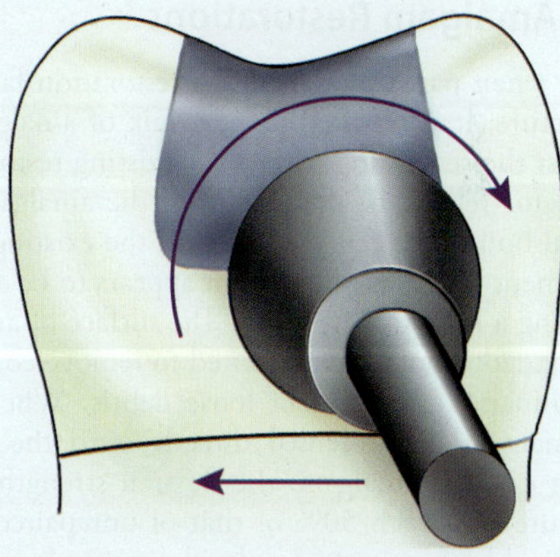

• **Fig. 8.27** Final finishing of an amalgam margin with a soft, unribbed prophylaxis cup and fine prophylaxis paste. The cup should be used with very light pressure to avoid flattening of anatomic contours.

Survival of Amalgam Restorations

Although many factors may contribute to the deterioration of dental amalgams, as noted in the prior sections, the ultimate test is the long-term survival of the well-placed dental amalgam restoration. The longevity of amalgam restorations depends on whether they were placed in general practices or in controlled clinical studies. The median survival times for posterior amalgam restorations were 7–15 years in general practices. Larger, more complex restorations fall within the lower end of this range.

Fig. 8.28 is based on 14 independent controlled clinical studies initiated between 1974 and 1983, in which the survival of amalgam restorations was rated in terms of their copper and zinc contents. Modern high-copper amalgams with Zn have the best overall survival of nearly 90% after 12 years. High-copper amalgams without Zn performed the next best with survival rates of approximately 80%. The survival curves for these two groups of amalgams could be distinguished only after approximately 6 years, when the better survival of the high-copper systems containing a small quantity of Zn became apparent. The next group comprised conventional low-copper amalgams with Zn. The worst performance was exhibited by low-copper amalgams that were Zn free. These systems exhibited failures in 50% of the restorations after only 10 years. The reasons for the differences seen in this study are not completely clear. However, the combined and perhaps synergistic effects of the additional Cu and Zn contents probably offered increased corrosion protection to the restorations.

Repaired Amalgam Restorations

Occasionally when part of an amalgam restoration fails, as from marginal fracture, it is repaired. A new mix of amalgam is condensed against the remaining part of the existing restoration. The important factor related to the quality of the amalgam repair is the interfacial bond between the new and the existing amalgam. Surface treatment of the aged amalgam appears to be a major factor in achieving a high-quality bond. The surface of an old amalgam to be bonded should be roughened to remove corrosion and saliva contaminants and freed of loose debris. When a freshly triturated amalgam is condensed directly onto the roughened surface of an existing amalgam, the flexural strength of the repaired structure can reach 50% of that of unrepaired amalgam. The repair should be attempted only if the area involved is one that will not be subjected to high stresses or one in which the two restoration parts are adequately supported and retained. It is worthwhile to note that rubbing mercury on the repair site before condensing new amalgam or increasing mercury content in the new amalgam can further improve the repair strength. Both approaches are discouraged as they increase the patient's exposure to mercury.

Making a slot on the existing amalgam to establish mechanical interlocking between the two materials also improves the quality of the repair joint. In vitro studies show that resin bonding agents appear to be effective when no mechanical roughening of the surface was performed, but yielding no benefit if adequate surface roughening of the existing amalgam had been carried out. Therefore, the use of resin bonding agents for amalgam repair is discouraged. It is important to point out that it is the reaction between the unreacted amalgam alloy in the old amalgam and the mercury in the new amalgam that provides the bonding. One may consider mercury as a bonding agent for amalgam repair.

Another repair option for areas that exhibit minor marginal breakdown—gaps that are 250 μm or less in width—is to etch the enamel adjacent to the restoration and, after rinsing and drying the marginal gap area, sealing the gap with a dentin bonding adhesive. There is evidence from a 10-year study (Mertz-Fairhurst, 1998) that bonded and sealed composite restorations placed directly over frank cavitated lesions extending into dentin arrested the clinical progress of these lesions for the duration of the study. Both sealed composite and conservative amalgam restorations exhibited superior clinical performance and longevity compared with unsealed amalgam restorations. This repair option is promising but needs more scientific evidence to prove that it can prevent secondary caries.

The clinical diagnosis of secondary (recurrent) caries is the main reason for replacing amalgam restorations; fracture is the second most common reason for failure of amalgam restorations.

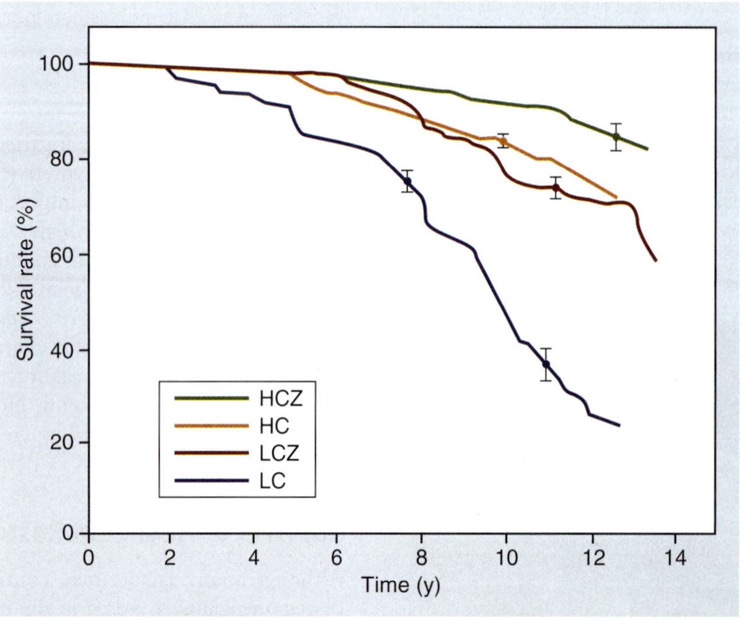

• **Fig. 8.28** Survival curves for amalgam restorations classified according to copper and zinc content. Both copper and zinc appear to provide protection to restorations. Thus, in these clinical trials, many more high-copper restorations containing zinc survived than low-copper restorations without zinc. HCZ, high-copper amalgam with zinc; HC, high-copper amalgam without zinc; LCZ, low-copper amalgam with zinc; and LC, low-copper amalgam without zinc.

When secondary caries is diagnosed, it inevitably requires the replacement of the restoration, but an alternative treatment is to remove part of the restoration to the full depth at the site of the defect. This is a recognized procedure to make a definitive diagnosis of the extent of the caries. Provided the main part of the restoration is satisfactory, the removed part of the restoration can then be filled with amalgam. The repair of an existing restoration is now considered a viable and cost-effective alternative to complete replacement.

CRITICAL QUESTION

A patient is concerned about the safety of amalgam fillings after hearing a news report on the toxicity of mercury. What quantifiable information can you provide to assure him that the levels of mercury vapor released from amalgam restorations are well below the known threshold levels for mercury toxicity?

Safety of Amalgam Fillings

The use of mercury in the oral environment has raised concerns ever since it was introduced in North America in 1833. Information on the biocompatibility of mercury and amalgam is presented in Chapter 17. The side-effects of mercury and reduction of mercury hazard in dental offices are discussed here to place the issue in perspective relative to the safety of amalgam. To understand the possible side effects of dental amalgam, the differences between allergy and toxicity must be discussed.

Allergy

Typically, allergic responses represent an antigen–antibody reaction marked by itching, rashes, sneezing, and difficulty in breathing, with swelling or other symptoms. Contact dermatitis or Coombs type IV *hypersensitivity* reactions represent the most likely physiologic side-effects to dental amalgam, but these reactions are experienced by less than 1% of the treated population. To confirm suspicions of true hypersensitivity, especially when a reaction has been sustained for 2 weeks or more, the patient should be evaluated by an allergist. A small percentage of people are allergic to mercury, just as a certain number of people are allergic to many other metallic elements. When such a reaction has been documented by an allergist, an alternative material, such as a composite or ceramic material, must be used. However, none of these materials has yet been proven to be *safer*, in all respects, than dental amalgam.

Toxicity

As defined in Chapter 17, toxicity is the relative ability of a material to cause injury to biological tissues, ranging from improper biochemical function, organ damage, and cell destruction to death. It is still sometimes conjectured that mercury toxicity from dental fillings is the cause of certain undiagnosed illnesses and that a real hazard may exist for the dentist or dental assistant when mercury vapor is inhaled during mixing, placement, and removal. In fact, fewer than 100 documented reports of mercury toxicity and allergy attributable to dental amalgam have been published over the past 70 years in the scientific literature. Of these cases, most of the affected individuals were dentists or assistants (nurses) in a dental clinic. Few such cases have been reported during the past several decades, presumably because of improvements in encapsulation technology, capsule design, scrap storage methods, and the elimination of carpets and other mercury retention sites. The matter has again come to the fore with recent concern over mercury pollution of the environment.

The patient's encounter with mercury vapor during insertion of the restoration is brief, and the total amount of mercury vapor released during occluding on amalgam restorations is far below the "no effect" level. The most reliable estimates suggest that mercury from dental amalgam does not contribute a significant amount to the total exposure of patients. Studies have shown that the magnitude of vapor exposure for a patient with 8–10 amalgam restorations is in the range of 1.1–4.4 μg per day. The threshold value for workers in the mercury industry is 350–500 μg per day. Thus, the toxicity threshold for patients receiving several amalgam restorations is far below the range of values established by the US government for occupational environments.

Mercury blood levels as measured in one study indicated that the average level in patients with amalgam was 0.7 ng/mL, compared with a value of 0.3 ng/mL for subjects with no amalgam. This difference was found to be statistically significant ($P < .01$). However, one should be aware of a study in Sweden demonstrating that one saltwater seafood meal per week raised average blood levels of mercury of the subjects from 2.3 to 5.1 ng/mL, a sevenfold increase (2.8 ng/mL) compared with the increase (0.4 ng/mL) associated with amalgam fillings. In fact, the normal daily intake of mercury is 15 μg from food, 1 μg from air, and 0.4 μg from water.

Undoubtedly small amounts of mercury are released during mastication. However, toxic reactions in the patient from these traces of mercury penetrating the tooth or sensitization from mercury salts dissolving from the surface of the amalgam are extremely rare.

Mercury Hygiene in Dental Offices

The potential hazards of mercury can be greatly reduced by attention to a few precautionary measures. The operatory should be well ventilated. All excess mercury—including waste, disposable capsules, and amalgam removed during condensation—should be collected and stored in well-sealed containers. Debris of amalgam from cutting and grinding can be trapped by installing amalgam particle separators in the dental wastewater stream. Proper disposal through reputable dental vendors is mandatory to prevent environment pollution. Increasing attention is being focused on correct disposal of potentially hazardous waste materials, including dental amalgams and mercury. Amalgam scrap and materials contaminated with mercury or amalgam should not be incinerated or subjected to heat sterilization. If mercury is spilled, it must be cleaned up as soon as possible. It is extremely difficult to remove mercury from carpets. Ordinary vacuum cleaners merely disperse the mercury further through the exhaust system. Mercury suppressant powders are helpful, but should be considered as temporary measures. If mercury comes in contact with the skin, the skin should be washed with soap and water.

As noted earlier, the reusable capsule utilized with a mechanical triturator should have a tightly fitting cap to avoid mercury leakage. When amalgam is being ground, a water spray and suction should be used. Eye protection, a disposable mask, and gloves are now standard requirements for dental practices.

The use of an ultrasonic amalgam condenser is not recommended. A spray of small mercury droplets has been observed surrounding the condenser tip during condensation. More detailed recommendations can be obtained by consulting the most recent reports of the ADA's Council on Scientific Affairs.

An important part of a program for handling toxic materials is periodic monitoring of actual exposure levels. Current recommendations suggest that this procedure be conducted annually. Several techniques are available. Instruments can be used that yield a time-weighted average for mercury exposure to sample the air in the operatory. Film badges are also available that can be worn by office personnel in a manner similar to radiation exposure badges. Biological determinations can be performed on office staff to measure mercury levels in blood or urine. The risk from mercury exposure to dental personnel cannot be ignored, but close adherence to simple hygiene procedures will help to ensure a safe working environment.

Regulation of Amalgam Use by Governments

Currently several countries are phasing out the use of dental amalgam because of environmental concerns as well as alleged side-effects that may be sustained by the patients who receive amalgam restorations. An important aspect of all of these actions is the conclusion that, from a medical point of view, there is no clinical evidence to suggest that amalgam is causing illness in the general population.

Denmark published draft orders in 1989 proposing to discontinue the sale of all mercury-containing products, including dental amalgam, by 1999. In 1992, the Swedish parliament approved a general plan to phase out mercury from all sources, including amalgam in children's primary teeth. The Swedish national health system stopped reimbursing patients for amalgam restorations in 1999. This decision greatly reduced the use of amalgam before the general ban in 2009. In 2008, Norway announced a general ban on the use of mercury in products, which include dental amalgam with a 3-year phase-out period. Sweden and Denmark announced similar bans in the same year.

In 2009, the FDA issued a final rule (FDA-2008-N-0163) classifying dental amalgam as a class II device. Class II devices are those for which general controls alone are insufficient to ensure safety and effectiveness and for which other methods are available to provide such assurances.

While the policy of dental amalgam use is being revised in several countries, a global discussion led by the United Nations Environment Programme (UNEP) on limiting the use of mercury products including dental amalgam was held between June 2010 and 2013. Following consultations with stakeholders and partners, a new global, legally binding instrument on mercury was developed, taking into account the challenges faced by both developed and developing countries.

The Minamata Convention

A "phase-out" of dental amalgam was first suggested by the Global Mercury Partnership, an organization formed by the UNEP. The terminology subsequently changed to "phase-down" and recognized that the complete cessation of the use of dental amalgam may be inappropriate as much needed to be achieved before this material can be completely replaced by alternatives.

The Minamata Convention on Mercury (2013) is an international legally binding treaty that aims to protect the human health and the environment from anthropogenic emissions and releases of mercury and mercury compounds. The convention addresses mercury-added products, including dental amalgam, which is made of approximately 50% of elemental mercury by weight, and proposes nine measures to phase down the use of dental amalgam. These measures show the interconnected and interdependent nature of phasing down dental amalgam, and reinforce the need for a multipronged approach as called for by WHO (Box 8 1).

Recently the International Association for Dental Research Policy (IADR) reaffirmed that, on the basis of the best available evidence, dental amalgam is safe to use for the general population without allergies to amalgam components or severe renal diseases.

The IADR further affirmed its support for the continuing use of amalgam when alternatives are less than optimal for clinical, economic, or practical reasons. At the same time they supported the phase-down strategy described in the Minamata Convention on Mercury. IADR emphasized the need, first, for increased oral disease prevention efforts to reduce the need for any kind of restorative material and, second, for further research on new biocompatible and environmentally friendly restorative materials and approaches that are proven to have equal or improved clinical longevity and cost-effectiveness when compared with amalgam restorations.

Even in affluent countries like the United Kingdom it has been seen that amalgam remains the material of choice for restoring posterior teeth in adults for NHS funded care. While dentists are knowledgeable and they embrace new techniques for posterior resin composite placement, funding arrangements in NHS dentistry appear to be a barrier to increasing use of resin composite in posterior teeth.

We should be careful before taking rash decisions on phasing out dental amalgam from a dental standpoint because if composite was the only choice available for long-term cost-effective treatment, it could put urgent dental care out of reach for the poor in developed countries like India and the general population in developing countries. Regardless of the outcomes of these sessions, the emphasis should remain on the need to educate patients and health providers about the benefits and risks of dental amalgam and to improve the care and consideration of patients who might benefit from treatment with amalgam fillings.

• BOX 8.1 Minamata Convention, Annex A, Part II4

Nine measures to phase down the use of dental amalgam

(i) Setting national objectives aiming at dental caries prevention and health promotion, thereby minimizing the need for dental restoration
(ii) Setting national objectives aiming at minimizing its use
(iii) Promoting the use of cost-effective and clinically effective mercury-free alternatives for dental restoration
(iv) Promoting research and development of quality mercury-free materials for dental restoration
(v) Encouraging representative professional organizations and dental schools to educate and train dental professionals and students on the use of mercury-free dental restoration alternatives and on promoting best management practices
(vi) Discouraging insurance policies and programs that favor dental amalgam use over mercury-free dental restoration
(vii) Encouraging insurance policies and programs that favor the use of quality alternatives to dental amalgam for dental restoration
(viii) Restricting the use of dental amalgam to its encapsulated form
(ix) Promoting the use of best environmental practices in dental facilities to reduce releases of mercury and mercury compounds to water and land

Acknowledgments

The authors wish to acknowledge Drs GW Marshall, Jr, and SJ Marshall for their previous contribution to this chapter.

Summary

- **Amalgam alloys**
  Before these alloys are reacted with mercury, they are known as **dental amalgam alloys** or alloys for dental amalgam. They are usually provided as:
  - Irregularly-shaped particles produced by milling or lathe-cutting a cast ingot of the amalgam alloy **(lathe cut)**
  - As spherical particles produced by atomizing the liquid alloy in a chamber filled with inert gas **(spherical)**, or
  - As a mixture of both lathe-cut and spherical particles **(admixed)**.
- **Composition**
  It is now customary to classify amalgam alloys as either,
  - Low-copper (conventional), or
  - High-copper alloys. In both types, the major components of the alloys are silver and tin.
- **Low-copper alloys**
  - Silver–tin alloys are quite brittle and difficult to blend uniformly unless a small amount of copper is substituted for silver. An increased copper content hardens and strengthens the silver–tin alloy.
  - The structure of these conventional alloys is dominated by Ag_3Sn (γ phase) with some Cu_3Sn (ϵ phase).
- **High-copper alloys**
  - The first high-copper alloy was formulated by mixing one part of silver–copper, spherical eutectic (Ag–Cu); 71.9% silver and 28.1% copper by weight) particles to two parts of Ag_3Sn, provided as lathe-cut particles. This modification raises the copper content to 11.8% by weight. This is often called "dispersed-phase alloy" or "admixed high-copper alloy."
  - Melting all components of the dispersed phase alloy makes a second type of high-copper alloy. This process yields a single-composition system. The copper content of this group of alloys can be as high as 30% by weight.
- **Powder configuration**
  - Lathe-cut powder
  - Atomized powder
- **Particle size**
  - The average particle sizes of modern powders range between 15 and 35 µm.
  - The particle size distribution can affect the character of the finished surface. A smaller average particle size tends to produce a more rapid hardening of the amalgam with greater early strength.
- **Lathe-cut powder versus spherical powder**
  - Amalgams made from lathe-cut powders or admixed powders tend to resist condensation better than amalgams made entirely from spherical powders.
  - Spherical alloys require less mercury than typical lathe-cut alloys.
- **Amalgamation**
  Modern dental amalgam alloys are based on the intermetallic compound Ag3Sn; therefore, the main reaction after trituration occurs between Ag3Sn and mercury. Other elements in the alloy, especially copper, also play a significant role in the final microstructures of set amalgams.
- **Clinical manipulation of amalgam for restorations**
- **Mercury/alloy ratio**
  - The amount of alloy and mercury to be used can be described as the mercury/alloy ratio, which signifies the number of parts by weight of mercury divided by the number of parts of alloy to be used for the particular technique.
  - The mercury content of the lathe-cut alloy is about 50% by weight and that for spherical alloys is 42% by weight.
- **Mechanical trituration**
  The objective of trituration is to provide proper amalgamation of the mercury and alloy. There is always an oxide layer of the alloy surface that hinders diffusion of mercury into the alloy. This film must be disrupted so that a clean surface of alloy can make intimate contact with the mercury. The oxide layer is removed by abrasion when the alloy particles and mercury are triturated.
- **Consistency of the mix**
  The proper time of mixing can be determined by observing the consistency of the mix. For example, the very grainy mix indicates undertrituration.
- **Condensation**
  - The goal of condensation is to compact the alloy into the prepared cavity so that the greatest possible density is attained.
  - The condenser tip, or face, is forced into the amalgam mass under hand pressure. Condensation is usually started at the center, and then the condenser point is stepped incrementally toward the cavity walls.
- **Carving and finishing**
  - After the amalgam has been condensed into the prepared cavity, it is carved to reproduce the proper tooth anatomy. The objective of carving is to simulate the anatomy rather than to reproduce extremely fine details.
  - Carving should not be started until the amalgam is hard enough to offer resistance to the carving instrument. A scraping or "ringing" sound should be heard when it is carved.
  - If the carving is started too soon, the amalgam may be so plastic that it may be pulled away from the margins, even by the sharpest carving instrument.
- **Properties of amalgam**
- **Dimensional stability**
- **Effect of moisture contamination**
- **Tarnish and corrosion resistance**
  - Amalgam restorations often tarnish and corrode in the oral environment.
  - The most common corrosion products found with conventional amalgam alloys are oxides and chlorides of tin.

The Minamata Convention

- *The Minamata Convention on Mercury (2013) is an international legally binding treaty that aims to protect the human health and the environment from anthropogenic emissions and releases of mercury and mercury compounds.*

Review Questions

1. Classify silver amalgam and write in detail about high-copper amalgam.
2. Classify silver amalgam. Discuss in detail composition, setting reaction and properties, and advantages of high-copper amalgam.
3. What is dental amalgam? Enumerate the functions of individual ingredients of dental amalgam. Differentiate between high-copper and low-copper amalgam alloys.
4. Define trituration. What are the different trituration methods for silver amalgam? Explain the amalgamation reactions of various types of dental amalgam.
5. Manufacturing of spherical silver alloy powder.
6. What is the role of silver and tin in dental amalgam?
7. Discuss the chemistry of setting of dental amalgam.
8. Discuss in brief trituration and condensation.
9. Zinc-free alloys.
10. Composition amalgamation reaction and properties of high-copper amalgam.
11. Unicompositional alloy.
12. Discuss in brief copper-rich amalgam alloy.
13. Admixed alloy.
14. Silver alloy–mercury ratio.
15. Describe the different methods of mulling dental amalgam.
16. What is the clinical significance of delayed expansion?
17. What is the effect of moisture contamination of amalgam?
18. What is the effect of creep on silver amalgam restoration?
19. Microleakage and its significance.
20. Discuss in brief mercury toxicity.

Selected Readings

Ajiboye AS, Mossey PA, Fox CH. International Association for Dental Research Policy and Position Statements on the Safety of Dental Amalgam. Journal of Dental Research. 2020;99(7):763-768. doi:10.1177/0022034520915878

Alexander G, Hopcraft MS, Tyas MJ, Wong RHK. Dental educators' attitudes towards the teaching of dental amalgam: A mixed methods analysis. Eur J Dent Educ. 2020;24:282-291. https://doi.org/10.1111/eje.12496

Anusavice K.J. Quality Evaluation of Dental Restorations: Criteria for Placement and Replacement. Quintessence: Chicago; Six chapters of the book written by various experts deal with clinical studies, methods of evaluation, and differences in diagnosis related to dental amalgam restorations. Evidence supporting a more conservative approach to replacement of the "ditched" amalgam restoration is presented.

Barbakow F.; Gaberthuel T.; Lutz F.; et al. Maintenance of amalgam restorations. Quintessence Int 19 861–870 (1988); A systematic procedure for recontouring, finishing, and polishing existing amalgam restorations is illustrated, along with proper selection of instruments.

Bauer J.G. A study of procedures for burnishing amalgam restorations. J Prosthet Dent 57 669–673 (1987); This report describes the combined factors of time from end of trituration, burnishing force, and number of burnishing strokes on margins, surface characteristics, and porosity for a high-copper admixed amalgam. Early times and minimal strokes gave the best results.

Bogacki R.E.; Hunt R.J.; del Aguila M.; et al. Survival analysis of posterior restorations using an insurance claims database. Oper Dent 27 488–492 (2002); This study found that composite restorations did not last as long as amalgam restoration based on insurance claim data collected between 1993 and 2000. The study also found changing dentists reduced the longevity of restorations by 30%.

Brownawell A.M.; Berent S.; Brent R.L.; et al. The potential adverse health effects of dental amalgam. Toxicol Rev 24 1–10 (2005); According to these authors, there is no convincing evidence pointing to any adverse health effects attributable to dental amalgam restorations besides hypersensitivity in some individuals.

Browning W.D.; Johnson W.W.; Gregory P.N. Clinical performance of bonded amalgam restorations at 42 months. J Am Dent Assoc 131 607–611 (2000); There were no differences in the clinical performance of amalgam with bonding agent or copal varnish.

Dodes J.E. The amalgam controversy. An evidence-based analysis. J Am Dent Assoc 132 348–356 (2001); Authoritative studies consistently have found that amalgam restorations are safe and effective. This review of the literature further supports this conclusion.

Duke E.S.; Cochran M.A.; Moore B.K.; et al. Laboratory profiles of 30 high-copper amalgam alloys. J Am Dent Assoc 105 636–640 (1982); The laboratory profiles identify the alloy systems and reflect the performance of the alloy. A classification for various types is presented.

Eames W.B. Preparation and condensation of amalgam with a low mercury/alloy ratio. J Am Dent Assoc 58 78–83 (1959); This technique revolutionized the procedure in constructing an amalgam restoration by use of minimal amounts of mercury in the original mix.

Fairhurst C.W.; Ryge G. X-ray diffraction investigation of the Sn-Hg phase in dental amalgam. In: (editor: Mueller W.M.) Advances in X-ray Analysis. Vol. 5 Plenum Press: New York; These investigators determined the of the Sn-Hg phase in dental amalgam to have hexagonal unit cell.

Fédération Dentaire Internationale, Technical Report 33. Safety of dental amalgam. Int Dent J 39 217 (1989); This authoritative organization reviewed the literature on mercury toxicity and concluded that there is no documented scientific evidence to show adverse effects from mercury in amalgam restorations except in rare cases of mercury hypersensitivity.

Ferracane J.L.; Mafiana P.; Cooper C.; et al. Time-dependent dissolution of amalgams into saline solution. J Dent Res 66 1331–1335 (1987); This study indicates that the rate of dissolution of ions from amalgams into saline is low once the amalgam has set, probably inhibited by formation of a surface film.

Fisher, J., et al. (2018). "The Minamata Convention and the phase down of dental amalgam." Bull World Health Organ 96(6): 436-438.

Gale E.N.; Osborne J.W.; Winchell P.G. Fracture at the margins of amalgam as predicted by creep, zinc content, and gamma-2 content. J Dent Res 61 678–680 (1982); The data suggest that equations based upon in vitro data to predict marginal breakdown for alloys might not be predictive for non-γ_2 alloys.

Innes D.B.K.; Youdelis W.V. Dispersion strengthened amalgams. Can Dent Assoc J 29 587–593 (1963); This research introduced the admix alloys.

Klausner L.H.; Green T.G.; Charbeneau G.T. Placement and replacement of amalgam restorations. A challenge for the profession. Oper Dent 12 105–112 (1987); A national survey assessed factors underlying the placement and replacement of amalgam restorations. The reactions to questions such as expected length of service and reasons for failure are interesting and a challenge to the profession is identified.

Letzel H.; Vrijhoef M.M.A. The influence of polishing on the marginal integrity of amalgam restorations. J Oral Rehabil 11 89–94 (1984); The effect of polishing on the marginal integrity of amalgam restorations continues to be a matter of some controversy, particularly with high-copper alloys. This study questions the necessity for polishing, at least in respect to marginal defects.

Letzel H.; van't Hof M.A.; Vrijhoef M.M.A.; et al. A controlled clinical study of amalgam restorations: Survival, failures, and causes of failure. Dent Mater 5 115–121 (1989); Bulk fracture or fracture at the marginal ridge was reported as the leading mode of failure. It is suggested that further improvements in mechanical properties and corrosion resistance are needed.

Letzel H.; van't Hoff M.A.; Marshall G.W.; et al. The influence of amalgam alloy on the survival of amalgam restorations: A secondary analysis of multiple controlled clinical trials. J Dent Res 76 1787–1798 (1997); An analysis of multiple clinical trials demonstrated the synergistic effects of copper and zinc content on the survival of amalgam restorations.

Lloyd C.H.; Adamson M. The fracture toughness of amalgam. J Oral Rehab 12 59–68 (1985); Admixed high-copper products have higher fracture toughness than those of a single-component powder, attributed to differences in microstructures.

Lynch, C. D., et al. (2018). "No more amalgams: Use of amalgam and amalgam alternative materials in primary dental care." Br Dent J **225**(2): 171-176.

Mahler D.B.; Adey J.D. Microprobe analysis of three high-copper amalgams. J Dent Res 63 921–925 (1984); The composition and structure of three high-copper amalgams before and after their reaction were studied.

Mahler D.B.; Van Eysden J. Dynamic creep of dental amalgam. J Dent Res 48 501–508 (1969); The first suggestion that creep may be a major factor in marginal breakdown of amalgam restorations. Although modern alloys have low creep values, the test is a useful screening tool in selecting commercial alloys.

Mahler D.B.; Adey J.D.; Marek M. Creep and corrosion of amalgam. J Dent Res 61 33–35 (1982); Corrosion was directly related to the amount of γ_2 phase present, while creep was either high or low, depending on the absence or presence of γ_2.

Mahler D.B.; Adey J.D.; Van Eysden J. Quantitative microprobe analysis of amalgam. J Dent Res 54 218–226 (1975); The presence of tin in the Ag-Hg phase (γ_1) was confirmed and Cu_3Sn was found in the original alloy particles. In the dispersant amalgam, little Sn-Hg phase (γ_2) was found and the reaction phase Cu_6Sn_5 was identified.

Mahler D.B.; Pham B.V.; Adey J.D. Corrosion sealing of amalgam restorations in vitro. Oper Dent 34 312–320 (2009); This in vitro study shows that gap sealing was influenced by the size of the initial gap as well as corrosion resistance of the amalgam, and zinc in the amalgam alloy resulted in the formation of zinc corrosion products in the gap. The latter might explain the reported reduction in marginal fracture of zinc-containing amalgams.

Mahler D.B.; Terkla L.G.; Van Eysden J.; et al. Marginal fracture versus mechanical properties of amalgam. J Dent Res 49 1452–1457 (1970); Two independent studies showed clinical superiority for the admixed alloy developed by Innes and Youdelis. These publications are classic, as they opened the vista of the high-copper alloy.

Marshall G.W. Jr.; Marshall S.J.; Letzel H.; et al. Microstructures of Cu-rich amalgam restorations with moderate clinical deterioration. Dent Mater 3 135–143 (1987); The large variations in porosity and corrosion products in clinically retrieved restorations are described. It also demonstrates a zinc-rich layer and other tin layers that form at the tooth-amalgam interface.

May K.N.; Wilder A.D.; Leinfelder K.F. Burnished amalgam restorations: A two-year clinical evaluation. J Prosthet Dent 49 193–197 (1983); Clinical behavior of amalgam restorations found that precarved burnishing improved the marginal integrity of lathe-cut alloys. Coupled with postcarved burnishing, it was suggested as a viable substitute for conventional polishing.

Mertz-Fairhurst E.J.; Curtis J.W. Jr.; Ergle J.W.; et al. Ultraconservative and cariostatic sealed restorations: Results at year 10. J Am Dent Assoc 130 1751–1757 (1999).

Minamata Convention on Mercury. Geneva: United Nations Environment Programme; 2013. Available from: http://www.mercuryconvention.org/Convention/tabid/3426/language/en-US/Default.aspx

Mitchell R.J.; Okabe T. Setting reactions in dental amalgam. Part 1. Phases and microstructures between one hour and one week. Crit Rev Biol Med 7 12–22 (1996); Two recent reviews of setting reactions are offered, covering microstructures of various amalgam types and their properties as related to clinical performance.

Mitchell R.J.; Koike M.; Okabe T. Posterior amalgam restorations usage, regulation, and longevity. Dent Clin North Am 51 573–589 (2007); Long-term studies have shown that under optimal conditions, posterior restorations of amalgam and resin composite last longer than reported previously and that amalgam restorations outlast composite restorations. In general practice settings, posterior amalgam and composite restorations both have lower longevities.

Mjör I.A. The safe and effective use of dental amalgam. Int Dent J 37 147–151 (1987); Many pertinent matters related to the amalgam restoration are discussed in this review, including mercury toxicity, longevity of the restoration, common causes for failure, and certain properties that relate to performance.

Mjör I.A.; Gordan V.V. Failure, repair, refurbishing and longevity of restorations. Oper Dent 27 528–534 (2002); This article advocates removing part of the restoration to the full depth to make a firm diagnosis regarding the extent of the lesion and the affected area that can be repaired or refurbished.

Okabe T.; Mitchell R.J.; Butts M.B.; et al. A study of high-copper amalgams. III. SEM observations of amalgamation of high-copper powders. J Dent Res 57 975–982 (1978); Third of a series of three publications defining the phases that occur in the setting reaction of the alloy and mercury and as influenced by parameters such as composition and particle configuration.

Opdam N.J.; Bronkhorst E.M.; Loomans B.A.; et al. 12-Year survival of composite vs. amalgam restorations. J Dent Res 89 1063–1067 (2010); This retrospective study shows that large composite restorations had a higher survival in the combined population and in the low-risk group, and three-surface amalgams exhibited better survival in high-risk patients.

Rogers K.D. Status of scrap (recyclable) dental amalgams as environmental health hazards or toxic substances. J Am Dent Assoc 119 159–166 (1989); A review presenting available evidence to show amalgam scrap is not a toxic substance or environmental health hazard; it also covers portions of the literature that indicate intraoral amalgams do not present an adverse health hazard.

Shen C.; Speigel J.; Mjör I.A. Repair strength of dental amalgams. Oper Dent 31 122–126 (2006); This study shows the need of condensing directly on the old amalgam to establish the bond between new and old amalgams.

Staninec M.; Eakle W.S.; Silverstein S.; et al. Bonded amalgam sealants: Two-year clinical results. J Am Dent Assoc 129 323–329 (1998); This study shows there is no difference in 2-year retention between bonded amalgams as pit and fissure sealants without mechanical preparation and resin-based pit and fissure sealants.

Söderholm K.J. An X-ray diffractometric investigation of the Sn-Hg binary system within the 0–40% Hg interval. J Dent Res 66 712–715 (1987); This study shows the presence of in the range of Sn-Hg used in dental amalgam.

Soncini J.A.; Maserejian N.N.; Trachtenberg F.; et al. The longevity of amalgam versus compomer/composite restorations in posterior primary and permanent teeth: findings From the New England Children's Amalgam Trial. J Am Dent Assoc 138 763–772 (2007); Compomer/composite restorations on posterior tooth surfaces in children may require replacement or repair at higher rates than amalgam restorations, even within five years of placement.

Sutow E.J.; Jones D.W.; Hall G.C. Correlation of dental amalgam crevice corrosion with clinical ratings. J Dent Res 68 82–88 (1989); Marginal breakdown and the corrosion behavior of γ_2 and γ_2-free amalgams were studied in vitro. The methodology is of particular interest.

Swartz M.L.; Phillips R.W. In vitro studies on the marginal leakage of restorative materials. J Am Dent Assoc 62 141–151 (1961); One of numerous studies demonstrating the reduction in microleakage as the amalgam restoration ages that is unique to restorative materials.

Vrihjoef M.M.A.; Vermeersch A.G.; Spanauf A.J. Dental Amalgam. Quintessence: Chicago; A comprehensive treatment of the various factors involved in the design of amalgam alloys, their properties, and the parameters that influence clinical behavior. The lifetime of an amalgam is determined by the material, the dentist and assistant, and the patient.

Walker R.S.; Wade A.G.; Iazzetti G.; et al. Galvanic interaction between gold and amalgam: Effect of zinc, time and surface treatments. J Am Dent Assoc 134 1463–1467 (2003); Galvanic interaction between cast gold and amalgam is reduced over time and surface treatments, but is increased considerably when the amalgam contains zinc.

PART III

Indirect Restorative Materials

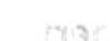

9

Metals

CHAPTER OUTLINE

KEY TERMS

Age hardening—The process of hardening certain alloys by controlled heating and cooling, which usually is associated with a phase change.

Annealing—The process of controlled heating and cooling that is designed to produce desired properties in a metal. Typically, the annealing process is intended to soften metals, increase their ductility, stabilize shape, and increase machinability (see *Stress Relief*).

Antiflux—A substance such as graphite that prevents the flow of molten solder on areas coated by the substance.

Base metal—A metal that readily oxidizes or corrodes. Important base metals for dental alloys are nickel, cobalt, iron, titanium, and chromium.

Cold welding—The metal-joining process by metallic bonding that does not rely on heating to achieve fusion but the pressure applied to the interface between parts to be joined; no liquid phase is produced within the interface joint.

CP Ti—Commercially pure titanium, which consists of 99 wt% or higher-purity titanium, with oxygen, carbon, nitrogen, and hydrogen dissolved interstitially.

Dislocation—An imperfection in the crystalline arrangement of atoms consisting of an extra partial plane of atoms (edge dislocation), a spiral distortion of normally parallel atom planes (screw dislocation), or a combination of the two types.

Flux—Compound applied to metal surfaces that dissolves or prevents the formation of oxides and other undesirable substances that may reduce the quality or strength of a soldered or brazed area.

Grain growth—The increase in the mean crystal size of a polycrystalline metal produced by a heat treatment process.

Grain refinement—The process of reducing the crystal (grain) size in a solid metal through the action of specific alloying elements or compounds; the process increases the yield strength of metals.

Lost wax technique—Process in which a wax pattern, prepared in the shape of missing tooth structure, is embedded in a casting investment and burned out to produce a mold cavity into which molten metal is cast.

Noble metal—Gold and platinum group metals (platinum, palladium, rhodium, ruthenium, iridium, and osmium), which are highly resistant to oxidation and dissolution in inorganic acids.

Precipitation hardening—The process of strengthening and hardening a metal by precipitating a phase or constituent from a saturated solid solution.

Recovery—A stage of heat treatment that results in the partial restoration of properties of a work-hardened metal without a change in the grain structure.

Recrystallization—The process of forming new stress-free crystals in a work-hardened metal through a controlled heat treatment process.

Soldering—Process of building up a localized area of a metal prosthesis with a molten filler metal or joining two or more metal components by heating them to a temperature below their solidus temperature and filling the gap between them using a molten metal with a lower liquidus temperature. If the melting temperature of the solder is greater than 450°C, the process is called *brazing*.

Springback—The amount of elastic strain that a metal can recover when loaded to and unloaded from its yield strength; an important property of orthodontic wires.

Strain hardening—The increase in strength and hardness and decrease in ductility of a metal that are caused by permanent deformation below its recrystallization temperature; also called *work hardening* or *cold working*.

Superelasticity—The ability of certain nickel–titanium alloys to undergo extensive elastic deformation resulting from a stress-assisted phase transformation, with the reverse transformation occurring on unloading; sometimes called *pseudoelasticity*.

Welding—Process of fusing two or more metal parts through the application of heat, pressure, or both, with and without a filler metal, to produce a localized union across an interface between the workpieces.

Working range—The maximum amount of elastic strain that an orthodontic wire can sustain before it permanently deforms.

Wrought alloy—A metal that has been permanently deformed to alter the shape of the structure and certain mechanical properties, such as strength, hardness, and ductility.

In his 1907 US Patent 865823, Taggart described a method of making gold inlays using the lost wax technique. The lost wax method of making metal objects involves pouring a molten metal into a mold that has been created with a wax pattern (Chapter 14). The process led to making custom precision casts for the restoration of missing tooth structure, such as onlays, crowns, multiple-unit fixed dental prostheses (FDPs), and frameworks for removable partial dentures (RPDs). Since the early 1980s, the number of dental alloys, along with new alloy systems, has increased dramatically as a result of the market price increase of noble metals, the performance of the same function at a lower cost, the need for increasingly specialized physical and mechanical properties, and the awareness of the importance of biological properties.

Objects of any design, intricate or simple, can be produced by using the lost wax technique as long as a wax pattern can be made and invested, and alloys can be melted, or by using alternative processing techniques such as computer-aided design/computer-aided manufacturing (CAD-CAM) milling and three-dimensional (3-D) printing. On the other hand, many ancillary dental materials and instruments are fabricated from initially cast alloys that have been subsequently rolled to form sheets or rods, drawn into wire or tubing, or forged into a finished shape. Rolling, drawing, and forging are major processes of permanently deforming metals.

Whenever a cast pure metal or alloy is permanently deformed to an intended shape in any manner, it is considered a wrought alloy. This permanent deformation alters the microstructure, and the alloy exhibits properties that are different from those it had in the as-cast state. The most significant change is the increase of *yield strength* with a reduction in ductility. The applications of wrought alloys in dentistry include orthodontic wires, clasps for RPDs, direct-filling gold (Chapter 8), root canal files and reamers, preformed crowns in pediatric dentistry, and surgical instruments. Most metal-based restorations and prostheses are cast and not wrought.

In the construction of dental appliances, there is often a need to join metal parts, cast or wrought, together using high heat. When wrought alloys are involved in such joining, the strength and fracture resistance of the wrought alloy will be compromised if the metal is exposed to the temperature range at which the wrought structure is diminished or lost. Such weakening can occur during the metal-joining process for stainless steel orthodontic appliances.

The ability to work with dental alloys and associated wrought alloys is dependent on the knowledge of these materials. The goal of this chapter is to become familiar with various types of casting alloys and associated wrought alloys. We will discuss the desirable properties and the relevant mechanical properties of dental alloys first. For casting alloys, the focus is the alloy classification and clinical applications of the alloys. For wrought alloys, the focus is the process of permanent deformation and its effect on the properties for their specific applications in dentistry. Several types of wrought alloys used in dentistry are described. The description of joining metals is like that for bonding presented in Chapter 6; the emphasis is on the principles and procedures of the process.

As previously done in Chapter 2, the terms *metal* and *alloy* are frequently used interchangeably.

In dentistry the most common casting alloys used for dental appliances and prostheses are based on a majority of one or more of the following metallic elements:

- Cobalt (Co)
- Gold (Au)
- Iron (Fe)
- Nickel (Ni)
- Palladium (Pd)
- Silver (Ag)
- Titanium (Ti)

Alloying is done for many reasons, typically to increase strength, increase corrosion resistance, or reduce costs.

Alloys are generally harder than pure metals. They are made up of atoms of different sizes, rather than being uniform. This means that the layers of atoms cannot slide over each other easily, making the whole alloy much stronger than any of the pure metals that the alloy contains in isolation. Alloys also tend to have better corrosion resistance than pure metals, and are more versatile for manipulating into different form.

Desirable Properties of Dental Alloys

Depending on the primary purpose of the prosthesis, the choice of casting alloy is made by the dentist in collaboration with a qualified dental laboratory technician or technologist. From the standpoint of patient safety and the risk of medicolegal issues, it is highly important to understand the following clinically important requirements and properties of dental casting alloys:

1. Biocompatibility—The alloy must tolerate oral fluids and not release any harmful products into the oral environment that might cause a toxic or allergic reaction. Biocompatibility will be covered in Chapter 17.
2. Tarnish and corrosion resistance—*Corrosion* is the physical deterioration of a material in the oral environment, and *tarnish* is a thin film that is adherent to the metal surface (Chapter 3). Both phenomena affect the durability and appearance of the prostheses.
3. Thermal properties—The melting range of the casting alloys must be low enough to form smooth surfaces with the mold wall of the casting investment (Chapter 14). For metal–ceramic prostheses, the alloys must have closely matching thermal expansion coefficients to be compatible with the given porcelains, and they must tolerate high processing temperatures without deforming via a creep process.
4. Strength requirements—The alloy must have sufficient strength for the intended application. For example, alloys for bridgework require higher strength than alloys for single crowns.
5. Fabrication—The molten alloy should flow freely into the investment mold, without any appreciable interaction with the investment material, and wet the mold to form a surface free of porosity. It should be possible to cut, grind, finish, and polish the alloy to obtain a prosthesis with a satisfactory surface finish.
6. Porcelain bonding—The alloy must be able to form a thin adherent oxide that enables chemical bonding to ceramic veneering materials.
7. Economic considerations—The cost of metals used for single-unit prostheses or as frameworks for FDPs or RPDs is a function of the metal density, fluctuations in metal prices, and the cost per unit mass.

Functional Mechanical Properties of Alloys

Mechanical properties are the measured responses of materials in the form of stress and strain under an applied force or distribution of forces. The relevant functional characteristics of casting and wrought alloys are described next.

CRITICAL QUESTION

What are two clinical disadvantages of cast metals that have lower elastic moduli? Why does a long-span bridge require alloys of high elastic modulus?

Elastic Modulus

One characteristic of a material with a high elastic modulus is its rigidity or stiffness. For a dental prosthesis, rigidity is equivalent to the resistance to flexure (bending). When a long-span FDP flexes during occluding of the pontic, the mesiodistal bending moment exerted on the abutment teeth can act as a dislodging force, lifting the mesial and distal aspects of the prosthesis. Furthermore, a flexing bridge can induce lateral forces on the abutment teeth, resulting in the loosening of these teeth. For a metal–ceramic prosthesis, the overlying brittle porcelain will fail catastrophically when the metal substructure flexes beyond the flexural limit of the ceramic. The elastic modulus is also important for the major connectors of an RPD, which must have enough rigidity to prevent flexure during the placement and function of the prosthesis. Resistance to flexure also allows the clasps of an RPD to fit into areas of minimal undercuts and still provide adequate retention.

CRITICAL QUESTION

Why is it that a cast prosthesis that is subjected to tensile stress above the alloy yield strength will not necessarily fracture?

Yield Strength (Proof Stress)

Recall the discussion in Chapter 4 that yield strength (YS), elastic limit, and proportional limit, by definition, are different properties, but all three terms have been used to reflect the capacity of a cast prosthesis to withstand mechanical stresses without permanent deformation. Ideally, dental alloys should have a high YS so that a large amount of stress must be applied before a permanent change in dimensions occurs. For an orthodontic appliance, it relates to the maximum force the wire can deliver. Generally, alloys with tensile YSs above 300 MPa function satisfactorily in the mouth.

CRITICAL QUESTION

How does the alloy ductility increase the fracture resistance of a margin of a cast metal crown or a clasp arm on an RPD?

Ductility (Percent Elongation)

Ductility represents the amount of permanent deformation under tensile stress that an alloy can undergo before it fractures. If the force applied is in a compressive mode, the property is called *malleability*. A reasonable amount of ductility and malleability is essential if a prosthesis requires adjustment to be functional, such as the bending of RPD clasps and the burnishing of crown margins. As discussed earlier, one needs to apply stress greater than the YS of the material to cause permanent deformation on a metal surface. Therefore, high ductility allows one to achieve more permanent deformation without fracture but does not indicate if burnishing or adjusting the prosthesis would be easier or more difficult in terms of the stress required.

CRITICAL QUESTION

Why is a harder metal more resistant to wear than a softer metal?

Hardness

Clinically, hardness reflects the resistance of the restoration to scratching and abrasion by the opposing tooth or restoration and the ability to maintain the smoothness of the prosthesis in the oral environment. However, a harder restoration surface can cause excessive wear of softer opposing dentition or restorations. In addition, harder surfaces are more difficult to cut, grind, finish, and polish because higher stress is required for each procedure.

Fatigue Resistance

Fatigue failure can occur when a material is subjected to repeated loading and unloading below its elastic limit. Most fractures of prostheses and restorations develop progressively over many stress cycles of loading and unloading. When the load is above a certain threshold, crack propagation is initiated from flaws within the prosthesis. Eventually a crack propagates to a critical size, and sudden fracture occurs. Common engineering expressions of fatigue fracture resistance are fatigue strength and endurance limit (Fig. 4.13). *Fatigue strength* (SNf) is defined as the stress at which failure occurs after a specific number of fatigue cycles. *Endurance limit* is the maximum stress that can be maintained without failure over an infinite number of cycles. Some alloys do not have a well-defined endurance limit.

Classification of Dental Casting Alloys

In 1932, the dental materials group at the National Bureau of Standards (now National Institute of Standards and Technology) classified dental gold alloys being used then by Vickers hardness number (VHN): type I (soft, VHN 50–90), type II (medium, VHN 90–120), type III (hard, VHN 120–150), and type IV (extra hard, VHN 150 and above). Since then, the number of alloy compositions and applications has increased vastly. They are now classified according to composition, intended usage, or mechanical properties.

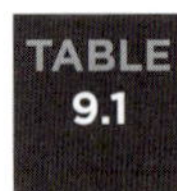

TABLE 9.1 Alloy Classification by Noble Metal Content—American Dental Association (2003)

Alloy Type	Total Noble Metal Content
High noble (HN)	Must contain ≥40% Au and ≥60% by weight of noble metal elements[a]
Noble (N)	Must contain ≥25% by weight of noble metal elements
Predominantly base metal (PB)	Contains <25% by weight of noble metal elements
Titanium and titanium alloys	Titanium ≥85% by weight

[a]Noble metal elements include Au, Pd, Pt, Rh, Ru, Ir, and Os.

Alloy Classification by Noble Metal Content

In 1984, the American Dental Association (ADA) proposed a simple classification for dental casting alloys based on the content of noble metals. Three categories were described: high noble (HN), noble (N), and predominantly base metal (PB). Subsequently, a fourth group of titanium and titanium alloys was added because of the unique characteristics of titanium. This classification is presented in Table 9.1. Noble metals comprise a group of seven metals that are resistant to corrosion and tarnish in the mouth. In order of increasing melting temperature, they include gold, palladium, platinum, rhodium, ruthenium, iridium, and osmium. These noble metals and silver are sometimes called *precious metals,* referring to their high economic value, but the term *precious* is not synonymous with *noble.* Silver is reactive in the oral cavity and is not a noble metal.

Based on this classification, the IdentAlloy program was established by manufacturers to provide documentation of certified alloys. Under this program, each alloy has a certificate (Fig. 9.1)

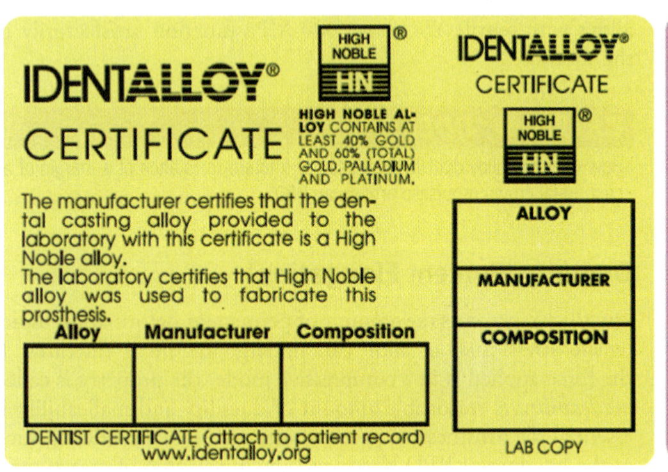

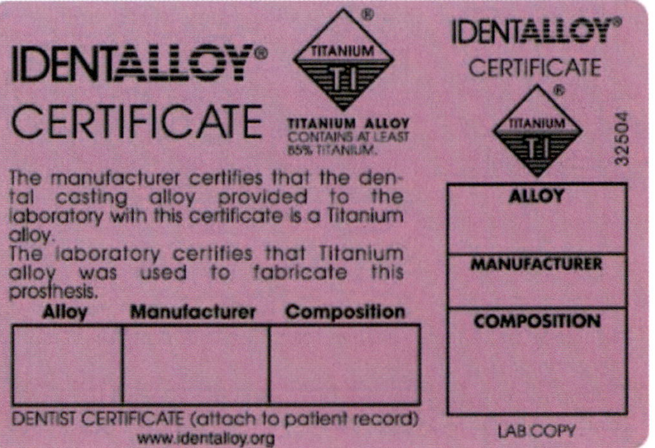

• **Fig. 9.1** Examples of IdentAlloy certificate.

that lists its manufacturer, alloy name, composition, and ADA classification. Some insurance companies use it as well to determine the cost of crown and bridge treatment. Keep in mind that this system certifies only the composition of alloys.

Alloy Classification by Mechanical Properties

The historic ADA Specification No. 5, which originally had composition ranges for the component elements in the four types of gold casting alloys, evolved to stipulating mechanical property requirements for YS, percentage elongation, and Vickers hardness. The relevant current standard is International Organization for Standardization (ISO) 22674:2016, which classifies metallic materials for fixed and removable restorations and appliances into six types according to YS and elongation, regardless of noble-metal contents (Table 9.2).

Alloy Classification by Principal Elements

Alloys may be classified based on the principal or most abundant element (e.g., a palladium-based alloy), or they may be named based on the two or three most important elements (e.g., Pd–Ag, Co–Cr, or Ni–Cr–Be alloys). The components are listed in decreasing order of weight percent. An exception to this rule is the identification of elements that substantially affect the properties of the alloy. For example, Ni–Cr–Mo–Be alloys are often designated as *Ni–Cr–Be alloys* because of the contributions of beryllium to the control of castability and surface oxidation at high temperatures and the relative health-hazard potential of beryllium compared with other metals. *Castability* refers to the ease of making quality castings. Excellent websites to view the wide range of dental alloy compositions include Argen at https://argen.com/.

Alloy Classification by Dental Applications

There are three categories of dental casting alloys designated by application: all-metal fixed prostheses, metal–ceramic prostheses, and RPDs. Each type of alloy classified by noble-metal content (Table 9.1) is available in all three categories. One may use high-noble and noble alloys intended for metal–ceramic prostheses to fabricate all-metal prostheses. However, alloys for all-metal restorations, which can deform or melt during porcelain firing, should not be used to make metal–ceramic restorations.

Base metal and titanium alloys, on the other hand, are often marketed for both all-metal and metal–ceramic prostheses because of their oxide formation at room temperature. In this chapter, dental alloys are discussed by their applications.

Alloys for All-Metal Prostheses

These alloys are discussed in three main categories: noble (includes high-noble alloys), predominantly base metal, and titanium and titanium alloys.

High-Noble and Noble Alloys

The compositions of selected high-noble and noble alloys are given in Table 9.3. Their physical and mechanical properties are shown in Table 9.4. Gold and palladium are the two major elements that make up the nobility of noble and high-noble alloys; these alloys are discussed in two categories: Au-based alloys and Pd-based alloys.

Gold-Based Alloys

Referring to Table 9.2, type I gold alloys are designed for inlays that are not subjected to substantial mastication forces. Type II alloys having greater mechanical properties than type I and are used for one-surface inlays. Type III alloys are used for constructing crowns, bridge abutments, and inlays, which are subjected to great stress during mastication. Type IV gold alloys are used in high-stress areas such as bridges and RPD frameworks (although the gold-based RPD is now rare). The alloys for bridge and RPD framework constructions must be sufficiently rigid to resist flexure, possess high YS to prevent permanent distortion, and be ductile enough for adjustment if the clasp of a framework has been distorted or needs adjustment.

Various elements have been incorporated into gold alloys to produce alloys with suitable properties. For example, platinum and palladium increase the hardness and elastic modulus of gold and raise the melting temperature of the alloy. A higher melting temperature is beneficial when components are to be joined by soldering. Copper in a sufficient quantity relative to the gold content renders the alloy heat treatable (Chapter 2) but can alter the color of the alloy. Silver forms solid solutions with gold and palladium and is effective in neutralizing the reddish color of copper in gold–copper alloys. Palladium has a good range of

TABLE 9.2 Classification of Metallic Materials for Dental Applications—ISO 22674 (2006)

Type	Yield Strength (MPa)	Elongation (%)	Examples of Applications
0[a]	—	—	Single-tooth fixed restorations—e.g., small veneered one-surface inlays, veneered crowns
1	80	18	Single-tooth fixed restorations, veneered or nonveneered one-surface inlays, veneered crowns
2	180	10	Single-tooth fixed restorations—e.g., crowns or inlays without restriction on the number of surfaces
3	270	5	Multiple-unit fixed restorations—e.g., bridges
4	360	2	Appliances with thin cross sections that are subjected to very high forces—e.g., RPDs, clasps, thin veneered crowns, wide-span bridges or bridges with small cross sections, bars, attachments, implant-retained superstructures
5	500	2	Thin RPDs, parts with thin cross-sections, clasps

ISO, International Organization for Standardization; RPD, removable partial denture.
[a]Metallic materials for metal–ceramic crowns produced by electroforming or sintering belong to type 0.

TABLE 9.3 Typical Compositions of High-Noble and Noble Alloys for All-Metal Prostheses

		ELEMENTAL COMPOSITION (PERCENT BY WEIGHT)						
Alloy Type	**Color**	**Au**	**Pd**	**Ag**	**Cu**	**Pt**	**In**	**Balance[a]**
1	Yellow	83	0.5	10	6	—	—	Zn; Ir
2	Yellow	82	—	—	—	18	—	Ir
	Yellow	77	1	13	8.5	—	—	Zn; Ir
3	Yellow	74.5	3.5	11	10.5	—	—	Zn; Ir
	Yellow	50	4	35	10	—	—	Zn; Ir
	Yellow	2	34.9	30	—	—	30	Zn:3; Ir
	White	—	25	71.5	—	—	2.5	Zn; Ru
4	Yellow	60	4	20.5	15	—	—	Zn; Ir
	Yellow	50	3	26	11.5	—	3	Zn:1; Ir
	Pale yellow	20	20	36	—	—	18	Zn:6; Ir
	White	4	30.3	45.7	18.5	—	—	Zn:1.5; Ir

[a]Elements without a value are less than 1% by weight.

TABLE 9.4 Physical and Mechanical Properties of Some Modern High-Noble and Noble Alloys for All-Metal Prostheses

Alloy Type	ADA Classification	Density (g/cm^3)	Yield Strength (MPa; soft/hard)	Hardness (VHN; soft/hard)	Elastic Modulus (GPa)	Elongation (%; soft/hard)
1	High noble	16.6	126	85	70	51
2	High noble	19.2	146	95	50	23
	High noble	15.4	221	120	109	54
3	High noble	15.5	207/276	121/182	76	39/19
	Noble	13.2	309/648	138/225	104	28/15
	Noble	10.5	297	180	51	5–6
	Noble	10.5	248/310	145/155	55	10/8
4	High noble	14.5	350/607	165/235	88	35/4
	Noble	13.2	428/683	180/255	86	28/16
	Noble	11.3	420/530	165/220	103	10/2
	Noble	10.6	460/700	195/265	116	10/3

ADA, American Dental Association; VHN, Vickers hardness number.

solubility with gold, silver, and copper, resulting in good mechanical properties and improvement of tarnish and corrosion resistance. Zinc acts as an oxygen scavenger during the melting and casting of noble and high-noble alloys.

CRITICAL QUESTION

What effects can the cooling rate of a heat-treated type III gold–copper alloy have on its hardness and ductility?

What happens within gold–copper alloys that are subjected to a prescribed heating–cooling cycle?

The underlying principles for heat treatment of these alloys have been discussed in Chapter 2. Briefly, the casting is placed in a furnace at 700°C for 10 minutes and then quenched in water to retain a disordered solid-solution phase with reduced YS and hardness but increased ductility. The process is called a **solution heat treatment**. The same casting is placed in a furnace with the temperature set between 200°C and 450°C for 15–30 minutes before quenching in water. The treatment produces regions of ordered solid-solution phase with increased YS and hardness but a reduction of elongation (Table 9.4). The process is called age hardening.

The softening heat treatment is indicated for prostheses that are ground or reshaped (permanent deformation) to a different form, either in or out of the mouth, to restore their ductility. Because the proportional limit is increased during age hardening, a considerable increase in the modulus of resilience can be expected. The hardening heat treatment is indicated for metallic RPDs, saddles, FDPs, and other similar structures where rigidity of the prosthesis is needed. For small structures, such as inlays, a hardening treatment is not usually required.

CRITICAL QUESTION

What characteristics of palladium make it a natural choice of element to replace gold for dental alloys?

Silver–Palladium Alloys

Silver–palladium alloys are often white and predominantly silver in composition and must contain at least 25% palladium to provide tarnish and corrosion resistance of the alloy. They may also contain copper and a small amount of gold to increase the ductility and improve the castability of the alloy for dental applications. Ag–Pd alloys can produce acceptable castings when close attention is paid to precise control of the casting and mold temperatures. Casting temperatures are in the range of those for yellow gold alloys. The copper-free Ag–Pd alloys may have physical properties similar to those of a type III gold alloy. With 15% or more copper, the alloy may have properties more like those of a type IV gold alloy.

As noted in Chapter 2, indium and palladium at 1:1 atomic ratio form a gold color intermetallic compound. When the content of indium in a Pd–Ag alloy is 18%–30% by weight, the alloy achieves a gold-like color. The colored phase of the Pd–In binary alloy system is hard and brittle and is not a strengthener. Iridium or ruthenium is added in small quantities to high-noble and noble alloy compositions for grain refinement because smaller grains improve the YS (Chapter 2).

CRITICAL QUESTION

What is the role of chromium in predominantly base metal alloys? How does beryllium improve the properties of nickel-based alloys?

Predominantly Base Metal Alloys

Currently there are two main groups of base metal dental alloys: nickel–chromium (Ni–Cr) and cobalt–chromium (Co–Cr). The Ni–Cr alloys can be further divided into those with and without beryllium, which improves castability and promotes the formation of a stable metal oxide for porcelain bonding. The majority of Ni–Cr alloys are used for small castings such as crowns and FDPs, and Co–Cr alloys are primarily used for casting RPDs for which a high elastic modulus and YS are needed. Table 9.5 lists the compositions and properties of selected base metal alloys for all-metal and metal–ceramic applications.

Chromium, a critical element of base metal alloys, oxidizes rapidly on the surface of the alloy to form a thin layer of chromium oxide, which prevents the diffusion of oxygen into the underlying metal and the corrosion process. Chromium in the bulk alloy also provides strengthening by solid-solution hardening. Molybdenum increases corrosion resistance and strength and

TABLE 9.5 Typical Compositions and Mechanical Properties of Base Metal Alloys for Crown, FDP, and Metal–Ceramic Applications

	COMPOSITION (% WT)					MECHANICAL PROPERTIES			
Alloy (Supplier)	Ni	Co	Cr	Mo	Balance[a]	Yield Strength (MPa)	Hardness (VHN)	Elastic Modulus (GPa)	Elongation (%)
IPS d.Sign 15 (Ivoclar)	58.7	1	25	12.1	Fe:1.9; Si:1.7; Ce	340	230	200	13
Rexalloy (Pentron Alloys/Argen)	67	—	14	8	Ga:8; Al; Fe; Si; Mn; Zr; Cu	300	177	191	27
Heraenium S (Heraeus Kulzer)	62.9	—	23	10	Si:2; Fe:15.5; Ce:0.5	310	220	224	29
NPX-III (CMP Industries)	76.5	*x*[b]	14	4.5	Al:2.5; Be:1.6; Ti	784	350	200	9
Argeloy Bond (Argen)	77	—	14	4.7	Mn; Fe; Si; C	630	370	207	10
Norex (Pentron Alloys/Argen)	—	55	25	—	W:10; Ru:5; Al; Nb; Y; Zr	621	350	204	7
Heraenium P (Heraeus Kulzer)	—	59	25	4	W:10; Si:1; Mn:0.8; N	650	330	200	8
Jelbond Supreme (Jelenko Alloys/Argen)	—	61	27	6	W:5; Mn; Si; Fe; C	475	365	223	8

FDP, fixed dental prosthesis; VHN, Vickers hardness number.
[a]Elements without a value are less than 1% by weight.
[b]*x* indicates trace amount.

decreases the thermal expansion coefficient of base metal alloys. Higher thermal expansion is beneficial for porcelain bonding and minimizes the risk of porcelain cracking or fracture. Some minor elements are incorporated to improve manipulation and mechanical properties. For example, beryllium lowers the fusion temperature of the alloys, which improves castability, and refines grain size, which increases strength. Manganese and silicon also improve the castability of the alloys. Carbon forms carbides with other elements in the alloy, increasing the hardness and YS with a reduction in ductility. The aluminum in Ni–Cr alloys forms a nickel–aluminum compound, Ni_3Al, which increases both the YS and the tensile strength. Nitrogen, which is incorporated in the alloy during casting in ambient air, also improves the overall qualities of the casting.

The manipulation and mechanical properties of base metal alloys are described in more detail in the following section on alloys for metal–ceramic prostheses and in the subsequent section on RPDs because base metals are used to a lesser extent for all-metal prostheses.

Titanium

Titanium has a high melting point (1668°C) and a high rate of oxidation above 900°C. It requires a special casting machine with high-temperature melting capability in a nonoxidizing chamber. For example, an argon arc with a nonconsumable tungsten electrode or high-frequency induction is used for melting titanium alloys in crucibles made of copper, magnesia, or carbon and in an argon or helium atmosphere. A casting investment consisting of oxides, such as MgO, ZrO_2, or Y_2O_3, which are more stable than titanium oxide, is used to ensure acceptable castability. Centrifugal force, casting pressure difference, and gas pressure have been used to force the molten metal flow into the mold. Titanium can react with the investment material during casting and forms a very hard surface layer called α-case, with a thickness up to 150 μm. The VHN of cast commercially pure titanium (CP Ti) increases from a bulk value of nearly 200 to approximately 650 at a depth of 25 μm below the surface. Special instruments are required in the dental laboratory for finishing and adjusting titanium castings.

Titanium derives its corrosion protection from a thin passivating oxide film (about 10 nm thick), which forms spontaneously with the surrounding oxygen. Titanium is considered the most biocompatible metal used for dental restorations and prostheses.

Commercially Pure Titanium

According to the American Society for Testing and Materials (ASTM) Standard F67, there are four unalloyed grades of CP Ti based on the concentration of impurities (Table 9.6). The elastic modulus of CP Ti is comparable to that of tooth enamel and noble alloys, but it is lower than that of other base metal alloys (Table 9.5). CP Ti is often selected for its excellent corrosion resistance, especially in applications for which high strength is not required. The major strengthening element is oxygen. Increasing the oxygen content of CP Ti increases not only the flexural strength but also the fatigue strength.

CRITICAL QUESTION

Why is a Ti–Al–V alloy with high strength not always preferred to the commercially pure titanium metal for dental prostheses? How do alloying elements affect the properties of titanium dental alloys?

Titanium Alloys

CP Ti undergoes an allotropic (polymorphic) transformation from a hexagonal close-packed (HCP) crystal structure (α phase) at 882°C to a more ductile body-centered crystal structure (β phase). By incorporating a combination of α- and β-phase stabilizers, four possible types of titanium alloys can be produced: α, near-α, α-β, and β. Alpha-phase stabilizers, such as aluminum, carbon, nitrogen, and gallium, raise the temperature for transforming α to β phase on heating. Beta-phase stabilizers, such as molybdenum, cobalt, nickel, niobium, copper, palladium, tantalum, and vanadium, lower the temperature for transforming β to α phase on cooling. Alpha alloys will form no β phase on cooling. Near-alpha alloys will form a limited amount of β phase on cooling. Alpha–beta alloys are metastable, which makes them heat treatable and will contain both phases at room temperature. Thermal treatment dictates the relative amount of α and β phases and mechanical properties. Beta alloys contain sufficient beta stabilizers to retain the β phase on cooling; they can be solution treated and aged to improve strength.

The most widely used titanium alloy in dentistry and for general engineering applications is Ti–6Al–4V, which is an α-β alloy. Although this alloy has greater strength than CP Ti, it is not as attractive for dentistry and biomedical applications because of

TABLE 9.6 Tensile Properties and Impurity Limits for Unalloyed (CP) Titanium (ASTM F67)[a]

	PHYSICAL PROPERTIES (MINIMUM)				IMPURITY LIMITS (MAX), PERCENT BY WEIGHT				
Designation	Tensile Strength (MPa)	Yield Strength (MPa)	Hardness (VHN)	Elongation (%)	N	C	H	Fe	O
Grade 1	240	170	126	24	0.03	0.08	0.015	0.20	0.18
Grade 2	340	280	178	20	0.03	0.08	0.015	0.30	0.25
Grade 3	450	380	221	18	0.05	0.08	0.015	0.30	0.35
Grade 4	550	480	263	15	0.05	0.08	0.015	0.50	0.40

ASTM, American Society for Testing Materials; VHN, Vickers hardness number.
[a]Elastic modulus is approximately 110 GPa for each type.

TABLE 9.7 Properties of Two α-β Titanium Alloys for Dental Prostheses

Alloy	Elastic Modulus (GPa)	Yield Strength (MPa)	Hardness (VHN)	Elongation (%)
Ti–6Al–4V	117	860	320	10–15
Ti–6Al–7Nb	105	795	330	10

VHN, Vickers hardness number.

some concerns about health hazards from the slow release of aluminum and vanadium. Vanadium in high doses is highly toxic, and aluminum has been reported to cause potential neurological disorders. Niobium has not been associated with any known toxic or adverse reactions in the body and belongs to the same group as vanadium in the periodic table. Replacing vanadium in Ti–6Al–4V with the same atomic percentage of niobium yields Ti–6Al–7Nb. Both alloys are considered to be acceptable for biomedical applications. The mechanical properties of the two alloys are similar (Table 9.7), and their corrosion resistance is similar to that of CP Ti. Their elastic moduli are similar to those of type IV alloys, and YSs range from those of type II to type V metallic materials, as described in ISO 22674 (Table 9.2).

CRITICAL QUESTION

Why does the manipulation of titanium alloys differ so much from that for Co–Cr and Ni–Cr alloys?

Manipulation of Titanium Alloys

The surface of titanium castings after divestment must be ground and polished to remove surface porosity and the α case for optimal functionality of the final prosthesis. The machinability of titanium and its alloys is generally considered poor because of several inherent properties of titanium, such as high chemical reactivity, relatively low thermal conductivity, high strength at high temperature, and low modulus of elasticity.

To eliminate the effect of oxygen during the fabrication of titanium prostheses, CAD-CAM has been used to produce fixed prosthesis frameworks.

CRITICAL QUESTION

How do alloys for all-metal prostheses differ from those required for metal–ceramic prostheses?

Alloys for Metal–Ceramic Prostheses

The chief objections to the use of *dental porcelain* as a restorative material are its low tensile strength and shear strength (Chapter 10). A method of minimizing this disadvantage is to bond the porcelain directly to a cast alloy substructure made to fit the prepared tooth. The process requires building on the metal substrate a tooth form with ceramic powder held together by a binder and subjecting the entire assembly to a heating process called *sintering*. Sintering densifies the packed ceramic particles to a solid firmly bonded to the metal substrate. This system is referred to as the *porcelain-fused-to-metal* (PFM) design. The preferred descriptive term for this composite system is *metal–ceramic,* and the metal is called *metal–ceramic alloy.* In this section, the requirements of metals, some representative alloy systems, and issues associated with these alloys are discussed.

Requirements of Alloys for Metal–Ceramic Applications

The alloys discussed in this section share at least three common features: (1) the potential to bond to dental porcelain, (2) solidus temperature sufficiently high to resist softening during sintering, and (3) coefficients of thermal contraction compatible with those of dental porcelain.

Porcelain Bonding to Metals

Porcelain bonding to metal substrate requires adherent oxides on the surface. The addition of a small quantity of an appropriate base metal to noble and high-noble alloys promotes oxide formation on the surface. For base metal alloys, some oxides may be poorly adherent to the metal substructure, which can result in porcelain delaminating from the metal substrate. However, the bond strengths for porcelain bonded to base metal alloys as determined in vitro have not generally been shown to be superior or inferior to those of noble metal alloys. Furthermore, clinical studies have not demonstrated a significant difference in the failure incidence between metal–ceramic restorations made from base metal alloys and those fabricated from high-noble or noble metal alloys. To produce the optimal metal oxide characteristics, the manufacturer's instructions must be followed precisely.

Solidus Temperature

When an alloy is heated close to its solidus temperature, it becomes susceptible to deformation under its own mass, which is known as *creep.* The degree of creep increases with the size of the prosthesis and the number of firings required for the porcelain. In the older literature, this creep process is referred to as the *sag* of the ceramic alloy (Fig. 9.2). All metal–ceramic alloys should have a solidus temperature that is substantially higher than the sintering temperature of the porcelain to minimize creep deformation.

CRITICAL QUESTION

How can differences in thermal contraction between a metal and its veneering ceramic affect the resistance to cracking or fracture of the veneer?

Why must a metal for metal–ceramic prostheses have its thermal contraction coefficient slightly higher than that of its veneering ceramic?

Thermal Compatibility of Metal–Ceramic Systems

The thermal expansion and contraction values of base metal alloys are generally similar to those of noble metal alloys. When a metal–ceramic prosthesis is cooled from the porcelain sintering temperature, the metal and its veneering ceramic contracts at different rates. Meanwhile, the chemical bond between the metal and the porcelain prevents the two components from separating; this condition forces the two components to adjust their respective dimensions during the cooling cycle. Thus the component that contracts more will be stretched by the adjacent component, which contracts less; together, the material that contracts less will be compressed by the other component. Such changes in dimension result in stresses that act on each of the two components. The

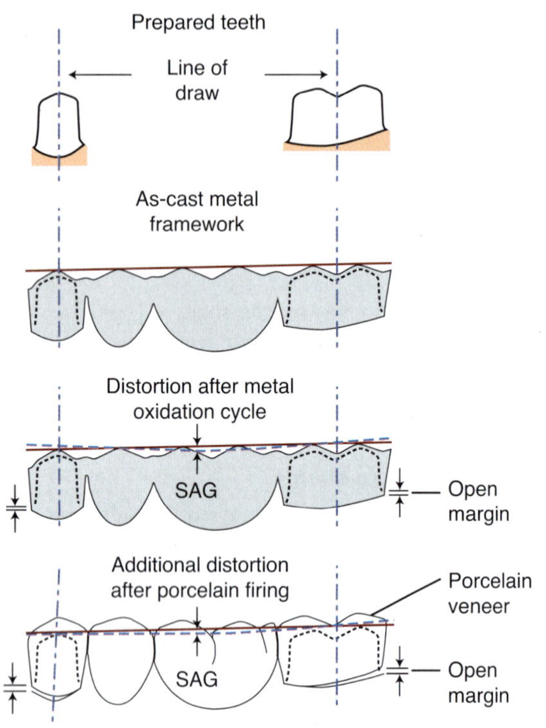

• **Fig. 9.2** Sag deformation in a fixed dental prosthesis (FDP) framework.

instantaneous stress at a given temperature during the cooling cycle is termed *transient stress,* and the stress distribution, which exists at room temperature, is called the *residual stress.* When the prosthesis is cooled, the tensile stress that develops in the porcelain is of concern. If the transient tensile stresses that develop within porcelain during cooling are insufficient to cause immediate cracking of the porcelain or delayed cracking after cooling to room temperature, the combination of a metal–porcelain system is considered thermally compatible. In fact, a slight thermal contraction mismatch, with a coefficient of thermal contraction of about 0.5×10^{-6}/°C higher for the metal, is preferred because the mismatch induces residual compressive stress in the porcelain along the bonded interface, which is protective in nature. This mechanism will be discussed in Chapter 10.

CRITICAL QUESTION

What are the benefits and drawbacks of the different types of alloys used for metal–ceramic prostheses?

High-Noble and Noble Alloys

Table 9.8 shows some typical high-noble and noble metal–ceramic alloys. The physical and mechanical properties of representative alloys are given in Table 9.9.

TABLE 9.8 Compositions of Representative High-Noble (HN) and Noble (N) Alloys for Metal–Ceramic Prostheses

		PRINCIPAL ELEMENTS (WEIGHT PERCENT)						
Alloy Type	**Typical Products (Supplier)**	**Au**	**Pt**	**Pd**	**Ag**	**Cu**	**Ga**	**Balance[a]**
Au–Pd–Pt/HN	SMG-3 (Dentsply Ceramco)[b]	81	6	11	—[a]	—	—	Re; Sn; Fe
Au–Pt–Pd/HN Au–Pt–Ag/HN	Argedent Y86 (Argen)[b]	86	10	2	—	—	—	In:2
	Degunorm (Dentsply Ceramco)[b]	74	9	—	9	4.4	—	Zn; In; Ir
Au–Pd–Ag/HN	Argedent 75 (Argen)[b]	75	—	12	10	—	—	In:1 ; Sn:1 ; Ir
	Aspire (Dentsply Ceramco)	52	—	26	17	—	—	Zn; In; Sn; Re
	Herabond (Heraeus-Kulzer)	52	—	27	18	0.2	—	Sn:2.7; In; Ir; Re
Au–Pd/HN	Olympia (Argen)	52	—	38	—	—	1.5	In:8.5; Ru
	Lodestar (Ivoclar Vivadent)	52	—	39	—	—	1.5	In:8.5; Re; Ru
	Argedent 65SF (Argen)	65	—	26	—	—	—	In:8.7
Pd–Au/N	Argedent 35SF (Argen)	35	—	57	—	—	4.8	Sn:3; Zn; Ru
Pd–Au–Ag/N	Argelite 52+ (Argen)	15	—	52.2	21.5	—	1	In:6; Sn:4
	Argelite 75+6 (Argen)	6	—	75	6.5	—	—	In:6; Ga:6
Pd–Ag/N	Albabond A (Heraeus-Kulzer)	—	—	57	33	—	—	Sn:6.8; In:3.4; Zn; Ir; Ru
	W-1 (Ivoclar Vivadent)	—	—	53	38	—	—	Sn:8.5; In; Ru; Li
Pd–Cu–Ga/N	Spartan Plus (Ivoclar Vivadent)	2	—	78.8	—	10	9	Ir; Ge; Li
Pd–Ga/N	Argebond 80 (Argen)	—	—	80	5	—	6.3	In:6.5; Sn; Zn:1
	Argelite 85 (Argen)	2	—	85	1.2	—	10	In:1.2; Ru

[a]Elements without value are less than 1% by weight.
[b]Yellow color alloy.

TABLE 9.9 **Physical and Mechanical Properties of Some High-Noble and Noble Metal–Ceramic Alloys in Table 9.8**

Alloy Type	Product Name	Density (g/cm^3)	Yield Strength (MPa; soft/hard)	Hardness (VHN; soft/hard)	Elastic Modulus (GPa)	Elongation (soft/hard) (%)
Au–Pt–Ag	Argedent Y86	18.4	405/469	160/195	76	12/9
Au–Pd–Ag	Herabond	14.5	520/600	220/260	134	12/8
Au–Pd	Olympia	14.4	550	250	124	30
Pd–Au	Argedent 35SF	13.9	510/572	245/245	124	25/20
Pd–Au–Ag	Argelite 75+6	11.4	565/600	250/265	111	32/30
Pd–Ag	Albabond A	11.4	460/540	205/235	122	26/18
Pd–Cu–Ga	Spartan Plus	11.0	740	310	140	10
Pd–Ga	Argebond 80	11.2	585/630	230/245	130	35/28

VHN, Vickers hardness number.

Gold–Platinum–Palladium Alloys

Gold–platinum–palladium alloys produced the first successful metal–ceramic restorations. Platinum raises the melting temperature. Rhenium (Re) is a grain refiner that increases hardness. Iron forms an oxide on the surface for porcelain bonding and increases the proportional limit and strength of the alloy by an $FePt_3$ precipitate. These alloys have adequate elastic modulus, strength, hardness, and elongation but are low in sag resistance. They are mostly used for making crowns and three-unit FDPs. Their use has decreased over time because more economical alloys have been developed with substantially better mechanical properties.

Gold–Palladium–Silver Alloys

Gold–palladium–silver alloys are economical alternatives to the Au–Pt–Pd or Au–Pd–Pt alloys. Their excellent tarnish and corrosion resistance and relative freedom from technique sensitivity have contributed to their long-term success. The higher palladium concentration above those of the Au–Pt–Pd alloys raises the melting ranges and improves resistance to creep deformation at elevated temperatures.

Gold–Palladium Alloys

These silver-free alloys are white in color and have a lower thermal contraction coefficient than that of either the Au–Pd–Ag or Pd–Ag alloys. When used with compatible low-expansion or low-contraction porcelains, Au–Pd alloys are considered nearly ideal compared with other noble metal alloys because these alloys contain no silver, and their surface oxide is virtually indiscernible. Thus the esthetic quality of metal–ceramic prostheses made with Au–Pd alloys is comparable to that obtained with Au–Pt–Pd alloys. The sag resistance of these alloys is somewhat better than that of Au–Pt–Pd alloys.

Palladium–Gold Alloys

The physical properties of palladium–gold alloys are generally similar to those of the Au–Pd alloys, and potential thermal contraction concerns for these alloys seem to have been resolved by changes in the porcelain composition. Few data are available on their laboratory and clinical performance.

Palladium–Gold–Silver Alloys

Palladium–gold–silver alloys are similar to the Au–Pd–Ag alloys in their potential for porcelain discoloration. They have a range of thermal contraction coefficients, which increase with an increase in silver content.

Palladium–Silver Alloys

This alloy type was the first gold-free noble alloy for metal–ceramic restorations. The replacement of gold by palladium raises the melting range but lowers the thermal expansion coefficient of the alloy. Silver, on the other hand, lowers the melting range but increases the thermal expansion coefficient. A proper balance of the two elements maintains a reasonably low casting temperature and a compatible thermal expansion coefficient. The thermal compatibility of these alloys is generally good except with certain low-expansion porcelains. The addition of tin and indium promotes oxide formation for porcelain bonding and yields precipitates for improving mechanical properties.

Adherence to porcelain is considered acceptable for most of the Pd–Ag alloys. However, Mackert et al. reported that one of these alloy products formed an internal oxide rather than the preferred external oxide. Instead, Pd–Ag nodules developed on the surface (Fig. 9.3) facilitate the retention of porcelain mechanically. This condition has not apparently produced clinical bond failures to warrant concern, and other Pd–Ag ceramic alloys have not been studied to determine whether they have similar oxidation behavior.

Because of their high silver content compared with that of gold-based alloys, the potential silver discoloration effect is most severe for these alloys. One should proceed with caution when light shades (higher values) of ceramic are desired.

Palladium–Copper–Gallium Alloys

Compositional differences for the Pd–Cu–Ga alloys result in a wide range of mechanical properties: YSs ranging from 520 to over 1200 MPa, percent elongation ranging from 7% to 30%, and VHN ranging from approximately 265 to over 400. Careful composition control by manufacturers has resulted in Pd–Cu–Ga alloys with VHNs of substantially less than 300.

The dark brown or black oxide formed during oxidation and subsequent porcelain sintering cycles makes it difficult for a technician to mask the color. Sometimes a thicker opaque porcelain layer is required to avoid excessive darkness (i.e., low value) with certain porcelains. An increase in oxide layer thickness occurs during the initial oxidation step for these alloys. To reduce the discoloration effect, the surface can be sandblasted prior to the application of opaque porcelain.

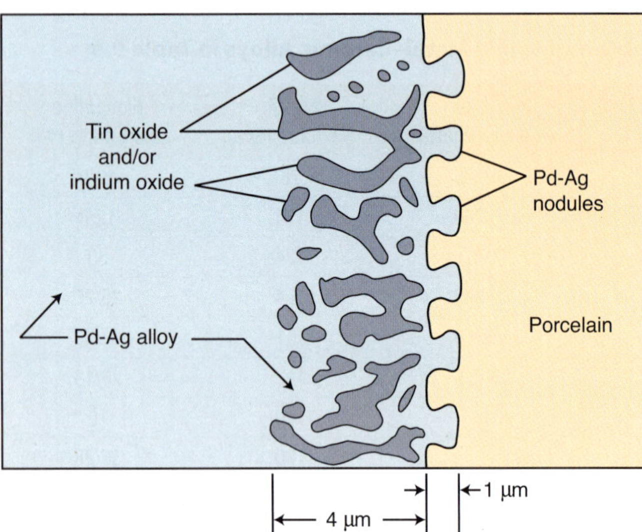

• **Fig. 9.3** Internal oxide formation and creep-induced nodule formation in a Pd–Ag alloy for metal–ceramic restorations.

Palladium–Gallium Alloys

The Pd–Ga alloys also have relatively dark oxides, which are somewhat lighter than those on the Pd–Cu–Ga alloys. Pd–Ga alloys generally tend to have relatively low thermal expansion coefficients, making the alloys more compatible with lower-expansion porcelains. The silver content is generally low and is not sufficient to cause significant porcelain "greening."

The effects of several dental laboratory variables (recasting old alloy, alternative oxidation cycle, stripping and rebonding of porcelain) on porcelain adherence were investigated for one Pd–Ga alloy, three Pd–Cu–Ga alloys, and one Au–Pd alloy. One finding was that remelting two and three times degraded porcelain adherence to the Pd–Ga alloy and one Pd–Cu–Ga alloy. Stripping of the original porcelain did not cause a significant decrease in adherence of the subsequently applied porcelain. An alternate oxidation procedure from the one recommended by the manufacturer significantly affected porcelain adherence to one Pd–Cu–Ga alloy and the Au–Pd alloy. Therefore, where there is doubt, the manufacturer should be asked to provide precise instructions to ensure sound metal–ceramic bonding.

CRITICAL QUESTION

What are the benefits and drawbacks of using a base metal casting alloy versus a noble metal casting alloy for a metal–ceramic restoration?

Predominantly Base Metal Alloys

Compared with other alloys for metal–ceramic prostheses, the base metal alloys (other than titanium and titanium alloys) generally are harder and stiffer (higher elastic modulus) (Tables 9.4 and 9.5); this enables the coping to be 0.1–0.2 mm thick without risking significant deformation under mastication stress or sagging of the metal framework at the porcelain-firing temperature. The higher melting temperatures make these alloys more difficult to cast than the high-noble and noble alloys.

Manipulation of Base Metal Alloys

Laboratory technicians fabricating base metal copings for metal–ceramic prostheses will face the following technical issues: casting condition, castability, finishing, and controlling oxide layers. The fusion temperatures of Ni–Cr and Co–Cr alloys are in the range of 1150–1500°C; an acetylene-oxygen flame or an electrical induction heating source is required for melting these alloys. The mold should be made of either phosphate- or silicate-bonded investment material, which maintains its surface integrity at the casting temperature of base metal alloys. The density of a base metal alloy is about half that of a gold-based alloy. The lower density not only reduces the force of gravity for bulky maxillary appliances on the supporting teeth but also reduces the thrust generated by the casting unit to force the molten base metal alloy to fill the mold. The use of a vent and a larger sprue size than that used for gold-based alloys may be needed (Chapter 14).

The castability of Co–Cr alloys is in the same range as that of Ni–Cr alloys without beryllium. Some noble and high-noble alloys were found to exhibit lower castability than Co–Cr alloys. In contrast, a study of the marginal accuracy of a high-noble alloy, four noble alloys, and a Ni–Cr–Be alloy revealed that for all alloys, marginal completeness was adequate, and marginal openings were considerably less than 50 μm. Some researchers claim that all alloys will theoretically produce complete castings under optimal burnout, melting, and casting conditions.

In general, the high hardness and high strength of these base metal alloys contribute to certain difficulties of adjusting prostheses. After casting, it is useful to sandblast the prosthesis to remove investment materials and excessive oxides. Grinding and polishing of fixed restorations to achieve proper occlusion will occasionally require more time at chairside. The removal of defective restorations may also require more time. The potential hazard of dust generated from the procedure is a concern and is discussed with the biological hazards of base metal alloys (Chapter 17).

The solidification shrinkages of base metal alloys are greater than those of gold-based alloys, which represent a challenge for technicians to obtain acceptable-fitting base metal castings. Using type V die stone for dies and enhancing the expansion of the investment mold during the setting of the investment are the most common practices to improve the fit of prostheses (Chapter 14).

The thickness of the oxide layer and the wetting of the oxide layer by porcelain are important factors in establishing the bonding of porcelain to the metal substrate. For the laboratory technician to produce optimal metal oxide characteristics, the manufacturer's instructions must be followed precisely. However, some instructions are relatively imprecise. For example, some alloys require a "light" sandblasting of the oxide layer formed during the initial oxidation step. The particle size of aluminum oxide abrasive is generally recommended, but neither the quality of abrasive nor the sandblasting pressure is usually specified. Contamination of the oxide layer with lower-purity abrasives could degrade the integrity of the interface between the metal oxide and the opaque porcelain. The ability of a laboratory technician to discriminate light from moderate sandblasting to reduce the thickness of these surface oxides is one example of the technique sensitivity of base metal alloys.

Mechanical Properties

The elastic modulus of base metal alloys is twice as much or greater than those for noble metal alloys. This property allows the technician to reduce the cross-sectional area of cast interproximal connectors. The rigidity of the prosthesis is proportional to the elastic modulus and the connector width (buccal-lingual dimension) but is proportional to the cube of the connector thickness (occlusal-gingival dimension). The cubic relationship with the connector thickness means that when an alloy with an elastic modulus that is twice as high is used, the connector thickness can be reduced by 20.6% while maintaining the same rigidity of the prosthesis. Using similar reasoning, a reduction of the coping thickness from 0.3 to 0.1 mm may increase the risk of porcelain fracture because of the increased coping flexibility. However, a finite element analysis of stresses induced in anterior metal–ceramic crowns under intraoral forces indicates that a reduction of base metal coping thickness (in veneered areas) from 0.3 to 0.1 mm exhibits only a slight effect on porcelain stresses.

It is a common practice to design the occlusal surface of metal–ceramic prostheses to be made from cast metal to avoid excessive wear of the opposing natural dentition. Compared with the same prostheses made of high-noble or noble alloys, the hardness of the base metal alloys makes the occlusal adjustment slightly more difficult to perform, and the resulting roughness can cause greater wear of the opposing tooth enamel. Repair of crowns with fractured porcelain veneers, which may be simply performed on noble metal substrates using pin-retained facings or metal–ceramic onlays, is more difficult to accomplish when the failed restoration has a framework cast with a nickel- or cobalt-based alloy.

Titanium-Based Alloys

As previously discussed, titanium undergoes a phase transformation at 882°C and exhibits a high rate of oxidation above 900°C. Therefore, a low-fusing ceramic with a sintering temperature below 800°C should be used to minimize oxidation and prevent any phase transformation during sintering. The high melting temperatures of CP Ti and titanium alloys make them highly resistant to sag deformation at porcelain-sintering temperatures, and the accompanying relatively low thermal expansion coefficient demands special low-expansion dental porcelains for bonding to titanium. Because of the α-case formation, caustic NaOH-based solutions or silicon nitride coatings have been employed to improve the bond between cast CP Ti and dental porcelain.

In general, in vitro bonding tests show that metal–ceramics fabricated from noble and base metal alloys exhibit higher bond strengths than those of low-fusing porcelain to titanium. However, a small number of studies show that the bond strengths are not statistically significantly different between the two groups. Differences in porcelain composition often require different firing temperatures, which may result in bond strength changes. However, there is no difference in porcelain bond strength between CP Ti and titanium alloys. Studies also show that surface treatment of CP Ti and titanium alloy before porcelain application can improve the bond strength. The treatments include silica deposition by magnetron sputtering; deposition of an intermediate metallic layer by silver plating; use of an admixture of titanium particles and porcelain as a bonding agent; incorporation of an intermediate ceramic layer; nitridation of the titanium surface; and surface roughening by a caustic bath, hydrochloric acid, or sandblasting. Although multiple firing has no effect on bond strength, firing in an argon atmosphere, which reduces oxide formation, improves the bond strength. It is believed that controlling the thickness and adherence of the oxide is the key to higher bond strength.

Properties of high-noble and base metal alloys (including CP Ti) for metal–ceramic prostheses are listed in Table 9.10.

CRITICAL QUESTION

Which factors must be considered by the dental laboratory and dentist for the preparation and adjustment of RPD frameworks that are cast from base metal alloys?

Alloys for Removable Partial Dentures

RPDs have four major metal components: connectors, rests, clasps, and mesh bases. Except for clasps, each component should be rigid and resist permanent deformation, which suggests a material of high elastic modulus and YS. Table 9.11 lists the compositions and mechanical properties of selected base metal alloys for RPDs. The density of these alloys ranges from 7.6 to 8.3 g/cm³. For clasps, the material must be resistant to permanent deformation, flexible to engage undercuts, and possess sufficient ductility to facilitate adjustment without fracture. Ideally, the clasps should be made of gold-based type IV alloy because of its lower elastic modulus, good ductility, and adequate YS (Table 9.4) and then soldered (discussed later) to the remaining framework made of a base metal alloy. This arrangement, however, inevitably promotes corrosion at the soldered (brazed) joint (Chapter 3). Although gold-based clasps can be embedded in the denture base resin to avoid corrosion at the solder joint, in practice, RPDs are cast in one piece using the same alloy. The effect of the high elastic modulus of the base metal alloy on the flexure and retention of the clasps can be adequately addressed by reducing the clasp thickness. The situation is similar to that discussed for FDPs.

TABLE 9.10 Comparative Properties of High-Noble Alloys and Base Metal Alloys for Metal–Ceramic Prostheses

Property	High-Noble Alloy	Co–Cr	Ni–Cr–Be	CP Ti
Biocompatibility	Excellent	Excellent	Fair	Excellent
Density	14 g/cm³	7.5 g/cm³	8.7 g/cm³	4.5 g/cm³
Elastic modulus (stiffness)	90 GPa	145–220 GPa	207 GPa	103 GPa
Sag resistance	Poor to excellent	Excellent	Excellent	Good
Technique sensitivity	Minimal	Moderately high	Moderately high	Extremely high
Bond to porcelain	Excellent	Fair	Good to excellent	Fair
Metal cost	High	Low	Low	Low[a]

[a]The dental laboratory costs for fabricating metal–ceramic prostheses are high for CP Ti, and few dental laboratories have the capability of producing Ti prostheses.

TABLE 9.11 **Compositions and Mechanical Properties of Selected Base Metal Alloys for Removable Partial Dentures[a]**

	ELEMENTAL COMPOSITION (WEIGHT PERCENT)					MECHANICAL PROPERTIES			
Alloy Name (Supplier)	Ni	Co	Cr	Mo	Balance[a]	Yield Strength (MPa)	Hardness (VHN)	Elastic Modulus (GPa)	Elongation (%)
Nobilstar (CMP Industries)	—	65	27.5	5.5	Si; Fe; Mn; C	640	430	193	9
Vitallium (Dentsply)	—	63.1	28.5	6	Mn; Si; C; N	600	410	200	9
JD (Jelenko Alloys/Argen)	—	63	28.5	6	Si; C; Mn; Fe; W	620	290	207	5
Heraenium EH (Heraeus Kulzer)	—	63.5	28	6.5	Si:1; Mn; C; N	620	310	228	7
Suprachrome + (Argen)	—	63	30	5	Mn; Si; C; N	745	390	200	13
Supercast (Pentron Alloys/Argen)	—	64	30	4	Mn; Si; C; N	655	340	228	3.5
Ticonium 100 (CMP Industries)	71.6	*x*[b]	16	5	Al:2.9; Mn:3.7; Be:0.8; Ti	790	360	186	7

VHN, Vickers hardness number.
[a]Elements without value are less than 1% by weight.
[b]*x* indicates trace amount.

Predominantly Base Metal Alloys

Cobalt–chromium–molybdenum alloy has been the primary metal for RPD prostheses. Cobalt increases the elastic modulus and strength. Inclusion of greater than 30% chromium by weight makes the alloy difficult to cast and forms the brittle σ phase. Molybdenum and manganese improve the corrosion resistance of the alloy. Carbide formation provides a high YS and hardness in the alloy but lowers ductility. Particular concerns are the higher hardness of some alloys, which can cause in vivo wear of the enamel; the need for special finishing in the dental laboratory; and the tendency of these alloys to undergo rapid work hardening.

Co–Cr alloy clasps are reported to be too retentive initially and to slowly lose this retention because of permanent deformation from repeated seating and removal of the appliance, which correspond to cyclic fatigue conditions. Caution is needed by the dental laboratory technician or the clinician in adjusting clasps on the cast framework to avoid fracture, even for RPD alloys that exhibit higher values of percent elongation.

Because of the high melting temperatures, these base metal alloys are induction melted and cast using phosphate- or silicate-bonded investments, as recommended by the manufacturer, to compensate for their high casting shrinkage and to minimize the potential for casting defects.

CRITICAL QUESTION

Because titanium alloy has an elastic modulus comparable to that of gold, how can the stiffness of an RPD made from this titanium alloy be increased to the same level of stiffness as a cobalt–chromium RPD?

Titanium-Based Alloys

CP Ti and titanium alloys have occasionally been used to make RPD frameworks because of the excellent biocompatibility, outstanding corrosion resistance, and good mechanical properties. Because of the low elastic modulus, compared with that of base metal alloys, the rigidity of the connector is often improved by increasing the thickness or changing the design. Increasing the rigidity also reduces debonding between the resin base and the metal framework. In addition, the lower YS and higher percent elongation of CP Ti suggest that cast clasps may be easily adjusted.

Laboratory casting of titanium remains a challenge because internal porosity within the clasp assemblies can lead to clasp fracture. The reaction layer on the surface must be removed chemically with hydrofluorosilicic acid or mechanically by sandblasting and rotary instruments.

The strong binding and high electrostatic character of the titanium surface oxide may result in higher plaque adherence to titanium frameworks compared with other base metal frameworks. A clinical survey of RPDs revealed gradual discoloration of titanium alloy frameworks, whereas those made with CP Ti and other base metal alloys did not discolor. It was hypothesized that aluminum segregates from the titanium alloy (Ti–6Al–4V) during casting and corrodes during service; further research is needed to verify this hypothesis. An in vitro study has also revealed that exposing titanium alloys to alkaline denture cleansers (pH greater than 11) causes discoloration. Laser welding of titanium has facilitated the repair of titanium frameworks because of the low thermal conductivity of titanium and localized heating during laser welding. This is also true for the Co–Cr and Ni–Cr alloys.

CRITICAL QUESTION

What are the merits and concerns of using alternative techniques other than casting for fabricating prostheses from dental alloys?

Alternative Technologies for Fabricating Prostheses

Shrinkage of the dental casting alloy in an investment mold occurs in three stages: (1) the thermal contraction of the liquid metal cooling to its liquidus temperature (Fig. 2.17), (2) the phase change from the liquid to the solid state (solidus temperature), and (3) the thermal contraction of the solid metal from the solidus temperature to room temperature. The linear solidification shrinkage of an alloy resulting from thermal contraction differs from the casting shrinkage for dental alloys because of the effect of the investment surrounding the solidifying casting.

The first-stage contraction is of no consequence to the final dimensions of the casting because the molten metal flows freely and fills the mold. For the second-stage contraction, the solidification starts at the walls of the mold, and the first layer of metal tends to adhere to the mold while the liquid metal continues to be fed from the reservoir, which results in no contraction of the casting relative to the investment mold. As the casting cools, it gains sufficient strength to contract independently of the mold. Any contraction of the casting from this point will affect the fit of the prosthesis. Finally, the casting shrinks thermally until it reaches room temperature. Because the thermal contraction coefficient of the metal casting is higher than that of the investment mold, the size of the final casting will be smaller than that of the investment mold, which is an accurate reproduction of the missing tooth structure. The difference in dimensions is called *casting shrinkage* and normally is compensated for by the setting and thermal expansion of the investment used (Chapter 14). Table 9.12 lists the linear solidification shrinkage of various alloys cast as smooth cylinders. Because the contraction of the alloy as it cools to room temperature dominates the casting shrinkage, the higher-melting alloys tend to exhibit greater shrinkage.

Technologies are currently available for fabricating metallic prostheses without metal melting and the associated casting shrinkage. Except for RPD frameworks, most metal prostheses can be made by one or more of the following methods: (1) sintering (or diffusion bonding) of burnished metal foil, (2) CAD-CAM processing of metal blocks, (3) copy milling of metal blocks, and (4) electroforming of metal copings. A fifth method, which has become highly popular worldwide, 3-D printing with selective laser melting of metal powder, can be used to fabricate most metal prostheses, including RPD frameworks.

Sintering of Burnished Foil

The most commonly used commercial foil system, Captek (Leach & Dillon, North Attleboro, MA), is used for making copings or frameworks for metal–ceramic prostheses. The protocol and guidelines for the Captek system are found in an article in the Selected Readings section. The main advantage of Captek crowns is their very low thickness, which ensures minimal tooth reduction or improved esthetics compared with conventional

TABLE 9.12 Linear Solidification Shrinkage of Casting Alloys

Alloy Type	Casting Shrinkage (%)
Type 1 (Au based)	1.56
Type 2 (Au based)	1.37
Type 3 (Au based)	1.42
Type 4 (Ni–Cr based)	2.30
Type 4 (Co–Cr based)	2.30

metal–ceramic crowns made with cast metal copings. For the construction of a multiple-unit FDP, a connector for the two abutment copings is waxed and cast with a recommended gold alloy. The copings are then joined with the connector using furnace soldering, electrical welding, or laser welding before the porcelain application.

CAD-CAM Processing

The dental application of CAD-CAM became available in the early 1980s to produce ceramic inlays and crowns during one chairside appointment. This technology has been improved and expanded, and computer-aided milling or grinding of a metal or a ceramic block can be performed accurately by a CAD-CAM process or by electrolytic or electrical discharge removal of metal. The CAD-CAM technique can be used to prepare prostheses from CP Ti or titanium alloy, which does not contain bulk casting defects or the hard α case found near the surface of cast titanium prostheses. More about the CAD-CAM process is provided in Chapter 15.

Copy Milling

The copy-milling process is based on the principle of tracing the surface of a resin prosthesis pattern, which is then replicated on a blank of ceramic, composite, or metal that is ground, cut, or milled by a rotating wheel whose motion is controlled by a link through the tracing device. The process is similar to that associated with cutting a key blank using a tracing of a master key. One commercial system of this type (Celay, Mikrona Technologies, Spreitenbach, Switzerland) has been in use since 1991. The pattern to be traced is made from a blue-colored resin-based composite (Celay-Tech, ESPE, Seefeld/Oberbay, Germany).

Electroforming

A master cast of the prepared tooth (teeth) is prepared and coated with a special die spacer to facilitate separation of the duplicating material. The dies are duplicated with a gypsum product that has a setting expansion of 0.1%–0.2%. After a conductive silver layer is applied to its surface, the die is connected to a plating head and then to a power source and placed in a plating solution. After a sufficiently thick layer of gold or other metal is deposited, the gypsum is removed, and the coping is sandblasted. The coping is then coated with a bonding agent during the wash bake, and subsequent ceramic layers are condensed and sintered in a conventional way.

As is true for the burnished foil system, a cast pontic is needed for joining electroformed copings to construct multiple-unit prostheses.

Three-Dimensional Printing

The process of 3-D printing is a form of additive manufacturing technology where a 3-D object is created by depositing successive layers of material. This technology is now being widely used with metal powders to fabricate dental restorations and prostheses. As described in Chapter 15, the metal powder is first spread across the working platform. A laser traces the outline of each part being printed, and metal powder is fused to the layer below it. As the platform is lowered, a new layer of material is spread across the platform, and the process is repeated until the printing process is completed. This process is called *selective laser melting* or *direct laser metal sintering*. For dental applications, the metal powder can be titanium, Co–Cr alloy, or a noble metal. The powder compositions for two Co–Cr alloys used for selective laser melting are

TABLE 9.13 Powder Compositions for Two Co–Cr Alloys Used for Selective Laser Melting

Manufacturer	Co	Cr	Mo	Si	Mn	Fe
SINT-TECH, France[a]	Balance (max. 62.5)	29	5.5	<1	<1	<1
Epson Atmix, Japan[b]	Balance (approx. 63.5)	29	6	<1	<1	<1

[a]Al Jabbari et al., 2019.
[b]Takaichi et al., 2013.

shown in Table 9.13, and it can be seen that these powder compositions are very similar to the compositions of the base metal casting alloys shown in Table 9.11. Additional technologies are discussed in Chapters 15 and 19.

Örtorp et al. reported the marginal and internal fit among three-unit Co–Cr-based FDPs using four fabrication techniques: (1) the traditional lost wax casting method, (2) CAD-CAM milling of a wax pattern followed by the lost wax casting method, (3) the CAD-CAM milling method, and (4) the direct laser metal sintering method. Initial results indicate that the best fit was exhibited by group 4, followed by groups 2, 1, and 3. A review published in 2020 shows that the total gap of single-crown soft milling had the highest accuracy, and for multiunit FDPs, additive manufactured restorations had the highest accuracy.

CRITICAL QUESTION

What are the differences between soldering, brazing, and welding?

Joining of Dental Alloys

There are three categories of metal-joining operations: soldering, brazing, and welding. The soldering and brazing processes for the metallic components (also called *substrate metals*) to be joined always employ a filler metal (usually called *solder*), along with a flux and a heat source. Brazing is conducted above 450°C, and soldering is conducted below that temperature. Both processes are performed below the solidus temperature of the substrate metal or metals; there is no melting at the workpiece surfaces. The term *soldering* is used in this section as a general term to describe both processes. Welding may not require a filler metal because the metal surfaces to be joined melt and fuse locally. The common characteristic of these operations is the achievement of bonding between the workpieces and/or the filler metals by a controlled heating procedure.

Metal-joining processes in dentistry have traditionally been dominated by the gold-based alloys, and soldering (or brazing) using a flame torch has been the main process. With the newer nongold alloys, the requirements of the metal-joining process differ among the alloys used. For example, titanium alloys oxidize readily at elevated temperatures, and an oxygen-free environment and a nonoxygen heating source are needed.

Spot welding based on electrical resistance has been used to weld alloys of low thermal conductivity, such as orthodontic appliances. New advances in the technology of heating sources have been adapted for orthodontic and other dental applications. They include the plasma torch, Nd:YAG laser, and tungsten inert gas (TIG) arc. The advantages of these technologies are that the area of heating is small—it can be 0.2 mm with the laser and TIG—and the duration of heating can be controlled. When the area of heating is very small, the thermal conductivity of the alloy can be of concern. High thermal conduction dissipates the thermal energy needed for melting the substrate metal. The very small area of heating is advantageous for Co–Cr and titanium alloys, which have lower thermal conductivities than gold-based alloys.

Although the advantages of modern heating sources have shifted the operation of metal joining in dental laboratories toward welding, gold soldering is a simpler procedure that can be conducted in the dental office.

CRITICAL QUESTION

Why should the flow of flux be restricted, and what kind of material is used?

Soldering Flux

A metal surface free of any contaminant, such as oxides, is essential for establishing metallic bonds between substrate metals. A flux is needed, and it has three primary functions: (1) dissolve surface oxides, (2) reduce existing oxides to pure elements, and (3) protect the surface from oxidation during soldering. The solder chosen must wet the metal substrate to be joined. To prevent the flow of molten solder onto adjacent areas, an antiflux, such as rouge mixed with chloroform or graphite, can be painted on these areas before heating the substrate metals.

Fluxes for use with noble metal alloys are generally based on boric acid, boric anhydride, and borax. Chromium oxides that form on base metal alloys are more stable, and fluoride-containing fluxes are needed to dissolve chromium, nickel, and cobalt oxides. Fluxes are also available for different temperature ranges to provide optimal activity.

The amount of flux used should be minimized because entrapment of flux within the filler metal can cause a weakened joint. Residual flux that is covered with porcelain can cause discoloration and bubbling of the porcelain. Flux combines with metal oxides and forms a glass during the soldering process, and the residue should be removed. After the soldering process, sandblasting the joint with alumina abrasive particles immediately after removal from the soldering investment and boiling in water are needed to remove glassy residue resulting from the reaction between the flux and oxides.

Filler Metal for Soldering

The filler metals should have acceptable color, adequate hardness and strength, and tarnish and corrosion resistance relative to the workpieces. Fillers and substrates do not need to have similar compositions, but the filler metals should have (1) a sufficiently low flow temperature, (2) the ability to wet the substrate metal, and (3) sufficient fluidity at the flow temperature.

Flow Temperature

When the filler metal melts, wets, and flows on the substrate metal, it bonds to this workpiece. The flow temperature of the filler metal is usually higher than its liquidus temperature to provide suitable viscosity and must be sufficiently lower than the solidus temperature of the substrate metal that melting of the substrate does not occur. For an alloy substrate that will be veneered with porcelain after soldering, the melting range of the filler metal should be higher than the sintering temperature of the porcelain to avoid sag deformation of the bridge framework during subsequent porcelain firing.

Wetting

Recall the discussion of the role of wetting in Chapter 2. Wetting of the substrate metal by the molten filler metal is essential to produce a metallic bond. Oxides have poor wettability characteristics; therefore, molten metal does not spread on the oxide layer of substrate metals. That is the reason why iron oxide is used as antiflux.

Fluidity

Molten filler metals should flow freely into the gap between the two substrate metals. When the surface of a metal prosthesis needs to be extended, such as for a deficient interproximal contact area, a filler metal can be used to build up the area. A filler metal with relatively sluggish fluidity then becomes desirable. This type of filler usually has a wide melting range, and flow can be controlled to well-defined areas.

CRITICAL QUESTION

How can one best assess if the quality of a solder joint is acceptable or not?

Heat Sources for Soldering

The most common instrument for the application of heat is a gas–air or gas–oxygen torch. All gases shown in Table 9.14 have potential flame temperatures high enough to melt any dental casting alloy currently in use. The thermal energy (heat content measured in calories per cubic meter of the fuel) from the combustion of the fuel must not only raise the temperature of both the substrate metal and the filler metal to the soldering temperature but also compensate for heat loss to the surroundings. Fuel with a lower heat content requires a longer period of heating at the desired temperature and is associated with an increased danger of oxidation during the soldering process.

Of the fuel gases in Table 9.14, the best choice is propane. Butane, which is more readily available in some parts of the world, has a similar flame temperature and heat content as propane. Both propane and butane have the advantage of being relatively pure compounds; therefore, they are uniform in quality, are virtually water free, and burn cleanly (provided that the torch flame is properly adjusted). With acetylene, which should only be used by an experienced dental laboratory technician, concerns are localized variations in flame temperature and the tendency for decomposition into carbon and hydrogen, with the incorporation of carbon in both nickel and palladium solders degrading the mechanical properties of the joints.

Another source of heating is a furnace that heats the assembled substrate metals along with flux and solder deposited at the joining site to an appropriate temperature for melting and flow of solder. Before the assembled substrate metals are placed into the oven, a uniform coating of a paste flux should be applied to the surface to be soldered. The advantage of furnace soldering is that every component can be heated and cooled uniformly in accordance with a precise schedule that prevents distortion, which might occur under localized heating, such as during soldering of metal–ceramic bridges.

TABLE 9.14 Thermal Characteristics of Fuel Gas Combustion

Fuel	Flame Temperature (°C)	Heat Content (kcal/m³)
Hydrogen	2,660	2,362
Natural gas	2,680	8,898
Propane	2,850	21,221
Acetylene	3,140	12,884

CRITICAL QUESTION

Which type of torch gas should be used for soldering noble alloys? Why is it not possible to use all torch gases?

Technique Considerations for Soldering

For fixed prostheses, where accurate alignment is needed, investment soldering is used, in which the parts to be joined are first indexed and joined by a temporary material, such as acrylic resin or sticky wax, and then mounted in a soldering investment, which holds the parts together during the soldering procedure. In contrast, freehand soldering is used for assembling orthodontic and some other appliances, in which the parts to be joined are manually held in contact during the soldering procedure. As soon as the filler metal has flowed to the desired position, the heating is discontinued, and the appliance is cooled.

The investment soldering technique involves several critical steps: (1) cleaning and preparing the surfaces to be joined, (2) assembling the parts to be joined, (3) preparation and fluxing of the gap surfaces between the parts, (4) maintaining the proper position of the parts during the procedure, (5) control of the proper temperature, and (6) control of the time to ensure adequate flow of solder and complete filling of the solder joint. Many of these steps are applicable to freehand soldering.

Other factors that may influence the result of soldering are discussed in the following.

Gap Width

The gap between the parts of the substrate metal to be joined must be sufficient to allow solder flow between the workpieces. If the gap is too great, the joint strength will be dictated by the strength of the filler metal. If the gap is too narrow, flux inclusions and porosity caused by incomplete flow of the filler metal may occur and lead to decreased strength. Inclusions or porosity can lead to distortion if any heating, such as porcelain application, takes place after the soldering operation. The ideal gap width is about 0.13 mm.

Flame

A torch flame can be divided into four zones, as shown in Figure 9.4. The portion of the flame used to heat the soldering assembly should be the tip of the reducing zone, in which the most efficient burning process occurs and the most heat is generated. An improperly adjusted torch or improperly positioned flame can lead to oxidation of the substrate or filler metal and result in a poor solder joint. It is also possible to introduce carbon into the substrate and filler metal by using the unburned gas portion of the flame. To prevent oxidation, the flame should not be removed once it has been applied to the joint area until the soldering process has been completed. The flame provides protection from oxidation, especially at the soldering temperature.

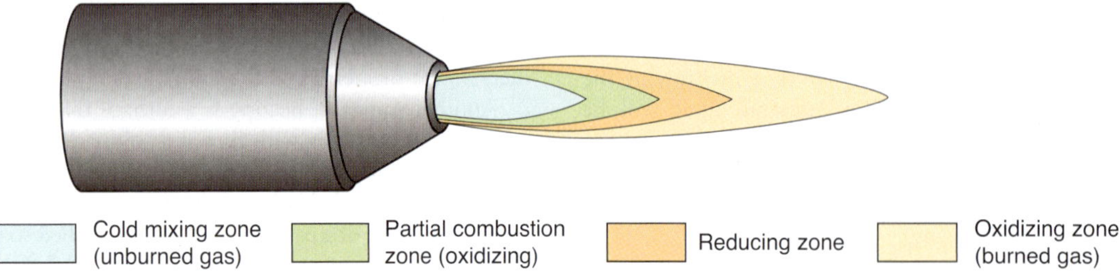

• **Fig. 9.4** Flame zones in a propane–oxygen torch flame.

Temperature and Time

The flame or furnace chamber should provide enough heat to the substrate metal to reach the flow temperature of the filler metal. Then the substrate metal will be hot enough to melt the filler metal as soon as it contacts the area to be joined.

Temperature and time control the diffusion of atoms across the filler–substrate interface. Alloying can take place by diffusion if the temperature remains constant for a sufficiently long time. An alloy formed at the interface of the substrate metal and filler metal through diffusion can have properties different from those of the filler metal and the substrate metal. Figure 9.5 shows such a soldered joint between two different substrate metals. On the left side, the filler–substrate interface is represented by a sharply defined plane. On the right side, the substrate metal appears to have alloyed with the solder at the joint surface adjacent to the nodular area (to the right of the solder boundary).

Therefore, the flame should be maintained in place until the filler metal has flowed completely into the connection and a short time longer to allow the flux or oxide to separate from the fluid filler metal.

CRITICAL QUESTION

What kind of heating source and surrounding environment are needed for joining titanium components?

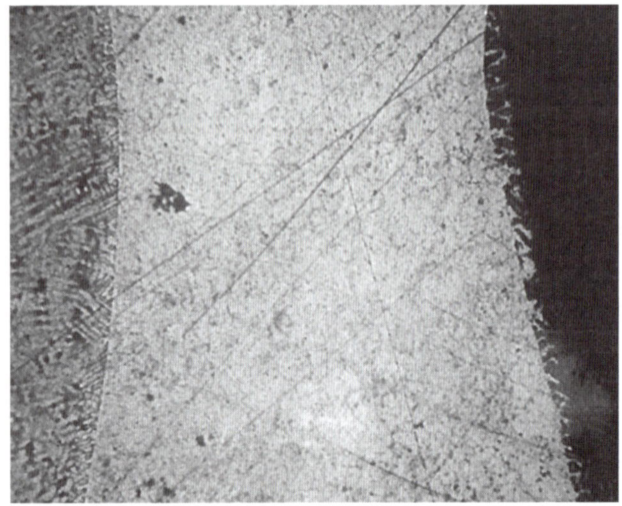

• **Fig. 9.5** Joining of two different substrate metals with the filler metal *(in center)*. **(Left)** Good bonding with no alloying between the filler metal and substrate metal. **(Right)** A nodular region of alloying that has occurred at the interface between the filler metal and another substrate alloy, which is not distinct in this micrograph. (Courtesy Clyde E. Ingersoll.)

Laser Welding of Commercially Pure Titanium

As previously noted, CP Ti is a highly reactive metal that oxidizes readily in air. At temperatures used for soldering procedures, the thickness of the titanium oxide layer increases, and it may spontaneously debond from the parent metal surface at temperatures exceeding 850°C. Thus the quality of the soldered joint is quite variable if a traditional torch-soldering or oven-soldering procedure is used.

Laser welding in an argon atmosphere is a method of choice for joining titanium components of dental prostheses because the coherent, high-intensity laser light can be focused on a small region and melt the substrate without extensive microstructural damage to the surrounding areas. An advantage of welding is that the joint will be composed of the same pure titanium as the substrate components, thereby preserving the excellent biocompatibility potential of CP Ti and avoiding the risk of galvanic corrosion effects within the prosthesis.

CRITICAL QUESTION

Why does the ductility of a pure metal depend on its crystal structure?

Wrought Alloys and Plastic Deformation of Metals

The term *wrought alloys* refers to solid cast alloys that have been mechanically shaped to specific configurations. The process causes alteration of the cast alloy microstructures and results in significant changes in the mechanical properties. The most notable changes are the increase of the YS or proportional limit with a reduction of ductility. This segment reviews the crystal structure of alloys, describes mechanisms of plastic deformation, and identifies correlations between microstructural features and mechanical properties.

Theoretical and Observed Shear Strengths of Metals

An atomic model illustrating permanent deformation of a metal having a perfect crystalline structure subjected to an applied shear stress is shown in Figure 9.6. Notice that the deformation or slip process requires the simultaneous displacement of plane 1 atoms relative to the plane 2 atoms. Studies have shown that theoretical shear strengths are much higher than those observed from mechanical testing of polycrystalline metals. For example, the differences for copper and iron are approximately 40 times greater and can be as much as 190 times greater for the ceramic SiC (Table 9.15). The table also shows that only whisker specimens, which are very thin single crystals of pure materials that achieve near perfection in their atomic lattice, exhibit shear strengths

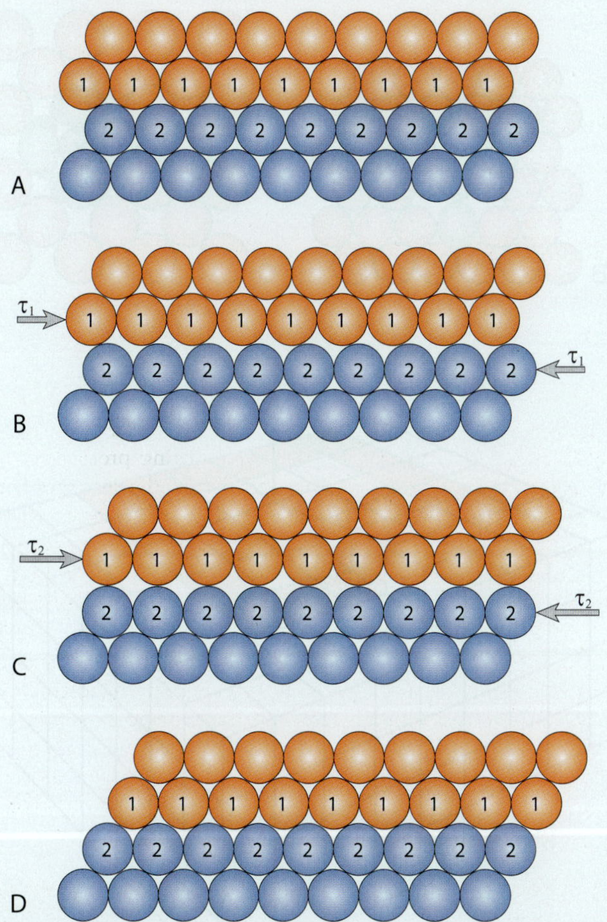

• **Fig. 9.6** Slip between adjacent planes of atoms. **(A)** The configuration of planes 1 (a atoms) and 2 (b atoms) when the solid is not stressed. **(B)** Application of a shear stress t1 causes plane 1 to move with respect to plane 2. **(C)** Increasing the shear stress to τ2 increases the relative lateral displacement of the two planes. This configuration corresponds to the state of maximum stored elastic energy. **(D)** The two planes have now been displaced by one interatomic distance with respect to each other. This configuration will be maintained if the load is removed. If the shear stress (τ2) remains, the planes will continue to slip past each other.

approaching their theoretical values. The key difference between whiskers and bulk polycrystalline specimens of the same material is the presence of crystal imperfections at the atomic level in the bulk material.

CRITICAL QUESTION

Why are the observed strengths of metals always lower than the theoretical strengths?

Crystal Imperfections

Recall Figure 2.16, which illustrates an ideal crystallization that leads to a polycrystalline structure. In reality, the growth is likely to be random and imperfect. When lattice positions have missing atoms, displaced atoms, or extra atoms, these sites are called *point defects.* The edge of an extra plane of atoms in the crystal is called a *line defect.* The grain boundaries on the external surface of the crystal are considered two-dimensional (2-D) imperfections in the crystal.

Point Defects

A *vacancy* or vacant atom site in a crystalline lattice may occur at a single site in the atomic arrangement (Fig. 9.7A), and two vacancies may condense as a divacancy (Fig. 9.7B); a trivacancy may also exist. An *interstitial atom* is illustrated in Figure 9.7C. All point defects are equilibrium defects, and a crystalline material that is in equilibrium will contain a certain number of these defects at a given temperature. The vacancies provide the principal mechanism for atomic diffusion in crystalline materials.

Line Defects (Dislocations)

The simplest type of line defect or dislocation, known as an *edge dislocation,* is illustrated in Figure 9.8A for a simple cubic structure. It can be noted that the atomic arrangement is regular except for the single vertical plane of atoms that is discontinuous. The edge dislocation (symbolized by ^^) is located at the edge of the partial plane. If the atoms have a helical arrangement around the dislocation line (analogous to spiral ramps in a parking garage), such arrangement is called *screw dislocation* (Fig. 9.9).

TABLE 9.15 Theoretical and Observed Shear Strengths

Materials	Shear Modulus (GPa)	OBSERVED SHEAR STRENGTH (GPA) Polycrystalline	OBSERVED SHEAR STRENGTH (GPA) Whisker	Calculated Shear Strength (GPa)
Copper	48	0.22	2.1	7.7
Iron	80	0.29	9.5	12.8
Nickel	76	0.48	2.7	12.1
Al_2O_3	170	—	14.6	27.1
BeO	140	0.28[a]	9.2	22.3
SiC	200	0.17[a]	14.6	31.8

[a]Measured in tension.

The tabulated values were calculated from tensile strength data given by Broutman IJ and Krock RH: *Modern Composite Materials,* Reading, MA, 1967, Addison-Wesley.

From Eisenstadt M: *Introduction to Mechanical Properties of Materials,* Upper Saddle River, NJ, 1971, Prentice Hall.

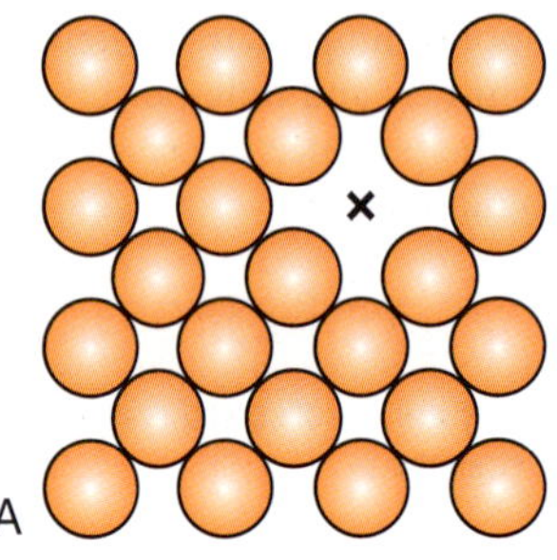

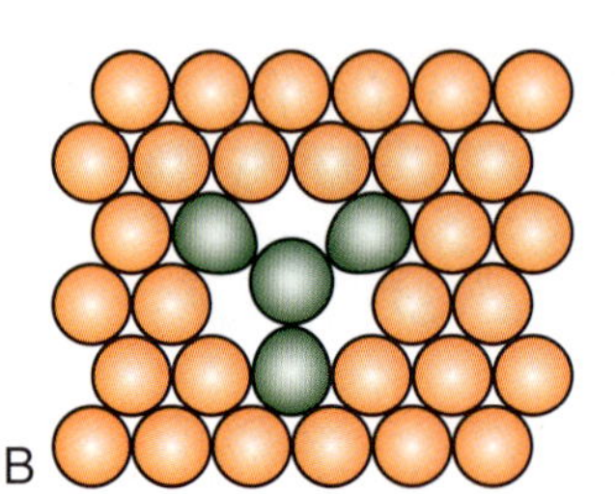

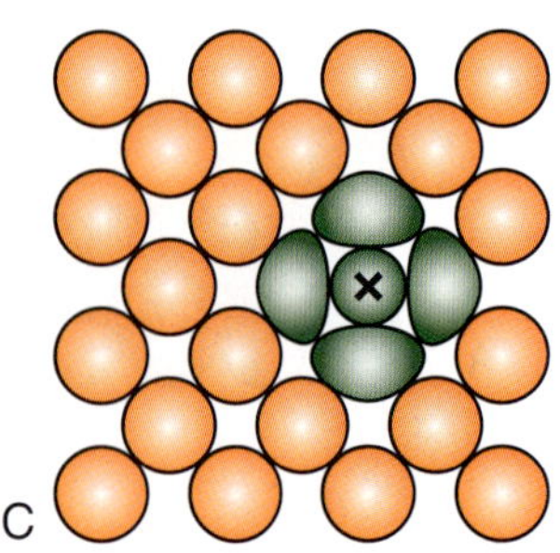

• **Fig. 9.7** Point defects. **(A)** Vacancy. **(B)** Divacancy (two missing atoms). **(C)** Interstitial (extra atom). Different colors are used to show that the atoms have been distorted by adapting to the space available. (Adapted from Van Vlack LH: *Elements of Materials Science,* ed 4, Reading, MA, 1980, Addison-Wesley.)

If a sufficiently large shear stress is applied across the top and bottom faces of the crystal containing the edge dislocation shown in Figure 9.8A, the bonds in the row of atoms adjacent to the dislocation will be broken, and new bonds with the next row will be established, resulting in movement of the dislocation by one interatomic distance, as indicated in Figure 9.8B. Continued application of this shear stress causes similar movements of one interatomic distance until the dislocation reaches the boundary of the crystal (Fig. 9.8C). The plane along which an edge dislocation moves is known as a *slip plane.* The result of this dislocation movement across the crystal is that the atomic planes on one side of the slip plane have been displaced one interatomic spacing with respect to the atomic planes on the other side of the slip plane. The crystallographic direction in which the atomic planes have been displaced is termed the *slip direction,* and the combination of a slip plane and a slip direction is termed a *slip system.* The screw dislocation is more difficult to visualize than the edge dislocation and is discussed in textbooks on engineering materials science. Dislocations in metallic materials often have a mixed character, consisting of both edge and screw components.

The inherent ability of a metal to deform plastically and exhibit ductility increase with the number of slip systems associated with the crystal structure. The number of slip systems in common crystal structures is in the decreasing order of face-centered cubic (FCC; e.g., gold, silver, copper, nickel, etc.), body-centered cubic (BCC; e.g., α-iron, chromium, etc.), and then HCP (e.g., cobalt, zinc, etc.).

Evidently, much less shear stress is required to initiate permanent deformation of the metal crystals that contain edge dislocations (Fig. 9.8) because only one row of atomic bonds is broken at a time, compared with the perfect crystal, where an entire row of atomic bonds across the two planes (Fig. 9.6) must be simultaneously broken

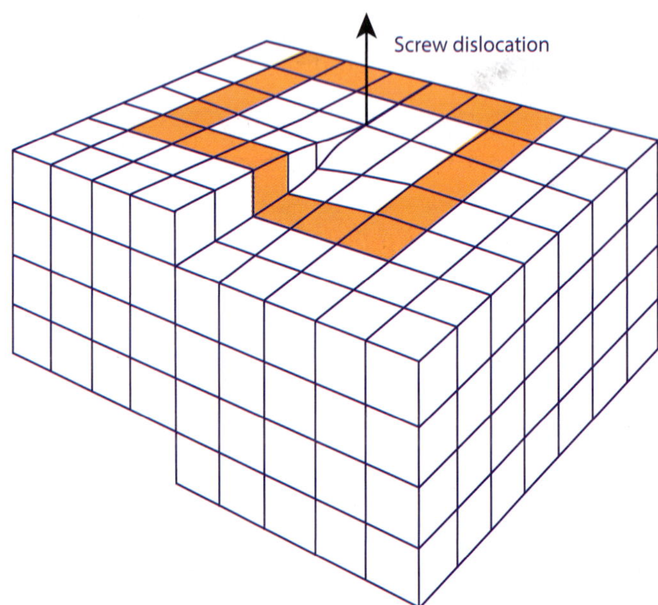

• **Fig. 9.9** Illustration of screw dislocation. A crystal defect characterized by a unit distortion of part of the crystal lattice in a particular direction such that the lattice planes perpendicular to that direction form continuous helical sheets.

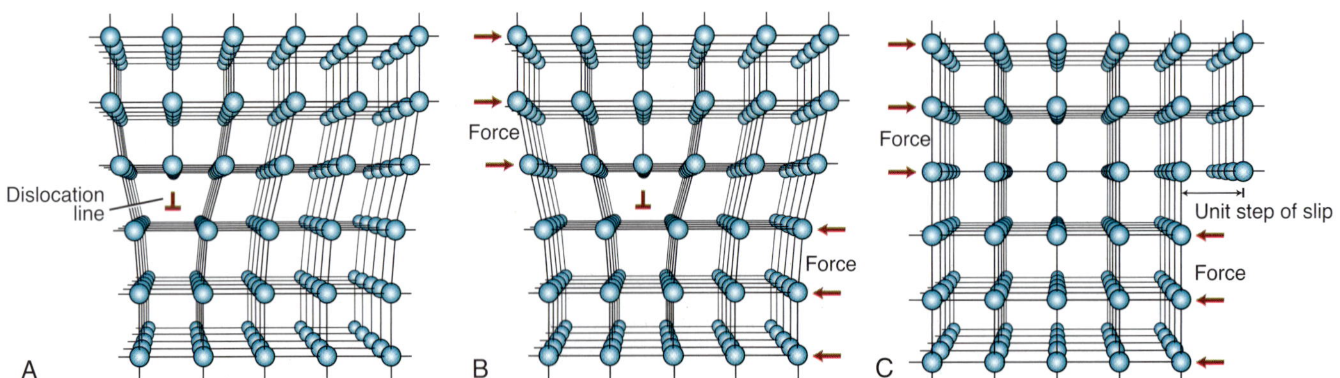

• **Fig. 9.8** Illustration and movement of edge dislocation. **(A)** An edge dislocation in a schematic cubic crystal structure. **(B)** The dislocation has moved one interatomic distance along the slip plane under the action of the shearing force indicated by the arrows. **(C)** The dislocation has reached the edge of the crystal, and a unit amount of slip has been produced. (Taken from Callister WD, Jr, Rethwisch DG: Materials science and engineering: an introduction, 8th ed, Hoboken, NJ, John Wiley & Sons, 2010.)

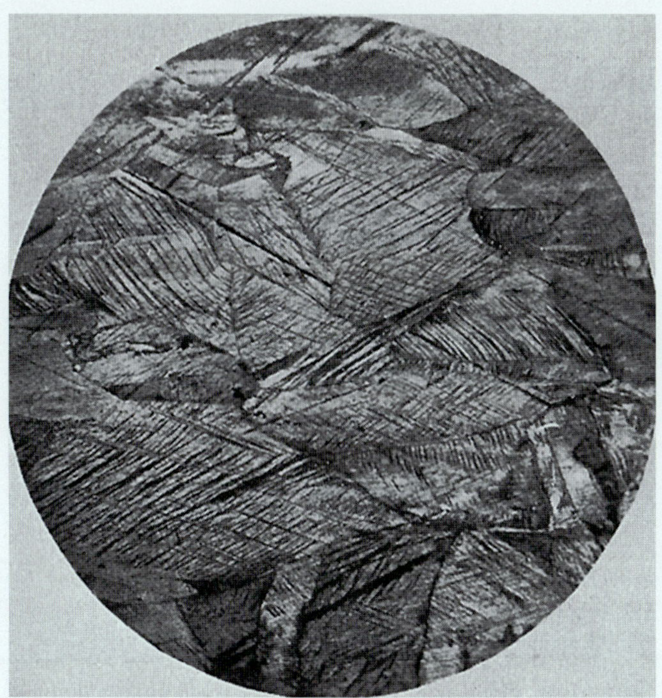

• **Fig. 9.10** Photomicrograph of cold-worked gold, showing deformed grains and slip lines (the parallel lines within grains) at surface offsets where dislocations have exited their slip planes (×100). (Courtesy S. D. Tylman.)

for shear deformation to occur. The proportional limit for a metal generally corresponds to the onset of significant movement of dislocations. The slip lines in Figure 9.10 correspond to slip planes where large numbers of dislocations have exited the metal, causing surface offsets that scatter the light used for observation. Thus one can conclude that permanent deformation of a metal is the result of dislocation movement and slip between atomic planes.

CRITICAL QUESTION

What fundamental strengthening mechanisms are available for alloys that are not possible for pure metals?

Dislocation Movement in Polycrystalline Alloys

Figures 9.8 and 9.11A illustrate one dislocation moving in a pure metal crystal; it appears that there is little hindrance of a moving dislocation along its slip plane. In reality, there are several scenarios in which dislocation movement can be impeded in pure metals and alloys. Alloys contain multiple phases, such as solid solutions and/or precipitates (Chapter 2), in addition to the numerous dislocations and grain boundaries found in pure metals. These crystal structural features represent obstacles that may be overcome by an application of increased stress to promote dislocation movement.

For solid–solution alloys, the atomic arrangement near solute atoms is locally distorted. The movement of dislocations along the slip plane will be impeded by the presence of such solute atoms (Fig. 9.11B). Precipitates can be coherent, where the atomic bonds are continuous across the interface with the solid–solution matrix, or incoherent, where interatomic bonds are not continuous across the interface. Coherent precipitates have the same crystal structure as the matrix phase and generate localized distortion in the atomic arrangement. Dislocations cannot move through incoherent precipitates but instead form loops of increasing size around these particles (Fig. 9.11C). Additional stress is needed to move dislocations through distorted regions, including coherent precipitates, or around incoherent precipitates.

Metals with a sufficient amount of ductility can be permanently deformed under mechanical stress at temperatures below their recrystallization temperatures (including room temperature), as discussed later. This process, also known as *cold working,*

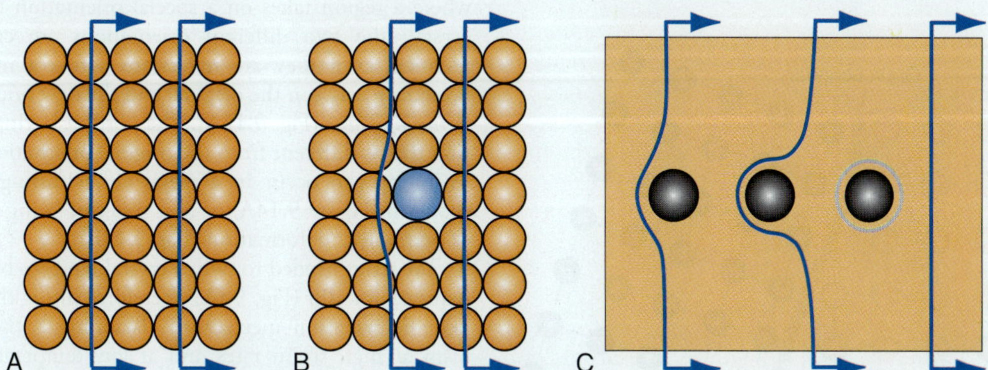

• **Fig. 9.11** Effect of precipitates on the movement of edge dislocation. The illustrations depict the view taken from the top of the three-dimensional (3-D) model shown in Figure 9.8. Each line with right-pointing arrows represents a line defect (dislocation) moving toward the right side of the grain. **(A)** A dislocation moves without any impediment within a grain; no extra effort is needed, and no strengthening effect occurs. **(B)** The darker and slightly larger sphere represents a solute atom or coherent precipitate that presents an obstacle to the movement of the dislocation; bending of the line defect implies that the movement has been impeded, and more stress is needed to pass through the obstacle. **(C)** The dark spheres represent incoherent precipitates, and the background simulates the rest of the grain. The dislocation cannot pass through the incoherent precipitate because it does not share the same lattice with the hosting grain. The first dislocation *(left)* bends as it moves close to the precipitate. The second dislocation *(middle)* continues to bend around the precipitate while the rest of the dislocation keeps moving toward the right. Finally, the dislocation *(right)* completes its encircling around the precipitate; the rest of the dislocation rejoins and moves on through the nonstrengthened area.

can create vast numbers of point defects and dislocations within the metals. These dislocations will interact with each other, mutually impeding their movements. Increased stress is required for further dislocation movement to continue the permanent deformation process.

The movement of a dislocation from one grain into another grain is unlikely, especially if the adjacent grain is misaligned (Fig. 9.12). Grain boundaries represent the ends of slip planes where dislocations cease to move and accumulate. As the grain size decreases, there will be more grain boundary area per unit volume to impede dislocation motion. Grain size can be controlled by rapid cooling or quenching or by the inclusion of a grain-refining element (Chapter 2), such as iridium in gold alloys. Cold working also alters the shapes of grains substantially (e.g., the grains are severely elongated parallel to the wire axis).

A higher stress, which is reflected in higher values of proportional limit, is needed for dislocations to overcome each impeding mechanism to continue moving along the slip plane. Therefore, these obstacles are considered mechanisms for the strengthening of metal alloys that include solid-solution strengthening, precipitation hardening, strain (or work) hardening, and grain-refinement strengthening. The elastic moduli of the wrought alloys remain the same as those of their cast counterparts because there are no changes in the crystalline structure. If a phase change has occurred in the alloy in the process, some change in the elastic modulus is expected.

CRITICAL QUESTION

Why does the clasp of an RPD fracture easily after a patient has bent it back and forth repeatedly to relieve discomfort?

Effects of Strengthening Metals

The ductility of the wrought alloys is decreased with each of the strengthening mechanisms just described. The corrosion resistance of the wrought alloys is also decreased because the

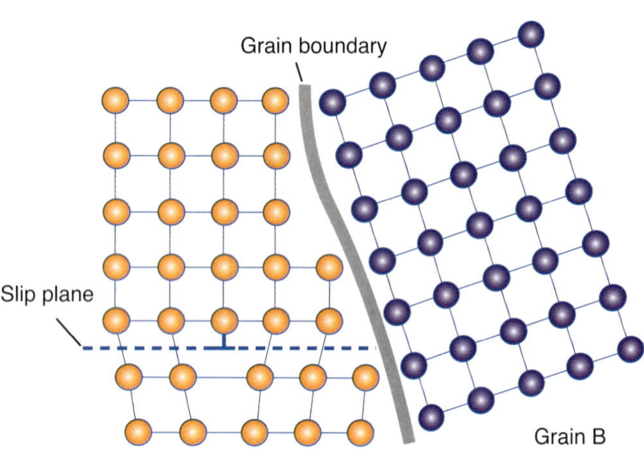

• **Fig. 9.12** This illustration shows the spatial lattices of two adjacent grains. Notice that the lattices are not aligned. There is a dislocation moving toward the grain boundary in grain A. Because of misalignment, the dislocation in grain A cannot move into grain B and is trapped at the grain boundary. In essence, the grain boundary is an obstacle to dislocation movement. Therefore, the greater the number of grain boundaries, the higher is the yield strength of the material.

dislocations produce localized regions of strain at the atomic level, which have higher energy than atomic arrangements in the undeformed metal. Corrosion is also a process that relieves stored energy (Chapter 3), and it can be minimized by stress relief (discussed later).

One can observe from the first row of photomicrographs of Figure 9.13 that the thinner the specimen becomes from rolling, as designated above each photomicrograph, the flatter or thinner the grains appear to be. Although brass is used in this example, the same effect would occur with wrought dental alloys. For the extreme example of a wire, the grains will be elongated parallel to the wire axis and resemble "strands of spaghetti" in a photomicrograph showing a longitudinal section.

Recall the example we used in the introduction of Chapter 4 regarding the adjustment of the retentive clasps. We can conclude that the crystal deformation generates dislocations, which can be moved with finger pressure on the clasp. The movements of the dislocations allow us to shape the clasp as needed. The region near the missing half-plane of the edge dislocation can be thought of as a linear vacancy within the crystal structure. These regions accumulate when there is an edge dislocation pileup at a grain boundary and grow to a flaw of critical size. Meanwhile, greater force is needed to overcome obstacles within the alloy. Eventually, the force applied is high enough to cause crack propagation and then fracture.

CRITICAL QUESTION

What is the difference between the twinning and dislocation movement mechanisms of plastic deformation?

Plastic Deformation Without Dislocation Movement

An alternative mode of permanent deformation in metals is twinning. *Twinning* refers to the atomic arrangement within a crystal where a region takes on a special orientation from the adjacent crystal; the two different orientations are crystallographically identical as if they are reflections across a mirror plane. This boundary between the original and the new orientation is called a *twinning plane* (Fig. 9.14A). The portion having a lattice orientation that is different from the original orientation is called a *twin.* Twinning can occur in a metal either during solidification, as shown in Figure 9.14A, or as a result of being stressed to a state of permanent deformation (Fig. 9.14B).

The stress needed to twin a crystal tends to be higher than that required for slip (Fig. 9.6). Therefore, slip is the normal permanent deformation mechanism. Twinning is the favored mechanism at high strain rates and at low temperatures, rather than dislocation movement, in metals having relatively few slip systems. One should note that permanent deformation by twinning is merely a reorientation of the lattice, and although the atoms in the twinned portion have moved, their positions relative to each other remain unchanged. On the other hand, permanent deformation by slip occurs along individual lattice planes for which the positions of atoms relative to each other have changed.

Twinning has significance for the permanent deformation of α-titanium alloys, which are highly important for some dental implants and are gaining interest for cast restorations. In the unit cell for α-titanium, the ratio of the lattice parameter (c) in the perpendicular direction to the basal plane and the lattice

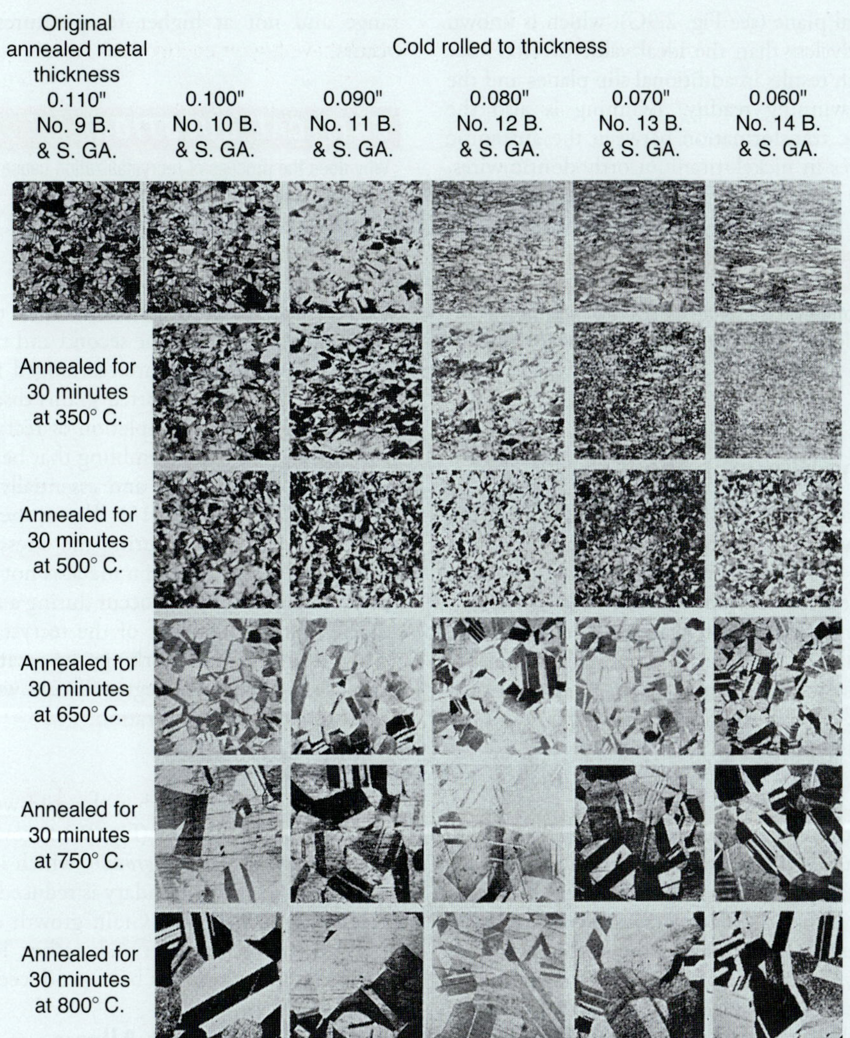

• **Fig. 9.13** Grain size and appearance of brass (copper 66%, zinc 34%) after cold working and annealing. Note that as the degree of cold working increases *(to the right in the figure),* the grains become more distorted. When the recrystallization proceeds, the grain size is inversely proportional to the degree of cold working (340). (Prepared by L. H. DeWald.)

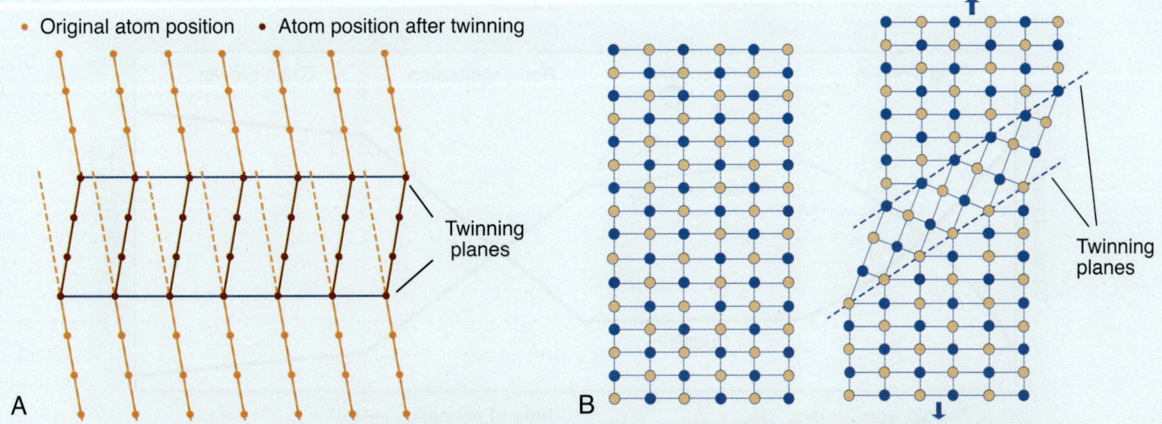

• **Fig. 9.14** Schematic illustration of twinning in a metal. **(A)** Atomic arrangement at the twinning planes in a face-centered cubic metal. The dashed lines show the orientation of the crystal if twinning had not occurred. Note that the atoms on either side of the two twinning planes have a mirror relationship. **(B)** A lattice structure before and after plastic deformation of a metal by twinning under tension. Note that the shape of the object has changed, but the relative position of the atoms remains unchanged. Also note that the atoms on either side of the twinning plane have a mirror relationship. The two colors of spheres provide a contrast of neighboring atoms.

parameter (*a*) in the basal plane (see Fig. 2.9G), which is known as the *c/a ratio,* is slightly less than the ideal value of 1.633 for the HCP structure, which results in additional slip planes and the tendency to undergo twinning readily. Twinning is also the mechanism for reversible transformation between the austenitic and martensitic structures in nickel–titanium orthodontic wires, which have considerable clinical significance.

CRITICAL QUESTION

Why must recrystallization of orthodontic wires be avoided when a stress-relief heat treatment is performed after manipulation to minimize fracture during placement?

Effects of Annealing Wrought Alloys

The effects associated with permanent deformation (e.g., strain hardening, decreased ductility, distorted grains, and increased dislocation density) can be reversed by simply heating the metal to an appropriate elevated temperature without melting it. This process is called annealing, and it takes place in three successive stages: recovery, recrystallization, and grain growth. The more severe the degree of cold working, the more rapidly the effects can be reversed by annealing. Also, the higher the melting point of the metal, the higher is the temperature needed for annealing.

Recovery

Heating increases atom diffusion and the initiation of annealing. As Figure 9.15 shows, there is a very slight decrease in tensile strength and no change in ductility during the recovery stage, which reduces the number of dislocations and relieves the internal strain energy resulting from cold working. Orthodontic appliances fabricated by bending wires are often subjected to a stress-relief anneal prior to their placement. This heat treatment stabilizes the configuration of the appliance and allows an accurate determination of the force that the appliance can deliver in the mouth. The elimination of residual stresses in the appliance also reduces the likelihood of fracture during clinical adjustments. It is essential that this heat treatment be performed in the recovery temperature range and not at higher temperatures where recrystallization occurs.

CRITICAL QUESTION

Why does the process of recrystallization cause a significant reduction in the tensile strength of the alloy?

Recrystallization

The recrystallization process involves a radical change in the microstructure, as seen in the second and third rows of Figure 9.13. The atoms at this stage are rearranged into a lower-energy configuration. The old, distorted grains disappear as new strain-free grains emerge. After completion of recrystallization, the alloy retains microstructures resembling that before cold working (upper left corner of Fig. 9.13) and essentially attains its original soft, ductile condition (Fig. 9.15). That is the reason why recrystallization must be avoided during the stress-relief heat treatment of orthodontic appliances. If a metal is not sufficiently cold worked, recrystallization may not occur during a typical annealing process.

The average grain size of the recrystallized structure depends on the degree of cold working; the greater is the number of such nuclei. The greater the degree of cold working, the smaller is the grain size after recrystallization.

Grain Growth

The grain size increases when the cold-worked alloy is annealed at an elevated temperature (Fig. 9.13, rows 4–6). This increase in grain size is called *grain growth,* which is a process by which the volume of the grain boundary is reduced; large grains grow at the expense of small grains. Grain growth does not proceed indefinitely to yield a single crystal; rather, it ceases after a relatively coarse grain structure has been produced.

Types of Wrought Alloys

Wrought alloys are used as wires by orthodontists for correcting displacements of teeth from proper occlusion and by prosthodontists and general dentists as clasps for the retention and stabilization

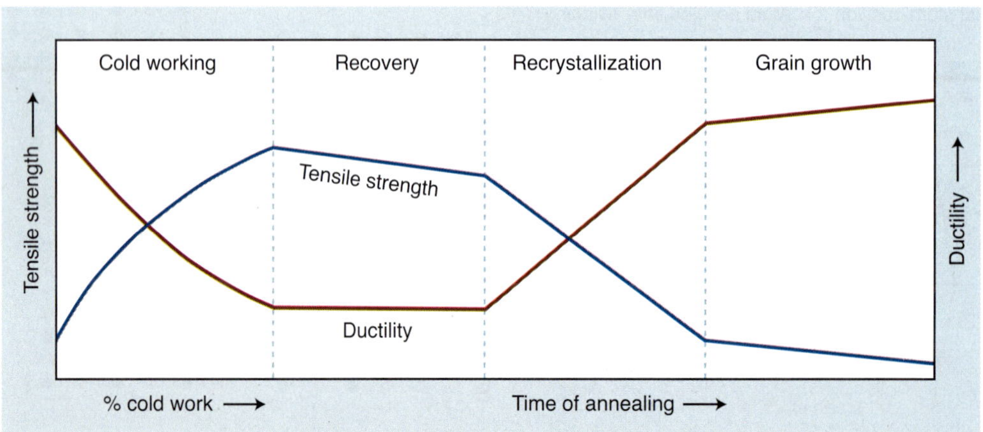

• **Fig. 9.15** Tensile strength and ductility of a metal as a function of the percentage of cold working and annealing time. Tensile strength increases during cold working, and ductility decreases. These properties change only slightly during recovery. During recrystallization, tensile strength decreases, and ductility increases rapidly. Only slight changes occur during grain growth. (Adapted from Richman MH: *Introduction to the Science of Metals,* Waltham, MA, 1967, Blaisdell.)

of RPDs. Wrought alloys are also made in the form of files and reamers for endodontists to clean and shape root canals or as prefabricated metal crowns for pedodontic patients.

Orthodontic wires are formed into various configurations or appliances to apply forces to move the teeth to a more desirable alignment. From the orthodontic viewpoint, as demonstrated by the loading of a cantilever beam (Fig. 9.16), the proportional limit (or YS) reflects the maximal amount of force a particular beam design can deliver. The elastic deflection (δ) of a cantilever beam under a load reflects the extent of tooth displacement that the designed appliance can deliver. The maximum elastic deflection is reached when the stress approaches the proportional limit and is called the working range of the beam. An obvious benefit of wrought wires is that they have a greater working range than their cast counterparts.

Physiologically, excessive forces acting on the tooth may cause root resorption, and insufficient forces yield no tooth movement. A properly designed orthodontic appliance applies appropriate amounts of force to the teeth. As the teeth move, the deflection of the device decreases. In response to the reduction in elastic deflection of the appliance, the level of force applied to the teeth is gradually reduced below the threshold level. When this happens, the appliance must be reactivated to increase the force level to its original value. Reactivation requires partial permanent deformation to obtain a suitable configuration for moving the teeth effectively.

The relationships for rectangular and round wires in Figure 9.16 show that the elastic deflection (δ) depends on the properties of metals selected (i.e., elastic modulus and proportional limit) and the dimensions of the beam (i.e., thickness, width, radius, and length). Thus, finding the optimal design for an appliance that will deliver the low, constant forces, which are biologically desirable for tooth movement, is possible. Practically, the working range of a material is considered to be the elastic strain at the YS of the wire, which is termed springback and defined as YS/E. The mechanical principles described here also apply to the design of retentive clasps and root canal files and reamers.

Wrought alloys used in dentistry, which include stainless steel, cobalt–chromium–nickel, nickel–titanium, and beta-titanium, are now discussed.

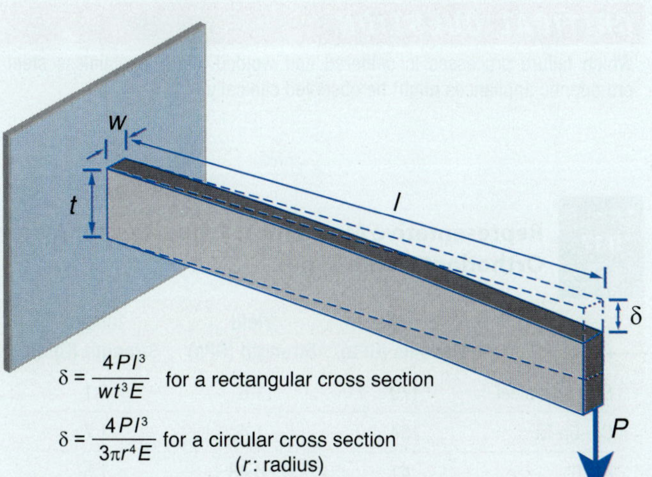

• **Fig. 9.16** Bending of a cantilever beam. δ, deflection; *t*, thickness; *w*, width; *l*, length; and *E*, elastic modulus.

CRITICAL QUESTION

What are the differences in the martensitic structures that form in plain carbon steels and austenitic stainless steels?

Stainless Steel Alloys

The metallurgy and terminology of stainless steels are closely related to the binary iron–carbon system, which yields the primary phases of carbon steel. Therefore, a brief outline of the carbon steels is presented here.

Carbon Steel

Carbon steels can be described simply as iron–carbon binary alloys that contain less than about 2.1% of carbon by weight. At room temperature, pure iron has a BCC structure that transforms into an FCC structure at 912°C. The solubility of carbon in BCC iron reaches a maximum of 0.02%, and this material is known as *ferrite.* The solid solution of carbon in FCC iron is called *austenite,* which has a maximal solubility of about 2.1% carbon. All carbon–steel compositions have the austenite structure at elevated temperatures.

When a plain carbon steel (only iron and carbon) containing 0.8% carbon is cooled slowly in the austenitic phase to 723°C, a solid-state eutectoid transformation occurs to yield a microstructural constituent called *pearlite,* which consists of alternating fine-scale lamellae of ferrite and iron carbide (Fe_3C). The Fe_3C phase is much harder and more rigid than austenite or ferrite. At temperatures below 723°C, when the carbon content is less than 0.8%, the carbon–steel microstructure consists of ferrite and pearlite, whereas plain carbon steels containing more than 0.8% carbon are much harder alloys with microstructures consisting of iron carbide and pearlite.

If austenite is cooled very rapidly (quenched), spontaneous transformation from the FCC structure to a body-centered tetragonal structure results in a new phase called *martensite,* which is very hard, strong, and brittle. The transformation occurs by small atomic displacements and does not involve elemental diffusion. The high hardness of martensite allows the grinding of a sharp edge, which is retained in extended use. Martensite is a metastable phase that transforms to ferrite and iron carbide when it is heated to elevated temperatures. This process is called *tempering;* it reduces the hardness of the alloy but increases its toughness.

Types of Stainless Steels

When approximately 12%–30% chromium by weight is added to carbon steel, the alloy is commonly known as *stainless steel.* The chromium in base metal alloys forms a very thin, transparent, adherent layer of Cr_2O_3, termed as *passivating oxide,* which prevents corrosion of the underlying alloy. If the oxide layer is ruptured by mechanical or chemical means, the passivating oxide layer eventually forms again in an oxidizing environment such as ambient air.

Based on the previously described crystal structures formed by iron and carbon atoms, there are three major types of stainless steels:

Ferritic Stainless Steels

These alloys provide good corrosion resistance at a low cost. They cannot be hardened by heat treatment or readily work hardened. Consequently, they have little application in dentistry.

Martensitic Stainless Steels

These alloys can be heat treated in the same manner as plain carbon steels, which results in a high YS and hardness for use in surgical and cutting instruments.

Austenitic Stainless Steels

The addition of nickel stabilizes the austenite phase on cooling of the alloy. The austenitic stainless steels are the most corrosion resistant of the three major types. Austenitic stainless steel is preferred for dental applications because it has the following properties: (1) greater ductility for more cold working without fracturing, (2) greater strength from cold work, (3) greater ease of welding, (4) ability to overcome sensitization, (5) less critical grain growth, and (6) comparative ease of reshaping.

The foregoing three classifications of stainless steels, with approximate compositions, are presented in Table 9.16.

CRITICAL QUESTION

How does austenitic stainless steel acquire its corrosion resistance? Can this protection be lost during the fabrication and normal use of a stainless steel appliance?

Corrosion Resistance of Austenitic Stainless Steel

Stainless steel can corrode under the conditions described in Chapter 3. For example, severe strain hardening produces highly stressed regions that are anodic to less stressed regions in the presence of saliva. Organic or inorganic deposits and any site of surface roughness on a metal may result in localized concentration cell corrosion. Therefore, a stainless steel orthodontic appliance should be polished so that it remains clean and less susceptible to tarnish or corrosion during use. When a stainless steel wire or a stainless steel appliance is abraded or cut with a carbon steel bur or similar steel tool, carbon steel debris from these tools becomes embedded in the stainless steel surface, causing dissimilar metal corrosion in vivo. Chlorine-containing cleansers should not be used to clean removable appliances fabricated from stainless steel.

When austenitic stainless steel is heated to between approximately 400°C and 900°C, chromium carbides precipitate along the grain boundaries, causing chromium near the grain boundaries to be depleted below the concentrations necessary for corrosion protection, which also weakens the alloy. This phenomenon is called *sensitization;* the stainless steel has become susceptible to intergranular corrosion. The temperature range of sensitization is within that used by the orthodontist for soldering and welding. In addition, filler materials that are employed for brazed or soldered joints in orthodontic appliances can also form galvanic couples in vivo.

The manufacturer can reduce the carbon content of the stainless steel to such an extent that carbide precipitation cannot occur or can severely cold work and heat the stainless steel within the sensitization temperature range to spread the formation of chromium carbide precipitates within the bulk grains instead of only at the grain boundaries. Elements such as titanium and tantalum, which preferentially form carbides, can be added to the stainless steel to preserve the level of chromium when the metal is exposed to elevated temperatures. This process is called *stabilization.*

TABLE 9.16 Compositions (Weight Percent) of Three Types of Stainless Steel[a] Based on Crystal Structure of Iron Atoms

Type of Stainless Steel	Chromium	Nickel	Carbon
Ferritic (BCC)	11.5–27.0	0	0.20 max.
Austenitic (FCC)	16.0–26.0	7.0–22.0	0.25 max.
Martensitic (BCT)	11.5–17.0	0–2.5	0.15–1.20

BCC, body-centered cubic; BCT, body-centered tetragonal; FCC, face-centered cubic.
[a]Silicon, phosphorus, sulfur, manganese, tantalum, and niobium may also be present in small amounts. The balance is iron.

Mechanical Properties of Austenitic Stainless Steel

The approximate values of the mechanical properties of a representative stainless steel orthodontic wire are listed in Table 9.17. Strength and hardness may increase with a decrease in cross-sectional dimensions because of the increased cold working that is required for forming smaller wires.

It is unfortunate that a stainless steel orthodontic wire can become fully annealed (recrystallized) after a few seconds at temperatures from 700°C to 800°C because soldering and welding of stainless steel wires are carried out in that temperature range. The YS of the wire and, thus, the working range necessary for a satisfactory orthodontic appliance are greatly reduced after such annealing. However, using low-fusing solders and minimizing the soldering and welding times can minimize the softening. Any softening that occurs under such conditions can be remedied considerably by contouring and polishing of the soldered areas.

An increase in the elastic properties of a stainless steel wire can be obtained by heating it to temperatures between 400°C and 500°C for 5–120 seconds after cold working. This *stress-relief heat treatment* promotes the recovery annealing stage, which removes the residual stresses introduced during manipulation of the wire. Thus it stabilizes the shape of the appliance. This is important clinically because such residual stresses can promote fracture when the appliance is being adjusted by the clinician.

CRITICAL QUESTION

Which failure processes in soldered and welded joints in stainless steel orthodontic appliances might be observed clinically?

TABLE 9.17 Representative Mechanical Properties for Major Orthodontic Wire Types

Alloy	Elastic Modulus (GPa)	Yield Strength (GPa)	Tensile Strength (GPa)
Stainless steel	179	1.6	2.1
Co–Cr–Ni	184	1.4	1.7
Ni–Ti	41	0.43	1.5
β-Ti	72	0.93	1.3

Soldering and Welding Stainless Steel

Stainless steel components are often joined by silver solders. Although such solders corrode in use because they are anodic to stainless steel, this is not objectionable in orthodontic appliances. These appliances are temporary structures, usually not worn in the mouth for more than 6–30 months, and frequent inspection by the orthodontist is necessary. As discussed earlier, a fluoride-containing flux is used to dissolve the passivating surface film formed by chromium.

Technical Considerations for Soldering

The freehand soldering of stainless steel is not greatly different from that of gold soldering, described earlier. A needle-like, nonluminous, gas-air flame may be used to minimize annealing of the metal surrounding the joint. The reducing zone of the flame should be used. The soldering should be observed in a shadow, against a black background, so that the temperature can be judged by the color of the workpiece. The color should never exceed a dull red.

Prior to soldering, the parts should be tack welded for alignment during the soldering procedure. Then flux should be applied, and the heavier gauge part should be heated first. Flux must cover all of the areas to be soldered before heat is applied. As soon as the flux fuses, the solder alloy should be added, and heating is then continued until the solder flows around and within the joint. After the solder has flowed, the work should be immediately removed from the heat source and quenched in water. From the preceding discussion on the sensitization of austenitic stainless steels, it should be evident that the objective during soldering is to use as little heat for as short a time as possible. Other heating techniques include the use of a hydrogen–oxygen torch, electric resistance heating, and indirect heating using a brass wire intermediary.

CRITICAL QUESTION

Does welding of stainless steel wires subject them to undesired annealing? What can be done to reduce the effect of annealing?

Welding

Flat structures such as bands and brackets are usually joined by spot welding, which produces a large electrical current that is forced by the electrode to flow through a limited area (spot) on the overlapped materials that are to be welded. The interfacial resistance of the materials to the current flow produces intense localized heating and fusion of the overlapped metals. No solder is employed. Ideally, melting is confined to the junction area, and a cast-type structure is formed. The grain structure of the surrounding wrought alloy should not be affected, but stress exists at the interface of the cast and wrought structures, which would be the most likely path of joint failure should fracture occur. The strength of the welded joint decreases with an increase in the area of recrystallization of the adjacent wrought structure, and the joint strength increases with the area of the weld. The welded joint is susceptible to corrosion, primarily because of the loss of passivation caused by sensitization and the localized stress at the interface between the weld area and the surrounding wrought structure.

Cobalt–Chromium–Nickel Alloys

Cobalt–chromium–nickel alloys were originally developed for use as watch springs (Elgiloy) and first marketed for use in orthodontic appliances during the 1950s. Elgiloy has excellent resistance to tarnish and corrosion in the oral environment, and it uses the same welding and soldering procedures used for stainless steel wires.

The manufacturer offers Elgiloy wires in four different tempers: soft, ductile, semiresilient, and resilient. The most widely used is the soft temper (Elgiloy Blue), which is easily manipulated and then heat treated to achieve increased resilience; other tempers are also responsive to heat treatment. The resulting changes in mechanical properties are associated with precipitation reactions. Clinicians can easily perform heat treatment using an electrical resistance welding apparatus and a special paste provided by the manufacturer to indicate the optimal period of time.

Because of their nearly identical values of elastic modulus (Table 9.17), the orthodontic force delivery for Elgiloy Blue and stainless steel orthodontic wires is essentially the same. Heat treatment of Elgiloy Blue orthodontic wires was found to increase the elastic modulus in tension from a range of 160–190 GPa for as-received wires to a range of 180–210 GPa, along with the springback (YS/E) increase from a range of 0.0045–0.0065 to a range of 0.0054–0.0074. Co–Cr–Ni wire products are also available from other manufacturers, but minimal mechanical property data have been reported in the literature.

Nickel–Titanium Alloys

A wrought nickel–titanium orthodontic wire alloy known as *Nitinol* (now *Nitinol Classic*) was introduced commercially during the 1970s. This wire alloy is noted for its much lower elastic modulus (Table 9.17) and much wider elastic working range compared with the stainless steel and Co–Cr–Ni wires. The alloy name *Nitinol* originally came from the two elements, nickel (Ni) and titanium (Ti), and the Naval Ordnance Laboratory where these alloys were developed.

The nickel–titanium alloys used in dentistry are based on the equiatomic intermetallic compound NiTi, which contains 55% nickel and 45% titanium by weight. Orthodontic wire alloys contain small amounts of other elements, such as copper and chromium. The microstructure consists predominantly of NiTi, but other very small precipitates having different compositions are also observed. The austenitic NiTi phase has a complex BCC structure, and the martensitic NiTi phase has been reported to possess a distorted monoclinic, triclinic, or hexagonal structure. The names *austenitic* and *martensitic* for these different crystallographic forms of NiTi have been taken from the metallurgical terminology for carbon steel and stainless steel.

Mechanical Properties

The approximate mechanical properties of Nitinol wire are shown in Table 9.17. The placement of permanent bends by the clinician in Nitinol wires is difficult because of their high resilience. Nitinol has high ductility, and its ability to undergo substantial work hardening is evident from the considerably higher tensile strength relative to the YS. The very low elastic modulus of Nitinol results in very low forces delivered by the appliance compared with similarly constructed and activated appliances from stainless steel and Co–Cr–Ni alloys, and the springback or elastic range available for tooth movement is much greater for Nitinol compared with these two alloys.

CRITICAL QUESTION

What are the clinical advantages of a shape memory nickel–titanium orthodontic wire compared with a stainless steel orthodontic wire?

Superelasticity and Shape Memory in Nickel–Titanium Orthodontic Wires

Transformation between the austenitic and martensitic forms of Nitinol alloys can be induced by both temperature and stress. Austenitic NiTi is the high-temperature, low-stress form, and martensitic NiTi is the low-temperature, high-stress form. Transformation between these phases occurs by a twinning process, which is reversible below the elastic limit and also results in changes in volume and electrical resistivity.

Figure 9.17 presents a highly schematic illustration of the stress–strain behavior for a certain type of NiTi wire in bending; the bending moment and the angular deflection are equivalent to the stress-versus-strain relationship tested in tension. Segment *a-b* corresponds to the initial elastic deformation of the wire, followed by segment *b-c,* where the austenitic structure transforms to the martensitic structure. After the transformation is completed at point *c* (typically at approximately 10% strain), further elastic deformation and plastic deformation occur with increasing bending moment along segment *c-d.* During unloading, this sequence of events is reversed, with segment *d-e* corresponding to loss of elastic strain (angular deflection) in the martensitic structure, followed by transformation back to the austenitic structure along segment *e-f,* and finally, loss of elastic strain in the austenitic structure along segment *f-g* as the bending moment decreases to zero. A small amount of permanent angular deflection remains in the wire because of the permanent deformation induced in segment *c-d.* This behavior in segments *b-c* and *e-f* is called superelasticity or *pseudoelasticity* in engineering materials science.

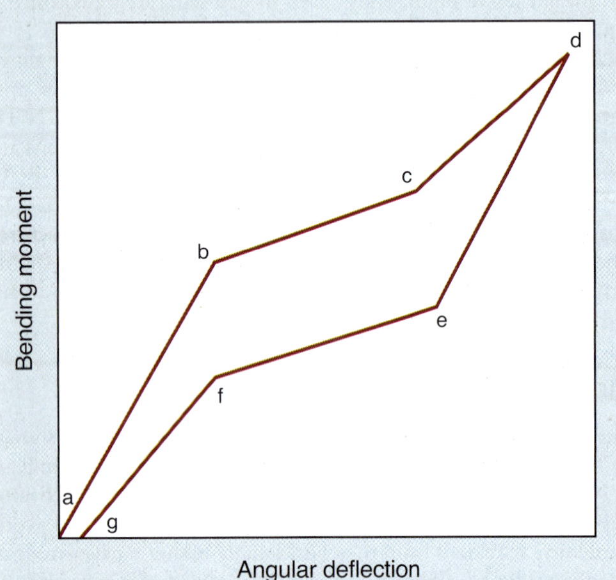

• **Fig. 9.17** Schematic bending movement versus angular deflection curve for a nickel–titanium orthodontic wire showing the regions of superelasticity: *b-c* during loading (activation) and *e-f* during unloading (deactivation). Such behavior imparts a large working range to the arch wire. Region *c-d* corresponds to permanent deformation during loading, and *d-e* corresponds to initial unloading of the permanently deformed arch wire. Regions *b-c* and *e-f* correspond to the forward and reverse directions, respectively, of the stress-induced transformation between the low-stress austenitic and high-stress martensitic structures. The final stage of unloading occurs along region *f-g*.

Segment *e-f* delivers a nearly constant force for tooth movement during deactivation (unloading), which does not occur with stainless steel or Co–Cr–Ni wires. When the superelastic wire is tested in tension, for which the stress and strain are uniform over the cross section, segments *b-c* and *e-f* are both horizontal (corresponding, respectively, to the stress-assisted transformation from austenite to martensite on loading and the reverse transformation on unloading). These two regions are referred to as the *upper superelastic plateau* and the *lower superelastic plateau,* respectively. There has been some question about whether the superelastic NiTi wires are activated sufficiently into the superelastic region under clinical conditions to take advantage of this property.

Tooth movement can also be achieved by another property of some NiTi wires. The shape of the appliance, such as an orthodontic arch wire, is first established when the alloy is heated at a temperature near 480°C to stabilize the austenitic structure (Fig. 9.18). When the appliance is cooled to room temperature, the alloy converts to the twinned martensitic phase and retains its shape. The appliance is then reshaped at room temperature by the clinician; the deformed martensitic structure is altered because of the stress induced by the deformation. When it is placed into brackets bonded to malpositioned teeth, exposure of the wire to body temperature will promote the deformed martensitic structure to revert back to the austenitic structure, and the appliance regains its shape established near 480°C, which allows for further tooth movement. This phenomenon is called *shape memory,* which is possessed at body temperature by some commercial NiTi wire products.

The temperature at which transformation from the martensitic structure to austenitic structure is completed is called the *austenite finish (Af) temperature.* This transformation temperature can be varied by elemental additions, such as copper and chromium, which are used for the commercial Copper Ni–Ti wires to achieve different activation temperatures (27°C, 35°C, and 40°C) in the oral environment. The Af temperature is a clinically relevant property of an NiTi orthodontic wire, and its measurement by differential scanning calorimetry (DSC) is included in ISO Standard 15841 (ADA Specification No. 32) on wires for use in orthodontics.

These standards subdivide orthodontic wires into type 1 and type 2, which display linear elastic and nonlinear elastic behavior, respectively, during unloading from 50°C. Stainless steel, cobalt–chromium–nickel, and β-titanium wires are type 1; nickel–titanium wires are type 2. Mechanical properties can be measured using the tension test or the three-point bending test, where the bending force during unloading is measured at 3-, 2-, 1-, and 0.5-mm deflections. Whereas type 1 wires can be tested at room temperature, type 2 wires are to be tested at 36 ± 1°C.

As noted previously, nickel–titanium orthodontic wires are difficult to reconfigure into clinical shapes, and they must be joined by mechanical crimps because the alloy can be neither soldered nor welded. In addition, nickel–titanium orthodontic wires have relatively rough surfaces, which result in high friction between arch wires and brackets; this can potentially prolong the time needed for clinical treatment.

CRITICAL QUESTION

What are the differences in the three general types of nickel–titanium orthodontic wires? Why is the superelasticity property of some NiTi alloys advantageous for endodontic applications?

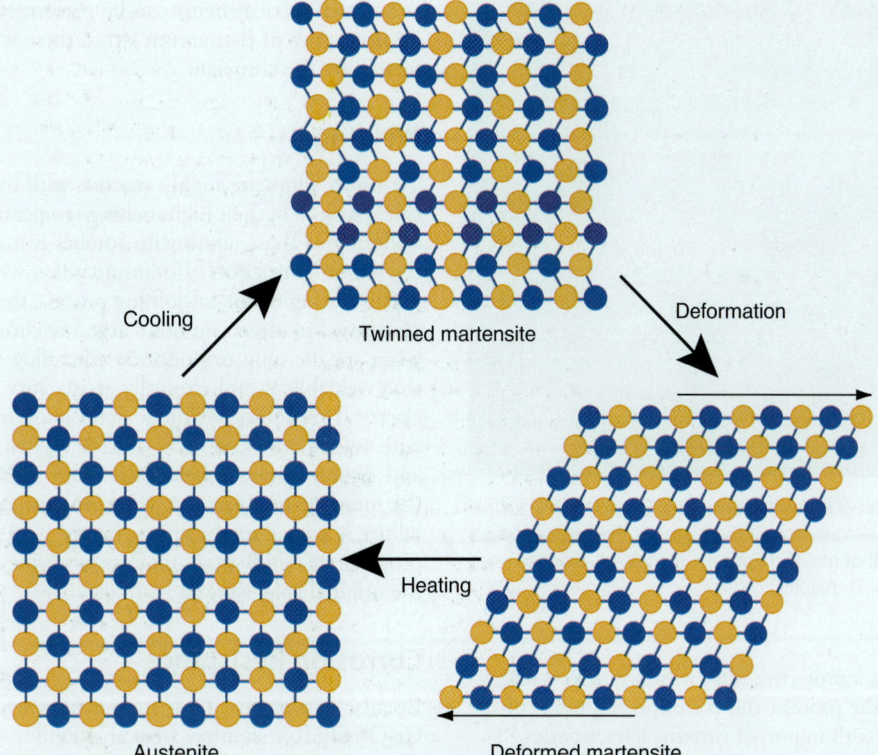

• **Fig. 9.18** Shape memory process. The austenite crystal is stable at a higher temperature and can be plastically deformed to some desired shape without altering its crystalline structure. When austenite is cooled to room temperature, it converts to a twinned martensite without undergoing a shape change. When the twinned martensite is deformed plastically under a stress, the structure detwins and takes up a new shape. Note that the overall shape of the object has changed, but the relative position between atoms did not change. Upon heating to body temperature (for orthodontic wire), the deformed martensite (detwinned martensite) will revert back to austenite and regain its original shape because there is no change in the relative position of the atom arrangement. Heating of twinned martensite will also recover the austenite structure.

Nickel–Titanium Endodontic Instruments

The outstanding property of the nickel–titanium alloy that resulted in its widespread use for endodontics is its much lower elastic modulus compared with the austenitic stainless steel that was formerly used for hand instruments. This allows the rotating NiTi file, used with an electric motor and reduction contra-angle handpiece, to negotiate curved root canals with facility. Although the pioneering article by Walia et al. investigated hand files fabricated from nonsuperelastic NiTi wire, subsequent NiTi alloys for rotary instruments were designed by manufacturers to have superelastic character with transformable austenite. The superelastic property enables the instrument to adapt along a sharply curving root canal during instrumentation, and the small increase in stress developed at the canal wall minimizes the risk for perforation of the canal. DSC studies have shown that the enthalpy change (ΔH) for transformation between martensite and austenite in rotary NiTi instruments is less than that for superelastic orthodontic wires, indicating that transformable austenite comprises a smaller proportion of the NiTi microstructure.

The drawback of the NiTi alloy is that nickel–titanium rotary endodontic instruments have generally been fabricated by machining the starting wire blanks, in contrast to stainless steel endodontic instruments, for which a special apparatus twists the tapered starting wire blank. However, rotary instruments have recently been introduced in which the NiTi wire blank is twisted (microstructure in the intermediate R-phase condition), rather than being machined. The machining process results in substantial permanent deformation (Fig. 9.19) at the edges of the cutting flutes and surface flaws that can lead to premature fracture of the instrument. It is likely that the NiTi alloy is inherently notch sensitive because the coexisting austenitic and martensitic NiTi phases have very different crystal structures.

Recently, new NiTi alloys, beginning with M-wire, have been introduced to endodontics, for which special manufacturer thermomechanical processing yields a largely martensitic microstructure. Rotary instruments fabricated by special proprietary protocols from these new alloys have improved fatigue resistance and have become widely used in practice. The novel products from one manufacturer are described as having the property of *controlled memory.*

Electropolishing is a method commonly used for surface finishing of many metallic medical appliances. This process has been used by some companies for NiTi root canal instruments. The instruments connected to an anode are immersed together with another electrode in a temperature-controlled bath of electrolytes, followed by passing direct electrical current into the solution. The metal at the anode is dissolved into the solution, whereas a reduction reaction will occur at the cathode. This process alters the surface composition and texture of the instrument and renders a more homogeneous

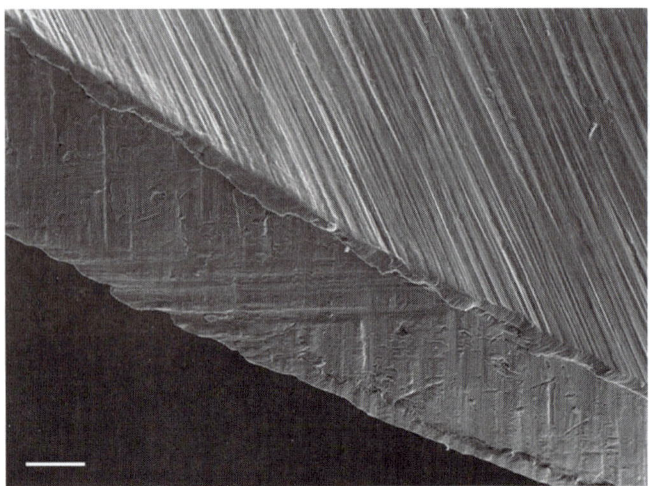

• **Fig. 9.19** Photomicrograph of a nickel–titanium rotary endodontic instrument, showing permanent deformation at the edges of the flutes (rollover) and other surface defects that resulted from the machining process used for fabrication. (Courtesy S. B. Alapati.)

surface oxide layer that is a protective film, with less defects and residual surface stress. In the process, the corrosion resistance of the metal is enhanced along with improved surface characteristics.

CRITICAL QUESTION

What is a potential clinical disadvantage of an orthodontic wire fabricated from β-titanium?

Beta-Titanium Alloys

The first commercial β-titanium orthodontic wires had an approximate composition (by weight) of 79% titanium, 11% molybdenum, 6% zirconium, and 4% tin. The addition of molybdenum stabilizes the BCC β-titanium structure at room temperature and yields an alloy of lower elastic modulus and higher ductility than those of the HCP α-titanium alloys. This means that β-titanium can easily be drawn into wires for orthodontic applications, but careful manufacturing attention to the drawing conditions is essential. Among all β-titanium orthodontic wires available, the original commercial alloy had the trade name of *titanium–molybdenum alloy* (TMA). This orthodontic alloy composition is very close to that of the engineering beta III titanium alloy.

Mechanical Properties of Beta-Titanium Wires

The elastic modulus of β-titanium wires is intermediate between that for stainless steel and Elgiloy wires and that for Nitinol wires (Table 9.17). The springback (YS/E) for β-titanium wires is much greater than that for the stainless steel and Elgiloy wires and very similar to that for the Nitinol wires. The β-titanium wires can be highly cold worked, and because of the BCC structure of the β phase, the wires have high formability, which is comparable to that of austenitic stainless steel, and can be readily bent into various orthodontic configurations.

Because of the high reactivity of titanium, careful control of the original cast ingot quality, the atmosphere, and other processing parameters during wire drawing is essential. (This is also true for manufacturing of the nickel–titanium orthodontic wires.) Whereas heat treatments can be performed to alter the mechanical properties of β-titanium wires, these wires should not be heat treated by the clinician.

Welding

Titanium alloys are highly reactive with oxygen at high temperature. Because of their high melting temperatures and this reactivity, soldering of these alloys with torches is not advisable. To prevent the potential reaction of titanium alloys with the oxygen in ambient air during the metal-joining process, these procedures are often performed in a vacuum or an argon environment. The β-titanium wires are the only orthodontic wire alloy type that demonstrates true weldability, and clinically satisfactory joints can be made by electrical resistance welding. Such joints need not be reinforced with solder, which is necessary for welded joints in stainless steel and Elgiloy wires. A weld made with insufficient heat will fail at the interface between the wires, whereas overheating may cause a failure adjacent to the joint. Figure 9.20 is a cross section of a properly welded β-titanium joint, showing minimum distortion of the original cold-worked structure.

Corrosion Resistance

Because of a passive TiO_2 surface film, which is analogous to the Cr_2O_3 film on stainless steel and Elgiloy wires, titanium and its alloys generally have excellent corrosion resistance and environmental stability. There has been some concern about the biocompatibility of orthodontic wires containing nickel, which may cause localized tissue irritation or an allergic reaction in some patients, and it should be noted that β-titanium is the only major orthodontic wire alloy that is nickel free.

Surface Property

The surface roughness of the β-titanium wires is much greater than that of the stainless steel and Elgiloy wires. Scanning electron microscopy observations suggest that the surface roughness originates from adherence of the titanium in the β-titanium alloys to the dies or rollers used in the wire-manufacturing process. Special proprietary lubricants must be used by the manufacturers to

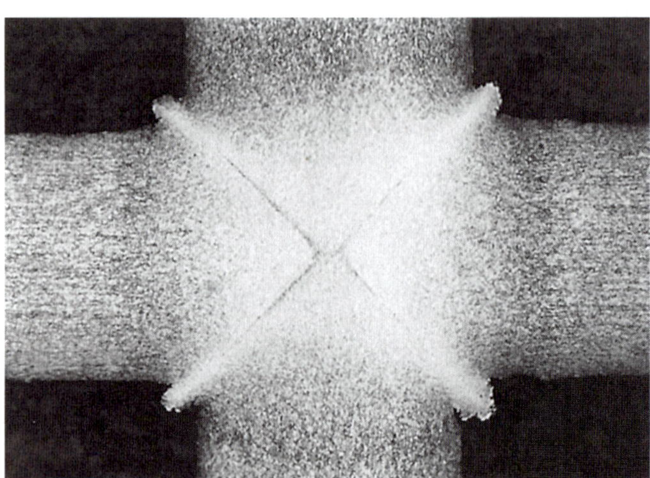

• **Fig. 9.20** Photomicrograph of a weld joint between two 0.43 × 0.63-mm β-titanium orthodontic wires showing minimum distortion of the original cold-worked microstructure. (Courtesy T. C. Labenski and A. J. Goldberg.)

alleviate this problem. During orthodontic treatment, the rough arch wire surfaces increase sliding friction, and localized cold welding of the arch wire alloy to the metal bracket has also been hypothesized.

Surface treatment of nickel–titanium and β-titanium orthodontic wires with nitrogen ion implantation has been performed to decrease adhesion between wires and brackets. One study reported significant differences for in vitro tooth movement with ion-implanted TMA and nickel–titanium wires, compared with their nonion-implanted counterparts. However, the results of a recent clinical study suggest that there were no significant differences for the rate of space closure when ion-implanted TMA, conventional TMA (not ion implanted), and stainless steel wires were used.

Additional Wrought Alloys

Noble metal wires are still occasionally employed in the construction of RPD clasps and orthodontic appliances and in retention pins for restorations and endodontic posts. The elastic modulus of these gold alloy wires is approximately 100–120 GPa, which is higher than that for titanium-based wrought alloys but considerably lower than those of stainless steel and Co–Cr–Ni wrought alloys. Table 9.18 shows the compositions of two types of noble metal wrought wires and the mechanical properties of two products: platinum–gold–palladium (P–G–P), which contains 40%–50% platinum, 25%–30% gold, and 25%–30% palladium by weight, and palladium–silver–copper (P–S–C), which consists of 42%–44% palladium, 38%–41% silver, 16%–17% copper, and 0%–1% platinum by weight. The high fusion temperature (hence high recrystallization temperature) of P–G–P wire would be especially useful for casting an RPD framework to this alloy. It is the high fusion temperatures of platinum and palladium that raise the fusion temperature of P–G–P wire. P–S–C wires have also been considered useful for dental applications because their fusion temperatures are higher than those of the gold-based alloy wires.

Wrought cobalt–chromium alloys for RPD clasps are also available. For example, a cobalt–chromium–tungsten–nickel wire (Ticonium) has a YS of approximately 920 MPa, a tensile strength of nearly 1400 MPa, and a percent elongation of 19%. This wrought alloy is not heat treatable and is designed for use with the lower-fusing nickel–chromium–beryllium casting alloy from the same manufacturer.

CRITICAL QUESTION

Pure gold can be used as a direct filling restorative material. What are the properties of gold that make this restorative material possible?

Direct Filling Gold

Pure gold is the noblest of all dental metals, rarely tarnishing or corroding in the oral cavity. It is inactive chemically, and it is not affected by air, heat, moisture, or most solvents. At room temperature, two thin sheets of atomically clean pure gold can be welded under pressure. The procedure is also called cold welding because it is conducted at room temperature. Pure gold is very soft (22 VHN), and the most ductile and malleable metal used in restorative dentistry. As a result, pure gold in the form of foil or powder can be adapted to the walls of a cavity preparation with only a minimal marginal gap. When the gold segments (like increments of amalgam or composite) are compacted with designated instruments to build up the bulk of material, the segments are bonded by metallic bonds (cold welding), and the bulk of material is work hardened by the pressure. Therefore, the final restoration retains characteristics of a wrought metal. The process of gold compacting is also known as condensation. After work hardening, its hardness (52–75 VHN) is equivalent to and may exceed that of type I gold alloy (50 VHN), and approaches that of type II gold alloy (90 VHN). This category of gold is also known as cohesive gold and direct filling gold for restorations.

Forms of Direct Filling Gold

Direct filling gold is supplied in three basic forms: foil (also known as fibrous gold), electrolytic precipitate (also called crystalline gold), and granular gold (also called powdered gold). They

TABLE 9.18 Physical Properties of Noble Metal Wires

Wire Type	Yield Strength Oven Cooled (MPa)	Tensile Strength Oven Cooled (MPa)	ELONGATION (%) Quenched	ELONGATION (%) Oven Cooled	Fusion Temperature (°C)
Formerly ANSI/ADA type I	860	930	15	4	960
Formerly ANSI/ADA type II	690	860	15	2	870
			MINIMUM ELONGATION (%)		
Wire Type	Proportional Limit (MPa)	Tensile Strength (MPa)	Quenched	Oven Cooled	Fusion Temperature (°C)
Platinum–gold–palladium	550–1030[a]	860–1240[a]	14–15	—	1500–1530
Palladium–silver–copper	690–790[b]	960–1070[b]	16–24	8–15	1040–1080

ADA, American Dental Association; ANSI, American National Standards Institute.
[a]Quenched (alloy does not age harden).
[b]Age hardened.
Data from *Dentists Desk Reference: Materials, Instruments and Equipment. Metals and Alloys: Precious Metal Wrought Wire,* Chicago, IL, 1981, American Dental Association; Lyman T: *Metals Handbook: Properties and Selection of Metals,* ed 8, Vol 1, Metals Park, OH, 1964, American Society for Metals.

can all be cold welded. However, the efficacy of restorations made from these materials is adversely affected by improper handling, contamination, deviations from established cavity design principles, inefficient placement methods, and faulty finishing techniques. With the exception of platinized foil and alloyed electrolytic precipitate, the chemical purity of most types of direct filling gold is 99.99% or higher.

Gold Foil

Gold foil is provided in sheets, which can also be transformed to other physical form like pellets, cylinders, ropes prepared by the dentist, or partially precondensed laminates of varying thickness produced by the manufacturer. Platinized gold foil is a laminated structure with one sheet of platinum foil between two gold foils. The objective of adding platinum to the gold foil is to increase the hardness and wear resistance of restorations made from this material. Standard No. 4 gold foil is supplied in 100 × 100 mm (4 × 4 inch) sheets that weigh 4 grains (0.259 g) and are about 0.51 μm thick. The numbering system refers to the weight of a standard sheet. The surface of gold foil is shown in the SEM image in Figure 9.21.

During storage, gold foil, like most metals, attracts gases to its surface from the environment, and any adsorbed gas film prevents the intimate atomic contact required for cold welding. To ensure the cleanness of the foil, most gold sheets are provided with an adsorbed protective gas film, such as ammonia. The ammonia-treated foil is called noncohesive foil. The volatile film on the foil is removed by heating immediately before inserting into the cavity preparation.

Electrolytic Precipitate Gold

Another form of direct filling gold is microcrystalline gold powder formed by electrolytic precipitation, which is sandwiched between sheets of gold foil and formed into strips. It is also called mat or sponge gold. The powder consists of dendritic crystals approximately 0.1 mm in length (Fig. 9.22).

This form of gold can be cut to a desired size and is often preferred for its ease in building up the internal bulk of the restoration. Mat gold made of electrolytic precipitate from gold, which is alloyed with a trace amount of calcium, can yield a further increase in hardness by dispersion strengthening without affecting the handling properties.

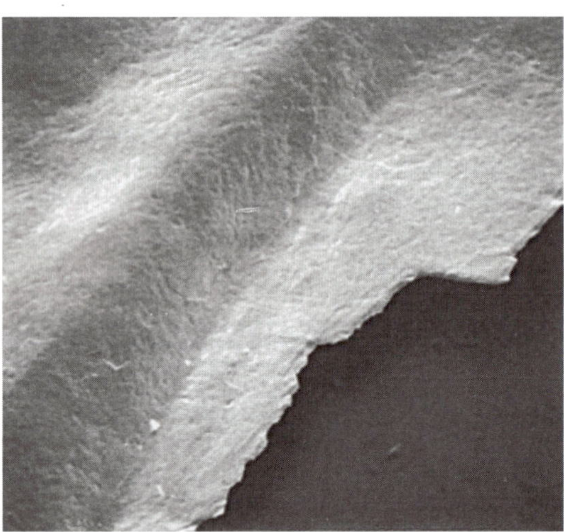

• **Fig. 9.21** Scanning electron micrograph of the surface of gold foil (×750). (Courtesy of CE Ingersoll.)

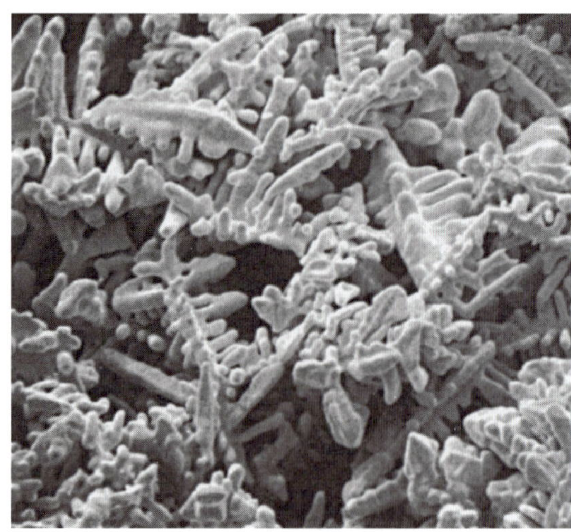

• **Fig. 9.22** Scanning electron micrograph of mat gold (×750). (Courtesy of CE Ingersoll.)

Granular (Powdered) Gold

Gold powders in agglomerated form can also be prepared by chemical precipitation or atomization from molten gold. To prevent agglomerates from disintegrating, the atomized and chemically precipitated powders are first mixed with a soft wax to form pellets. These wax-gold pellets are wrapped with foil. The resulting pellets are cylindrical in shape and are available in several diameters and lengths. Heating to burn away wax is mandatory before insertion into the prepared cavity.

CRITICAL QUESTION

Why do direct filling golds have to be flamed before insertion in cavity preparation?

Preparation of Direct Filling Gold for Restoration

Prior to placing direct filling gold in the cavity preparation, the dentist heats the material to remove the protective coating or wax introduced by the manufacturer, or contaminants on the surface acquired during storage and packaging. Individual pellets can be held over an open flame of pure alcohol, or a group of pellets or other gold forms can be placed on a so-called annealing plate heated by electricity. This step is commonly called annealing, heat treatment, or **degassing**. A more appropriate term would be ***desorption*** (a phenomenon whereby a substance is released from a surface; opposite of sorption).

Proper desorption is a matter of heating long enough at a temperature that removes contaminants and, in the case of powdered gold, that burns away the wax. Heating times vary depending on the size and configuration of the gold segment. Powdered gold pellets may take 15–20 seconds, whereas gold foil pellets and electrolytic gold pellets may require only 1 or 2 seconds. Underheating can compromise cohesion between segments. Overheating can lead to excessive sintering and possibly contamination by the tray, instruments, or flame. The result may be incomplete cohesion, embrittlement of the portion being heated, and poor compaction characteristics.

Powdered gold must be heated in a flame to ensure the complete elimination of the wax. When heating in bulk on a tray, an excessive amount of gold should be avoided because of the difficulties that prolonged and repeated heating can create. Care should be taken to handle pieces with stainless steel wire points or similar instruments that will not contaminate the gold.

Regardless of the type of direct gold used, flame desorption of surface contaminates will occur when the gold segment has exhibited a dull-red glow. The fuel for the flame may be alcohol or gas, but alcohol is preferred because there is less danger of contamination. The alcohol should be pure methanol or ethanol without colorants or other additives. Advantages of flame desorption include the selection of a piece of appropriate size, desorption of only those pieces used, and reduced exposure to contamination.

Compaction of Direct Filling Gold

Two of the main processes that control the quality of the final direct gold restoration are cold welding and wedging. *Wedging* refers to the pressurized adaptation of the gold form within the space between tooth structure walls and corners that have been slightly deformed elastically.

A totally dry cavity is mandatory throughout the compaction process to ensure complete cohesion. The increments of gold must be of a proper size for insertion and in the proper "atomically clean" condition for condensing or compacting. The first segment must be sufficiently large that it is secured by compacting it within the prepared cavity. The second and subsequent segments must cold weld to each other, and this will occur only if the surface is free of contaminants and moisture.

Condensers

The condenser can be straight, curved, angled, round, square, or rectangular, and the surface of the tip can be smooth or serrated. The tip can be flat faced or convex faced. The condenser tip should also be kept atomically clean.

Size of the Condenser Tip

As in condensation of amalgam, the force distribution to the gold depends on the area of the point working surface of the instrument. It follows that small condenser tips are indicated to achieve the desired compaction at lower forces than those that might damage oral structures. The lower limit of the condenser tip size is based on the tendency of the tip to penetrate an area of the condensed foil.

Compaction Method

The gold segments can be compacted by hand pressure alone, by hand pressure combined with a hand mallet, or by a mechanical device that is activated by a spring, pneumatic pressure, or electronically (using an electromallet). The direction of force application, the amount of applied pressure, and the compaction pattern are critically important factors controlling the quality of the gold restoration.

Condenser penetration should be less than the thickness of each segment that is compacted. The depth of each cold-welded mass is usually between 0.2 and 0.3 mm. The final density is controlled by the direction and the magnitude of the compaction force and by the size and shape of the condenser tip. The condenser tip must be stepped in a controlled overlapping pattern with the condenser tip placed approximately the distance of the tip radius away from the last area to be compacted. Porosity is likely to occur in all direct gold restorations. Each type of gold requires a slight variation in technique to avoid either closed pores or open pores that intersect the surface.

A small amount of excess material is provided to ensure a proper contour and an adequate surface finish. The excess material is trimmed away with sharp gold knives and files of suitable shapes and sizes, and with abrasive disks, stones, and strips. Whenever the strips are used, cooling water spray must be applied to dissipate heat and reduce trauma to the pulpal tissue.

CRITICAL QUESTION

Pure gold has a density of 19.3 g/cm^3. Why is the apparent density of the direct filling gold restoration after condensation often less than 16 g/cm^3?

Physical Properties of Compacted Gold

Table 9.19 shows some representative property values of various methods of compacting golds. Transverse (bending) strength reflects three types of stresses: compressive, tensile, and shear (see Chapter 4). In direct filling golds, the failure usually occurs from tensile stress because of incomplete cohesion. Bending strength represents an indirect indicator of cohesive strength. Hardness indicates the overall quality of compacted gold.

The maximal density of gold is 19.3 g/cm^3. The density values shown in Table 9.19 indicate the presence of voids in all direct gold restorations. Apparently, voids are inevitable, but they should be kept to a minimum to achieve the maximal strength attainable.

Hardness may not be a valid measure of the effectiveness of a particular restorative material for its intended purpose of restoring the tooth. It may, however, indicate the overall quality of compacted gold.

There is no evidence that the differences in physical properties among the various forms of gold are clinically significant. The physical properties of the compacted gold (restoration) are probably more greatly influenced by the competence of the dentist in manipulating and placing the gold material.

Direct Gold Restoration

Restorations made with the direct filling golds do not exhibit the high strength and hardness of those made with dental casting alloys. The use of direct filling golds is generally limited to areas where they simply "fill" a space (such as pits and small class I, II, III, V, and VI restorations) and for repairing casting margins. The concerns for possible damaging effects on the pulp have been disputed. Apparently direct gold that is compacted properly into sound tooth structure produces only a minimal pulpal response.

High-quality direct gold restorations can be ensured only when four principal conditions are satisfied: (1) the appropriate gold form is used for each specific clinical situation, (2) the material is used only where it is indicated, (3) a perfectly dry and clean field is provided, and (4) the material is properly manipulated with the correct instruments. Obviously these conditions can be satisfied only if the clinician has acquired the necessary knowledge, skills, and experience. The cavity preparation is critically important, since it must provide adequate access form, retention, adequate support, well-defined finish lines, and adequate pulp

TABLE 9.19 Representative Physical Properties of Direct Filling Golds

Materials and Technique	Transverse Strength (MPa)	KHN	Apparent Density (g/cm³)[a]
Mat gold			
Hand	161	52	14.3
Mechanical	169	62	14.7
Combined	169	53	14.5
Powdered gold			
Hand	165	55	14.4
Mechanical	155	64	14.5
Combined	190	58	14.9
Gold foil			
Hand	296	69	15.9
Mechanical	265	69	15.8
Combined	273	69	15.8
Mat gold and gold foil			
Hand	196	70	15.0
Mechanical	206	71	15.1
Combined	227	75	15.0

KHN, Knoop hardness number.
[a]Density is calculated by dividing the weight of the specimen by its volume.
Data from Richter WA, Cantwell KR: A study of cohesive gold. *J Prosthet Dent* 15:722, 1965.

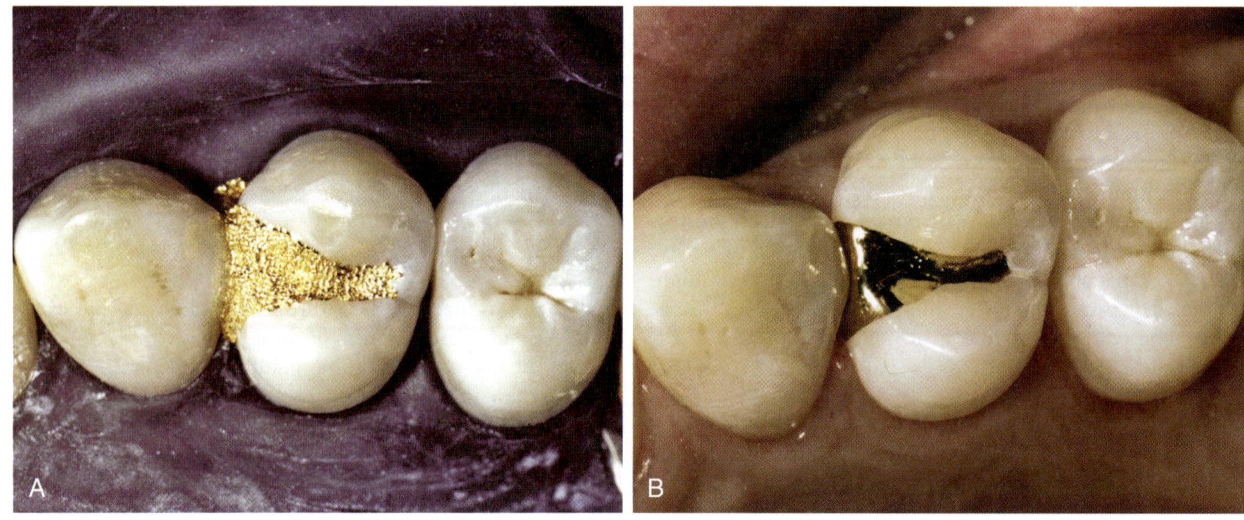

• **Fig. 9.23** Clinical example of direct gold foil restoration. **(A)** Class II MO preparation filled with cohesive gold foil. **(B)** Finished gold foil restoration. (Courtesy of Dr Richard D Tucker and Dr John Sechena.)

protection. The chief disadvantages of using direct filling gold are its yellow metallic color, high thermal conductivity, and technical difficulties in forming a dense restoration.

The American Academy of Gold Foil Operators posts clinical cases by their members at its website (http://www.aagfo.org/Procedures.html and http://www.goldfoil.org/Procedures.htm). Note that these restorations were placed under rubber dam isolation. The use of a rubber dam is essential to minimize the risk of contamination by saliva, water, and other contaminants during placement. Figure 9.23 is a clinical example of a class II gold foil restoration.

Acknowledgments

The author wishes to acknowledge Dr Paul Cascone, Dr Kenneth Anusavice, and Dr A. Jon Goldberg for their previous contributions to this chapter. The author also wants to thank Dr Danna Mota Morena, Faculty of Dentistry, University Center Christus (Unichristus), Fortaleza, Brazil, for reviewing and providing valuable information for this chapter.

Summary

- **Metal** is "an opaque lustrous chemical substance that is a good conductor of heat and electricity and, when polished, is a good reflector of light."
- Pure metal has specific melting point and boiling point, and has basic physical and mechanical properties.
- **Alloys** are prepared by fusion of the elements above their melting points.
- Alloying of metals is done to improve castability, ductility, strength, hardness, tarnish resistance, and corrosion resistance.
- To resist tarnish and corrosion of metals in the oral environment and to optimize their passivity, alloying is done to provide passivation of the alloy through the formation of a thin surface layer of oxide.
- **Noble metals** are highly resistant to corrosion and oxidation and do not require alloying elements for protection in corrosive environments.
- **Oxidizable elements** such as tin and indium are added to high noble (HN) and noble (N) alloys used for metal–ceramic prostheses to promote bonding between the ceramic veneer and the metal oxide on the metal surface.
- All pure metals and alloys used as restorative materials in dentistry are **crystalline solids**.
- A unique characteristic of metals is that they are generally excellent thermal and electrical conductors.
- Generally metal alloys are stronger and more dense than nonmetallic structures.
- Gallium and mercury—liquid at body temperature but when alloyed, they become a component of the solid alloy at oral temperature.
- **Grade 2 CP titanium** is used widely because of its ease of forming into different shapes, its moderately high strength (equal to or greater than 275 MPa), and its excellent corrosion resistance.
- Two nonwhite metals in the periodic table are gold and copper. High gold content alloy is yellow in hue and high concentration of copper gives a reddish-yellow hue to the alloy.
- Cobalt-, nickel-, palladium-, or silver-based dental alloys are "white" or silver in appearance.
- Compared with ceramics, polymers, and composites, metals have greater **fracture toughness (KIc)**—that is, the ability to absorb energy and inhibit crack extension under an applied tensile stress.
- Free electrons of metal act as conductors of both thermal energy and electricity.
- **Metallic bonding** is also responsible for the luster of polished metals and their typical ability of undergoing significant permanent deformation under mechanical stresses above their elastic limits or yield points.
- **Solid solution:** When two metals are completely soluble in each other, in the solid state the structure will appear to be entirely homogeneous, since only one phase is formed during solidification.
- When two metals are not completely soluble in each other, the solid state is a mixture of two or more phases, for example, eutectic and peritectic alloys.
- The temperature-versus-composition graphs for such alloys are referred to as "isomorphous phase diagrams."
- The thermal expansion coefficient (TEC) of palladium is too low for it to be used with most commercial porcelains, so elements such as silver are needed to raise the TEC of palladium alloys.
- **Palladium** whitens gold alloys markedly. It raises the melting range of gold alloys as well as their elastic modulus, strength, and hardness.
- **Gallium** in Pd-based PFM alloys strengthens the alloy and decreases their melting range.
- **Platinum (Pt)** is used primarily in yellow-gold PFM alloys to increase the melting range, hardness, strength, and elastic modulus.
- Silver is added to Au–Ag–Cu casting alloys to offset the reddish hue contributed by Cu and also improves the flow of casting alloy, but it causes greening of the porcelains.
- Copper strengthens and reddens Au–Ag–Cu crown and bridge alloys but it can discolor porcelain by the formation of dark-colored oxide.
- Zinc is added to crown and bridge alloys as an oxygen scavenger, thereby reducing gas porosity in castings.
- **Grain refiners**—iridium, rhenium, and ruthenium.
- Latent heat of solidification is defined as the number of calories of heat liberated from 1 g of a substance when it transforms from a liquid to a solid.
- During the supercooling process, crystallization of the pure metal begins.
- Atoms of a metal migrate in the liquid state at a rapid rate that is related to its diffusion coefficient of approximately 10^{-5} cm^2/s.
- **Solidification** begins with the formation of embryos in the molten metal, that is, small clusters of atoms that form nuclei of crystallization that have the same arrangement as the long-range atomic order found in the solidified metal.
- The grain boundaries in a solidified metal are revealed by polishing and etching of the cast metal surface by a specific solution for a given time.
- The regular atom arrangement in a cast metal becomes discontinuous at a grain boundary, so the movement of dislocations along the atomic slip planes during permanent deformation of ductile dental alloys continues until the dislocations meet a grain boundary.
- The **grain boundaries** are the final sites at which a molten metal solidifies during the formation of an equiaxed grain structure.
- The grain boundaries accumulate low-melting phases, precipitate, and porosity is also seen in interdendritic regions of dental alloys with a **cast dendritic microstructure.**
- **Substitutional solid solution:** The atoms of the solute metal occupy the positions in the crystal structure that are normally occupied by the solvent atoms in the pure metal.
- **Interstitial solid solution:** The solute atoms are present in random positions (interstices) between the atoms in the crystal structure of the solvent metal.

- In the cored structure, the dendrites (core) have higher melting temperatures and the interdendritic regions (matrix), have lower melting temperatures.
- **Eutectic alloys** correspond to a composition with the lowest melting point in an alloy system used for joining metal components through a process of brazing or soldering.
- The temperature at which the eutectic composition melts is lower than the fusion temperature of pure parent metals (eutectic means "lowest melting").
- **Casting alloys** are classified based on their noble metal alloy content, mechanical properties, principal element, and dental application.
- The **American Dental Association (ADA)** classified dental casting alloys based on the content of noble metals into three categories: high-noble (HN), noble (N), and predominantly base metal (PB).
- Casting alloys should be biocompatible, tarnish, and corrosion resistant, have sufficient strength, allow porcelain bonding, and be economical.
- Compared with other alloys for metal–ceramic prostheses, base metal alloys generally have a higher hardness and elastic modulus (stiffness).
- The **fusion temperatures** of Ni–Cr and Co–Cr alloys are in the range of 1150–1500°C. The investment mold should be made of either phosphate- or silicate-bonded investment material, which maintains its surface integrity at the casting temperature of base metal alloys.
- The density of a base metal alloy is 7.6–8.3 g/cm^3, about half that of a gold-based alloy which is 14.5 gm/cm^3.
- **Cobalt–chromium–molybdenum alloy** has been the primary metal for partial denture prostheses.
- Co–Cr clasps are reported to be too retentive initially and slowly lose this retention because of plastic deformation.
- Recent methods employed to reduce the casting/processing errors or shrinkage are, sintering of burnished metal foil, CAD-CAM processing of metal blocks, copy milling of metal blocks, electroforming of metal copings, and three-dimensional printing with metal powder followed by sintering.
- **Stereolithography** is a form of additive manufacturing technology where a three-dimensional object is created by depositing successive layers of material.
- Allergy with the metal substances can be due to one of the following reasons, viz. (1) leaching from an alloy into the oral environment by dissolution; (2) particles released to the environment during grinding and polishing; (3) propagated by vapor during casting.
- **Allergens** can be harmful for the patient, clinician as well as technician.
- There are three categories of metal-joining operations: **soldering, brazing**, and **welding**.
- The primary difference between soldering and brazing is that brazing requires a heating temperature above 450°C and soldering is conducted below that temperature.
- Welding may not require a filler metal since the metal surfaces to be joined will melt and fuse locally.
- **Spot welding** based on electrical resistance has been used to weld orthodontic appliances.
- Recent advances in the technology of heating sources include the plasma torch, Nd:YAG laser, and tungsten inert gas (TIG) arc.
- A **flux** is used to reduce the metal oxide, which is essential for the molten solder to wet the substrate metals. **Antiflux** is used to prevent flow of molten solder onto adjacent areas.
- Based on their use, fluxes are of three types viz. protecting the surface from oxide layer formation, reducing the oxide, dissolving the oxide layer.
- Heat sources for soldering are hydrogen, natural gas, acetylene, propane, and furnace soldering.
- **Plastic deformation** occurs when the applied stress increases above the elastic limit.
- Only the elastic strain is recovered after loading is released from a metal that has been loaded beyond its proportional limit.
- **Point defects** are lattice positions with either missing, displaced, or extra atoms.
- Defects like **vacancies** are the principal mechanism for atomic diffusion in crystalline materials.
- The plane along which an edge dislocation moves is known as a **slip plane** and its direction is known as **slip direction**.
- Plastic deformation of metal is due to the dislocation movement and slip between atomic planes.
- Permanent deformation of metals under mechanical stress below their recrystallization temperatures is known as **cold working**.
- The effects associated with plastic deformation can be reversed by heating the metal to a temperature that is approximately half the melting point on the **absolute temperature scale**.
- Commercially pure titanium exists in a stable hexagonal close-packed crystal structure at temperatures below 882°C (α-titanium) and a stable body-centered cubic structure above that temperature (β-titanium).
- **Soldering** of titanium alloys with torches is not advised, as they are highly reactive with oxygen at high temperatures.

Review Questions

Write short notes on:

1. Cast base metal alloys
2. Heat treatment of noble metal alloys
3. Eutectic alloys
4. Solidification defects in casting
5. Eutectic and peritectic alloys
6. Classification of alloys
7. Cooling curve
8. Grain refinement and grain size
9. Solid solution
10. Phase diagram
11. Describe the composition and properties of commonly used base metal alloys.
12. Describe in detail the various metals and alloys used for the fabrication of removable partial denture (RPD) framework.
13. Enumerate the difference between soldering, brazing, and welding.
14. Properties of orthodontic wires.
15. Eutectic and peritectic alloys.
16. Precipitated gold.
17. Karat and fineness.
18. Annealing and degassing and their purpose.
19. How is casting of titanium and its alloys different from others?

Selected Readings

Akova T, Ucar Y, Tukay A, et al.: Comparison of the bond strength of laser-sintered and cast base metal dental alloys to porcelain. *Dent Mater* 24:1400–1404, 2008. The bond strength to porcelain was not significantly different for cast Ni–Cr, cast Co–Cr, and laser-sintered Co–Cr alloys. Compositions of the Co–Cr alloys for casting and laser sintering are compared.

Alapati SB, Brantley WA, Iijima M, et al.: Metallurgical characterization of a new nickel-titanium wire for rotary endodontic instruments. *J Endod* 35:1589–1593, 2009. TEM, TMDSC, and Micro-XRD analyses of the M-wire for rotary endodontic instruments.

Brantley W, Berzins D, Iijima M, et al.: Structure/property relationships in orthodontic alloys. In Eliades T, Brantley WA (editors): Orthodontic Applications of Biomaterials: A Clinical Guide. Elsevier, 2017. This chapter in a recently published book provides a comprehensive account of current orthodontic alloys used for wires, brackets, and other appliances. Another chapter discusses the use of nickel–titanium products in orthodontic practice.

Brantley WA, Guo W, Clark WAT, et al.: Microstructural studies of 35°C copper Ni-Ti orthodontic wire and TEM confirmation of low-temperature martensite transformation. *Dent Mater* 24:204–210, 2008. TEM examination revealed that the very low-temperature transformation in NiTi wires is twinning in the martensite structure. Optical microscope, SEM and TEM images, along with important electron diffraction patterns, were presented.

Bridgeport DA, Brantley WA, Herman PF: Cobalt-chromium and nickel-chromium alloys for removable prosthodontics: Part 1. Mechanical properties of as-cast alloys. *J Prosthodon* 2:144–150, 1993. This article presents more recent measurements of the mechanical properties of removable partial denture alloys and contains relevant SEM photographs of the fracture surfaces.

Gatto E, Matarese G, Di Bella G, et al.: Load-deflection characteristics of superelastic and thermal nickel-titanium wires. *Eur J Orthod* 35:115–123, 2013. Three-point bending plots for seven NiTi wires tested in a manner similar to the current ISO wire standard. Composition information is provided for the different NiTi alloys.

Papazoglou E, Brantley WA, Johnston WM, et al.: Effects of dental laboratory processing variables and in vitro testing medium on the porcelain adherence of high-palladium casting alloys. *J Prosthet Dent* 79:514–519, 1998.

Setcos JC, Babaei-Mahani A, Silvio LD, et al.: The safety of nickel containing dental alloys. *Dent Mater* 22:1163–1168, 2006. This paper reviews papers published after 1985 in regard to biological reactions to nickel in dentistry. It is concluded that nickel-containing dental alloys do not pose a risk to patients or members of the dental team.

Shen Y, Zhou HM, Zheng YF, et al.: Metallurgical characterization of controlled memory wire nickel-titanium rotary instruments. *J Endod* 37, 1566–1571, 2011. SEM examination, XRD analyses, and Vickers hardness measurements were performed for controlled memory NiTi rotary instruments. The low risk for these instruments fracturing in the root canal is noted.

Shoher I, Whiteman A: Captek—A new capillary casting technology for ceramometal restorations. *Quintessence Dent Technol* 18:9–20, 1995. This paper describes the technology of the Captek system.

10

Ceramic-Based Materials

CHAPTER OUTLINE

KEY TERMS

Ceramic, CAD–CAM—Ceramic that is formulated for the production of the whole or part of a ceramic prosthesis through the use of a computer-aided design, computer-aided manufacturing process.

Ceramic, castable—Glass or other ceramic specially formulated to be cast into a refractory mold as a core coping or framework for a ceramic prosthesis.

Ceramic, core—Opaque or semitranslucent crystalline dental ceramic material that provides sufficient strength, toughness, and stiffness to support overlying layers of veneering ceramics.

Ceramic, dental—Inorganic compound with nonmetallic properties typically consisting of oxygen and one or more metallic (or semimetallic) and/or nonmetallic elements, such as aluminum, calcium, lithium, magnesium, potassium, silicon, sodium, tin, titanium, and zirconium. Ceramic frits that are provided in a powder form for veneering (layering) ceramics are typically composed of a mixture of glass and crystalline particles.

Ceramic, glaze—Specially formulated ceramic powder that, when mixed with a liquid, applied to a ceramic surface, and heated to an appropriate temperature for a sufficient time, forms a smooth glassy layer on a dental ceramic surface.

Ceramic, hot pressed (pressable ceramic)—Ceramic that can be heated to a flow temperature and forced under isostatic pressure to fill a cavity in a refractory mold.

Ceramic, stain—Mixture of one or more pigmented metal oxides and a low-fusing glass that can modify the shade of the ceramic-based restoration; this mixture is dispersed in an aqueous medium, applied to the surface of porcelain or other dental ceramic, and heated to the vitrification temperature of this material for a specific time.

Glass–ceramic—Ceramic consisting of at least one glass phase and at least one crystalline phase that is produced by a controlled crystallization of the glass.

Glass-infiltrated core ceramic—A partially sintered core ceramic with a porous structure that is densified by the capillary inflow of a molten glass.

Green state—Term referring to an as-pressed or minimally sintered condition prior to final sintering.

Metal–ceramic prosthesis—A partial crown, full crown, or fixed partial denture made with a metal substructure to which porcelain is bonded for aesthetic enhancement via an intermediate metal oxide layer. The terms porcelain fused to metal (PFM), porcelain bonded to metal (PBM), porcelain to metal (PTM), and ceramometal are also used to describe these prostheses, but metal–ceramic (MC) is the term accepted internationally.

Porcelain—A relatively dense, white ceramic material produced by sintering a mixture of feldspar, kaolin, quartz, and other substances, strictly referring to those containing kaolin.

Porcelain, feldspathic—Ceramic composed of a glass matrix phase and one or more crystalline phases, such as leucite ($KAlSi_2O_6$), sanidine ($KAlSi_3O_8$), and apatite [$Ca_5(PO_4)_3(F, Cl, OH)$]. Most commercial dental porcelains designed for metal–ceramic restorations are partially crystallized feldspathic glasses that consist of tetragonal leucite ($K_2O{\cdot}Al_2O_3{\cdot}4SiO_2$) crystals in a glass-phase matrix.

Sintering—Process of heating closely packed particles below the melting point of the main component to densify and strengthen a structure as a result of bonding, diffusion, and flow phenomena.

Slip casting—Process used to form "green" ceramic shapes by applying a slurry of ceramic particles and water or a special liquid to a porous substrate (such as a die material), thereby allowing capillary action to remove water and densify the mass of deposited particles.

Spinel or spinelle—Crystalline mineral composed of mixed oxides such as $MgO{\cdot}Al_2O_3$.

Thermal compatibility—Condition of low transient and residual tensile stress in ceramic adjacent to a metal or ceramic core that is associated with a small difference in the coefficients of thermal contraction between the core material and the veneering ceramic.

Transformation toughening—A ceramic-strengthening mechanism that occurs through transformation of crystalline structure. For example, the stress-activated tetragonal (t) to monoclinic (m) transformation in yttria-stabilized zirconia causes slight volume expansion at the crack tip that keeps the crack from propagating and raises the stress needed to keep the crack propagation to fracture the prosthesis.

CRITICAL QUESTION

Which property best describes the fracture resistance of dental ceramics?

What Are Ceramics?

Dental ceramics consist of silicate glasses, **porcelains**, **glass–ceramics**, or highly crystalline solids. They exhibit chemical, mechanical, physical, and thermal properties that distinguish them from metals, acrylic resins, and resin-based composites. Silicate glasses differ from nonsilicate glasses in that silicone is the central divalent cation that is bound to four relatively large oxygen anions that link in a random order to other tetrahedra to form polymeric-type $(SiO_2)_n$ chains. In silica-based ceramics, each oxygen atom invariably connects two SiO_4 tetrahedra only at the corners, and no edges and faces of tetrahedra are shared. The properties of ceramics are customized for dental applications by precisely controlling the types and amounts of the components used in their production. Ceramics are more resistant to corrosion than plastics. Ceramics do not react readily with most liquids, gases, alkalis, and weak acids. They also remain stable over long time periods. They exhibit good to excellent strength and fracture toughness. One of the strongest and toughest ceramics, zirconium dioxide, has a flexural strength similar to that of steel, but its fracture toughness is much lower than that of steel. However, metals are tougher than either ceramics or plastics. Although ceramics are strong, temperature resistant, and resilient, these materials are brittle and may fracture without warning when flexed excessively or when quickly heated and cooled (i.e., under thermal shock conditions). Most dental ceramics are compounds of oxygen with metals or semimetals (metalloids) that have some properties of both metals and nonmetals, but, all ceramic products are nonmetallic in nature.

Most ceramics are characterized by their biocompatibility, esthetic potential, refractory nature, high hardness, low to moderate fracture toughness, excellent wear resistance, susceptibility to tensile fracture, and chemical inertness. For dental applications a ceramic with a hardness less than that of tooth enamel and an easily polishable surface are desirable to minimize the wear damage that can be produced on enamel by the ceramic surface. However, adequate fracture resistance is an important requirement of any dental ceramic. In this regard, the fracture toughness is the most critically important property because it is a measure of the resistance to crack growth under a state of tensile stress.

CRITICAL QUESTION

If tensile strength is not a reliable property of dental ceramics, which property is a better measure of the material's fracture resistance?

The susceptibility to tensile fracture is a drawback, particularly when flaws and tensile stress coexist in the same location within a ceramic prosthesis. However, the tensile strength of ceramics is not a useful parameter to describe their fracture resistance for several reasons. Strength is not an inherent property of ceramics because it varies with specimen size, specimen length, specimen shape, loading rate, surface preparation methods, and the environment. For example, the strength of silica-based ceramics increases with a decrease in specimen thickness, an increase in stressing rate, and a smoother surface. Such variability indicates that strength is not necessarily a bulk property since surface conditions can significantly alter the mean strength as well as the spread of experimental values, as indicated by the Weibull modulus and the coefficient of variation. In comparison, fracture toughness is a true material property that is a measure of the resistance to crack propagation.

It is generally believed that dental ceramics fail primarily because of their brittleness and poor ductility or elongation. In general, the major reason for fracture of ceramics is their inability to suppress crack growth by deforming plastically in areas adjacent to crack tips that are subjected to tensile stress. Since there is no other property that directly expresses brittleness, except perhaps for the reciprocal of percent elongation, two fracture mechanics properties may better explain this behavior.

- Fracture toughness or plane strain fracture toughness, which is designated as K_{Ic}, describes the critical stress intensity factor based on a mode I (tensile loading perpendicular to the crack plane) crack opening under tensile stress. For dental ceramics, K_{Ic} varies between 0.75 $MPa{\cdot}m^{1/2}$ for **feldspathic porcelain** and 8 $MPa{\cdot}m^{1/2}$ or more for yttria-stabilized **zirconia**, or ceria-stabilized alumina–zirconia ceramic. In comparison, the K_{Ic} values for enamel, dentin, and resin composites are 0.7 to 1.3, 3.1, and 0.8 to 2.5 $MPa{\cdot}m^{1/2}$, respectively.
- Another property that is used to describe the brittle fracture resistance of ceramics is the critical strain energy release rate, which is designated as G. The energy release rate failure criterion is that a crack will grow when the energy release rate is greater than or equal to a critical value, Gc, which is referred to as the fracture energy. This property is a measure of the unit strain energy that is released per unit increase in crack area as a ceramic with flaws or cracks is loaded progressively. Comparative values of K_{Ic} ($MPa{\cdot}m^{1/2}$) and G_c (kJ/m^2) for different types of materials are (1) glass, 0.7 versus 0.007; (2) PMMA, 1.1 versus 0.5; and (3) steel, 150 versus 107, respectively.

Chemical inertness is an important characteristic because it ensures that the chemically stable surface of dental restorations does not release potentially harmful elements, and it reduces the risk for surface roughening and increased abrasiveness or increased susceptibility to bacterial adhesion over time. Other important attributes of dental ceramics are their potential for matching the appearance of natural teeth, their thermal insulating properties (low thermal conductivity and low thermal diffusivity), and their freedom from galvanic effects (low electrical conductivity). Because the metal atoms transfer their outermost electrons to the nonmetallic atoms and stabilize their highly mobile electrons, ceramics are excellent thermal and electrical insulators.

CRITICAL QUESTION

What roles do oxygen, potassium, and leucite play in the structure and properties of feldspathic veneering (layering) ceramics?

Dental ceramics are nonmetallic, inorganic structures, primarily containing compounds of oxygen with one or more metallic or semimetallic elements (aluminum, boron, calcium, cerium, lithium, magnesium, phosphorus, potassium, silicone, sodium, titanium, and zirconium). Many dental ceramics contain a crystal phase and a silicate glass matrix phase. Their structures are characterized by

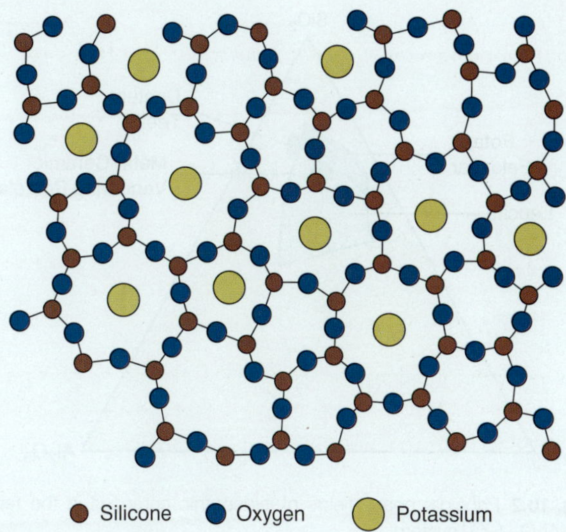

• **Fig. 10.1** Two-dimensional amorphous structure of potassium silicate glass.

chains of $(SiO_4)^{4-}$ tetrahedra in which Si^{4+} cations are positioned at the center of each tetrahedron with O^- anions at each of the four corners (Fig. 10.1). The resulting structure is not close packed and it exhibits both covalent and ionic bonds. The SiO_4 tetrahedra are linked by sharing their corners. They are arranged as linked chains of tetrahedra, each of which contains two oxygen atoms for every silicone atom. The primary structural unit in all silicate structures is the negatively charged silicone–oxygen tetrahedron $(SiO_4)^{4-}$. It is composed of a central silicone cation (Si^{4+}) bonded covalently to four oxygen anions located at the corners of a regular tetrahedron. For feldspathic veneering porcelains, alkali ions such as sodium or potassium occupy sites that allow them to bond to electrons from unbalanced oxygen ions (see Fig. 10.1). Alkali cations such as potassium or sodium tend to disrupt silicate chains and increase the thermal expansion of these glasses. The thermal expansion coefficient (TEC) can be further increased by including crystalline particles such as tetragonal leucite ($K_2O{\cdot}Al_2O_3{\cdot}4SiO_2$ or $KAlSi_2O_6$), whose TEC ranges from 22 to 30 × 10^{-6}/K. Two of the primary phase fields (potash feldspar and leucite) that are found in commercial feldspathic veneering ceramics are shown in a ternary section of the $K_2O{\cdot}Al_2O_3{\cdot}SiO_2$ phase diagram in Figure 10.2. Sanidine ($KAlSi_3O_8$), a potassium aluminosilicate phase, exists at high temperatures although it may be retained on cooling in the form of monoclinic crystals.

VITABLOCS Mk II is the only known dental ceramic with sanidine as the primary crystal phase. The glass matrix phase in these porcelains is formulated from one or more forms of the mineral feldspar ($KAlSi_3O_8$, $NaAlSi_3O_8$, and $CaAl_2Si_2O_8$). Many of the veneering ceramics (also called porcelains) are derived from potash feldspar ($K_2O{\cdot}Al_2O_3{\cdot}6SiO_2$ or $KAlSi_3O_8$), although some may be based on soda feldspar or a combination of both types. Compositions of some dental ceramics are listed in

.1. In industry, the term *porcelain* is generally associated with ceramics produced with a significant amount of kaolinite [$Al_2Si_2O_5(OH)_4$ or $Al_2O_3{\cdot}2SiO_2{\cdot}2H_2O$]. Kaolinite is a form of kaolin, which is a type of clay. None of the modern low-fusing or ultralow-fusing porcelains contains any clay product such as kaolinite. However, it may be used in the formulations for high-fusing porcelain and ceramic denture teeth (see Fig. 10.2). Thus, these ceramics are technically not porcelains and they can

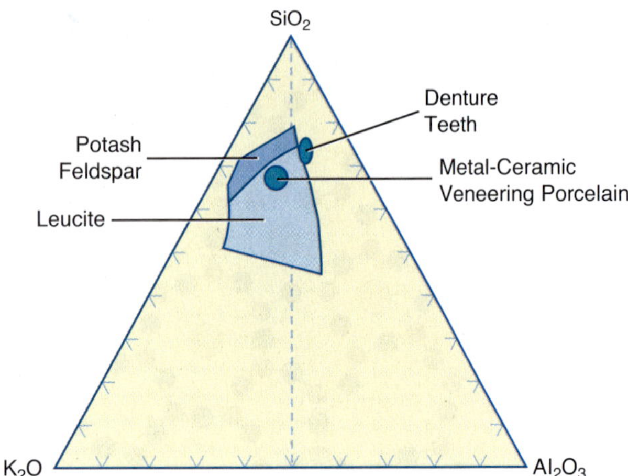

• **Fig. 10.2** Principal phase fields of feldspathic ceramics in the ternary K_2O–Al_2O_3–SiO_2 system.

be considered a type of glass (e.g., leucite glass, fluorapatite glass, or feldspathic glass). However, until the international community sees the need to change our terminology from *porcelain* to *glass*, we will continue to use the term *porcelain*.

Ceramics are composed of metallic and nonmetallic elements that form crystalline and/or noncrystalline compounds. They may form binary compounds such as **alumina** (Al_2O_3) and zirconia (ZrO_2) by the bonding of metals, which release their positive valence electrons to nonmetals that can accept or share electrons (negative ions). The free energy for bonding of positive metal ions to negative nonmetal ions must be sufficiently low so that the metallic ions preferentially attract nonmetallic ions rather than their own ions or other positive ions. Molecules with one oxygen atom (such as Na_2O, K_2O, or CaO) are useful in dental porcelain as fluxes. They may also act as opacifiers. Molecules that contain three oxygen atoms for every two other atoms (such as Al_2O_3) are used as stabilizers. They are also added as crack blockers or toughening crystals. Silica (SiO_2) is the main glass-forming structure used in all dental veneering ceramics. All silicates of dental interest are derived from silica tetrahedral structures that can be linked as chains, double chains, or three-dimensional distributions of tetrahedra. Fluxing cations such as K^+ or Na^+ neutralize the negative charges of the silicate backbones and disrupt the continuity of silicate networks (see Fig. 10.1), leading to lower **sintering** temperatures and increased coefficients of thermal expansion.

Zirconia is of major dental importance because of its high fracture toughness. However, pure ZrO_2 is not useful because cracks occur during sintering as a result of transformation from the tetragonal to the monoclinic phase. This transformation can be fully or partially suppressed by the addition of certain oxides such as MgO, Y_2O_3, CaO, or CeO. Most of the current zirconia ceramic materials for dental prostheses are based on tetragonal zirconia particles (TZP) that are fully stabilized with yttria (Y_2O_3). The addition of yttria to pure zirconia replaces some of the Zr^{4+} ions in the zirconia lattice with Y^{3+} ions. This produces oxygen vacancies, since three O^{2-} ions replace four O^{2-} ions. For several dental zirconia products, approximately 0.25% of Al_2O_3 is added to prevent the leaching of yttria (Y_2O_3).

Multicomponent or mixed oxide structures may also be useful for dental applications. Three examples of this class of ceramics include $MgO{\cdot}Al_2O_3$ (**spinel**), $3Al_2O_3{\cdot}2SiO_2$ (mullite, which is located along the right-side border of Fig. 10.2), and Al_2TiO_5 or $Al_2O_3{\cdot}TiO_2$ (aluminum titanate). The spinel structure is used in a **glass-infiltrated ceramic** (In-Ceram Spinell [ICS]) for applications in which greater translucency is required. Most nonoxide ceramics are not of practical use in dentistry either because of their high processing temperatures, complex processing methods, or their unesthetic color and opacity. Such ceramics include borides (TiB_2, ZrB_2), carbides (B_4C, SiC, TiC, WC), nitrides (AlN, BN, Si_3N_4, TiN), selenide (ZnSe), silicide ($MoSi_2$), sialon (Si_3N_4 with Al_2O_3), and syalon (Si_3N_4 with Al_2O_3 and Y_2O_3).

Glass–ceramics are partially crystallized glasses that are produced by nucleation and growth of crystals in the glass matrix phase. An example of such a product that has been used in dentistry is Dicor glass–ceramic, which was based on the growth of tetrasilicic fluormica crystals in a glass matrix. This material was originally supplied in a glass ingot form. The glass ingots, which contained a nucleating agent, were melted and cast into a refractory mold and subsequently processed thermally to produce the crystal phase of the glass–ceramic core material. Casting of glass forms is no longer performed for producing dental prostheses. Hot pressing and CAD–CAM processing are now used to produce glass–ceramic core frameworks for crowns and bridges.

CRITICAL QUESTION

Which property of bilayer ceramics is used as a measure of the **thermal compatibility** of ceramic materials?

Dental ceramics are formed into prosthetic shapes and configurations through a variety of processes including sintering, casting, hot isostatic pressing, **copy-milling**, and CAD–CAM machining. The components of the ceramics are based on metal oxides and glasses that are formulated for each particular application. For example, ceramics made as veneering structures on metal frameworks must be capable of bonding to the surface oxide of the metal substructure or to other veneering ceramic layers. *The coefficient of thermal expansion (CTE) and coefficient of thermal contraction (CTC) of the ceramic layers must be matched to that of the metal framework in such a way that crack-initiating tensile stresses in the ceramic are avoided or minimized during cooling.* The CTEs and CTCs of the veneering ceramics are controlled by varying their composition. In this chapter the calculated TEC differences between two bonded materials are used to describe thermal compatibility between adjacent structural materials.

Other component oxides are included to modify the esthetic or appearance characteristics of the final prosthesis, including the hue, value, chroma, opacity, and luminescence. Dental ceramic prostheses may also be used without a metal substructure when ceramic teeth are used in dentures or when all-ceramic crowns and fixed dental prostheses (FDPs) are used to satisfy optimal esthetic or biocompatibility requirements.

This chapter describes the composition, microstructure, properties, manipulation procedures, and performance characteristics of ceramic materials used for producing metal–ceramic (MC) and all-ceramic prostheses cemented on prepared teeth, on implant abutments, or on other material substrates used in the construction process. Although ceramics made from kaolin, feldspar, and quartz have been used for many centuries, major improvements in dental ceramics have occurred only within the past century. To understand the current state of materials science and technology, dental students, graduate students, and practicing dentists should be familiar with the terminology. The Glossary section provides the definitions required to facilitate an understanding of ceramic science and technology as they relate to dental prosthetic applications and the clinical performance of MC and ceramic–ceramic restorations.

Applications of Ceramics in Dentistry

Dental ceramic science and technology represent the fastest growing areas of dental materials research and development. During the past two decades numerous types of ceramics and processing methods have been introduced. Some of these materials can be formed into inlays, onlays, veneers, crowns, and more complex FDPs. Several of the core ceramics can be resin bonded micromechanically to tooth structure.

This chapter describes the ceramics used for MC prostheses and the new generation of ceramic products, such as Cercon, Lava, IPS e.max ZirCAD, In-Ceram Zirconia, IPS e.max CAD, Denzir, BruxZir, Procera AllCeram, and Procera Zirconia, which are being used currently for ceramic prostheses in dental practices. Previous glass–ceramics were produced either by crystallization of tetrasilicic fluormica or leucite crystals. However, further increases in strength and fracture toughness occurred subsequently with lithium disilicate–based products such as IPS Empress 2 and IPS e.max Press, among others. Introduced later were products such as In-Ceram Alumina, a glass-infiltrated **alumina core** ceramic; In-Ceram Zirconia, a glass-infiltrated zirconia–alumina core ceramic; Lava, a partially sintered or fully sintered zirconia core that is formed by a true CAD–CAM process (by scanning dies without the need for a wax pattern); and Cercon, a partially sintered zirconia ceramic that is milled to an enlarged size in the **green state** based on scanning of a wax pattern. It is also possible to scan prepared teeth and mill a prosthesis using the Cerec system (Sirona Corp., Germany). The Cerec 1 system was introduced in the mid-1980s and improvements in software and hardware led to the Cerec 2 and Cerec 3 systems for production of ceramic inlays, onlays, and veneers, and the commercial InLab system for large-scale processing of ceramic copings, frameworks, and monolithic ceramic prostheses.

Dental ceramics are used primarily for the production of FDPs. Although ceramics such as zirconia can be used for endodontic posts and implant abutments, their primary applications are for crowns and bridges. Because of its lack of translucency, zirconia is better suited for applications involving posterior teeth or for elderly patients whose teeth have lost much of their original translucency. Each family of dental ceramics has specific indications and contraindications for which it is best suited or not suited. The characteristics and uses of the range of dental ceramics are described in this chapter.

CRITICAL QUESTION

Which two inventions dramatically increased the success and survival probability of metal–ceramic restorations?

History of Dental Ceramics

Ceramic-like tools have been used by humans since the end of the Old Stone Age around 10,000 BCE to support the lifestyles and needs of fisher-hunter-gatherer civilizations. During the Middle Stone Age (10,000–5500 BCE) ceramics were important materials, and they have retained their importance in human societies ever since. Stone Age craftsmen took rocks and shaped them into tools and artifacts by a process called flaking and flintknapping, whereby stone chips could be fractured away from the surfaces of hard, fine-grained, or amorphous materials including chert, flint, ignimbrite, indurated shale, lava, obsidian, quartz, and silicified limestone. For example, craftsmen of the Paleo-Indian culture, from 10,000 to 6000 BCE, made arrowheads, spear points, and flaking tools from a variety of natural rock materials. Such rocks contained mineral phases such as feldspar, mica, and quartz, which have since been used in dental ceramics.

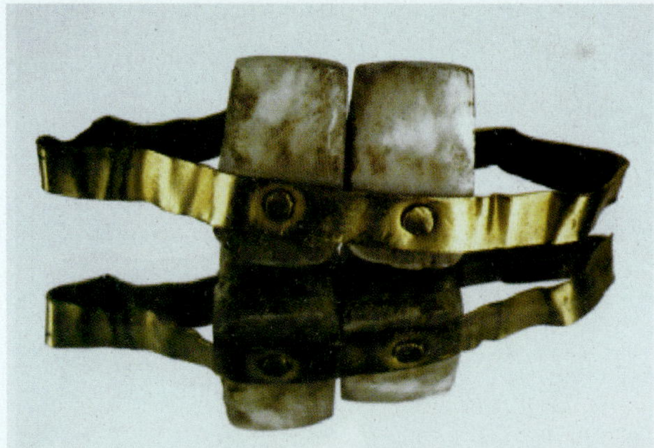

• **Fig. 10.3** Copy of Etruscan denture recovered from a tomb in Etruria, Italy, circa 700 BCE. Gold bands of this type held human or animal teeth (possibly oxen) that were fastened by means of gold rivets. (Courtesy of the Science Museum, London.)

Because natural minerals are not tooth colored, subsequent civilizations used a variety of materials to produce simulated teeth. In approximately 700 BCE, the Etruscans made artificial teeth of ivory and bone, human teeth, and animal teeth (possibly oxen) that were held in place by gold wires or flat bands and rivets (Fig. 10.3). Animal bone and ivory from hippopotami and elephants were used for many years thereafter.

Human teeth that were sold by the poor and teeth obtained from the dead were also used for centuries thereafter, but dentists generally avoided this option. One of the first sets of dentures made for the US President George Washington (Fig. 10.4) contained extracted teeth but later his dentures were made of hippopotamus ivory. The ivory tooth forms were supported in the maxillary denture by a gold palatal plate and the dentures were retained by pressure applied by coiled springs attached to the sides of the denture bases. President Washington was inaugurated in 1789 with one remaining tooth. He suffered from poor oral health (although it is reported that he had brushed his teeth regularly with tooth powder). His poor-fitting dentures caused him much discomfort during his presidency (1789−1797) and until his death, in 1799, at the age of 67. None of his dentures were ever made of wood, contrary to erroneous reports circulated since his death.

The first porcelain tooth material was patented in 1789 by de Chemant, a French dentist in collaboration with Duchateau, a French pharmacist. This product, an improved version of the "mineral paste teeth" produced in 1774 by Duchateau, was introduced in England soon thereafter by de Chemant. However, this baked compound was not used to produce individual teeth, since there was no effective way at that time to attach the teeth to a denture base material.

In 1808, Fonzi, an Italian dentist, invented a "terrometallic" porcelain tooth held in place by a platinum pin or frame. Planteau, a French dentist, introduced porcelain teeth to the United States in 1817, and Peale, an artist, developed a baking process in Philadelphia for these teeth in 1822. Commercial production of these teeth by Stockton began in 1825. In England, Ash developed an improved version of the porcelain tooth in 1837. In

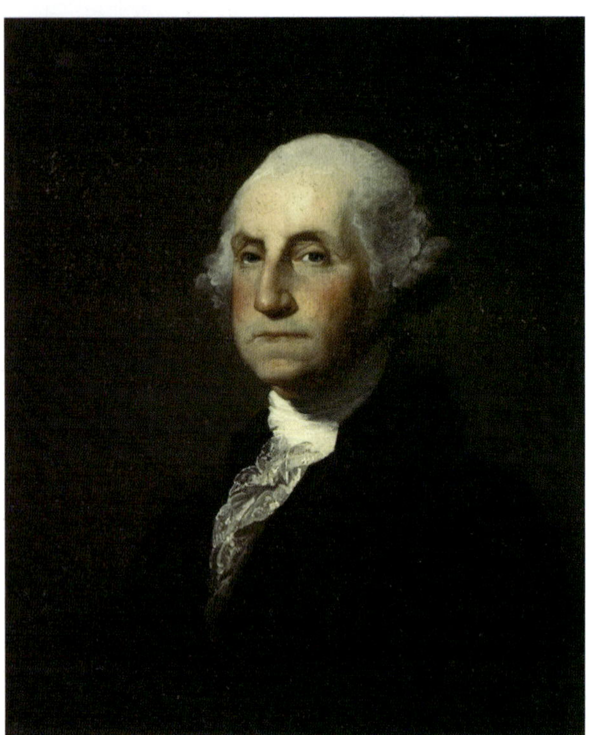

• **Fig. 10.4** Portrait of President Washington, who died on December 14, 1799. Technology for producing porcelain denture teeth was not available until 1825, although these prostheses were not refined until vulcanized rubber denture bases were developed in 1839.

Germany, Pfaff in 1756 developed a technique to make impressions of the mouth using plaster of Paris, but it was not until 1839 that the invention of vulcanized rubber allowed porcelain denture teeth to be used effectively in a denture base. In 1844, the nephew of Stockton founded the SS White Company, which became active in the further refinement of the design and mass production of porcelain denture teeth.

Charles Land introduced one of the first ceramic crowns to dentistry in 1903. Land, the grandfather of aviator Charles Lindbergh, published in the *Independent Practitioner* in 1886 and 1887 a technique for preparing the tooth cavity for an inlay, making a platinum foil matrix, and fabricating a ceramic inlay using high-fusing feldspathic porcelain. The sintering temperature was empirically determined as reported by Gilbert ("Notes on Dental Porcelain," Harvard University Dental School, 1906), who described the temperature required to "set" the inlay as one that was between the melting point of pure gold (1084°C) and the maximum temperature recommended for the porcelain muffle (1370°C).

These crowns exhibited excellent esthetics, but the low flexural strength of porcelain resulted in a high incidence of fracture. Since the 1960s, feldspathic porcelains with reliable chemical bonding have been used in MC prostheses. However, feldspathic porcelains have been considered too weak to be used reliably in the construction of all-ceramic crowns without a tougher ceramic core, a cast-metal core, or metal-foil coping. Furthermore, their firing shrinkage results in significant discrepancies in fit and adaptation of margins unless correction firings are performed.

Two of the most important breakthroughs responsible for the long-standing superb esthetic performance and clinical survival probabilities of MC restorations are described in the patents of Weinstein and Weinstein (1962) and Weinstein et al. (1962). One of these patents identified the formulations of feldspathic porcelain that enabled the systematic control of the sintering temperature and CTE. The other patent described the components that could be used to produce alloys that bond chemically to and that are thermally compatible with the feldspathic porcelains. The first commercial porcelain was developed by VITA Zahnfabrik in about 1963. Although the first VITA porcelain products were known for their esthetic properties, the subsequent introduction of the more versatile Ceramco porcelain led to thermal expansion behavior that allowed this porcelain to be used safely with a wider variety of alloys.

A significant improvement in the fracture resistance of all-porcelain crowns was reported by McLean and Hughes in 1965, when they introduced a dental **aluminous** core ceramic consisting of a glass matrix containing between 40% and 50% Al_2O_3 by weight. Because of the inadequate translucency (**opaque**, chalky white appearance) of the aluminous porcelain core materials, a feldspathic porcelain veneer was required to achieve acceptable esthetics. The flexural strength (modulus of rupture) of the core material was approximately 131 MPa. McLean (1979) reported a low 5-year fracture rate of only 2% for anterior crowns but an unacceptably high fracture rate of 15% when aluminous porcelain was used for molar crowns. Another deficiency of the aluminous porcelain crown was the large sintering shrinkage (approximately 15%–20%) of the core material at its high firing temperature. Because of their relatively high fracture rate in posterior sites, the principal indication for the use of aluminous porcelain crowns was the restoration of maxillary anterior crowns where esthetics was of paramount importance. Since the introduction of aluminous porcelain crowns in the early 1900s and methods to produce durable MC crowns in the 1960s, improvements in the composition of ceramics and the method of forming the ceramic core of ceramic crowns have greatly enhanced our ability to produce better-fitting fracture-resistant crowns made entirely of ceramic material.

Significant developments in MC properties, design, and performance—such as opalescence, specialized internal staining techniques, greening-resistant porcelains, porcelain butt-joint margins, and **shoulder porcelains**—have significantly enhanced the overall appearance and "vitality" of MC crowns and bridges and the clinical survivability of these restorations. Improvement in all-ceramic systems developed by controlled crystallization of a glass (Dicor) was demonstrated by Adair and Grossman (1984). This glass was melted and cast into a refractory mold and subsequently crystallized to form the Dicor glass–ceramic containing tetrasilicic fluormica crystals in a glass matrix. A further development was the introduction of a machinable glass–ceramic version (Dicor MGC), which had a tetrasilicic fluormica crystal volume of approximately 70%. In the early 1990s a pressable glass–ceramic (IPS Empress), containing approximately 34% leucite by volume, was introduced. IPS Empress had a strength and marginal adaptation similar to those of Dicor glass–ceramic, but it required no specialized crystallization treatment. Neither of these materials was indicated for producing **fixed dental prostheses.** A more fracture-resistant, pressable glass–ceramic (IPS Empress 2) containing approximately 70% lithia disilicate crystals by volume was introduced in the late 1990s. This core ceramic has been used for three-unit FDPs as far posterior as the second premolar. The fracture toughness of IPS Empress 2 glass–ceramic (3.3 $MPa{\cdot}m^{1/2}$) is more than twice that of its predecessor, IPS Empress glass–ceramic (1.3 $MPa{\cdot}m^{1/2}$).

These improvements in the composition of ceramics and the method of forming the core of all-ceramic crowns and bridges have greatly enhanced our ability to produce more accurate and fracture-resistant all-ceramic crowns. Significant progress has been made toward the goal of developing less abrasive veneering ceramics. In 1992 Duceram LFC (low-fusing ceramic) was marketed as an ultralow-fusing ceramic with three unique features: (1) it was based on a hydrothermal glass in which water was incorporated into the silicate glass structure to produce nonbridging hydroxyl groups that disrupt the glass network, thereby decreasing the glass transition temperature, viscosity, and firing temperature, and increasing the CTE to allow its use as a veneer for certain low-expansion metals; (2) these types of ceramics were also claimed to be "self-healing" through a process of forming a 1-μm thick hydrothermal layer along the ceramic surface; and (3) the extremely small size of the crystal particles (400–500 nm) enhanced the opalescence of the ceramic by reflecting blue light hues from the surface and yellow hues from the interior of the ceramic. Other ultralow-fusing ceramics (sintering temperatures below 850°C) now commonly referred to as low-fusing ceramics have been introduced with a veneering glass; these materials were claimed to be kinder to opposing tooth enamel either because they were predominantly a glass phase material or because they contained very small crystal particles.

Classification of Dental Ceramics

In this chapter dental ceramics are divided into two main categories:

1. Ceramics used to veneer metal frameworks for MC—that is, porcelain-fused-to-metal (PFM) prostheses. Shown in Figure 10.5 is a cross-sectional view of a MC crown.
2. Ceramics used to produce all-ceramic prostheses.

Dental ceramics can be classified according to one or more of the following parameters:

1. Uses or indications (anterior and posterior crown, veneer, post and core, **fixed dental prosthesis**, **ceramic stain**, **glaze**)
2. Composition
3. Principal crystal phase and/or matrix phase (silica glass, leucite-based feldspathic porcelain, leucite-based glass–ceramic, lithia disilicate–based glass–ceramic, aluminous porcelain, alumina, glass-infused alumina, glass-infused spinel, glass-infused alumina/zirconia, and zirconia
4. Processing method (casting, sintering, partial sintering and glass infiltration, **slip casting** and sintering, hot-isostatic pressing, CAD–CAM milling, and copy-milling)
5. Firing temperature (ultralow fusing, low fusing, medium fusing, and high fusing) (Table 10.1)
6. Microstructure (amorphous glass, crystalline, crystalline particles in a glass matrix)
7. Translucency (opaque, translucent, transparent)
8. Fracture resistance (low, medium, high)
9. Abrasiveness (comparison relative to tooth enamel against tooth enamel)

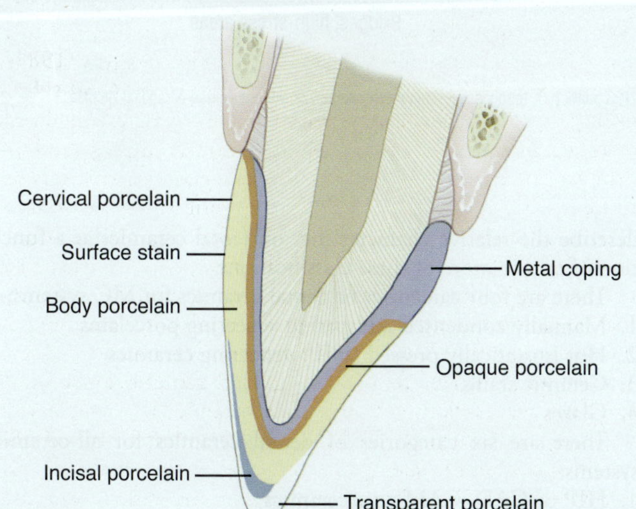

• **Fig. 10.5** Schematic illustration of a metal–ceramic (porcelain fused to metal) crown.

TABLE 10.1 Classification of Dental Ceramics by Sintering Temperature

Class	Applications	Sintering Temperature Range
High fusing	Denture teeth, and fully sintered alumina and zirconia core ceramics	>1300°C (>2372°F)
Medium fusing	Denture teeth, presintered zirconia	1101–1300°C (2013–2372°F)
Low fusing	Crown and bridge veneer ceramic	850–1100°C (1562–2012°F)
Ultralow fusing	Crown and bridge veneer ceramic	<850°C (<1562°F)

To allow a clinician to select the best material for a given clinical situation, the following sections describe the relative characteristics of dental ceramics as a function of one or more of these classifications. Table 10.2 lists the types of dental ceramics by their recommended indications for and contraindications against their use. Although manufacturers and dental laboratory owners usually list the indications for use of ceramic products, they do not typically state their contraindications. Only after clinical evidence of adverse events occur do the indications change and contraindications become more clearly specified. Table 10.2 reflects a relatively conservative perspective on uses of each type of ceramic based in part on evidence from clinical studies. The information presented does not guarantee success nor is it predictive of failure, because many variables are involved that may shift the balance of risk from low to high. *Note that bruxism is a typical contraindication for most ceramics because of the higher risk for fracture as well as the increased risk for wear of opposing tooth enamel surfaces.* An example of severe wear of enamel by ceramic is shown in Figure 10.6. Although the extreme abrasion damage shown in this figure may not have occurred primarily because of bruxism, it was related to increased stresses that developed because posterior teeth were not present to distribute the applied mastication forces over posterior teeth as well.

Dental ceramics can be classified by composition. It is not feasible to discuss the compositions of the numerous existing dental products. However, it is useful to be familiar initially with some representative compositions of feldspathic porcelains and an aluminous porcelain. The compositions of typical products are given in Table 10.3. *Note that the major component in most of these ceramics is silica, which is the basis of the glass matrix phase of feldspathic porcelains used as a veneering or layering structure of both*

TABLE 10.2 General Indications and Contraindications for Use of Dental Ceramics

Type	Primary Application	Secondary Applications	Contraindications
Feldspathic porcelain	Metal–ceramic veneers Anterior laminate veneers	Single-surface inlays/low-stress sites High translucency needed	Inlays, onlays, crowns, and bridges (except as metal–ceramic veneers) Bruxism
Aluminous porcelain	Core ceramic for anterior crowns	Low-stress premolar crowns	Molar crowns Bridges Bruxism
Leucite glass–ceramic	Anterior single-unit crowns Anterior laminate veneers	Low-stress premolar inlays and crowns High translucency needed	High-stress situations Bridges Bruxism
Lithia disilicate glass–ceramic	Anterior and premolar crowns Anterior three-unit bridges Premolar crowns	Anterior laminate veneers Posterior three-unit bridges to second premolar	High-stress posterior situations Bridges involving molar teeth Bruxism
Alumina	Core ceramic for crowns Low-stress anterior bridges	Low-stress posterior bridges	Anterior veneers High-stress posterior bridges Bruxism
Glass-infiltrated spinel	Anterior crowns	High translucency needed	Anterior bridges Posterior crowns and bridges Bruxism
Glass-infiltrated alumina	Anterior and posterior crowns	Anterior bridge substructures up to three units	Anterior veneers Posterior crowns and bridges High translucency needed Bruxism
Glass-infiltrated alumina/zirconia	Posterior crowns Posterior bridge substructures up to three units	Anterior bridge substructures up to three units	Anterior veneers and crowns Where high translucency needed Bruxism
Zirconia (Y-TZP) (with veneering ceramic)	Posterior crowns Posterior bridge substructures up to five units		Anterior veneers, crowns, and bridges High translucency is needed Bruxism
Zirconia (3Y-TZP) (monolithic, without veneering ceramic)	Posterior crowns and bridges (limited clinical data available)	Posterior core ceramic bridges	Anterior veneers, crowns, and bridges High translucency is needed Bruxism
Ce-TZP/Al2O3	Posterior crowns and bridge substructures (no clinical data available)	—	Anterior veneers, crowns, and bridges High translucency is needed Bruxism
4Y-PSZ	Anterior crowns, posterior crowns, veneers, onlays		Bridges, high-stress areas
5Y-PSZ	Anterior crowns, posterior crowns, veneers, onlays		Bridges, high-stress areas

4Y-PZE, 5 mol% Y_2O_3 partially stabilized zirconia; 5Y-PZE, 5 mol% Y_2O_3 partially stabilized zirconia; 3Y-TZP, 3 mol% Y_2O_3 tetragonal zirconia polycrystal; Y-TZP, yttria-stabilized tetragonal zirconia polycrystal.

MC and all-ceramic prostheses. These veneering ceramics provide hue, value, chroma, and translucency characteristics to the final restoration. In addition, the fine-grain varieties may cause less wear of opposing enamel or tooth restorations than coarse-grain ceramics.

Classification by processing method is also informative because it is likely that many of the ceramics that fall within a specific type of processing requirement will behave similarly in a clinical setting, particularly with respect to marginal fit, polishability, failure mechanisms, esthetic potential, wear resistance, abrasiveness, and survivability. A classification of materials by processing method is presented in Table 10.4. To allow a clinician to select the best material for a given clinical situation, the following sections describe the relative characteristics of dental ceramics as a function of one or more of these classifications.

There are four categories of dental ceramics for MC systems:

1. Manually condensed feldspathic veneering porcelains
2. Hot isostatically pressed (HIP) veneering ceramics
3. Ceramic stains
4. Glazes

There are six categories of dental ceramics for all-ceramic systems:

1. HIP or CAD–CAM core ceramics
2. Manually condensed veneering ceramics
3. Hot-pressed veneering ceramics
4. Liners

5. Ceramic stains
6. Ceramic glazes

These material categories are discussed in this chapter.

The compositions of these ceramics are generally classified by the principal crystal phases controlling their properties.

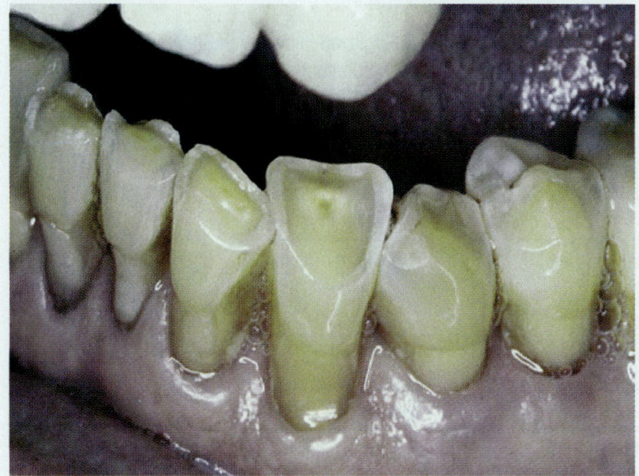

• **Fig. 10.6** Excessive wear of mandibular teeth abraded by opposing porcelain surfaces. (Courtesy of Dr Henry Young.)

The most common crystal phases are

- Leucite
- Lithia disilicate
- Alumina
- Combinations of alumina and zirconia
- Zirconia
- Apatite

Leucite crystals are included in veneering porcelains for MCs to opacify and strengthen these glass-matrix materials and to control their thermal expansion and contraction coefficients. Leucite crystals also play similar roles in the formulation of HIP and CAD–CAM core structures of all-ceramic prostheses. Note that although most of the dental literature emphasizes the TEC, the thermal contraction coefficient is more relevant for analyzing stresses in veneering ceramic that develop during cooling. This difference is most significant for glass-phase ceramics.

Lithia disilicate glass–ceramics, alumina/zirconia, and zirconia are used exclusively for the core structure of the all-ceramic applications. Total core ceramic restorations (also known as Full Contour restorations) of posterior crowns and bridges made from either lithia disilicate glass–ceramic or zirconia ceramic have been used to eliminate veneer chipping, gross fracture of veneering (layering) ceramics, and to maximize the size of connectors in FDPs (bridges) in order to reduce connector fractures. One of the main concerns on the use of core ceramic prostheses is their potential for increased wear of opposing tooth

TABLE 10.3 Composition (Percentage by Weight) of Selected Ceramics

	LOW-FUSING VACUUM PORCELAIN			METAL–CERAMIC PORCELAIN			HIP GLASS–CERAMIC	HAP/GLASS
				LOW FUSING				
Component	Aluminous Porcelain	Dentin	Enamel	Dentin	Enamel	Ultralow Fusing	IPS e.max Press (Based on $Li_2O{\cdot}2SiO_2$)	IPS e.max Ceram Veneer Ceramic
SiO_2	35.0	66.5	64.7	59.2	63.5	60–70	57–80	45–70
Al_2O_3	53.7	13.5	13.9	18.5	18.9	5–10	0–5	5–22
CaO	1.1	2.1	1.8	—	—	1–3.0	—	1–11
Na_2O	2.8	4.2	4.8	4.8	5.0	10–15	—	4–13
K_2O	4.2	7.1	7.5	11.8	12.3	10–13	0–13	3–9
B_2O_3	3.2	6.6	7.3	4.6	0.1	0–1.0	—	—
ZnO	—	—	—	0.6	0.1	—	0–8	—
ZrO_2	—	—	—	0.4	0.1	0–1.0	0–8	—
BaO, Y_2O_3	—	—	—	—	—	0–0.2	—	—
SnO_2	—	—	—	—	—	0–0.2	—	—
Li_2O	—	—	—	—	—	0–1.0	11–19	—
F	—	—	—	—	—	0–1.0		0.1–2.5
P_2O_5	—	—	—	—	—	—	0–11	0.5–6.5
Sb_2O_3	—	—	—	—	—	0–1.0	—	—
CeO_2	—	—	—	—	—	0–0.2	—	—
TiO_2	—	—	—	—	—	1–3.0	—	—
Pigments/other	—	—	—	—	—	—	0–8/0–10	0–3
Sintering/firing temperature (°C)	980	980	950	900	900	650–700	945	750

TABLE 10.4 **Methods of Processing the Ceramic Core Component of a Ceramic Prosthesis**

Initial Forming Method	Examples	Initial Material Form	Second Processing Step	Subsequent Form	Final Steps
Condensation	Ceramco, VITA VMK, Duceram LFC, IPS d.Sign	Powder and mixing liquid	Sintering of core ceramic	Dense core ceramic with less than 5 vol% porosity	Veneer, glaze
Hot pressing	IPS Empress 2, OPC 3G, Finesse Pressable	High-quality ceramic ingot	Stain only or stain and glaze (inlays), or veneering ceramic	Stained/glazed inlay or veneered core	Stain and/or glaze for crowns and FPDs
Casting	Dicor (obsolete)	Glass core	Crystallization heat treatment (ceramming)	Glass–ceramic core containing a glass phase and tetrasilicic fluormica crystals	Shading porcelain (obsolete)
Slip casting	In-Ceram Alumina, In-Ceram Spinell, In-Ceram Zirconia	Powder and mixing liquid	Partial sintering	Partially sintered core	Glass infiltration, trimming of excess glass, veneer, glaze
Computer-aided milling (CAM) of fully sintered form	Cerec VITABLOCS, In-Denzir, BruxZir	High-quality ceramic ingot	Margin repair (if necessary)	High-quality core possibly with repaired margin	Veneer, glaze (except for BruxZir)
Computer-aided milling (CAM) of partially sintered form	Cercon, Lava, e.max ZirCAD	Partially sintered ceramic block	Final sintering of machined/ground core and margin repair (if necessary)	Fully sintered core possibly with repaired margin	Veneer, glaze
Copy-milling	Variety of ceramic products	High-quality ceramic block	Margin repair (if necessary	High-quality core possibly with repaired margin	Veneer, glaze
Machining, grinding of dry-pressed powder on enlarged die	Procera AllCeram	Dry pressed and machined alumina block	Sintering	High-quality core containing 99.9% alumina	Veneer, glaze

enamel. Although the surfaces of these prostheses can be glazed to minimize enamel wear, the long-term durability of glaze layers continues to be evaluated.

Metal–Ceramic Systems: Composition and Properties

Benefits of Metal–Ceramic Prostheses

The chief limitation to the use of an all-porcelain crown in fixed prosthodontics is its lack of tensile and shear strength. A method for minimizing this disadvantage is to bond the porcelain directly to a metal coping that fits the prepared tooth. The MC restoration has a facial metal thickness of 0.3–0.5 mm. It is veneered with opaque porcelain approximately 0.3 mm in thickness. The body porcelain is about 1 mm thick.

Several clinical studies over the past 50 years confirm the high overall survival percentages of MC prostheses. One clinical study revealed that the fracture rate of MC crowns as well as bridges made from a high noble alloy was as low as 2.3% over 7.5 years of service. The most outstanding advantage of MC restorations is their resistance to fracture. With metal occlusal surfaces, the fracture rate in posterior sites could be reduced further. Another potential advantage of MC restorations over total-ceramic restorations is that less tooth structure needs to be removed to provide the proper bulk for the crown, especially if thinner (<0.1 mm) layered noble foil metal is used, where metal alone is used on occlusal surfaces and lingual cusps or porcelain butt-joint margins are used on facial and buccal surfaces. Such designs also cause less wear of antagonist enamel than occurs when enamel is opposed by a ceramic surface.

There are relatively few disadvantages to MC restorations compared with all-ceramic choices. One of the most frequently mentioned disadvantages is the potential for metal allergy. However, such allergic reactions are very rare except possibly when nickel-containing alloys are used. Although MC restorations have accounted recently for about 60%–70% of all fixed restorations, an MC crown is not the best esthetic choice for restoring a single maxillary anterior tooth. An all-ceramic crown offers a greater potential for success in matching the appearance of the adjacent natural tooth, especially when a relatively high degree of translucency is desired.

A dark line at the facial margin of an MC crown associated with a metal collar or metal margin is a significant esthetic concern when gingival recession occurs (Fig. 10.7A and B). This adverse esthetic effect can be minimized by designing the crown with a ceramic margin or by using a very thin knife-edge margin of metal veneered with opaque shoulder porcelain. This ceramic margin should be polished and/or glazed to avoid a rough surface at the margin. The use of MC crowns with porcelain shoulder or butt-joint margins or with knife-edge metal margins is successful procedure for improving the esthetics of MC prostheses.

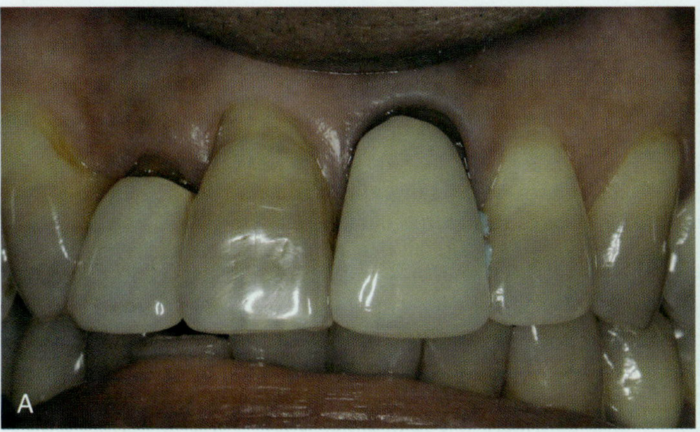

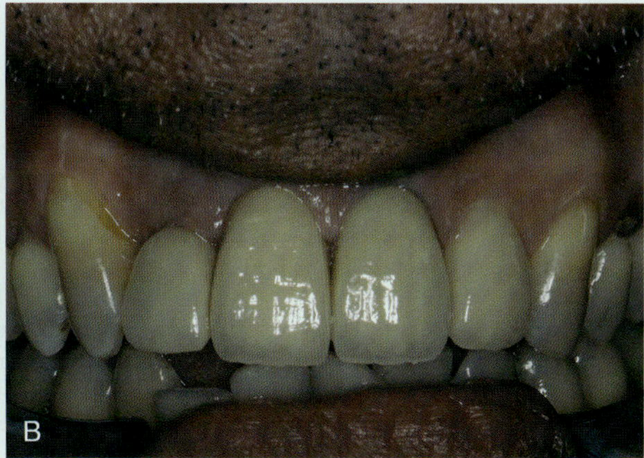

• **Fig. 10.7** **(A)** Esthetic issues caused by gingival recession and exposure of dark metal collar in metal–ceramic restoration. **(B)** Significant improvement in esthetics can be achieved by replacing the metal–ceramic crowns with all ceramic prosthesis.

CRITICAL QUESTION

Which components of ceramics can cause excessive wear of tooth enamel?

Ceramic Composition

Conventional dental porcelain is a vitreous ceramic based on a silica (SiO_2) network and potash feldspar ($K_2O{\cdot}Al_2O_3{\cdot}6SiO_2$), soda feldspar ($Na_2O{\cdot}Al_2O_3{\cdot}6SiO_2$), or both. The ternary diagram in Figure 10.2 for the K_2O–Al_2O_3–SiO_2 system shows the approximate composition ranges of feldspathic porcelain products used for MC prostheses and denture teeth. This diagram is based on the use of potash feldspar ($K_2O{\cdot}Al_2O_3{\cdot}6SiO_2$) rather than soda feldspar ($Na_2O{\cdot}Al_2O_3{\cdot}6SiO_2$), which is also used in some products. Pigments, opacifiers, and glasses are added to control the fusion temperature, sintering temperature, CTC, and solubility. The feldspars used for dental porcelains are relatively pure and colorless. Thus, pigments must be added to produce the hues of natural teeth or the color appearance of tooth-colored restorative materials that may exist in adjacent teeth.

Feldspathic porcelains contain, by weight, a variety of oxides including a SiO_2 matrix (52–65%), Al_2O_3 (11–20%), K_2O (10–15%), Na_2O (4–15%), and certain additives, including B_2O_3, CeO_2, Li_2O, TiO_2, and Y_2O_3. These ceramics are called porcelains because they contain a glass matrix and one or more crystal phases, although the term *porcelain* traditionally refers in industry to products produced from kaolin as a major component. They cannot be classified as glass–ceramics because crystal formation does not occur through controlled nucleation, crystal formation, and growth.

There are four types of veneering ceramics. Feldspathic porcelains include:

- Ultralow- and low-fusing ceramics (feldspar-based porcelain, nepheline syenite—based porcelain, and apatite-based porcelain)
- Low-fusing specialty ceramics (shoulder porcelains and wash-coat ceramics)
- Ceramic stains
- Ceramic glazes (autoglaze and **overglaze**)

The compositions of two typical low-fusing veneering porcelains for MC prostheses are listed in Table 10.3.

The particle type and crystal particle size may greatly influence the potential abrasiveness of the ceramic prosthesis. The abrasiveness of the finished surface will depend on the thickness of the veneer and the presence or absence of crystalline particles. Excessive wear of enamel may occur by direct two-body contact against core ceramics of all-ceramic restorations or opaque porcelain of MC restorations, but core ceramics that are veneered are unlikely to contact opposing enamel except in situations where inadequate tooth reduction or excessive occlusal reduction has occurred.

CRITICAL QUESTION

How does the leucite content of veneering porcelain for MC prostheses control the cracking resistance of the porcelain?

Silicate glass represents the matrix phase of feldspathic porcelains. Silica (SiO_2) can exist in four different forms: crystalline quartz, crystalline cristobalite, crystalline tridymite, and noncrystalline fused silica. Fused silica is a high-melting material whose melting temperature is attributed to the three-dimensional network of covalent bonds between silica tetrahedra, the basic structural units of the glass network. Fluxes (low-fusing glasses) are often included to reduce the temperature required to sinter the porcelain powder particles at sufficiently low temperatures so that the alloy to which it is fired does not melt or sustain sag (flexural creep) deformation.

Potassium and sodium feldspars are naturally occurring minerals composed of potash (K_2O) or soda (Na_2O), alumina (Al_2O_3), and silica (SiO_2). They are used in the preparation of many dental porcelains designed for MC crowns and many other dental glasses and ceramics. When potassium feldspar is mixed with various metal oxides and fired to high temperatures, it can form leucite and a glass phase that will soften and flow slightly. The softening of this glass phase during porcelain firing allows the porcelain powder particles to coalesce. For dental porcelains, the process by which the particles coalesce is called liquid-phase sintering, a process controlled by diffusion between particles at a temperature sufficiently high to form a dense solid. The driving force for sintering is the decrease in energy caused by a reduction in surface area.

Another important property of feldspar is its tendency to form crystalline leucite ($K_2O{\cdot}Al_2O_3{\cdot}4SiO_2$) when it is melted. Leucite is a potassium–aluminum–silicate mineral with a high CTE (20–25 $\times$ 10^{-6}/K) compared with feldspar glasses that have much lower coefficients of thermal expansion (8.6 $\times$ 10^{-6}/K). When feldspar is heated at temperatures between 1150°C and

1530°C, it undergoes incongruent melting to form crystals of leucite in a liquid glass. Incongruent melting is the process by which one material melts to form a liquid plus a different crystalline material. This tendency of feldspar to form leucite during incongruent melting controls thermal expansion during the use of porcelains for metal bonding. Some dental glasses do not contain leucite as a raw material. Since feldspar is not essential as a precursor to the formation of leucite, these glasses are modified with additions of leucite to control their CTC.

The compositions of the veneering (layering) ceramics used for MC restorations (see Table 10.3) generally correspond to those used previously for veneering aluminous porcelain core ceramic except for increased concentrations of K_2O and Na_2O. For MC porcelains, specific concentrations of soda, potash, and/or leucite are necessary to reduce the sintering temperature and to increase the thermal expansion to a level compatible with that of the metal coping. The opaque porcelains also contain relatively large amounts of metallic oxide opacifiers to conceal the underlying metal and to minimize the thickness of the opaque porcelain layer.

Veneering ceramics ("porcelains") for metals have higher expansion and contraction coefficients than the ceramics used to veneer alumina or zirconia core ceramics. They should not be subjected to nonessential repeated firings, because this may lead to devitrification and an increased risk of cloudiness within the porcelains as well as potential changes in their CTE (α_e) and CTC (α_c). It is imperative that a proper matching of these thermal properties of the alloy and porcelain be ensured to reduce the risk for chipping or cracking of the ceramic veneers either during cooling from the sintering or glazing temperatures or at some later time in clinical service.

Metal Composition

Single-unit crowns and bridges may be made from MC systems (combinations of metal substructure and veneering ceramic). In this chapter the term *metal-ceramic* (MC) is used synonymously with *porcelain fused to metal* (PFM), although the former term (MC) is the most internationally accepted descriptor for these types of prosthetic material systems.

Many alloys are available to be veneered with low-fusing and ultralow-fusing porcelains. The compositions of these high-noble, noble, predominantly base metal alloys control the castability, bonding ability to porcelain, the esthetics of the MC restoration, and the magnitudes of stresses that develop in the porcelains during cooling from the sintering temperature. A typical list of alloy types of one manufacturer is presented in Table 10.5. Some important properties of these alloys are listed. Of particular importance to the section in the following is the CTE or CTC, which must match closely to that of the veneering porcelain to be used.

The compositions of the high-noble alloys, titanium and titanium alloys, noble alloys, predominantly base metal alloys CPTi, Ti alloys used for MC restorations are discussed further in Chapter 9. The reader is referred to this chapter for a description of these systems and of the effects and purposes of the constituent metals.

Ultralow-Fusing Ceramics for Metal–Ceramic Prostheses

Most of the ultralow-fusing ceramics (sintering temperatures below 850°C) have microstructures that exhibit either a well-distributed dispersion of small crystal particles or few or no crystals. Initial results of wear studies are promising in several cases relative to the enamel wear (see Fig. 10.6) caused by these ceramics, although not all ultralow-fusing ceramics exhibit this decreased level of abrasiveness. Ultralow-fusing ceramics contain less Al_2O_3 and increased concentrations of CaO, K_2O, Li_2O, and Na_2O.

Ultralow-fusing porcelains generally contain, by weight, 20.1–22.6% tetragonal leucite and 0–2.6% cubic leucite, although one product contains 11.5–11.6% tetragonal leucite and 2.9–4.6% cubic leucite. The conventional **frits** have been reported to be admixtures of three kinds of glass frits. One of these ultralow-fusing frits exhibits very small (less than 1 μm) leucite crystals.

Ultralow-fusing dentin and enamel ceramics may be easier to polish and may yield smoother and less abrasive surfaces than conventional low-fusing and medium-fusing porcelains. Because of their lower concentration of leucite crystals compared with conventional porcelains, they have lower expansion and contraction coefficients. Their lower sintering temperatures provide opportunities for use with alloys that have lower fusion temperatures, such as type II and type IV gold alloys, whose compositions have been modified to ensure proper chemical bonding and matched thermal expansion and contraction coefficients.

Glass Modifiers

The sintering temperature of crystalline silica is too high for its use as a veneer on cast dental alloys. At such temperatures the alloys would melt. In addition, the CTC of crystalline silica is too low for these alloys. Bonds between the silica tetrahedra can be broken by the addition of alkali metal ions such as sodium, potassium, and calcium. These ions are associated with the oxygen atoms at the corners of the tetrahedra and interruption of oxygen–silicone bonds. As a result, the three-dimensional silica network contains many linear chains of silica tetrahedra that are able to move easily at lower temperatures than the atoms that are locked into the three-dimensional structure of silica tetrahedra. This ease of movement is responsible for the increased fluidity (decreased viscosity), lower softening temperature, and increased thermal expansion conferred by glass modifiers. However, too high a modifier concentration reduces the chemical durability (resistance to attack by water, acids, and alkalis) of the glass. In addition, if too many tetrahedra are disrupted, the glass may crystallize (devitrify) during porcelain firing operations. Hence, a balance between a suitable melting range and good chemical durability must be maintained.

Manufacturers employ glass modifiers to produce dental porcelains with different firing temperatures. Dental porcelains are classified according to their firing temperatures. A typical classification is given in Table 10.1. Other metallic oxides also can be introduced, as indicated in Table 10.3. Boric oxide (B_2O_3) can behave as a glass modifier to decrease viscosity, to lower the softening temperature, and to form its own glass network. Because boric oxide forms a separate lattice interspersed with the silica lattice, it still interrupts the more rigid silica network and lowers the softening point of the glass. The role of alumina (Al_2O_3) in glass formation is complex. Alumina is not a true glass former, but it can take part in the glass network to alter the softening point and viscosity.

Pigmenting oxides are added to obtain the various shades needed to simulate natural teeth. These coloring pigments are produced by fusing metallic oxides with fine glass and feldspar and then regrinding to a powder. These powders are blended with the unpigmented powdered frit to provide the proper hue and chroma. Examples of metallic oxides and their respective color contributions to porcelain include iron or nickel oxide (brown); copper oxide (green); titanium oxide (yellowish brown); manganese oxide (lavender); and cobalt oxide (blue). Opacity may be

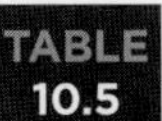

Composition and Properties of Typical Alloys for Metal–Ceramic Prostheses

	COMPONENTS AND PROPERTIES								
Alloy Product	Principal Elements	Noble Metal (wt%)	ADA Class	2% Proof Stress (MPa)	Elongation (%)	Hardness (VHN)	Elastic Modulus (GPa)	CTE (25–500°C) 10^{-6}/K	CTE (25–600°C) 10^{-6}/K
Brite Gold	Au–Pt–In	99.0	HN	230	15.0	100	79	14.8	15.0
Brite Gold XH	Au–Pt	97.9	HN	355–427	11.0	180	107	14.4	14.7
Golden Ceramic	Au–Pt–Pd	97.4	HN	360	12.0	165	64	14.6	14.7
Aquarius Hard	Au–Pt–Pd	97.2	HN	455	12.0	205	88	14.5	14.8
Aquarius	Au–Pt–In	97–98	HN	320	12.0	160	79	14.6	14.8
IPS d.SIGN 98	Au–Pt	98.0	HN	510	8.0	220	80	14.3	14.6
Y	Au–Pt–Pd	96.8	HN	320	12.0	160	81	14.6	14.8
Aquarius XH	Au–Pt–Pd	96.8	HN	510	7.0	220	83	14.1	14.4
Y-2	Au–Pt–Pd	94.6	HN	380	12.0	155	83	15.0	15.1
Y-Lite	Au–Pd–Ag	93.8	HN	500	14.0	225	88	13.9	14.1
Sagittarius	Au–Pd–Pt	95.8	HN	580	10.0	245	94	14.0	14.3
Y-1	Au–Pd–Pt	87.4	HN	340	15.0	185	99	14.8	15.0
IPS d.SIGN 96	Au–Pd–Pt	87.7	HN	405	15.0	214	92	14.3	14.5
IPS d.SIGN 91	Au–Pd–In	90.6	HN	570	31.0	250	136	14.2	14.4
W	Au–Pd–Ag	80.4	HN	455	21.0	220	113	14.2	14.5
W-5	Au–Pd–Ag	78.2	HN	530	20.0	255	118	14.0	14.2
Lodestar	Au–Pd–In	90.0	HN	495	20.0	240	98	14.1	14.3
W-3	Au–Pd–In	88.3	HN	495	17.0	225	128	13.9	14.1
W-2	Au–Pd–Ag	85.3	HN	640	20.0	205	113	14.2	14.6
Evolution Lite	Au–Pd–In–Ag	89.6	HN	375	11.0	280	130	14.2	14.5
Capricorn	Pd–In–Ga–Au	84.1	N	525	21.0	260	101	14.3	14.5
IPS d.SIGN 84	Pd–In–Au–Ag	84.2	N	485	29.0	295	117	13.8	14.0
IPS d.SIGN 67	Pd–Ag–Sn–Au	66.7	N	545	15.0	240	104	13.9	14.2
Spartan Plus	Pd–Cu–Ga–Au	80.8	N	795	20.0	310	97	14.3	14.6
Capricorn 15	Pd–Ag–Au–Pd	66.9	N	490	21.0	255	101	14.3	14.5
Aries	Pd–Ag–Sn	63.7	N	415	46.0	185	98	14.7	14.8
IPS d.SIGN 59	Pd–Ag–Sn	59.2	N	490	14.0	230	139	14.5	14.8
IPS d.SIGN 53	Pd–Ag–Sn–In	53.8	N	545	13.0	250	132	14.8	14.9
W-1	Pd–Ag–Sn	53.3	N	485	11.0	240	114	15.2	15.4
Calisto CP+	Co–Pd–Cr–Mo	25.0	N	640	10.0	365	180	14.4	14.9
Pisces Plus	Ni–Cr–W	0	PB	600	10.0	280	183	14.1	14.4
IPS d.SIGN 15	Ni–Cr–Mo	0	PB	340	13.0	200	200	13.9	14.2
IPS d.SIGN 30	Co–Cr–Mo	0	PB	520	6.0	375	234	14.5	14.7

achieved by the addition of cerium oxide, zirconium oxide, titanium oxide, or tin oxide.

Medium- and high-fusing porcelains are used for the production of denture teeth. The low-fusing and ultralow-fusing types are used as veneering ceramics for crown and bridge construction. Some of the ultralow-fusing porcelains are used for titanium and titanium alloys because of their low-contraction coefficients that closely match those of the metals and because the low firing temperatures reduce the risk for growth of the metal oxide. However, some of these ultralow-fusing porcelains contain enough leucite to raise their CTC as high as those of conventional low-fusing porcelains.

To ensure adequate chemical durability, a self-glaze of porcelain is preferred to an add-on glaze. A thin external layer of glassy material is formed during a self-glaze firing procedure at a temperature and time that cause localized softening of the glass phase. The add-on glaze slurry material that is applied to the porcelain surface for an overglaze procedure contains more glass modifiers and thus has a lower firing temperature. However, a higher proportion of glass modifiers tend to reduce the resistance of the applied glazes to leaching by oral fluids.

Another important glass modifier is water, although it is not an intentional addition to dental porcelain. The hydronium ion, H_3O^+, can replace sodium or other metal ions in a ceramic that contains glass modifiers. This fact accounts for the phenomenon of "slow crack growth" of ceramics exposed to tensile stresses and moist environments. It also may account for the occasional long-term failure of porcelain restorations after several years of service.

Ceramic Processing Methods

The processing stages of the ceramic core for the production of ceramic prostheses are summarized in Table 10.4. The quality of the final ceramic prosthesis is dependent on each stage of the fabrication process. Machining or grinding of the core structure is of particular importance, since flaws or minute cracks can be introduced that can possibly be propagated to the point of fracture during subsequent intraoral stressing cycles. The use of computer-aided manufacture (CAM) processes is most likely to induce such damage, although ceramics with higher fracture toughness are less likely to sustain such damage. It is possible that subsequent sintering or veneering procedures can reduce the potential for crack propagation of cracks in the prostheses while in service. Although reheating tends to seal surface cracks, it does not necessarily "heal" subsurface cracks.

- **Veneered and stained:** Feldspathic porcelains that are used to make traditional MC restorations, some aluminous porcelains (Vitadur-N, Vitadur Alpha, Hi-Ceram), and pure alumina ceramic (Procera AllCeram) are condensed by vibration and sintered at high temperatures.
- **Hot-pressed ceramics** (IPS Empress, IPS Empress 2, Finesse All-Ceramic, and OPC-3G) are heated, injected under pressure into a mold, and then veneered or stained.
- **Cast and cerammed crowns**, such as Dicor, an obsolete glass–ceramic, were made using the lost-wax technique. The glass was cast into a mold, heat treated to form a glass–ceramic, and colored with shading porcelain and surface stains.
- For **slip-cast ceramics** (In-Ceram, ICS, In-Ceram Zirconia), a slurry of liquid and particles of either alumina, magnesia–alumina silicate (spinel), or zirconia and alumina are placed on a dry refractory die that draws out the water from the slurry. The slip-cast deposit is sintered on this die, which creates a porous coping. This is then coated with a slurry of a glass-phase layer. During firing, the glass melts and infiltrates the porous ceramic core. Translucent porcelain veneers are then fired onto the core to provide final contour and color.
- For **CAD–CAM** processes, the ceramic block materials (Dicor MGC, VITA Cerec Mk I, and VITA Cerec Mk II) are shaped into inlays, onlays, or crowns using a CAD–CAM system (Cerec). *CAM* refers to computer-aided machining (or milling). These blocks can also be used in copy-milling devices (Celay) that mill or machine blocks into core shapes in a manner similar to that for cutting a key from a key blank—that is, by tracing over a master die of the shape to be produced out of the ceramic. CAD–CAM processing is described further in the section "All-Ceramic Systems."

CRITICAL QUESTION

How is the degree of sintering controlled and what parameter defines complete sintering?

Fabrication of Metal–Ceramic Prostheses

The MC restoration shown schematically in Figure 10.5 has a facial metal thickness of 0.3–0.5 mm. It is veneered with opaque porcelain approximately 0.3 mm in thickness. The body porcelain is about 1 mm thick.

Since a ductile metal is used as an inner core of an MC crown, cracks will not propagate in the metal, but they can progress through the veneering ceramic or within the interfacial region. With proper design and physical properties of the porcelain and metal, the porcelain is protected by a residual compressive stress so that brittle fracture of the veneer can be avoided or at least minimized. Although most MC restorations involve cast metal copings, several novel noncast approaches (electrodeposition, milling, swaging, and burnishing) for the fabrication of metal substructures have been developed in recent years. The fracture resistance of MC prostheses made from these core metals is less reliable compared with those made from traditional cast metal copings and frameworks.

CRITICAL QUESTION

What condition is required of cast metals to achieve ionic and/or covalent bonding to veneering porcelain?

Cast Metal for Metal–Ceramic Prostheses

The development of the MC restoration was the result of advances in the formulation of both alloys and porcelains. To bond to alloys suitable for the copings, porcelains must have a sufficiently low sintering temperature and they also must have CTEs and CTCs that are closely matched to those of the alloys.

A metal oxide is necessary to promote chemical bonding. The gold alloys developed for porcelain bonding have higher melting ranges than typical gold alloys for all-metal prostheses; the higher melting ranges are necessary to prevent sag, creep, or melting of the coping or framework during the sintering and/or glazing of porcelain. These gold alloys contain small amounts (about 1%) of base metals such as iron, indium, and tin, as discussed in Chapter 9. A wide range of high-noble and noble alloys is summarized in Table 10.5. The base metals form a surface oxide layer during the oxidation treatment, and this surface oxide is responsible for development of a bond with porcelain. This process is sometimes called degassing, which is a misnomer, because the primary purpose is to produce an adherent metal oxide on the surface to facilitate bonding to porcelain. This porcelain–metal bond is primarily ionic and chemical in nature and is capable of forming even when the metal surface is smooth and little opportunity exists for mechanical interlocking. The chemical bonding may be primarily ionic but is likely to have a covalent component as well.

CRITICAL QUESTION

Why should a metal coping or framework have a higher expansion coefficient than its veneering porcelain?

The alloys and porcelains used for the construction of such restorations have a number of stringent requirements. For example, the metal framework must not melt during porcelain firing and also must resist high-temperature "sag" deformation. Sag or flexural creep occurs only at high temperatures. It does not occur at oral temperatures. Both the metal and the ceramic must have CTE and CTC that are closely matched such that the metal must have a slightly higher value to avoid the development of undesirable residual tensile stresses in the porcelain. If the contraction coefficients are not nearly equal, stresses may occur that weaken both the porcelain and the bond. For example, a difference in the CTC of 1.7×10^{-6}/K can produce a shear stress of 280 MPa in porcelain next to the metal–porcelain interface when the porcelain is cooled from 954°C to room temperature. Because the shear resistance to failure is far less than 280 MPa, these thermal stresses would likely cause spontaneous bond failure or cracking of the veneering ceramic.

High tensile stresses in the veneering ceramic develop from a contraction coefficient mismatch between alloy and porcelain in which the porcelain contracts more than the metal. The tensile stresses induced within the restoration by occlusal forces would be added to the residual thermal tensile stresses. However, for metal–porcelain systems that have an average contraction coefficient difference of 0.5×10^{-6}/K or less (between 600°C and room temperature), fracture is unlikely to occur except in cases of extreme stress concentration or extremely high intraoral forces. These are known as *thermally compatible systems.* Many restorations made from metal and porcelain combinations having contraction coefficient differences between 0.5 and 1.0×10^{-6}/K are known to survive for many years. These results are explainable by survival probability analyses, which assume that the maximum biting force on anterior crowns rarely exceeds 890 N (200 lb) and the maximum force on posterior crowns rarely exceeds 2224 N (500 lb). However, the *Guinness Book of Records* (1993) cites the maximum clenching force ever recorded for posterior teeth as 4337 N (975 lb) sustained for 2 seconds. The second highest bite force ever recorded was 2447 N (550 lb). Most patients generate typical bite forces of 400–800 N (90–180 lb) between molar teeth and much lower forces between premolars and between anterior teeth. Thus, a rather small number of patients have bite force capabilities likely to cause fracture of MC crowns or bridges even when residual thermal incompatibility stresses are present. As a rule, lower forces are generated by younger children, female patients, a more closed bite, occlusion between natural teeth, a complete denture, and an FDP. Chipping fractures have been reported at greater frequencies in veneers of zirconia prostheses compared with MC prostheses. There are several possible causes, including thermal incompatibility, inadequate substrate design, and contact (Hertzian) stresses.

Another equally important property of MC systems is the relatively high proportional limit and high modulus of elasticity of these materials. Alloys with a high modulus of elasticity share a greater proportion of stress than the adjacent porcelain.

Technical Aspects of Metal–Ceramic Products

Cast Metal Copings and Frameworks

Copings and frameworks for MC prostheses are produced by casting of molten metal, CAD–CAM machining, electrolytic deposition techniques, or swaged metal processes. The most common method is the melting and casting of specialized metals, and this process is highlighted as the principal process in this chapter. For the casting process, the relatively high melting temperatures of most alloys can break down gypsum-bonded investments at the casting temperatures, so the more refractory phosphate-bonded investment must be used.

Each casting should be carefully cleaned to ensure a strong bond to the porcelain. For example, an alloy such as Olympia (Heraeus Kulzer), a gold–palladium, silver-free alloy, is heated in the porcelain furnace to a temperature of 1038°C to burn off any remaining impurities to form a thin oxide layer. This so-called degassing treatment does not actually degas the interior structure of the alloy. Instead, it produces an oxide layer on the alloy surface that is essential for the formation of the porcelain–metal bond.

The need for a clean metal surface cannot be overemphasized. Metal oxidation is necessary for all gold–porcelain systems. Oil from fingers and other sources such as air lines represents a possible contaminant. The surface may be cleansed adequately by finishing with clean ceramic-bonded stones or sintered diamonds, which are used exclusively for finishing. Final sandblasting with high-purity alumina abrasive before oxidation ensures that the porcelain will be bonded to a clean and mechanically retentive surface.

Frameworks for MC bridges must be designed such that the framework will not be deformed at porcelain sintering temperatures, and the connectors must be large enough to resist flexural strains that may cause cracking under intraoral loading.

Opaque porcelain is condensed on the oxidized surface at a thickness of approximately 0.3 mm (see Fig. 10.5) and is then fired to its sintering temperature. Translucent porcelain is then applied, and the tooth form is created. Porcelain powder is applied by the condensation methods previously described. The unit is again fired. Several cycles of porcelain application and firing may be necessary to complete the restoration. A final glaze is then produced either by self-glazing (Fig. 10.8) or firing an overglaze layer.

CRITICAL QUESTION

True or false? Creep deformation of a high-noble alloy framework for a four-unit bridge occurs at an elevated temperature and continues to increase as the framework cools rapidly to room temperature.

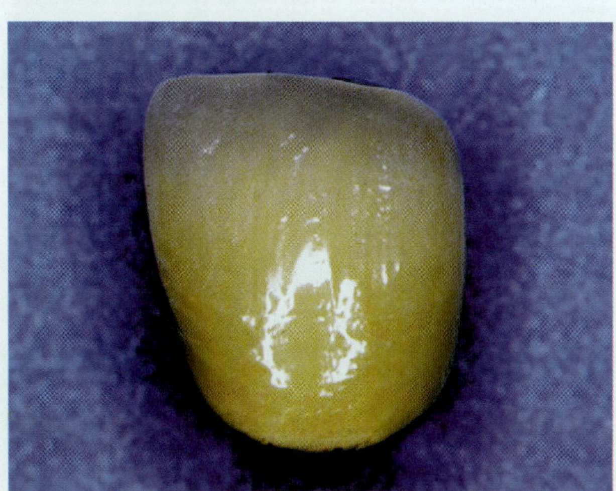

• **Fig. 10.8** Autoglazed veneer ceramic.

Creep or Sag

Creep can be reduced if the metal has the proper composition, so that a dispersion strengthening effect occurs at an elevated temperature. When certain gold alloys are heated to approximately 980°C, a second phase is precipitated that can harden or strengthen the alloy. Such creep has been reduced in some of the commercial alloys, but it apparently cannot be eliminated. The solidus temperature (the lower end of the melting range) of base metal alloys, such as nickel–chromium, is higher than that of gold alloys; hence, base metal alloys are less susceptible to sag deformation than are gold-based alloys. High-temperature *creep* or *sag* of some high-noble and noble alloys occurs when the temperature approaches 980°C. Once the alloy temperature decreases by 100°C or more, no further creep deformation occurs. For "high-noble" yellow-hued alloys, the spans of fixed partial dentures should not exceed three units, since the mass of the prosthesis may increase the bending stress to the point where permanent deformation occurs at the porcelain sintering temperature.

CRITICAL QUESTION

True or false? The marginal adaptation and fit of a cast crown are equivalent to those of a swaged foil crown.

Metal–Ceramic Crowns and Bridges Based on Swaged Metal Foil Laminates

The most widely used product of this type has been Captek (Precious Chemicals Co., Inc., Altamonte Springs, FL), which is an acronym for "capillary assisted technology." The product is designed to fabricate the metal coping of an MC crown without the use of a melting and casting process. It is a laminated gold alloy foil sold as a metal strip. Strips of P (Au–Pt–Pd) and G (Au–Ag) metals are applied to a die with a swaging instrument, burnished with a hand instrument or a "P-Press" on the die, and then heated sequentially (P layer followed by the G layer) in a porcelain oven to form a coping with moderate strength. A "bonder" layer is applied and fired, the coping is then veneered with condensed porcelain, and the porcelain is sintered at typical porcelain firing temperatures. Examples of Captek components and a finished bridge are shown in Figure 10.9. For bridges, the pontics are made typically from a palladium-based alloy that is gold coated. The technology is based on the principle of capillary action to produce a gold-based composite metal. Captek P and G metals can yield thin metal copings for crowns or frameworks for MC bridges. The maximal span length recommended for Captek–porcelain bridges is 18 mm, which allows space for up to two pontics. The completed metal coping or framework is a composite metal structure consisting of a gold matrix and small particles of a Pt–Pd–Au alloy with a resulting grain size in the range of 15–20 μm. The outer surfaces of the copings contain approximately 97% gold.

The process begins with the preparation of a master refractory die that replicates the prepared tooth. The original gypsum die is sprayed with a surface tension–reducing agent to facilitate flow of the impression material and to reduce bubble formation. Die spacer is applied and undercuts are blocked out. The master die is placed in a duplication flask and silicone impression material is poured into the flask and around the master die. The resulting master impression (mold) is poured with a refractory material (Capvest) to produce a refractory die. The die is heat treated, and the margins are marked with a red pencil. Captek adhesive is applied to the die to enhance adhesion to the Captek metal and to enhance capillary action.

After heat treatment, Captek P metal, a malleable Au–Pt–Pd alloy, is adapted to the surface. This metal layer provides a three-dimensional capillary network that will subsequently be filled with Captek G metal (97.5% Au, 2.5% Ag by weight) to form an alloy with a high gold content. After this composite material is burnished on the die and the margins are trimmed, it is sintered in a porcelain furnace. The metal copings and Pd–Ag pontics (if needed) are then coated with a slurry of Au, Pt, and Pd powder (Capbond) and liquid, resulting in a thin coating of gold to

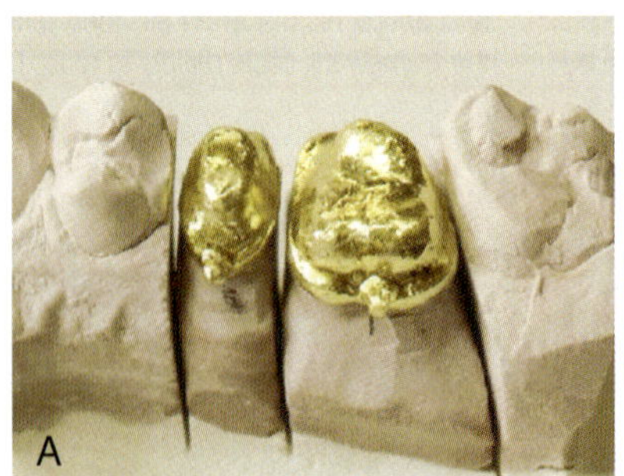

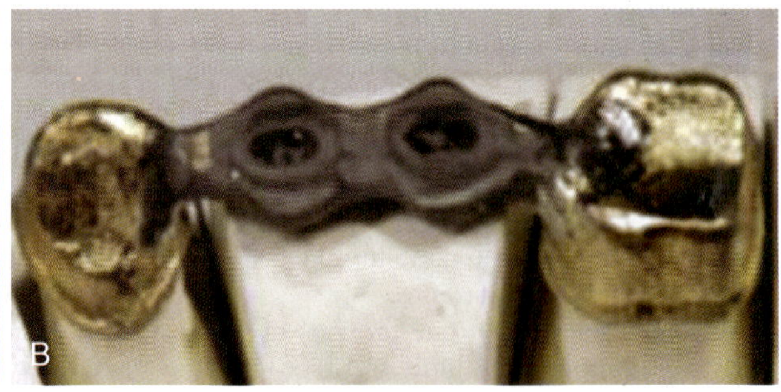

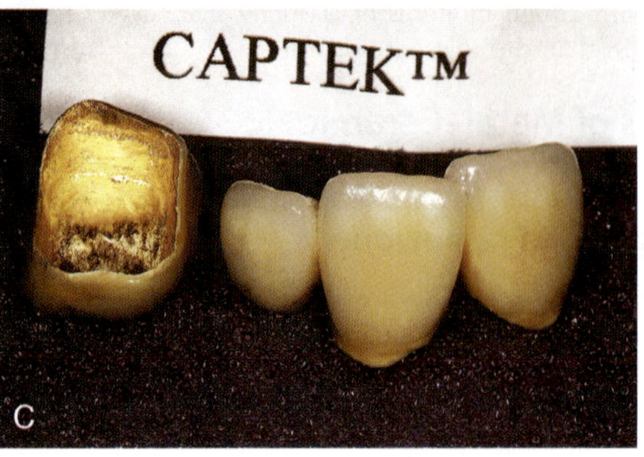

• **Fig. 10.9** **(A)** Captek noble metal copings. **(B)** Pontic section attached to two noble metal copings. **(C)** Interior surface of finished Captek crown (*left*) and finished three-unit FDP (*right*). Captek three-unit bridge.

enhance areas of Captek P that have been ground during adjustment and to provide a gold color similar to that of areas that have not been ground. The completed copings have a thickness of approximately 0.25 mm. Thus, this method provides thinner metal copings than those (0.50 mm) typically produced by the cast metal process. The metal surfaces are veneered with two thin coats of an opaque porcelain and additional layers of translucent porcelains.

Compared with cast metal margins formed from the lost-wax process, the accuracy of marginal adaptation for Captek crowns is highly dependent on the skill of the dental technician in trimming the burnished metal copings. In addition, the atomic bonding of veneering ceramics to Captek copings and frameworks is controlled by a special bonder layer, while bonding of ceramics to cast metal is controlled by oxidizable elements within the alloy surface. Another potential concern for the Captek system is the difficulty of bonding the dissimilar metals in the coping and the pontic surfaces. Clinical data for Captek crowns and bridges are very limited. Thus, caution must be exercised in using this system for crowns and bridges in high-stress areas.

Porcelain Condensation

Porcelain for ceramic and MC prostheses as well as for other applications is supplied as a fine powder designed to be mixed with water or another liquid and condensed into the desired form. The powder particles are of a particular size distribution to produce the most densely packed porcelain when they are properly condensed. If the particles are of the same size, the density of packing would not be nearly as high. Proper and thorough condensation is also crucial in obtaining dense packing of the powder particles. This provides two benefits: lower firing shrinkage and less porosity in the fired porcelain. This packing, or condensation, may be achieved by various methods, including the vibration, spatulation, and brush techniques.

- The first method uses mild vibration to pack the wet powder densely on the underlying framework. The excess water is blotted away with a clean tissue and condensation occurs toward the blotted area.
- In the second method, a small spatula is used to apply and smooth the wet porcelain. This smoothing action brings the excess water to the surface, where it is removed.
- The third method employs the addition of dry porcelain powder to the surface to absorb the water. The dry powder is placed by a brush to the side opposite from an increment of wet porcelain. As the water is drawn toward the dry powder, the wet particles are pulled together.

Whichever method is used, it is important to remember that the surface tension of the water is the driving force in condensation and that the porcelain must not be allowed to dry out until condensation is complete.

Sintering Procedure

The thermochemical reactions between the porcelain powder components are virtually completed during the original manufacturing process. Thus, the purpose of firing is to sinter the particles of powder together properly for a specific time and temperature combination to form the prosthesis. Some chemical reactions occur during prolonged firing times or multiple firings. Of particular importance are the observed changes in the leucite content of the porcelains designed for fabrication of MC restorations. As stated earlier, leucite is a high-expansion and high-contraction crystal phase whose volume fraction in the glass matrix can greatly affect the CTC of the porcelain. Changes in the leucite content can cause the development of a CTC mismatch between the porcelain and the metal and thus can produce stresses during cooling that are sufficient to cause crack formation in the porcelain.

The condensed porcelain mass is placed in front of or below the muffle of a preheated furnace at approximately 650°C for low-fusing porcelain. This preheating procedure permits the remaining water to evaporate. Placement of the condensed mass directly into even a moderately warm furnace results in a rapid production of steam, thereby introducing voids or fracturing large sections of the veneer. After preheating for approximately 5 minutes, the porcelain is placed into the furnace and the firing cycle is initiated.

The size of the powder particles influences not only the degree of condensation of the porcelain but also the soundness or apparent density of the final product. At the initial firing temperature, the voids are occupied by the atmosphere of the furnace. As sintering of the particles begins, the porcelain particles bond at their points of contact and the structure shrinks and densifies. As the temperature is raised, the sintered glass gradually flows to fill the air spaces. However, air becomes trapped in the form of voids because the fused mass is too viscous to allow all of the air to escape. An aid in the reduction of porosity in dental porcelain is *vacuum firing*. Complete sintering is accomplished when the structure achieves 100% of its theoretical density. However, this is unlikely to occur even in the presence of a vacuum, since it is very unlikely that all porosity will be eliminated under typical dental sintering conditions.

Vacuum firing reduces porosity in the following way. When the porcelain is placed into the furnace, the powder particles are packed together with air channels around them. As the air pressure inside the furnace muffle is reduced to about one-tenth of atmospheric pressure by the vacuum pump, the air around the particles is also reduced to this pressure. As the temperature rises, the particles sinter together, and closed pores are formed within the porcelain mass. The air inside these pores is isolated from the furnace atmosphere. At a temperature about 55°C below the sintering temperature, the vacuum is released and the pressure inside the furnace increases by a factor of 10, from 0.1 to 1 atm. Because the pressure is increased by a factor of 10, the pores are compressed to one-tenth of their original size, and the total volume of porosity is accordingly reduced. Not all of the air can be evacuated from the furnace. Therefore, a few bubbles are present, but they are markedly smaller than those obtained with the usual air-firing method. At a condition of 95%–99% theoretical density, the dental veneering ceramic is claimed to be mature or fully sintered. A list of some veneering ceramics for MC prostheses is given in Table 10.6.

Cooling

The proper cooling of a porcelain-veneered prosthesis from its firing temperature to room temperature is the subject of considerable importance. The catastrophic fracture of glass that has been subjected to sudden changes in temperature is a sufficiently familiar experience so that most lab technicians are cautious about exposing dental porcelain to extremely rapid cooling (thermal shock) after firing. The cooling of dental porcelain, however, is a complex matter, particularly when the porcelain is bonded to a metallic substrate. Multiple firings of a **metal–ceramic prosthesis** can cause the CTC of the leucite-containing porcelain to increase and actually make it more likely to crack or craze because of tensile stress development.

TABLE 10.6 Veneering Ceramics for Metal–Ceramic Prostheses

Veneering Ceramic	Compatible Alloys	Manufacturer
Synspar	Most alloys	Jeneric/Pentron
Pencraft Plus	Most alloys	Jeneric/Pentron
Finesse Low Fusing	Most alloys	DENTSPLY Ceramco
Ceramco II	Most alloys	DENTSPLY Ceramco
Ceramco II Silver	Silver-containing alloys	DENTSPLY Ceramco
Ceramco 3	Most alloys	DENTSPLY Ceramco
Duceragold (hydrothermal)	Degunorm type IV gold alloy for metal–ceramics	Degussa
SymbioCeram (hydrothermal)	Most alloys	Degussa
Duceram Plus	Most alloys	Degussa
Duceram LFC	Most alloys	Degussa
Excelsior	Most alloys	Ney
Porcelfina	Most alloys	Ney
IPS d.SIGN	Most alloys	Ivoclar Vivadent Inc.
IPS Classic V	Most alloys	Ivoclar Vivadent Inc.
VITA Response	Degunorm (Degussa) and Mainbond A (Heraeus), type IV gold alloys for metal–ceramics	VITA Zahnfabrik
VITA VMK 95	Most alloys	VITA Zahnfabrik
VITA Omega	Most alloys	VITA Zahnfabrik
VITA Omega 900 (low-fusing)	Most alloys	VITA Zahnfabrik

CRITICAL QUESTION

What three conditions control the durability of ceramic bonding to an oxidized metal coping?

Bonding Porcelain to Metal

The primary requirement for the success of an MC restoration is the development of a durable bond between the porcelain and the metal oxide. For an MC bond to be maintained over time, there should be minimal residual tensile stresses in the porcelain after cooling from the sintering temperature. An unfavorable stress distribution during the cooling process can result in immediate or delayed cracking of the porcelain. Thus, for a successful MC restoration to be achieved, both a strong interface bond and thermal compatibility are required.

Three factors control the durability of MC bonding: (1) mechanical interlocking or interatomic bonding at the interface between porcelain and the metal oxide; (2) interatomic bonding across the oxide–porcelain interface; and (3) the type and magnitude of residual stress in the veneering ceramic. Atomic or chemical bonding is primarily responsible for metal–porcelain adherence. However, there is some evidence to support MC bonding through a mechanical interlocking mechanism. One Pd–Ag alloy formed an internal oxide but not an external oxide. However, metal nodules were formed on the surface via a creep mechanism. These nodules presumably provided sufficient mechanical retention of porcelain for clinical use, since this alloy has been used for many years without noted problems.

The oxidation behavior of these alloys largely determines their potential for bonding with porcelain. Research into the nature of metal–porcelain adherence has indicated that those alloys that form adherent oxides during the oxidation cycle also form a good bond to porcelain, whereas those alloys with poorly adherent oxides or poor wetting porcelain to the oxide (Fig. 10.10) form poor bonds.

Glazes and Stain Ceramics

CRITICAL QUESTION

How should the strength of a ceramic three-unit FDP with a polished and glazed porcelain veneer compare with that of an FDP with a highly polished veneer without a glazed surface?

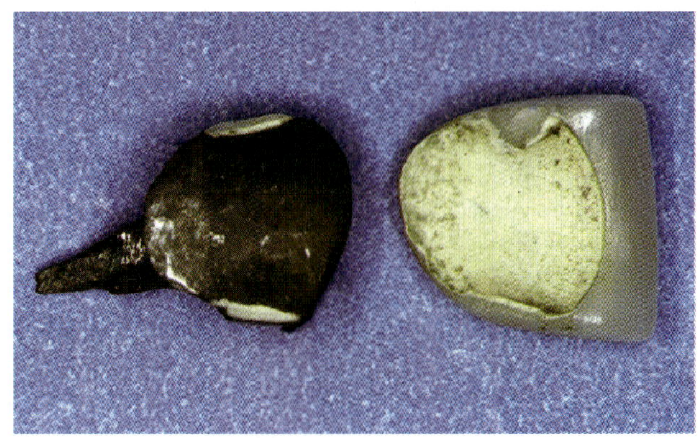

• **Fig. 10.10** Bond failure of metal–ceramic post and core prosthesis.

The esthetics of porcelains for MC and ceramic prostheses, veneers, and denture teeth may be enhanced through the application of stains and glazes to provide a more life-like appearance and color match to adjacent teeth or restorations. The fusing temperatures of glazes are reduced by the addition of glass modifiers, typically alkali oxides, which reduce the chemical durability of glazes. Stains are simply tinted glazes that are also exposed to the same chemical durability problems. However, most of the currently available glazes appear to have adequate durability when they are produced in thicknesses of 50 μm or more.

One method for ensuring that the applied characterizing stains will be permanent is to use them internally. Internal staining and characterization can produce a life-like result, particularly when simulated enamel craze lines and other features are built into the porcelain rather than merely applied on the surface. The disadvantage of internal staining and characterization is that the porcelain must be stripped completely if the color or characterization is unacceptable.

Autoglazed feldspathic porcelain is stronger than unglazed porcelain. The glaze is effective in sealing surface flaws and reducing stress concentrations. Shown in Figure 10.8 is an MC crown with a properly fired autoglazed porcelain surface. If the glaze is removed by grinding, the transverse strength may be only half that of the sample with the glaze layer intact. However, some studies indicate that porcelains with highly polished surfaces have strengths comparable to those of specimens that were polished and glazed. This observation is of clinical importance. After the porcelain restoration is cemented in the mouth, it is common practice for the dentist to adjust the occlusion by grinding the surface of the porcelain with a diamond bur. This procedure can weaken the porcelain if the glaze is removed and the surface is left in a rough condition. This can cause increased wear of enamel. For this condition, an acceptable solution is to polish the surface with Sof-Lex (3M, Minneapolis, MN) finishing disks, a Shofu (Shofu, Kyoto, Japan) porcelain laminate polishing kit, or other abrasive system. A smoother surface also reduces the abrasion damage caused to opposing teeth or restorations.

It is generally believed that glazing of feldspathic porcelain eliminates surface flaws and produces a smoother surface. However, an optimal method of producing the smoothest surface in the shortest time has not been established. It is logical to assume that fine polishing of a roughened surface followed by glazing produces smoother surfaces than polishing alone, sandblasting followed by glazing, or diamond grinding followed by glazing. However, even though one polishes and/or glazes a porcelain veneer surface, the surface will either slowly or markedly break down in the presence of solvents in our everyday diets, which include citric acid, acetic acid, and alkalis. Further degradation will occur during exposure of glass-phase ceramics such as porcelain to acidulated phosphate fluoride (APF) gel, as shown in Figure 10.11.

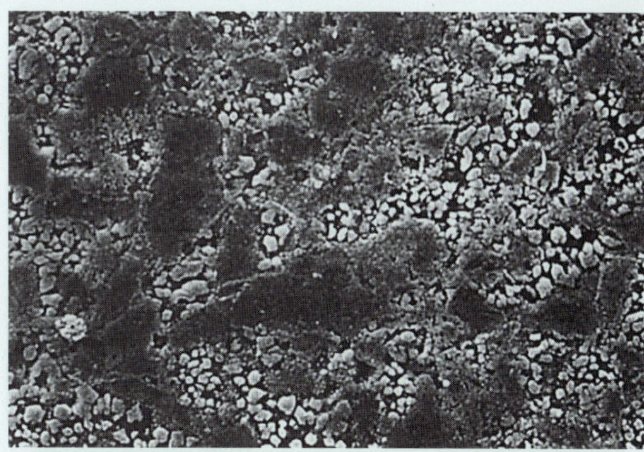

• **Fig. 10.11** Surface of feldspathic gingival (body) porcelain after a 30-minute exposure to 1.23% acidulated phosphate fluoride. Most of the degradation has occurred in the glass matrix rather than in the crystal phase.

Benefits and Drawbacks of Metal–Ceramic Restorations Compared with All-Ceramic Restorations

A properly made MC crown is more fracture resistant and durable than most all-ceramic crowns and bridges. This technology is well established compared with technologies required of the most recent all-ceramic products. Although the biocompatibility of some metals used for copings and frameworks may be a concern for patients who have known allergies to those metals, these situations are rare. A metal coping or framework provides an advantage compared with zirconia-based ceramic prostheses when endodontic access openings through crowns are required. Temporary repairs for ceramic fractures that extend to the metal framework are possible without the need for intraoral sandblasting treatment by using current resin bonding agents. All-ceramic crowns may be more susceptible to chipping fracture and to bulk fracture in posterior sites. Fractures of ceramic connectors represent another disadvantage of all-ceramic prostheses, especially when the manufacturers' recommendations for connector shape and size cannot be satisfied because of limited space. Overall, the esthetic appearance of an all-ceramic restoration is generally superior to that of an MC restoration for anterior as well as posterior situations (Fig. 10.12A and B However, properly designed MC crowns are highly esthetic when adequate tooth reduction principles are satisfied. In addition, metal coping designs such as those with thinner facial metal (0.1–0.5 mm) and/or knife-edge facial metal margins or collarless metal margins can further enhance the esthetic potential of these anterior crowns.

CRITICAL QUESTION

What causes stress concentrations? How can they promote fracture of all-ceramic prostheses in the presence of low occlusal forces?

Methods for Strengthening Ceramics

Minimizing the Effect of Stress Concentrations

Why do dental ceramic prostheses fail to exhibit the strengths that we would expect from the high interatomic bond forces? The answer is that numerous minute scratches and other flaws are present on the surfaces of these materials. These surface flaws behave as sharp slits whose tips may be as narrow as the spacing between several atoms in the material. Under intraoral loading, tensile stresses that develop within the ceramic structure are greatly increased and concentrated at the tips of these flaws. This stress concentration geometry at the tip of each surface flaw can increase the localized stress to extremely high levels even though a relatively low average stress exists throughout the bulk of the structure. When the induced tensile stress exceeds the nominal strength of the material structure, the bonds at the notch tip rupture, forming a crack. This stress concentration phenomenon explains how materials fail at stresses far below their theoretical

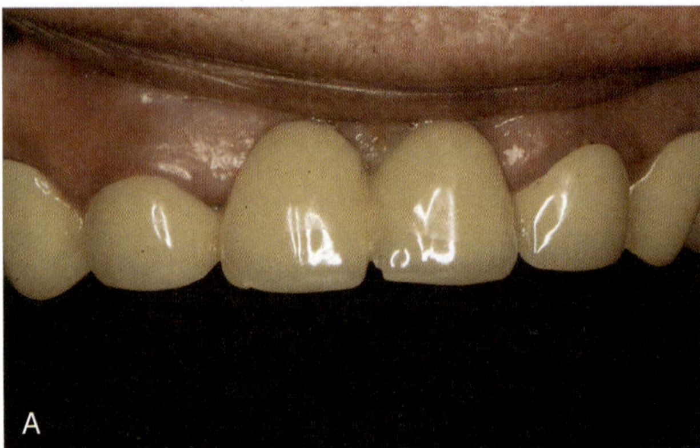

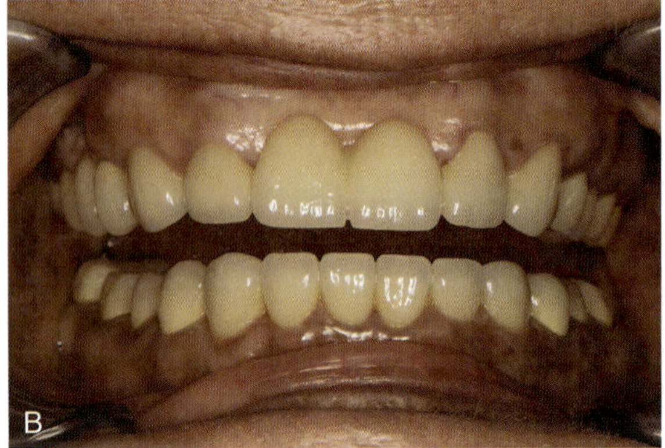

• **Fig. 10.12 (A)** Full mouth rehabilitation showing poorly fabricated metal–ceramic restorations. **(B)** All-Ceramic restorations showing a higher degree of esthetics.

strength. However, there are other variables that affect the magnitude of these stresses, including prosthesis design, load orientation, loading rate, microstructure, and residual processing stresses. These variables are discussed in other chapters.

Stress raisers are discontinuities in ceramic structures and in other brittle materials that cause a stress concentration in these areas. The design of ceramic dental restorations should be carefully planned with sufficient bulk and a minimum of sharp angular changes to avoid stress raisers in the ceramic. *Abrupt changes in shape or thickness in the ceramic contour can act as stress raisers and make the restoration more prone to failure.* For example, the **incisal** line angles on an anterior tooth prepared for a ceramic crown should be well rounded and the occlusal reduction for molar teeth should provide sufficient bulk for the ceramic product under consideration.

The brittle fracture behavior of ceramics and their low tensile strengths compared with those predicted from bonds between atoms can be understood by considering stress concentration around surface flaws. Because ceramics, unlike metals, tend to have no mechanism for yielding to stress without fracture, cracks may propagate through a ceramic material at low average stress levels. As a result, ceramics and glasses have tensile strengths that are much lower than their compressive strengths. In the oral environment, tensile stresses are usually created by bending forces, and the maximal tensile stress created by the bending forces occurs within the surface of a restoration or prosthesis. It is for this reason that surface flaws are of particular importance in determining the strength of ceramics.

As the crack propagates through the material, the stress concentration is maintained at the crack tip unless the crack moves completely through the material or until it meets another crack, pore, or crystalline particle, which may reduce the localized stress. The removal of surface flaws or a reduction in their size and number can produce a very large increase in strength. Reducing the depth of surface flaws in the surface of a ceramic is one of the reasons that polishing and glazing of dental porcelain are so important.

The fracture resistance of ceramic prostheses can be increased through one or more of the following seven options:

1. Select stronger and tougher ceramics.
2. Develop residual compressive stresses within the surface of the material by thermal tempering.
3. Develop residual compressive stress within interfacial regions of weaker, less tough ceramic layers by properly matching coefficients of thermal expansion and contraction.
4. Reduce the tensile stress in the ceramic by appropriate selection of stiffer supporting materials (greater elastic moduli).
5. Minimize the number of firing cycles for feldspathic porcelains.
6. Design the ceramic prosthesis with greater bulk and broader radii of curvature for connectors in areas of potential tensile stress to minimize stress concentrations and the magnitude of tensile stresses that can develop during function.
7. Adhesively bond the ceramic crowns to the tooth structure.

In all-ceramic crowns, several conditions can produce stress concentrations. For Captek-type crowns, creases or folds of the platinum or gold foil substrate that become embedded in the porcelain leave notches that act as stress raisers. Sharp line angles in the preparation also create areas of stress concentration in the restoration. Shown in Figure 10.13 is an MC pontic that has fractured because of a poor framework design. Large changes in porcelain thickness, a factor that is also determined by the tooth preparation, can create areas of stress concentration.

A small particle of porcelain along the internal porcelain margin of a crown also induces locally high tensile stresses. A stray particle that is fused within the inner surface of a shoulder porcelain margin of an MC crown can cause localized tensile stress concentrations in porcelain when an occlusal force is applied to the crown.

Even though an MC restoration is generally more fracture resistant than most ceramic crowns of the same size and shape, care must be taken to avoid subjecting the porcelain in an MC prosthesis to loading that produces large localized stresses. If the occlusion is not adjusted properly on a porcelain surface, contact points rather than contact areas will greatly increase the localized stresses in the porcelain surface as well as within the internal surface of the crown. These contact stresses can lead to the formation of the

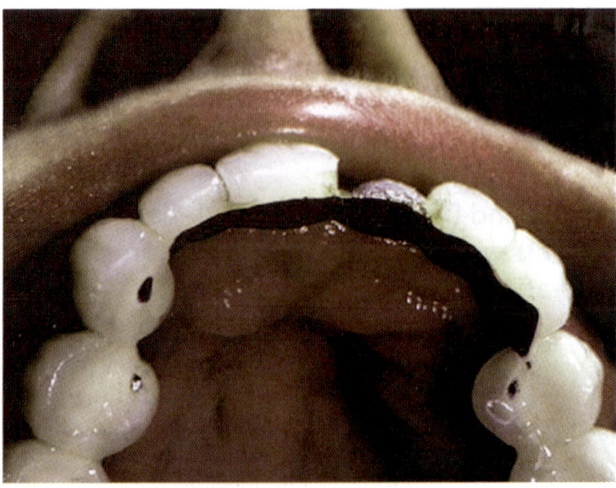

• **Fig. 10.13** Porcelain debonding from a metal pontic substrate of a long-span metal–ceramic bridge.

so-called Hertzian cone cracks, which may lead to chipping of the occlusal surface.

Fracture mechanics is a science that allows scientists to analyze the influence of flaw/stress interactions on the probability of crack propagation through an elastic, brittle solid. The principles of linear elastic fracture mechanics were developed in the 1950s by Irwin (1957). This pioneering research on fracture phenomena was based on earlier investigations by Griffith (1920) and Orowan (1944, 1949, 1955). Irwin found that when a brittle material was subjected to tensile stresses, specific crack shapes in certain locations were associated with greatly increased stress levels. He also recognized the importance of determining the fracture toughness of these materials as a measure of their ability to resist fracture. The fracture toughness (K_{Ic}) of a material represents the resistance of a material to rapid crack propagation in a stress field. In contrast, the strength of a material depends primarily on the size of the initiating crack that is present. The strength of dental ceramics and other restorative materials is controlled by the size of the cracks or defects that are introduced during processing, production, and handling. In this chapter a description is given of the processing methods used to produce ceramic prostheses and the potential of these methods to introduce flaws or cracks that may limit their clinical survival.

CRITICAL QUESTION

True or false? Residual compressive stress develops in the veneering ceramic of an all-ceramic crown in the same way as it does in an MC crown.

Development of Residual Compressive Stresses

The fabrication of MC and all-ceramic prostheses usually involves sintering the ceramic at high temperature or hot pressing a veneering ceramic onto the metal or core ceramic. The process of cooling to room temperature offers the opportunity to take advantage of mismatches in CTC of adjacent materials in the ceramic structure. However, if the porcelain veneer contracts more than the metal coping or framework, axial and hoop tensile stresses develop that can cause cracking of the ceramic (Fig. 10.14). Ideally, the ceramic veneer should sustain slight compression in the final restoration. As stated previously, a self-glazed surface layer can also set up compressive stress on cooling. Shown in Figure 10.15 is an overglazed glass–ceramic three-unit FDP.

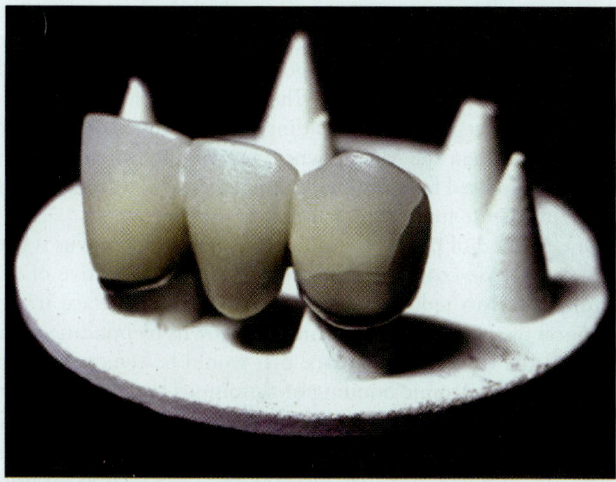

• **Fig. 10.14** Crack in metal–ceramic crown after cooling of a three-unit bridge.

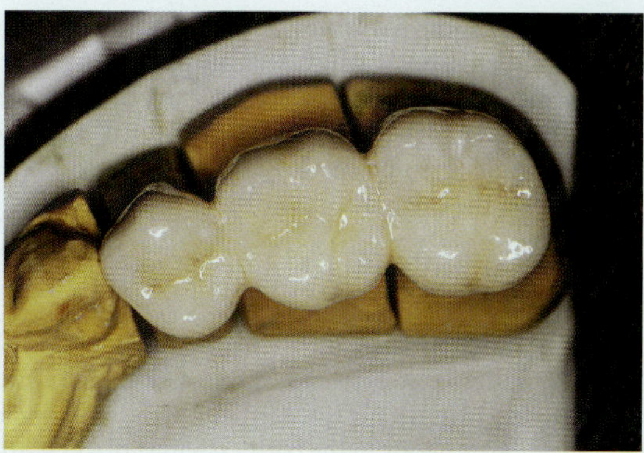

• **Fig. 10.15** Overglazed surface on the veneering ceramic of a three-unit FPD produced with a lithia disilicate–based glass–ceramic framework.

To prevent fracture of a ceramic prosthesis, one must prevent tensile stresses from occurring. Of course, this is an unrealistic requirement. Instead, if one could produce a significant amount of compressive stress in the area of the ceramic structure, a greater level of offsetting tensile stress would need to be developed during oral function for the prosthesis to reach the tensile stress needed to cause fracture. One method of introducing residual compressive stresses within the ceramic is to choose veneering ceramics whose thermal expansion or contraction coefficient is slightly less than that of the core ceramic.

Consider three layers of porcelain, the outer two of the same composition and CTC and the inner layer of a different composition with a higher CTC. Suppose that the layers were bonded together and the bonded structure was allowed to cool to room temperature. The inner layer would have a higher CTC and tend to contract more as it cooled. Thus, on cooling to room temperature, the inner layer would produce axial and hoop compressive stresses in the adjacent outer layer. In this way the protective compressive stress of the ceramic structure would increase its fracture resistance and survival probability.

Another procedure is to rapidly cool the prosthesis by removing the prosthesis and cooling it on the benchtop rather than slowly cooling the prosthesis in the furnace. This is especially useful for MC prostheses, since the thermal conductivity and diffusivity of metal lead to increased compression in the veneer.

We can apply the same principle to an MC system as well. The metal and porcelain should be selected with a slight mismatch in their CTC (the metal CTC being slightly higher) so that the metal contracts slightly more than the porcelain on cooling from the firing temperature to room temperature. This mismatch leaves the porcelain adjacent to the metal in a state of residual compression, which effectively protects the MC restoration against fracture of the veneering ceramic.

Minimizing the Number of Firing Cycles

The purpose of porcelain firing procedures is to densely sinter the particles of powder together and produce a relatively smooth, glassy layer (glaze) on the surface. In some cases, a stain layer is applied for shade adjustment or for characterization, such as stain lines or fine cracks. Several chemical reactions occur over time at porcelain firing temperatures; of particular importance are increases in the concentration of crystalline leucite in the porcelains designed for fabrication of MC restorations. Leucite, $K_2O{\cdot}Al_2O_3{\cdot}4SiO_2$, a high-expansion crystal phase, can increase the CTC of the porcelain. Changes in the leucite content caused by multiple firings can alter the CTC of some porcelain products. Some porcelains undergo an increase in leucite crystals after multiple firings, which will increase their CTE. If the expansion coefficient increases above that for the metal, the expansion mismatch between the porcelain and the metal can produce stresses during cooling sufficient to cause immediate or delayed crack formation in the porcelain.

Ion Exchange

The technique of ion exchange is an effective method of introducing residual compressive stresses into the surface of a ceramic. If a sodium-containing glass article is placed in a bath of molten potassium nitrate, potassium ions in the bath exchange places with some of the sodium ions in the surface of the glass article and remain in place after cooling. Since the potassium ion is about 35% larger than the sodium ion, the diffusion of the potassium ion into the place formerly occupied by the sodium ion creates residual compressive stresses in the surface. Increases of 100% or more in flexural strength of feldspathic porcelains have been achieved with several ion exchange products containing a significant concentration of small sodium ions. However, the depth of the compression zone is less than 100 μm. Therefore, this strengthening effect may be lost if the porcelain or glass–ceramic surface is ground, worn, or eroded by long-term exposure to certain inorganic acids.

Thermal Tempering

Perhaps the most common method for strengthening glasses is by thermal tempering, which creates residual surface compressive stresses by rapidly cooling the surface of the object while it is hot and in the softened (molten) state. This rapid cooling produces a skin of rigid glass surrounding a soft (molten) core. As the molten core solidifies, it tends to shrink, but the outer skin remains rigid. The pull of the solidifying molten core, as it shrinks, creates residual tensile stresses in the core and residual compressive stresses within the outer surface.

Thermal tempering is used to strengthen glass for uses such as automobile windows and windshields, sliding glass doors, and diving masks. Often the rapid cooling of the outer skin is accomplished by jets of air directed at the thermally softened glass surface. If one observes the rear window of an automobile through polarized sunglasses, one can see a regular pattern of spots over the entire window. This pattern of spots corresponds to the arrangement of the air jets employed by the manufacturer in the tempering process. For dental applications, it is more effective to quench hot glass-phase ceramics in silicone oil or other special liquids rather than using air jets that may not uniformly cool the surface. This thermal tempering treatment induces a protective region of compressive stress within the surface. However, this process is technique sensitive, since large counterbalancing tensile stresses may develop when excessive cooling rates occur during the tempering process.

Dispersion Strengthening and Toughening

Reinforcement of ceramics with a dispersed phase of a different material can prevent or inhibit propagation of cracks. This process is referred to as dispersion strengthening. When small, tough crystals are homogeneously distributed in a glass, the ceramic structure is toughened and strengthened because cracks cannot penetrate the fine particles as easily as the glass. This technique was applied many years ago in the development of aluminous porcelains (in which Al_2O_3 particles were dispersed in a glassy porcelain matrix) for all-porcelain crowns. Many current dental veneering ceramics have a glassy matrix that is reinforced by a dispersed crystal phase. Glass matrices in dental ceramics have been strengthened and toughened by a variety of dispersed crystalline phases including leucite, lithia disilicate, alumina, and tetrasilicic fluormica.

Almost all of the modern higher strength ceramics derive their improved fracture resistance from the crack-blocking ability of the crystalline particles. Hot-pressed core ceramics and veneering glass–ceramics contain a glass phase strengthened with crystalline particles of leucite ($K_2O{\cdot}Al_2O_3{\cdot}4SiO_2$), lithia disilicate ($Li_2O{\cdot}2SiO_2$), alumina ($Al_2O_3$), magnesia–alumina spinel ($MgO{\cdot}Al_2O_3$), and other types of crystals. Some crystal phase additions are not as effective as others in toughening the ceramics. Toughening depends on the crystal type, its size, its volume fraction, the interparticle spacing, and its relative CTE relative to the glass matrix.

All-Ceramic Systems

Based on a 1994 survey, MC crowns and bridges were used for approximately 90% of all fixed restorations. Over the next couple of decades these perceptions changed significantly. A 2016 survey based on ceramic material preferences showed that the top three choices for anterior crowns were lithium disilicate (54%), layered zirconia (17%), and leucite-reinforced glass ceramic (13%). The top three choices for posterior crowns were all-zirconia (32%), PFM (31%), and lithium disilicate (21%).

Newer developments in ceramic products with improved fracture resistance, advanced CAD–CAM technology, and excellent esthetic capability have led to a significant increase in the use of all-ceramic products. Ceramic crowns and bridges have been in widespread use since the beginning of the 20th century.

One of the first HIP core ceramics was IPS Empress, a leucite-based glass–ceramic. Because of its relatively low flexural strength and fracture toughness, this glass–ceramic was limited to anterior single-unit restorations. Other ceramics that were limited to single-unit restorations were Vitadur N aluminous porcelain, Cerestore magnesia–alumina shrink-free ceramic, and Dicor, a tetrasilicic-fluormica-based glass–ceramic. Although these materials had reasonably good success rates for a few years, their limitations slowly but surely led to the development of stronger and tougher ceramics that allowed for a broader range of uses.

Aluminous Porcelain

Until the 1960s, high-fusing feldspathic porcelains had been used to produce all-ceramic crowns. The relatively low strength of this type of porcelain prompted McLean and Hughes (1965) to develop an alumina-reinforced porcelain core material for the fabrication of ceramic crowns. The alumina-reinforced crowns were generally regarded as providing slightly better esthetics for anterior teeth than the MC crowns. However, the strength of the core porcelain used for alumina-reinforced crowns was inadequate to warrant its use for posterior teeth.

One method of producing aluminous porcelain crowns was to form a tin oxide coating on platinum foil. The objective of this technique was to reduce the weakening effect of surface irregularities on the inner surface of porcelain crowns by bonding a thin platinum foil to the inner surface that would be cemented to the prepared tooth. Atomic bonding of aluminous porcelain was promoted by electroplating the platinum foil with a thin layer of tin and oxidizing it in a furnace to provide a continuous film of tin oxide. The rationale was that the bonded foil served as an inner skin on the fit surface to reduce subsurface porosity and the formation of microcracks in the porcelain, thereby increasing the fracture resistance of the restoration. The clinical performance of these crowns was excellent for anterior teeth, but approximately 15% of molar crowns fractured within 7 years after they were cemented with a glass ionomer cement.

Glass–Ceramics

A glass–ceramic is a material that is formed into the desired shape as a glass and then subjected to a heat treatment to induce partial devitrification—that is, loss of glassy structure by crystallization of the glass. Crystalline particles, needles, or plates formed during this ceramming process interrupted the propagation of cracks in the material when an intraoral force was applied, thereby promoting increased strength and toughness. The use of glass–ceramics in dentistry was first proposed by MacCulloch in 1968. He used a continuous glass-molding process to produce denture teeth. He also suggested that it should be possible to fabricate crowns and inlays by centrifugal casting of molten glass.

The first commercially available castable ceramic material for dental use, Dicor, was developed by Corning Glass Works and marketed by Dentsply International. Dicor was a castable glass formed into an inlay, facial veneer, or full-crown by a lost-wax casting process similar to that employed for metals. After the glass casting core or coping was recovered from the casting investment the glass was sandblasted to remove the residual casting investment and the sprues were cut away. The glass was then covered by a protective "embedment" material and subjected to a heat treatment that caused microscopic plate-like crystals of tetrasilicic fluormica to grow within the glass matrix. This crystal nucleation and growth process is called ceramming. Once the glass was cerammed, it was fit on the prepared dies, ground as necessary, and coated with veneering porcelain and a stain and glaze layer to match the shape and appearance of adjacent teeth. Dicor glass–ceramic was capable of producing remarkably good esthetics, perhaps because of the "chameleon" effect, in which part of the color of the restoration was picked up from the adjacent teeth as well as from the tinted cements used for luting the restorations.

When used for posterior crowns, the Dicor glass–ceramic crowns were more susceptible to fracture than anterior crowns. Shown in Figure 10.16 is the stress pattern (colored areas) computed by finite element analysis in a 0.5-mm thick molar Dicor crown loaded on the occlusal surface, just within the marginal ridge area. The maximum tensile stress (73 MPa) is shown by the larger red area within the internal surface directly below the point of applied force (above the small white area in the occlusal surface) and just above the 50-μm thick layer of resin cement (designated by the arrow in Fig. 10.16).

More recently, glass–ceramics based on leucite, lithium disilicate, and hydroxyapatite have been used. These ceramics are available as powders or as solid blocks that can be machined through CAD–CAM processes or hot pressed either as a core ceramic or as a veneering ceramic. The powders are added to a liquid that allows the mixture to be applied as a thick slurry in which the particles are consolidated into a relatively dense mass by a process called condensation. The condensed mass is then sintered at an elevated temperature. These materials are described further in subsequent sections.

CRITICAL QUESTION

Which processing technique is most likely to generate the deepest flaws in a ceramic core framework?

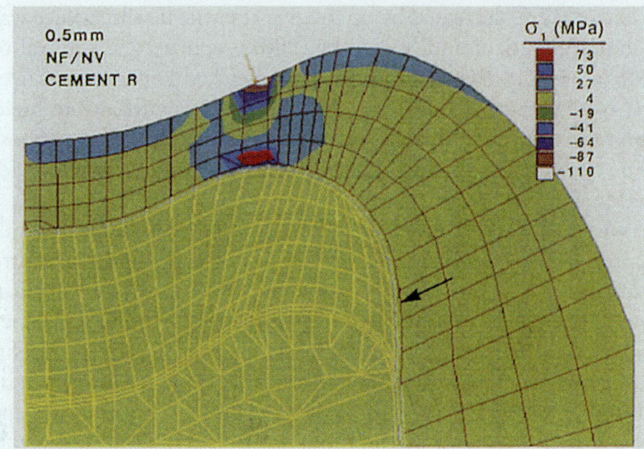

• **Fig. 10.16** Stress distribution resulting from loading (close to the marginal ridge area) of the occlusal surface of a finite element model of a ceramic crown with an occlusal thickness of 0.5 mm. The maximal principal tensile stress of 73 MPa is located directly below the point of occlusal loading (red line) within the internal surface of the crown adjacent to the 50-μm thick layer of resin cement (*arrow*).

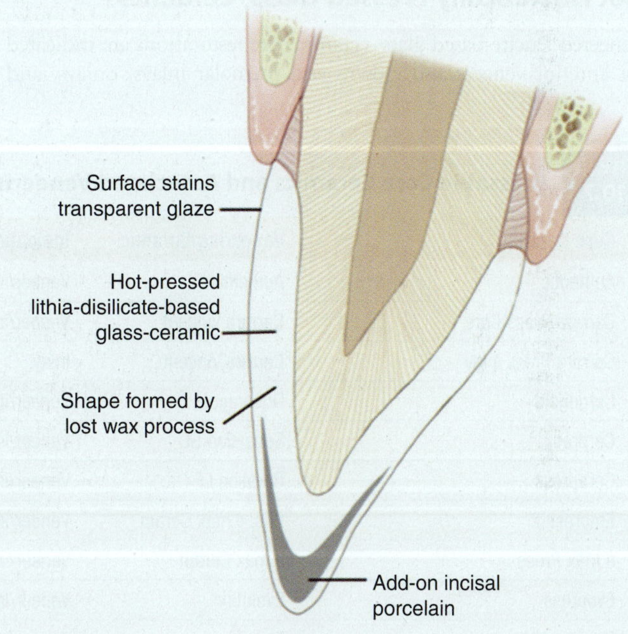

• **Fig. 10.17** Cross-sectional illustration of cemented Empress 2 ceramic crown with a lithia disilicate–based ceramic core.

This type of ceramic is characterized by the controlled crystallization (termed *ceramming*) of a glass through the presence of one or more nucleating agents. Dicor, a glass–ceramic that contained 55% by volume of tetrasilicic fluormica ($KMg_{2.5}Si_4O_{10}F_2$), was developed by Corning Glass Works and sold through Dentsply International. This product was derived from the quaternary ceramic system, K_2O–MgF_2–MgO–SiO_2. Dicor was the first castable glass used for dental prosthetic applications. Besides its relatively low flexural strength (110–172 MPa) and low fracture toughness (1.6–2.1 $MPa{\cdot}m^{1/2}$), the original cast form was colorless and prostheses had to be colored by the application of a thin layer of shading porcelain. Subsequent products were provided as dark and light shades of machineable glass–ceramic (MGC). The flexure strength of Dicor MGC decreased by up to 88% after the tensile surface was ground. Malament and Socransky (2001) reported the survival of 43% of nonacid-etched and 75% of acid-etched Dicor crowns over a 16-year period. Survival was greater for crowns that were luted with resin cement compared with either glass ionomer or zinc phosphate cement. Dicor and Dicor MGC glass–ceramics are no longer used in dentistry.

We have learned much from the studies of Malament et al. regarding the variables that play a major role in the fracture susceptibility of one type of glass–ceramic. Additional clinical data have been obtained from many other studies of other ceramics as well. At this point in the chapter, it may be useful to consider some of the general indications for use of different ceramic products based on existing data. A conservative approach to these recommendations is presented in Tables 10.7 and 10.8. Manufacturers of these products may recommend other applications as possible uses of their ceramics, but the probability of clinical fracture is not provided to give the user an indication of the time-dependent probability of clinical fracture. Thus, a conservative approach is recommended until validated clinical evidence supports these applications.

Hot Isostatically Pressed Glass–Ceramics

Veneered leucite-based glass–ceramic core restorations are indicated for anterior veneers and crowns and premolar inlays, onlays, and crowns. Hot-pressed leucite-containing glass–ceramics have been used for many years. The technology of hot-pressing leucite-based and lithia disilicate–based glass–ceramics is well established, and this technology has recently been applied to the hot pressing of veneer ceramics on metals and zirconia core ceramics. The most widely used leucite-based products are IPS Empress (Ivoclar Vivadent), Cerpress SL (Leach and Dillon), Finesse (DENTSPLY Ceramco), and IPS e.max CAD (Ivoclar Vivadent). These glass–ceramics contain approximately 35 vol% of leucite ($K_2O{\cdot}Al_2O_3{\cdot}4SiO_2$) crystals. The glass-matrix layering ceramic for these core materials also contains leucite. These glass–ceramics have relatively low flexure strength (≤112 MPa) and fracture toughness (1.3 MPa·m$^{1/2}$), so they are not recommended for molar crowns or bridges. A partial listing of HIP core ceramics is given in Table 10.7.

IPS Empress 2 (Ivoclar Vivadent), IPS Eris (Ivoclar Vivadent), and Optec OPC 3G (Pentron Laboratory Technologies) contain approximately 65–70 vol% of lithia disilicate ($Li_2O{\cdot}2SiO_2$) as the principal crystal phase. The lithia disilicate materials that are used as glass–ceramics have a narrow sintering range, which makes the processing of ceramic prostheses very technique sensitive. Figure 10.17 shows a schematic cross-section of an all-ceramic crown made with a lithia disilicate core ceramic. This glass–ceramic is composed of approximately 70 vol% of lithia disilicate and 30 vol% glass. This glass base contains at least 4% ZrO_2, which could account for this material's improved strength. This ceramic is fairly translucent but is somewhat opaquer (Fig. 10.18) and a stronger

TABLE 10.7 Pressable Core Ceramics and Associated Veneering Ceramics for All-Ceramic Prostheses

Core Ceramic	Veneering Ceramic	Indications	Manufacturer
Authentic	Authentic	Veneer/inlay/onlay/anterior crown	Ceramay
Carrara Press Core	Carrara Vincent	Veneer/inlay/onlay/anterior crown	Elephant
Carrara Press Inlay	Carrara Vincent	Inlay	Elephant
Cergogold	Duceragold	Veneer/inlay/onlay/anterior crown	Degussa
Cerpress	Sensation SL	Veneer/inlay/onlay/anterior and posterior crown	Dentagold
Cerapress	Creation LF	Veneer/inlay/onlay/anterior crown	Girrbach
Empress 2	Eris, e.max Ceram	Veneer/inlay/onlay/anterior and posterior crown/anterior FPD	Ivoclar Vivadent
e.max Press	e.max Ceram	Veneer/inlay/onlay/anterior and posterior crown/anterior FPD	Ivoclar Vivadent
Evopress	Evolution	Veneer/inlay/onlay/anterior crown	Wegold
Finesse All Ceramic	Finesse	Veneer/inlay/onlay/anterior crown	DENTSPLY Ceramco
Fortress Pressable	—	—	Mirage Dental
Magic Coating Caps Schicht-Pressing	Magic Ceram 2	Veneer/inlay/onlay/anterior crown	D.T.S. Denta TechnoStore
Magic Easy Press Colorier-Pressing	—	Veneer/inlay/onlay/anterior crown	D.T.S. Denta TechnoStore
Nuance Presskeramik	Nuance 750	Veneer/inlay/onlay/anterior crown	Schutz Dental Group
Optec OPC Low Wear	Optec OPC Low Wear	Veneer/inlay/onlay/anterior and posterior crown	Jeneric Pentron
Optec OPC 3G	Optec OPC 3G Porcelain	Veneer/inlay/onlay/crown/anterior FPD	Jeneric Pentron
Trendpress	Trendkeramik LFC	Veneer/inlay/onlay/anterior crown	Binder Dental
PLATINApress	Platina M	Veneer/inlay/onlay/anterior crown	Heimerle + Meule
Vision Esthetic	Vision Esthetic	Veneer/inlay/onlay/anterior crown	Wohlwend
VITAPress	VITA Omega 900	Veneer/inlay/onlay	Vident

Adapted from Kappert HF, Krah MK: Keramiken—eine Übersicht. *Quintessenz Zahntech* 27(6):668–704, 2001.

TABLE 10.8 Indications for Use of VITA In-Ceram, VITABLOCS, and VM 9 Ceramics

	OXIDE CERAMICS					FELDSPAR-BASED CERAMICS			
	GLASS-INFILTRATED VITA IN-CERAM CORE CERAMICS (SLIP/GRIND)			VITA IN-CERAM CORE CERAMICS (SINTER/GRIND)		VITABLOCS (GRIND)		VITA PM 9 (PRESS)	
Indications for Use	**Spinel**	**Alumina**	**Zirconia (Alumina/Zirconia**	**AL**	**YZ**	**Mk II**	**TriLuxe/TriLuxe Forte**	**Overpressing Technique**	**Substructure-Free Layering Technique**
Inlay									
Onlay									
Veneer									
¾ Crown									
Anterior crown	X	X		X	X	X	X	X	X
Anterior three-unit FDP		X	X	X	X			X	
Anterior four-unit FDP					X				
Posterior crown		X	X	X	X	X	X	X	
Posterior three-unit FDP			X	X	X			X	
Posterior four-unit FDP					X				
Veneering ceramic	VITA VM 7	VITA VM 7	VITA VM 7	VITA VM 7	VITA VM 9	VITA VM 9 (individualize only)	VITA VM 9 (individualize only)	VITA VM 9	VITA VM 9

FDP, fixed dental prosthesis.
Adapted from VITA In-Ceram Professionals. http://www.vita-vip.com/index.php?site=VITA_EN_ZT_materials_indicators

core ceramic than the leucite-based glass–ceramic (Empress). The mean flexural strength of lithia disilicate is approximately 350 MPa compared with the 112 MPa strength of leucite-based glass–ceramics. This strength and a fracture toughness of 3.3 MPa·m$^{1/2}$ for lithia disilicate–based glass–ceramics are generally sufficient for most anterior and posterior crowns and for anterior three-unit bridges even though the flexural strength and fracture toughness of their layering ceramics are substantially lower. Although the core ceramic fracture resistance is moderately high, veneered prostheses have been reported to be susceptible to chipping, which may require replacement or recontouring of the affected prostheses. Examples of cracking and chipping of these prostheses are shown in Figures 10.19–10.21. A follow-up material to lithia disilicate is lithia silicate material, with minimal change to the physical properties. The latest iteration of these silicate glasses is the addition of lithia metasilicate to the lithia disilicate crystals with the inclusion of 10% ZrO_2 in the glass matrix.

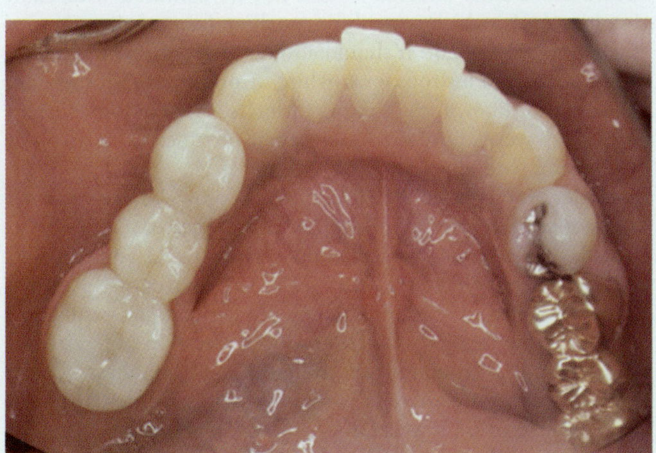

• **Fig. 10.18** A three-unit ceramic posterior fixed dental prothesis (tooth numbers 19–21; Fédération Dentaire Internationale tooth numbers 34–36) produced with a lithia disilicate–based core ceramic.

Hot-pressed ceramics (IPS Empress, IPS Empress 2, Finesse All-Ceramic, and OPC-3G) are made by creating a wax pattern, which is invested. Similar to the lost-wax technique, this investment is heated and injected under pressure into the investment mold. This technique can also be used to veneer MC prostheses, as mentioned earlier. These materials have numerous advantages as found listed in Box 10.1, but need to be used cautiously given that there are some disadvantages as well.

Fluorapatite Glass–Ceramic

Nano-fluorapatite glass–ceramic veneer, such as e.max Ceram, has a relatively low CTE ($\sim 9.5 \times 10^{-6}$/K) and is matched to that of lithia disilicate glass–ceramic core material and to some alumina and zirconia ceramics. Thus, because of the higher expansion coefficients of conventional feldspathic porcelain veneers,

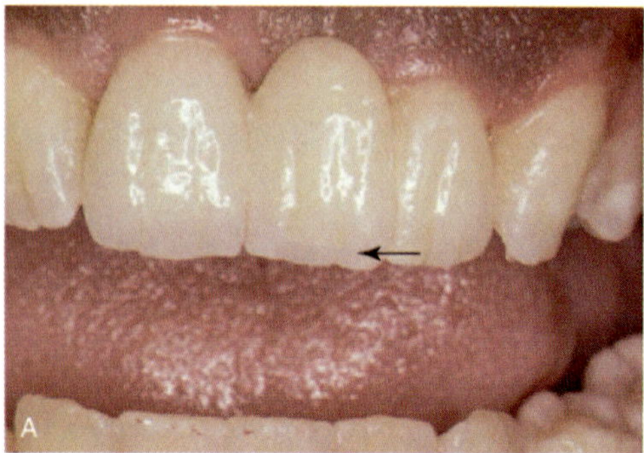

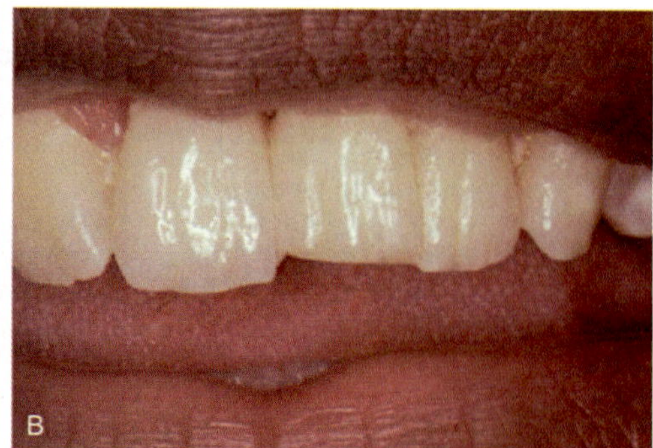

• **Fig. 10.19** Cracking and fracture of a crown. **(A)** Crack *(black arrow)* in crown of a three-unit bridge made with a lithia disilicate–based glass–ceramic core. **(B)** Fracture of the crown shown.

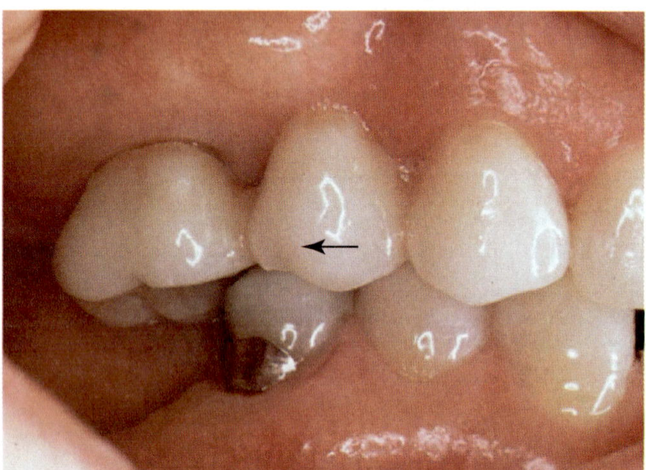

• **Fig. 10.20** Chipping of veneer ceramic on the pontic of a three-unit bridge made with a lithia disilicate–based glass–ceramic core.

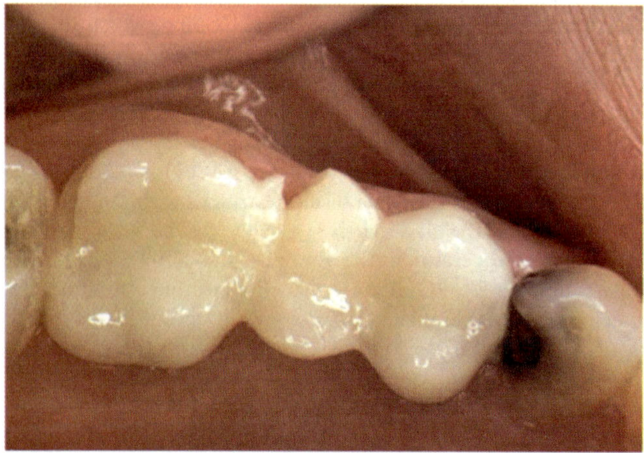

• **Fig. 10.21** Chipped veneer ceramic on a pontic of a bridge made with a lithia disilicate–based core ceramic. Also note the crack in the distal area of the posterior crown.

they cannot be used on lithia disilicate core frameworks. However, the fluorapatite-based layering glass–ceramics are thermally compatible with these core glass–ceramics. Because of their sufficiently high-volume fraction of glass-matrix phase, these

• BOX 10.1 Lithium Disilicate—Pros and Cons

Pros
- Excellent optical characteristics and good mechanical properties
- Clinical versatility
- Biocompatibility
- Favorable abrasiveness
- Marginal accuracy and internal fit
- High strength of adhesion to the substrate
- Monolithic and layered

Cons
- Glaze coating and fluorapatite ceramic veneering can increase wear
- Critical to adjust intraorally
- Chipping of the veneering ceramics

ceramics can be acid etched and bonded to resin cement using well-established procedures.

Yttria-Stabilized Zirconia

Zirconia has been used as a biomaterial since the 1970s. It has been widely used as a hip replacement material and has been used in dentistry for crown and bridge applications since 2004. Zirconium dioxide (ZrO_2), or zirconia, is a white crystalline oxide of zirconium. Dental zirconia should not be confused with cubic zirconia, ZrO_2, which is a cubic crystalline form of zirconia used as a diamond simulant. It should also not be confused with zirconium, which is a lustrous, gray-white, strong transition metal, or zircon (also known as zirkon), which is zirconium silicate, $ZrSiO_4$. However, pure zirconium can be obtained from zircon by purification with chlorine.

Under atmospheric pressure, pure zirconia can exhibit three different crystal structures. At temperatures greater than 2367°C, zirconia has a cubic structure. Between 1167°C and 2367°C, zirconia is tetragonal, and below 1167°C the structure is monoclinic. The tetragonal to monoclinic phase transition results in a 3–5% volume increase, which produces cracks in bulk zirconia samples and a reduction in strength and toughness. Under this condition pure zirconia would be useless for dental restorative applications. However, if one modifies the composition by doping with Mg, Ca, Sc, Y, or Nd, the high-temperature tetragonal phase can be stabilized at room temperature. In this way, the tetragonal to monoclinic phase transformation stresses are avoided, microcracks are prevented, and the positive mechanical properties of the tetragonal phase are preserved.

Another possibility for stabilizing the high-temperature tetragonal phase at room temperature is to reduce the crystal size to less than 10 nm.

Zirconia is a nonmetal with an extremely low thermal conductivity—about 20% as high as that of alumina (Al_2O_3). It is chemically inert and highly corrosion resistant. Pure ZrO_2 has a monoclinic crystal structure at room temperature and transforms to tetragonal and cubic zirconia at elevated temperatures. The large volume expansion that occurs during the transformation of nondoped zirconia from cubic to tetragonal and tetragonal to monoclinic phases leads to structural expansion and high tensile stresses that cause zirconia to crack during cooling from the processing temperatures. To solve this problem, stabilizing oxides such as magnesium oxide (MgO), yttrium oxide (Y_2O_3), calcium oxide (CaO), and cerium oxide (Ce_2O_3) are added to zirconia. The stability of single-phase tetragonal zirconia is enhanced by highly soluble trivalent stabilizers such as yttria, which induce vacancies, or tetravalent stabilizers such as ceria, which are oversized or undersized with respect to zirconium. The most common stabilizer for dental applications is yttria (Y_2O_3). The addition of 3–5 mol% of Y_2O_3 results in a stabilized core ceramic referred to as yttria-stabilized zirconia or yttria-stabilized tetragonal zirconia polycrystals (Y-TZP). Magnesia (MgO) has also been used to produce an Mg-PSZ core ceramic (Denzir-M, Dentronic AB, Skellefteå, Sweden). Ceria (Ce_2O_3) is used as a stabilizer in a Ce-TZP/Al_2O_3 core ceramic (NanoZir, Panasonic, Japan).

Stabilized Zirconia

If a larger concentration of stabilizer (i.e., more than 8 mol% yttria) is added, the zirconia becomes all cubic phase and is called *FSZ*, which is the component of cubic zirconia and devices such as oxygen sensors and fuel cells. The increase in volume does not occur in FSZ. The most common stabilizer for dental applications is yttria in the quantities of 3–5 mol%. At that concentration, the oxide-doped zirconia is known as *PSZ* or *TZP*, depending on the microstructure. The PSZ consists of nanosized metastable tetragonal particles that have precipitated out in cubic phase matrix approximately 50 μm in grain size during tempering of cooling cycle. Metastable tetragonal crystallites below a critical size (far below 1 μm) can be maintained in this form in a densely sintered structure down to room temperature. These crystallites allow for sintering a highly dense structure termed *TZP*, with each single crystallite that is almost 100% metastable tetragonal crystallites at room temperature. Normally, the material is designated by the quantity of stabilizer before the abbreviation of the stabilizer and then the type of microstructure. Therefore *3Y-TZP* refers to 3 mol% Y_2O_3 tetragonal zirconia polycrystal, and 5Y-PSZ has 5 mol% Y_2O_3 partially stabilized zirconia. Magnesia has also been used to produce an Mg-PSZ core ceramic (ZirMagnum, Cad.esthetics AB, Skellefteå, Sweden). Ceria is used as a stabilizer in a Ce-TZP/Al_2O_3 core ceramic (KZR-CAD NANOZR, Yamakin Co. Ltd., Osaka, Japan).

High strengths were discovered to correlate with a high tetragonal phase content, whereas a high amount of monoclinic phase leads to low strengths. For example, the fracture toughness of a 92% dense nondoped monoclinic zirconia has been reported to be 2.1 MPa·m$^{1/2}$, and the fracture toughness of tetragonal 3Y-TZP is approximately 8–10.3 MPa·m$^{1/2}$. This improvement was identified to have been caused by a tetragonal to monoclinic transformation, which will be discussed in the following section.

CRITICAL QUESTION

Which microstructural changes occur in 3Y-TZP ceramic for transformation toughening to occur at the tip of cracks in the presence of tensile stress? Through what mechanism does transformation toughening increase the resistance of yttria-stabilized zirconia to fracture?

Transformation Toughening

The structural stabilization of zirconia by yttria results in a significant proportion of metastable tetragonal phase. This metastable tetragonal phase strengthens and toughens the structure by a localized transformation to the monoclinic phase when tensile stresses develop at crack tips. The resulting volume expansion adjacent to the crack tips produces a high local compressive stress around the crack tips, which increases the localized fracture toughness and inhibits the potential for crack propagation. This phenomenon of transformation toughening increases the flexural and tensile fracture resistance of stabilized zirconia prostheses and presumably the survival probabilities of zirconia-based restorations. Although surface grinding may increase surface toughening in principle through the tetragonal to monoclinic phase transformation, excessive grinding by instruments with coarse abrasives or large flutes is not recommended by most zirconia suppliers because deep flaws may offset any advantage presented by localized compressive stresses. The fracture toughness of a 92.2% dense nondoped monoclinic zirconia has been reported to be 2.06 MPa·m$^{1/2}$. An extrapolation to full density yields a value of 2.6 MPa·m$^{1/2}$. In comparison, the fracture toughness of tetragonal 3Y-TZP is approximately 8–10.3 MPa·m$^{1/2}$.

When pure ZrO_2 is heated to a temperature between 1470°C and 2010°C and cooled, its crystal structure begins to change from a tetragonal to a monoclinic phase at approximately 1150°C. During cooling to room temperature, a volume increase of several percent occurs when it transforms from the tetragonal to monoclinic crystal structure (Fig. 10.22). As stated previously, this polymorphic transformation can be prevented with certain dopant additives such as 3 mol% yttrium oxide (Y_2O_3 or yttria). This ZrO_2 ceramic material is designated as 3Y-TZP (tetragonal zirconia polycrystals). The volume increase in this case is constrained if the zirconia crystals are sufficiently small and the microstructure is strong enough to resist the resulting stresses. This material is extremely strong (flexural strength, 900 MPa) and tough (fracture toughness, K_{Ic}, ranges from 8 to 10.3 MP·m$^{1/2}$). Many Y-TZP products are available in dentistry for CAD–CAM processing.

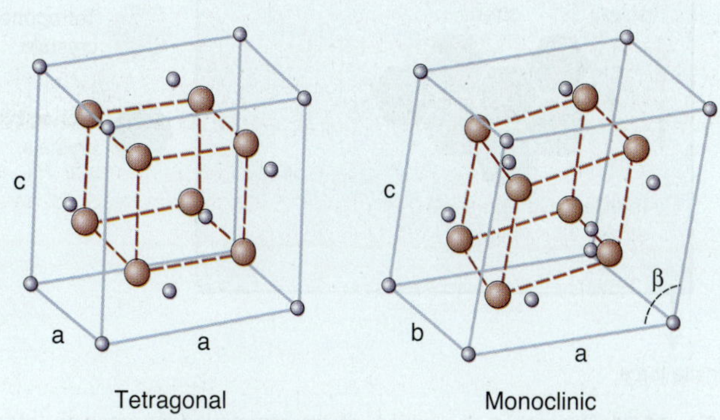

• **Fig. 10.22** Tetragonal and monoclinic unit cell structures.

These Y-TZP products fall into three groups:

1. Products that are milled in the green (compacted) state
2. Products that are milled in a partially sintered state
3. Products that are milled in the fully sintered state

Product names are given in the following CAD–CAM section.

The "transformation toughening" mechanism of crack shielding results from the controlled transformation of the metastable tetragonal phase to the stable monoclinic phase. Several types of crack shielding processes are possible including microcracking, ductile zone formation, and transformation zone formation. By controlling the composition, particle size, and the temperature versus time cycle, zirconia can be densified by sintering at a high temperature and the tetragonal structure can be maintained as individual grains or precipitates as it is cooled to room temperature. The tetragonal phase is not stable at room temperature and it can transform to the monoclinic phase and a corresponding volume increase. When sufficient stress develops in the tetragonal structure and a crack in the area begins to propagate, the metastable tetragonal crystals (grains) or precipitates next to the crack tip can transform to the stable monoclinic form. In this process a 3% expansion by volume of the ZrO_2 crystals or precipitates occurs that places the crack under a state of compressive stress (Fig. 10.23) and crack progression is arrested. To advance this crack further, additional tensile stress would be required. Because of this strengthening and toughening mechanism, the yttria-stabilized zirconia ceramic is sometimes referred to as "ceramic steel." A cross-sectional view of a Lava crown with a Y-TZP core is shown in Figure 10.24A, and four veneered, Lava zirconia crowns are shown in Figure 10.24B.

A regeneration heat treatment of machined or superficially ground Y-TZP at 900°C for 1 hour or for less time at 900–1000°C converts the monoclinic phase within the surface back to the tetragonal phase. Thus, if veneer firing occurs after a grinding procedure, the thermal treatment can induce the reverse transformation of monoclinic to the tetragonal phase in the ground areas of the zirconia structure.

Box 10-2 traces the steps in the development of commercially used zirconia.

Monolithic Zirconia

One approach for reducing the fracture susceptibility of ceramic restorations is to use only core ceramic (monolithic zirconia) and no veneering ceramic. Table 10.9 lists some properties of several core ceramics including a Y-TZP product and its veneering ceramic. Monolithic zirconia may be especially useful in the most posterior areas where high occlusal clenching forces or parafunctional forces are applied. Of course, the most effective way to accomplish this task is to eliminate the veneering ceramic. Several all-zirconia products of this type were marketed in 2010, including Crystal Diamond Zirconia (Crystal, Scottsdale, AZ), BruxZir Solid Zirconia (Glidewell Labs, Newport Beach, CA), Opalite All-Zirconia (The Aurum Group, Calgary, Alberta, Canada), and KZ3 Zirconia (Keller Laboratories, St. Louis, MO). Although the fracture resistance of all-zirconia crowns is exceptionally high, the risk for catastrophic wear of opposing enamel and dental restorations is one of the major potential challenges to the effective, safe use of solid zirconia prostheses. Clinical studies have confirmed that properly polished monolithic zirconia does not cause excessive wear of opposing enamel. This is in contrast to glazed monolithic zirconia, which has been shown to cause excessive wear of enamel, especially after the glaze has worn off. Two other disadvantages of an all-zirconia crown are the difficulty in adjusting occlusion when significant premature contacts are present and the cutting difficulty and heat generated in removing defective crowns or when making an endodontic access opening with diamond burs.

Increasing the translucency of zirconia

Another disadvantage of monolithic zirconia is the opaque nature of this material. Translucency of zirconia is dependent on:

- The size and shape of the constituent crystals,
- The quantity and type of additives,
- The heating methods,
- Temperature and atmospheric conditions used for sintering, and

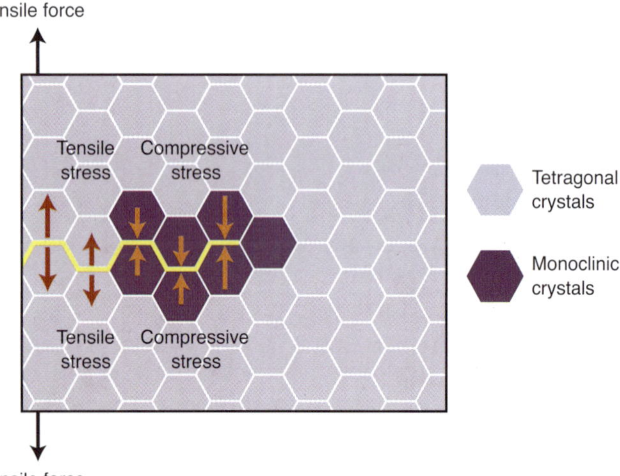

• **Fig. 10.23** Schematic illustration of transformation toughening of a Y-TZP ceramic.

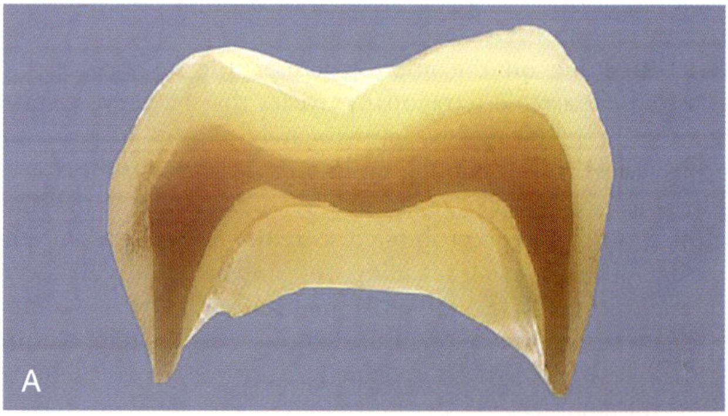

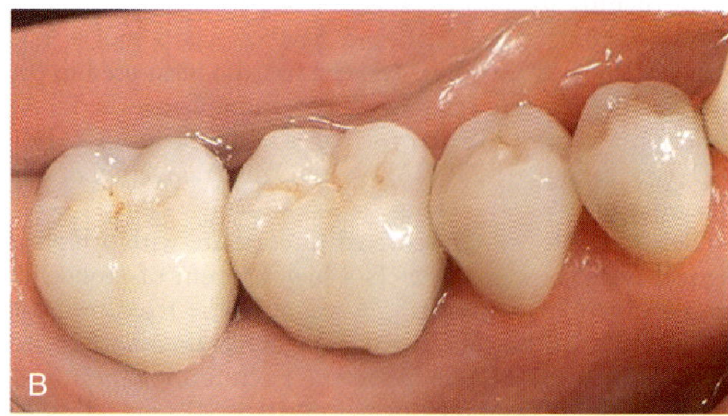

• **Fig. 10.24** Crowns with Lava zirconia-based core. **A,** Cross-section of a veneered crown. **B,** Four veneered crowns. (Images provided courtesy 3M ESPE, St. Paul, MN, and Dr. J. Sorensen.)

• BOX 10.2 Various Types of Zirconia Available for Use in Dental Applications

1. The first generation, tetragonal zirconia polycrystals (3Y-TZP), consists of 5.2 wt% or 3 mol% Y_2O_3 dopants and 0.25 wt% Al_2O_3 and has a small grain size (0.3–0.5 μm), high fracture toughness (9–10 MPa/m²), high flexural strength (900–1200 MPa), and a Young modulus of 210 GPa at room temperature. It is relatively sintered at a low temperature. Recently, advanced protocols have been developed to reduce the opacity of zirconia and make it more translucent by intensifying the heat treatment conditions.
2. The second generation, partially stabilized zirconia (3Y-PSZ), is doped with 3 mol% of Y_2O_3, but the sintering aid (0.25 wt% Al_2O_3) is eliminated, and the sintering temperature and/or duration is increased. The grain size of 3Y-PSZ is increased to 0.5–0.7 μm, and the cubic phase content is increased from 6%–12% to 20%–30%. As a consequence, the translucency is increased to TP = 24–31, and the biaxial strength is decreased to 900–1150 MPa.n additional approach that can be used is to replace tetragonal zirconia grains with optically isotropic cubic zirconia particles by increasing the yttria content to diminish the grain boundary light scattering to yield fully stabilized zirconia.
3. The third generation, 4–5Y-PSZ, incorporates more optically isotropic cubic zirconia (50%–80%), has a grain size of 1–4 μm and is produced by increasing the Y_2O_3 dopants to 4–5 mol% and increasing the sintering temperature and/or duration more than that of the second generation. However, cubic zirconia is weaker and more brittle than its tetragonal counterpart, which jeopardizes the strength of the zirconia. The translucency is increased to TP = 30–43, and the biaxial strength is decreased to 450–740 MPa.
4. Other types of zirconia include zirconia-toughened ceramics and alumina-toughened zirconia. Additional experimental novel zirconia types with improved translucency have been developed, including graded zirconia and nanostructured zirconia.

- The inclusion of pores which influence light scattering.

Different methods have been introduced that focus on creating a more isotropic index of refraction that decreases the birefringent effect.

- One approach is to decrease the amount of alumina from 0.25 to 0.10 wt% or 0.05 wt%; however, the hydrothermal stability is then lowered, as well.
- Another method of improving the translucency level is increasing the yttria content and adding cubic-phase zirconia. Manufacturers increased the yttria content with the production of 4Y-PSZ and 5Y-PSZ, where the tetragonal phase is lowered to about 75% and 50%, respectively, with the balance as cubic phases. With increase of cubic phase and their larger grain size, these zirconia materials exhibit greater translucency, thereby improving esthetics. However, reducing the volume of the tetragonal phase leads to less transformation toughening and lower strength and fracture toughness of the zirconia. For example, one company increased the yttria content in its zirconia from 5.2 to 9.32 wt%38. As a result, however, the bending strength (flexural strength) dropped from 1100 to 600 MPa and the fracture toughness decreased from 5 to 2.4 MPa (Fig. 10.25).
- The translucency of zirconia is also affected by the sintering temperature and atmospheric conditions during sintering.
- The heating method and temperature determine the density, porosity, and grain size of zirconia, thereby influencing the scattering of light.

These translucent zirconia ceramics have strengths similar to lithia disilicate and are therefore indicated for single-unit restorations only (Fig. 10.26).

Shading of Monolithic Zirconia

Zirconia is an opaque monochromic material. Therefore, two principal techniques have been developed for coloring zirconia restorations to overcome esthetic problems and to decrease zirconia opacity.

- One technique involves the use of "precolored zirconia," which is based on adding metal oxides to the Y-TZP powder before pressing the milling blocks and then sintering them at high temperature.
- The other technique involves the immersion of milled zirconia restorations in coloring liquids, such as chloride solutions (rare earth elements), before sintering to achieve the desired shade.

Fracture Strength of Zirconia

For zirconia, the fracture toughness tends to increase with increasing grain size. Therefore, the influence of grain size on transformation toughening is contrary to the increase in fracture strength for the small grain sizes seen in many other materials. One study of the influence of grain size on three-point bending strength and Vickers fracture toughness revealed that the fracture

TABLE 10.9 Physical Properties of Alumina, Zirconia-Toughened Alumina, and 3Y-TZP

Property	Alumina	Zirconia-Toughened Alumina (ZTA)	Zirconia (Y-TZP)
Density (g/cm³)	3.95	4.10	6.07
Vickers hardness (VHN; GPa)	1175; 11.5	1750; 17.2	1300; 12.8
Flexural strength (MPa)	330	760	≥900
Average grain size (μm)	1–5	1.5	≤0.5
Modulus of elasticity (GPa)	300	310	200
Poisson ratio	0.25	0.26	0.30
Fracture toughness (MPa·m½)	3.5	5–7	9–13
CTE (10^{-6}/K)	8.1	8.1	10.3
Thermal conductivity (W/m·K)	24	21	2.5–2.8

CTE, coefficient of thermal expansion; 3Y-TZP, 3 mol% Y_2O_3 tetragonal zirconia polycrystal; Y-TZP, yttria-stabilized tetragonal zirconia polycrystal.

The 3, 4, 5 mole % Yttria-Zirconia Continuum

3 Y-TZP: Opaque Zirconia	4 Y-TZP: Largely Opaque	5 Y-TZP: Most Translucent
Highest mechanical properties	Highest mechanical properties	Lower mechanical properties
White opaque	Some translucency	Moderate translucency
Mainly tetragonal phase	Tetragonal and cubic phases	More cubic, less tetragonal phase

• **Fig. 10.25** Relative properties of different types of stabilised zirconia.

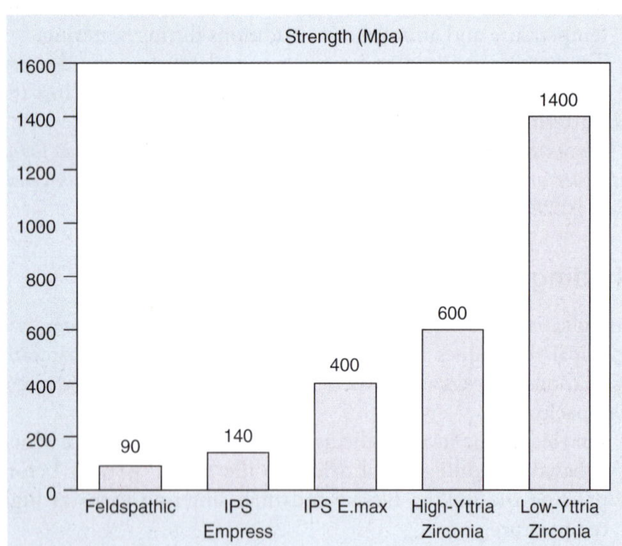

• **Fig. 10.26** This graph represents the difference in flexural strength of commonly used contemporary ceramic materials. (Adapted from Donovan TE, Alraheam IA, Sulaiman TA. An evidence-based evaluation of contemporary dental ceramics. Dental Update. 2018;45(6):541–546.)

strength increases linearly for 3Y-TZP from 650 MPa for a 0.9-μm grain size up to 1000 MPa for a critical grain size of 1.4 μm, after which this decreases to 750 MPa for a mean grain size of 1.8 μm. The change in fracture strength is mainly governed by the change in fracture toughness for the grain size between 0.9 and 1.8 μm. However, this relationship probably does not apply to nanocrystalline (~100-nm grain size) zirconia used in dentistry because the mean grain size is much smaller than the extrinsic defects, such as cracks caused by grinding. Thus, the dependence of fracture strength on grain size should be small for dental CAD–CAM zirconia. The decrease in strength caused by very large grain sizes is likely caused by premature transformation, which causes microcracking. Kosmač et al. reported that grinding reduced the monoclinic content and the flexural strength of fine-grained zirconia, but grinding did not affect the flexural strength of coarse-grained zirconia. Curtis et al. reported that grinding with coarse-grit burs decreased the flexural strength of zirconia, but grinding with fine-grit burs did not cause a statistically significant change. Other studies listed in the reference section may present conflicting results because of differences in the initial microstructure, composition, particle size distribution, maximum flaw sizes, and flaw size distribution. The relative advantages and disadvantages of zirconia restorations are listed in Box 10.3.

• BOX 10.3 Zirconia

Pros
- Excellent mechanical characteristics and good optical properties
- Excellent biocompatibility and low plaque retention
- Favorable wear behavior
- Implant abutments for esthetic sites
- Crack-hindering potential (through PTT)
- Marginal accuracy and internal fit
- Monolithic and layered

Cons
- Opacity
- Unetchable with conventional methods
- Low temperature degradation and aging
- Critical to adjust intraorally
- Glaze coating and fluorapatite ceramic veneering can increase wear
- Chipping of the veneering ceramics

Hydrothermal Degradation

The long-term performance of Y-TZP may be compromised by this material's susceptibility to hydrothermal degradation. Although hydrothermal effects have been generally reported between 200°C and 400°C, longer exposure times at oral temperatures may also degrade zirconia, resulting in increased surface roughness, fragmented grains, and microcracks. The degradation process is initiated by a transformation of the surface to the monoclinic phase, which spreads through the surface grains and into adjacent grains by stresses that develop during this process. The controlling mechanism is unknown, although OH^- groups are thought to be responsible for breaking the atomic bonds at the surface, which produces residual stresses and the initial transformation from the tetragonal to monoclinic phase.

Glass-Infiltrated Core Ceramics

To minimize sintering shrinkage and to ensure adequate fit of ceramic prostheses, three **glass-infiltrated core ceramic** systems have been developed, one based on partially sintered alumina, one based on a magnesia–alumina **spinel** ($MgAl_2O_4$), and one with a zirconia–alumina core. Each of these partially sintered ceramics can be infiltrated with a lanthanum glass without any significant dimensional change.

VITA In-Ceram Alumina contains approximately 85 vol% of alumina. The partially sintered framework is formed by a slip-casting process, which produces dense packing of particles against a porous die. After firing at 1120°C for 10 hours or more, a partially sintered structure is formed. This porous core ceramic

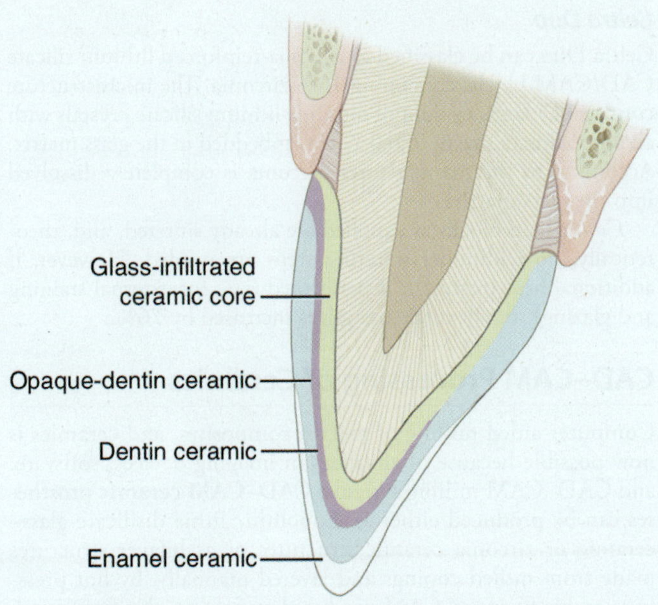

• **Fig. 10.27** Cross-sectional illustration of an In-Ceram crown with a glass-infiltrated core ceramic.

framework is then infused with molten lanthanum glass. A schematic illustration of a cross-section of an In-Ceram Alumina crown is shown in Figure 10.27.

The same type of process can also be applied to ICS, which is a magnesia–alumina spinel ($MgAl_2O_4$) core ceramic, and In-Ceram Zirconia. After glass infiltration, ICS ceramic is more translucent than In-Ceram Alumina or In-Ceram Zirconia, but the mean strength is significantly lower (~350 MPa vs. ~600 MPa). The mean flexure strength of In-Ceram Zirconia (~620 MPa) is only slightly greater than that of In-Ceram Alumina.

A summary of the indications for the use of VITA In-Ceram core ceramics, VITABLOCS Mk II feldspathic ceramic, and VITA VM 9 feldspathic ceramic is presented in Table 10.8. These are the proposed uses that are recommended by the manufacturer. The survivability of ceramic prostheses depends on many factors, some of which are controllable by the dentist and others that are not. For example, evidence of high caries risk, extensive periodontal disease, or severe bruxism is a contraindication for all dental ceramic prostheses, and under such conditions previously listed indications for ceramics (see Table 10.2) do not apply.

Alumina Core Ceramic

Procera AllCeram (Nobel Biocare) is an alumina-core ceramic that is indicated for anterior and posterior crowns. To produce these crowns, a die is first produced from an impression and digitized using a mechanical profiling device; then a computer converts the coordinates of the die surface into a digital database. An oversized die is then produced onto which pure alumina is dry pressed. The oversize green alumina body is then sintered, and the resulting shrinkage yields the desired size and shape onto which a feldspathic porcelain veneer is applied and sintered. The Procera AllCeram core is more translucent than In-Ceram Zirconia and has comparable strength (620–700 MPa). Because alumina cannot be acid etched to produce micromechanical retention, the surface is sandblasted with silica-coated alumina particles by a Rocatec system (3M ESPE Minneapolis, MN), which is required to ensure sufficient resin bonding. Figure 10.28 A shows a fractured three-unit alumina-based bridge whose retentive flanges were dimpled to promote micromechanical bonding. The fracture surface in Figure 10.28B shows a relatively large void that may have contributed to the fracture.

Zirconia-Toughened Alumina (ZTA)

ZTA is composed, by weight, of 70%–90% alumina and 10%–20% zirconia. The core of In-Ceram Zirconia before glass infiltration, by weight, is approximately 62% alumina, 20% zirconia, and 18% glass. Thus, it is not strictly a ZTA ceramic. Similar to the toughening of Y-TZP, ZTA is toughened by a stress-induced transformation mechanism. In ZTA microstructures, stress-induced transformation toughening occurs from uniform internal strain that causes the zirconia structure to crack and the zirconia particles to undergo phase transformation. During this process the number of zirconia particles increases and this change induces compressive stress within the alumina structure. The result of this process is that the strength of alumina is doubled and the toughness is increased two to four times. The properties of alumina, ZTA, and Y-TZP are summarized in Table 10.9. The ZTA properties are based on an 85% alumina/15% zirconia product (ZTA-96, Astro Met, Inc. Cincinnati, OH).

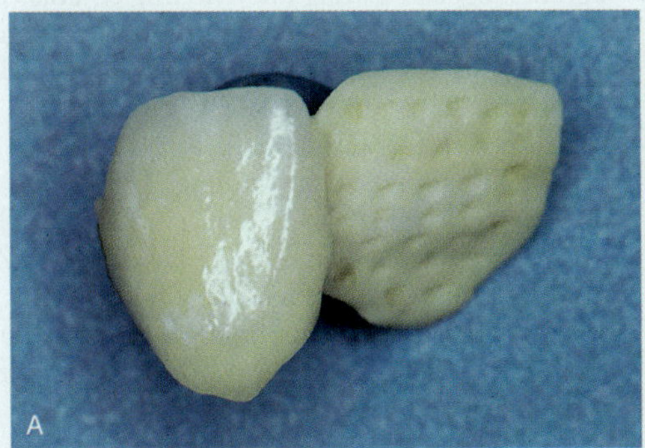

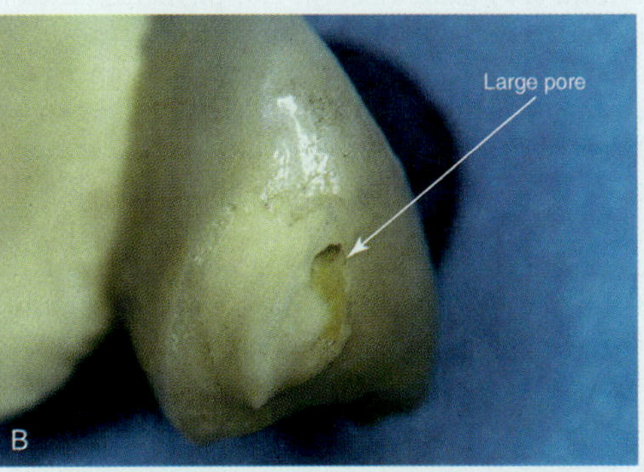

• **Fig. 10.28** Fractured connector of a three-unit resin-bonded bridge made with an alumina core ceramic. **(A)** Dimples on the retaining flange indicating poor wetting of the adhesive. **(B)** A void within the connector to the other flange.

CAD/CAM Zirconia-Reinforced Lithium Silicate Glass–Ceramic

Two zirconia-reinforced lithium silicate ceramics are available for CAD/CAM restorations: VITA Suprinity (VITA Zahnfabrik) and Celtra Duo (Dentsply). Both materials rely on the addition of 10% by weight zirconium oxide to lithium silicate glass compositions to improve their mechanical and optical properties. Zirconia-reinforced lithium silicate glass–ceramics have mechanical properties comparable with those of lithium disilicate glass–ceramics. After crystallization, a dual microstructure is obtained of lithium metasilicate and lithium disilicate crystals embedded in glassy matrix containing zirconium oxide.

Incorporation of ZrO_2 particles into the glass matrix is an effective method to improve the mechanical properties of glass–ceramics. In addition to the crack deflection effect, the glass–ceramic is also strengthened by ZrO_2 transformation toughening. The expansion in the volume of the ZrO_2 grain accompanying the phase transition produces compressive stress on the crack, or microcracks around the crack, both consuming the energy of the main crack and thereby increasing the fracture resistance of the glass–ceramic.

The content of ZrO_2 plays an important role in the strengthening effect of ZrO_2 in lithium disilicate glass–ceramic. When the ZrO_2 content was below 10 wt%, ZrO_2 acted as nucleation agent and $Li_2Si_2O_5$ crystals have a spherical morphology, instead of rod-like structure. This results in the loss of interlocking effect of $Li_2Si_2O_5$ crystals and the decrease of mechanical strength. The addition of 15 wt% ZrO_2 strengthens and toughens the glass–ceramic, with flexural strength increasing from 310 (ZrO_2 free) to 340 MPa (ZrO_2 reinforced), and fracture toughness increasing from 2.2 to 3.5 MPa $m^{1/2}$.

Although the addition of ZrO_2 particles improved the mechanical strength of lithium silicate glass–ceramic, the addition of ZrO_2 particles causes some manufacturing problems. Unfortunately ZrO_2-reinforced lithium silicate exhibits poor machinability with high tangential and normal grinding forces and energy. ZrO_2-reinforced lithium silicate is the most difficult to machine compared with feldspar, leucite, and lithium disilicate glass–ceramics. Edge chipping damage was found during milling. Thus, the manufacturing of high-strength ZrO_2-reinforced lithium silicate is still a technical challenge.

VITA Suprinity

VITA Suprinity CAD/CAM blocks are composed of silicon dioxide (SiO_2), lithium oxide (Li_2O), potassium oxide (K_2O), phosphorus pentoxide (P_2O_5), aluminum oxide (Al_2O_3), zirconium dioxide (ZnO_2), cerium (IV) oxide (CeO_2), and pigments. These CAD/CAM blocks are produced in three distinct stages. Initially, zirconium dioxide, silicon dioxide, lithium oxide, and other ceramic components are heated at a temperature of 1500°C to melt all components. After creating a homogenous solution, the melted glass is poured into molds to form blocks. The resulting glass block is brittle and not suited for the CAD/CAM milling process; thus, a second heating treatment is necessary. In the second heating stage (from 500 to 600°C), the crystals within the glass matrix form lithium metasilicate and the glass block achieves adequate mechanical properties to withstand the stresses of the milling process. The resulting translucent glass–ceramic block is then made commercially available.

After milling, the translucent glass–ceramic restoration must be recrystallized at a temperature of 840°C for 8 minutes. The crystallization forms a homogeneous structure of lithium disilicate with a subsidiary crystal phase containing zirconium oxide.

Celtra Duo

Celtra Duo can be classified as zirconia-reinforced lithium silicate CAD/CAM blocks containing 10% zirconia. The microstructure consists of a large amount of ultrafine lithium silicate crystals with an approximate size of 0.5–0.7 μm embedded in the glass matrix. According to the manufacturer, zirconia is completely dissolved into the glass matrix.

Celtra Duo blocks as supplied are already sintered, and, theoretically, no additional sintering steps are needed. However, if additional heat treatment is performed (i.e., for external staining and glazing), the flexural strength is increased by 76%.

CAD–CAM Processing of Ceramics

Computer-aided milling of metals, composites, and ceramics is now possible because of advances in imaging devices, software, and CAD–CAM milling systems. **CAD–CAM ceramic** prostheses can be produced either as monolithic lithia disilicate glass–ceramic or zirconia ceramic structures or as bilayer structures made from milled copings and layered manually, by hot pressing, or by fusing a CAM-produced veneer to the framework (CAD-on method). A ceramic veneer that is pressed on a metal is referred to as the POM method. CAD–CAM prostheses can be produced either by industrial milling processes or by chairside milling units. The industrial CAD–CAM systems are very expensive with typical costs in excess of several hundred thousand USD. However, they are capable of processing multiple jobs with a high level of accuracy and reproducibility. Chairside systems are limited in their processing speed and their ability to process large cases.

Layered zirconia prostheses can be produced from partially sintered ceramics and shaped by carbide burs to enlarged dimensions that compensate for sintering shrinkage. Fully sintered ceramics are shaped by diamond disks and burs to the precise dimensions derived from a scanned image of the prepared teeth. Typically, the external surface must be ground and polished manually, although some CAD–CAM systems are capable of milling the external surface. Shown in Figure 10.29 is a simulated digitized image of a crown to be produced from a ceramic blank and an adjacent image of a partially milled crown. Shown in Figure 10.30 is Cerec ceramic block, a milled inlay form, and the final inlay.

As mentioned previously, zirconia ceramics can be milled in the green state, in the partially sintered state, or in the fully sintered state. A four-unit Cercon core ceramic framework can be milled in the green state (Fig. 10.31), after simulated try-in (Fig. 10.32), and after sintering, staining, and glazing the veneering ceramic (Fig. 10.33). Representative products that fall into each of these categories are as follows:

1. Green-state milling: Cercon (Degudent/DENTSPLY Ceramco), Lava (3M ESPE), ZirkonZahn (USA), Hint-Els Zirkon TPZ-G (DigiDent)
2. Partially sintered-state milling: IPS e.max ZirCAD (Ivoclar Vivadent), VITA In-Ceram YZ Cubes (VITA Zahnfabrik), Everest (Kavo Dental), Hint-Els Zirkon TZP-W (Digident), DC-Shrink (DCS), Precident DCS (DCS)
3. Fully sintered-state milling: Denzir Premium HIP Zirconia (Etkon USA), Zirkon Pro 50 (Cynovad), Kavo Everest ZH Blanks (Kavo Dental)

This is by no means a complete list, since new products are introduced each year. For example, the family of ceria-stabilized ceramics has only recently been introduced. Shown in Figure 10.34 is a schematic illustration of the crystalline nanoparticles in a Ce-TZP/Al_2O_3 core ceramic that has a very high fracture toughness

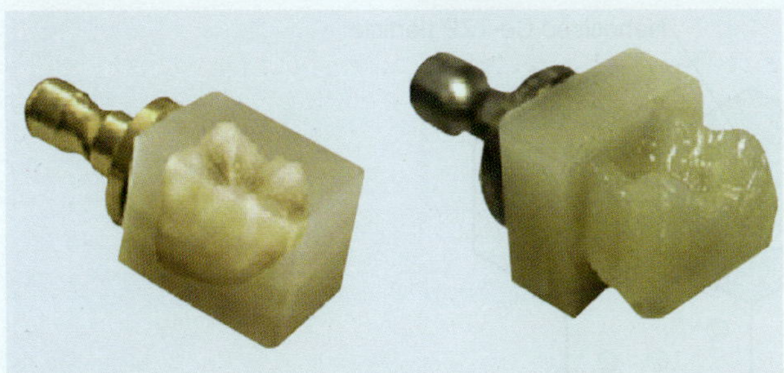

• **Fig. 10.29** (*Left*) Simulated digitized image, (*right*) partially milled feldspathic ceramic (VITABLOCS TriLuxe Forte) processed by the Sirona inLab CAD–CAM system.

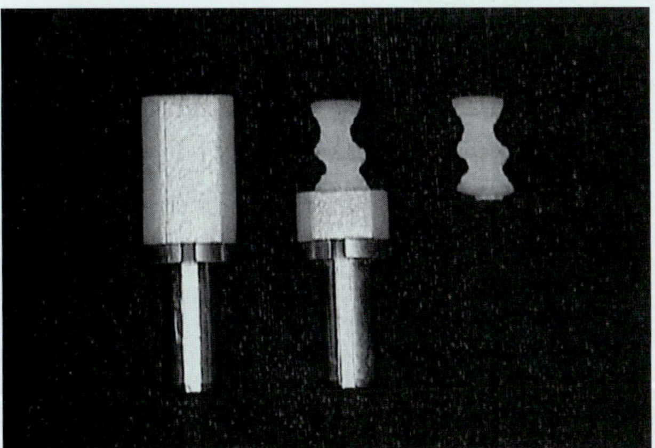

• **Fig. 10.30** (*Left*) CAD–CAM ceramic block before milling. (*Center*) An intermediate stage of milling. (*Right*) After removal of the inlay from the mounting stub.

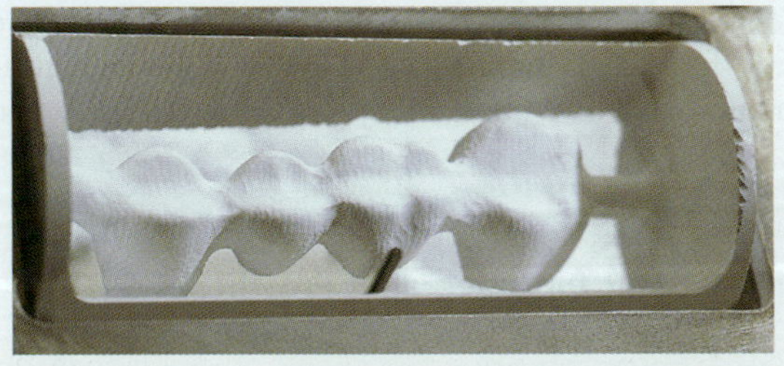

• **Fig. 10.31** Cercon zirconia core ceramic after initial milling of the "green state" ceramic. (Courtesy of Dentsply Ceramco, Burlington, NJ.)

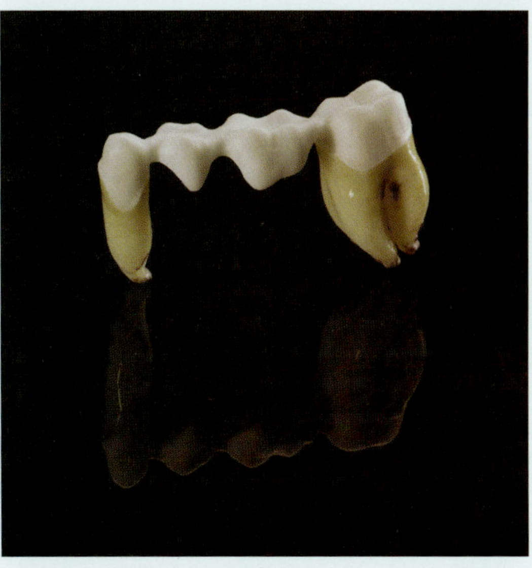

• **Fig. 10.32** Finished FDP framework made with Cercon core ceramic placed on teeth. (Courtesy of Dentsply Ceramco, Burlington, NJ.)

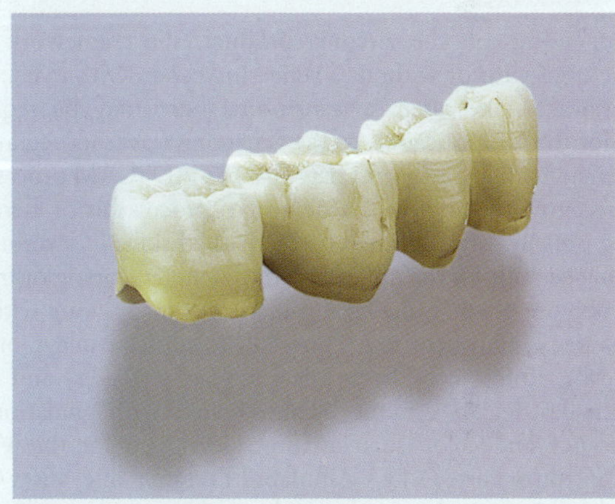

• **Fig. 10.33** Final Cercon FDP with veneering ceramic and stain characterization. (Courtesy of Dentsply Ceramco, Burlington, NJ.)

and flexure strength. No validated clinical data on this product are yet available. One of the products of this type that has been introduced in Japan is called NanoZir (Panasonic). However, the list is indicative of the emerging market for dental ceramics and for CAD–CAM systems.

A typical procedural sequence for producing ceramic prostheses by a CAD–CAM system using partially sintered blanks is as follows:

1. Set the blank in the milling machine holder according to the manufacturer's instructions.
2. Set the enlargement factor to compensate for sintering shrinkage. The factor will vary according to the overall size of the prosthesis.
3. Insert the appropriate machining/milling tool.
4. After machining is completed, remove the framework and residual blank.
5. Cut the framework from the blank using a diamond disk.
6. Clean the partially sintered framework completely.
7. Dry the framework completely.
8. Place the framework in the isothermal hot zone of the sintering furnace.
9. Set the thermal processing conditions according to the sintering instructions for the specific product.
10. Sinter the framework to achieve optimum density.
11. After cooling, remove the sintered framework.
12. Inspect the framework for surface and subsurface flaws using fiberoptic transillumination.
13. Evaluate the framework for adequacy of wall thickness, ease of seating, and marginal fit.
14. If necessary, use a water-cooled diamond tool to perform minor adjustment corrections.
15. Rinse the framework thoroughly with water and dry it completely.

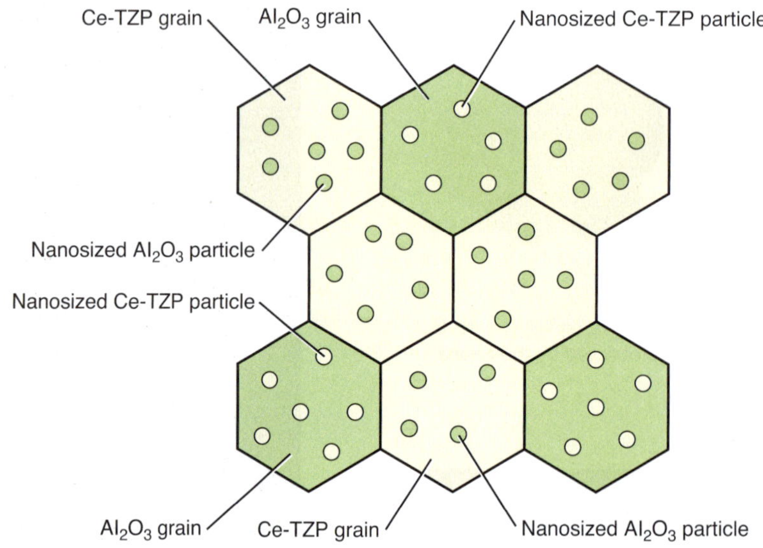

• **Fig. 10.34** Schematic illustration of nanostructure crystalline particles in a Ce-TZP/Al_2O_3 core ceramic that has recently been introduced for dental applications.

16. Depending on the zirconia product, the framework may be used with or without a veneering ceramic. If a veneering ceramic is indicated, a transitional liner may be required prior to the application of the veneering (layering) ceramic.

Chairside milling is the ultimate goal of CAD–CAM processing. Until recently, the ability of a dentist to process his or her own ceramic prostheses was limited by the lack of skills in layering the veneering ceramic on the milled and fully sintered coping or framework. Because of the experience gained over many years with the Cerec system, many dentists are now able to fabricate inlays, onlays, and crowns from leucite-based ceramic blanks (ingots) and lithia disilicate–based glass–ceramic blanks. Blanks with gradations of translucency and color, such as those developed for the VITABLOCS Triluxe Forte (VITA Zahnfabrik) ceramic line, allow clinicians to produce single-unit finished prostheses without the need for skills in layering of a veneering porcelain. The weak link in all-ceramic prostheses is the relatively low fracture resistance of the veneering ceramics (Table 10.10).

The quality and precision of the more costly commercial imaging, designing, and milling systems has increased markedly since the 1980s because of advances in the software that controls these variables. Thus, it is likely that lab-operated CAD–CAM systems will continue to support crown and bridge needs well into the future.

Copy-Milling Technology

A copy-milling technique has also been used to machine porcelain. This technology was made possible by means of the Celay system (Mikrona Technologies, Spreitenbach, Switzerland). This system was based on a mechanical device that is used to trace the

TABLE 10.10 Properties of Three Types of Core Ceramics and a Veneering Ceramic for All-Ceramic Prostheses

	PRINCIPAL CRYSTAL FORM			
Property	Leucite	Lithium Disilicate	Zirconia (Y-TZP)	Ceramic With HAP Nanocrystals for Veneering Y-TZP
Crystallinity (vol%)	35	70	≥97.5 (may also include crystalline HfO_2, Al_2O_3, Na_2O, SiO_2, Fe_2O_3, etc.)	N/A
Flexural strength (MPa)	85–112	215–400	900	85–110
Fracture toughness (MPa·m$^{1/2}$)	1.3–1.7	2.2–3.3	8–10.3	0.75–1.0
Vickers hardness (GPa)	5.9	6.3	8.8–11.8	4.8–5.4
Expansion coefficient (10^{-6}/K)	15.0–15.4	9.7–10.6	10.0–11.0	9.8
Elastic modulus (GPa)	65–86	95–103	210	65
Chemical durability[a] (μg/cm^2)	100–200	30–50	30	10–20

Y-TZP, yttria-stabilized tetragonal zirconia polycrystal.
[a]ISO 6872.

surface of a prefabricated pattern of the designed restoration made from a blue resin-based composite (Celay-Tech, ESPE, Seefeld-Oberbayern, Germany). The resin pattern can be produced directly on prepared teeth or indirectly on dies made from impressions. As the tracing tool passes over the pattern, a milling machine duplicates these movements as it grinds a copy of the pattern from a block of alumina or other ceramic material. Currently, it is possible to machine Celay In-Ceram or ICS material and then infiltrate the pattern with a sodium-lanthanum glass in a manner similar to that used for conventional In-Ceram crown cores or bridge frameworks. Both types of glass-infiltrated alumina are veneered with Vitadur Alpha porcelain. No long-term clinical data are yet available for Celay-produced restorations. Because the accuracy of the copy-milled crowns is dependent on the care, time, and the profile tracing ability of the technician, the marginal quality of crowns made from the copy-milling technique is likely to be inferior to that of copings made from the hot-pressing method. Listed in Table 10.11 are some ceramics that can be processed by copy-milling or by CAD–CAM procedures.

Effect of Design on Fracture Susceptibility of Metal–Ceramic and All-Ceramic Restorations

There are many examples of atypical designs that lead to ceramic fracture of MC prostheses. One of these involves bridges with cast-joined connectors that are used occasionally to avoid soldering bridge framework components that do not fit the prepared teeth. Shown in Figure 10.35 is a four-unit MC cast-joined bridge with two connector fractures at the two cast-joined sections in the metal framework. Tougher, stronger ceramics can sustain higher tensile stresses before cracks develop in areas of tensile stress. Conventional feldspathic porcelains should not be used as the core of ceramic crowns, especially in posterior areas, because occlusal

TABLE 10.11 CAD–CAM and Copy-Milled Ceramics Used for All-Ceramic Prostheses

Ceramic Block	Core/Veneer Processing	Ceramic Veneer	Indications	Core/Veneer Supplier
CerAdapt	Highly sintered Al_2O_3	AllCeram	Implant superstructure	Nobel Biocare
Cercon Base	Presintered ZrO_2; postsintered after milling	Cercon Ceram S	Crowns and FPDs	DENTSPLY Ceramco
DC-Kristall	Leucite based	Triceram	Crowns	DCS Dental AG/Esprident
DC-Zirkon	Presintered ZrO_2; hot isostatic postcompaction	Vitadur D Triceram	Crowns and FPDs	DCS Dental AG/VITA/Esprident
Denzir	Densely sintered; hot isostatic overpressing	Empress 2	Crowns and three-unit FPDs	Decim, Ivoclar
IPS ZirCAD	Presintered ZrO_2; hot isostatic postcompaction	IPS ZirPress	Crowns and FPDs	Ivoclar Vivadent
LAVA Frame	ZrO_2; presintered and postsintered	LAVA Ceram	Crowns and FPDs	3M ESPE
ProCad	Leucite based	Maltechnik	Veneers, inlays, onlays, and crowns	Ivoclar Vivadent
Procera AllCeram	Al_2O_3; presintered and postsintered	AllCeram	Crowns and FPDs	Nobel Biocare
Procera Zirconia	Al_2O_3/ZrO_2; presintered and postsintered	AllCeram	Crowns and FPDs	Nobel Biocare
Synthoceram	Al_2O_3 reinforced; pressed and postsintered	Sintagon	Crowns	Elephant
VITABLOCS Mark II	Feldspathic porcelain block	VITA VM9 (partial veneer only)	Veneers, inlays, onlays, and crowns	VITA Zahnfabrik
VITABLOCS Real Life	Feldspathic porcelain block	VITA VM9 (partial veneer only)	Anterior veneers and crowns	VITA Zahnfabrik
VITABLOCS Alumina	Sintered Al_2O_3: followed by glass infiltration	Vitadur AlphaVintage AL	Crowns and FPDs	VITA ZahnfabrikShofu Inc
VITABLOCS Spinell	Sintered $MgO–Al_2O_3$ spinel followed by glass infiltration	Vitadur Alpha	Crowns	VITA Zahnfabrik
VITABLOCS Zirconia	Sintered Al_2O_3/ZrO_2 followed by glass infiltration	Vitadur AlphaVintage ZR	Crowns and FPDs	VITA ZahnfabrikShofu Inc
VITABLOCS TriLuxe for Cerec	Feldspathic porcelain block	VITA VM9 (partial veneer only)	Anterior veneers and crowns	VITA Zahnfabrik
Zircagon	ZrO_2; presintered and postsintered	Zircagon	Crowns	Elephant

Modified from Kappert HF, Krah MK, Keramiken—eine Übersicht, *Quintessenz Zahntech* 27(6):668–704, 2001, and from Mantri SS, Bhasin AS. CAD-CAM in dental restorations: An overview. *Ann Esss Dent*II(3):123–128 2010.

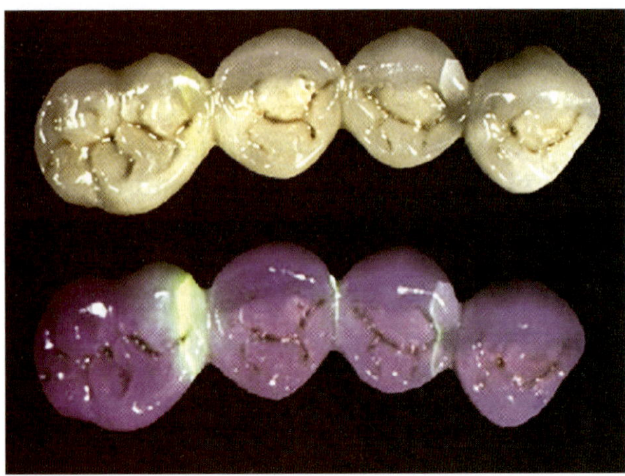

• **Fig. 10.35** Cast-joining fractures in terminal connectors of a four-unit metal–ceramic bridge. Cast-joining designs. The cracks in each of the connectors are highlighted with fluorescent dye in the lower photo.

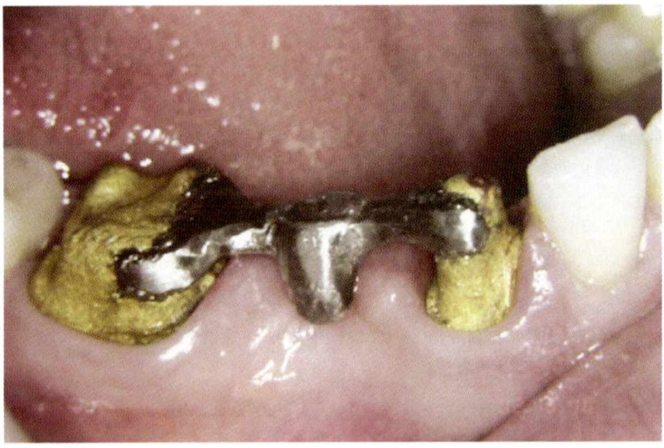

• **Fig. 10.36** Framework of gold "galvanometal" copings and a base metal pontic. (Courtesy of Dr Renata Faria.)

forces can easily subject them to tensile stresses that exceed the tensile strength of the ceramic. Of major concern are tensile stresses that are concentrated within the inner surface of posterior ceramic crowns (see Glass–Ceramic section). Shown in Figures 10.36 and 10.37 is a framework on two galvanometal copings and a fractured three-unit FDP, respectively. The copings were made using a "galvanometal" process to electrodeposit pure gold onto dies. To minimize the cost of gold used in the process, a base metal pontic was bonded to the copings and it was also coated with a gold layer. As the photos illustrate, cracking of porcelain has occurred at the junctions of the pontic with the crowns and porcelain has also debonded from the gold surface, as is expected, since pure gold cannot form an oxide that is needed for chemical bonding to porcelain.

When fractures occur, a sketch of the observed fracture surface is helpful in determining the cause of fracture. An illustration of the main crack patterns that can develop in an MC crown is shown in Figure 10.38. Some cracks travel along the metal–metal oxide interface and others may propagate along the interface between the metal oxide and opaque porcelain. The third type can occur cohesively entirely within the porcelain. The first two types are indicative of a material processing error and the third may be indicative of a crown design error, excessive loading, or other uncontrollable factors.

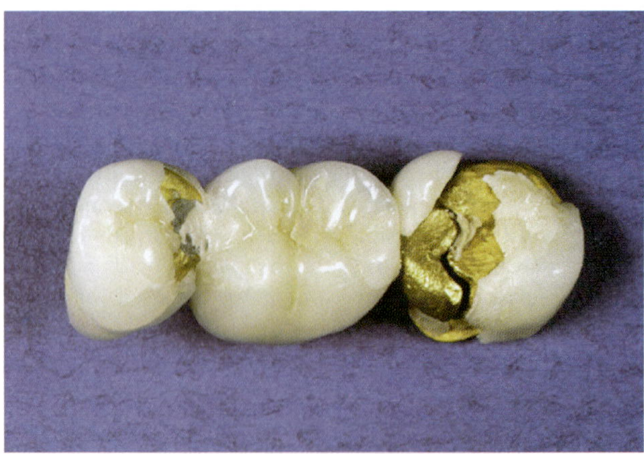

• **Fig. 10.37** Fractures of metal–ceramic bridge made with gold "galvanometal" copings and a base metal pontic. (Courtesy of Dr Renata Faria.)

Although ceramic and MC prostheses are susceptible to design errors, some variations in design have minimal effects on stress levels generated during loading. For example, the MC crown designs shown in Figure 10.39 have quite different metal thicknesses in the facial area, yet finite element analyses reveal no significant differences in the maximum principal tensile stresses that develop under simulated loading.

Sharp line angles in the preparation will also create areas of stress concentration in the restoration, primarily where a tensile component of bending stress develops. A small particle of ceramic along the internal porcelain margin of a crown can induce locally high tensile stresses during try-in or final cementation. Furthermore, when grinding of this surface is required for adjustment of fit, one should use the finest grit abrasive that will accomplish the task. This precaution will reduce the probability of forming microcracks and reduce the depth of microfissures produced by the abrasive particles. Grinding flaws in the inner surface of ceramic crowns represents the greatest damage that can be produced in ceramics by processing techniques.

Because the forces on anterior teeth are relatively small, low to moderate tensile stresses can be supported by ceramic crowns more safely. However, if there is a great amount of vertical overlap (overbite) with only a moderate amount of horizontal overlap (overjet), high tensile stresses can be produced.

CRITICAL QUESTION

Describe four ways in which control of tooth preparations and the design of crowns and bridges can increase the resistance to fracture of all-ceramic crowns.

Most ceramics should be designed in such a way as to overcome their weaknesses—that is, the relatively low fracture toughness and tensile strength of the veneering ceramic and its susceptibility to crack formation in the presence of surface flaws. The design should avoid exposure of the ceramic to high tensile stresses. Knife-edge margins should be avoided because of the risk of cracking or chipping during the try-in phase. The tensile stresses in a ceramic FPD can be reduced by using greater connector heights (Fig. 10.40). However, a connector height greater than 4 mm makes the anatomic form in the buccal area of a posterior FPD too bulky and unesthetic (Fig. 10.41). Broadening the

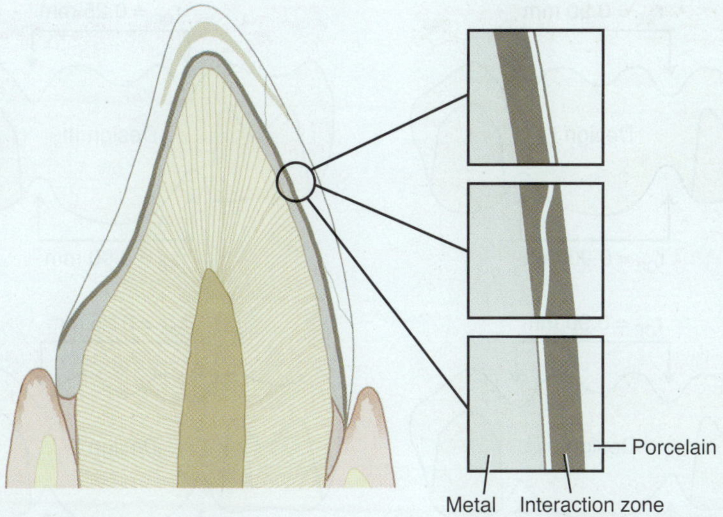

• **Fig. 10.38** Cross-sectional illustration of three principal types of interfacial zone fractures.

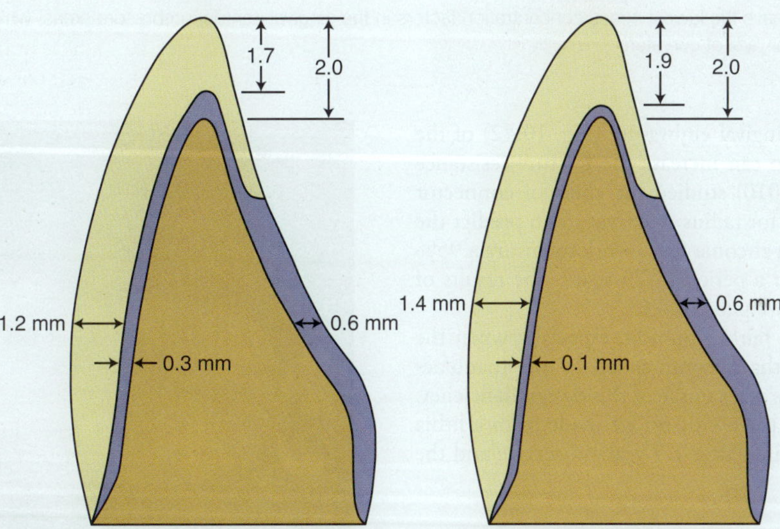

• **Fig. 10.39** Cross-sectional illustrations of metal–ceramic crown designs with reduced metal thickness. Metal is represented by a blue color and porcelain by yellow. (*Left*) Facial metal thickness of 0.3 mm. (*Right*) Facial metal thickness of 0.1 mm represents a more esthetic option.

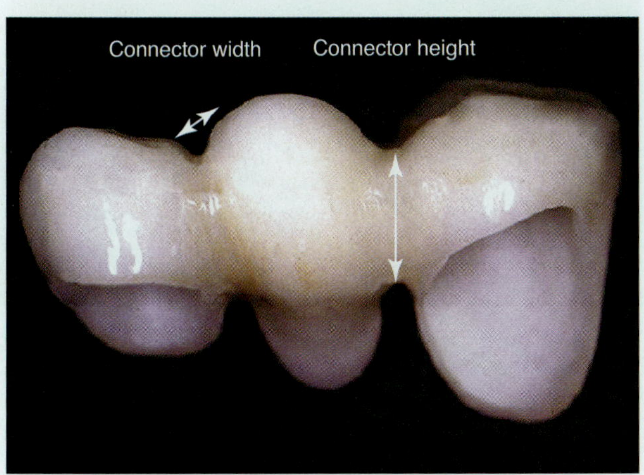

• **Fig. 10.40** Connector dimensions for a three-unit ceramic bridge.

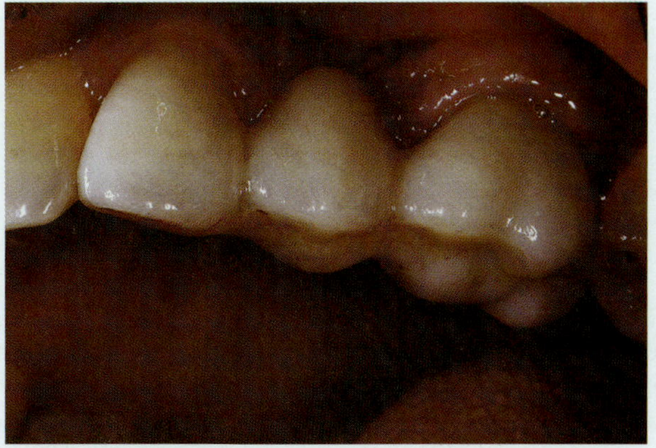

• **Fig. 10.41** A three-unit ceramic anterior–posterior produced totally with a lithia disilicate-based core ceramic. Note the relatively large connector (4 mm in height) necessary to resist fracture in posterior areas.

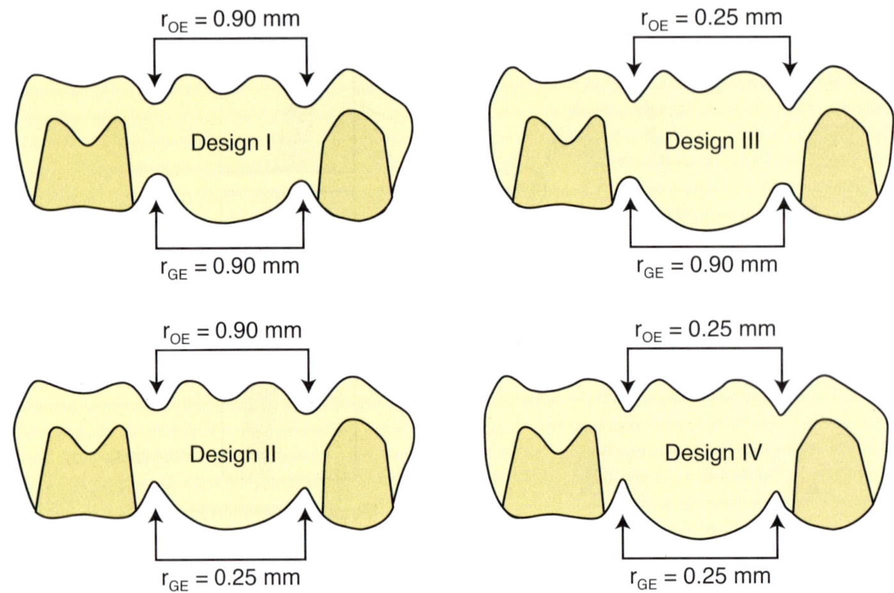

• **Fig. 10.42** Ceramic bridges with various radii of curvature in occlusal and gingival embrasures. Designs I and III have the lowest stress concentration factors in the gingival (tensile) embrasure areas, which have the larger radii of curvature.

radius of curvature of the gingival embrasure (Fig. 10.42) of the interproximal connector also can increase the fracture resistance of an FDP. Quinn et al. (2010) studied the effect of connector diameter rather than connector radius of curvature to predict the minimal connector size for a zirconia framework to ensure a 95% survival against fracture over a period of 20 years. The results of this analysis are presented in Figure 10.43.

Fractured connectors are fairly common, especially when the connector size is less than that recommended by the manufacturer. Figure 10.44 illustrates an example of this design deficiency. The distal connector of the three-unit bridge made from a lithia disilicate core ceramic fractured after 1.5 years in service and the

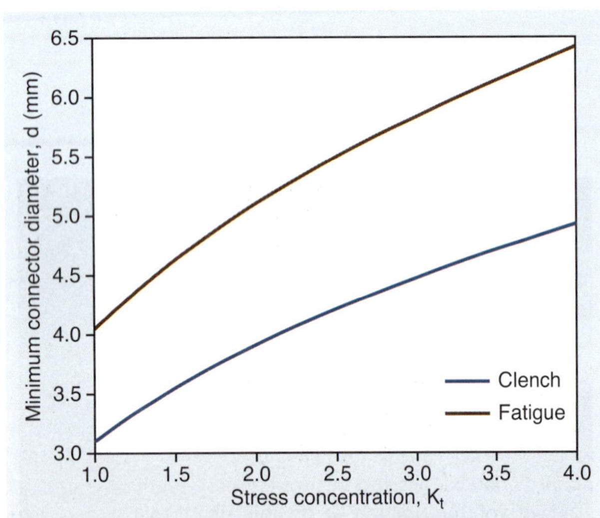

• **Fig. 10.43** Predicted minimum connector diameter for four-unit ceramic bridge made from 3Y-TZP to ensure a survival of 95% for at least 20 years. (Adapted from Quinn GD, Studart AR, Hebert C, VerHoef JR, Arola D: Fatigue of zirconia and dental bridge geometry: Design implications. *Dent Mater* 26(12):1133–1136, 2010.)

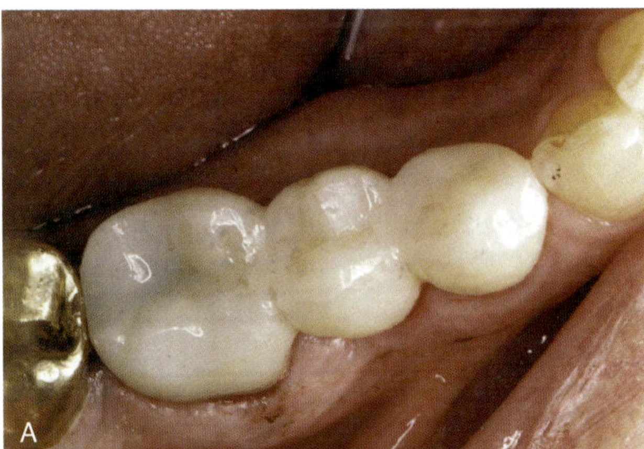

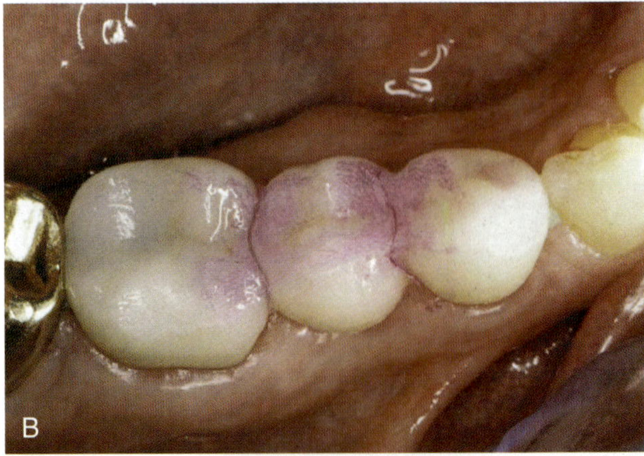

• **Fig. 10.44 (A)** Postcementation photo of three-unit ceramic bridge made with a lithia disilicate–based core ceramic. **(B)** Fractured connectors of the bridge after approximately 1.5 years. The posterior connector height was found to be 3.5 mm, which was 0.5 mm less than that recommended by the manufacturer.

mesial connector fractured later. The height of the distal connector was only 3.5 mm, or 0.5 mm less than was recommended.

Bonding of Resin to Dental Ceramics

Bonding to prosthetic ceramics is important for three reasons: (1) resin-based composite cements are believed to increase the retention of all-ceramic prostheses, (2) resin-based composite cements are believed to increase the fracture resistance and survivability of ceramic restorations, and (3) resin-based composite is the material of choice for repair of chipped or fractured core or veneer ceramic. However, silane-based coupling does not bond chemically to all ceramics. For example, as previously shown in Figure 10.36, the framework of the fractured resin-bonded bridge made with an alumina framework could not be etched. The dimpled area on one of the retained flanges of the bridge suggests that macromechanical bonding to the resin cement had been chosen. The clean separation of this framework from the resin-based cement indicates inadequate bonding. In addition, examination of the fractured flange indicates the presence of a large void that may have contributed to the fracture of the connector.

The mechanism of silane-based primer bonding to a silica network of silica-based ceramics is well known. In addition, abrasive blasting and acid etching of the glass matrix of these ceramics create surface irregularities that can further enhance the retention of the resin cement. The penetration of the adhesive resin into the macroscopic irregularities, combined with chemical bonding, may also inhibit water access to the ceramic surface, thereby enhancing the durability of bonded ceramic prostheses. Furthermore, acid etching can blunt the tips of microcracks within the ceramic surface. This blunting process reduces the stress concentration at the crack tips. If any voids are trapped within the interface between the crown and cement in the occlusal area, occlusal loads above this site can generate tensile stresses in the ceramic that may cause crack formation or fracture.

Silane primers or coupling agents have dual functionality, including an unsaturated group for polymerizing to adhesive resins and resin-based composites and methoxy groups (–OCH_3) that are hydrolyzed to silanols (Si–OH) for bonding to inorganics such as silica-based ceramics or metal oxide substrates through the formation of siloxane (–Si–O–Si–) bonds or (–Si–O–M–) bonds on other metal oxide substrates. Silane primers provide covalent bonds that promote adhesion at the interface between polymers and hydrolytically stable silica-based substrates, assuming that the substrate is free of contaminants. Figure 10.45 shows a schematic illustration of the bonding stage of silane primer or adhesive to a silica-based ceramic.

The reaction of silanes with silica-based ceramics involves four stages: hydrolysis, condensation, hydrogen bonding, and bond formation. After hydrolysis of the methoxy groups, condensation to oligomers occurs, and the oligomers then hydrogen bond with –OH groups of the substrate. Then, during curing, covalent links are formed with the substrate, with simultaneous loss of water. These reactions typically occur simultaneously after the initial hydrolysis stage.

Although a monolayer of silane-based primer is preferred, multilayer adsorption generally occurs. Estimated thicknesses from deposition of a 0.25% silane solution onto glass range from three to eight molecular layers. Kitayama et al. reported that silane-based monomers produced the best bonding to silica-based ceramic, and monomers that are based on either phosphate ester or phosphonic acid monomers produce better bonding to zirconia. These bonding mechanisms are described further in Chapter 6.

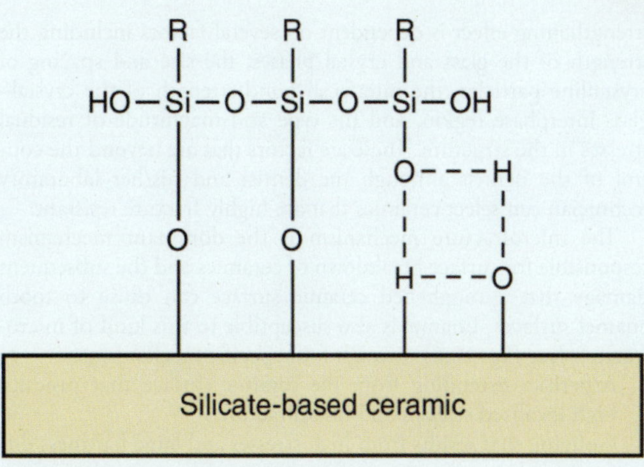

• **Fig. 10.45** Schematic illustration of silane bonding to silica-based ceramic.

CRITICAL QUESTION

How can the potential abrasive damage of tooth enamel that opposes ceramic surfaces be minimized? Why is the hardness of a ceramic not a good predictor of wear?

Abrasiveness of Dental Ceramics

Ceramics are generally considered the most biocompatible, durable, and esthetic materials available for rehabilitation of teeth, occlusal function, and facial appearance. Currently available products exhibit variable mechanical properties (hardness, flexure strength, fracture toughness, and elastic modulus), physical properties (index of refraction, color parameters, translucency, chemical durability, and thermal compatibility of core and veneering ceramics), and ability to be bonded to tooth structures and other substrates. In spite of their overall excellence in meeting the ideal requirements of a prosthetic material, dental ceramics have one major drawback: these materials can cause catastrophic wear of opposing tooth structure under certain conditions. The most extreme damage occurs when a roughened surface contacts tooth enamel or dentin under extraordinarily high occlusal forces. This may occur because of bruxing, premature occlusal contacts, and/or inadequate occlusion adjustments. When cuspid-guided disocclusion is ensured, the wear of opposing enamel and dentin will be greatly reduced. The abrasive wear of opposing tooth structure can be reduced further by periodically refinishing the occlusal surface after frequent exposures to carbonated beverages and/or APF.

Abrasive wear mechanisms for dental restorative materials and tooth enamel include (1) adhesion (metals and composites) in which localized bonding of two surfaces occurs, resulting in pull-out, and transfer of matter from one surface to the other, and (2) microfracture (ceramics and enamel), which results from gouging, asperities, impact, and contact stresses that cause cracks or localized fracture. For ceramic and enamel, two-phase brittle structures are involved. The ceramic consists of a glass matrix that contains variable levels and sizes of crystals. Tooth enamel consists of a small volume fraction of organic phase matrix and a high-volume fraction of hydroxyapatite crystals. The wear of either material depends on the ease with which cracks can propagate through the structure. If microscopic cracks are forced to pass around the crystal particles rather than through them, the material will usually be more fracture and abrasion resistant. The relative strengthening effect is dependent on several factors including the strength of the glass and crystal phases, the size and spacing of crystalline particles, the interfacial bond strength of the crystal–glass interphase region, and the type and magnitude of residual stresses in the structure. These are factors that are beyond the control of the dentist although the dentist and his/her laboratory technician can select ceramics that are highly fracture resistant.

The microfracture mechanism is the dominant mechanism responsible for surface breakdown of ceramics and the subsequent damage that a roughened ceramic surface can cause to tooth enamel surfaces. Enamel is also susceptible to this kind of microfracture (see Fig. 10.6) through four specific mechanisms:

1. Asperities extending from the ceramic surface that produce high localized stresses and microfracture.
2. Gouging that results from high stresses and large hardness differences between two surfaces or particles extending from these surfaces.
3. Impact or erosion that occurs through the action of abrasive particles carried in a flowing liquid such as saliva.
4. Contact stress microfracture that increases localized tensile stress and also enhances the damage caused by asperities, gouging, and impact or erosion.

Because of microfracture mechanisms, it may be necessary to polish the ceramic surface periodically to reduce the height of asperities and to minimize enamel wear rates. Of major concern is the potential catastrophic damage that can be incurred by enamel in contact with polycrystalline asperities having high fracture toughness (K_{Ic}) values such as alumina (3.5–4.0 MPa·$m^{1/2}$), magnesium-stabilized zirconia (9–12 MPa·$m^{1/2}$), yttrium-stabilized zirconia (8.0–10.3 MPa·$m^{1/2}$), or cerium-stabilized zirconia (10–16 MPa·$m^{1/2}$). In contrast, glass, which has a fracture toughness of only 0.75 MPa·$m^{1/2}$, should cause less gouging, contact stress, and impact damage to contacting enamel surfaces.

The abrasiveness of ceramics against enamel is affected by numerous factors and properties of the crystal phase particles and the glass matrix (if present). These include hardness, tensile strength, fracture toughness, fatigue resistance, particle–glass bonding, particle–glass interface integrity, chemical durability, exposure frequency to corrosive chemical agents (APF, carbonated beverages), abrasiveness of foods, residual stress, subsurface quality (voids or other imperfections), magnitude and orientation of applied forces, chewing patterns, bruxing frequency, contact area, lubrication by saliva, and duration of exposure to abrasive particles. As a general rule, the larger the hardness difference between two sliding surfaces, the greater is the degree of wear. However, this simple principle does not explain the wide variation in wear rates that are exhibited by different patients under apparently similar conditions. Thus, it is easy to understand why the hardness of the ceramic is not a good predictor of the potential wear of enamel surfaces by a ceramic.

Wear Rates of Ceramics Compared With Other Materials

To minimize enamel abrasion by a contacting ceramic structure, one should use a ceramic that exhibits uniform surface microfracture at the same rate as tooth enamel under the same conditions of loading, antagonist structure, food substance abrasiveness, applied forces, and degree of lubrication. The breakdown of the ceramic surface should be uniform so that asperities such as large crystalline inclusions do not project out of the surface.

These asperities produce high stress concentration areas within the opposing enamel surface that lead to gouging, troughing, and greater localized microfracture of the enamel structure. If such nonuniform surface wear of ceramics occurs during oral function, the only solutions available to reduce enamel wear are to reduce the occlusal load by occlusal adjustment or to polish the ceramic surface periodically to reduce stress concentrations and the height of these asperities. However, polishing of ceramics is a relatively slow process and care must be taken to minimize the generation of heat in the process.

Wear of Enamel by Ceramic Products and Other Restorative Materials

Another factor that can increase the wear of enamel by ceramics is the nonuniform clustering of crystals. IPS Empress after hot pressing at 1180°C exhibits clusters of relatively large (5–10 μm) leucite crystals ($KAlSi_2O_6$) with cracks between the crystal agglomerates. This noninterlocking arrangement of leucite crystals also occurs in the veneering ceramic after it is sintered at 910°C. In contrast, IPS Empress 2 core ceramic exhibits a uniform dispersion of smaller lithia disilicate ($Li_2Si_2O_5$) crystals after hot pressing at 920°C and veneering at 800°C.

One should expect greater wear of enamel by IPS Empress compared with IPS Empress 2. IPS Empress ceramic contains 35 ± 51% by volume of leucite crystals that are formed in a noninterlocking particle cluster pattern (Höland et al., 2000). The core microstructure of IPS Empress 2 is quite different from that of IPS Empress, as evidenced by elongated lithia disilicate crystals 0.5–4 μm in length and a smaller concentration of lithium orthophosphate crystals (Li_3PO_4) approximately 0.1–0.3 μm in diameter (Höland et al., 2000). An in vitro study involving 50,000 wear cycles in a poppy seed/PMMA-bead slurry revealed significantly greater three-body wear of enamel by IPS Empress veneer ceramic (6.06 mm^2) compared with IPS Empress 2 veneer ceramic (1.82 mm^2). This represents a 238% increase in surface area lost because of ceramic abrasiveness. Enamel wear volume losses caused by other materials were as follows: Vita Omega (4.44 mm^2), Procera AllCeram (4.97 mm^2), Finesse (5.23 mm^2), and Vitadur Alpha (6.61 mm^2), which is an aluminous porcelain.

Studies of ultralow-fusing ceramics have generally revealed significantly lower enamel wear rates than those produced by conventional porcelains. However, the results of one study suggest that one of these ceramics, Duceram LFC, caused significantly more enamel wear (0.197 mm^3) than Creation porcelain (0.135 mm^3) or Vitadur Alpha porcelain (0.153 mm^3), presumably because of the higher void volume within the surface layer of Duceram LFC (Magne et al., 1999). In this study, the combined enamel/ceramic wear rates were significantly greater for Duceram LFC (0.363 mm^3) and Vitadur Alpha (0.333 mm^3) compared with that for Creation porcelain (0.260 mm^3). Veneering ceramics contain either large crystalline filler particles or a glass structure with no crystals or very small crystals such as nanocrystalline fluorapatite.

The results from another study (Al-Hiyasat, 1999) of enamel wear (after 25,000 simulated chewing cycles) by ceramics using a cornmeal slurry (three-body condition) revealed greater relative wear depth in enamel by Duceram LFC (0.74 mm) and Vitadur Alpha (0.80 mm) compared with Vita Cerec Mk II (0.48 mm). The result for Duceram LFC is in contrast with two-body wear data (Al-Hiyasat et al., 1998) indicating significantly less enamel wear in distilled water without an abrasive food medium by Duceram LFC (0.54 mm after 25,000 simulated chewing cycles) and Vita Mk II (0.65 mm) and a gold alloy (0.09 mm) compared with

Vitadur Alpha porcelain (0.93 mm) and Vita Omega porcelain (0.96 mm). The wear rate of enamel by gold alloy was significantly less than that produced by the four ceramics. The explanation given for the higher wear rate of enamel by Duceram LFC was the presence of porosity within the surface of the ceramic.

One would expect the latter types of ceramics to cause minimal wear of enamel. The results of one study (Metzler et al., 1999) indicate that the relative enamel loss was less for two ultralow-fusing ceramics, Finesse (0.56) and Vita Omega 900 (0.60), compared with Dentsply Ceramco II porcelain (0.85), a large particle leucite-based porcelain.

Krejci et al. (1994) reported significantly lower estimated 5-year enamel wear rates for amalgam (50 μm) and a new Cerec CAD–CAM ceramic, Vita Cerec Mk II V7K (95 μm), compared with the original Vita Cerec Mk I ceramic (225 μm). In comparison, the wear of enamel by enamel was 107 μm. Hacker et al. (1996) found considerably lower enamel wear rates for a gold–palladium alloy (9 μm) compared with AllCeram veneer ceramic (60 μm) and Dentsply Ceramco porcelain (230 μm).

Jagger et al. (1995) reported the following wear depths of dentin after wear by restorative materials: amalgam (0 μm), microfilled composite (7 μm), gold alloy (16.7 μm), conventional composite (31.7 μm), and Vitadur N aluminous porcelain (100 μm). These results indicate that direct filling materials are less abrasive to dentin than aluminous porcelain. This result is not surprising. What is of importance is the significant potential benefit of amalgam and microfilled composite as the least abrasive restorative materials for situations in which opposing dentin is exposed.

Al-Hiyasat et al. (1998) investigated the effect of a carbonated beverage (Coca-Cola) on the wear of human enamel and three dental ceramics: Vitadur Alpha (feldspathic porcelain), Duceram LFC (ultralow-fusing porcelain), and Vita Mark II, a machinable ceramic. Tooth-ceramic specimens were tested in a wear machine under a load of 40 N, at 80 cycles per minute, for a total of 25,000 cycles. The test was performed in distilled water or with intermittent exposure to a carbonated beverage (Coca-Cola). When tested in water, Vitadur Alpha porcelain caused significantly more enamel wear and also exhibited greater wear than Duceram LFC and Vita Mark II. However, after exposure to the carbonated beverage, the enamel wear produced by Duceram LFC did not differ significantly from that produced by Vitadur Alpha porcelain. Vita Mark II produced the least amount of enamel wear. Exposure to the carbonated beverage significantly increased the enamel wear. The wear of Duceram LFC and Vita Mark II increased with exposure to the carbonated beverage. It was concluded that exposure to the carbonated beverage accelerated the enamel wear produced by Duceram LFC and Vita Mark II ceramics. Overall, Vita Mark II was the most resistant to wear and it was also significantly less abrasive than Vitadur Alpha porcelain.

CRITICAL QUESTION

Why does glazing sometimes not decrease the abrasive potential of ceramic crowns?

Reducing Abrasiveness of Ceramics by Polishing and Glazing

In theory, the smoothest surface should cause the least wear damage to opposing surfaces. Depending on the initial surface roughness of the ceramic surface, glazing the surface may not adequately decrease the surface roughness since the glassy layer may be of insufficient thickness to fill in scratches and grooves within the ground surface. Thus, under certain conditions, polishing or polishing followed by glazing may be required.

Jagger and Harrison (1994) reported that the amount of enamel wear produced by both glazed (28.8 μm) and unglazed Vitadur N aluminous porcelain (29 μm) was similar; however, wear produced by polished porcelain (12 μm) was substantially less. Polished or glazed porcelain caused significantly less wear than unglazed porcelain. Polishing was accomplished with 3M Sof-Lex disks and Shofu rubber points.

After 25,000 cycles of abrasion testing of various porcelain surfaces on human enamel in vitro, Al-Hiyasat et al. (1997) reported no significant difference between the enamel wear of glazed and polished groups, but wear produced by the unglazed groups was significantly higher ($P < .05$). Sixty pairs of tooth–porcelain specimens were tested under load in distilled water with and without intermittent exposure to a carbonated beverage. Wear of enamel and Vitadur Alpha porcelain specimens was determined after 5000, 15,000, and 25,000 cycles. Exposure to a carbonated Coca-Cola and Schweppes beverages significantly increased the amount of enamel wear produced by all porcelain surfaces ($P < .001$). The finish of the porcelain surface did not influence wear.

Guidelines for Minimizing Excessive Wear of Enamel by Dental Ceramics

To minimize the wear of enamel by dental ceramics, the following steps should be taken:

1. Ensure cuspid-guided disocclusion
2. Eliminate occlusal prematurities
3. Use metal in functional bruxing areas
4. If occlusion is in ceramic, use ultralow-fusing ceramics
5. Polish functional ceramic surfaces
6. Repolish ceramic surfaces periodically
7. Readjust occlusion periodically if needed

Ceramic and opposing surfaces should be examined periodically for evidence of excessive wear. Occlusal adjustment and polishing of the ceramic surfaces should be performed to reduce the risk for further surface degradation. Noble metal surfaces are especially indicated for individuals who exhibit evidence of severe bruxing since the wear rates of gold alloys are very low compared with the wear damage caused by either traditional ceramics or recent ultralow-fusing ceramics. A rough ceramic surface that is in hyperocclusion with opposing enamel is very likely to cause great abrasive wear of tooth surfaces. To minimize the risk of such wear damage to tooth enamel or other surfaces, the smoothest possible ceramic surface should be produced. This can be accomplished by (1) polishing only, (2) polishing followed by glazing, or (3) glazing only. The second choice is preferred. Glazing is recommended whenever possible prior to cementation of a prosthesis. If this is not possible, polishing alone is acceptable. Glazing of a very rough ceramic surface may not sufficiently reduce the surface roughness to minimize wear damage. However, it is reasonable to assume that a glazed rough surface is better than a rough, nonglazed surface since the troughs are filled in with glass, which reduces the surface roughness. It is not always possible to polish a ceramic surface in the clinic. Because of the heat generated during polishing of ceramic-based prostheses, the increased temperature of pulpal tissue may lead to irreversible pulpitis. This is especially true when the tooth has been greatly reduced in size and the pulp chamber is within 0.5 mm of the external surface of the prepared tooth.

There are several clear indications for polishing ceramic surfaces. Polishing of ceramic prostheses should be performed when they cannot be autoglazed. Polishing of ceramic restorations that have functional occlusal pathways or subgingival extensions will ensure optimal smoothness. All CAD–CAM inlays or other ceramic prostheses that will not receive veneering ceramic should also be polished.

Intraoral instrumentation can produce a smoother surface than an autoglazing procedure. Highly polished porcelain may also be naturally glazed or overglazed without significantly increasing the surface roughness. Increased time or cycles of glazing will decrease surface roughness.

Polishing instruments should be selected according to the type of ceramic, type of restoration, and level of smoothness desired. If the crown was ground with a 100 μm grit diamond, the first polishing abrasive should be 75 μm or less. If the abrasive is too fine, more time will be needed to polish the surface. Hulterstrom and Bergman (1993) found that two of the best polishing systems were Sof-Lex disks (3M Dental) and Shofu porcelain laminate polishing kit followed by diamond paste. Polishing is preferred over glazing as a procedure to reduce abrasion damage of enamel. Ceramic surfaces should be refinished periodically after acid exposure, especially APF. The Shofu porcelain polishing kit followed with diamond paste or Sof-Lex disks (3M) without a diamond paste follow-up is useful as effective finishing products.

For the Sof-Lex disks, one should start with the disk that is the most effective at removing the initial grinding patterns. If the abrasive grit size on the disk is too small, it will take too long to decrease the roughness. If the grit size is too large (e.g., extra coarse or coarse), the surface will become rougher. Also, if the polishing procedure is performed in the mouth, care should be taken to avoid heat build-up. Sof-Lex disks are made to be used in a wet environment, so water coolant should be used whenever possible.

The Shofu kit contains a series of rubber point abrasives and rubber wheels. The shank of the rubber tips is color coded to distinguish the abrasive grit characteristic. The diamond paste is expressed from a tube or removed from a jar and applied to the ceramic surface using either a Robinson Wheel brush or a felt wheel. This paste is more amenable to use for extraoral polishing of dental ceramics.

Clinical Performance of All-Ceramic Restorations

Malament and Socransky (1999) reported survival probabilities for acid-etched Dicor and nonetched Dicor restorations of 76% and 50%, respectively, after 14 years ($P < .001$). Nonetched (nonbonded) Dicor crowns exhibited a 2.2 times greater risk of failure than acid-etched restorations ($P < .01$). Ceramic crown survival was greatest for incisor teeth and decreased progressively to a maximum failure level for second molar crowns. All lateral incisor crowns survived during the 14-year study. Survival of acid-etched and resin-bonded Dicor crowns for subjects 33–52 years of age was 62% at 14 years compared with 82% for those 52 years of age and older.

Tooth preparation for all-ceramic crowns is virtually the same as that required for MC restorations. Occlusal surfaces and incisal edges must be reduced about 1.5–2.0 mm. Axial surfaces should be reduced at least 1.0 mm circumferentially, although the guidelines for one all-ceramic product indicate that an axial reduction of 0.8 mm is sufficient. The preparation should be either a shoulder with a rounded gingivoaxial line angle or a 120° chamfer (deep chamfer). Knife-edge margins should never be chosen for any ceramic product.

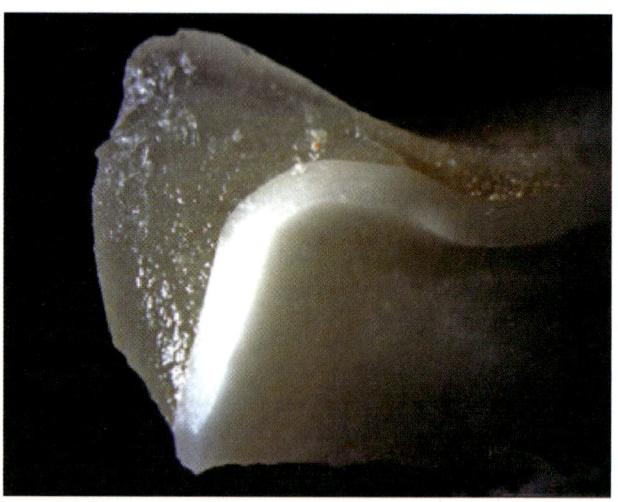

• **Fig. 10.46** Fracture of overextended veneering ceramic.

Clinicians have experienced fractures of crowns during initial seating because of knife-edge margins, overextension of veneering porcelain beyond the support area of the core ceramic (Fig. 10.46), undetected or incompletely removed ceramic particles on the internal surface, distortion of impressions or trays, undercut areas on the tooth that were not properly blocked out, and inadequate occlusal or connector thickness under hyperocclusion conditions.

A light seating force combined with internal inspection and correction of these irregularities is indicated as a routine procedure. For cementation, a resin cement is indicated for the weaker products, such as OPC-3G, Finesse All-Ceramic, IPS Empress, IPS Empress 2, and ICS. Etching of ceramics with a glass matrix creates micromechanical retention areas on the internal surface. A dual-curing or self-curing cement is recommended. A vibratory instrument or a light tapping procedure will ensure complete seating since some of these cements are quite viscous or behave in a thixotropic manner (increased flow under vibratory or light tapping action). The excess cement should be removed completely immediately after seating. After polymerization, residual resin can be removed with abrasive disks, stones, or burs. For any ceramic crown, large voids in the cement must be minimized since the tensile stresses in the unsupported areas of a ceramic crown will be increased under occlusal forces.

A systematic review by Morimoto (2016) showed estimated survival rates for glass–ceramics and feldspathic porcelain were between 92% and 95% at 5 years and 91% at 10 years. Failures were related to fractures/chipping (4%), followed by endodontic complications (3%), secondary caries (1%), debonding (1%), and severe marginal staining (0%). Ceramic inlays, onlays, and overlays showed high survival rates at 5 years and 10 years, and fractures were the most frequent cause of failure.

A long-term evaluation (Malament, 2020) of the performance of pressed acid-etched e.max lithium disilicate glass–ceramic complete and partial coverage restorations in posterior teeth showed that the 16.9-year estimated cumulative survival was 96.49%. The estimated cumulative survival of posterior complete and posterior partial coverage restorations was 96.75% at 10.5 years and 95.27% at 16.9 years.

Carvalho (2018) found that the estimated survival rate of CAD–CAM fabricated restorations was around 89.7% at 5 years. A meta-analysis by Sailer (2018) revealed an estimated 5-year survival rate of 98.7% for MC implant-supported FDPs, and of 93.0% for zirconia–ceramic implant-supported FDPs.

Sulaiman (2020) evaluated a total of 188,695 (51,751 lithium disilicate and 136,944 zirconia) restorations and found an overall fracture rate of 1.35%. Lithium disilicate monolithic single crowns had a fracture rate of 0.96%, which was significantly lower than that of layered single crowns at 1.26%. When the different types of lithium disilicate restorations were compared, fixed partial denture (monolithic and layered) fracture rates were significantly higher than those of single crowns. Monolithic zirconia single crowns (0.54%) fractured at a lower rate than layered zirconia single crowns (2.83%) and monolithic fixed partial dentures (1.83%), while layered single crowns (2.83%) had a higher fracture rate than that of layered fixed partial dentures (1.93%). Monolithic anterior and posterior zirconia restorations fractured at a lower rate than layered anterior and posterior zirconia restorations. Posterior monolithic zirconia restorations fractured at a lower rate than anterior restorations, while posterior layered zirconia restorations fractured at a higher rate than anterior zirconia restorations.

Box 10.4 describes the clinical factors involved in choosing the right ceramic material for a given clinical situation.

Ceramic Veneers

The success rate of etched and bonded porcelain veneers has been well established since the concept of acid etching of porcelain was established in 1981. However, limited long-term data are available to compare the longevity of these restorations with the survival times and probabilities for MC or ceramic crowns.

A recent meta-analysis found that the estimated cumulative survival for feldspathic porcelain veneers was 95.7% at 5 years and ranged from 64% to 95% at 10 years across three studies. A post hoc meta-analysis indicated that the 10-year best estimate may approach 95.6%. They found that the partial bonding of porcelain veneers to reduced enamel may be associated with decreased estimated cumulative survival rates (Layton, 2012). The same group however found that there was limited evidence available about the survival of nonfeldspathic veneers, and the 5-year survival rate could be around 90% (Layton, 2013). Furthermore, crowns that are made from alumina or zirconia core ceramics should not be used for ceramic veneers because of their opacity and their inability to be etched and bonded effectively to tooth enamel.

The importance of preparation technique and bonding cannot be overstated when it comes to veneers. Gurel (2013) found a survival rate of 99% for veneers with preparations confined to enamel and 94% for veneers with enamel only at the margins. They concluded that laminate veneers have high survival rates when bonded to enamel and provide a safe and predictable treatment option that preserves tooth structure.

Ceramic veneers represent a more conservative approach than the use of full crowns. The control of esthetics is technique sensitive since the resin cement, whose color may change over time, plays a key role in the overall appearance. In addition, resin-bonded veneers and crowns that extend into the root area of patients with poor oral hygiene have been associated with leakage and secondary caries caused by improper cementation.

Several products are available for porcelain veneers. Most of these ceramics have relatively high translucency and most are sold with a bonding kit and instructions for etching with hydrofluoric acid (HF) or ammonium bifluoride (NH_4HF_2) gels. Do not etch the ceramic with phosphoric acid from a conditioning kit for composite. Read the instructions carefully. Some ceramics require sandblasting instead of etching when using the bonding kit. An appropriate technique for bonding ceramic veneers is provided in Chapter 7 (Box 7.3).

• BOX 10.4 Clinical Indications of Various Types of Ceramics

The following indications for ceramic system use are based upon the best available clinical evidence:

1. Fixed partial dentures: metal–ceramic should be the material of choice for FPDs, but monolithic zirconia FPDs can be considered if economics is a consideration.
2. Single anterior crowns: layered lithium disilicate provides the best combination of aesthetic outcomes and survivability. With bruxing patients, layered zirconia with polished zirconia on the palatal surface provides reasonable aesthetics, along with lack of wear to the opposing dentition.
3. Premolars: depending on the aesthetic demands and parafunctional activity of the patient, monolithic lithium disilicate or zirconia, and layered zirconia could be considered.
4. Molars: monolithic zirconia crowns provide the best combination of minimal tooth reduction, economics, and lack of opposing wear with acceptable aesthetics.
5. Mandibular incisors: monolithic zirconia crowns are indicated primarily because of the possibility of minimal tooth reduction.
6. Bonded ceramic onlays and partial veneers: etched, bonded lithium disilicate restorations are the clear winners. The most important data presented in this article is that, at 45 months, lithium disilicate onlays had a failure rate of 1.1%. With the prevailing philosophy of minimally invasive dentistry and the call for additive versus subtractive procedures, it is clear that many teeth previously restored with crowns can now be effectively restored with conservative bonded ceramic materials. This also greatly improves the efficacy of in-office CAD–CAM procedures.

Donovan, T. E., et al. (2018). An evidence-based evaluation of contemporary dental ceramics. Dental Update **45***(6): 541-546.*

Chemical Attack of Glass-Phase Ceramics by Acidulated Phosphate Fluoride

Topical fluorides are routinely used for caries control. The effect of such agents on the surface of ceramic restorations has been studied. APF, one of the most commonly used fluoride gels, is known to etch glass by selective leaching of sodium ions, thereby disrupting the silica network. When glazed feldspathic porcelain is exposed to 1.23% APF or by 8% stannous fluoride, a surface roughness is produced within 4 minutes. As can be seen in Figure 10.10, a 30-minute exposure to 1.23% APF gel appears to preferentially attack the glass phase (areas with white precipitate particles) of a gingival (body) porcelain. Obviously this roughness leads to staining, plaque accumulation, and further breakdown of the structure. However, the use of lower concentrations, such as 0.4% stannous fluoride and 2% sodium fluoride, has no significant effect on the ceramic surface. Dentists should be aware of these long-term clinical effects of fluorides on ceramic and composite restorations (because of their glass filler particles) and avoid the use of APF gels when composites and ceramics are present. APF gels should not be used on glazed porcelain surfaces. If such a gel is used, the surface of the restoration should be protected with petroleum jelly, cocoa butter, or wax.

Porcelain Denture Teeth

The manufacture of denture teeth constitutes virtually the sole current use for high-fusing or medium-fusing dental porcelains. Their composition is slightly higher in the alumina content as shown in Figure 10.2. Denture teeth are made by packing two or more porcelains of differing translucencies for each tooth into metal molds. They are fired on large trays in high-temperature ovens. Porcelain teeth are designed to be retained on the denture base by mechanical interlocking. The anterior teeth are made with projecting metal pins that become surrounded with the denture base resin during processing, whereas the posterior teeth are molded with diatoric spaces into which the denture base resin may flow.

Either porcelain or acrylic resin denture teeth can be employed in the fabrication of complete and partial dentures. Porcelain teeth are generally considered to be more esthetically satisfactory than acrylic teeth. They are also much more resistant to wear, although the development of new polymers has improved the wear resistance of acrylic teeth. Porcelain teeth also have the advantage of being the only type of denture teeth that allow the denture to be rebased (replacement of the entire acrylic denture base).

Compared with acrylic resin teeth, the disadvantages of porcelain teeth are their brittleness, the need for mechanical retention, the extra time required to grind and contour the surfaces, and the clicking sound produced on contact with the opposing teeth. Porcelain teeth also require a greater interridge distance because they cannot be ground as thin in the ridge lap area as acrylic teeth without destroying the diatoric channels that provide their only means of retention to the denture base resin.

Factors Affecting the Color Appearance of Ceramics

In addition to their biocompatibility and chemical inertness, another principal reason for the choice of ceramics as restorative materials is their esthetic qualities in matching the adjacent tooth structure in translucency, color, and chroma. Color phenomena and terminology are discussed in Chapter 3. Perfect color matching is extremely difficult and demands exceptional skill and experience on the parts of the dentist and lab technician. The structure of the tooth influences its color. Dentin is more opaque than enamel and reflects light very well. Enamel represents a predominantly crystalline layer over the dentin and is composed of tiny prisms or rods cemented together by an organic substance. The indices of refraction of the rods and the cementing substance are different. As a result, light rays are dispersed by varying proportions of absorption, transmission, scattering, and reflection to produce a resulting translucent effect. This creates a sensation of depth as the scattered light ray reaches the eye. As the light ray strikes the tooth surface, part of it is reflected, and the remainder penetrates the enamel and is scattered. Any light reaching the dentin is either absorbed or partially reflected to the eye and partially scattered within the enamel. If dentin is not present, as in the tip of an incisor, some of the light ray may be transmitted into the oral cavity. As a result, this area may appear to be more translucent than that toward the gingival area. Because the law of energy conservation must apply, the following relationship shows the five energy components that are derived from the energy (E) of the incident light:

$$E_{incident} = E_{scattered} + E_{reflected} + E_{absorbed} + E_{transmitted} + E_{fluoresced}$$

Although some of the absorbed light may be converted into heat, some may be transmitted back to the eye as fluorescent energy. Light rays can also be dispersed, giving a color or shade that varies in different teeth. The dispersion can vary with the wavelength of the light. Therefore, the appearance of the teeth may vary according to whether they are viewed in direct sunlight, reflected daylight, tungsten light, or fluorescent light. This phenomenon is called metamerism. The dentist and laboratory technician must reproduce the esthetic characteristics sufficiently such that the appearance of a ceramic prosthesis is discernible only to the trained eye.

Dental porcelains are pigmented by the inclusion of oxides to provide desired shades. Specimens of each shade are distributed in a specific order in shade guides to assist the clinic team in selection of the best match to adjacent natural teeth or other ceramic or resin composite restorations. The colors of dentin (body) porcelain and opaque porcelain vary among manufacturers for a given shade. What are the reasons for this variation? Each manufacturer designs a specific system for developing shades of opaque and dentin porcelains. Ambiguity in the true color of a shade arises from differences among shade guides. Apparently each manufacturer interprets what a given shade should be. Anatomically contoured shade guides are made manually to combine an opaque, dentin, and incisal porcelain on each tab. The porcelains used are uniquely made for shade guides and they are not always produced from dental porcelains. The manual process leads to variations among manufacturers and among shade guides for any shade.

Shade guides are produced by dental ceramic manufacturers to assist dentists and lab technicians in selecting optimum ceramic shades and for communicating the desired prosthesis appearance to each other and the laboratory technician. Shade guides made of porcelain are used most often by dentists to describe a desired appearance of a natural tooth or ceramic prosthesis. However, there are several deficiencies of shade guides.

- Shade guide tabs are much thicker than the thickness of ceramic that is used for dental crowns or veneers, and they are more translucent than teeth and ceramic crowns backed by a nontranslucent dentin substructure or veneering ceramics backed by an opaque core ceramic, or a metal framework.
- Much of the incident light is transmitted through a tab. In contrast, most of the incident light on a crown is reflected except at the incisal edge and at proximal incisal areas.
- Furthermore, the necks of shade tabs are made from a deeper hue—that is, higher chroma—and this region tends to distract the observer's matching ability in the gingival third of the tab. To avoid this situation, some clinicians grind away the neck area of a set of shade tabs.

The production of color sensation with a pigment is a physically different phenomenon from that obtained by optical reflection, refraction, and dispersion. The color of a pigment is determined by selective absorption and selective reflection. For example, if white light is reflected from a red surface, all the light with a wavelength different from that of red is absorbed and only the red light is reflected. It follows, then, that if a red hue is present in a ceramic crown but the red hue of the same wavelength is not present in the light beam, the tooth will appear as a different shade. If the tooth or restoration surface is rough, most of the light will be scattered and little will penetrate its structure.

Ceramic Veneers, Inlays, and Onlays

The success rate of etched and bonded porcelain veneers has been well established since acid etching of porcelain was established in 1981. The estimated cumulative survival for feldspathic porcelain veneers was 95.7% at 5 years and ranged from 64% to 95% at 10 years across three studies. The 5-year cumulative estimated survival for etchable nonfeldspathic porcelain veneers is over 90%. Ceramic veneers represent a more conservative approach than the use of full crowns. The control of esthetics is technique sensitive because the conventional acid–base cements or resin-based luting cements play a key role in the overall appearance.

The discovery that dental porcelains and glass–ceramics can be etched with HF or other acids to create retentive micromechanical irregularities similar to those in acid-etched enamel has led to the development of resin-bonded, acid-etched ceramic restorations. One must be extremely careful in handling HF (see Chapter 7) because even short-term contact can cause catastrophic injury to affected tissues. An emergency management plan for laboratories that use HF should be established.

Ceramic veneers are used primarily for esthetic improvement of stained or hypoplastic anterior teeth. Resin-bonded, acid-etched ceramic inlays and onlays are also used for posterior restorations. A resin cement is used for bonding to the etched metal and enamel. The long-term clinical performance of ceramic veneers and resin-bonded inlays and onlays has been well documented. Their esthetic characteristics are excellent. However, one should be aware of the potential for ceramic veneers to abrade opposing teeth excessively. Thus, the surface of the ceramic restorations should be polished to as smooth a surface finish as possible after they have been adjusted into the desired incisal function prior to cementation.

Critical Observation and Analysis of Fractures

Clinical fractures of MC restorations, although rare, still occur, especially when a new alloy or veneering porcelain is being used or a new technology (such as POM veneer ceramic for metal frameworks) has been adopted. As is generally true for all dental materials, a learning curve is associated with the initial use of new products. When fractures occur, it is extremely useful to make a vinyl polysiloxane impression of the fracture site as soon as possible for future fractographic analysis. All information on the crown or bridge should be recorded, including the visual appearance of the fracture site, the location, the approximate size, and occlusion (Anusavice, 2012). A photograph is also very helpful in analyzing the potential cause of fracture. Although there are an infinite number of fracture paths that may occur, three types are of particular importance in diagnosing the cause of fracture. Shown in Figure 10.40 are fracture paths that have occurred primarily at three sites in an MC crown: (1) along the interfacial region between opaque porcelain (P) and the bonding zone (I) between porcelain and the metal substrate (top), (2) within the bonding zone (center), and (3) between the metal and the bonding zone (bottom). For conventional MC crowns made from cast copings, the bonding zone is synonymous with the metal oxide layer. For copings made using atypical methods such as the technologies associated with the Captek system (Leach and Dillon), and electroforming processes, bonding to porcelain is achieved through the formation of an intermediate layer of material such as the Capbond MC "bonder" (bonding agent) for the Captek foil crown system or some other bonding agent.

To characterize the principal site of fracture, a low-magnification examination of the fracture surface may be sufficient in a few cases. However, a magnification of 3–100 times is required more often because minute microstructural details such as pores may reveal wake hackle patterns that clearly show the direction of crack propagation in these areas. Each of the three principal fracture paths in Figure 10.40 is indicative of excessive tensile stress, a material defect, or a processing factor. The location and shape of a fracture surface are major factors used to determine the cause of fracture. For fractures confined to the occlusal surface of posterior crowns, a cone-crack type of fracture (apex of the cone at the fracture surface and the base of the cone extending into the veneer) suggests that localized loading at small contact areas may be the cause. Fractures that occur in the proximal occlusal area of the crowns may be caused by inadequate support of the veneer by the core framework material. Fractures that occur well away from the sites of loading may be caused by thermal incompatibility stresses. The procedures for obtaining evidence from fractured all-ceramic restorations are the same as those used for MC restorations. As proposed by Heintze and Rousson (2010), fractures of ceramic–ceramic prostheses can be classified by whether they should be polished (grade 1), repaired (grade 2), or replaced (grade 3).

What is the purpose of the impression? It allows a replica of the fracture surface to be made from an epoxy resin. The replica allows fractographic observations of the fracture surface to be made, and these models can then be examined by a fractography expert under low magnification using optical microscopy and stereoscopic microscopy, followed by scanning electron microscopy. The location of the critical flaw indicates the origin of the fracture. Fracture surface markings observed on the replica assist the expert in determining the origin and to confirm the suspected cause of fracture. Shown in Figure 10.47A, is a residual section of a fractured Procera AllCeram alumina-based crown with a glass-phase veneer that fractured after 4 years of clinical service. The cause of fracture can be assessed by visual inspection, characterization of principal fracture features, detailed examination of optical microscopy and stereomicroscopy images, and, if necessary, scanning electron microscopy images. These analyses for the fractured crown on the left side of Figure 10.47 revealed fracture paths that are shown by black arrows on Figure 10.47B. These paths suggest that fracture started from an initial crack at the mesial margin (1), propagating 2 mm upward (2), until catastrophic fracture occurred by spreading laterally to areas (4) and area (5), which exhibit an example of compression curl. Area 3 represents another fracture initiation site that is not involved in the bulk fracture process. It illustrates incidental surface damage in an area where crack propagation was localized only in the veneer ceramic.

The fractographic procedures described previously are based on the assumption that the prosthesis was free of cracks during try-in and during cementation. However, dentists are not typically trained to inspect prostheses received from the lab using fiberoptic transillumination. Examination under such lighting can reveal surface and subsurface cracks that may exist in the ceramic and MC prostheses either before or after try-in for fit. Shown in Figure 10.48 is a laboratory technician who is using a fiberoptic light source to inspect a ceramic prosthesis for cracks that may be hidden from typical fluorescent or incandescent light sources.

Many factors are associated with the fracture of all-ceramic prostheses. These factors fall into one of eight categories:

1. Inherent surface defects
2. Processing defects
3. Loading (bite force and load orientation)
4. Design
5. Material properties
6. Residual stress
7. Procedural errors
8. Diet

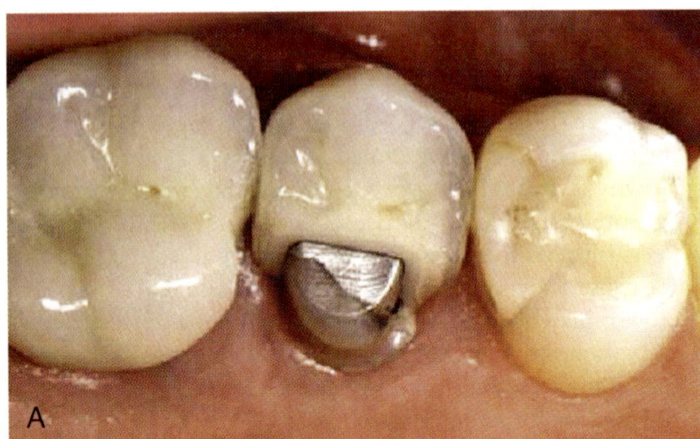

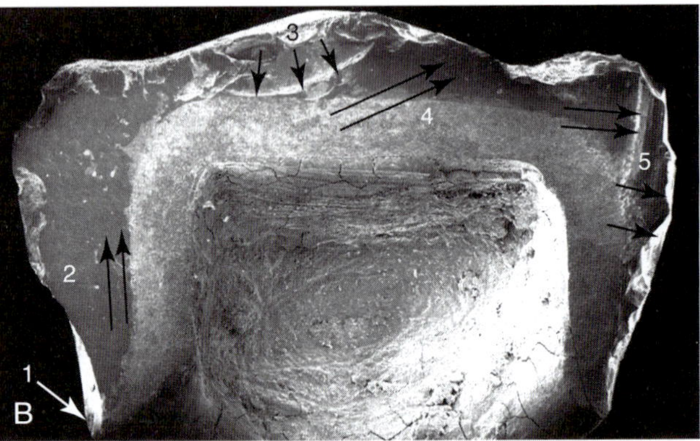

• **Fig. 10.47** **(A)** Fractured Procera AllCeram premolar crown. **(B)** SEM image of the retrieved fractured segment. The initiating crack occurred near the mesial margin (1) and propagated upward approximately 2 mm before crown fracture occurred in areas (2) and (4), terminating in the compression curl area (5). Area (3) represents contact damage within the occlusal veneering ceramic that does not extend into the alumina core ceramic. (From Scherrer SS, Quinn GD, Quinn JB: Fractographic failure analysis of a Procera AllCeram crown. *Dent Mater* 24:1107–1113, 2008.)

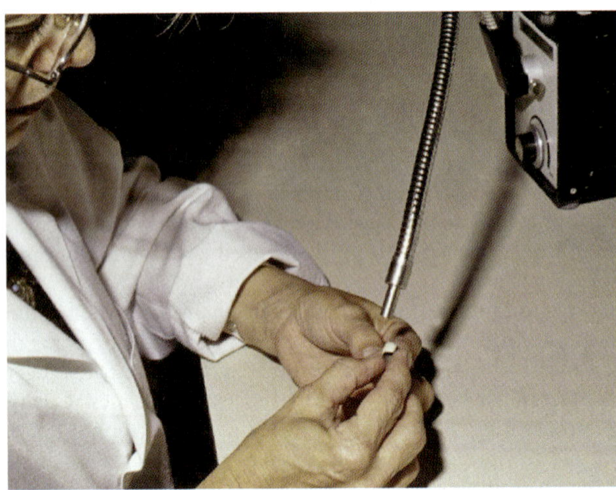

• **Fig. 10.48** Inspection for cracks using fiberoptic transillumination.

Within these categories the following variables may contribute to crack initiation, crack propagation, chipping, and bulk fracture: surface treatment, excessive loading during try-in, bruxing loads, loading location, load distribution, load magnitude, transient cooling stresses, residual cooling stresses, inadequate tooth preparation, improper core framework design, inadequate crown thickness, inadequate core thickness, improper connector size, quality of the cement layer, bond quality of ceramic veneer to core ceramic, voids in the cement layer or at the cement/ceramic interface, and the elastic moduli of component and supporting substrate materials. To reduce the risk for ceramic fracture, sufficient tooth reduction, sufficient thickness of the ceramic, adequate prosthesis design, distributed vertical loading, and meticulous attention to the recommended manufacturers' procedures are required.

Principles for Selection of Dental Ceramics

A properly made MC crown is more fracture resistant and more durable than most all-ceramic crowns and bridges. This technology is well established compared with the technologies required for the most recent all-ceramic products. Although the biocompatibility of some metals used for copings and frameworks may be a concern for patients who have known allergies to those metals, these situations are rare. A metal coping or framework provides an advantage compared with zirconia-based ceramic prostheses when endodontic access openings through crowns are required. Temporary repairs for ceramic fractures that extend to the metal framework are possible, without the need for intraoral sandblasting treatment, by using current resin bonding agents. All-ceramic crowns can be more susceptible to chipping fracture and to bulk fracture in posterior sites. Fractures of ceramic connectors represent another disadvantage of all-ceramic prostheses, especially when the manufacturer's recommendations for connector shape and size cannot be applied. Overall, the aesthetic appearance of an all-ceramic restoration is generally superior to that of an MC restoration for anterior and posterior situations. However, properly designed MC crowns are highly aesthetic when adequate tooth-reduction principles are satisfied. In addition, metal coping designs, such as thinner facial metal (0.1–0.5 mm) and/or knife-edge facial metal margins, or collarless metal margins can further enhance the aesthetic potential of these anterior crowns.

Although an all-ceramic crown exhibits superb aesthetics, some all-ceramic bridges are not as aesthetic because the connectors must be sufficiently thick to minimize the risk for fracture, or the core ceramic is excessively opaque. Some all-ceramic crowns will not be aesthetic if the tooth preparations are inadequate, particularly when insufficient tooth structure has been removed. Not all patients will benefit from the placement of all-ceramic crowns or bridges. Some individuals exhibit certain characteristics that would allow only a metal or MC bridge to be used. For example, if an individual bruxes frequently and with great force, an all-ceramic bridge would not be likely to survive. A ceramic bridge should not be placed in patients who have a long span across the pontic site because the higher stresses under function could lead to premature fracture. There are several clear indications and contraindications that should be kept in mind when treatment planning crown and bridge cases made with a ceramic system. Therefore, all-ceramics are preferred over MCs when aesthetics is a prime concern, when MC aesthetics is unacceptable, or when a history of metal hypersensitivity exists. Contraindications for all-ceramic prostheses include severe bruxism, extensive wear of tooth structure or restorations, excessive bite-force capability, and a previous history of all-ceramic inlay or crown fractures.

The toughest and strongest core ceramics have opaque cores that are veneered with layers of translucent ceramic. The prediction of the most durable ceramic should be based on the fracture resistance of the entire bilayer or trilayer system, not simply of the core ceramic itself. In the absence of randomized, controlled clinical data, in vitro tests of the monolithic ceramic materials and of layered ceramics that simulate the designs used in clinical practice are highly desirable. For example, Figure 10.49 shows the mean fracture loads across three strength ranges of three-unit bridges made using four ceramic materials. If more bridges had been tested, Weibull analyses could have been performed on the data to determine the reliability and fracture probabilities over time. More importantly, finite element models can be developed for any prosthesis design that can be applied with dynamic fatigue data for the component ceramic materials using Life Ceramics Analysis and Reliability Evaluation software (CARES; NASA) to predict the time-dependent probabilities for fracture.

The success or failure of ceramic restorations can be related to material-, dentist-, lab-, technician-, and patient-related factors. The specific cause of failure often results from failure to follow the manufacturer's guidelines. For example, feldspathic porcelain must be supported by a metal coping or high-strength ceramic core to resist occlusal loading and prevent excessive flexural strain and should not be used as the core ceramic for a ceramic–ceramic crown. The comparative fracture toughness values of ceramics are listed in Tables 10.8 and 10.12. Another cause of fracture is inadequate occlusal reduction on premolar and molar teeth. A minimum of 1.5-mm reduction is recommended for MC crowns in molar areas, compared with a thickness of 2.0 mm for most ceramic crowns. However, the introduction of monolithic zirconia crowns suggests that occlusal reductions as low as 0.6 mm may be adequate in some cases. For any ceramic product, the tooth preparation guidelines recommended by the manufacturer should

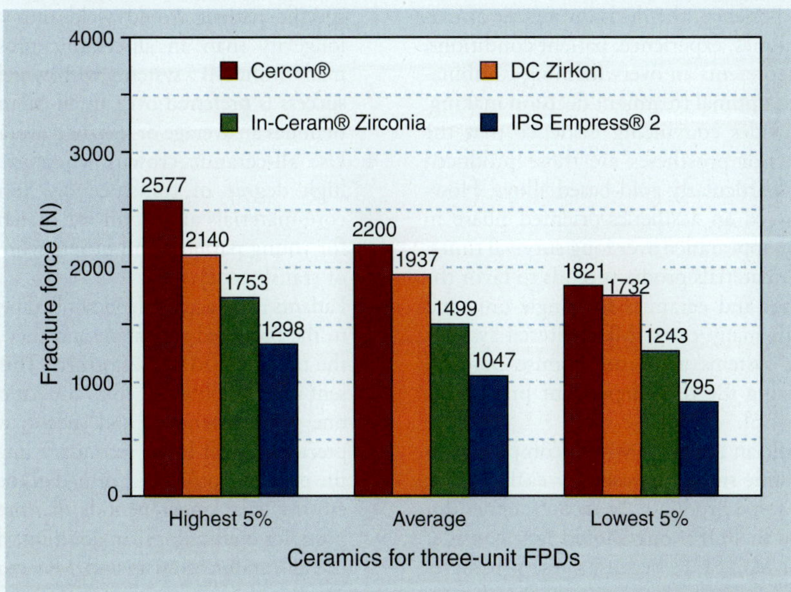

• **Fig. 10.49** Average loads (N) required to fracture at midpontic of three-unit bridges made from four ceramics in which the core ceramic thickness was 0.8 mm, the veneer thickness was 0.7 mm, and the connector height was 4 mm. The differences between the weakest and strongest ceramic bridges in each grouping were 99%, 110%, and 129%, respectively. The core ceramics for the four products are as follows: Cercon and DC Zirkon-Ceram are zirconia-based ceramics, In-Ceram Zirconia is glass-infiltrated zirconia-reinforced alumina ceramic, and Empress 2 is a lithia disilicate–based ceramic. (Adapted from Tinschert J., et al.: Fracture resistance of lithium disilicate-, alumina-, and zirconia-based three-unit fixed partial dentures: A laboratory study. *Int J Prosthodont* 14:231–238, 2001.)

TABLE 10.12 **Properties of Veneering Ceramics for Zirconia Core Materials**

Veneering Ceramic	Cercon Ceram S	Lava Ceram	Tri-Ceram	VITA VM9	Cerabien CZR
CTE (100–400°C)	9.6	9.6	8.2	9.1	9.1
Tg (°C)	488	549	561	>590	561
Strength (MPa)	63 ± 8	81 ± 12	81 ± 22	96 ± 8	66 ± 5
Sintering temperature (°C)	830	810	755	910	930

CTE, coefficient of thermal expansion.

be followed for the specific ceramic that will be used. These guidelines should be discussed with the lab technician to ensure that standardized procedures are followed.

When a dentist writes a prescription for an MC or ceramic prosthesis, specific information is required on the material to be used and the design that is needed. How should these decisions be made by a competent clinician? The intraoral conditions and optimal treatment options must first be considered. For missing teeth, restoring the dentition to occlusal function may be accomplished with implants and crowns or FDPs. The aesthetic needs, expectations, and financial resources of the patient are the next criteria to be considered. The treatment choice is then made on the basis of anticipated success rates, survival times, and minimization of risk factors that are determined from published clinical studies and the previous experience of the clinician, the dental lab technician, and their colleagues. For recent dental school graduates, the previous experience is often based on the materials and techniques learned in dental school. For well-established dentists, experiences in dental practices complement their dental school and advanced education training. Although one may have developed an extensive base of experience, the decision matrix of materials, design options, techniques, experience, patient conditions, and predicted success rates represents an overwhelming combination of variables to factor into optimal treatment decision making.

The dental literature provides convincing evidence that the most durable types of posterior prostheses are those produced from high-noble cast alloys, particularly gold-based alloys. However, the profession has entered an aesthetics-oriented phase in which decisions tend to favor appearance over long survival times. Thus, the selection of dental materials products tends to favor the use of resin-based composites and ceramics for single-unit and multiple-unit restorations. In many cases, MC material systems are chosen over all-ceramic systems as a compromise between aesthetic needs and minimizing the time-dependent probability of failure or maximizing survival.

The dentist and lab technician are faced with a complex challenge of deciding which ceramic should be used for each specific clinical situation. Although some products are recommended for posterior three-unit to five-unit FDPs, one should first consider the use of all-metal FDPs or MC FDPs because these prostheses will have a much greater life expectancy. *It is imperative that the dentist should familiarize himself with the various options available and not depend on the technician for recommendations. The choice of material should be based on an implicit understanding of the material and the clinical scenario with inputs from the technician.*

Only when a patient is highly resistant to accepting metallic components during the treatment-planning discussions should all-ceramic FDPs be used because the fracture resistance of posterior all-ceramic FDPs is based on (1) the strength and fracture toughness of the ceramic components, (2) the connector dimensions (minimum height of 4 mm), (3) connector shape (gingival embrasures must have broad radii of curvature), and (4) the patient's biting force. Thus, the selection of a ceramic for these prostheses is a very risky proposition because optimal conditions for their success are not yet known. An indicative list of recommendations for different clinical scenarios is presented in Box 10.4.

Before a decision is made to use an all-ceramic crown, six criteria should be considered to minimize the risks of poor esthetics, clinical failures, remakes, and possible disagreements and misunderstandings between dentists, patients, technicians, and manufacturers.

1. The dentist should not consider all-ceramic crowns for patients with evidence of extreme bruxism, clenching, or malocclusion. The use of all-zirconia crowns has been proposed but no randomized, controlled clinical trials of all-ceramic and MC restorations have been reported. In this case, MC or all-metal prostheses should be used.
2. The experience of the laboratory technician should be extensive to ensure a success rate of at least 98% over a 3-year period. This is the success rate for MC crowns and bridges after 7.5 years. Only technicians who demonstrate meticulous attention to detail should be selected. Such technicians are reluctant to accept impressions with unreadable margins.
3. The dentist should judge whether previous esthetic success with MC prostheses combined with the esthetic demands of the specific patient would yield more predictable outcomes and longevity than an all-ceramic prosthesis. An MC prosthesis made from MC systems with which one had previous clinical success is preferred over an all-ceramic prosthesis when the patient has an average or less than average appreciation of esthetics.
4. Use all-ceramic crowns when the adjacent teeth exhibit a high degree of translucency. Several relatively translucent core materials are useful for matching adjacent tooth shades for young patients and others who may exhibit a high degree of translucency.
5. Patients must accept the described benefits, risks, and alternatives to the proposed treatment and they must give their consent for the treatment to be performed. This means that informed consent must be obtained from the patient, preferably in writing. As one gains experience and success with these restorations, this precaution will be of secondary importance. Initially, however, the patient should be informed of the higher success rates of MC crowns over longer periods of time, especially when used for posterior applications. In addition, the cost differential between the all-ceramic crowns and MC crowns should be considered. The initial cost and the expenses associated with remakes for the all-ceramic crowns will be higher than those associated with MC crowns. The patient should again be informed of the relative cost of these restorations and their consent should be obtained for the proposed material of choice.
6. The skill of the dentist is of paramount importance in producing perfect impressions derived from smooth preparations free of undercuts with continuous, well-defined margins, and with adequate total tooth reduction. If this performance cannot be consistently maintained without a significant increase in preparation time compared to preparations for MC prostheses, the use of the all-ceramic crowns is contraindicated. As stated in criterion 2, a reputable technician should not accept impressions with incomplete or unreadable margins.

Summary

- **Dental ceramics** are attractive because of their biocompatibility, long-term color stability, chemical durability, wear resistance, and ability to be formed into precise shapes, although in some cases, they require costly processing equipment and specialized training for lab technicians. Dental ceramics consist of silicate glasses, **porcelains**, **glass–ceramics**, or highly crystalline solids. They exhibit chemical, mechanical, physical, and thermal properties that distinguish them from metals, acrylic resins, and resin-based composites.

- It is generally believed that dental ceramics fail primarily because of their brittleness, which is inversely related to its ductility or percent elongation.
- In general, the major reason for fracture of ceramics is their inability to suppress crack growth by deforming plastically in areas adjacent to crack tips that are subjected to tensile stress.
- Fracture toughness or plane strain fracture toughness, which is designated as KIc, describes the critical stress intensity factor based on a crack opening under tensile stress.
- Another property that is used to describe the brittle fracture resistance of ceramics is the critical strain energy release rate, which is designated as G.
- **Methods for strengthening ceramics**
  - **Minimizing the effect of stress concentrations**
    The fracture resistance of ceramic prostheses can be increased through one or more of the following seven options:
    - Select stronger and tougher ceramics.
    - Develop residual compressive stresses within the surface of the material by thermal tempering.
    - Develop residual compressive stress within interfacial regions of weaker, less tough ceramic layers by properly matching coefficients of thermal expansion and contraction.
    - Reduce the tensile stress in the ceramic by appropriate selection of stiffer supporting materials (greater elastic moduli).
    - Minimize the number of firing cycles for feldspathic porcelains.
    - Design the ceramic prosthesis with greater bulk and broader radii of curvature for connectors in areas of potential tensile stress to minimize stress concentrations and the magnitude of tensile stresses that can develop during function.
    - Adhesively bond the ceramic crowns to the tooth structure.
- **Classification of dental ceramics**
  Dental ceramics can be classified according to one or more of the following parameters:
  - Uses or indications (anterior and posterior crown, veneer, post and core, **fixed dental prosthesis, ceramic stain, glaze**).
  - Composition:
    - Principal crystal phase and/or matrix phase (silica glass, leucite-based feldspathic porcelain, leucite-based glass-ceramic, lithia disilicate-based glass-ceramic, aluminous porcelain, alumina, glass-infused alumina, glass-infused spinel, glass-infused alumina/zirconia, and zirconia.
  - Processing method (casting, sintering, partial sintering and glass infiltration, **slip casting** and sintering, hot-isostatic pressing, CAD-CAM milling, and copymilling).
  - Firing temperature (ultralow fusing, low fusing, medium fusing, and high fusing).
  - Microstructure (amorphous glass, crystalline, crystalline particles in a glass matrix).
  - Translucency (opaque, translucent, transparent).
  - Fracture resistance (low, medium, high).
  - Abrasiveness (comparison relative to tooth enamel against tooth enamel).
- **Ceramics used to veneer metal frameworks for metal-ceramic (MC)—that is, porcelain-fused-to-metal prostheses**
  There are four categories of dental ceramics for metalceramic systems:
  1. Manually condensed feldspathic veneering porcelains
  2. Hot isostatically pressed (HIP) veneering ceramics
  3. Ceramic stains
  4. Glazes.
- **Ceramics used to produce all-ceramic prostheses**
  There are six categories of dental ceramics for all-ceramic systems:
  1. HIP or CAD-CAM core ceramics
  2. Manually condensed veneering ceramics
  3. Hot-pressed veneering ceramics
  4. Liners
  5. Ceramic stains
  6. Ceramic glazes.

The compositions of these ceramics are generally classified by the principal crystal phases controlling their properties.

The most common crystal phases are

- Leucite
- Lithia disilicate
- Alumina
- Combinations of alumina and zirconia
- Zirconia
- Apatite

Lithia disilicate glass–ceramics, alumina/zirconia, and zirconia are used exclusively for the core structure of the all-ceramic applications.

- **Ceramic composition**
  Conventional dental porcelain is a vitreous ceramic based on a silica (SiO_2) network and potash feldspar ($K_2O•Al_2O_3•6SiO_2$), soda feldspar ($Na_2O•Al_2O_3•6SiO_2$), or both.
- **Ceramic processing methods**
- Sintering: Feldspathic porcelains that are used to make traditional metal–ceramic restorations are condensed by vibration and sintered at high temperatures.
- Hot-pressed ceramics are heated, injected under pressure into a mold, and then veneered or stained.
- Cast and cerammed crowns, glass is cast into a mold, heat treated to form a glass–ceramic, and colored with shading porcelain and surface stains.
- Slip cast sintering.
- CAD–CAM systems.
- **Hot isostatically pressed (HIP) glass–ceramics**
  Veneered leucite-based glass-ceramic core restorations are indicated for anterior veneers and crowns and premolar inlays, onlays, and crowns. This glass-ceramic is composed, by volume, of approximately 70% lithium disilicate and 30% glass.
- **Glass-infiltrated core ceramics**
  To minimize sintering shrinkage and ensure adequate fit of ceramic prostheses, three glass-infiltrated core ceramic systems have been developed, one based on partially sintered alumina, one based on a magnesiaalumina spinel ($MgAl_2O_4$), and one with a zirconiaalumina core. Each of these partially sintered ceramics can be infiltrated with a lanthanum glass without any significant dimensional change.
- **Alumina core ceramic**
  To produce these crowns, a die is first produced from an impression and digitized using a mechanical profiling device

and a computer that converts the coordinates of the die surface into a digitized database. An oversized die is then produced onto which pure alumina is drypressed. The oversize green alumina body is then sintered and the resulting shrinkage yields the desired size and shape, onto which a feldspathic porcelain veneer is applied and sintered.

- **Yttria-stabilized zirconia**
  A partially stabilized tetragonal zirconia (stabilized either by ceria or yttria) that is used for producing the core veneered framework or substructure for crowns or bridges. The "transformation toughening" mechanism of crack shielding results from the controlled transformation of the metastable tetragonal phase to the stable monoclinic phase.
- **CAD–CAM processing of ceramics**
  CAD-CAM ceramic prostheses can be produced either as monolithic lithia disilicate glass-ceramic or zirconia ceramic structures or as bilayer structures made from milled copings and layered manually, by hot pressing, or by fusing a CAM-produced veneer to the framework.
- **Abrasiveness of dental ceramics**
  In spite of their overall excellence in meeting the ideal requirements of a prosthetic material, dental ceramics have one major drawback. These materials can cause catastrophic wear of opposing tooth structure under certain conditions.
  - Asperities extending from the ceramic surface that produce high localized stresses and microfracture.
  - Gouging that results from high stresses and large hardness differences between two surfaces or particles extending from these surfaces.
  - Impact or erosion that occurs through the action of abrasive particles carried in a flowing liquid such as saliva.
  - Contact stress microfracture that increases localized tensile stress and also enhances the damage caused by asperities, gouging, and impact or erosion.

Review Questions

1. Classify ceramics and discuss in detail ceramics for metal–ceramic restorations.
2. Discuss in detail metal–ceramic restorations and metal alloy used for the same.
3. Discuss in detail strengthening of ceramics.
4. Discuss in brief bisque stages of ceramics.
5. Discuss in brief HIP (pressable) ceramics.
6. Discuss in brief transformation toughening.
7. Discuss in brief role of zirconia in ceramic restorations.
8. Discuss in brief bonding of ceramic to metal.
9. Discuss in brief DICOR.
10. Discuss in brief glazing of dental porcelain.
11. Discuss in brief CAD–CAM ceramic restorations.
12. Classify ceramics by fabrication techniques and discuss sintering in detail.
13. Discuss in brief feldspathic porcelains.
14. Discuss in brief aluminous porcelain.
15. Discuss in brief wear of enamel due to ceramics.
16. Discuss in brief metal alloys used in metal–ceramic restorations.
17. Discuss in brief core ceramics.
18. Classify ceramics by use and discuss in brief glazes and stains.
19. Classify ceramics by use, method of fabrication, and melting range.
20. Discuss in brief glass–ceramics.
21. Discuss in brief low-fusing and ultralow-fusing ceramics.
22. Creep and sag related to PFM restorations.
23. Discuss in brief uses of ceramics in dentistry.
24. Discuss in brief vacuum firing for dental ceramics.
25. Discuss in brief techniques for condensing feldspathic porcelain.
26. Discuss in detail fabrication of metal–ceramic prostheses.
27. Discuss in detail composition of metal-free ceramics used in dentistry.
28. Discuss in brief principles governing selection of dental ceramics for clinical use.
29. Discuss in detail strengthening of ceramics with emphasis on dispersion strengthening.
30. Enumerate advantages and disadvantages of ceramic restorations.
31. What are the factors influencing the fracture of ceramic restorations?
32. Discuss in detail physical properties of dental ceramics.
33. Discuss in brief factors affecting color and optical properties of dental ceramics.
34. Discuss in brief materials used for fabrication of ceramic veneers.
35. Discuss in brief influence of surface finish on wear caused by dental ceramics.

Selected Readings

Aboushelib M.N.; de Kler M.; van der Zel J.M.; et al. Microtensile bond strength and impact energy of fracture of CAD-veneered zirconia restorations. J Prosthodont 18 (3) 211–216 (2009).

Ahmed WM, Troczynski T, McCullagh AP, Wyatt CCL, Carvalho RM. The influence of altering sintering protocols on the optical and mechanical properties of zirconia: A review. J Esthet Restor Dent. 2019;31(5):423-30.

Albakry M.; Guazzato M.; Swain M.V. Biaxial flexural strength, elastic moduli, and x-ray diffraction characterization of three pressable all-ceramic materials. J Prosthet Dent 89 374–380 (2003).

Albakry M.; Guazzato M.; Swain M.V. Fracture toughness and hardness evaluation of three pressable all-ceramic dental materials. J Dent 31 181–188 (2003).

Albakry M.; Guazzato M.; Swain M.V. Influence of hot pressing on the microstructure and fracture toughness of two pressable dental glass-ceramics. J Biomed Mater Res B: Appl Biomater 71 99–107 (2004).

Anusavice K.J.; Hojjatie B. Effect of thermal tempering on strength and crack propagation of feldspathic porcelain. J Dent Res 70 1009–1013 (1991); A study that showed a 158% increase in biaxial flexure strength of a porcelain subjected to thermal tempering.

Anusavice K.J.; Hojjatie B.; Chang T.-C. Effect of grinding and fluoride-gel exposure on strength of ion-exchanged porcelain. J Dent Res 73 (8) 1444–1449 (1994); A study that demonstrated the weakening of an ion-exchanged porcelain by grinding to a depth of 100 μm or more.

Anusavice K.J.; Kakar K.; Ferree N. Which mechanical and physical testing methods are relevant for predicting the clinical performance of ceramic-based dental prostheses? Clin Oral Implants Res 18 (Suppl 3) 218–231 (2007).

Anusavice K.J.; DeHoff P.H.; Hojjatie B.; et al. Influence of tempering and contraction mismatch on crack development in ceramic surfaces. J Dent Res 68 1182–1187 (1989); A study of the application of thermal tempering to strengthen dental porcelain.

Anusavice K.J.; Shen C.; Vermost B.; et al. Strengthening of porcelain by ion exchange subsequent to thermal tempering. Dent Mater 8 149 (1992); The influence of ion exchange and tempering on strengthening of porcelain.

Anusavice K.J. Standardizing failure, success, and survival decisions in clinical studies of ceramic and metal-ceramic fixed dental prostheses. Dent Mater 28 (1) 102–111 (2012).

ASTM-C1161. Standard test method for flexural strength for advanced ceramics at ambient temperature. American Society for Testing Materials: West Conshohocken, PA.

ASTM-C1368. Standard test method for determination of slow crack growth parameters of advanced ceramics by constant stress-rate flexural testing at ambient temperature. American Society for Testing Materials: West Conshohocken, PA.

ASTM-F394–78. Standard test method for biaxial flexure strength (modulus of rupture) of ceramic substrates. American Society for Testing Materials: West Conshohocken, PA.

ASTM-C1239. Reporting uniaxial strength data and estimating Weibull distribution parameters for advanced ceramics. American Society for Testing Materials: West Conshohocken, PA.

Ban S.; Anusavice K.J. Influence of test method on failure stress of brittle dental materials. J Dent Res 69 1791–1799 (1990).

Barinov S.M.; Ivanov N.V.; Orlov S.V.; et al. Influence of environment on delayed failure of alumina ceramics. J Eur Ceram Soc 18 2057–2063 (1998).

Beuer F.; Edelhoff D.; Gernet W.; et al. Three-year clinical prospective evaluation of zirconia-based posterior fixed dental prostheses (FDPs). Clin Oral Invest (2009).

Binns D.B. Some physical properties of two-phase crystal-glass solids. In: (editor: Stewart G.H.) Science of Ceramics. Vol. 1 Academic Press: London, p. 315; A classic paper on the reinforcement of glasses with crystalline particles.

Bulpakdi P.; Taskonak B.; Yan J.H.; et al. Failure analysis of clinically failed all-ceramic fixed partial dentures using fractal geometry. Dent Mater 25 (5) 634–640 (2009).

Cattani-Lorente M.; Scherrer S.S.; Ammann P.; et al. Low temperature degradation of a Y-TZP dental ceramic. Acta Biomater (2010).

Cattell M.J.; Clarke R.L.; Lynch E.J. The biaxial flexural strength and reliability of four dental ceramics. Part II. J Dent 25 409–414 (1997).

Cattell M.J.; Clarke R.L.; Lynch E.J. The transverse strength, reliability and microstructural features of four dental ceramics. Part I. J Dent 25 399–407 (1997).

Cattell M.J.; Chadwick T.C.; Knowles J.C.; et al. Flexural strength optimisation of a leucite reinforced glass ceramic. Dent Mater 17 21–33 (2001).

Cesar P.F.; Soki F.N.; Yoshimura H.N.; et al. Influence of leucite content on slow crack growth of dental porcelains. Dent Mater 24 1114–1122 (2008).

Cesar P.F.; Yoshimura H.N.; Miranda W.G. Jr.; et al. Relationship between fracture toughness and flexural strength in dental porcelains. J Biomed Mater Res B: Appl Biomater 78 265–273 (2006).

Chevalier J.; Gremillard L.; Deville S. Low-temperature degradation of zirconia and implications for biomedical implants. Annu Rev Mater Res 37 1–32 (2007).

Coornaert J.; Adriaens P.; De Boever J. Long-term clinical study of porcelain-fused-to-gold restorations. J Prosthet Dent 51 (3) 338–342 (1984); A 7.5-year study survival level of 97.7% for metal-ceramic crowns and FPDs.

Davidge R.W.; McLaren J.R.; Tappin G. Strength-probability-time (SPT) relationships in ceramics. J Mater Sci 8 1699–1705 (1973).

de Kler M, de Jager N, Meegdes M, et al.: *Influence of thermal expansion mismatch and fatigue loading on phase changes in porcelain veneered Y-TZP zirconia discs. J Oral Rehabil* 34:841-847, 2007.

DeHoff P.H.; Anusavice K.J. Analysis of tempering stresses in bilayered porcelain discs. J Dent Res 71 (5) 1139–1144 (1992); Paper demonstrating the feasibility of air blasting a porcelain to induce surface compression.

DeHoff P.H.; Anusavice K.J. Viscoelastic finite element stress analysis of the thermal compatibility of dental bilayer ceramic systems. Int J Prosthodont 22 (1) 56–61 (2009).

de Kler M.; de Jager N.; Meegdes M.; et al. Influence of thermal expansion mismatch and fatigue loading on phase changes in porcelain veneered Y-TZP zirconia discs. J Oral Rehabil 34 (11) 841–847 (2007).

Della Bona A.; Kelly J.R. The clinical success of all-ceramic restorations. J Am Dent Assoc 139 (Suppl 9) 8S–13S (2008).

Della Bona A.; van Noort R. Shear vs. tensile bond strength of resin composite bonded to ceramic. J Dent Res 74 (9) 1591–1596 (1995).

Della Bona A.; Anusavice K.; Mecholsky J. Jr. Failure analysis of resin composite bonded to ceramic. Dent Mater 19 (8) 693–699 (2003).

Denry I.L.; Holloway J.A. Microstructural and crystallographic surface changes after grinding zirconia-based dental ceramics. J Biomed Mater Res Part B: Appl Biomater 76 (2) 440–448 (2006).

Denry I.L.; Kelly J.; Donovan T.E. State of the art of zirconia for dental applications. Dent Mater 24 (3) 299–307 (2008).

Denry I.L.; Peacock J.J.; Holloway J.A. Effect of heat treatment after accelerated aging on phase transformation in 3Y-TZP. J Biomed Mater Res B: Appl Biomater 93 (1) 236–243 (2010).

Factors essential for successful all-ceramic restorations. J Am Dent Assoc 139 (Suppl 9) 14S–18S (2008).

Donovan TE: Factors essential for successful all-ceramic restorations. *J Am Dent Assoc* 139(suppl 9):14S–18S, 2008.

Dorsch P. Thermal compatibility of materials for porcelain-fused-to-metal (metal-ceramic) restorations. Ceramic Forum International/Ber Dt Keram Ges 59 1 (1982); This paper identifies key factors involved in porcelain–metal compatibility.

Drummond J.L. In vitro aging of yttria-stabilized zirconia. J Am Ceram Soc 72 675–676 (1989).

Ebrahimi M.E.; Chevalier J.; Fantozzi G. Slow crack-growth behavior of alumina ceramics. J Mater Res 15 142–147 (2000).

El Attaoui H.; Saadaoui M.; Chevalier J.; et al. Static and cyclic crack propagation in Ce-TZP ceramics with different amounts of transformation toughening. J Eur Ceram Soc 27 (2–3) 483–486 (2007).

Eliasson A.; Arnelund C.F.; Johansson A. A clinical evaluation of cobalt-chromium metal-ceramic fixed partial dentures and crowns: A three- to seven-year retrospective study. J Prosthet Dent 98 (1) 6–16 (2007).

Esquivel-Upshaw J.F.; Anusavice K.J. Ceramic design concepts based on stress distribution analysis. Compend Contin Educ Dent 21 649–652 (2000). 654; quiz 656; A review of design concepts based on finite element analyses of stresses in ceramic crowns.

Esquivel-Upshaw J.F.; Young H.; Jones J.; et al. Four-year clinical performance of a lithia disilicate-based core ceramic for posterior fixed partial dentures. Int J Prosthodont 21 (2) 155–160 (2008).

Esquivel-Upshaw J.; Rose W.; Oliveira E.; Yang M.; Clark A.E.; Anusavice K. Randomized, controlled clinical trial of bilayer ceramic and metal-ceramic crown performance. J Prosthodontics 22 (3) 166–173 (2012 Sep 14).

Fairhurst C.W.; Lockwood P.E.; Ringle R.D.; et al. Dynamic fatigue of feldspathic porcelain. Dent Mater 9 269–273 (1993).

Fairhurst C.W.; Anusavice K.J.; Hashinger D.T.; et al. Thermal expansion of dental alloys and porcelains. J Biomed Mater Res 14 435 (1980); Thermal expansion data are provided for alloys and porcelains, and changes in porcelain thermal expansion that can be caused by multiple firings are described.

Fischer J.; Stawarczyk B. Compatibility of machined Ce-TZP/Al_2O_3 nanocomposite and a veneering ceramic. Dent Mater 23 (12) 1500–1505 (2007).

Fischer H.; Weber M.; Marx R. Lifetime prediction of all-ceramic bridges by computational methods. J Dent Res 82 238–242 (2003).

Fischer J.; Stawarczyk B.; Trottmann A.; et al. Impact of thermal properties of veneering ceramics on the fracture load of layered Ce-TZP/A nanocomposite frameworks. Dent Mater 25 (3) 326–330 (2009).

Gibbs CH, Anusavice, KJ, Young HM, et al.: Maximum clenching force of patients with moderate loss of posterior tooth support: A pilot study. 88(5):498–502, 2002.

Gonzaga C.C.; Cesar P.F.; Miranda W.G. Jr.; et al. Slow crack growth and reliability of dental ceramics. Dent Mater 27 (4) 394–406 (2011).

Gonzaga C.C.; Yoshimura H.N.; Cesar P.F.; et al. Subcritical crack growth in porcelains, glass-ceramics, and glass-infiltrated alumina composite for dental restorations. J Mater Sci Mater Med 20 1017–1024 (2009).

Gonzaga C.C.; Okada C.Y.; Cesar P.F.; et al. Effect of processing induced particle alignment on the fracture toughness and fracture behavior of multiphase dental ceramics. Dent Mater 25 1293–1301 (2009).

Gregg A. Helvey, D., MAGD, CDT (2017). What is in your Zirconia? Compend Contin Educ Dent 38(4): 213-218.

Guazzato M.; Proos K.; Sara G.; et al. Strength, reliability, and mode of fracture of bilayered porcelain/core ceramics. Int J Prosthodont 17 142–149 (2004).

Griffith A.A. The phenomenon of rupture and flow in solids. Phil Trans Roy Soc Lond A 221 163–198 (1921); Griffith was one of the pioneers who contributed to the field of fracture mechanics.

Guazzato M.; Walton T.R.; Franklin W.; et al. Influence of thickness and cooling rate on development of spontaneous cracks in porcelain/zirconia structures. Aust Dent J 55 (3) 306–310 (2010).

Heintze S.D.; Rousson V. Survival of zirconia- and metal-supported fixed dental prostheses: A systematic review. Int J Prosthodont 23 (6) 493–502 (2010).

Heuer A.H. Transformation toughening in ZrO_2-containing ceramics. J Am Ceram Soc 70 (10) 689–698 (1987).

Irwin G.R. Analysis of stresses and strains near the end of a crack traversing a plate. J Appl Mech 24 361–364 (1957); Another pioneer in fracture mechanics.

Höland W.; Schweiger M.; Frank M.; et al. A comparison of the microstructure and properties of the IPS Empress 2 and the IPS Empress glass-ceramics. J Biomed Mater Res 53 (4) 297–303 (2000); The KIc value was measured as 3.3 ± 0.3 MPa for IPS Empress 2 and 1.3 ± 0.1 MPa for IPS Empress. The authors concluded that IPS Empress 2 can be used to fabricate three-unit bridges up to the second premolar.

Höland W.; Schweiger M.; Frank M.; et al. A comparison of the microstructure and properties of the IPS Empress 2 and the IPS Empress glass-ceramics. J Biomed Mater Res 53 297–303 (2000).

Holm C.; Tidehag P.; Tillberg A.; et al. Longevity and quality of FPDs: A retrospective study of restorations 30, 20, and 10 years after insertion. Int J Prosthodont 16 283–289 (2003).

Hulterstrom A.K.; Bergman M. Polishing systems for dental ceramics. Acta Odontol Scand 51 (4) 229–234 (1993); Two products were superior in their polishing effectiveness.

Hummel M.; Kern M. Durability of the resin bond strength to the alumina ceramic Procera. Dent Mater 20 (5) 498–508 (2004).

Kappert H.F.; Krah M.K. Keramiken—eine Übersicht. Quintessenz Zahntech 27 (6) 668–704 (2001); An excellent overview of ceramic products in use at the end of the twentieth century.

Karl M.; Fischer H.; Graef F.; et al. Structural changes in ceramic veneered three-unit implant-supported restorations as a consequence of static and dynamic loading. Dent Mater 24 (4) 464–470 (2008).

Kelly J.R. Dental ceramics: What is this stuff anyway? J Am Dent Assoc 139 (Suppl 4) 4S–7S (2008).

Kelly J.R.; Denry I. Stabilized zirconia as a structural ceramic: An overview. Dent Mater 24 (3) 289–298 (2008).

Kelly J.R.; Nishimura I.; Campbell S.D. Ceramics in dentistry: Historical roots and current perspectives. J Prosthet Dent 75 18–32 (1996).

Kelly J.R.; Rungruanganunt P.; Hunter B.; et al. Development of a clinically validated bulk failure test for ceramic crowns. J Prosthet Dent 104 (4) 228–238 (2010).

Kitayama S.; Nikaido T.; Ikeda M.; et al. Internal coating of zirconia restoration with silica-based ceramic improves bonding of resin cement to dental zirconia ceramic. Biomed Mater Eng 20 (2) 77–87 (2010).

Kitayama S.; Nikaido T.; Takahashi R.; et al. Effect of primer treatment on bonding of resin cements to zirconia ceramic. Dent Mater 26 (5) 426–432 (2010). Epub Jan 25.

Kohorst P.; Herzog T.J.; Borchers L.; et al. Load-bearing capacity of all-ceramic posterior four-unit fixed partial dentures with different zirconia frameworks. Eur J Oral Sci 115 (2) 161–166 (2007).

Kosmač T.; Oblak C. Ageing and fatigue behaviour of surface treated Y-TZP dental ceramics. Key Eng Mater 817–820 (2008).

Kosmač T.; Oblak C.; Marion L. The effects of dental grinding and sandblasting on ageing and fatigue behavior of dental zirconia (Y-TZP) ceramics. J Eur Ceram Soc 28 (5) 1085–1090 (2008).

Kosmač T.; Oblak Č.; Jevnikar P.; et al. Strength and reliability of surface treated Y-TZP dental ceramics. J Biomed Mater Res 53 (4) 304–313 (2000); Grinding and sandblasting various Y-TZP ceramics containing 3 mol% yttria revealed that grinding lowered the mean strength and Weibull modulus, whereas sandblasting provided a powerful method for strengthening, but at the expense of reduced reliability.

Land C. Porcelain dental arts. Dental Cosmos 45 615–620 (1903); A historic article describing one of the first ceramic crowns made in dentistry.

Larsson C, Holm L, Lovgren N, et al.: Fracture strength of four-unit Y-TZP FPD cores designed with varying connector diameter. An in-vitro study, *J Oral Rehabil* 34(9):702-709.

Layton D.M.; Clarke M.; Walton T.R. A systematic review and meta-analysis of the survival of feldspathic porcelain veneers over 5 and 10 years. Int J Prosthodont 25 (6) 590–603 (2012 Nov).

Layton D.M.; Clarke M. A systematic review and meta-analysis of the survival of non-feldspathic porcelain veneers over 5 and 10 years. Int J Prosthodont 26 (2) 111–124 (2013 Mar).

Lee J.J.; Kwon J.Y.; Bhowmick S.; et al. Veneer vs. core failure in adhesively bonded all-ceramic crown layers. J Dent Res 87 (4) 363–366 (2008).

Lehmann F.; Kern M. Durability of resin bonding to zirconia ceramic using different primers. J Adhes Dent 11 (6) 479–483 (2009).

Lohbauer U.; Petschelt A.; Greil P. Lifetime prediction of CAD/CAM dental ceramics. J Biomed Mater Res 63 780–785 (2002).

Lohbauer U.; Amberger G.; Quinn G.D.; et al. Fractographic analysis of a dental zirconia framework: A case study on design issues. J Mech Behav Biomed Mater 3 (8) 623–629 (2010).

Lohbauer U.; Kramer N.; Petschelt A.; et al. Correlation of in vitro fatigue data and in vivo clinical performance of a glass ceramic material. Dent Mater 24 39–44 (2008).

Luthardt R.; Holzhuter M.; Rudolph H.; et al. CAD/CAM-machining effects on Y-TZP zirconia. Dent Mater 20 (7) 655–662 (2004).

MacCulloch W.T. Advances in dental ceramics. Br Dent J 124 361 (1968); The first description of the use of glass ceramics for dental applications.

Mackert J.R. Jr.; Butts M.B.; Fairhurst C.W. The effect of the leucite transformation on dental porcelain expansion. Dent Mater 2 32 (1986).

Mackert J.R. Jr.; Butts M.B.; Morena R.; et al. Phase changes in a leucite-containing dental porcelain frit. J Am Ceram Soc 69 C-69 (1986); The susceptibility of porcelains to phase changes during heat treatment is described.

Mackert J.R. Jr.; Ringle R.D.; Parry E.E.; et al. The relationship between oxide adherence and porcelain-metal bonding. J Dent Res 67 474 (1988); Quality of porcelain bond is dependent on adherence of the metal oxide.

Makhija, S. K., et al. (2016). Dentist material selection for single-unit crowns: Findings from the National Dental Practice-Based Research Network. J Dent **55**: 40-47.

Magne P.; Oh W.-S.; Pintado M.R.; et al. Wear of enamel and veneering ceramics after laboratory and chairside finishing procedures. J Prosthet Dent 82 (6) 669–679 (1999).

Malament, K. A., et al. (2020). Comparison of 16.9-year survival of pressed acid etched e.max lithium disilicate glass ceramic complete and partial coverage restorations in posterior teeth: Performance and outcomes as a function of tooth position, age, sex, and thickness of ceramic material. J Prosthet Dent.

Malament K.A.; Socransky S.S. Survival of Dicor glass-ceramic dental restorations over 14 years: Part I. Survival of Dicor complete coverage restorations and effect of internal surface acid etching, tooth position, gender, and age. J Prosthet Dent 81 (1) 23–32 (1999); This study demonstrated greater fracture rates of posterior Dicor crowns, maxillary crowns, crowns in male patients, and crowns in patients between the ages of 33 and 52 years.

Malament K.A.; Socransky S.S. Survival of Dicor glass-ceramic dental restorations over 16 years. Part III: Effect of luting agent and tooth or tooth-substitute core structure. J Prosthet Dent 86 (5) 511–519 (2001).

Mantri S.S.; Bhasin A.S. CAD/CAM in dental restorations: An overview. Ann Esss Dent II (3) 123–128 (2010); A useful overview of CAD/CAM systems.

Manziuc M-M, Gasparik C, Negucioiu M, Constantiniuc M, Burde A, Vlas I, et al. Optical properties of translucent zirconia: A review of the literature. The Euro Biotech Journal. 2019;3(1):45-51.

McCabe J.F.; Carrick T.E. A statistical approach to the mechanical testing of dental materials. Dent Mater 2 139–142 (1986); A useful review of Weibull statistical parameters and their interpretation.

Mecholsky J.J. Jr. Fracture mechanics principles. Dent Mater 11 (2) 111–112 (1995); A useful review of the principles of the fracture behavior of brittle materials.

Mecholsky J.J. Fractography—determining the sites of fracture initiation. Dent Mater 11 (2) 113–116 (1995).

Mitov G.; Lohbauer U.; Rabbo M.A.; et al. Investigations of subcritical crack propagation of the Empress 2 all-ceramic system. Dent Mater 24 267–273 (2008).

Miyazaki T, Nakamura T, Matsumura H, Ban S, Kobayashi T. Current status of zirconia restoration. J Prosthodont Res. 2013;57(4): 236-61.

Molin M.K.; Karlsson S.L. Five-year clinical prospective evaluation of zirconia-based Denzir 3-unit FPDs. Int J Prosthodont 21 (3) 223–227 (2008).

Morena R, Beaudreau GM, Lockwood PE, et al.: Fatigue of dental ceramics in a simulated oral environment. J Dent Res 65:993.

Morena R.; Lockwood P.E.; Evans A.L.; et al. Toughening of dental porcelain by tetragonal ZrO_2 additions. J Am Ceram Soc 69 C75 (1986); The use of partially stabilized zirconia to increase the toughness of dental porcelains is explored via a process termed transformation toughening.

Morimoto, S., et al. (2016). Survival rate of resin and ceramic inlays, onlays, and overlays: A systematic review and meta-analysis. J Dent Res **95**(9): 985-994.

Myers M.L.; Ergle J.W.; Fairhurst C.W.; et al. Fatigue failure parameters of IPS-Empress porcelain. Int J Prosthodont 7 549–553 (1994).

Myers M.L.; Ergle J.W.; Fairhurst C.W.; et al. Fatigue characteristics of a high-strength porcelain. Int J Prosthodont 7 253–257 (1994).

In: (editor: Nassau K.) The fifteen causes of color. In The Physics and Chemistry of Color. Wiley: New York, pp. 1–454; An excellent review of the principles of color and color perception.

Neimar Sartori, G. T. and K. T. Jin-Ho Phark, Richard Lin, Sillas Duarte, Jr, (2015). CAD/CAM high-strength glass-ceramics. Quintessence of Dental Technology: 39-54.

Odman P.; Andersson B. Procera AllCeram crowns followed for 5 to 10.5 years: A prospective clinical study. Int J Prosthodont 14 504–509 (2001); Clinical survival rates of 97.7% and 93.5%, respectively, were reported for Procera AllCeram crowns after 5 and 10 years, respectively. However, the failure rate after 10 years was 7%. Thus one should distinguish between the survival rate and failure.

Oilo M.; Gjerdet N.R.; Tvinnereim H.M. The firing procedure influences properties of a zirconia core ceramic. Dent Mater 24 (4) 471–475 (2008).

Orowan E. Energy criteria of fracture. Weld J Res Suppl 20 157s (1955).

Orowan E. Fracture and strength of solids. Rep Prog Phys 12 185 (1949).

Orowan E. The fatigue of glass under stress. Nature 154 341–343 (1944).

Ozcan M.; Niedermeier W. Clinical study on the reasons for and location of failures of metal-ceramic restorations and survival of repairs. Int J Prosthodont 15 299–302 (2002); These authors report a survival level for repaired metal–ceramic crowns with previous porcelain fractures of 89% after 3 years.

Pinto M.M.; Cesar P.F.; Rosa V.; et al. Influence of pH on slow crack growth of dental porcelains. Dent Mater 24 814–823 (2008).

Pjetursson B.E.; Sailer I.; Zwahlen M.; et al. A systematic review of the survival and complication rates of all-ceramic and metal-ceramic reconstructions after an observation period of at least 3 years. Part I: Single crowns. Clin Oral Implants Res 18 (Suppl 3) 73–85 (2007).

Quinn G.B. Fractography of ceramics and glasses. NIST recommended practice guide. Special publication 960–916 National Institute of Standards and Technology: Washington, DC; A superb guide to fractography with detailed explanations of experimental procedures.

Quinn G.B.; Morrell R. Design data for engineering ceramics; a review of the flexure test. J Am Ceram Soc 74 2037–2066 (1991).

Quinn J.B.; Quinn G.D. A practical and systematic review of Weibull statistics for reporting strengths of dental materials. Dent Mater (2009).

Ritter J.E. Critique of test methods for lifetime predictions. Dent Mater 11 147–151 (1995).

Ritter J.E. Predicting lifetimes of materials and material structures. Dent Mater 1 142–156 (1995).

Sagirkaya E.; Arikan S.; Sadik B.; Kara C.; Karasoy D.; Cehreli M. A randomized, prospective, open-ended clinical trial of zirconia fixed partial dentures on teeth and implants: Interim results. Int J Prosthodont 25 (3) 221–231 (2012 May).

Sailer I.; Feher A.; Filser F.; et al. Five-year clinical results of zirconia frameworks for posterior fixed partial dentures. Int J Prosthodont 20 (4) 383–388 (2007).

Salazar Marocho S.; Studart A.; Bottino M.; et al. Mechanical strength and subcritical crack growth under wet cyclic loading of glass-infiltrated dental ceramics. Dent Mater 26 (5) 483–490 (2009).

Scherrer S.S.; Cattani-Lorente M.; Vittecoq E.; et al. Fatigue behavior in water of Y-TZP zirconia ceramics after abrasion with 30 μm silica-coated alumina particles. Dent Mater (2010).

Scherrer S.S.; Quinn G.D.; Quinn J.B. Fractographic failure analysis of a Procera AllCeram crown using stereo and scanning electron microscopy. Dent Mater 24 (8) 1107–1113 (2008).

Seghi R.R.; Denry I.; Brajevic F. Effects of ion exchange on hardness and fracture toughness of dental ceramics. Int J Prosthodont 5 (4) 309–314 (1992).

Shah K, Holloway JA, Denry IL. Effect of coloring with various metal oxides on the microstructure, color, and flexural strength of 3Y-TZP. J Biomed Mater Res B Appl Biomater. 2008;87:329-337.

Shahmiri R, Standard OC, Hart JN, Sorrell CC. Optical properties of zirconia ceramics for esthetic dental restorations: A systematic review. J Prosthet Dent. 2018;119(1):36-46.

Sjögren G.; Molin M.; van Dijken J. A 10-year prospective evaluation of cad/cam-manufactured (Cerec) ceramic inlays. Int J Prosthodont 17 (2) 241–246 (2004).

Spear F.; Holloway J. Which all-ceramic system is optimal for anterior esthetics? J Am Dent Assoc 139 (Suppl 9) 19S–24S (2008).

Stawarczyk B, Keul C, Eichberger M, Figge D, Edelhoff D, Lumkemann N. Three generations of zirconia: From veneered to monolithic. Part I. Quintessence Int. 2017;48(5):369-80.

Stawarczyk B, Keul C, Eichberger M, Figge D, Edelhoff D, Lumkemann N. Three generations of zirconia: From veneered to monolithic. Part II. Quintessence Int. 2017;48(6):441-50.

Studart A.R.; Filser F.; Kocher P.; et al. In vitro lifetime of dental ceramics under cyclic loading in water. Biomaterials 28 (17) 2695–2705 (2007).

Suansuwan N.; Swain M. Adhesion of porcelain to titanium and a titanium alloy. J Dent 31 (7) 509–518 (2003); Reported maximum marginal discrepancies of 161 μm for In-Ceram crowns compared with 83 μm and 63 μm for Procera AllCeram and IPS Empress crowns, respectively.

Sulaiman TA, Abdulmajeed AA, Delgado A, Donovan TE. Fracture rate of 188695 lithium disilicate and zirconia ceramic restorations after up to 7.5 years of clinical service: A dental laboratory survey. The Journal of Prosthetic Dentistry. 2020;123(6):807-10.

Suputtamongkol K.; Anusavice K.J.; Suchatlampong C.; et al. Clinical performance and wear characteristics of veneered lithia-disilicate-based ceramic crowns. Dent Mater 24 (5) 667–673 (2008).

Swain M.V. Toughening mechanisms for ceramics. Mater Forum 13 237–253 (1989).

Swain M.V. Unstable cracking (chipping) of veneering porcelain on all-ceramic dental crowns and fixed partial dentures. Acta Biomater 5 (5) 1668–1677 (2009).

Taskonak B.; Yan J.; Mecholsky J.J. Jr.; et al. Fractographic analyses of zirconia-based fixed partial dentures. Dent Mater 24 (8) 1077–1082 (2008).

Taskonak B.; Griggs J.A.; Mecholsky J.J. Jr.; et al. Analysis of subcritical crack growth in dental ceramics using fracture mechanics and fractography. Dent Mater 24 700–707 (2008).

Teixeira E.C.; Piascik J.R.; Stoner B.R.; et al. Dynamic fatigue and strength characterization of three ceramic materials. J Mater Sci Mater Med 18 (6) 1219–1224 (2007).

Tholey M.J.; Swain M.V.; Hiel N. SEM observations of porcelain Y-TZP interface. Dent Mater (2009).

Tinschert J.; Natt G.; Mohrbotter N.; et al. Lifetime of alumina- and zirconia ceramics used for crown and bridge restorations. J Biomed Mater Res B: Appl Biomater 80 317–321 (2007).

Tinschert J.; Zwez D.; Marx R.; et al. Structural reliability of alumina-, feldspar-, leucite-, mica- and zirconia-based ceramics. J Dent 8 529–535 (2000).

Tinschert J.; Natt G.; Mautsch W.; et al. Fracture resistance of lithium disilicate-, alumina-, and zirconia-based three-unit fixed partial dentures: A laboratory study. Int J Prosthodont 14 (3) 231–238 (2001).

Tinschert J.; Natt G.; Mautsch W.; et al. Marginal fit of alumina and zirconia-based fixed partial dentures produced by a CAD/CAM system. Oper Dent 26 (4) 367–374 (2001).

Tinschert J.; Schulze K.A.; Natt G.; et al. Clinical behavior of zirconia-based fixed partial dentures made of DC-Zirkon: 3-year results. Int J Prosthodont 21 (3) 217–222 (2008).

Tsalouchou E.; Cattell M.J.; Knowles J.C.; et al. Fatigue and fracture properties of yttria partially stabilized zirconia crown systems. Dent Mater (2007).

Tsitrou E.A.; Northeast S.E.; van Noort R. Brittleness index of machinable dental materials and its relation to the marginal chipping factor. J Dent 35 (12) 897–902 (2007); The machinability of four restorative materials was estimated by calculating their brittleness indexes (BI) and a marginal chipping factor (CF).

Valandro L.; Ozcan M.; Bottino M.; et al. Bond strength of a resin cement to high alumina and zirconia-reinforced ceramics. J Adhes Dent 8 (3) 175–181 (2006).

Vergano P.J.; Hill D.C.; Uhlmann D.R. Thermal expansion of feldspar glasses. J Am Ceram Soc 50 59 (1967); One of the first studies that demonstrated the influence of the high-expanding leucite phase on the thermal expansion of feldspar glasses.

Wachtman J.B. Jr.; Capps W.; Mandel J. Biaxial flexure test of ceramic substrates. J Mater 7 188–194 (1972).

Wagner W.C.; Chu T.M. Biaxial flexural strength and indentation fracture toughness of three new dental core ceramics. J Prosthet Dent 76 140–144 (1996).

Wang H.; Aboushelib M.N.; Feilzer A.J. Strength influencing variables on CAD/CAM zirconia frameworks. Dent Mater 24 (5) 633–638 (2008).

Wassermann A.; Kaiser M.; Strub J.R. Clinical long-term results of VITA In-Ceram Classic crowns and fixed partial dentures: A systematic literature review. Int J Prosthodont 19 (4) 355–363 (2006).

Weibull W. A statistical distribution function of wide applicability. J Appl Mech 18 293–297 (1951).

Weinstein M., Weinstein A.B.: Porcelain-covered metal-reinforced teeth, US Patent No. 3,052,983, September 11, 1962; This patent and the following patent describe the development of high-expanding porcelains suitable for fusing with dental alloys. These patents provided the basis for modern metal-ceramic restorations.

Weinstein M., Katz S., Weinstein A.B.: Fused porcelain-to-metal teeth, US Patent No. 3,052,982, September 11, 1962; One of the major advances in ceramics used for metal-ceramic restorations is documented here.

Wen M.Y.; Mueller H.J.; Chai J.; et al. Comparative mechanical property characterization of 3 all-ceramic core materials. Int J Prosthodont 12 534–541 (1999).

Yoshimura H.N.; Cesar P.F.; Soki F.N.; et al. Stress intensity factor threshold in dental porcelains. J Mater Sci Mater Med 19 1945–1951 (2008).

Yoshimura H.N.; Narita N.E.; Molisani A.L.; et al. High temperature flexural strength and fracture toughness of AlN with Y_2O_3 ceramic. J Mater Sci 44 5773–5780 (2009).

Yoshimura H.N.; Molisani A.L.; Narita N.E.; et al. Porosity dependence of elastic constants in aluminum nitride ceramics. Mater Res 10 127–133 (2007).

Yoshimura H.N.; Cesar P.F.; Miranda W.G.; et al. Fracture toughness of dental porcelains evaluated by IF SCF, and SEPB methods. J Am Ceram Soc 88 1680–1683 (2005).

Zhang Y.; Lawn B.; Rekow E.; et al. Effect of sandblasting on the long-term performance of dental ceramics. J Biomed Mater Res B Appl Biomater 71 (2) 381–386 (2004).

Zhu Q.; deWith G.; Dortmans L.J.; et al. Subcritical crack growth behavior of Al_2O_3-glass dental composites. J Biomed Mater Res B: Appl Biomater 65 233–238 (2003).

Zarone F, Di Mauro MI, Ausiello P, Ruggiero G, Sorrentino R. Current status on lithium disilicate and zirconia: A narrative review. BMC Oral Health. 2019;19(1):134.

Kontonasaki E, Rigos AE, Ilia C, Istantsos T. Monolithic Zirconia: An update to current knowledge. Optical properties, wear, and clinical performance. Dent J (Basel). 2019;7(3).

Zhang Y, Lawn BR. Novel zirconia materials in dentistry. Journal of Dental Research. 2017;97:002203451773748.

Donovan TE, Alraheam IA, Sulaiman TA. An evidence-based evaluation of contemporary dental ceramics. Dental Update. 2018;45(6):541-6.

Fu L, Engqvist H, Xia W. Glass-ceramics in dentistry: A review. Materials (Basel). 2020;13(5).

Guth JF, Stawarczyk B, Edelhoff D, Liebermann A. Zirconia and its novel compositions: What do clinicians need to know? Quintessence Int. 2019;50(7):512-20.

11

Prosthetic Polymers and Resins

CHAPTER OUTLINE

KEY TERMS

Acrylic resins—polymers of acrylic acid, methacrylic acid, or acrylonitrile; any group of thermoplastic resins made by polymerizing esters of acrylic or methylmethacrylate acids.

Chemically activated polymerization—a chemical reaction in which a tertiary amine activates an initiator, such as benzoyl peroxide, which will react with the methylmethacrylate monomer to form polymethylmethacrylate;

Cold-cure resin—a resin formed when polymerization occurs as a result of a chemical

Complete dentures—complete denture is a removable or fixed dental prosthesis that replaces the entire dentition and associated structures of the maxillae or mandible

Denture—an artificial substitute for missing natural teeth and adjacent tissues;

Denture base—the part of a denture that rests on the foundation tissues and to which teeth are attached;

Denture liner—The polymeric material used to replace the tissue-contacting (intaglio) surface of an existing denture. A denture liner may be hard or soft, short or long term.

Denture processing—the means by which the denture base materials are polymerized to the form of a denture

Denture resin packing—filling and pressing a denture base material into a mold within a refractory flask

Denture tooth—a term commonly referring to an artificial tooth used in the fabrication of a resin-based prosthesis

Flexible resin removable denture—a metal-free removable denture constructed using one or more thermoplastic flexible resins including acetal resins, polycarbonates, acrylic resins and polyamides (nylons) and polyaryletherketones, including polyetheretherketone

Heat-activated resin—resin formed by thermal activation of smaller molecular chain molecules to form a larger molecular chain

Injection molding—the adaptation of a plastic material to the negative form of a closed mold by forcing the material into the mold through appropriate gateways

Long-term resilient soft liner—A resilient polymeric material that is bonded to the tissue-contacting surface of a denture for cushioning and/or improved retention. Such liners typically are heat-processed, and thus, they are more durable than chemical-activated, short-term soft liners and tissue conditioners.

Maxillofacial prosthesis—any prosthesis used to replace part or all of any stomatognathic

Monomer—a chemical compound that can undergo polymerization; any molecule that can be bound to a similar molecule to form a polymer

Relining—The process of replacing the tissue-contacting surface of an existing denture.

Removable partial denture—a removable partial denture that restores a partially edentulous arch;

Resilient soft denture liner—A polymeric material that is placed on the tissue-contacting surface of a denture base to absorb some of the mastication impact energy by acting as a type of "shock absorber" between the occlusal surfaces of a denture and the underlying oral tissues. A denture soft liner may also be used to engage natural or prosthetic undercuts so as to provide retention, stability, and support. These materials may be placed chairside (directly) or in the dental laboratory (indirectly).

Short-term soft liner (tissue conditioner)—A resilient polymeric material that is employed for brief periods (up to 14 days) to absorb masticatory impact and adapt to changing ridge contours (e.g., following the extraction of teeth or surgical alteration of an edentulous or partially edentulous ridge). Such materials are typically chemical-activated polymers and tend to degrade more rapidly than heat-activated resins.

Dentures and Denture Base Resins

The Glossary of Prosthodontic Terms - 9 (The Academy of Prosthodontics, 2017) defines a complete denture as a fixed or removable dental prosthesis that replaces the entire dentition and associated structures of the maxillae or mandible. Such a prosthesis is composed of artificial teeth attached to a denture base. In turn, the denture base derives its support through contact with the oral tissues, teeth, or dental implants.

Although individual denture bases can be formed from metals, the majority of denture bases are fabricated using common polymers. Such polymers are chosen based on availability, dimensional stability, handling characteristics, color, and compatibility with oral tissues.

A description of commonly used denture base polymers is presented in this chapter. Considerable attention is given to individual processing systems and polymerization techniques. In addition, methods for improving the fit and dimensional stability of resin-based prostheses are provided.

Fabrication of Dentures

Since the mid-1940s, the majority of denture bases have been fabricated using polymethyl methacrylate (PMMA) resins. PMMA is a colorless transparent solid. To facilitate its use in dental applications, the polymer can be tinted with pigments, dyes, fillers, and fibers to provide almost any color, shade, and degree of translucency. Its color, optical characteristics, and dimensional properties remain stable under normal intraoral conditions, and its physical properties have proven to be adequate for dental applications.

One established advantage of PMMA is the relative ease with which this material can be processed. PMMA denture base material is commonly supplied as a powder–liquid system (Fig. 11.12). The liquid contains mostly methyl methacrylate monomers, dimethacrylate or trimethacrylate cross-linking agents (Fig. 11.13), and an inhibitor, and the powder contains predominantly PMMA resin in the form of microsized beads (or spheres). When the liquid and powder are mixed in the proper proportions, a workable mass is formed. The material is introduced into a properly formed mold cavity and polymerized. Recall from Chapter 2 that polymerization can be activated by chemical, heat, and light energy. Microwave energy may also be used for polymerization. In addition, computer-aided design/computer-aided manufacturing (CAD-CAM) technologies of milling PMMA pucks and three-dimensional (3-D) printing using methacrylate-based monomers (Chapter 15) are also available.

General Technique of Denture Base Fabrication

Several processing techniques are available for the fabrication of denture bases (Figs 11.4 to 11.11). Each technique requires a suitable impression of the associated dental arch, followed by the fabrication of an accurate gypsum cast. In turn, a resin record base is fabricated on the cast. Wax is added to the record base, and prosthetic teeth are positioned in the wax (Fig. 11.14A). The prosthetic teeth are related to the opposing dentition and evaluated in the patient's mouth before proceeding.

In the laboratory, a bronze denture flask is used, and the completed tooth arrangement is encased in a suitable investing medium (usually gypsum). A plastic denture flask is mandatory if microwave energy is used. Subsequently, the denture flask is opened, and the wax denture base is eliminated in a hot water bath, leaving the prosthetic teeth in place. After a thorough cleansing of the mold, an appropriate separator is applied to the gypsum surface. In turn, a resin denture base material is introduced into the mold cavity and polymerized under pressure. Following polymerization, the denture is recovered and prepared for clinical placement.

Not all denture base processing requires flasks. When light-activated resin or CAD-CAM processing is used, no flask is needed. In this chapter, we will discuss commonly available denture base materials and the properties and additional applications of denture base resins.

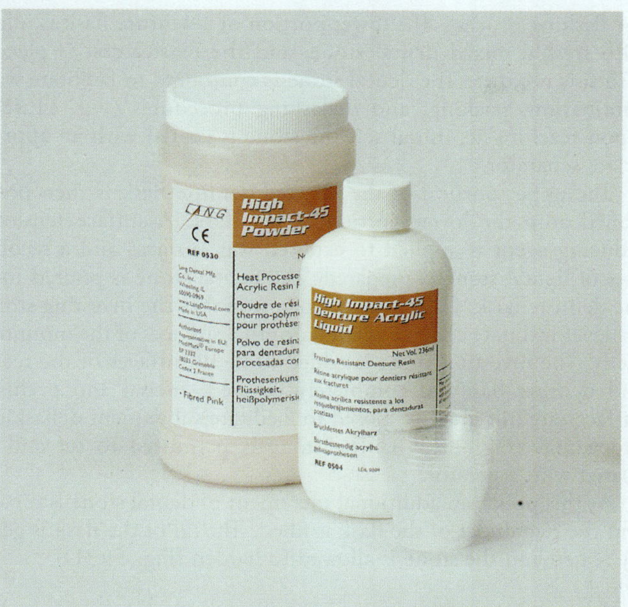

• **Fig. 11.1** A representative heat-activated resin. The majority of heat-activated resins are supplied as powder–liquid systems. (Courtesy of Lang Dental Mfg. Co., Inc. Wheeling, IL.)

Heat-Activated Denture Base Resins

Heat-activated materials are used in the fabrication of nearly all denture bases. The thermal energy required for polymerization of such materials can be provided with a water bath or microwave oven. The emphasis in this chapter is on heat-activated systems because of the prevalent use of these resins.

COMPOSITION

- As previously noted, most PMMA resin systems include powder and liquid components (Fig. 11.1). The powder consists of prepolymerized spheres of PMMA and a small amount of benzoyl peroxide, termed the *initiator,* which is responsible for starting the polymerization process. The liquid is predominantly nonpolymerized methyl methacrylate monomer with small amounts of hydroquinone. Hydroquinone is added as an ***inhibitor***, which prevents undesirable polymerization or "setting" of the liquid during storage. Inhibitors also retard the curing process and thereby increase the working time.
- A *cross-linking agent,* glycol dimethacrylate can also be added to the liquid. Glycol dimethacrylate is chemically and structurally similar to methyl methacrylate. Therefore, it can be incorporated in the growing polymer chains (Fig. 11.2). One should note that methyl methacrylate possesses one carbon–carbon double bond per molecule and glycol dimethacrylate possesses two double bonds per molecule. As a result, an individual molecule of glycol dimethacrylate can participate in the polymerization of two separate polymer chains and unite the two polymer chains. If sufficient glycol dimethacrylate is included in the mixture, several interconnections can be formed. These interconnections yield a net-like structure that provides increased resistance to deformation. Cross-linking agents are incorporated into the liquid component at a concentration of 1%–2% by volume.

Powder
- Prepolymerized spheres of PMMA
- Benzoyl peroxide – *initiator*
- Pigments – salts of cadmium/iron/organic dyes

Liquid
- Nonpolymerized methyl methacrylate monomer
- Glycol dimethacrylate – *cross-linking agent*
- Hydroquinone – *inhibitor*

CLASSIFICATION OF DENTURE BASE POLYMERS (ISO – 1567)

Type 1 – Heat polymerizable polymers
- Class 1 – Powder and liquid
- Class 2 – Plastic cake

Type 2 – Autopolymerizable polymers
- Class 1 – Powder and liquid
- Class 2 – Powder and liquid pour type resins

Type 3 – Thermoplastic blank or powder
Type 4 – Light-activated materials
Type 5 – Microwave-cured materials

Storage

Manufacturers of heat-activated resin systems generally recommend specific temperature and time limits for the storage of powder and liquid components. Strict observance of such recommendations is

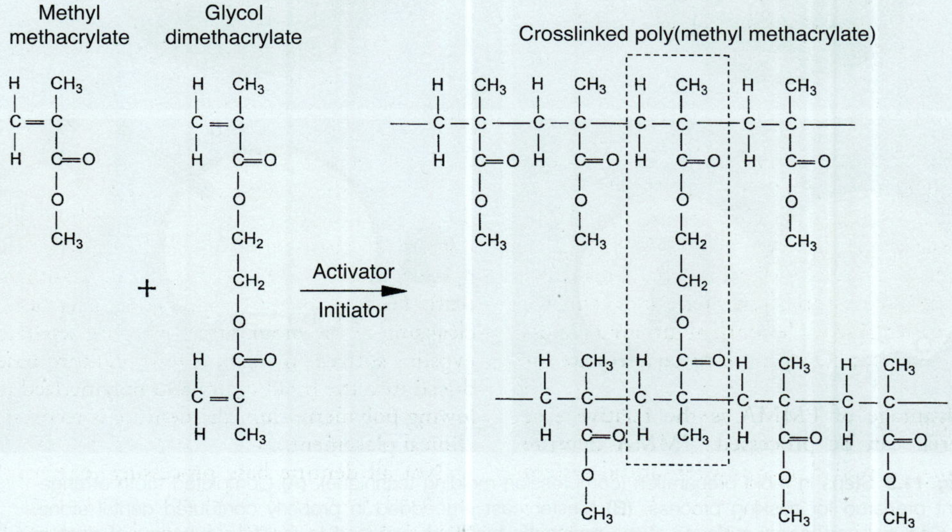

Methyl methacrylate + Glycol dimethacrylate —(Activator / Initiator)→ Crosslinked poly(methyl methacrylate)

• **Fig. 11.2** Chemical basis for the formation of cross-linked polymethyl methacrylate. Glycol dimethacrylate is incorporated into polymethyl methacrylate chains and may "bridge" or "interconnect" such chains.

essential or else components can undergo changes that may affect the working properties as well as the chemical and physical properties of the processed denture bases.

Compression Molding Technique

As a rule, heat-activated denture base resins are shaped via compression molding. Therefore, the compression molding technique is described in detail in the following text.

Preparation of the Mold

Before mold preparation, prosthetic teeth must be selected and arranged in a manner that will fulfill both esthetic and functional requirements. In turn, the completed tooth arrangement is sealed to the master cast.

At this stage, the master cast and completed tooth arrangement are removed from the dental articulator (Fig. 11.3A). The master cast is coated with a thin layer of separator to prevent adherence of dental stone to the base of the master cast during the flasking process. The lower portion of a denture flask is filled with freshly mixed dental stone, and the master cast is placed into this mixture. The dental stone is contoured to facilitate wax elimination, packing, and deflasking procedures (Fig. 11.3B). Upon reaching its initial set, the stone is coated with an appropriate separator.

The upper portion of the selected denture flask is then positioned atop the lower portion of the flask. A surface tension-reducing agent is applied to exposed wax surfaces and a second mix of dental stone is prepared. The dental stone is poured into the denture flask. Care is taken to ensure that the investing stone achieves intimate contact with all external surfaces of the mounted teeth. The investing stone is added until all surfaces of the teeth and denture base are completely covered. Incisal and occlusal surfaces are minimally exposed to facilitate subsequent deflasking procedures (Fig. 11.3C). The stone is permitted to set and is coated with separator.

At this point, an additional increment of dental stone is mixed and the remainder of the flask is filled. The lid of the flask is gently seated and the stone is allowed to harden (Fig. 11.3D).

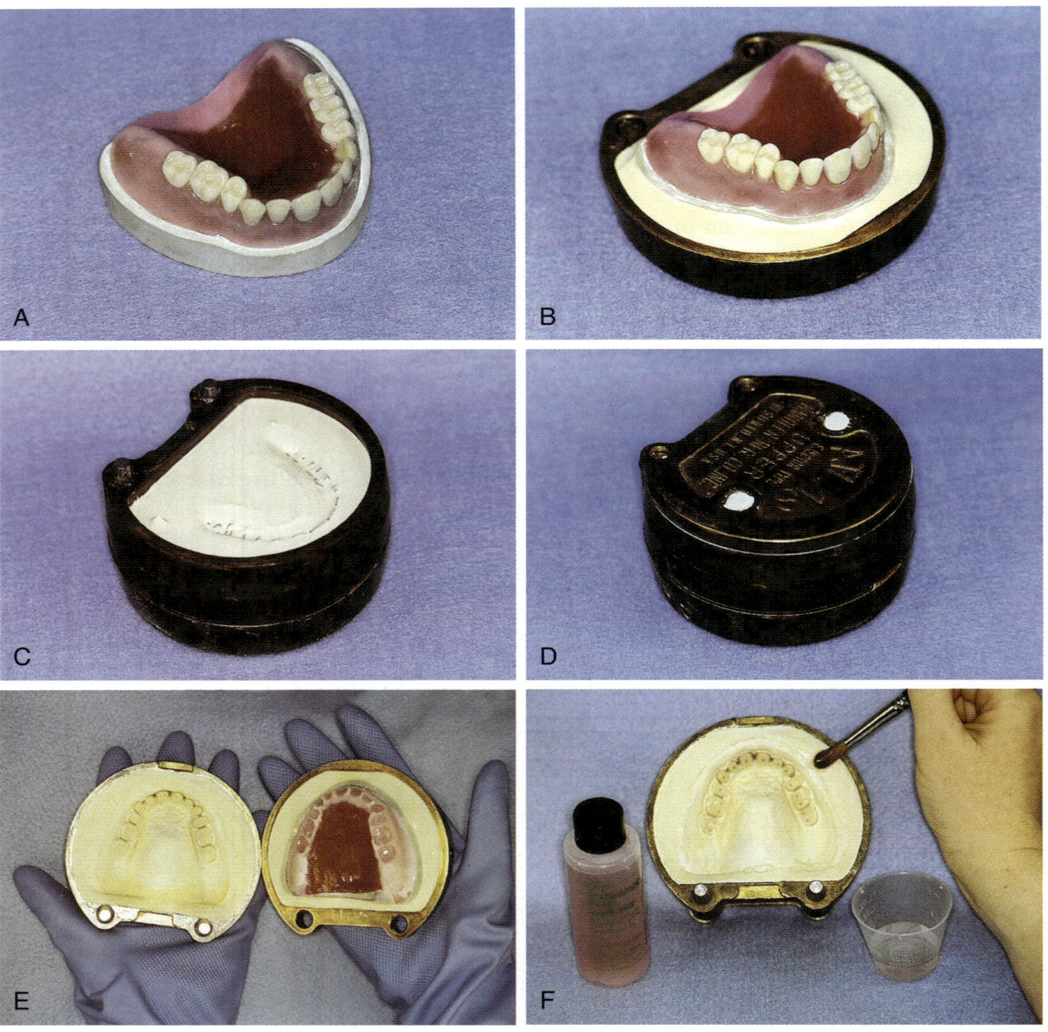

• **Fig. 11.3** Steps in mold preparation (compression molding technique). **(A)** Completed tooth arrangement prepared for flasking process. **(B)** Master cast embedded in properly contoured dental stone. **(C)** Occlusal and incisal surfaces of the prosthetic teeth are exposed to facilitate subsequent denture recovery. **(D)** Fully flasked complete maxillary denture. **(E)** Separation of flask segments during wax elimination process. **(F)** Placement of alginate-based separating medium.

After the stone has hardened, the record base and wax must be removed from the mold. To accomplish this task, the denture flask is immersed in boiling water for 4 min. The flask is then removed from the water and the appropriate segments are separated. The record base and softened wax remain in the lower portion of the denture flask while the prosthetic teeth remain firmly embedded in the investing stone of the remaining segment (Fig. 11.3E). The record base and softened wax are carefully removed. Residual wax is removed from the mold cavity using hot water. The mold cavity is subsequently cleaned with a mild detergent solution and rinsed with boiling water.

CRITICAL QUESTION

What is the purpose of a separating medium that is used during denture base fabrication? What is the chemical basis for popular separating media?

Selection and Application of a Separating Medium

The next step in denture base fabrication involves the application of an appropriate separating medium onto the surfaces of the mold cavity. This medium must prevent direct contact between the denture base resin and the mold surface. Failure to place an appropriate separating medium can lead to two major difficulties: (1) If water is permitted to diffuse from the mold surface into the denture base resin, it can affect the polymerization rate as well as the optical and physical properties of the resultant denture base. (2) If dissolved polymer or free monomer is permitted to soak into the mold surface, portions of the investing medium can become fused to the denture base. These difficulties often produce compromises in the physical and esthetic properties of processed denture bases. Hence, the importance of employing an appropriate separating medium should not be overlooked.

The most popular separating agents are water-soluble alginate solutions. When applied to dental stone surfaces, these solutions produce thin, relatively insoluble calcium alginate films and prevent direct contact of denture base resins.

A small quantity of separator is dispensed into a disposable container and with a fine brush spread the separating medium onto the exposed surfaces of a warm, clean stone mold (Fig. 11.3F). Separator should not be permitted to contact exposed portions of acrylic resin teeth, since its presence interferes with chemical bonding between acrylic resin teeth and denture base resins. Subsequently, the mold sections are oriented to prevent “pooling” of separator, and the solution is permitted to dry.

CRITICAL QUESTION

Why do denture base resin systems contain polymer beads? How does the inclusion of polymer beads affect volumetric shrinkage?

Polymer-to-Monomer Ratio

Proper polymer-to-monomer ratio is of considerable importance in the fabrication of well-fitting denture bases with desirable physical properties. The following paragraphs are intended to provide practical, unambiguous information.

The polymerization of denture base resins results in volumetric and linear shrinkage. This is understandable when one considers the molecular events occurring during the polymerization process.

Envision two methyl methacrylate molecules. Each molecule possesses an electrical field that repels nearby molecules. Consequently, the distance between molecules is significantly greater than the length of a representative carbon-to-carbon bond. When the methyl methacrylate molecules are chemically bonded, a new carbon-to-carbon linkage is formed. This produces a net decrease in the space occupied by the components.

Research indicates that the polymerization of methyl methacrylate to form PMMA yields a 21% decrease in the volume of material. As might be expected, a volumetric shrinkage of 21% would create significant difficulties in denture base fabrication. To minimize dimensional changes, resin manufacturers prepolymerize a significant fraction of the denture base material. This can be thought of as “preshrinking” the selected resin fraction.

In practice, the prepolymerized fraction is supplied as a powder, and is commonly referred to as *polymer*. The nonpolymerized fraction is supplied as a liquid, and is termed a *monomer*. When the powder and liquid components are mixed in the proper proportions, a dough-like mass results. Commercial products generally use a polymer-to-monomer ratio of approximately 3:1 by volume. This ratio provides sufficient monomer to thoroughly wet the polymer particles but does not contribute excess volume that would produce polymerization shrinkage. Using a 3:1 ratio, the volumetric shrinkage can be limited to approximately 7%. The initial setting expansion of the gypsum mold and swelling of the polymerized acrylic resin after exposure to water in the denture flask and later, further compensate this shrinkage. The polymerization shrinkage of denture base resin is discussed in depth later in the chapter.

CRITICAL QUESTION

What are the five physical stages through which properly mixed denture base resins pass? During which stage should compression molding be initiated?

Polymer–Monomer Interaction

When monomer and polymer are mixed in the proper proportions, a workable mass is produced. Upon standing, the resultant mass passes through five distinct stages. These stages can be described as:

(1) sandy,
(2) stringy,
(3) dough like,
(4) rubbery or elastic, and
(5) stiff.

During the sandy stage, little or no interaction occurs on a molecular level. Polymer beads remain unaltered, and the consistency of the mixture can be described as “coarse” or “grainy.” Later, the mixture enters a stringy stage. During this stage, the monomer attacks the surfaces of individual polymer beads and is absorbed into the beads. Some polymer chains are dispersed in the liquid monomer. These polymer chains uncoil, thereby increasing the viscosity of the mix. This stage is characterized by “stringiness” or “stickiness” when the material is touched or drawn apart.

Subsequently, the mass enters a dough-like stage. On a molecular level, an increased number of polymer chains enter the solution. Thus, monomer and dissolved polymer are formed. It is important to note that a large quantity of swollen, but undissolved polymer also remains. Visibly the mass behaves as a pliable dough. It is no longer tacky and does not adhere to the surfaces of the mixing jar or spatula. The physical and chemical characteristics exhibited during the later phases of this stage are ideal for compression molding.

Hence, the material should be introduced into the mold cavity during the latter phases of the dough-like stage.

Following the dough-like stage, the mixture enters a rubbery or elastic stage. This is because monomer is dissipated by evaporation and by further penetration into remaining polymer beads. The mass rebounds when compressed or stretched. Because the mass no longer flows freely to assume the shape of its container, it cannot be molded by conventional compression techniques.

Upon standing for an extended period, the mixture becomes stiff. This can be attributed to continued evaporation of unreacted monomer. From a clinical standpoint, the mixture appears very dry and is resistant to mechanical deformation.

Dough-Forming Time

The time required for the resin mixture to reach a dough-like stage is termed *the dough-forming time*. American National Standards Institute/American Dental Association (ANSI/ADA) Standard No. 139—Dental Base polymers: 2020 requires that this consistency be attained in less than 40 min from the start of the mixing process. Majority of denture base products reach a dough-like consistency in less than 10 min.

Working Time

Working time is defined as the time a denture base material remains in the dough-like stage. This period is critical to the compression molding process. ANSI/ADA Specification No. 12 requires the dough to remain moldable for at least 5 min.

The ambient temperature affects the working time. Hence, the working time of a denture resin can be extended via refrigeration. A significant drawback associated with this technique is that moisture may condense on the resin when it is removed from the refrigerator, which may degrade the physical and esthetic properties of a processed resin. Moisture contamination can be avoided by storing the resin in an airtight container. Following removal from the refrigerator, the container should not be opened until it reaches room temperature.

Packing

The placement and adaptation of denture base resin within the mold cavity are termed *packing*. This process represents one of the most critical steps in denture base fabrication. It is essential that the mold cavity be properly filled at the time of polymerization. The placement of too much material yields a denture base that exhibits excessive thickness and resultant malpositioning of prosthetic teeth. Conversely, the use of too little material leads to noticeable denture base voids or porosity. To minimize these difficulties, the mold cavity is packed in a well-defined sequence.

While in a dough-like state, the resin is removed from its mixing jar and rolled into a rope-like form. Monomer is painted over the necks of the denture teeth to promote bonding to the denture base. Subsequently, the resin rope is bent into a horseshoe shape and placed into the portion of the flask that houses the prosthetic teeth (Fig. 11.4A). Two thin polyethylene/cellophane separator sheets are placed over the master cast, and the flask is reassembled. If a single sheet is placed, it might possibly tear during packing.

The flask assembly is placed into a specially designed press and pressure is applied incrementally (Fig. 11.4B). Slow application of pressure permits the resin dough to flow uniformly throughout the mold space. Excess material is displaced eccentrically. The application of pressure is continued until the denture flask is fully closed. Next, the flask is opened and the polyethylene/cellophane packing sheet is removed from the surface of the resin with a rapid, continuous tug. Cellophane sheet is moistened by dipping it in water for 30 minutes to prevent adhesion with the resin.

Excess resin will be found on the relatively flat (land) areas surrounding the mold cavity. This excess resin is called *flash*. Using a sharp blade, the flash is carefully separated from the body of resin that occupies the mold cavity (Fig. 11.4C). Care is taken not to chip the gypsum surfaces of the mold. Pieces of gypsum that have become dislodged must be removed so that they are not incorporated into the processed denture base.

A fresh polyethylene/cellophane sheet is placed between the major portions of the flask, and the flask assembly is once again placed in the press. Trial closures are repeated before the elapse of working time and until no flash is observed.

When flash is no longer apparent, the mold is closed for the last time with no polyethylene sheet interposed. The mold sections are properly aligned and placed in the flask press. Again, pressure is incrementally applied. Following definitive closure, the flask is transferred to a flask carrier (Fig. 11.4D). The flask carrier maintains pressure on the flask assembly during denture base processing. A cross-sectional representation of the denture flask assembly is presented in Figure 11.5.

Injection Molding Technique

In addition to compression molding techniques, denture bases can be fabricated via injection molding using specially designed flasks. One half of the flask is filled with freshly mixed dental stone, and the master cast is settled into this mixture. The dental stone is appropriately contoured and permitted to set. Subsequently, sprues or ingates are attached to the wax denture base, which leads to an inlet or pressure port (Fig. 11.6A). The remaining half of the flask is positioned, and the investment process is completed (Fig. 11.6B). Wax elimination is performed as previously described (Fig. 11.6C), and the flask is reassembled. Subsequently, the flask is placed into a carrier that maintains pressure on the assembly during resin introduction and processing.

Upon completion of the foregoing steps, resin is mixed and injected into the mold cavity (Fig. 11.6D). The flask is then placed into a water bath for polymerization of the denture base resin if a heat-curing resin is used. Upon completion, the denture is recovered, adjusted, finished, and polished.

Currently there is some debate regarding the comparative accuracy of denture bases fabricated by compression molding and those fabricated by injection molding. Available data and clinical information indicate denture bases fabricated by injection molding can provide slightly improved clinical accuracy.

However, the advantages of injection molding are not straightforward. For example, although tooth movement is minimized, resin viscosity must be lower than that used in compression molding in order to facilitate injection.

This requires a substantially smaller polymer-to-monomer ratio, and consequently results in increased curing shrinkage. Hence, the palatal fit is compromised. This is illustrated in Figure. 11.12D, in which a greater opening at the posterior palatal seal area is shown for injection molding than for any of the other molding processes. From a clinical perspective, this requires greater (i.e., deeper) preparation of the postpalatal seal area (on the dental cast) to ensure contact of the polymerized denture base with the patient's palatal tissues. However, certain studies have proved that the injection molding method has the advantage of dimensional accuracy over the conventional molding technique (Jafar Gharechahi et. al).

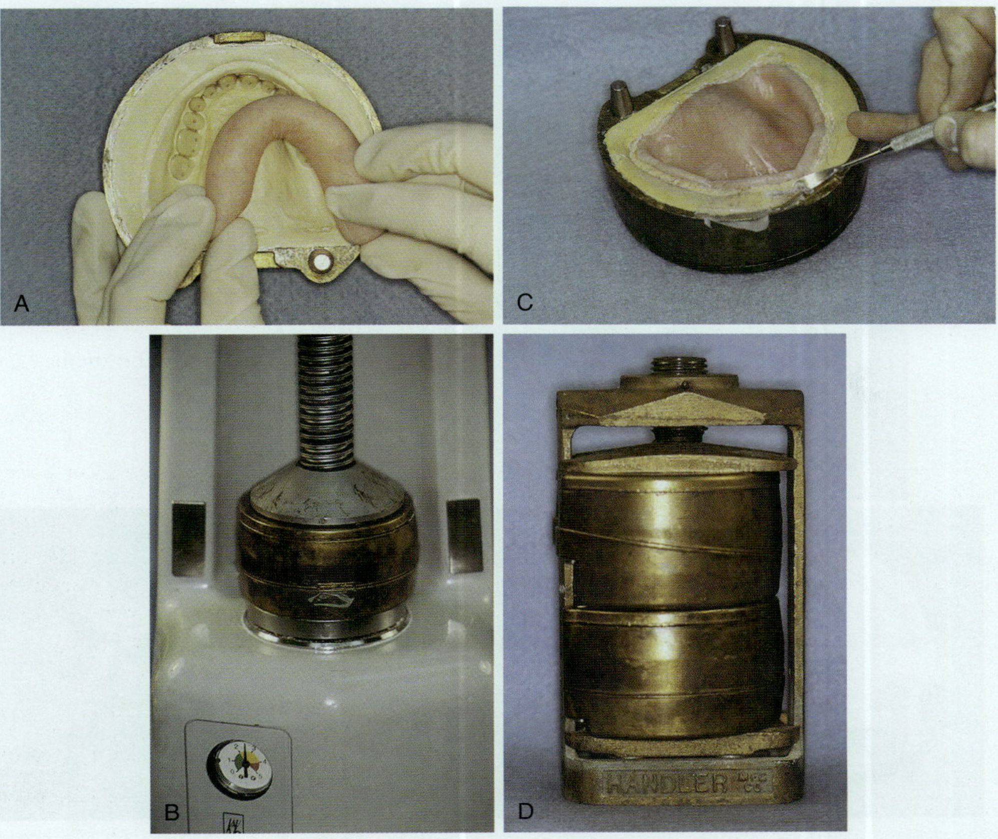

• **Fig. 11.4** Steps in resin packing (compression molding technique). **(A)** Properly mixed resin is bent into a horseshoe shape and placed into the mold cavity. **(B)** The flask assembly is placed into a flask press, and pressure is applied. **(C)** Excess material is carefully removed from the flask. **(D)** The flask is transferred to a flask carrier, which maintains pressure on the assembly during processing.

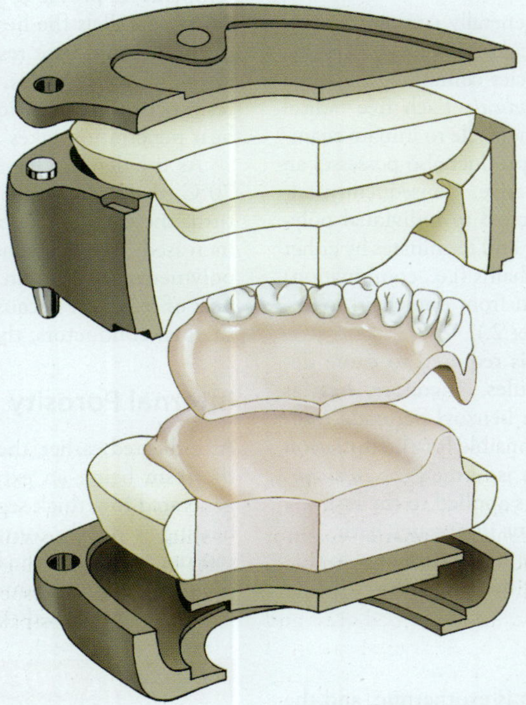

• **Fig. 11.5** A cross-sectional representation of the denture flask and its contents.

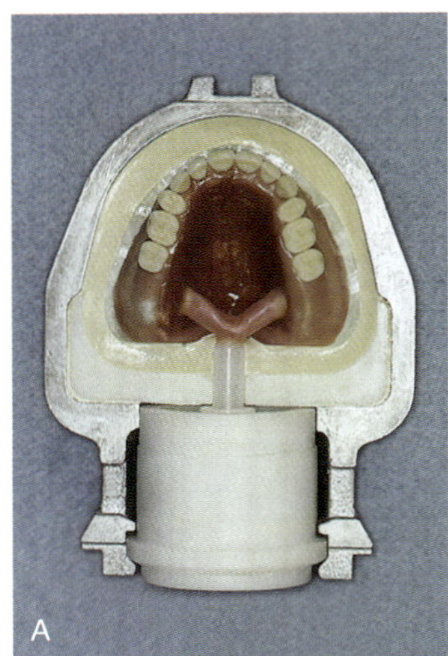

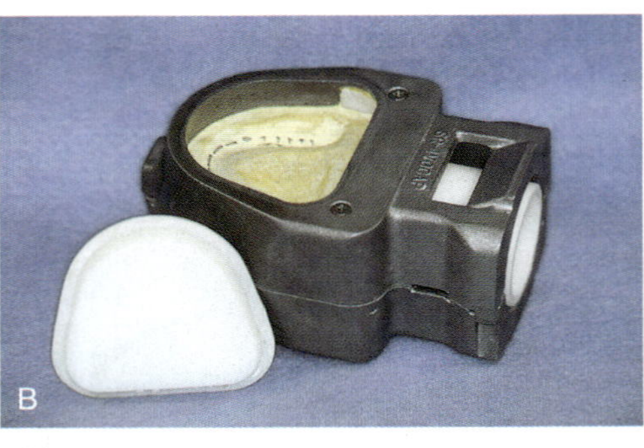

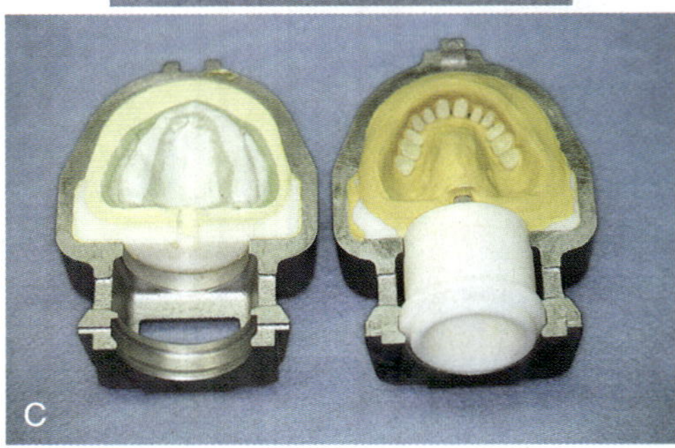

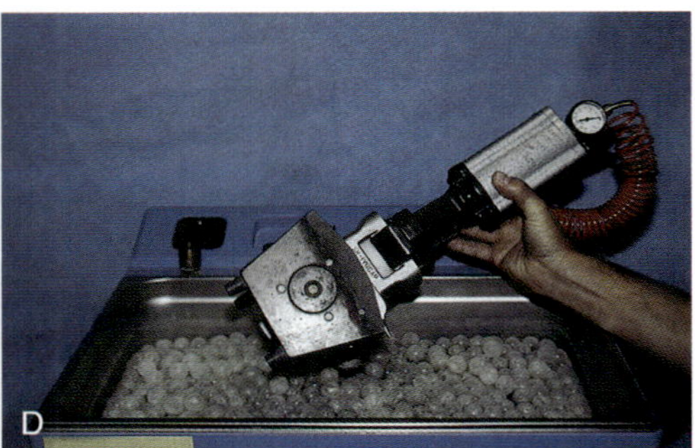

• **Fig. 11.6** Steps in mold preparation (injection molding technique). **(A)** Placement of sprues for introduction of resin. **(B)** Occlusal and incisal surfaces of the prosthetic teeth are exposed to facilitate denture recovery. **(C)** Separation of flask segments during wax elimination process. **(D)** Injection of resin and placement of assembly into water bath.

Polymerization Procedure

As previously noted, denture base resins generally contain benzoyl peroxide. When heated above 60°C, molecules of benzoyl peroxide decompose to yield electrically neutral species containing unpaired electrons. These species are termed *free radicals*. Each free radical rapidly reacts with an available monomer molecule to initiate chain-growth polymerization. Since the reaction product also possesses an unpaired electron, it remains chemically active. Consequently, additional monomer molecules become attached to individual polymer chains. This process occurs very rapidly and terminates by either (1) the direct connection of two growing chains (i.e., combination) or (2) the transfer of a single hydrogen ion from one chain to another. (See also Figs 2.31 to 2.36 in Chapter 2.)

In the system under discussion, heat is required to cause decomposition of benzoyl peroxide molecules. Therefore, heat is termed the *activator*. Decomposition of a benzoyl peroxide molecule yields two free radicals that are responsible for the initiation of chain growth. Hence, benzoyl peroxide is termed the *initiator*.

During denture base fabrication, heat is applied to the resin by immersing a denture flask and flask carrier in a water bath. The water is heated to a prescribed temperature and maintained at that temperature for a period suggested by the manufacturer.

Temperature Rise

The polymerization of denture base resins is exothermic, and the amount of heat evolved can affect the properties of the processed denture bases. Representative temperature changes occurring in water, investing stone, and resin are presented in Fig. 11.7. The temperature profile of the investing stone (identified as "plaster") closely parallels the heating curve for the water. The temperature of the denture base resin lags somewhat during the initial stages of the heating process. This can be attributed to the fact that the resin occupies a position in the center of the mold and therefore heat penetration takes a longer time.

As the denture base resin attains a temperature slightly above 70°C, the temperature of the resin begins to increase rapidly. In turn, the decomposition rate of benzoyl peroxide is significantly increased. This sequence of events leads to an increased rate of polymerization and an accompanying increase in the exothermic heat of reaction. Because resin and dental stone are relatively poor thermal conductors, the heat of reaction cannot be dissipated.

Internal Porosity

As indicated earlier, the polymerization process is exothermic and the resin being an extremely poor thermal conductor, the heat generated in a thick segment of resin cannot be dissipated. When heating is poorly controlled, the peak temperature of this resin can rise well above the boiling point of monomer (100.8°C). This causes boiling of unreacted monomer and produces porosity within the processed denture base.

CRITICAL QUESTION

What causes porosity in denture bases? How can these defects be minimized?

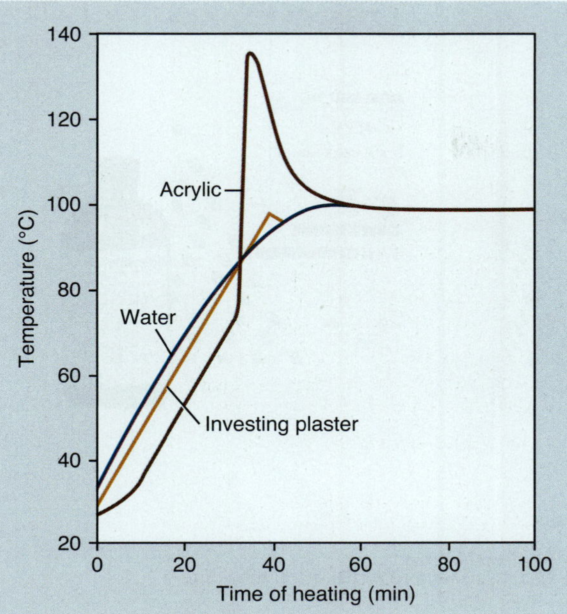

• **Fig. 11.7** Temperature–time heating curves for the water bath, investing plaster, and acrylic resin during the polymerization of a 25.4 mm cube of denture resin. (Modified from Tuckfield WJ, Worner HK, Guerin BD: Acrylic resins in dentistry. *Aust Dent* J 47:119–121, 1943. Reproduced with permission from the Australian Dental Journal.)

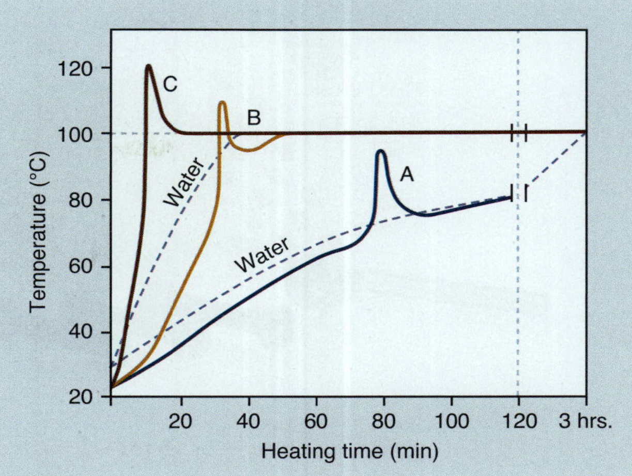

• **Fig. 11.8** Temperature changes in acrylic resin when subjected to various curing schedules. (Modified from Tuckfield WJ, Worner HK, Guerin BD: Acrylic resins in dentistry. *Aust Dent J* 47:119–121, 1943. Reproduced with permission from the Australian Dental Journal.)

Polymerization Cycle

The heating process used to control polymerization is termed the *polymerization cycle* or *curing cycle*. This process should be carefully regulated to avoid the effects of uncontrolled temperature rise.

The curing cycle presented in Fig. 11.7 is unsatisfactory because of the marked temperature increase during the early stages of polymerization. Rapid heating of the resin mass may cause the monomer to boil, producing porosity within the polymerized denture base. Fortunately, this process can be controlled by heating the resin more slowly during the polymerization cycle.

The relationship between the rate of heating and temperature rise within the denture base resin is illustrated in Fig. 11.8. The polymerization cycle represented by curve C probably would yield porosity in thick portions of the denture, since the temperature of the resin exceeds the boiling point of the monomer (100.8°C). On the other hand, the polymerization cycle represented by curve A probably would result in the presence of unreacted monomer since the resin temperature fails to reach the boiling temperature of the monomer (100.8°C). Thus, it is logical to assume that an optimum polymerization cycle lies somewhere between curves A and C.

Research has led to the development of guidelines for polymerization of denture base resins. The resultant polymerization cycles have been quite successful for denture bases of various sizes, shapes, and thicknesses.

One technique involves processing the denture base resin in a constant temperature water bath at 74°C (165°F) for 8 h or longer, with no terminal boiling treatment. A second technique consists of processing in a 74°C water bath for 8 h and then increasing the temperature to 100°C for 1 h. A third technique involves processing the resin at 74°C for approximately 2 h and increasing the temperature of the water bath to 100°C and processing for 1 h.

Researchers have observed that the pressure built up within the mold during processing would elevate the boiling temperature of the monomer, thereby preventing the occurrence of porosity due to vaporization of monomer. Possibly this is the reason why porosity is not seen even if the technicians are not strictly adhering to curing cycles (Yau WFE et al).

Following completion of the chosen polymerization cycle, the denture flask should be cooled slowly to room temperature. Rapid cooling can result in distortion of the denture base because of differences in thermal contraction of resin and investing stone. To minimize potential difficulties, the flask should be removed from the water and bench cooled for 30 min. Subsequently, the flask should be immersed in cool tap water for 15 min. The denture base can then be deflasked and prepared for delivery. To decrease the probability of unfavorable dimensional changes, the denture should be stored in water until it is placed in the oral cavity.

PROPERTIES OF DENTURE BASE RESINS (ISO 1567)

Type	Flexural strength	Flexural modulus	Residual monomer	Water sorption	Solubility
	MPa	*GPa*	*wt%*	*μg/mm³*	*μg/mm³*
1, 3, 4, 5	65	2.0	2.2	32	1.6
2	60	1.5	4.5	32	8.0
	(minimum)	(mini)	(max)	(max)	(max)

Polymerization via Microwave Energy

PMMA resin can be polymerized using microwave energy. This technique employs a specially formulated resin and a nonmetallic flask (Fig. 11.9). A conventional microwave oven is used to supply the thermal energy required for polymerization.

The major advantage of this technique is the speed wi th which polymerization can be accomplished, but overheating can occur

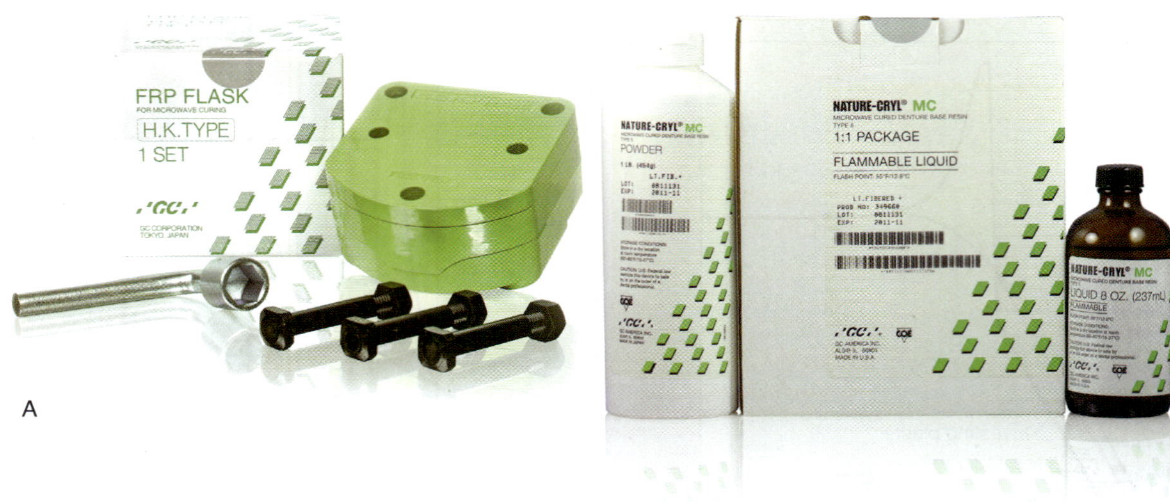

• **Fig. 11.9** A representative nonmetallic microwave flask **(A)** and microwave resin **(B)**. (Courtesy of GC America, Inc. Alsip, IL.)

in thick sections, causing the monomer to boil and produce porosity. It should also be noted that although the polymerization time is reduced, the required technician time is unaffected. Available information indicates that the physical properties of microwave resins are comparable to those of conventional resins. Furthermore, the fit of denture bases polymerized using microwave energy is comparable to those processed via conventional compression molding techniques.

CAD-CAM Procedures in Denture Base Fabrication

Although the first CAM software program was developed by Dr Patrick Hanratty in the 1950s, it was not until the 1990s that CAD-CAM technologies were used to generate complete dentures. The first English-language account of computer-aided technology in the fabrication of complete dentures was published by Maeda et al. in 1994. The authors employed stereolithography to generate complete dentures in a proof-of-concept effort. Beginning in 1995, Goodacre employed a series of procedures intended to facilitate the fabrication of complete dentures using subtractive techniques. In the ensuing years, Kawahata et al. and Kanazawa et al. used computer numerical control (CNC) milling to advance and refine previous efforts. CNC is an automated control of machining and 3-D printers by means of a computer. In 2012, Goodacre et al. published the first clinical account of CAD-CAM dentures milled from prepolymerized PMMA.

Advantages associated with CAD-CAM fabrication of complete dentures include enhanced material properties and improved dimensional stability of the resultant prostheses. PMMA "pucks" are fabricated at increased pressures and under strictly controlled thermal conditions. Consequently, these materials display decreased porosity, increased polymerization, and a diminished residual monomer content. Moreover, the prepolymerized resins used in current subtractive processes are approximately 8% more dense than their conventionally processed counterparts. These factors are likely to yield enhanced clinical performance and decreased surface colonization by undesirable species such as *Candida albicans.*

Machining of prepolymerized PMMA specimens also affects the clinical adaptation and the dimensional stability of completed denture bases. As previously noted, dentures fabricated via compression molding techniques are subject to polymerization shrinkage during the fabrication process. In addition, compression-molded prostheses are susceptible to distortion upon recovery from the mold. Corresponding changes are not observed in machined specimens because polymerization shrinkage and stress relaxation occur before the machining process. As a result, milled denture bases exhibit improved adaptation to the underlying ridges upon clinical placement and are less susceptible to distortion because relaxation has occurred prior to the machining process.

Currently, the most common CAD-CAM techniques for the fabrication of complete dentures employ milling technologies. Clinicians are responsible for accurately capturing the anatomical ridge forms, identifying critical landmarks (e.g., incisal edge position, facial midline, lip line, etc.), recording desired ridge/arch relationships, and determining appropriate tooth shades and forms. This information is transferred to the dental laboratory or manufacturer responsible for prosthesis fabrication. Design is accomplished in a virtual environment (CAD) and subsequently exported to a milling device for production (CAM).

CRITICAL QUESTION

What are the benefits associated with the chemical-activated processes compared with heat-activated processes?

In the existing environment, dominant systems employ two-component manufacturing processes. The required denture base is manufactured as one component, and the corresponding teeth are manufactured as a separate yet continuous monolithic component. The denture base and tooth forms may be joined in a variety of ways, and the prosthesis is finished, polished, and prepared for clinical placement.

Chemically Activated Denture Base Resins

As already noted, heat and microwave energy can be used to induce denture base polymerization. The application of thermal energy leads to decomposition of benzoyl peroxide and the production of free radicals. The free radicals formed as a result of this process initiate polymerization.

Chemical activators can also be used to induce denture base polymerization. Chemical activation does not require the application of thermal energy. Therefore, it can be completed at room temperature. As a result, chemically activated resins often are referred to as *cold-curing, self-curing,* or *autopolymerizing* resins.

As discussed in Chapter 2, in most instances, chemical activation is accomplished through the addition of a tertiary amine, such as dimethyl-para-toluidine, to the denture base liquid (i.e., monomer). Upon mixing of the powder and liquid components, the tertiary amine causes decomposition of benzoyl peroxide. As a result, free radicals are produced and polymerization is initiated. Polymerization progresses in a manner similar to that described for heat-activated systems.

It should be noted that the fundamental difference between heat-activated resins and chemical-activated resins is the method by which benzoyl peroxide is divided to yield free radicals. All other factors in this process (e.g., initiator and reactants) remain the same.

As might be expected, denture bases fabricated using chemically activated resins and heat-activated resins are quite similar. Nonetheless, chemically activated resins exhibit certain advantages and disadvantages that are worthy of discussion.

As a general rule, the degree of polymerization achieved using chemically activated resins is not as complete as that achieved using heat-activated systems. This indicates that there is a greater amount of unreacted monomer in denture bases fabricated via chemical activation. This unreacted monomer creates two major difficulties. First, it acts as a plasticizer, resulting in decreased transverse strength of the denture resin. Second, the residual monomer serves as a potential tissue irritant, thereby compromising the biocompatibility of the denture base.

From a physical standpoint, chemically activated resins display slightly less shrinkage than their heat-activated counterparts. This imparts greater dimensional accuracy to chemically activated resins.

The color stability of chemically activated resins generally is inferior to the color stability of heat-activated resins. This property is related to the presence of tertiary amines within the chemically activated resins. Such amines are susceptible to oxidation and accompanying color changes that affect the appearance of the resin. Discoloration of these resins can be minimized via the addition of stabilizing agents that prevent such oxidation.

Technical Considerations

Chemically activated denture base resins are most often molded using compression techniques. Therefore, mold preparation and resin packing are essentially the same as those described for heat-activated denture resins.

Polymer and monomer are supplied in the form of a powder and a liquid, respectively. These components are mixed according to the manufacturer's directions and permitted to attain a dough-like consistency. The working time for chemically activated resins is shorter than for heat-activated materials. Therefore, special attention must be paid to the consistency of the material and rate of polymerization.

A lengthy initiation period is desirable since this provides adequate time for trial closures. One method for prolonging the initiation period is to decrease the temperature of the resin mass. This can be accomplished by refrigerating the liquid component and/or mixing vessel before the mixing process. When the powder and liquid are mixed, the polymerization process slows down. As a result, the resin mass remains in a doughy stage for an extended period and the working time is prolonged.

Mold preparation and resin packing are accomplished in the same manner described for heat-activated resins. In cases of chemically activated resins with minimal working times, it is doubtful that more than two trial closures can be made. Therefore, extreme care must be taken to ensure that a proper amount of resin is employed and a minimal number of trial closures are needed.

Processing Considerations

Following definitive closure of the denture flask, pressure must be maintained throughout the polymerization process. The time required for polymerization will vary with the material chosen.

Initial hardening of the resin generally will occur within 30 min but polymerization continues for an extended period. To ensure sufficient polymerization, the flask should be held under pressure for a minimum of 3 h.

The polymerization of chemically activated resins is never as complete as the polymerization of heat-activated materials. Resins polymerized via chemical activation generally display 3–5% free monomer, whereas heat-activated resins exhibit 0.2–0.5% free monomer. Therefore, it is important that the polymerization of chemically activated resins be as complete as possible. Failure to achieve a high degree of polymerization will predispose the denture base to dimensional instability and can lead to tissue irritation.

Heat-Activated Versus Chemically-Activated Denture Base

The residual monomer in chemical-activated denture base materials creates two difficulties. First, the residual monomer acts as a plasticizer, resulting in decreased transverse strength of the denture resin. Second, the residual monomer serves as a potential tissue irritant, thereby compromising the biocompatibility of the denture base.

From a physical standpoint, chemical-activated resins display slightly less shrinkage than their heat-activated counterparts. This imparts greater dimensional accuracy to chemical-activated resins.

The color stability of chemical-activated resins generally is inferior to the color stability of heat-activated resins. This property is related to the presence of tertiary amines within the chemical-activated resins. Such amines are susceptible to oxidation and accompanying color changes that affect the appearance of the resin. Discoloration of these resins can be minimized via the addition of stabilizing agents that prevent such oxidation.

Fluid Resin Technique

The fluid resin technique employs a pourable, chemically activated resin for the fabrication of denture bases. The material is supplied in the form of powder and liquid components. When mixed in the proper proportions, these components yield a low-viscosity resin. This resin is poured into a mold cavity, subjected to increased atmospheric pressure, and allowed to polymerize at ambient temperature. Laboratory aspects of the fluid resin technique are described in the following paragraphs.

Tooth arrangement is accomplished using accepted prosthodontic principles. The completed tooth arrangement is then sealed to the underlying cast and placed in a specially designed flask (Fig. 11.10A). The flask is filled with a reversible hydrocolloid

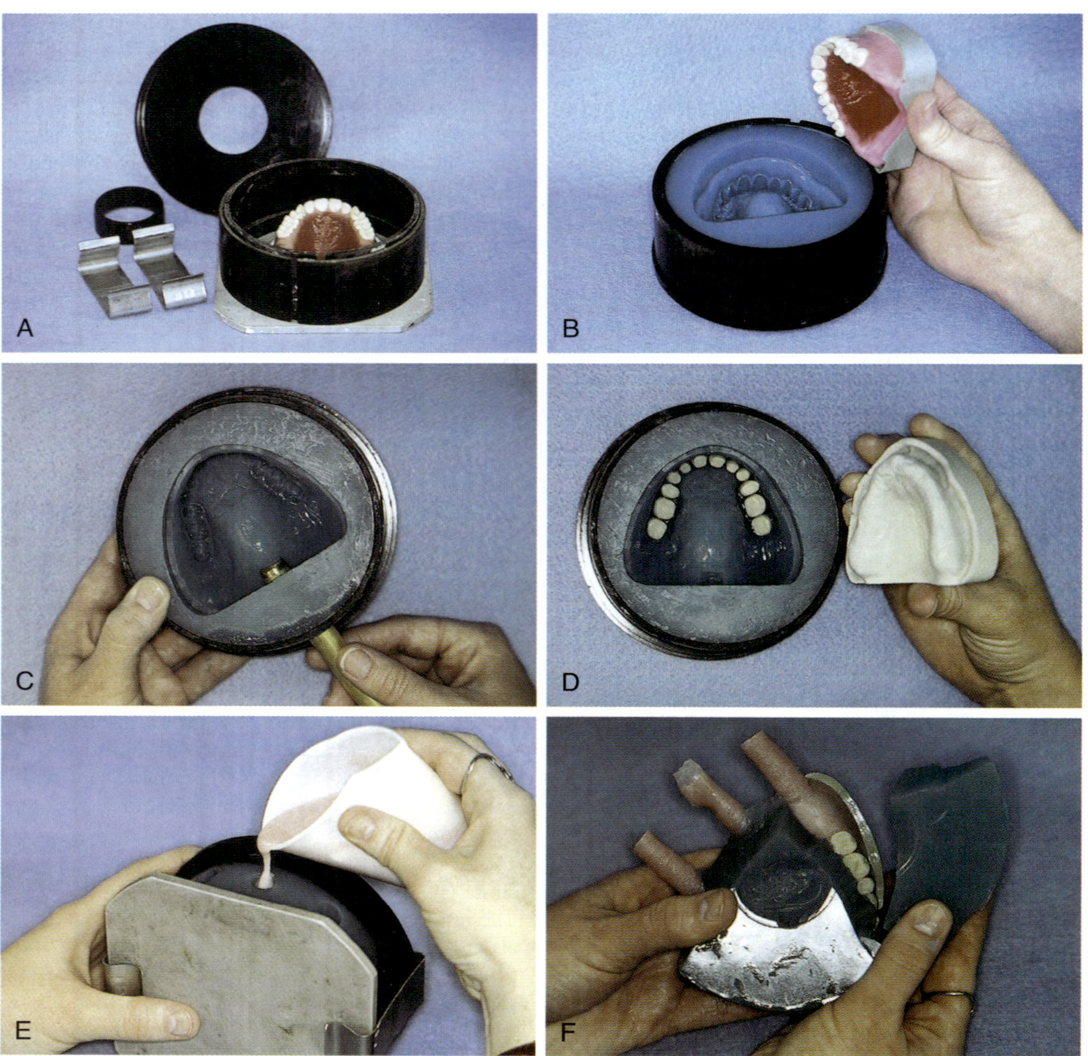

• **Fig. 11.10** Steps in mold preparation (fluid resin technique). **(A)** Completed tooth arrangement positioned in a fluid resin flask. **(B)** Removal of tooth arrangement from reversible hydrocolloid investment. **(C)** Preparation of sprues and vents for the introduction of resin. **(D)** Repositioning of the prosthetic teeth and master cast. **(E)** Introduction of pour-type resin. **(F)** Recovery of the completed prosthesis.

investment medium, and the assembly is cooled. (See the section on Agar [Reversible Hydrocolloid] in Chapter 13.) Following gelation of the hydrocolloid, the cast with the attached tooth arrangement is removed from the flask (Fig. 11.10B). At this stage, sprues and vents are cut from the external surface of the flask to the mold cavity (Fig. 11.10C).

Wax is eliminated from the cast with hot water. The prosthetic teeth are retrieved and carefully seated in their respective positions within the hydrocolloid investing medium. Subsequently, the cast is returned to its position within the mold (Fig. 11.10D).

The resin is mixed according to the manufacturer's directions and poured into the mold via the sprue channels (Fig. 11.10E). The flask is then placed in a pressurized chamber (i.e., a pressure pot) at room temperature and the resin is permitted to polymerize. According to available information, only 30–45 min are required for polymerization. Nevertheless, a longer period is recommended.

Following completion of the polymerization process, the denture is retrieved from the flask (Fig. 11.10F) and the sprues are removed. The denture/cast assembly is returned to the articulator for correction of processing changes. Subsequently, the denture base is finished and polished. After finishing and polishing, the denture should be stored in water to prevent dehydration and distortion.

Advantages claimed for the fluid resin technique are:

- improved adaptation to underlying soft tissues,
- decreased probability of damage to prosthetic teeth and denture bases during deflasking,
- reduced material costs, and
- simplification of the flasking, deflasking, and finishing procedures.

Potential disadvantages of the fluid resin technique include:

- noticeable shifting of prosthetic teeth during processing,
- air entrapment within the denture base material,
- poor bonding between the denture base material and acrylic resin teeth, and
- technique sensitivity.

In general, denture bases fabricated in this manner exhibit physical properties that are somewhat inferior to those of conventional

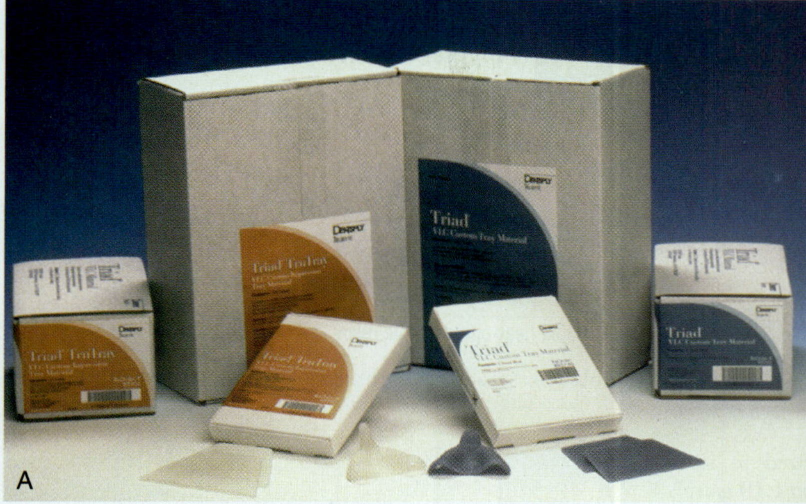

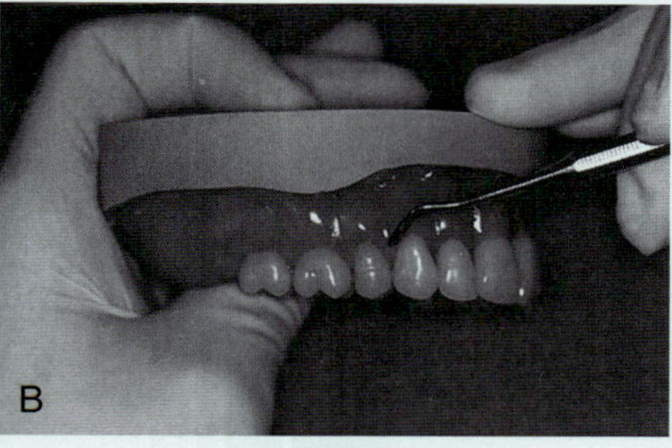

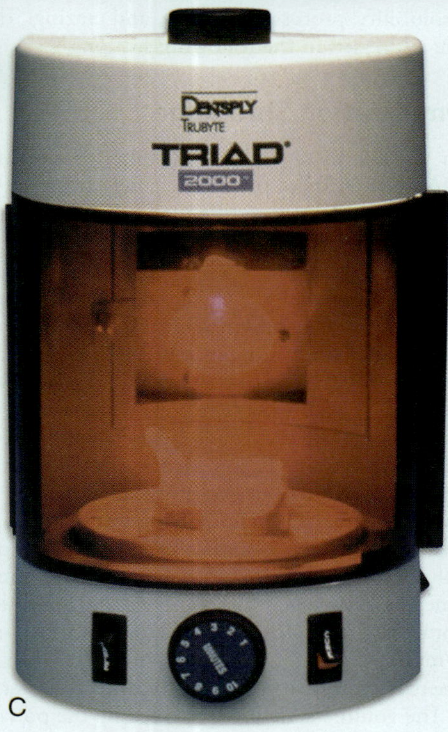

• **Fig. 11.11** Steps in denture fabrication (light-activated denture base resins). **(A)** Representative light-activated denture base resin. Sheet and rope forms are supplied in light-proof pouches to prevent inadvertent polymerization. **(B)** Teeth are arranged and the denture base sculpted using light-activated resin. **(C)** The denture base is placed into a light chamber and polymerized according to the manufacturer's recommendations. (Parts A and C courtesy of Dentsply International, York, PA.)

heat-processed resins. Nonetheless, clinically acceptable dentures can be obtained using fluid resins.

Light-Activated Denture Base Resins

Visible light-activated denture base resins have been available to the dental community for several years. These materials have been described as resin-based composites having matrices of urethane dimethacrylate (Chapter 5, Fig. 5.14), microfine silica, and high–molecular-weight acrylic resin monomers. Acrylic resin beads are included as organic fillers. Blue light is the activator, while a photosensitizing agent such as camphorquinone serves as the initiator for polymerization. Single-component denture base resins are supplied in sheet and rope forms and are packed in lightproof pouches to prevent inadvertent polymerization (Fig. 11.11A).

Denture base fabrication using a light-activated resin is significantly different from that of heat-activated or chemically activated resin. A light-activated resin cannot be flasked in a conventional manner since the opaque investing media prevent the penetration of light. Instead, the denture base is molded on an accurate cast and subsequently the teeth are positioned (Fig. 11.11B). In turn, the denture base is exposed to a high-intensity visible light source for an appropriate period (Fig. 11.11C). Following polymerization, the denture is removed from the cast, finished, and polished in a conventional manner.

The most recent generation of light-activated denture base resins consists of three resins; that include:
(1) a base-forming resin,
(2) a tooth-setting resin, and
(3) a contouring resin.

The base-forming resin is adapted to the dental cast. The cast and denture base are placed into a high-intensity light chamber to induce polymerization. Subsequently, the tooth-setting resin is used to attach the prosthetic teeth to the polymerized base. A high-intensity light source is used to polymerize the tooth-setting resin, thereby maintaining prosthetic teeth in the desired positions.

Next, a contouring resin is used to generate the desired final surface form. The resultant prosthesis is placed into the light chamber to complete the denture base fabrication process. The denture is then removed from the cast, finished, and polished in a conventional manner.

Physical Properties of Denture Base Resins

The physical properties of denture base resins are critical to the fit and function of removable dental prostheses. Characteristics of interest include polymerization shrinkage, porosity, water absorption, solubility, processing stresses, and crazing. These characteristics are addressed in the following sections.

Polymerization Shrinkage

When methyl methacrylate monomer is polymerized to form PMMA, the density of the mass changes from 0.94 to 1.19 g/cm^3. This change in density results in a volumetric shrinkage of 21%. When a conventional heat-activated resin is mixed at the suggested powder-to-liquid ratio, about one-third of the mass is liquid monomer. The remainder of the mass is prepolymerized PMMA. Consequently, the volumetric shrinkage exhibited by the polymerized mass should be approximately 7%. This figure is in agreement with values observed in laboratory and clinical investigations.

There are several possible reasons why materials exhibiting such high volumetric shrinkages can be used to produce clinically satisfactory denture bases. It appears the shrinkage exhibited by these materials is distributed uniformly to all surfaces. Hence, the adaptation of denture bases to underlying soft tissues is not significantly affected, provided the materials are manipulated properly.

Volumetric proportion of polymer to monomer used is 3:1. Volumetric shrinkage that happens during the conversion of monomer to polymer is 21%. Polymer cannot shrink further and only monomer can undergo shrinkage. When monomer and polymer are mixed together, no visible volumetric change happens. The volume is mainly provided by the polymer powder and not the monomer liquid. Hence, the net shrinkage will only be 7% because the 21% is shared by the polymer volume.

In addition to volumetric shrinkage, one must also consider the effects of linear shrinkage. Linear shrinkage exerts significant effects upon denture base adaptation and cuspal interdigitation.

By convention, the magnitude of linear shrinkage is determined by measuring the distance between two predetermined reference points in the second molar regions of a completed tooth arrangement. Following polymerization of the denture base resin and removal of the prosthesis from the master cast, the distance between these reference points is measured once again. The difference between prepolymerization and postpolymerization measurements is recorded as linear shrinkage. The greater the linear shrinkage, the greater is the discrepancy observed in the initial fit of a denture.

CRITICAL QUESTION

Why is the relatively high volumetric shrinkage of a denture base resin not usually considered as a significant clinical problem?

Based on a projected volumetric shrinkage of 7%, an acrylic resin denture base should exhibit a linear shrinkage of approximately 2%. In reality, linear shrinkage rarely exceeds 1% (Table 11.1).

Examination of the polymerization process indicates thermal shrinkage of resin is primarily responsible for the linear changes observed in heat-activated systems. During the initial stages of the cooling process, the resin remains relatively soft. Consequently, the resin mass contracts at about the same rate as the surrounding dental stone.

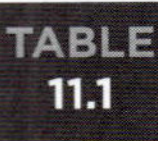

Polymerization Shrinkage of Maxillary Denture Bases

Material	Linear Shrinkage (%)
High-impact acrylic resin	0.12
Vinyl acrylic resin	0.33
Conventional acrylic resin	0.43
Pour-type acrylic resin	0.48
Rapid heat-cured acrylic resin	0.97

Data from Stafford GD, Bates JF, Huggett R, Handley RW: A review of the properties of some denture base polymers. *J Dent* 8:292, 1960.

As cooling proceeds, the soft resin approaches its glass transition temperature, Tg (see Chapter 6, Dental Polymers). The glass transition temperature is a thermal range in which the polymerized resin passes from a soft, rubbery state to a rigid, glassy state. Cooling the denture base resin beyond the glass transition temperature yields a rigid mass. As might be expected, this rigid mass contracts at a rate different from that of surrounding dental stone. The shrinkage occurring below the glass transition temperature is thermal in nature and varies according to the composition of the resin.

To illustrate the effect of thermal shrinkage, consider the following example. The glass transition temperature for PMMA is approximately 105°C. Room temperature is 20°C. The generally accepted value for linear coefficient of thermal expansion, α, for PMMA is 81 ppm/°C. Therefore, as the denture base resin cools from the glass transition temperature to room temperature, it undergoes a linear shrinkage, which can be expressed as:

$$\text{Linear shrinkage} = \alpha\,\Delta T = (81\ \text{ppm}/^\circ\text{C})(105^\circ\text{C} - 20^\circ\text{C}) = (100\%) = 0.69\% \quad (1)$$

This value is in agreement with linear shrinkages of 0.12%–0.97% reported for various commercial denture resins (see Table 11.1).

Glass transition temperature Tg of different types of methacrylate resins (°C):

Methyl	125
Ethyl	65
n-Propyl	38

Commercially available denture resins have Tg between 65°C and 105°C because it has different copolymers.

Complete dentures constructed using chemically activated resins generally display better adaptation than those constructed using heat-activated resins. This phenomenon can be attributed to the negligible thermal shrinkage displayed by chemically activated resins. Processing shrinkage has been measured as 0.26% for a chemically activated resin, compared with 0.53% for a heat-activated resin.

Given the preceding information regarding polymerization shrinkage and denture base adaptation, chemically activated resins appear to provide significant advantages over heat-activated resins. However, there are several other factors that affect the overall dimensional characteristics of processed denture bases including the type of investing medium, method of resin introduction, and temperature used to activate the polymerization process.

On completion of the polymerization process, individual denture bases and master casts are retrieved and returned to their respective dental articulator(s). Dimensional changes are assessed with respect to the proposed vertical dimension at occlusion.

Fluid resin techniques used in conjunction with hydrocolloid investing media generally yield decreases in vertical dimension. Conversely, dentures processed using heat-activated or chemically activated resins in conjunction with compression molding techniques usually display increases in overall vertical dimension. Minimal increases in vertical dimension are considered desirable since they permit a return to the proposed occlusal vertical dimension via occlusal grinding procedures. Dimensional changes occurring in denture bases fabricated from various resins are illustrated in Figure 11.12. Additional dimensional factors include setting expansion of the gypsum product used to make the master cast and investing component and expansion from water sorption of the cured acrylic resin after polymerization is complete.

CRITICAL QUESTION

What are the causes of porosity when fluid resin denture fabrication techniques are used? How can these difficulties be minimized?

Porosity

The presence of surface and subsurface voids can compromise the physical, esthetic, and hygienic properties of a processed denture base. It has been noted that porosity is likely to develop in thicker portions of a denture base. Such porosity results from the vaporization of unreacted monomer and low–molecular-weight polymers when the temperature of a resin reaches or surpasses the boiling points of these species. Nonetheless, this type of porosity may not occur equally throughout the affected resin segments.

To facilitate our understanding of these effects, consider the specimens in Figure 11.13A, no porosity, and Figure 11.13B, localized subsurface porosity. Specimens B and C were flasked in such a manner that the section displaying porosity was nearer the center of the investment mass, whereas the nonporous section was nearer the surface of the metal flask. As might be expected, the metal of the flask conducts heat away from the periphery with sufficient rapidity to prevent a substantial temperature rise. As a result, the low–molecular-weight species does not boil and porosity does not develop. In contrast, resin specimens occupying central positions in the mold are surrounded by larger amounts of gypsum. Because gypsum is a poor thermal conductor, heat is not readily dissipated. Consequently low–molecular-weight species are vaporized and noticeable porosity is produced.

Porosity can also result from inadequate mixing of powder and liquid components. If this occurs, some regions of the resin mass will contain more monomer than others. During polymerization, these regions shrink more than adjacent regions, and the localized shrinkage tends to produce voids (Fig. 11.13D).

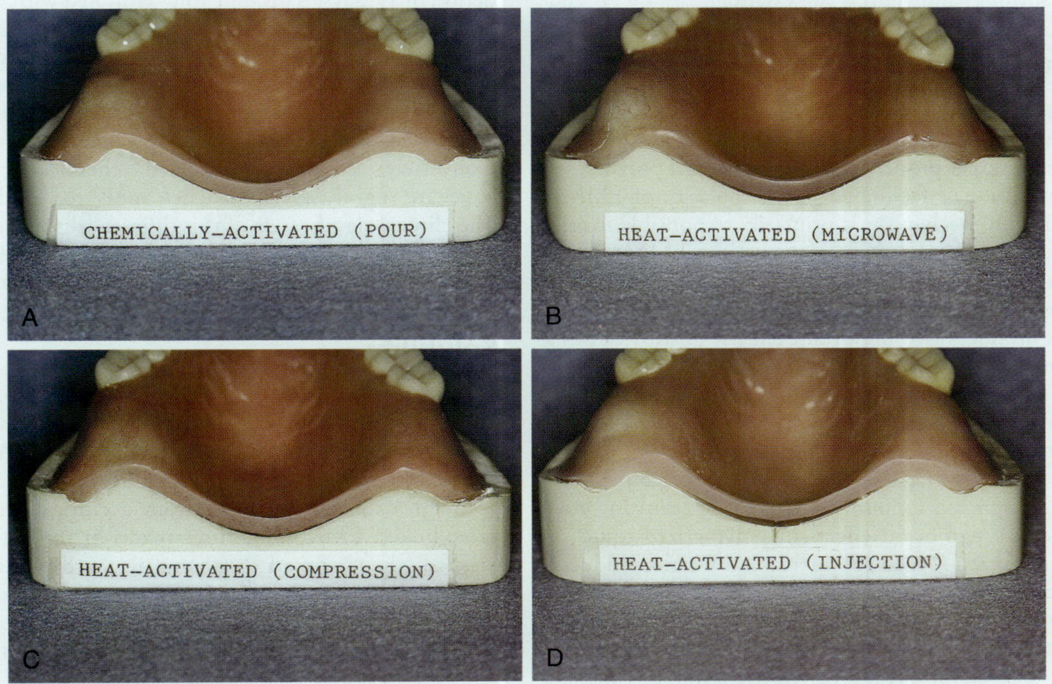

• **Fig. 11.12** Dimensional changes resulting from polymerization. **(A)** Chemically activated resin, pour technique. **(B)** Microwave resin, compression molding. **(C)** Conventional heat-activated resin, compression molding. **(D)** Heat-activated resin, injection molding. (Demonstration and photographs courtesy of Dr Rodney Phoenix.)

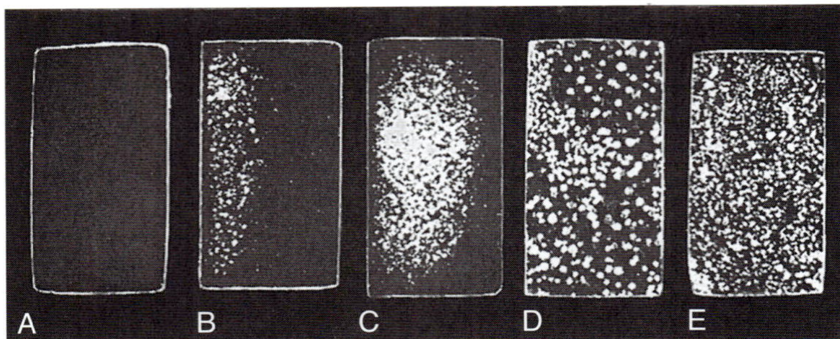

• **Fig. 11.13** Heat-activated denture base resin exhibiting different types and degrees of porosity. **(A)** Properly polymerized; no porosity. **(B)** and **(C)** Rapid heating, relatively small subsurface voids. **(D)** Insufficient mixing of monomer and polymer; large voids resulting from localized polymerization shrinkage. **(E)** Insufficient pressure during polymerization; relatively large, irregular voids. (From Tuckfield WJ, Worner HK, Guerin BD: Acrylic resins in dentistry. *Aust Dent J* March 1943.)

The occurrence of such porosity can be minimized by ensuring the greatest possible homogeneity of the resin. Proper polymer-to-monomer ratio and well-controlled mixing procedures are essential. Because the material is more homogeneous in the dough-like stage, it is wise to delay packing until this consistency has been reached.

A third type of porosity can be caused by inadequate pressure or insufficient material in the mold during polymerization (Fig. 11.13E). Voids resulting from these inadequacies are not spherical; they assume irregular shapes. These voids may be so abundant that the resultant resin appears significantly lighter and more opaque than its intended color.

A final type of porosity is most often associated with fluid resins. Such porosity results from air entrapment during mixing and pouring procedures. If air inclusions are not removed, sizable voids may be produced in the resultant denture bases. Therefore careful mixing, spruing, and venting are essential.

Water Absorption

PMMA absorbs small amounts of water when placed in an aqueous environment. This water exerts significant effects on the mechanical and dimensional properties of the processed polymer.

Although absorption is facilitated by the polarity of PMMA molecules, a diffusion mechanism is primarily responsible for the ingress of water. As water molecules penetrate the PMMA mass, they occupy positions between polymer chains. Consequently, the affected polymer chains are forced apart. The introduction of water molecules produces two important effects. First, it causes a slight expansion of the polymerized mass. Second, water molecules interfere with the entanglement of polymer chains and thereby act as plasticizers (see the section, *Solvation and Dissolution Properties* in Chapter 2, Structure of Matter).

PMMA can exhibit water sorption value up to 32 $\mu g/mm^3$ (ISO 1567). Although this amount of water may seem inconsequential, it produces significant effects in polymerized resins. It has been estimated that for each 1% increase in weight produced by water absorption, acrylic resin exhibits a linear expansion of 0.23%. Laboratory trials indicate the linear expansion caused by water absorption is approximately equal to the thermal shrinkage encountered as a result of the polymerization process. Hence, these processes very nearly offset one another.

As previously noted, water molecules can also interfere with entanglement of polymer chains and thereby change the physical characteristics of the resultant polymer. When this occurs, polymer chains generally become more mobile. This permits the relaxation of stresses incurred during polymerization. As stresses are relieved, polymerized resins may undergo changes in shape. Fortunately, these changes are relatively minor and do not exert significant effects on the fit or function of the processed bases.

Because the presence of water adversely affects the physical and dimensional properties of denture base resins, diffusion coefficients also warrant consideration. The diffusion coefficient (D) of water in representative heat-activated denture acrylic resin is 0.011×10^{-6} cm²/s at 37°C.

For a representative chemically activated resin, the diffusion coefficient is 0.023×10^{-6} cm²/s. Since the diffusion coefficients of water in representative denture resins are relatively low, the time required for a denture base to reach saturation can be considerable. This is dependent upon the thickness of the resin as well as the storage conditions. A typical denture base may require a period of 17 days to become fully saturated with water. The results of laboratory investigations indicate that there are very slight differences in the dimensions of heat-activated and chemical-activated denture bases following prolonged storage in water. Compression-molded heat-activated denture bases are slightly undersized when measured from second molar to second molar. Conversely, compression-molded chemical-activated denture bases are slightly oversized when measured in the same regions. The clinical significance of this difference is negligible. According to the specification ANSI/ADA Standard No. 139, weight gain following immersion must not be greater than 0.8 mg/cm^2.

Solubility

Although denture base resins are soluble in a variety of liquids, they are virtually insoluble in the fluids commonly encountered in the oral cavity. According to the specification ANSI/ADA Standard No. 139 weight loss must not be greater than 0.04 mg/cm^2.

Such a loss is negligible from a clinical perspective. Non–cross-linked PMMA dentures made in the 1940s swelled and warped when exposed to ethanol in the diet. Addition of cross-linking agents (see Fig. 2.23, Chapter 2, Structure of Matter) to the resin composition has solved this problem.

CRITICAL QUESTION

What are the causes of processing stresses? What are the clinical implications of these stresses if any?

Processing Stresses

Whenever a natural dimensional change is inhibited, the affected material sustains internal stresses. If stresses are released, distortion of the material can occur. This principle has important ramifications in the fabrication of denture bases, since stresses are always induced during processing.

Consider the events that occur during denture base polymerization. A moderate amount of shrinkage occurs as individual monomers are linked to form polymer chains. During this process, it is possible that friction between the mold walls and soft resin may inhibit normal shrinkage of these chains. As a result, the polymer chains are stretched and tensile stresses exist within the material.

Stresses are also produced as a result of thermal shrinkage. As a polymerized resin is cooled below its glass transition temperature, the resin becomes relatively rigid. Further cooling results in thermal shrinkage. The clinician must remember that a denture base resin generally is encased in a rigid investing medium, such as dental gypsum, during this process. Since denture base resins and dental stone contract at markedly different rates, a contraction differential is established. This disparity in contraction rates also yields stresses within the resin. Additional factors that may contribute to processing stresses include improper mixing and handling of the resin and poorly controlled heating and cooling of the flask assembly.

Crazing

When dimensional changes alone cannot relieve internal stresses, hairline microcracks may develop as a means of dissipating energy and completing relaxation. The production of such flaws, or microcracks, is termed *crazing.*

In a clinical setting, crazing is evidenced by small linear cracks that appear to originate at a denture's surface. Crazing in a transparent resin imparts a "hazy" or "foggy" appearance. In a tinted resin, crazing imparts a whitish appearance. In addition to esthetic effects, these surface cracks predispose a denture resin to fracture.

From a physical perspective, crazing may result from stress application or from partial dissolution by a solvent. Tensile stresses are most often responsible for crazing in denture base applications. It is believed that crazing is produced by mechanical separation of individual polymer chains that occurs upon application of tensile stresses.

Crazing generally begins at the surface of a resin and is oriented at right angles to tensile forces. Microcracks formed in this manner subsequently progress internally. An example of crazing is presented in Figure 11.14.

As noted, crazing can also be produced as a result of solvent action. Microcracks produced in this manner are oriented more randomly than those depicted in Figure 11.14. Solvent-induced crazing generally results from prolonged contact with liquids such as ethyl alcohol. The development of improved acrylic resin teeth and cross-linked denture base resins has resulted in a decreased incidence of denture base crazing.

CRITICAL QUESTION

What variables reduce the strength of acrylic resin denture bases? What processing method is most likely to produce denture bases with decreased fracture resistance?

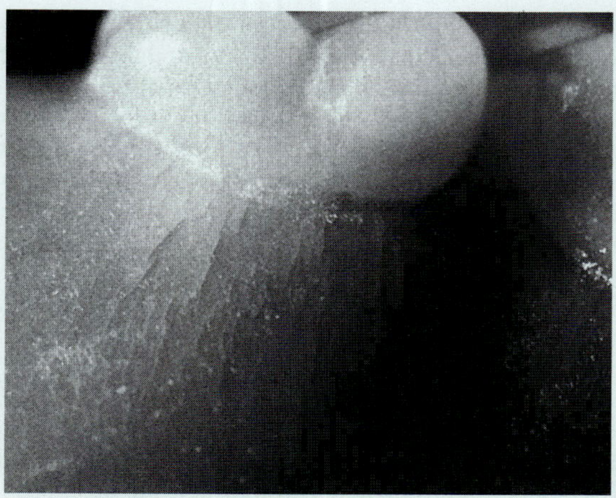

• **Fig. 11.14** Crazing around porcelain teeth.

Strength

Strength of an individual denture base resin is dependent on the composition, processing technique, and conditions presented by the oral environment.

To provide acceptable physical properties, denture base resins must meet or exceed the standards presented in ANSI/ADA Specification No. 12 (ISO 1567). A transverse test is used to evaluate the relationship between the applied load and resultant deflection in a resin specimen of prescribed dimensions. Typical deflection-load results are presented in Figure 11.15.

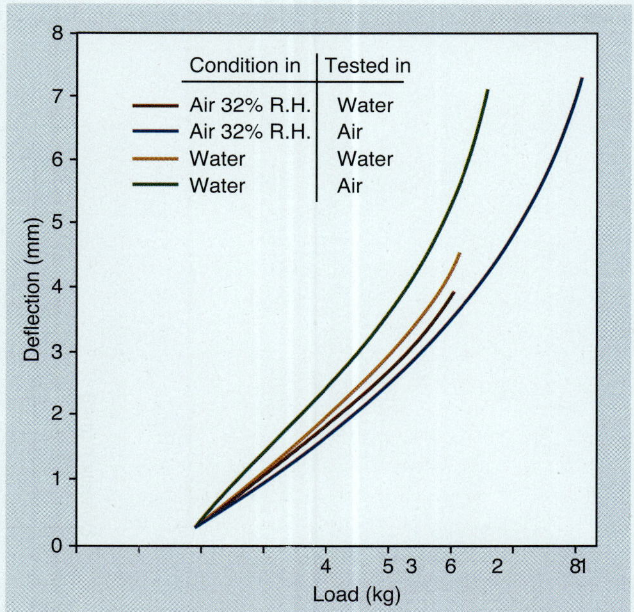

• **Fig. 11.15** Transverse deflection-load curve for a typical denture base resin, showing the influences of different conditioning procedures and testing environments. All specimens were conditioned for 3 days as indicated before testing. R.H., relative humidity. (Data from Swaney AC, Paffenbarger GC, Caul HJ, Sweeney WT: American Dental Association Specification No. 12 for denture base resin, ed. 2, *J Am Dent Assoc* 46(1):54–66, 1953. Reprinted by permission of ADA Publishing, a Division of ADA Business Enterprises, Inc.)

Inspection of Figure 11.15 reveals a curvature to each component of the deflection load plot. Since no straight-line portion is evident, one may assume that plastic deformation (i.e., irreversible deformation) occurs during the loading process. Some elastic deformation (i.e., recoverable deformation) also occurs. From a clinical standpoint, this means that load application produces stresses within a resin and a change in the overall shape of the denture base. When the load is released, stresses within the resin are released and the denture base begins to return to its original shape. Nevertheless, plastic deformation prevents complete recovery and some permanent deformation will remain.

Perhaps the most important determinant of resin strength is the degree of polymerization exhibited by the material. As the degree of polymerization increases, the strength of the resin also increases. In this regard, the polymerization cycle employed with a heat-activated resin is extremely important. Figure 11.16 reveals the effects that processing cycles exert upon deflection-load properties. Note that increased duration of the polymerization cycle appears to yield improved physical properties.

In comparison with heat-activated resins, the chemically activated resins generally display lower degrees of polymerization. As a result, chemically activated resins exhibit increased levels of residual monomer as well as decreased strength and decreased stiffness. Despite these characteristics, heat- and chemically activated resins display similar elastic moduli.

Impact Strength and Hardness

The Charpy impact strength for a heat-activated denture resin can range from 0.98 to 1.27 J, whereas that for a chemically activated resin is 0.78 J. The impact strength of high-impact resins such as Lucitone 199 can be twice as high as the values reported for conventional PMMA resins. Increased impact strength of these products is associated with the addition of a rubbery, branched comonomer such as butyl acrylate. Clinicians should recognize that these figures are useful only for comparison of products, since the energy absorbed by an individual specimen is dependent on specimen size and geometry, distance between specimen supports, and the presence or absence of notching.

The Knoop hardness for heat-activated resin is 20, whereas chemically activated resin is between 16 and 18.

Creep

Denture resins display viscoelastic behavior. In other words, these materials act as rubbery solids. When a denture base resin is subjected to a sustained load, the material may exhibit deformation with both elastic (recoverable) and plastic (irrecoverable) components. If this load is not removed, additional plastic deformation can occur over time. This additional deformation is termed *creep*.

The rate at which this progressive deformation occurs is termed the *creep rate*. This rate can be elevated by increases in temperature, applied load, residual monomer, and the presence of plasticizers. Although creep rates for heat-activated and chemically activated resins are very similar at low stresses, creep rates for chemically activated resins increase more rapidly as stresses are raised.

Biological Properties of Denture Base Resins

Infection-Control Procedures

Care should be taken to prevent microbial and viral cross-contamination between patients and dental personnel, including personnel in the dental laboratory. New appliances should be disinfected before leaving the dental laboratory. Existing prostheses should be disinfected before entering the laboratory and following completion of laboratory procedures. All materials used for finishing and polishing should be handled according to

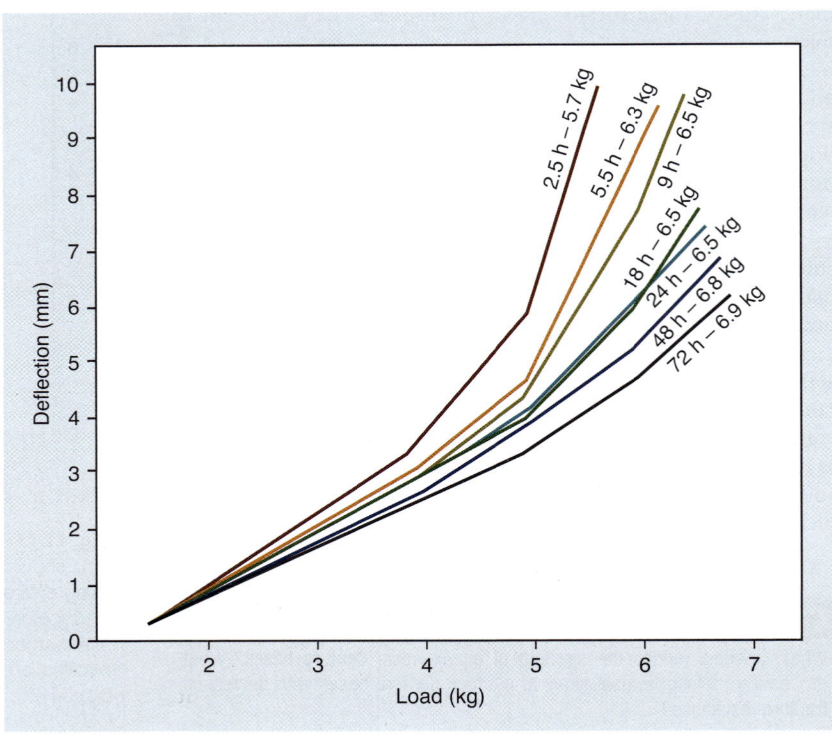

• **Fig. 11.16** Deflection-load curves for samples of polymethyl methacrylate polymerized for different periods at 71°C (160°F). Processing times and fracture loads are noted on individual curves. (Data from Harman IM: Effects of time and temperature on polymerization of a methacrylate resin denture base. *J Am Dent Assoc* 38(2):188–203, 1949. Reprinted by permission of ADA Publishing, a Division of ADA Business Enterprises, Inc.)

established infection-control guidelines. Items such as rag wheels should be autoclaved, and materials such as pumice should be used according to unit-dose recommendations.

CRITICAL QUESTION

Which components of denture resins are most likely to cause an allergic reaction?

Allergic Reactions

Possible toxic or allergic reactions to PMMA have long been postulated. Reactions can occur following contact with the polymers, residual monomers, benzoyl peroxide, hydroquinone inhibitor, pigments, or a reaction product between some component of the denture base and its environment. Despite the foregoing concerns, adverse reactions are more commonly related to uninterrupted denture wear.

Clinical experience indicates that true allergic reactions to acrylic resins seldom occur in the oral cavity. Irritation is slightly more common and is related to residual monomer. Irritation reactions are relatively rare because the residual monomer content of a properly processed denture is less than 1%. Furthermore, surface monomer is completely eliminated following storage in water for at least 17 h.

Reactions to residual monomer should occur shortly after prosthesis delivery. However, the majority of patients reporting sore mouth resulting from denture wear have worn the offending prostheses for months or even years. Clinical evaluation of these cases indicates that tissue irritation is commonly related to continuous intraoral wear, fungal colonization, poor oral hygiene, trauma secondary to ill-fitting denture bases, and/or suboptimal denture occlusion.

Repeated or prolonged contact with monomer can also result in contact dermatitis. Personnel involved in the manipulation of denture resins most commonly experience this condition. Hence, dental laboratory personnel should refrain from handling such materials with bare hands. The high concentration of monomer in freshly mixed resins may produce local irritation and serious sensitization of the fingers.

Finally, it should be noted that inhalation of monomer vapor may be detrimental. Therefore the use of monomer should be restricted to well-ventilated areas.

Toxicology

There is no evidence that commonly used dental resins produce systemic toxic effects in humans. As previously noted, the amount of residual monomer in processed PMMA is extremely low. To enter the circulatory system, residual monomer must pass through the oral mucosa and underlying tissues. These structures function as barriers that significantly diminish the volume of monomer reaching the bloodstream.

Residual monomer that does reach the bloodstream is rapidly hydrolyzed to methacrylic acid and excreted. It is estimated that the half-life of methyl methacrylate in circulating blood is 20–40 min.

Metal oxide (cadmium/selenium) red pigments were used for many years to color denture base resins. Although toxic in all concentrations, the pigments are locked within the denture base polymer network and used in very small concentrations. Nevertheless, most manufacturers have switched to organic pigment systems (e.g., Cromophtal red BRN) to avoid such toxic effects.

CRITICAL QUESTION

What is the optimal technique for repairing a fractured acrylic denture base?

Additional Procedures Associated With Dentures

Denture Repair Resins

Despite the favorable physical characteristics of denture base resins, denture bases sometimes fracture. In most instances, these fractures can be repaired using compatible resins. Repair resins may be light, heat, or chemically activated.

To accurately accomplish repair of a fractured prosthesis, the clinician must realign and lute components together using an adherent wax or cyanoacrylate glue. When this has been accomplished, a repair cast is generated using dental gypsum or silicone putty (putty is indicated in cases where severe undercuts are present). The denture is then removed from the cast and the luting medium is eliminated. Then, the fracture surfaces are trimmed to provide sufficient space for repair material. The gypsum cast is coated with separating medium to prevent adherence of repair resin, and the denture base sections are repositioned and affixed to the cast.

At this point a repair material is chosen. Chemically activated resins are generally preferred over heat- and light-activated resins despite the fact that chemically activated resins display lower transverse strengths. The principal advantage of chemically activated resins is that they can be polymerized at room temperature. Heat- and light-activated repair materials must be placed in water baths and light chambers, respectively. Heat generated by water baths and light chambers often causes stress release and distortion of previously polymerized denture base segments.

The following sequence is employed to accomplish denture base repair using a chemically activated resin. A small amount of monomer is painted onto the prepared surfaces of the denture base to soften and swell the old resin and thereby facilitate bonding of the repair material. Increments of monomer and polymer are added to the repair area using a small sable-hair brush or suitable substitute. Mixed material can also be added with an instrument. A slight excess of material is placed at the repair site to account for polymerization shrinkage. The assembly is placed in a pressure chamber and allowed to polymerize. The repair site is then shaped, finished, and polished using conventional techniques.

CRITICAL QUESTION

Why are denture reliner materials considered temporary-use products?

Relining Resin Denture Bases

During the service the contour of the ridge changes and it is sometimes necessary to alter tissue surfaces of prostheses to ensure proper fit. In some instances, this can be achieved by selective grinding procedures. In other instances, tissue surfaces must be replaced by **relining** the existing dentures.

Relining involves replacement of the tissue surface of an existing denture. An impression of the soft tissues is made using the existing denture as an impression tray. A gypsum cast is generated in the impression, and the resultant assembly is invested in a brass denture flask. Subsequently, the flask is opened and prepared for the introduction of resin.

If the denture is to be relined, the impression material is removed from the denture. The tissue surface is cleaned to enhance bonding between the existing denture base and the reline material. Next, an appropriate resin is introduced and shaped using a compression molding technique.

For relining, a low polymerization temperature is desirable to minimize distortion of the remaining denture base. Hence, a chemically activated resin is usually chosen. The selected material is mixed according to the manufacturer's recommendations, placed into the mold, compressed, and permitted to polymerize. Finally, the denture is recovered, finished, and polished.

Several manufacturers offer chemically activated resins for relining dentures intraorally. Unfortunately many of these materials generate enough heat to injure oral tissues. To receive ADA approval, materials must comply with ANSI/ADA Specification No. 17, which places limits on the rate of temperature rise and maximum acceptable temperature. A rise in temperature by 5°C during curing in the mouth is well tolerated.

Some materials are marketed for home use. Unfortunately, majority of the patients do not possess adequate knowledge to manipulate these materials correctly; therefore the use of such products can result in damage to the oral tissues. Thus, the purchase and use of such products should be discouraged.

CRITICAL QUESTION

Under what conditions might soft denture *liners* be used rather than rebasing an acrylic denture base?

Short- and Long-Term Soft Denture Liners

The purpose of a soft denture liner is to absorb some of the energy produced by masticatory impact. Hence, a soft liner serves as a "shock absorber" between the occlusal surfaces of a denture and the underlying oral tissues. The most commonly used liners are plasticized acrylic resins. These resins can be heat activated or chemically activated and are based on familiar chemistry described previously. Additional materials include silicone rubber, plasticized vinyl polymers and copolymers, polyphosphazene fluoropolymers, and fluoroethylene and polyvinyl siloxane addition-cured silicones.

All soft denture liners exhibit glass transition temperatures that are lower than body temperature to allow sustained resilience. Most of the commonly used materials gain that property by incorporating plasticizers. Chemically activated soft liners generally employ PMMA or polyethyl methacrylate as principal structural components. These polymers are supplied in powder form and subsequently are mixed with liquids containing 60%–80% of a plasticizer. The plasticizer commonly used is a large molecular species such as dibutyl phthalate or an alcohol for **short-term tissue conditioners**. The distribution of large plasticizer molecules reduces entanglement of polymer chains, thereby permitting individual chains to "slip" past one another. This slipping motion permits changes in the shape of the soft liner and provides a cushioning effect for the underlying tissues. It is important to note that the liquids used in such applications do not contain acrylic monomers. Consequently the resultant liners are considered short-term soft liners or tissue conditioners.

Unlike chemically activated soft liners, heat-activated materials generally are more durable and can be considered **long-term soft liners**. Nonetheless, these materials degrade over time and should not be considered as permanent.

A number of heat-activated soft liners are supplied as powder–liquid systems. The powders are composed of acrylic resin polymers and copolymers, whereas the liquids consist of appropriate acrylic monomers and plasticizers. When mixed, these materials form pliable resins exhibiting glass transition temperatures (Tg) below mouth temperature.

Although plasticizers impart flexibility, they also present certain difficulties. Plasticizers are not bound within the resin mass. Therefore, they may be "leached out" of soft liners. As this occurs, soft liners become progressively more rigid. Consequently, it is advantageous to use liners that are less prone to leaching phenomenon.

In recent years the phthalate ester plasticizers have raised concerns, as they mimic estrogenic hormones in the body after they are released from the liner. Alternatives are now in use, including trimellitates, aliphatic dibasic esters, phosphates, benzoates, citrate esters, polymeric plasticizers, sulfonic acid, chloroparaffins, and sorbitol.

As PMMA is replaced by higher methacrylates (e.g., ethyl, *n*-propyl, and *n*-butyl), the Tg becomes progressively lower. As a result, less plasticizer is required and the effects of leaching can be minimized.

Vinyl resins have also been used in soft liner applications. Unfortunately, plasticized polyvinyl chloride and polyvinyl acetate are subject to leaching and will harden during sustained use.

Perhaps the most successful materials for soft liner applications have been the silicone rubbers. These materials are not dependent upon leachable plasticizers; therefore, they retain their elastic properties for prolonged periods. Unfortunately, silicone rubbers may lose adhesion to underlying denture bases.

Silicone rubbers may be chemically activated or heat activated. Chemically activated silicones are supplied as two-component systems that polymerize via condensation reactions.

Processing Resilient Soft Denture Liners

Placement of chemically activated soft liners is not complicated. The denture base is relined to permit an acceptable thickness of the chosen material. A special adhesive is then applied to the surface of the denture base to facilitate bonding. The resilient material is mixed, applied to the denture base via compression molding, and permitted to polymerize. Then, the denture is recovered, finished, and polished. As with all resilient liners, the use of rotary instruments that rotate from the liner toward the denture base to prevent the initiation of peeling is important.

Heat-activated silicones are one-component systems supplied as pastes or gels. These materials are applied and contoured using compression molding techniques. Heat-activated silicones can be applied to polymerized resin bases, or they can be polymerized in conjunction with freshly mixed resins.

To promote adhesion between silicone soft liners and rigid denture base materials, rubber-PMMA cements are often used. These cements serve as adhesive intermediates that bond to both soft liners and denture resins.

At least one silicone liner does not require an adhesive when it is cured together with an acrylic denture base material. This material is actually a silicone copolymer that contains components capable of bonding with acrylic resins.

Laboratory procedures for heat-activated silicones are similar to those described for other chemically activated materials. Bases are invested and mold spaces prepared as required. Relief is provided to permit an acceptable thickness of the chosen material(s). Packing, compression molding, and processing are performed in accordance with manufacturer's recommendations. The denture is then recovered, finished, and polished.

Care of Denture Resilient Soft Liners

All soft liners display certain shortcomings. For instance, silicone liners are poorly adherent to denture base resins. Many resilient soft liners bond well to denture bases but become progressively more rigid as plasticizers are lost to the oral environment. Hardening rates for these liners are associated with the initial plasticizer content. As the plasticizer content is increased, the probability of plasticizer loss is increased. Hence, materials with a high initial plasticizer content tend to harden rather rapidly.

Soft liners also exert significant effects on associated denture bases. As the thickness of a soft liner is increased, the thickness of the accompanying denture base must be decreased, and this results in decreased strength of the denture base. Furthermore, materials used in conjunction with soft liners (e.g., adhesives and monomers) may cause partial dissolution of denture bases. This can result in fracture during clinical service.

Perhaps the greatest difficulty associated with long- and short-term silicone soft liners is that these materials cannot be cleaned effectively. As a result patients often report disagreeable tastes and odors related to these materials. Research indicates that the liners themselves do not support mycotic growth, but such growth is supported by debris accumulating in the pores of these materials. The most common fungal growth that develops on soft liners is *Candida albicans*.

Several cleaning regimens have been used in conjunction with soft liners; however, these regimens have met with limited success. Both oxygenating and hypochlorite-type denture cleansers have been employed. Unfortunately, these agents can cause color change and significant damage to soft liners, especially the silicone materials.

Mechanical cleaning of soft liners may lead to damage, but such debridement is often necessary. If mechanical cleaning is undertaken, a soft brush should be used in conjunction with a mild detergent solution or nonabrasive dentifrice. Ultrasonic cleaning can also be tried.

In attempts to address potential problems, antimycotic agents have been incorporated into soft liners. Although this approach is promising, the limited duration of antimycotic activity is far from ideal. Therefore additional research is warranted.

Based on the preceding information, none of the soft liner materials discussed earlier are completely satisfactory for other than short-term applications. However, a material suitable as a permanent soft liner was introduced in 1989 (Gettleman et al., 1989; Gettleman, 2004) following extensive NIH-supported research and clinical trials. This soft liner material uses a polyphosphazene fluoroelastomer (PNF, a polymer with –[–P=N–]– as the main chain, and fluorocarbon side groups). PNF forms an interpenetrating network with difunctional and trifunctional cross-linking acrylics, formulated with barium sulfate filler for radiopacity. The liner material is compression molded in the laboratory, polymerized in hot water, and bonded to new or existing acrylic denture bases. It has no plasticizers that can leach out of the liner surface. Therefore, the liner stays soft permanently, provides comfort by absorbing chewing forces due to its high-energy damping, is nonporous to resist fungus growth, and is easily adjusted to customize fit. (Novus™ Resilient Liner, Lang Dental Manufacturing Co, Wheeling, IL.)

The manufacturers of NOVUS claim the following benefits for their product:

- Shock absorption during chewing.
- Permanent softness with no plasticizers to leach out.
- Resistance to surface and subsurface fungal growth.
- Low surface tension with excellent wetting.
- Easy adjustment and polishing with rotary instruments.
- Engagement of deep anatomical undercuts.
- Moldable around implant heads and bars.
- Excellent bonding to acrylic denture bases.
- Radiopaque (can be identified if parts are swallowed or inhaled).
- Unlimited shelf life of the single-component paste if refrigerated.
- Use of standard dental laboratory compression molding processing steps.

Resin Impression Trays and Tray Materials

Resin trays are often used in dental impression procedures. Unlike stock trays, resin impression trays are fabricated to fit the arches of individual patients. Therefore, resin impression trays are commonly called as custom trays.

The overwhelming majority of custom trays are fabricated using light-activated and chemically activated resin systems. Each system has advantages and disadvantages. Light-activated materials eliminate methyl methacrylate exposure, but are more expensive and require high-intensity light units for polymerization. Chemically activated resins are less expensive but have been associated with contact dermatitis, particularly in laboratory personnel. Because each material exhibits advantages and disadvantages, the choice of custom tray material is commonly based upon individual preference.

The steps in custom tray fabrication are described as follows: A preliminary impression is made using a stock tray and an appropriate impression material. In turn, a gypsum cast is generated. A suitable spacer is placed on the stone cast to provide the desired relief. Subsequently a separating medium is applied to the surface of the cast. At this stage, fabrication techniques for light-activated materials and chemically activated materials become divergent.

Light-activated resins are supplied in sheet and gel forms. Sheet forms are preferred for custom tray fabrication because of their favorable handling characteristics. Individual sheets are pliable and can be adapted to the associated casts and spacers with relative ease. A handle is added to facilitate removal of the tray from the mouth and the entire assembly is placed in a light chamber and the resin is polymerized.

Chemically activated resins typically are PMMAs and are supplied as powder–liquid systems. The components are mixed to form a dough-like mass. The dough is then rolled into a sheet approximately 2 mm thick, adapted to the diagnostic cast with a handle as above, and allowed to polymerize.

Upon completion of the fabrication process, both light-activated and chemically activated custom trays are removed from the associated casts and mechanically trimmed. The peripheries are rounded to make sure that patients will not be harmed by sharp or irregular edges. At this point, trays can be evaluated intraorally and refined as required.

Denture Cleansers

Patients use a wide variety of agents for cleaning artificial dentures. These include dentifrices, proprietary denture cleansers, mild detergents, household cleansers, bleaches, and vinegar.

The most common commercial products are based upon immersion techniques. These cleansers are marketed in powder and tablet forms containing alkaline compounds, detergents, sodium perborate, and flavoring agents. Dissolved in water, sodium perborate decomposes to form an alkaline peroxide solution. This solution subsequently releases oxygen, which loosens debris via mechanical means.

Household bleaches (hypochlorites) also are used in denture cleaning applications. Dilute bleach solutions can be used to remove certain types of stains. Unfortunately, prolonged use of bleach-containing solutions can remove color from denture base and relining materials.

Bleaches and bleach solutions should not be used for cleaning metal prostheses such as removable partial denture frameworks. These solutions produce significant darkening of base metals and can damage the serviceability of affected prostheses irreparably.

The use of brushes and abrasive cleansers can produce a range of effects on resin surfaces. Toothbrushes alone produce minimal wear of resin surfaces. Toothbrushes in conjunction with most commercial dentifrices, mild detergents, and soaps also appear to be relatively nondestructive. Conversely, household cleansers, such as kitchen and bathroom abrasives, are definitely contraindicated. Prolonged use of such cleansers may cause noticeable wear of resin surfaces and adversely affect the function and esthetics of these prostheses. Therefore, patients should be educated regarding the care and cleaning of resin prostheses.

Thermoplastic Denture resins (Flexible Dentures)

Four types of thermoplastic resins – known as flexible denture resins – are popularly used: polyamides, polyesters, polycarbonates and acrylics.

Polyamides (Nylon)

Nylon is a generic name given to a class of thermoplastic polymers known as polyamides. These polyamides are produced by the condensation reactions between a diamine NH_2-(CH_2)6-NH_2 and a dibasic acid, CO_2H-(CH_2)4-COOH. Nylon is a crystalline polymer, whereas PMMA is amorphous. This crystalline effect accounts for the lack of solubility of nylon in solvents, as well as high heat resistance and high strength coupled with ductility. The manufacturers of modern dental nylon systems, such as *Bioplast, Valplast, FlexStar V, Biotone, Lucitone FRS, Sunflex* recommend their use for the fabrication of partial dentures and small-to-medium size complete dentures. Nonmetal clasp dentures (NMCD) are becoming very popular among dentists.

Nylon denture base resins first became available in the 1950s. Nylon's flexible nature facilitates the fabrication of both the denture base and the clasps from the same material. Nylon has fairly good acceptance by patients owing to their light weight, flexible nature, and the provision of clasps that are similar in color to the gingiva. Nylon was developed by Wallace Carothers and associates, of the Du Pont Chemical Co, in the 1930s.

The type of nylon or the additives in their formulations have not been divulged by the manufacturers of nylon denture base materials. Nylons which have been documented in the literature belong to 6.6, 6.10, 11, and 12. These numbers indicate the number of building blocks used in the production of the material (carbon atoms in the structure) and have an influence on their properties such as melting point and tensile strength.

The first generation denture bases showed high rates of shrinkage because of the processing technique. Nylon is resistant to common solvents and hence it cannot be dough molded as followed in acrylics. Nylon in the molten form is injected into the flask under pressure. The continuous replenishment of molten material (270–300°C) during injection molding compensates for the shrinkage.

Flexural strength of different brands of polyamides ranges from 27 to 98 MPa. Elastic modulus ranges from 540 to 1600 MPa and tensile strength 60–70 MPa according to the manufacturer's data. Other properties are as follows:

Density 1.02–1.06 (g/cm^3)
Molding temperature 240–288°C
Glass transition temperature 50–155°C
Shrinkage 0.8%
Solubility 0–2 $\mu g/mm^3$
Water absorption 17–30 $\mu g/mm^3$
Surface roughness 0.21–0.24 µM
Shear bond strength with acrylic 2.5–3.3 MPa
Shear bond strength after surface treatment 16.5–19.6 MPa

Penetration of water molecules into the structure has a lowering effect on the modulus of elasticity in polyamide. The necessity of storage in wet conditions needs further investigations for its endorsement. There are no significant differences in surface roughness between PMMA and polyamide. Ra values of polyamide ranged between 0.20 and 0.24 µm while that of PMMA ranged between 0.20 and 0.28 µm. Clinically accepted surface roughness value of denture bases is (Ra) 0.2 µm.

Polyamide has a comparable toxicity profile with the conventional PMMA denture base materials. Although the flexural strength and modulus of elasticity and rigidity of nylon (polyamide) denture base materials are relatively low, they demonstrate great impact strength, toughness, and resistance to fracture. Addition of glass fibers to polyamides, can improve the stiffness and other mechanical properties. Polyamides do not bond to self-curing resins and hence doing repair and reline is difficult and must be done in a laboratory. However, a number of methods are currently being tried out.

Polyesters

Polyester is a kind of plastic used for making man-made fibers. Polyester resin that has polyethylene terephthalate copolymer is the main ingredient of *EstheShot*, a popular polyester-based denture resin. *EstheShot Bright*, another brand has polyester; polycycloalkylene terephthalate copolymer as the main ingredient. Both the products have safety, esthetics, and functionality. Properties of the former products are as follows:

Flexural strength 76 MPa
Elastic modulus 2000–2200 MPa
Density 1.12 g/cm^3
Molding temperature 230–240°C
Water absorption 10.72 $\mu g/mm^3$
Shear bond strength with acrylic resin 17.5 MPa

Polycarbonates

Polycarbonate resin has been used clinically as a denture material for nearly two decades. Polycarbonates behave almost similar to acrylic resin. Reigning and Reigning N are popular brands of denture resins. Physical attributes of polycarbonates are almost equal to those of polyester resin. Polycarbonates have lower water absorbency and better abradability than other resins used for NMCDs. Properties of polycarbonate denture resins are as follows:

Flexural strength 70–80 MPa
Elastic modulus 2300–2400 MPa
Density 1.20 g/cm^3
Molding temperature 300–340°C

Acrylic resin

Acry-Tone is the only acrylic resin currently used for nonmetallic clasp dentures. This is flexible, fully reparable and relinable, and translucent. Acry-Tone comes as solidified ingots, ready for injection in any system. It is hypoallergenic and has five times less residual monomers than conventional heat-cured dentures. The material's pink shade matches 95% of patients' tissue color. This product uses an acrylic resin that is much softer than other thermoplastic resins. Information on its physical attributes is limited.

Density 1.15 g/cm^3
Molding temperature 260–270°C
Shrinkage 0.4–0.7%
Water absorption 22 μg/mm^3
Shear bond strength with acrylic resin 17.1 MPa

Information available on the thermoplastic resins about the physical and mechanical properties and clinical usage are at present very limited except for polyamides but may be made available in the future.

CRITICAL QUESTION

What precautions should be taken in using porcelain teeth in a denture? What are the clinically relevant differences between porcelain teeth and acrylic resin teeth?

Resin Teeth for Prosthetic Applications

Majority of preformed artificial teeth sold is made of acrylic or vinyl acrylic resins. As might be expected, the majority of resin teeth are based on PMMA compositions.

PMMA resins used in the fabrication of prosthetic teeth are very similar to those used in denture base construction. The degree of cross-linking at the occlusal and incisal surfaces of prosthetic teeth is much greater than that exhibited by the polymerized denture base materials. The increased cross-linking of prosthetic teeth in conjunction with the addition of inorganic filler yields enhanced stability, increased wear resistance, and improved clinical properties.

Cervical portions of prosthetic teeth often exhibit reduced cross-linking. This facilitates chemical bonding with denture base resins. Additional retention may be achieved by removing the glossy "ridge-lap" surfaces of resin teeth preparing mechanical undercuts.

Chemical bonding between resin teeth and heat-activated denture base materials has proven extremely effective. Nevertheless, bond failures can occur if ridge-lap surfaces are contaminated by residual wax or misplaced separating media. To optimize bonding, gypsum molds must be flushed with hot water and the exposed cervical portions of prosthetic teeth must be thoroughly cleaned with mild detergent solutions. Separating media must be applied only to gypsum mold surfaces and should not extend onto the exposed surfaces of resin teeth. As a final measure, ridge-lap surfaces should be wet with monomer immediately before denture base resin introduction.

More recently, manufacturers have introduced "hybrid" teeth to enhance the wear resistance of prosthetic dentitions. These teeth include composite resin and PMMA components. Composite resins are found primarily on occlusal and incisal surfaces of the prosthetic teeth, and are intended to provide improved wear resistance. Unfortunately, chemical bonding between composites and heat-activated denture base materials is inferior to that which occurs between resin teeth and such denture base materials. To address this shortcoming, manufacturers have incorporated PMMA at the ridge-lap and lingual surfaces of hybrid teeth. The presence of PMMA on these surfaces facilitates predictable bonding with heat-activated PMMA denture base resins. Nevertheless, operators must be certain not to eliminate the PMMA surfaces while setting the prosthetic teeth.

As might be expected, the laboratory steps prescribed for hybrid teeth in conjunction with heat-activated resins are identical to those prescribed for resin teeth used in combination with heat-activated resins. Despite shared chemistries, chemically activated PMMA denture base resins and their heat-activated counterparts display distinct differences. Notably, mechanical retention is the primary method for securing resin teeth to chemically activated denture base materials. While chemical bonding also may be used, it requires a distinct modification of the fabrication process. To achieve predictable chemical bonding, a mixture of equal volumes of methylene chloride and chemically activated methyl methacrylate monomer is applied to the necks of resin teeth for approximately 5 min. Excess solution is then removed. This treatment softens and swells the resin and facilitates development of an interpenetrating network between the denture teeth polymers and those of the denture base during polymerization. The resultant bond strengths are similar to those obtained between resin teeth and heat-activated denture base resins.

Despite the current emphasis on resin teeth, prosthetic teeth also can be fabricated using dental vacuum- or pressure-fired porcelains. Hence, a comparison of resin and porcelain teeth is provided in the following paragraphs.

Resin teeth display greater impact resistance and ductility than porcelain teeth. As a result, resin teeth are less likely to chip or fracture on impact, as when a denture is dropped. Furthermore, resin teeth are easier to adjust and display greater resistance to thermal shock. In comparison, porcelain teeth display better dimensional stability and increased wear resistance. Unfortunately, porcelain teeth often cause significant wear of opposing enamel, metal, and resin tooth surfaces, especially when contacting surfaces have been roughened. Therefore, porcelain teeth should not oppose such surfaces, and if they are used, they should be polished periodically to reduce abrasive damage.

As a final note, resin teeth are capable of chemical bonding with commonly used denture base resins. Porcelain teeth, however, do not form chemical bonds with denture resins and must be retained by bonded pins, mechanical undercuts, and/or silanization. Leakage at the tooth-denture base junction can be seen as a dark line when food and microbes penetrate the interface.

CRITICAL QUESTION

What are the benefits and drawbacks of materials used in the construction of maxillofacial prostheses?

Materials for Maxillofacial Prosthetics

For centuries, prostheses have been used to mask maxillofacial defects. The ancient Egyptians and Chinese used waxes and resins to reconstruct missing portions of the craniofacial complex. In the 16th century, the French surgeon Ambroise Paré described a variety of simple prostheses used for the cosmetic and functional replacement of maxillofacial structures. During subsequent years, restorative techniques and materials were improved and refined.

Casualties in World Wars I and II established an increased need for maxillofacial prosthetics, and the dental profession assumed a major role in maxillofacial reconstruction and rehabilitation processes.

Despite improvements in surgical and restorative techniques, the materials used in maxillofacial prosthetics are far from ideal. An ideal material should be inexpensive, biocompatible, strong, and stable. In addition, the material should be skin like in color and texture. Maxillofacial materials must exhibit resistance to tearing, and should be able to withstand moderate thermal and chemical challenges. Currently, no material fulfills all of these requirements. A brief summary of maxillofacial materials is included in the following paragraphs.

Ideal properties of a material used for maxillofacial prosthesis:

- high resistance to tearing
- high tensile strength and resulting elongation
- hardness similar to the missing facial tissue
- resist water, saliva, and sweat absorption
- easy to manipulate and process
- nontoxic, nonallergenic, and biocompatible
- easy color matching

Acrylics

Autopolymerizing acrylic resin can be used to fabricate facial prosthesis. Acrylic in different shades viz. pink, clear, and tooth colored can be blended and pigments can be added to the monomer to obtain a favorable color match to Indian skin.

Latexes

Latexes are soft, inexpensive materials that can be used to create life-like prostheses. Unfortunately, these materials are weak, degenerate rapidly, and exhibit color instability. Therefore, the use of latexes is restricted to make up industry.

Vinyl Plastisols

Plasticized vinyl resins sometimes are used in maxillofacial applications. Plastisols are thick liquids composed of small vinyl particles dispersed in a plasticizer. Colorants are added to these materials to match individual skin tones. Subsequently, vinyl plastisols are heated to impart desired physical characteristics. Unfortunately, vinyl plastisols harden with age as a result of plasticizer migration. Ultraviolet light also has an adverse effect on these materials. For these reasons, the usefulness of vinyl plastisols is limited.

Silicone Rubbers

Silicones were introduced in the mid-1940s and have been used in maxillofacial applications since the 1950s. Both heat-curing and room-temperature–curing silicones are in use today, and both exhibit advantages and disadvantages.

Room-temperature–curing silicones are supplied as single-component materials that cure by evaporation of acetic acid. They are "characterized" by a natural flesh-like appearance by using dyed rayon fibers, dry earth pigments, and/or oil paints. Prostheses are polymerized by bulk packing in two- or three-part gypsum molds made from the sculpting of the facial part, but more durable molds have been made from epoxy resins or metals.

Heat-curing silicones are supplied as semisolid or putty-like materials that require milling, packing in two- or three-part molds under pressure, and a 30-min heat application cycle at 180°C. Pigments are milled into these materials. Thus intrinsic color can be achieved. Heat-curing silicones display better strength and color stability than room-temperature–curing silicones. All of the silicones are susceptible to fungus growth and fraying at the feather-edge margins, so a process of bonding to a sheet of polyurethane on the tissue surface has been developed. This process not only enhances prosthesis longevity but also improves the effectiveness of skin adhesives.

The major disadvantage of heat-curing silicones is the requirement for a milling machine and a press. Furthermore, a metal mold normally is used, and fabrication of the mold is a lengthy procedure. A stone mold may be housed within a brass denture flask, but this increases the risk of damage to the silicone material during deflasking.

Polyurethane Polymers

Polyurethane also can be used in maxillofacial prosthetics. Fabrication of a polyurethane prosthesis requires accurate proportioning of three components. The material is placed in a stone or metal mold and allowed to polymerize at room temperature. Although a polyurethane prosthesis has a natural feel and appearance, it is susceptible to rapid deterioration and fungus growth.

Chlorinated Polyethylene

In an effort to overcome the deficiencies of the latex, vinyl plastisol, silicone, and polyurethanes as maxillofacial materials, a thermoplastic elastomer based on chlorinated polyethylene (CPE) was investigated in the 1970s and 1980s. With further development, CPE was shown to provide higher edge strength, permanent elasticity, and minimal fungus growth (Gettleman, 1992). In a recent randomized, controlled clinical trial, it was found that the material was equally preferred by patients who had never worn facial prostheses before, but patients who had worn silicone rubber prostheses in the past favored that material in the trial. Methods of layering the prosthetic material in the molds to develop color at depth were also reported, which may be useful in future maxillofacial prosthetic applications.

Additional information may be found in a review by Lemon et al. (2005), which presents current concepts regarding facial prosthetic rehabilitation of patients with head and neck cancer and facial prosthetic biomaterials.

Incorporation of CAD/CAM technology and 3-D printing will greatly improve the quality of maxillofacial prosthetic treatment.

Summary

- Denture base resins can be **heat activated, chemically activated,** or **light activated**.
- Denture base resins are supplied as powder and liquid or as sheet and rope forms.
- **For heat-activated resins:**
  Powder consists of prepolymerized polymethyl methacrylate in the form of spheres and benzoyl peroxide as the initiator.
  Liquid consists of predominantly nonpolymerized methyl methacrylate monomer, hydroquinone as inhibitor and glycol dimethacrylate as cross-linking agent.
- **For chemically activated resins:**
  Powder composition is the same as above.
  Liquid consists of dimethyl para toluidine apart from other ingredients.
- **Visible light-activated denture base resins** have been described as resin-based composites having matrices of urethane dimethacrylate, microfine silica, and high–molecular-weight acrylic resin monomers. Acrylic resin beads are included as organic fillers. Visible light is the activator, while a photosensitizing agent such as camphorquinone serves as the initiator for polymerization.
- The polymerization of methyl methacrylate to form polymethyl methacrylate yields a 21% decrease in the volume of material. Using a 3:1 ratio of polymer to monomer, the volumetric shrinkage can be limited to approximately 7%.
- When monomer and polymer are mixed in the proper proportions, a workable mass is produced which passes through five distinct stages viz. (1) sandy, (2) stringy, (3) dough like, (4) rubbery or elastic, and (5) stiff.
- The time required for the resin mixture to reach a dough-like stage is termed the **dough-forming time.** This consistency may be attained in less than 40 min from the start of the mixing process.
- **Working time** is defined as the time a denture base material remains in the dough-like stage (at least 5 min).
- The placement and adaptation of denture base resin within the mold cavity is termed **packing**.
- The heating process used to control polymerization is termed the **polymerization cycle** or **curing cycle**.
- The unreacted monomer in chemically activated resins creates two major difficulties. First, it acts as a plasticizer, resulting in decreased transverse strength of the denture resin. Second, the residual monomer serves as a potential tissue irritant.
- Resins polymerized via chemical activation generally display 3–5% free monomer, whereas heat-activated resins exhibit 0.2–0.5% free monomer.
- Denture base resins can be shaped or molded via compression molding, injection molding, or fluid resin technique.
  - **Relining** involves replacement of the tissue surface of an existing denture.
- **Denture liners** can be either short term (chemically activated) or long term (heat activated). The most commonly used liners are plasticized acrylic resins. The plasticizer commonly is a large molecular species such as dibutyl phthalate or an alcohol.
- **Denture cleansers** include dentifrices, proprietary denture cleansers, mild detergents, household cleansers, bleaches, and vinegar. These cleansers are marketed in powder and tablet forms containing alkaline compounds, detergents, sodium perborate, and flavoring agents.
- Toothbrushes in conjunction with most commercial dentifrices, mild detergents, and soaps are relatively nondestructive means of cleaning a denture.
- **Hybrid teeth** include composite resin-based and polymethyl methacrylate components. Composite resins are found primarily on occlusal and incisal surfaces of the prosthetic teeth and polymethyl methacrylate at the ridge-lap and lingual surfaces of hybrid teeth.
- The different materials used for maxillofacial prosthesis are: latexes, vinyl plastisols, silicone rubbers, polyurethane polymers, and chlorinated polyethylene.

Review Questions

1. Describe the ideal requirement of denture base resins. Give the composition and curing cycles of heat cure acrylic denture base resins.
2. Classify dental resins. Discuss manipulation, curing procedure of heat cure acrylic resin.
3. Compare self-cure and heat cure acrylic resins.
4. Write a brief note on denture reliners (resilient liners).
5. Curing cycle of heat cure acrylic resin.
6. Composition of heat cure acrylic resin.
7. Injection molding technique.
8. Porosity and its effects on denture base resins.
9. A brief note on separating media.
10. Denture cleansers.
11. Uses of chemically activated acrylic resin.

Selected Readings

Arima T.; Murata H.; Hamad T. The effects of cross-linking agents on the water sorption and solubility characteristics of denture base resins. J Oral Rehabil 23 476 (1996).

Bartoloni J.A.; Murchison D.F.; Wofford D.T.; et al. Degree of conversion in denture base materials for varied polymerization techniques. J Oral Rehabil 27 488 (2000).

Blagojevic V.; Murphy V.M. Microwave polymerization of denture base materials: A comparative study. J Oral Rehabil 26 804 (1999).

Caswell C.W.; Norling B.K. Comparative study of the bond strengths of three abrasion-resistant plastic denture teeth bonded to a cross-linked and a grafted, cross-linked denture base material. J Prosthet Dent 55 701 (1986).

Chai J.; Takahashi Y.; Takahashi T.; et al. Bonding durability of conventional resinous denture teeth and highly crosslinked denture teeth to a pour-type denture resin. Int J Prosthodont 13 112 (2000).

Clancy J.M.S.; Boyer D.B. Comparative bond strengths of light-cured, heat-cured, and autopolymerizing denture resins to denture teeth. J Prosthet Dent 61 457 (1989).

Compagnoni M.A.; Barros Barbosa D.; de Souza R.F.; et al. The effect of polymerization cycles on porosity of microwave-processed denture base resin. J Prosthet Dent 91 281 (2004).
Cunningham J.L.; Benington I.C. An investigation of the variables which may affect the bond between plastic teeth and denture base resin. J Dent 27 129 (1999).
Dhir G.; Berzins D.W.; Dhuru V.B.; et al. Physical properties of denture base resins potentially resistant to *Candida* adhesion. J Prosthodont 16 465 (2007).
Gettleman L.M. Chlorinated polyethylene and polyphosphazenes. In L. Gettleman & Z. Khan, Cochairs. J. Setcos, Editor: Materials research in maxillofacial prosthetics, Trans Acad of Dental Mater 5 (1) 156–172 (1992).
Gettleman L.M. Uses of polyphosphazene in dentistry. Chapter 2 In: (editors: Mario G.; Roger D.) Applicative Aspects of Poly (organophosphazenes). Nova Science Publishers: New York, pp. 33–47.
Gettleman L.M.; Vargo J.M.; Goist K.C.; et al. Laboratory and clinical testing of a polyphosphazene resilient denture liner vs. a silicone rubber liner. In: (editor: Kawahara H.) Oral Implantology and Biomaterials. Progress in Biomedical Engineering Series. Vol. 7 Elsevier: Amsterdam, pp. 15–20.
Kiat-amnuay S.; Jacobs R.F.; Chambers M.S.; et al. Clinical trial of chlorinated polyethylene for facial prosthetics. Int J Prosthod 23 263–270 (2010).
Jagger D.C.; Jagger R.G.; Allen S.M.; et al. An investigation into the transverse and impact strength of "high strength" denture base acrylic resins. J Oral Rehabil 29 263 (2002).
Jorge J.H.; Giampaolo E.T.; Machado A.L.; et al. Cytotoxicity of denture base acrylic resins: A literature review. J Prosthet Dent 90 190 (2003).
Jorge J.H.; Giampaolo E.T.; Vergani C.E.; et al. Cytotoxicity of denture base resins: Effect of water bath and microwave postpolymerization heat treatments. J Prosthet Dent 92 568 (2004).
Kiat-amnuay S.; Jacob R.F.; Chambers M.S.; et al. Clinical trial of chlorinated polyethylene for facial prosthetics. Int J Prosthodont 23 (3) 263–270 (2010).
Lemon J.C.; Kiat-amnuay S.; Gettleman L.M.; et al. Facial prosthetic rehabilitation: Preprosthetic surgical techniques and biomaterials. Current Opinion in Otolaryngology and Head and Neck Surgery 13 (4) 255–262 (2005);
This review presents current concepts regarding facial prosthetic rehabilitation of patients with head and neck cancer and facial prosthetic biomaterials.
Levin B.; Sanders J.L.; Reitz P.V. The use of microwave energy for processing acrylic resins. J Prosthet Dent 61 381 (1989).
Machado C.; Sanchez E.; Azer S.S.; et al. Comparative study of the transverse strength of three denture base materials. J Dent 35 930 (2007).
Monsenego P.; Baszkin A.; deLourdes Costa J.; et al. Complete denture retention, wettability studies on various acrylic resin denture base materials. J Prosthet Dent 62 308 (1989).
Phoenix R.D.; Mansueto M.A.; Ackerman N.A.; et al. Evaluation of mechanical and thermal properties of commonly used denture base resins. J Prosthodont 13 17 (2003).
Rached R.N.; Powers J.M.; Del Bel Curry AA: Repair strength of autopolymerizing, microwave, and conventional heat-polymerized acrylic resins. J Prosthet Dent 92 79 (2004).
Sanders J.L.; Levin B.; Reitz P.V. Porosity in denture acrylic resins cured by microwave energy. Quintesence Int 18 453 (1987).
Sarac Y.S.; Sarac D.; Kulunk T.; et al. The effect of chemical surface treatments of different denture base resins on the shear bond strength of denture repair. J Prosthet Dent 94 259 (2005).
Shlosberg S.R.; Goodacre C.J.; Munoz C.A.; et al. Microwave energy polymerization of poly (methyl methacrylate) denture base resin. Int J Prosthodont 2 453 (1989).
Stafford G.D.; Bates J.F.; Huggett R.; Handley R.W. A review of the properties of some denture base polymers. J Dent 8 292 (1960).
Swaney A.C.; Paffenbarger G.C.; Caul H.J.; Sweeney W.T. American Dental Association Specification No. 12 for denture base resin, ed. 2. J Am Dent Assoc 46 (1) 54–66 (1953).
Takahashi Y.; Chai J.; Takahashi T.; et al. Bond strength of denture teeth to denture base resins. Int J Prosthodont 13 59 (2000).
Takamata T.; Setcos J.C. Resin denture bases: Review of accuracy and methods of polymerization. Int J Prosthodont 2 555 (1989).
The Academy of Prosthodontics. The glossary of prosthodontic terms, 8th edition (GPT-8). J Prosthet Dent 94 10–92 (2005). PMID: 16080238.
Tsuchiya H.; Hoshino Y.; Tajima K.; et al. Leaching and cytotoxicity of formaldehyde and methyl methacrylate from acrylic resin denture base materials. J Prosthet Dent 71 618 (1994).
Tuckfield W.J.; Worner H.K.; Guerin B.D. Acrylic resins in dentistry. Aust Dent J 47 119–121 (1943).
Wong D.; Cheng L.Y.Y.; Chow T.W.; et al. Effect of processing method on the dimensional accuracy and water sorption of acrylic resin dentures. J Prosthet Dent 81 300 (1999).
Zappini G.; Kammann A.; Wachter W. Comparison of fracture tests of denture base materials. J Prosthet Dent 90 578 (2003).

Further Reading: Thermoplastic Denture resins (Flexible Dentures)

Mieszko Wieckiewicz, Volker Opitz, Gert Richter, Klaus W. Boening: Physical Properties of Polyamide-12 versus PMMA Denture Base Material, Hindawi Publishing Corporation, BioMed Research International, Volume 2014, Article ID 150298, 8 pages, http://dx.doi.org/10.1155/2014/150298
Vivek.R, Polyamides as a Denture Base Material – A Review, IOSR Journal of Dental and Medical Sciences, Volume 15, Issue 12 Ver. VIII (December. 2016), PP 119-121
Fueki K et al. Clinical application of removable partial dentures using thermoplastic resin. Part II: Material properties and clinical features of non-metal clasp dentures. Journal of Prosthodontic Research (2014), 58:71–84
Jafar Gharechahi, Nafiseh Asadzadeh, Foad Shahabian, Maryam Gharechahi: Dimensional changes of acrylic resin denture bases: Conventional versus injection-molding technique, Journal of Dentistry, Tehran University of Medical Sciences, (2014); Vol. 11, No. 4: 398-405.
Yau WFE et al.: Pressure and temperature changes in heat cured acrylic resin during processing, Dental Materials (2002), 18:622-629.

12 Dental Implants

CHAPTER OUTLINE

KEY TERMS

Alloplastic—Related to implantation of an inert foreign body.

Ankylosis—A condition of joint or tooth immobility resulting from oral pathology, surgery, or direct contact with bone.

Biointegration—A condition that occurs when ceramic implant materials are used and there is no space between the bone and dental implant.

Bioacceptance—The ability to be tolerated in a biological environment in spite of adverse effects.

Bioactive—Capable of promoting the formation of hydroxyapatite and bonding to bone.

Endosteal implant—A device placed into the alveolar and/or basal bone of the mandible or maxilla that transects only one cortical plate.

Epithelial implant—A device placed within the oral mucosa.

Implantation—The process of grafting or inserting a material such as an inert foreign body (alloplast) or tissue within the body.

Micromotion—The displacement of the implant root relative to the bone when the implant is loaded as a result of lack of friction or bone integration.

Osseointegration—The process by which living bony tissue forms to within 100 Å of the implant surface without any intervening fibrous connective tissue.

Osteoinductive—Ability to promote bone formation through a mechanism that induces the differentiation of osteoblasts.

Replantation—Reinsertion of a tooth back into its jaw socket soon after intentional extraction or accidental removal.

Subperiosteal implant—A dental device that is placed beneath the periosteum and overlies cortical bone.

Transosteal implant—A device that penetrates both cortical plates and the thickness of alveolar bone.

History of Dental Implants

The restoration and replacement of missing teeth are important aspects of modern dentistry. As teeth are lost due to decay, gum disease, and trauma, there is a demand for improvement of esthetics and restoration of function.

Conventional methods of restoration include removable complete dentures, removable partial dentures, fixed prosthesis, or combination of these. There are different indications for each method, with associated advantages and disadvantages. Removable dentures have long been considered problematic because of their varying stability that happens over a period of time and the inconvenience of removing them each day. Also, many removable dentures were bulky, complicated the chewing. Fixed prostheses were considered more esthetic and comfortable for the patient, but they involved the preparation of adjacent teeth and they were associated with problems such as secondary decay or irreversible pulpitis. If the adjacent teeth did not have restorations, the decision to prepare them for a fixed prosthesis was difficult because two or more natural teeth would have to be surgically altered to provide retention for one or more artificial teeth (a bridge).

For centuries people have attempted to replace missing teeth by implanting synthetic and natural substances. ***Implantation*** has been defined as the insertion of any object or material, such as an **alloplastic** substance or other tissue, either partially or completely, into the body for therapeutic, diagnostic, prosthetic, or experimental purposes. Implantation is usually differentiated from other, similar procedures such as **replantation** and transplantation. *Replantation* refers to the reinsertion of a tooth back into its jaw socket after its accidental or intentional removal, whereas transplantation is the transfer of a body part (homogeneous or heterogeneous) from one host to another.

CRITICAL QUESTION

How did the concept of implantation evolve into a widely used restorative technique in dentistry?

Dental implants began as far back as the early Greek, Etruscan, and Egyptian civilizations, employing different designs and materials ranging from jade and other stones and metals to bone and ivory. Some of the design concepts used then have evolved into the implants of today.

Seashells were used in place of teeth in CE 600, evidence of which was found in Honduras, and tooth restorations made of jade and turquoise, were found in Mayan skulls. Albucasis de Condue (936–1013) of France used ox bone to replace missing teeth; this was one of the early documented placements of implants. Through the centuries various tooth transplants made of either human or animal teeth were tested. These transplants became status symbols and they quickly replaced other artificial alternatives for restoring missing teeth. Toward the 18th century, Pierre Fauchard and John Hunter further documented tooth transplantation and specified conditions for the success of this procedure. They claimed that success was greater with anterior teeth, premolar teeth, and transplants placed in young people with healthy tooth sockets. Failure was believed to be the result of the incompatibility of the type of tooth used or the lack of conformity of the tooth to the socket.

The recognition of failure rates of transplants increased interest in the implantation of artificial tooth roots. In 1809 Maggiolo fabricated gold roots that were fixed to teeth by means of a spring. These gold implants were placed into fresh extraction sites, although they were not truly submerged into bone. The crowns were placed after healing had occurred around the implant. Many attempts followed. Harris (1887) proposed the use of a platinum post coated with lead. The post was shaped like a tooth root, and the lead was roughened for retention in the socket. Bonwell (1895) implanted gold or iridium tubes to restore a single tooth or to support complete dentures. Payne (1898) implanted a silver capsule as a foundation for a porcelain crown that was cemented after weeks. Scholl (1905) demonstrated a porcelain corrugated root-shaped implant that lasted for 2 years and was anchored to adjacent teeth by pins. Greenfield (1913) introduced and patented a hollow "basket" implant made of a meshwork of 24-gauge iridium-platinum wires soldered with 24-karat gold. This device was used to support single implants as well as fixed dental prostheses comprising as many as eight implants.

Consistent problems with these artificial implant designs and materials supported the need for a scientific approach to implant selection and placement. Some have proposed that the "modern era" started in 1925. In 1937 Venable et al. analyzed the interactions of cobalt-based alloy and other available metals and alloys with bone. They concluded that certain metals produced a galvanic reaction, which led to corrosion when these metals contacted tissue fluids. They proposed the use of Vitallium, a cast alloy, which was composed of cobalt, chromium, and molybdenum. This alloy was considered to be relatively inert, compatible with living tissue, and resistant to the adverse reactions with body fluids. Vitallium has also been used in different forms of surgical devices, such as dental **subperiosteal implant** and orthopedic plates, screws, nails, and joints. Early evaluations documented Vitallium implants with survival times of 10 or more years.

The background of research, development, and applications of biomaterials for dental implants began with the application of available substances, often of metallic origin. Some separate the period before 1950 as an era of applications driven by need and availability. Examples include the early use of wires, pins, and rods fabricated from gold and other noble metals and alloys. In the 1950s, the cobalt-based alloys were cast and finished for subperiosteal and some root-form designs. The austenitic iron-based stainless steels constituted from iron–chromium and nickel (sometimes with molybdenum as well) were also utilized in wrought and machined conditions. Within a decade, titanium and other reactive-group metals—plus carbons, ceramics, and eventually polymers—were considered.

The more "modern" era of biomaterials arose by the 1970s, when materials known and tested in many disciplines were constituted, fabricated, and finished as biomaterials. Consensus standards rapidly evolved for these biomaterials, which resulted in more consistent control of their properties. A very important aspect of this evolution—which included biomaterials, designs, and clinical application—was the clinical research led by PI Brånemark in Sweden. His studies utilized unalloyed titanium, a root-form design and very controlled conditions for surgery, restoration, and maintenance. Data presented in literature reviews and consensus conferences over the period 1972–2002 have demonstrated significant improvements in dental implant survival statistics. When outcomes were evaluated by objective criteria, the average survival at 5 years was about 50% in the 1970s. In the 2000s, average survival at 10 years was above 90%.

Classification of Implants

Implants can be classified according to anatomic location, device design, implant properties, or implant attachment mechanism. In a broad context, there are four implant design types that can be classified by anatomic location and they have evolved over centuries of development.

Implant Design

The first and most commonly used type of design is the endosteal (also called endosseous) implant, a device placed into an alveolar and/or basal bone of the mandible or maxilla that usually transected only one cortical plate. These implants were formed in many different shapes, such as root-form cylindrical cones or screws or thin plates called plate or blade forms, and they were used in all areas of the mouth. One example of an **endosteal implant** was called the blade implant (Fig. 12.1), which was developed independently in 1967 by two groups led initially by Roberts (1970) and Linkow (1968). Endosteal blade implants consisted of thin plates placed into bone; they were most commonly used for narrow anatomic structures such as posterior edentulous areas after significant resorption of bone. Because of various issues with blade implants, their application in more recent implantology has decreased. Another example of an endosteal implant was the ramus frame implant, a horseshoe-shaped stainless steel device inserted into the ascending rami (bilateral) and the anterior symphysis area of the mandible. As with the blade implants, the number of applications has been limited. The most popular endosteal implant has been the root form (Fig. 12.2), which was designed initially to

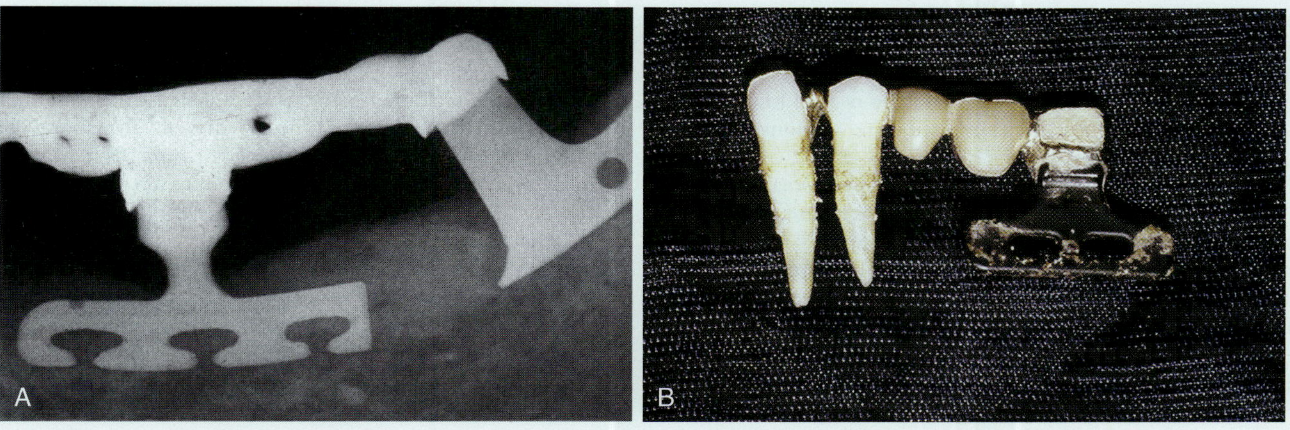

• **Fig. 12.1** **(A)** Blade implants embedded in bone, with some bone loss. **(B)** Failed blade implant prosthesis that was also attached to natural teeth. (Courtesy of Dr Mickey Calverley.)

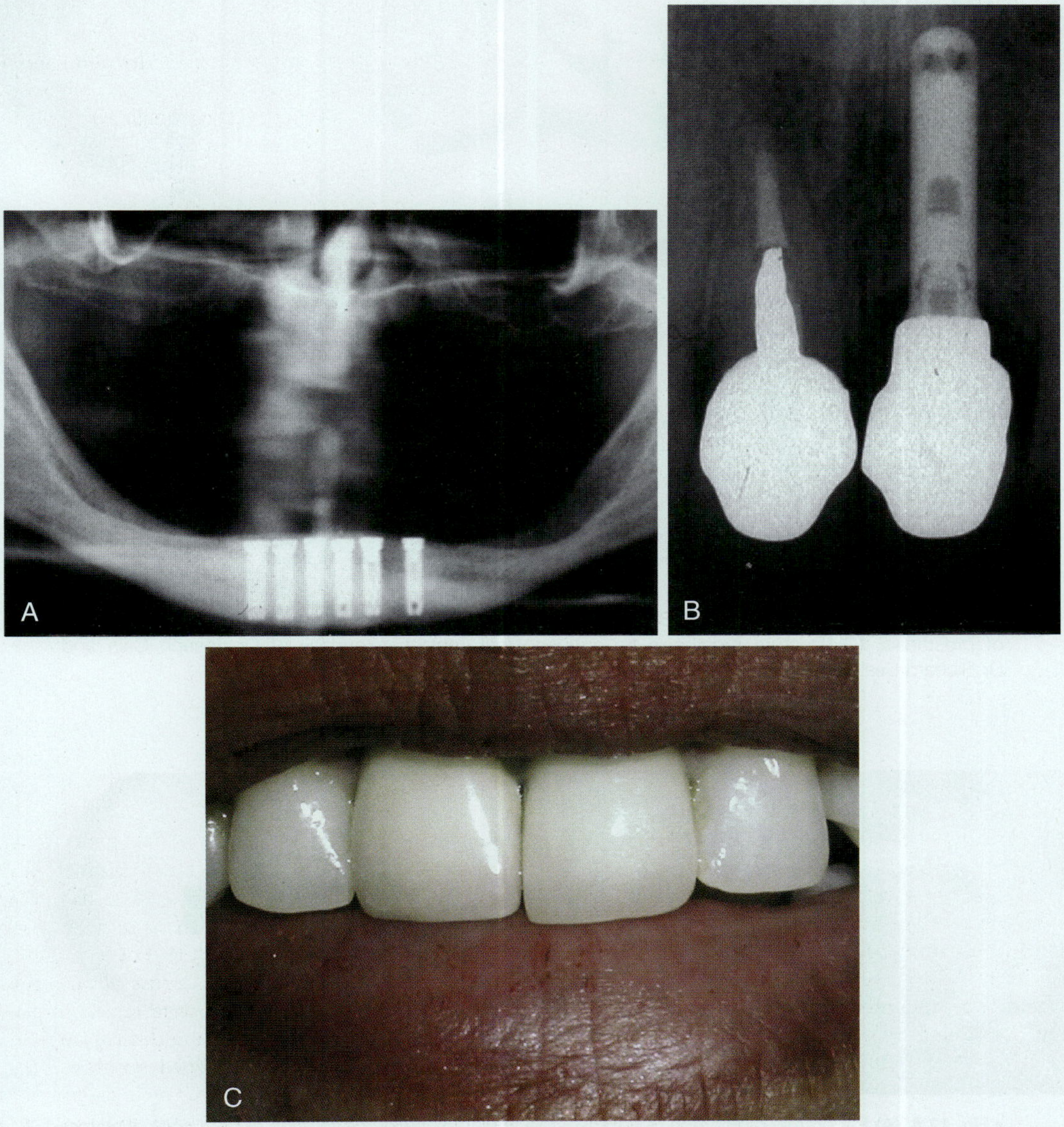

• **Fig. 12.2** **(A)** Endosteal implants are placed directly into bone; they mimic root forms for proper placement and location in bone. **(B)** and **(C)** Restored anterior implant blending well with adjacent teeth.

mimic the shape of tooth roots for directional load distribution as well as for positioning in bone. In longitudinal studies, the root-form implant has the most documentation of the endosteal implants, although several surgical stages may be needed for completion. Zygomatic and pterygoid implants are versions of long endosteal implant designs.

The second implant design was the **subperiosteal implant** (Fig. 12.3), which employed an implant substructure and superstructure. The custom-cast frame was placed directly beneath the periosteum overlying and fitting along the bony cortex. This implant was first developed by Dahl (1943) and refined by Berman (1950), who used a direct bone impression technique. These devices were used to restore partially dentate or completely edentulous jaws when there was inadequate bone for endosseous implants. Use of the subperiosteal implant has been limited because of numerous considerations, including the difficulty of retrieval.

The third design was the **transosteal implant** (Fig. 12.4), which combined subperiosteal and endosteal components. This type of implant penetrated both cortical plates and passes through the full thickness of the alveolar bone. Use of the transosteal implant has been restricted to the anterior area of the mandible and provides support for tissue-borne overdentures. The concept of transosseous implants was first conceived in Germany in the early 1930s; early examples were made of a cobalt alloy. Small (1968) developed the mandibular staple implant made of a titanium alloy, which was modified by Bosker (1983), who produced the transmandibular implant made of a gold alloy. Other names for transosteal implants have included

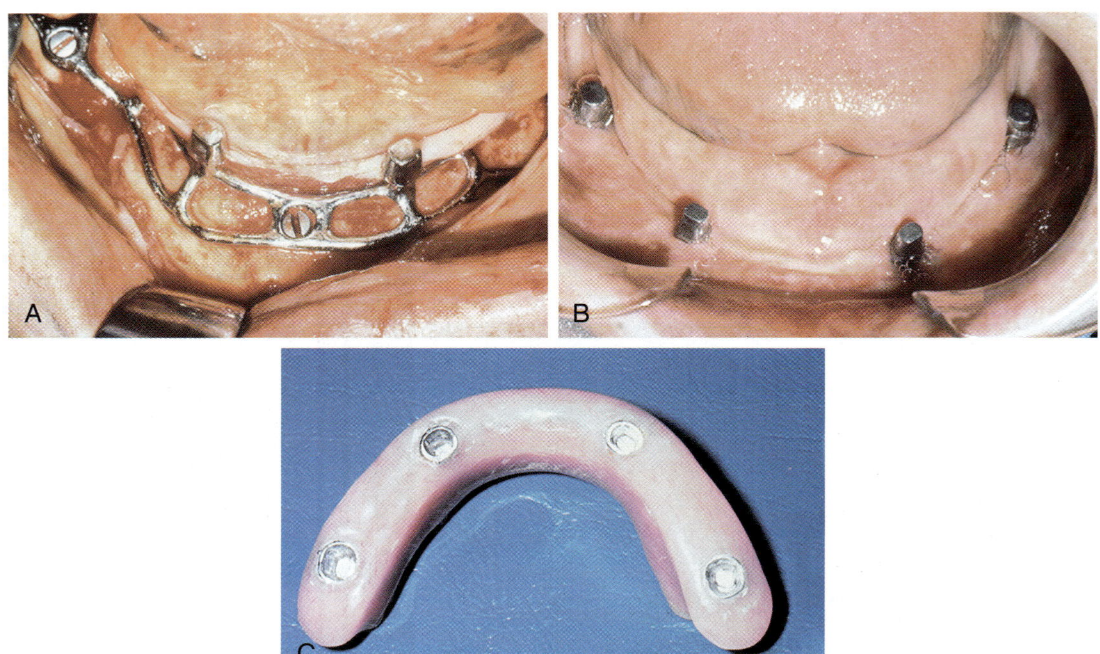

• **Fig. 12.3** **(A)** Subperiosteal implant positioned beneath the periosteum. Impression making often requires a difficult surgical technique. **(B)** Superstructure for subperiosteal implant allowing for attachment of prosthesis. **(C)** Denture prosthesis for subperiosteal implant. (Courtesy of Dr Joseph Cain and Dr Richard Seals.)

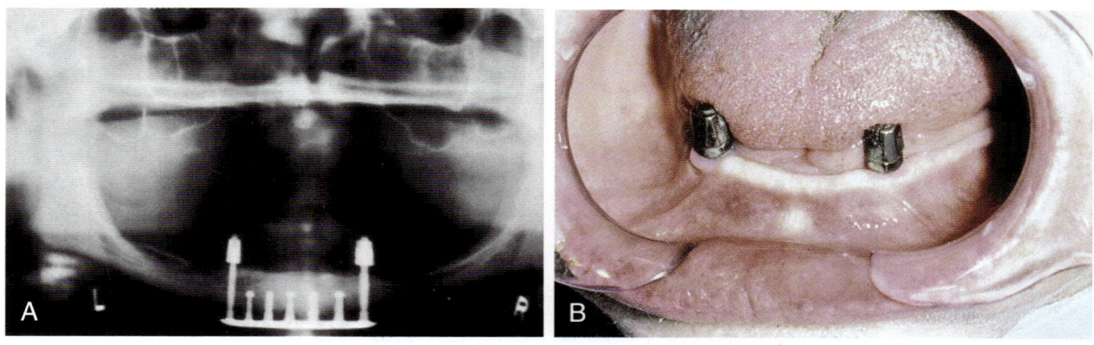

• **Fig. 12.4** **(A)** Panoramic radiograph of a transosteal implant showing perforation of both cortical plates, hence the name *staple implant*. **(B)** Transmucosal abutment for transosteal implant allowing for placement of denture restoration. (Courtesy of Dr Joseph Cain and Dr Richard Seals.)

staple bone implant, mandibular staple implant, and *transmandibular implant.*

The fourth implant design was the **epithelial implant**, which was inserted into the oral mucosa. This type was associated with a simple surgical technique where the mucosa was used as an attachment site for multiple metal inserts placed into an acrylic denture. Several disadvantages were associated with the epithelial implant, most notably a painful healing process, unpredictable long-term success, and a requirement for continuous wear. The current use of "mucosal inserts" or epithelial implants is very limited.

Some oral implantologists also include the endodontic stabilizer as an anatomy-specific application system. These smooth or threaded pins (or screws) were placed through endodontically treated teeth with the implant extending into the bone. They were constructed from alloys or ceramics made of alumina or zirconia. Reported difficulties included sealing the transition zone from tooth to bone and the limited strength of small-diameter pins or screws.

From a historical and applications perspective, these systems were reviewed in the early 1970s by Natiella et al (1972) and subsequently in each decade by researchers who participated in professional society–based consensus conferences. To summarize the various biomaterials and designs tested for dental implants, examples of devices received for examination prior to 1990 are shown in Figures 12.5–12.7.

Implant Design

- Endosteal implant
- Subperiosteal implant
- Transosteal implant
- Epithelial implant

Implant Properties

Implant biomaterials can also be classified according to their composition and their physical, mechanical, chemical, electrical, and biological properties. These classifications often include ranked comparisons of properties such as elastic moduli, tensile strength, and ductility to determine optimal clinical applications (Table 12.1). These properties are used to aid in the design and fabrication of the prosthesis. For example, the elastic modulus of the implant is inversely related to the strain transferred across the implant–tissue interface during loading of the implant; that is, the greater the elastic modulus of an implant, the greater is the stress in the implant and the lower is the stress transferred to bone. This effect is known as stress shielding, which eventually results in bone loss. The phenomenon of stress shielding can be explained as follows: In healthy individuals, loads or stresses are continuously being passed through the body in the form of fluctuations of pressure and tension. The viscoelastic properties of the entire connective tissue system allow for these stress fluctuations to pass through layers of tissues. Implant that is made of a harder element will have a tendency to absorb the stresses which are being transmitted to the specific body area. When the tissues surrounding an implant are "shielded" from stress impact by the harder material, the surrounding bone tissue will not receive enough stress or loads and the density of the bone begins to deteriorate (osteopenia). Stresses are necessary for maintenance of normal bone structure.

An implant with an elastic modulus comparable to that of bone should be selected to produce a more uniform stress distribution across the interface. Metals possess high strength and ductility, whereas the ceramics and carbons are brittle materials. Ductility is also important because it relates to the potential for permanent deformation of abutments or fixtures in areas of high tensile stress.

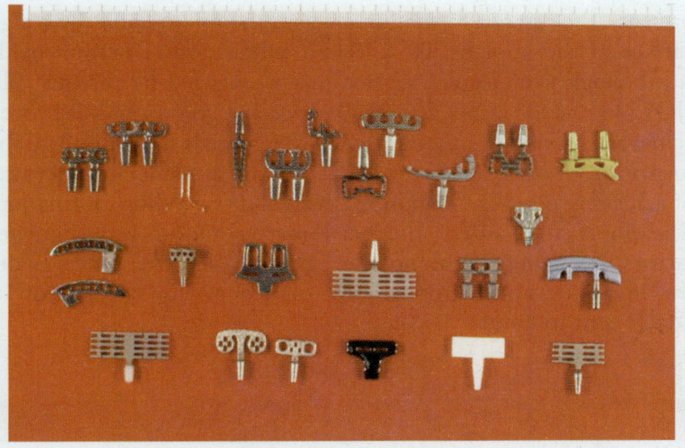

• **Fig. 12.5** Collection of endosteal blade implant designs for restoring single or adjacent teeth.

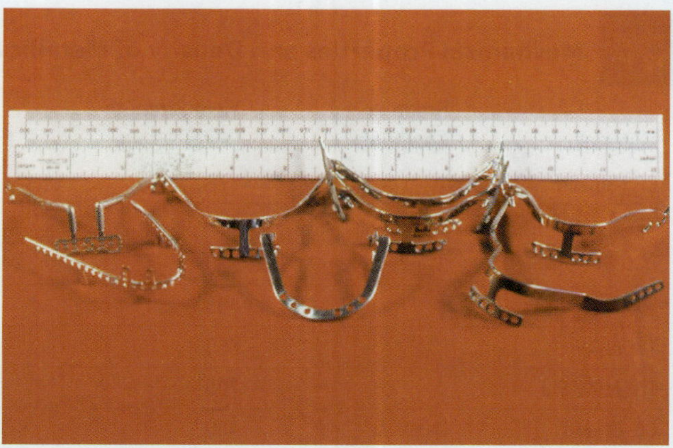

• **Fig. 12.6** Collection of endosteal implants for partial arch restorations.

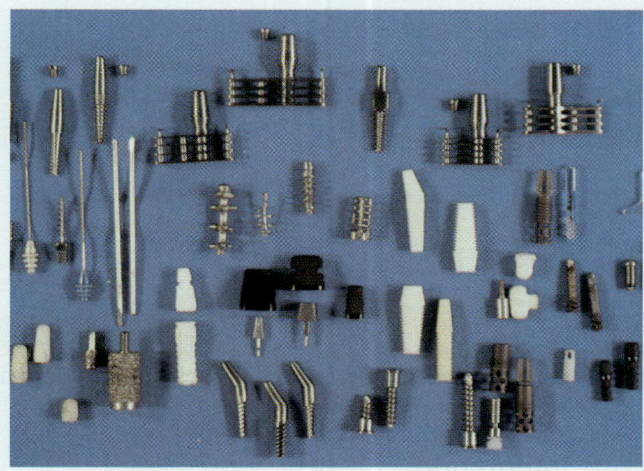

• **Fig. 12.7** Collection of different designs and materials used for endosseous implants.

TABLE 12.1 Mechanical Properties and Density of Metallic and Ceramic Implant Materials

Material	Grade or Condition	Yield Strength (MPa)	Elongation (%)	Modulus of Elasticity (GPa)	Tensile Strength (MPa)	Density (g/cm^3)
CP titanium	1	170	24	102	240	4.5
	2	275	20	102	345	4.5
	3	380	18	102	450	4.5
	4	483	15	104	550	4.5
Ti-6Al-4V		860	10	113	930	4.4
Ti-6Al-4V ELI		795	10	113	860	4.4
Co–Cr–Mo	Cast	450	8	240	700	8.0
Stainless steel	Annealed	190	40	200	490	8.0
	Cold worked	690	12	200	860	8.0
Aluminum oxide	Polycrystalline	400[a] (500/flexure)	0.1	380	220	3.96
Zirconium oxide	Y_2O_3 (stabilized)	1200 (flexure)	0.1	200	350	6.0
Cortical bone		N/A	1	18	140	0.7
Dentin		N/A	0	18.3	52	2.2
Enamel		N/A	0	84	10	3.0

[a]ASTM standard, minimum values.

CRITICAL QUESTION

What is the preferred implant-to-tissue interaction? How has this influenced the popularity of implant applications?

Tissue Integration

Another way of classifying implants is through interactions at the implant-to-tissue interface. Periodontal structures, which attach teeth to bone, consist of highly differentiated fibrous tissue. These fibers are replete with numerous cells and nerve endings that allow for functional force transfer, sensory function, bone formation, and tooth movements. Although this is the ideal form of integration, there are no known implant biomaterials or designs at present that can stimulate the growth of these fibers and fully mimic the function of the periodontal ligament and a natural tooth.

Historically, implant interactions occurred through fibrous connective tissue, and this was accepted as a measure of successful implant function (the pseudoligament concept). This type of interaction was reported to be very susceptible to acute or chronic inflammatory responses, which were accompanied by pain and eventual loss of the implant. Such an implant has also been called a pseudoperiodontium. These pseudoperiodontium fibers orient parallel to the implant's surface, suspending the implant rather than connecting the implant to the bone. However, periodontal ligament (horizontal and oblique fibers) connects the tooth to the bone, thus transmitting stresses to bone due their orientation. Despite numerous reports of implant success, clinical studies indicate that this type of interaction is susceptible to a greater amount of progressive loosening and infection, with subsequent loss of the implant construct.

The implant-to-bone interaction (called **osseointegration**) is characterized by direct contact between bone and the surface of a functional implant after 1 year. This central theme of the Brånemark group was called "direct anchorage to bone" and had become a major attribute of dental implants. This mode is described as the direct adaptation of bone to implants without any other intermediate nonbony tissue and has been described by some as similar to tooth **ankylosis**, where no periodontal ligament or fibrous tissue exists. The strength of this contact has been shown to be stable, which is advantageous compared with the soft tissue interface described previously.

This type of osseous interface has been described extensively and includes a process wherein bone-producing cells migrate along the implant surface through the connective tissue scaffolding that forms adjacent to the implant surface. Much of the contact is formed by osseous cellular hemidesmosome (JOI glossary of terms 2016). Integration at the implant interface is highly dependent on the implant surface's chemistry and design. Bone apposition has been reported at higher rates when microscopic surface ridges are present. The osseous formation engages the microscopically rough surface of the implant like a Velcro connection. Titanium oxide is a biological molecular surface that is engaged by osseous cells (JOI glossary of terms 2016). Osseous integration has also been achieved through the use of **bioactive** materials that stimulate the formation of bone along the surface of the implant. Another way of achieving osseous integration involves de novo bone formation, wherein a mineralized interfacial matrix and/or active growth factors are deposited along the implant's surface. Once again, the implant's surface topography influences the strength of its attachment to bone.

CRITICAL QUESTION

What is the implication of having direct bone contact and the absence of a periodontal ligament on the prosthetic superstructure?

Implant-supported restorations differ from tooth-supported restorations in that the former lack periodontal ligament, which reduces shear stress and strain, provides shock absorption, and reduces the development of dangerously high occlusal forces. These benefits of the periodontal ligament reduce the potential for inadvertent damage to the tooth or restoration. With the increased popularity of all-ceramic restorations, the effect of no periodontal ligament attachment in implant-supported restorations must be established. Ceramic materials are brittle by nature and because of inherent processing flaws; they cannot withstand any stress above their yield point, which is equivalent to their tensile strength. These stresses can be generated during occlusal loading. Implants, on the other hand, are directly anchored to the bone and cannot readily flex laterally under extremely high occlusal loads to relieve some of the excessive loading. Based on an in vitro study, Vult von Steyern et al. (2005) analyzed the fracture strength of all-ceramic prostheses on abutment teeth and implants. They concluded that implant-supported ceramic prostheses fractured at higher loads than those supported by natural teeth because of the lack of a periodontal ligament. To date, there are no clinical studies comparing the performance of ceramic FDPs supported by implants and natural teeth.

Conversely, studies have analyzed whether the type of prosthetic material can affect the longevity of an implant. Brånemark and Skalak advocated the use of acrylic for the prosthetic superstructure to act as a shock absorber and essentially dissipate the load on the implants and the bone surrounding them. To date, acrylic, gold, and ceramic are being used in implant superstructures. In the absence of a periodontal ligament, minimizing the load along the bone–implant interface is logical. However, there is no evidence to associate the use of any prosthetic material with the longevity and survival of the implants.

- Implant-supported ceramic prostheses fractured at higher loads than those supported by natural teeth because of the lack of periodontal ligament.
- There is no evidence to associate the use of any prosthetic material with the longevity and survival of the implants.

CRITICAL QUESTION

What is the purpose of pretreating implant surfaces?

Implant Components

To understand the material characteristics and function of an implant, one must first be knowledgeable about its numerous component parts. Although each implant system varies, the parts are basically consistent. The body of the implant (called a fixture for the Brånemark system) (Fig. 12.8A) is the component that engages with bone. Depending on the implant system, the body section can have different surfaces, namely, macroscopic (implant design) and microscopic features. Macroscopic features include thread design, namely press-fit design, threads (square, buttress reverse buttress, and "V" shaped), fins, grooves, and slots. Microscopic features are mainly sandblasted, large grit, acid-etched implant surface (SLA), plasma sprayed or coated. These surface characteristics are often classified as subtraction (acid etch) or addition (coating) types. Each surface type is meant to serve a particular purpose—for example, increased surface area enhances bone integration, and better implant design improves cortex engagement which plays an important role in immediate and long-term bone anchorage. The coated or plasma-sprayed biomaterials, discussed later in this chapter, are used to enhance attachment to bone. The second component (Fig. 12.8B) is the transmucosal abutment, which provides the connection between the implant body and the intraoral prosthesis to be fabricated (Fig. 12.8C), which will provide intraoral function. The abutment is usually connected to the implant body by means of a screw; however, it can also be cemented or connected by a Morse taper-type design. Abutments can become engaged to the implant body either by an internal or external connection (initially a hexagon) within the implant body, which also serves as an antirotation device and is particularly important for single-unit restorations. The last part of an implant is the prosthesis. This can be attached to the abutments through the use of screws, cement, precision attachments, locator attachments, magnets, or other designs, such as those used for removable implant overdentures.

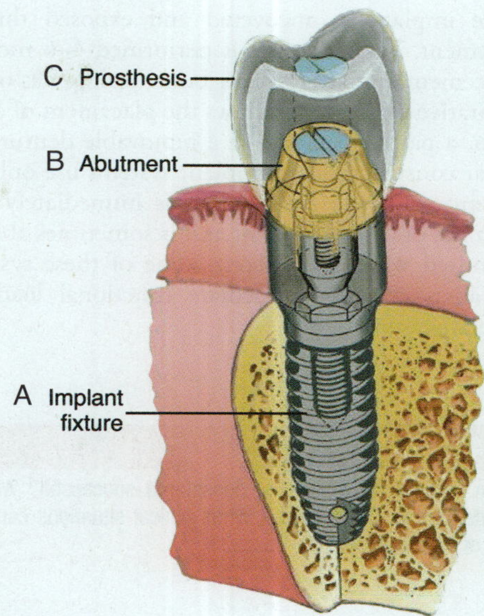

• **Fig. 12.8** Diagram of implant components. **(A)** The implant fixture (endosteal root form). **(B)** Transmucosal abutment serving as the attachment between fixture and the actual prosthesis. **(C)** The actual prosthesis, which can either be cemented, screwed, or swaged.

Implant Components
- The body of the implant (fixture)
- Transmucosal abutment, which provides the connection between the implant body and the prosthesis
- The prosthesis

Implant Surgical Placement

Placement and restoration of implants intended to integrate with bone are usually performed in stages. The first stage, or stage 1, occurs when the implant is surgically placed into the bone. The implant is left within the bone (passive) for a period of months, depending on the bone quality, and allowed to heal and become integrated. A secondary surgery, or stage 2, is sometimes required whereby the implant is uncovered and exposed through the oral environment. This exposure is performed 4–6 months after implant placement and after proper bone healing has occurred.

The restorative phase then follows the placement of abutments and a crown, a partial denture, or a removable denture, with or without a bar construct. Some implant systems use only one surgical intervention, where the implant is immediately placed in contact with the oral environment and is sometimes able to function in a limited way within days. Some of these systems have even been advocated for immediate functional loading, with reports of relative success.

CRITICAL QUESTION

When can an implant restoration be considered successful? What criteria are used to determine this success? What clinical situations can affect the success rate of dental implants?

Evaluation of Clinical Success

There have been several long-standing debates about what is considered successful in implant dentistry. Some consider that the encapsulation of an implant with a pseudoperiodontium is a successful implant condition. The most frequently cited success criteria from the 1970s are those in the publication edited by Schnitman and Schulman (1979). More recently, summaries from Cochran and Fritz (1996) and Albrektsson et al. (1986 and 1991) are often cited. Proposed early requirements included:

1. implant mobility less than 1 mm when tested clinically;
2. no evidence of X-ray radiolucency;
3. bone loss less than one-third the height of the implants;
4. absence of infection, damage to structures, and violation of body cavities—inflammation, if present, must be amenable to treatment; and
5. a success rate of 75% or more after 5 years of functional service using objective criteria for evaluation.

As an example, these conditions were somewhat different from the criteria of Albrektsson et al. (1986), which included the following:

1. the implant must be immobile when tested clinically;
2. there must be no evidence of periapical X-ray radiolucency;
3. vertical bone loss should be less than 0.2 mm annually following the implant's first year;
4. absence of signs and symptoms such as pain, infections, neuropathies, paresthesias, or violation of the mandibular canal; and
5. a success rate of 85% or more at the end of a 5-year observation period and 80% at the end of a 10-year period when evaluated by objective criteria for success.

Smith and Zarb (1989) recommended an addition to Albrektsson's criteria by stating that the patient's and dentist's satisfaction should be the primary consideration and that esthetic conditions should be met. Patient satisfaction and patient attitude toward the prosthesis have been included in some subsequent lists of criteria for success. Although these criteria have become more stringent in recent years, success in implant dentistry is still difficult to quantify.

In 2008, the International Congress of Oral Implantologists arrived at a consensus for rating implant success, survival, and failure. The scale ranges from 1 to 4, with 1 being deemed successful and optimal health and 4 as clinical failure. The consensus evaluates the presence of pain or tenderness, mobility, bone loss, and exudate history.

Standardized criteria for success should continue to evolve to enable proper evaluation of implant dentistry as the systems and treatments change over time.

Evaluation of Failure

Most recently, there has been much focus on peri-implant diseases because the diagnosis of these has never been fully established. As such, implant failures resulting from peri-implantitis range anywhere from 11% to 55%, and the true prevalence of this disease is elusive. *Peri-implantitis* and *perimucositis* are defined as mucosal inflammation surrounding the implant with or without 2 mm or more of bone loss after restoration (implant loading). The incidence of perimucositis and peri-implantitis on patients who receive implants varies from 20% to 90% within a period of 5–11 years. There are no definitive interventions associated with successful therapy of peri-implant disease. With more and more implants being placed in lieu of traditional fixed and removable dental prosthesis to replace missing teeth, peri-implantitis is becoming a major dental health issue. In 2017 the World Workshop on the Classification of Periodontal and Peri-Implant Diseases and Conditions was convened to outline proper identification of peri-implant diseases. Although the causes of peri-implantitis and peri-mucositis are still being investigated, there is a strong link between the incidence of the disease and chronic periodontitis, poor plaque control, and absence of regular implant maintenance. The links between systemic risk factors, such as smoking and diabetes, were found to be inconclusive.

CRITICAL QUESTION

What is the primary mechanism of failure involved with dental implants?

Longevity of Dental Implants

The popularity of dental implants to restore full or partial edentulism has been the result of predictable outcomes with high success rates. Success rates of 96%–98% are reported for mandibular implants and 94%–96% for maxillary implants, depending on the quality of bone, surgical technique, and primary implant stability. Implant failure can occur at an early stage or a late stage. Early-stage failures occur prior to loading or placement of the prosthesis and are most commonly associated with poor surgical techniques or inability to achieve primary stability. The use of efficient surgical drills and irrigation plays a crucial role in temperature rise, leading to bone necrosis. Protective coatings with boron nitride, titanium boron nitride, and diamond-like carbon (DLC) have significantly improved drill performance and durability. The recent addition of DLC burs is superior in mechanical properties, enhancement in corrosion resistance, and wear resistance compared to conventional stainless steel drills. However, the delamination of coatings can affect peri-implant healing. Osseodensification burs based on modified flute design and drilling protocol can significantly influence dental implants' stability in the softer bone.

Brånemark and Albrektsson reported strict protocols required to achieve proper osseointegration. These include following proper aseptic techniques and allowing the bone to heal around the implant for a period of 4–6 months. The healing process allows the bone to be generated around the implant free from bacteria and micromovements, which can disrupt bone deposition around the implant. Micromovements above 150 μm have been shown to encourage soft tissue deposition and eventual encapsulation of the implant body with fibrous tissue. This occurrence is classified as a failure of osseointegration. Allowing the bone surrounding the implant to heal necessitates a two-step surgical technique in implant placement. Stage 1 occurs when the implant is surgically placed into the bone. A flap is reflected and the implant is screwed into the bone (Fig. 12.9). The soft tissue is placed over the implant body to allow healing of the bone to occur. Stage 2 or the uncovering stage occurs when the soft tissue is removed to expose the implant to the oral cavity (Fig. 12.10). This exposure is performed 4–6 months after implant placement and after proper bone healing has occurred.

In 1990 Schnitman et al. reported on the success of immediate loading of dental implants. This technique eliminates the need for a second surgery and allows the implant to be used immediately to support a temporary or permanent prosthesis (Fig. 12.11). There are mixed results regarding the success rates between immediately loaded and conventionally loaded implants. While the success rates vary, there is consensus that immediate loading constitutes a more technique-sensitive process and patient-selective endeavor. Researchers conclude that if these guidelines are followed, the success rates for immediately loaded implants are more favorable. As

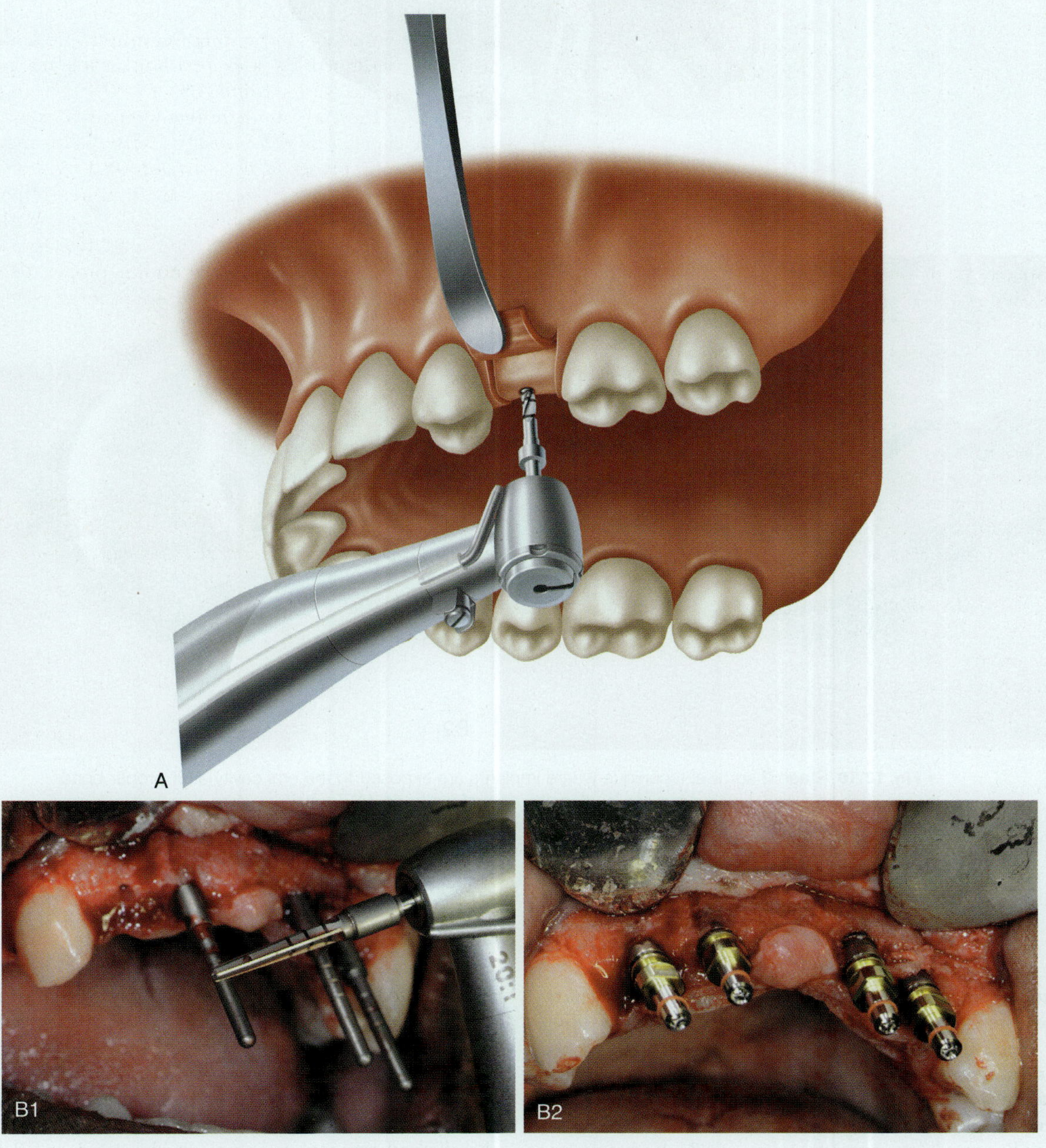

• **Fig. 12.9** Stage 1 surgery for implant dentistry involves placing the implant in bone. **(A)** Several drills are needed to accommodate the size of the implant in bone. **(B)** Osteotomies must be double checked for parallelism and proper positioning. Multiple implants being placed must be verified with placement pins. (Part A ©2012 Zimmer Dental Inc., all rights reserved. Part B from Garg AK: *Implant Dentistry,* ed 2, St. Louis, Mosby, 2010.)

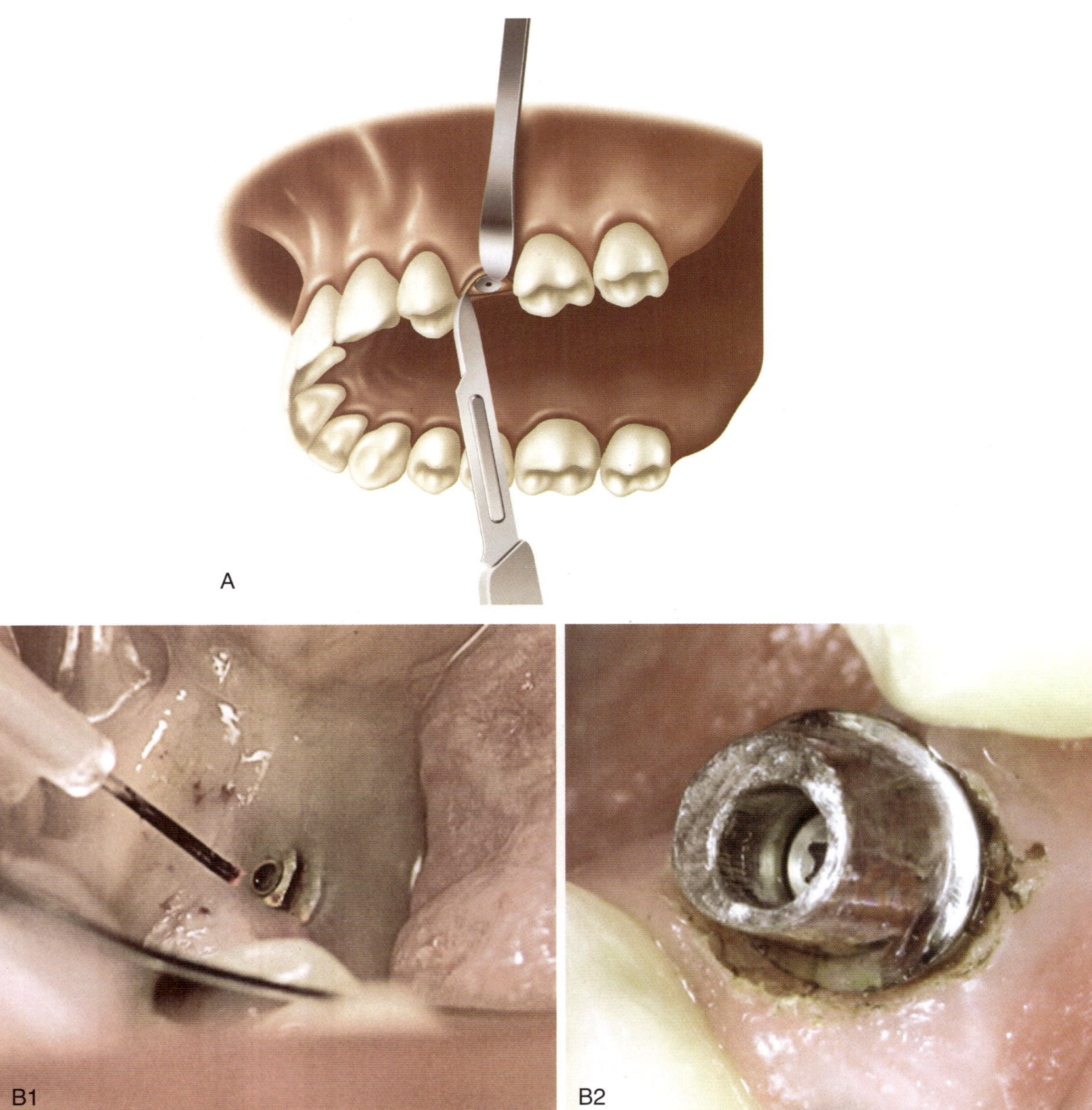

• **Fig. 12.10** Stage 2 surgical technique where implants are exposed to the oral cavity after proper bone healing has occurred. Uncovering can be done by several methods. **(A)** Technique using standard incision. **(B)** Stage 2 technique utilizing laser surgery. (Part A ©2012 Zimmer Dental Inc., all rights reserved. Part B from Garg AK: *Implant Dentistry,* ed 2, St. Louis, Mosby, 2010.)

with conventional implants, primary stability is important in achieving proper osseointegration. The problem with immediately loading implants is that micromovement can occur and jeopardize the bone formation around the implant body. However, research has shown that there is a range of allowable micromovement from 30 to 150 μm, where bone deposition is not hindered. The advantages of immediate loading are shorter treatment times, which lead to greater patient convenience and comfort by reducing the number of surgeries and allowing the immediate placement of a prosthesis.

Late-stage failures occur after loading or placement of a prosthesis and can be the result of complications stemming from uncontrolled peri-implant disease or overloading of the implant. Overloading can be due to lateral or oblique forces exerted on the prosthesis from improper occlusal loading or parafunctional habits. Bone is susceptible to microfractures or fatigue fractures, depending on the type and amount of occlusal load being exerted. Once the bone reaches the tolerance limit for the occlusal loads, these fractures can occur and can lead to implant failure. Excessive bone deformation has been shown to occur between 2000 and 3000 microstrain units, and pathological overloading can be seen at over 4000 microstrain units (a microstrain unit equals the strain that produces a deformation of one part per million).

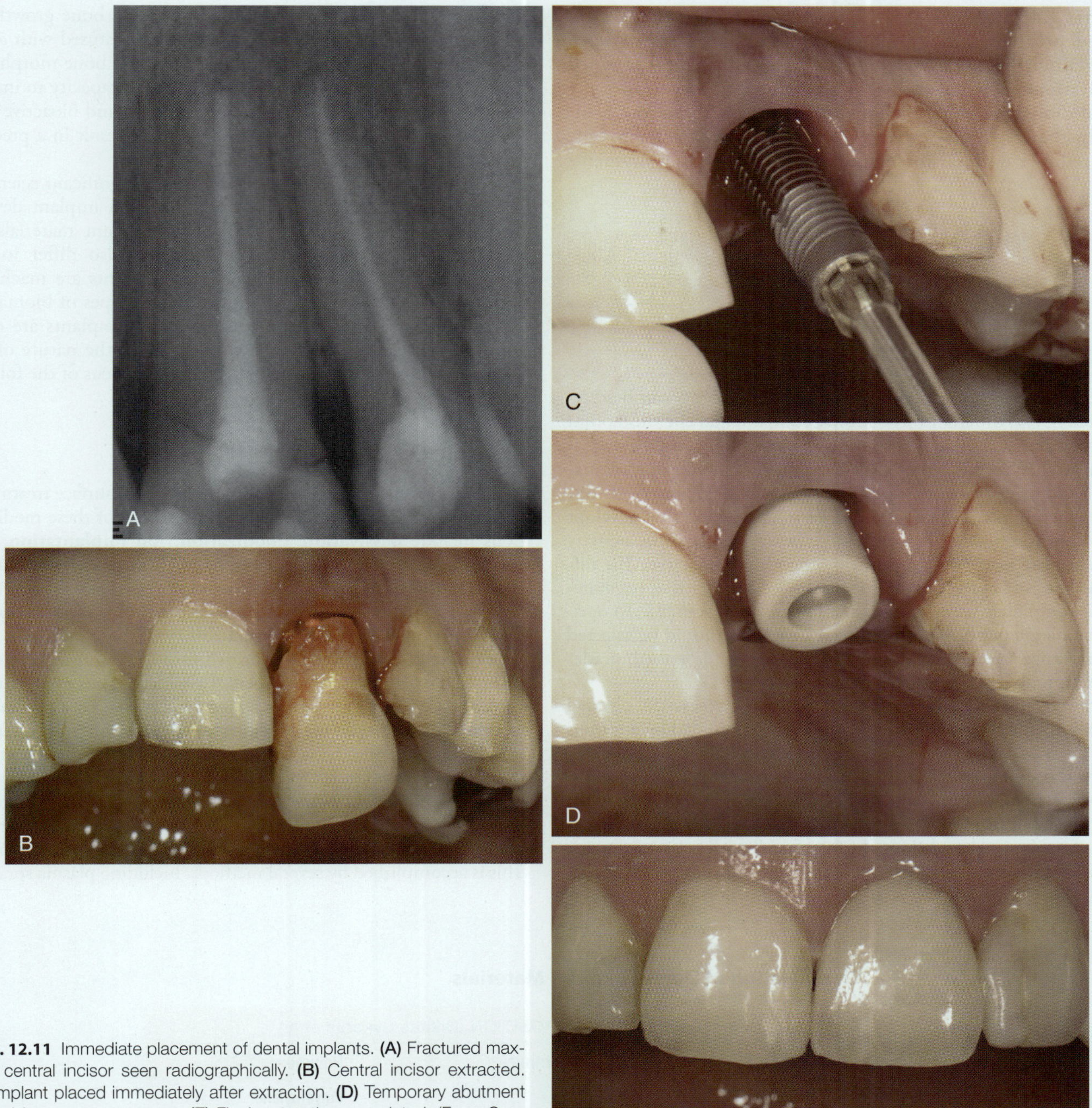

• **Fig. 12.11** Immediate placement of dental implants. **(A)** Fractured maxillary central incisor seen radiographically. **(B)** Central incisor extracted. **(C)** Implant placed immediately after extraction. **(D)** Temporary abutment placed for temporary crown. **(E)** Final restoration completed. (From Garg AK: *Implant Dentistry,* ed 2, St. Louis, Mosby, 2010.)

CRITICAL QUESTION

Which factors in the implant and prosthesis design affect the load transfer to bone?

A delicate balance must be achieved in load transfer from implant to bone to maintain proper bone health. Excessive occlusal forces lead to overloading of the bone surrounding the implant, which can, in turn, lead to bone resorption and microfracture. Conversely, minimal load transfer to bone can lead to bone atrophy from disuse. Rough surfaces along the implant are typically conducive to transferring more load to the bone due to the increased surface area contact. This reduction in localized stress decreases the strain around the implants. On the other hand, smooth-surfaced implants have the opposite effect, as evidenced by resorption along the marginal areas, where there is a smooth transition from the implant to bone.

The type of prosthesis used can also have an effect on how the forces are transferred along the implants. Prosthesis design should minimize long cantilever arms so as to avoid offset loads or high bending moments on the implants. Lateral forces are not tolerated as well as direct axial loading. Cement-retained prostheses have been found to be more favorable in maintaining proper axial loading as opposed to screw-retained restorations. The absence of a screw hole allows proper occlusal design for the prosthesis to adequately direct the loading to the implant. Conversely, the presence of a screw hole will redirect occlusal forces and introduce bending moments to the implant.

CRITICAL QUESTION

Which biomaterial is best for certain types of implants?

Implant Biomaterials

Materials used for the fabrication of dental implants can be categorized in two different ways. From a fundamental chemical point of view, dental implants fall into one of the following three primary groups: metals, ceramics, and polymers. In addition biomaterials can be classified based on the type of biologic response they elicit when implanted and the long-term interaction that develops with the host tissue. Three major types of biodynamic activity have been reported: biotolerant, bioinert, and bioactive. The different levels of biocompatibility emphasize the fact that no material is completely accepted by the biologic environment. To optimize biologic performance, artificial structures should be selected to minimize the negative biologic response while ensuring adequate function (Table 12.2).

Biotolerant materials are those that are not necessarily rejected when implanted into living tissue, but are surrounded by a fibrous layer in the form of a capsule. Bioinert materials allow close apposition of bone on their surface, leading to contact osteogenesis. Bioactive materials also allow the formation of new bone onto their surface, but ion exchange with host tissue leads to the formation of a chemical bond along the interface (bonding osteogenesis). Bioinert and bioactive materials are also called *osteoconductive*, meaning that they can act as scaffolds allowing bone growth on their surfaces. *Osteoconductive* should not be confused with *osteoinductive* materials, such as recombinant human bone morphogenetic protein 2 (rhBMP-2), which refers to the capacity to induce bone formation de novo. Biotolerant, bioinert, and bioactive materials are all biocompatible by definition and result in a predictable host response in specific application.

Today, implant materials are subjected to significant scientific scrutiny, which includes regulatory approval of implant devices used in vivo. The most commonly used implant materials are made from metallic biomaterials. Implants also differ in the nature of their surface condition. Some implants are machined and finished; others are coated with different types of biomaterials. Of the four types of implants, endosteal implants are most commonly used for dental applications. Thus, the nature of the biomaterials used for these devices is a central focus of the following discussion.

Metallic Implants

Metallic implants undergo one or more of several surface treatments prior to final packaging for implantation. Some of these modifications include **passivation**, **anodization**, **ion implantation**, and **texturing** by several different methods. *Passivation* refers to the enhancement of the oxide layer to minimize the release of metallic ions as a result of surface transfers. The minimization of ion release contributes to the **biocompatibility** of these materials. Passivation treatments can be performed through immersion in 40% nitric acid or anodization, a process by which an electrical current is passed through the implant when it is placed in a specialized solution. The former method of treatment minimally increases the thickness of the oxide layer, whereas the latter treatment can result in a thicker oxide layer, which has been shown to be beneficial in enhancing corrosion resistance. Surface texturing increases the surface area of the implant and enhances tissue interactions by increasing the area through which stresses are transferred to bone. This is accomplished by several methods, including plasma spraying

TABLE 12.2 Classification of Dental Implant Materials

Biodynamic Activity	CHEMICAL COMPOSITION (Nikitas Sykaras et al)		
	Metals	Ceramics	Polymers
Biotolerant	Gold Cobalt–chromium alloys Stainless steel Zirconium Niobium Tantalum		Polyethylene Polyamide Polymethylmethacrylate Polytetrafluoroethylene Polyurethane
Bioinert	Commercially pure titanium Titanium alloy (Ti-6Al-4V)	Aluminum oxide Zirconium oxide	
Bioactive		Hydroxyapatite Tricalcium phosphate Tetracalcium phosphate Calcium pyrophosphate Fluorapatite Brushite Carbon: vitreous, pyrolytic Carbon–silicon Bioglass	

with titanium, acid etching, and blasting with aluminum oxide or another ceramic or resorbable blast material. It is important that the increased implant surface area remains passive, because a greater surface area influences the overall release of metallic ions. Another surface modification for the implant is ion implantation, which consists of bombarding the surface of the implant with high-energy ions up to a surface depth of a few micrometers. This procedure has been claimed to increase the corrosion resistance of the metal through the formation of a titanium nitride TiN surface layer if the ion is nitrogen.

Titanium and Titanium Alloy

The most popular implant biomaterials in use today are titanium, titanium alloy, and calcium phosphate–coated materials. One result of the current extensive research focus is that titanium has become one of the most popular implant biomaterials. Titanium exists in nature as a pure element with an atomic number of 22. With an atomic weight of 47.9, titanium makes up about 0.6% of the earth's crust and is a million times more abundant than gold. This metal exists as rutile (TiO_2) or ilmenite ($FeTiO_3$) compounds and requires specific extraction methods to be recovered in its elemental state. The Kroll process involves reduction of $TiCl_4$ by magnesium, whereas the iodide process involves formation of titanium iodide through the reaction of titanium with iodine. The titanium iodide is later decomposed on a heated titanium wire. Titanium has several favorable physical properties, which include low density of 4.5 g/cm^3 and relatively high flexure strength comparable to that of cast forms of cobalt and stainless steel alloys. Titanium is also very resistant to corrosion; as a result of this property, a thin layer of titanium oxide, which is formed instantly on its surface, can passivate it. This metal has the ability to form an oxide layer of nanometer thickness within a millisecond, and this oxide reforms if lost because of mechanical removal. If left unchecked, this oxide layer can become thicker over time. Pure titanium has the ability to form several oxides, including TiO, TiO_2, and Ti_2O_3. Of these, TiO_2 is considered the most stable and is found after exposure to physiological conditions.

The most commonly used titanium products are grades 1–4 of unalloyed Ti. Titanium alloys, namely, Ti-6Al-4V and Ti-6Al-7Nb, are used in extra low interstitial (ELI) grades. The ELI contains low levels of oxygen dissolved in interstitial sites in the metal. Lower amounts of oxygen and iron improve the ductility of the ELI titanium alloy, which can be alloyed with different elements to modify its properties. For example, titanium undergoes a transformation from a hexagonal close-packed alpha phase to a body-centered cubic beta phase at 883°C. Alloying elements can be added to stabilize either phase. Ti-6Al-4V is one of the titanium alloys more commonly used. Aluminum acts as an alpha stabilizer for the purpose of increasing strength and decreasing density. Vanadium is a beta-phase stabilizer, which is used to minimize the formation of $TiAl_3$ to approximately 6% or less and to decrease the alloy's susceptibility to corrosion. With the exception of pure titanium, the modulus of elasticity of Ti-6Al-4V is closer to that of bone than that of any other widely used metallic implant biomaterial. Newer titanium alloys have been developed, including Ti-13Nb-13Zr and Ti-15Mo-2.8Nb. These alloys utilize other phase stabilizers instead of aluminum and vanadium, and they may exhibit greater strength and corrosion resistance.

As listed earlier, commercially pure (CP) Ti comes in different grades, from CP grades I to IV. The compositions of these metals in weight percentage are given in Table 12.3. The strength of CPTi is less than that of Ti-6Al-4V alloy, although the modulus of elasticity values is comparable. The elastic modulus of a typical Ti alloy (113 GPa) (see Table 12.1) is only slightly higher than that for the CP grade IV Ti (102 GPa). The yield strength of Ti-6Al-4V ELI and Ti-6Al-4V alloys (795 and 860 MPa, respectively) is 65–78% greater than that for CPTi. Ti alloys are able to maintain the fine balance between sufficient strength to resist fracture under occlusal forces and to retain a lower modulus of elasticity for more uniform stress distributions across the bone–implant interface.

Stainless Steel

Another alloy used for surgical implants is stainless steel. Used in the form of surgical austenitic steel, these metals have 18% chromium for corrosion resistance and 8% nickel to stabilize the austenitic structure. Stainless steel is most often used in the wrought and heat-treated state and possesses high strength and ductility. Despite its low cost and ease of fabrication, this alloy is not widely used in implant dentistry because of a potential allergic response to nickel as well as a susceptibility to crevice and pitting corrosion. The corrosion products for stainless steel contain iron, chromium, nickel, and molybdenum. These elements or their ions can accumulate in the tissues surrounding the implant and subsequently be transported to different parts of the body to produce a potentially unfavorable response. Surface treatments such as surface passivation and ion implantation are used to improve the corrosion resistance, although austenitic stainless steels are still prone to localized attack in long-term applications.

TABLE 12.3 Composition of CP Titanium and Alloys (Percent by Weight)[a]

Titanium	N	C	H	Fe	O	Al	V	Ti
CP grade I	0.03	0.08	0.015	0.20	0.18	—	—	Balance
CP grade II	0.03	0.08	0.015	0.30	0.25	—	—	Balance
CP grade III	0.05	0.08	0.015	0.30	0.35	—	—	Balance
CP grade IV	0.05	0.08	0.015	0.5	0.4	—	—	Balance
Ti-6Al-4V alloy	0.05	0.08	0.015	0.3	0.2	5.50–6.75	3.50–4.50	Balance
Ti-6Al-4V (ELI alloy)	0.05	0.08	0.012	0.25	0.13	5.50–6.50	3.50–4.50	Balance

[a]ASTM Standard, minimum values.

Cobalt–Chromium–Molybdenum Alloy

Cobalt–chromium–molybdenum cast alloys generally consist of 63% cobalt, 30% chromium, and 5% molybdenum with small amounts of carbon, manganese, and nickel. Molybdenum is a stabilizer; chromium provides the passivating effect to ensure corrosion resistance; and carbon serves as a hardener. Vitallium was introduced by Venable in the late 1930s and is part of the Co–Cr–Mo alloy family. This metal was initially shown to lack electrochemical activity and any tissue reaction. Ticonium, a Ni–Cr–Mo–Be alloy, was also used as a dental implant material, although this alloy revealed some adverse issues related to corrosion and biocompatibility. In later studies, Vitallium was associated with chronic inflammation and no osseous integration for several endosteal and subperiosteal designs. In an attempt to improve implant performance, inert biomaterials in the form of aluminum oxide and other ceramics were deposited on alloy surfaces. Aluminum oxide and zirconium oxide coated on cobalt alloys were found to have no effect on improving biological acceptability of the implants evaluated. Co–Cr–Mo alloys have a high elastic modulus and resistance to corrosion. The additions of ceramic coatings such as calcium phosphate did not significantly alter the bulk portions of the alloy. Studies of cobalt alloys have shown that their lower ductility is a result of the agglomeration of compounds rich in carbon, chromium, and molybdenum. Also, studies have shown that reducing the carbon content and controlling the processing of the alloy improve ductility. Co–Cr–Mo and stainless steel alloy continue to be used for some implants, such as subperiosteal and transosteal implants and ramus frames, because of their castability, mechanical properties, and lower cost.

Ceramic and Ceramic-Like Coated Implant Systems

Several synthetic and biological materials have been used specifically for the treatment of bone defects, ridge augmentation, and osteoporotic lesions. These biomaterials are also used to coat metallic implants to produce ceramic-like surfaces, which can be more thermodynamically stable, hydrophilic, and nonconductive of heat and electricity, thereby producing a high-strength integration with bone and the surrounding tissues. These ceramics can either be plasma sprayed or coated onto the metallic implant to produce a bioactive surface. The term *bioactive* refers to a variety of inorganic biomaterials that can enhance integration with bone. These are generally brittle and may have high elastic moduli and low tensile strengths.

Ceramic implants can withstand only relatively low tensile or shear stresses induced by occlusal loads, but they can tolerate quite high levels of compressive stress. Aluminum oxide (Al_2O_3) is used as a standard biomaterial for ceramic implants because of its inertness (biostability), with no evidence of adverse in vivo reactions. Zirconia (ZrO_2) has also demonstrated a high degree of inertness, although alumina (Al_2O_3) has shown a higher surface wettability compared with other surfaces, such as those of metallic implants. These types of ceramic implants are not bioactive in that they do not promote the formation of bone. They have high strength, stiffness, and hardness and function very well for some designs of dental implants. There are certain limitations for zirconia implants like low tensile strength and modulus of elasticity. However, further research and long-term evidence are recommended for two-piece zirconia implants. Table 12.1 lists the mechanical properties of different metallic biomaterials, including ceramic implant biomaterials.

Of the synthetic types of materials, calcium phosphates are the most successful for grafting and bone augmentation. This performance is probably associated with the fact that bone is composed of 60–70% calcium phosphate. These materials are nonimmunogenic and are biocompatible with host tissues. The two most commonly used calcium phosphates are hydroxyapatite (HA), or $Ca_{10}(PO_4)_6(OH)_2$, and tricalcium phosphate (TCP), $Ca_3(PO_4)_2$. HA and TCP are used as bone graft materials in granular or block form to serve as a template for the formation of new bone. Because these materials are known to promote and achieve a direct bond of the implant to hard tissues, they are classified as bioactive. Both also promote vertically directed bone growth as well as a relatively strong bond to bone. Calcium phosphate and HA particles are utilized as resorbable blast media. The residue of resorbable blast media does not elicit an immunological response to the implant surface compared to other blast medium residues like Al_2O_3. They may elicit an osteogenic response.

Biointegration is defined in the seventh edition of the *Glossary of Prosthodontic Terms* as "the benign acceptance of a foreign object by living tissue." More specifically, the biointegration of bone with an implanted material indicates the bond of bone to HA. HA, TCP, and other calcium phosphates are bioactive in part as a result of the release of calcium and phosphate ions within the surrounding tissue. Studies have revealed several differences in the tissue response to these materials following implantation. The beta form of TCP is resorbed more rapidly than HA and results in a breakdown of TCP. Some have reported a replacement of mesenchymal cells with features resembling osteoprogenitor cells. Studies have also shown that after 4 weeks of implantation, osteocytes accumulate adjacent to HA granules, indicating the possibility of osteogenesis with these implants. This is one of the justifications for using calcium phosphate compounds for coatings on implants placed into bone.

Use of these calcium phosphates as coating biomaterials for metallic implants is directly related to their physical and chemical properties. The more crystalline the HA coatings, the more resistant they are to clinical dissolution. A minimum of 50% crystalline HA is considered a preferable concentration for coatings. Implants coated with HA have shown a wide range of properties, from 85% crystalline HA and 15% TCP to 97% crystalline HA. Dissolution of the coating occurs at a higher rate with the more amorphous structural conditions. Heat treatment after the deposition process improves the crystallinity of HA. The major advantage of these ceramic-like coatings is that they can stimulate the adaptation of bone and very often exhibit a more intimate bone-to-implant contact compared with a metallic surface. The amount of bone integration has been compared between metallic implants and ceramic-coated implants in numerous studies, which suggest that there is a greater bone-to-implant integration with the HA-coated implants. However, other studies indicate that there is no significant difference between the HA-coated and the uncoated implants after months of integration, which implies that early integration may be quite different.

Bioglasses (SiO_2–CaO–Na_2O–P_2O_5–MgO) are another form of bioactive ceramic biomaterials. These materials are known to form a carbonated HA layer in vivo as a result of their calcium and phosphorus content. Formation of this layer is initiated by the migration of calcium, phosphate, silica, and sodium ions into tissue as a result of external pH changes. A silica-rich gel layer forms on the surface as elements is released. The silicone depletion initiates a migration of calcium and phosphate ions to the silica gel layer from both the bioglass surface and tissue fluids. This results in the formation of a calcium–phosphorus layer that stimulates osteoblasts to proliferate. These osteoblasts produce collagen fibrils that become incorporated into the calcium–phosphorus layer and are later anchored by the calcium–phosphorus crystals. This layer is 100–200 μm thick and has been shown to form a strong bone–bioglass interface. Bioglasses are classified as bioactive materials because they stimulate the formation of bone. They are more often used as grafting materials for ridge augmentation or bony defects than as coating materials for metallic implants because the interfacial bond strength of bioglasses with the metallic substitute and other ceramic substrates is weak and is subject to dissolution in vivo. Despite their favorable **osteoinductive** ability, bioglasses are also very brittle, which makes them unsuitable for use for some stress-bearing implant applications.

Other Implant Materials

Carbon and a carbon compound (C and SiC) were introduced in the 1960s for use in dental implantology. Vitreous carbon, which elicits a very minimal response from host tissues, is one of the most biocompatible materials. Studies have confirmed that the morphology of the bone–implant interface is similar to that associated with an HA implant. Compared with the metallic implants, carbon is more inert under physiological conditions and has a modulus of elasticity similar to that of dentin and bone. Thus, carbon deforms at a rate similar to those tissues, enhancing the transmission of biomechanical forces. However, carbon is susceptible to fracture under tensile and stress conditions because of its brittleness and its susceptibility to fracture under tensile stress in the presence of surface flaws, which is usually generated as a component of flexural loading. Carbon-based biomaterials have also been used for ceramic-like coatings on metallic implants.

Polyetheretherketone (PEEK) is an organic synthetic polymeric tooth-colored material which has the potential to serve as an esthetic dental implant material. It has excellent chemical resistance and biomechanical properties. In its pure form, Young modulus of PEEK is around 3.6 GPa. Meanwhile, Young modulus of carbon-reinforced PEEK is around 18 GPa which is close to that of cortical bone. Hence, PEEK could exhibit lesser stress shielding when compared to titanium. However, PEEK has less potential for osteoblast differentiation, compared to titanium. PEEK is a bioinert material and it does not possess any inherent osseoconductive properties. PEEK can be coated and blended with bioactive particles to increase the osseoconductive properties and surface roughness. However, high temperatures involved in plasma spraying can deteriorate PEEK. Furthermore, thick calcium phosphate coatings on PEEK can delaminate because of their limited bond strength when compared to coated titanium implants. Combining PEEK with particles in the size range of micrometers can reduce its mechanical properties. Hence considerable research has been initiated to modify PEEK by coating or blending it with nanosized particles and producing nanolevel surface topography.

CRITICAL QUESTION

What are the indications for the use of mini-implants in dental practice?

Mini-implants have been gaining wide popularity in recent years. More notably, their use in orthodontics for appliance anchorage has increased. Other uses include overdenture retention in areas where there is minimal bone available or in areas that are narrow. They can also be used to anchor temporary prostheses in the case of overdentures on an arch with newly extracted teeth. These implants were initially used as temporary implants, which helped anchor the prosthesis while the larger-diameter implants were left alone to osseointegrate. They could then be removed once the final prosthesis was fabricated. Over time, the success of these mini-implants has led to their evolution as final restorations for compromised cases. The diameter of mini-implants ranges from 1.8 to 2.9 mm (Fig. 12.12). Most mini-implants can be placed without having to reflect a flap in the gingival tissue because of their small diameter. Mini-implants are also designed for immediate loading, offering the convenience of few visits and allowing the patients to have teeth right away. Although these implants are essentially made from the same material as the larger standard implants and are constructed as root-form implants, the main difference lies in their smooth surface without any surface characterization and smaller diameter. This smaller size allows placement of these implants in areas where standard implants would normally require a bone grafting procedure, which results in additional trauma and expense to patients. As the applications of mini-implants continue to grow, they are slowly being incorporated for use with fixed dental prostheses, adding additional support along the pontic areas.

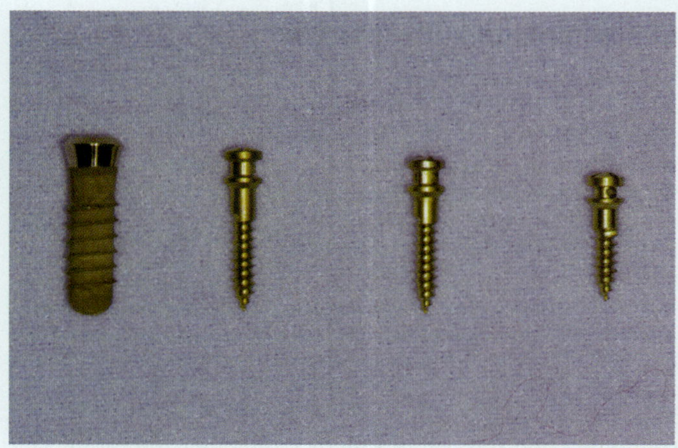

• **Fig. 12.12** Mini-implants used for orthodontic anchorage, showing 2 mm diameter of the mini-implants as compared with the 4 mm diameter of standard implants.

CRITICAL QUESTION

With the abundance of implant materials to choose from, how does a clinician know which biomaterial is best for a particular implant application?

Selecting an Implant Biomaterial

Because of the abundance of different implant biomaterials and implant systems, it is important to know the indications for their use. Perhaps the most important consideration is the strength of the implant biomaterial and the type of bone in which the implant will be placed. The other factors to consider are the implant design, abutment choices, abutment availability, surface finish, and biomechanical considerations of restorative treatments.

Characteristics of the Material

The strength of an implant is often a consideration, depending on its area of placement. If the implant is located in a zone of higher force transfer (e.g., in the posterior area of the arch), the clinician might consider using a higher-strength material such as grade-IV CP titanium or one of the titanium alloys. Some controversy exists as to which titanium metal or alloy to use, because some researchers believe that aluminum and vanadium can be **toxic** if released in sufficient quantities. Other considerations for selection include a history of implant fracture in the placement area of interest, the use of narrower implants, and a history of occlusal or parafunctional habits. Anterior implants, which are designated for use in narrow spaces, have smaller diameters, in the range of 3.25 mm or less. The wall thickness of narrow two-piece internal connection implants will be thin, requiring more robust implant material to resist fracture. Esthetic demand, especially in thin biotype mucosa, may recommend the use of Zirconia implants. Conversely, single implants placed in posterior areas have larger diameters, up to 7 or 8 mm. The selection of implant biomaterial must also be evaluated in terms of the abutment and intraoral biomaterials and dental materials. Electrochemical studies of the corrosion of metals now provide lists of acceptable and unacceptable combinations under conditions where parts touch one another and galvanic corrosion might exist. In general, the titanium and cobalt alloys are relatively stable and both have been combined electrochemically with the high noble dental alloys. Base metal and amalgam combinations are a concern.

The selection of abutment material on titanium implants may also play a crucial role in the long-term stability of implant–abutment junction. Metal abutments have significantly fewer mechanical failures compared to zirconia abutments. Zirconia abutments are reliable for anterior esthetic zones. Zirconia abutments with the internal connection of metal component two-piece zirconia abutments have fewer fracture rates than full-zirconia one-piece abutments. Alternative abutment materials like PEEK are still in limited use and are at the research stage.

CRITICAL QUESTION

How do implant characteristics and the quality and quantity of bone affect the survival time of implants?

As previously stated, the type of bone in which the implant will be placed is of critical importance. Bone for implantation has been classified into four types: type I consists of mostly homogeneous compact bone; type II consists of a thick layer of compact bone surrounding a core of dense trabecular bone; type III is a thin layer of cortical bone surrounding a core of dense trabecular bone; and type IV is composed of a thin layer of cortical bone with a core of low-density trabecular bone (Fig. 12.13). Type IV bone is by far the most compromised bone environment for implant stability because of its inadequate quality and quantity.

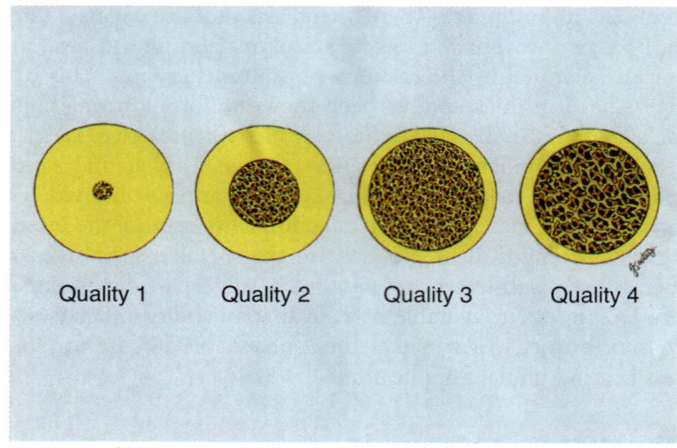

• **Fig. 12.13** Four qualities of bone.

Characteristics of Hydroxyapatite Coating

There has been much debate about when to use metallic or HA-coated implants. As mentioned earlier, HA-coated implants stimulate bone growth and have been shown to have a greater percentage of bone-to-implant integration. However, there are also some studies showing that HA is a very unstable implant material under some conditions (inflammation, infections, micromotion) and can prove detrimental to bone and tissues in the long term. Gottlander and Albrektsson (1991) examined the bone-to-implant contact area both at 6 weeks and 12 months for HA-coated and CPTi implants and concluded that the bone-to-implant contact area at 6 weeks was 65% for HA and 59% for Ti. However, at 12 months, Ti exhibited a 75% contact area versus 53% for HA. As mentioned earlier, HA can also be subjected to dissolution, and higher crystallinity must be maintained to minimize this occurrence. Unfortunately some amount of amorphous biomaterial is often present during plasma spray processing of the coating, and this substance is susceptible to dissolution.

Some studies have shown that the survival rate of HA-coated implants is initially higher than that for titanium plasma–sprayed implants, but in one study, the survival rate significantly decreased after 4 years. Failures were associated with inflammation of the surrounding tissues, with delamination and exfoliation of the implant. The delamination of surface coatings would be more due to excessive torsional forces while inserting in dense bone than softer bone. Thus, HA-coated surfaces are recommended for posterior maxilla with softer bone qualities. Some implants were retrieved before failure; these revealed partial loss of the HA coating, with flattening and thinning in some areas as well as an increase in local Cl and Mg ions. The implications of these factors relative to clinical implant failure remain unknown. Another concern is the adherence of microorganisms to the HA surface. A study of failed titanium and HA-coated implants revealed a colonization of coccoid and rod-shaped bacteria on HA implants, possibly as a result of the bioreactivity of HA. The roughened surface of the HA implants can also contribute to plaque growth, peri-implantitis, and dissolution once the coating is exposed. This can decrease the chance of long-term survival. Clinically it is highly challenging to decontaminate an exposed HA surface than SLA or acid-etched surfaces. Currently, there is no internationally established protocol to manage the infected HA surface.

In spite of all its possible disadvantages, HA has multiple indications for implant applications. Studies reporting on the biological response to both the coated and uncoated implants suggest that HA-coated implants were interfaced intimately with bone and that the mineralized matrix extended into the microporosity of the HA coating. Numerous osteocytes were found along the periphery of HA-coated implants, which indicates that these implants are a better option for areas of poor bone quality such as the maxilla. In one study, Brånemark-type titanium implants were evaluated in type IV bone and a survival rate of 63% was found for mandibular implants and 56% for maxillary implants. These values are lower than the survival rates of 90% or more when these implants were placed in type I and II bone.

HA-coated implants can be used in fresh extraction sites, owing to the initial stability afforded by these types of implants. Implant placement can sometimes be performed immediately after an extraction. Initial stability has been reported to be difficult to obtain in some of these cases, and this could lead to implant loss. A comparison of the survival rate of HA-coated implants, metallic implants, and hollow basket implants was made after 7 years of immediate implant placement. Survival rates of 95%, 90%, and 82% were found, respectively. The implant–bone interface contact area was also shown to be 62% for HA-coated implants and 29% for metallic implants after 28 days of placement.

Further advances in the field of dental surgery have allowed placement of implants in areas where bone was not normally present or had been lost. Maxillary and nasal sinus lifts are commonplace in partially dentate individuals who need an implant-based reconstruction. Bone grafts have enabled placement of a sinus lift in posterior areas where bone is deficient. Unfortunately, the quality of bone produced from these bone grafts is of lower quality, and an implant needs a substantial implant–bone contact area for function. Most of these implant sites oppose fully dentate arches, which normally exert a higher amount of masticatory force. Thus, initial stability, enhanced bone integration, and higher strength are important implant properties for these locations. Studies have revealed that HA-coated implants exhibited a push shear bond strength of 7 MPa versus 10 MPa for titanium metallic implants after a period of 10 weeks. After 32 weeks, HA-coated implants continued to have shear strengths five times greater than those of metallic surface implants.

- Quality of bone produced from bone grafts is of lower quality.
- HA-coated implants have shear strengths five times greater than those of metallic surface implants (32 weeks).

Another study compared the torsional strength of CPTi, Ti-6Al-4V, and HA-coated implants. Tensile strength for a period of up to 4 months ranged from 74 Ncm for the uncoated implants to 186 Ncm (HA-coated implants). These torsion-resistance values reflect the rotational shear resistance of the implant. Thus, HA-coated implant surfaces in this circumstance provided greater implant–bone interface area, higher shear tolerance, and higher torsional strengths in areas where a sinus lift procedure had been conducted.

A meta-analytic review was reported on the overall performance of coated and uncoated implants. It suggests that the survival rates are similar for both and that the HA coating did not compromise the long-term survival of these implants. Indications from reviews supporting the selection of HA-coated implants over titanium- or metal-surfaced implants include: (1) the need for greater bone–implant interface contact area, (2) the ability to place the implant in type IV bone, (3) fresh extraction sites, and (4) newly grafted sites. It has also been shown that the advantages of HA-coated implants are mainly short term in nature and are related to the initial stability of the implant, which most often determines its prerestorative success or failure.

Recent trends suggest SLA and other subtractive surfaces also produce long-term predictable success in various clinical scenarios. Active implant surfaces have shown improved implant surface wettability, promoting better adhesion to plasma proteins helping in faster healing. Active surfaces are produced by rinsing modified sandblasted/acid-etched surfaces under an N_2 atmosphere. It is then submerged in an isotonic NaCl solution. A wide range of implant surfaces showed promising results in the last decade, increasing clinicians' challenges to choose better surface characterization.

CRITICAL QUESTION

Several types of biocompatibility test data may be useful in selecting an appropriate implant. What is the principal factor on the basis of which an implant material should be selected as suitable or unsuitable for osseointegration?

Biocompatibility of Implants

The concept of biomaterial biocompatibility does not refer to total inertness but rather to the ability of a material to perform with an appropriate response in a specific application. Biocompatibility is affected by the intrinsic nature of the material as well as its design and construction. Therefore the state of biocompatibility may be specific to a particular situation or function. The American Dental Association outlines some acceptance guidelines for dental implants, including the following: (1) evaluation of physical properties that ensure sufficient strength; (2) demonstration of ease of fabrication and sterilization potential without material degradation; (3) safety and biocompatibility evaluation, including cytotoxicity testing, and tissue interface characteristics; (4) freedom from defects; and (5) at least two independent longitudinal prospective clinical studies demonstrating efficacy.

The primary surface interactions between an implant material and its host take place at the surface of the implant within a region of approximately the size of one water molecule (about 0.1–1.0 mm). However, this does not mean that the implant–tissue interactions are isolated to this interface. Some studies have reported high titanium levels in both the spleen and lungs of rabbits immediately following surgery, but these concentrations were well within normal limits. In humans, Ti levels have been reported at 50 ppm, but they can reach levels of up to 200 ppm in tissues surrounding some titanium implants. At this level tissue discoloration may be visible, but it is still well tolerated by the body. Kasemo and Lausmaa (1991) demonstrated the dissolution of corrosion products into the bioliquid and adjacent tissues. Thus the outermost atomic layers of an implant are critical regions associated with biochemical interactions of the implant–tissue interface. These reports emphasize the importance of process controls and a high degree of standardization and surface cleanliness in the production of implants.

Acceptance Guidelines for Dental Implants

1. Evaluation of physical properties that ensure sufficient strength;
2. Demonstration of ease of fabrication and sterilization potential without material degradation;
3. Safety and biocompatibility evaluation, including cytotoxicity testing, and tissue interface characteristics;
4. Freedom from defects; and
5. At least two independent longitudinal prospective clinical studies demonstrating efficacy.

CRITICAL QUESTION

What are the important considerations for intraoral prosthesis design and material?

Biomechanics

The integration of bone with implants serves as the basis for the biomechanical analyses performed for dental implants. Close approximation of bone-integrated conditions with the surface of an implant permits the transfer of forces and site-specific stresses with elastic displacement of the bone and implant. The stresses that are generated are highly affected by four main considerations: (1) masticatory factors (frequency, bite force, the direction of load, and mandibular movements); (2) support for the prosthesis (implant supported, implant tissue supported, implant tooth supported; (3) the mechanical properties of the materials involved in the implant restoration (elastic modulus, ductility, fracture strength, etc.); and (4) the design of the implant body and the associated intraoral prostheses. One of the most important variables affecting the close apposition of bone to the implant surface is the relative movement, or micromotion. It has long been documented that movement shortly after implantation prevents the formation of bone and encourages the formation of fibrous connective tissue around the implant surface. This collagen-rich connective tissue is known to be of lower modulus and strength and function is likely to change over time. This is the reason that a delay of months for intraoral restoration has been recommended before loading after surgery. As mentioned previously, success has been reported with immediate loading of implants depending on bone quality, patient selection, implant stability, and short-term controls of intraoral function. The key issue is control of implant-to-tissue micromotion during the initial healing of bone.

Numerous studies have defined the relationships for the response of bone to the types of biomechanical stresses and strains and their magnitudes. The results have been summarized as the "frost paradigm," where microstrain magnitudes are correlated with bone conditions of disuse atrophy (less than 500 $\mu\epsilon$), normal function (500–1500 $\mu\epsilon$), and microtrauma (more than 1500 $\mu\epsilon$). This concept is depicted schematically in Figure 12.14. This paradigm affords opportunities to evaluate implant and construct designs on a relative basis using finite element models and analyses. Once again, this literature is well developed.

Two main types of loading conditions can occur at an implant site. These are represented by axial forces and bending moments caused by noncentric loading conditions. A bending moment can best be demonstrated by visualizing a cantilever beam design in which the maximum bending moment is located at the fixed base of support and is calculated as force (perpendicular to the beam) times the length of the lever arm. These bending moments become highly significant depending on the type and design of implant restoration planned.

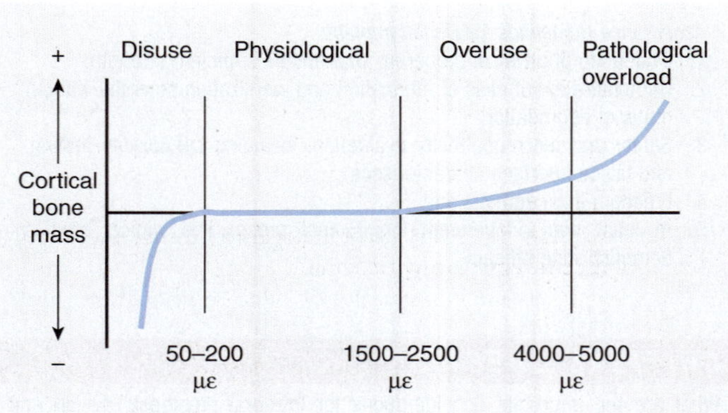

• **Fig. 12.14** Schematic diagram of Frost paradigm.

Rangert (1989), Skalak (1983), and Brunski (1988) analyzed the theoretical effects of cantilever length, number of implants, arrangement of implants, and prosthesis design. Their models were based on the initial Brånemark hybrid prosthesis for the atrophic mandible (Fig. 12.15). This type of restoration usually involves four to six implants confined to the area between the mental foramen of the mandible, with cantilevers extending from the most distal implant. These were restored with acrylic resin and denture teeth, which were attached to a metallic superstructure by the use of several types of attachment methods. The most significant aspect of these studies is the optimal ratio of the cantilever length to the interfixture distance, commonly termed as AP spread.

When two or more implants are placed in a straight line, the bending moment will be distributed proportionately to the implants provided that the intraoral prosthesis is designed to be sufficiently rigid. Placement of the implants in an offset manner has been suggested for more favorable positioning because it redistributes oblique forces during implant loading. However, some recent studies have shown that tripodization of implants does not necessarily minimize stresses as much as the use of wider-diameter implants placed in a straight line. An increase in the anteroposterior placement of implants is also recommended to minimize the off-axis loading of the implant components. The load is greatest at the most distal implant when an anteriorly positioned cantilever prosthesis exists. Thus, the distance between the most terminal abutment and the one adjacent to it should be increased to reduce the stress and stain induced within the most distal abutment.

Another important factor to consider is the passive fit of the prosthesis on the implant. A misfit will lead to a nonuniform distribution of load, with the unit closest to the load bearing most of the forces. For well-integrated implants, the weakest link in the early systems of Brånemark was the gold or abutment screw, which was regarded as the safety feature for these restorations. The external loads were transferred through the gold screw if an inaccurate fit or overload existed, and the screw would deform and fracture. These screws were fairly retrievable and were easy to replace. The ultimate tensile strength of the gold screw was designed to function within the normal ranges of occlusal force in the molar region.

Some guidelines include computing the anteroposterior span of all the implants and allowing a distance of 1.5 times any cantilever distance while limiting the maxilla to a maximal cantilever of 8 mm because of the limitations of bone quality. Any cantilever length over 7 mm causes a significant increase in microstrain within both the framework and bone. Therefore, for any length over 7 mm, ideal functional conditions should be considered, or the decision to proceed under less ideal conditions should be approached with extreme caution.

Another area of debate is the attachment of implants to natural teeth. The consensus seems to be that attaching implant prostheses to natural teeth should be limited. This issue stems from the different nature of attachments to bone between the implant and the tooth. The implant is integrated with bone (rigid), meaning that it has a direct connection with bone. On the other hand, a tooth is attached to bone through the periodontal ligament, which provides sensory functions to the tooth and also deforms in response to masticatory loads. Bone formation or resorption is determined by the tension or compression within the periodontal ligament. A concern associated with attachment of an implant to

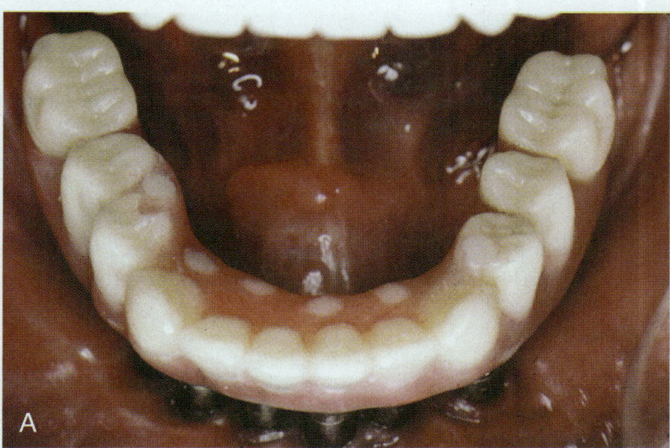

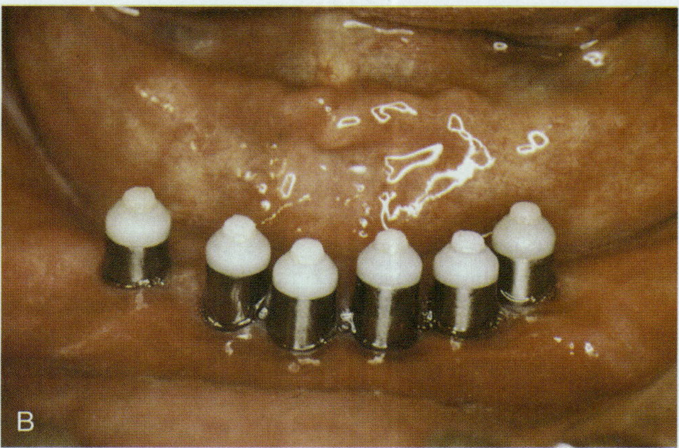

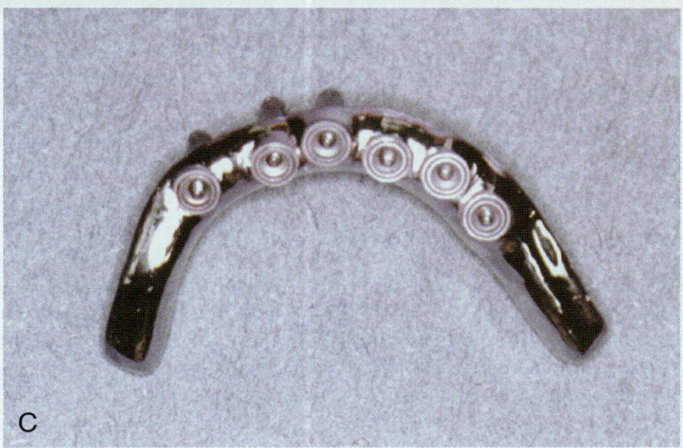

• **Fig. 12.15** **(A)** The original Brånemark hybrid prosthesis designed to accommodate severely atrophic mandibles. **(B)** The hybrid prosthesis usually utilizes four to six implants. **(C)** Corresponding superstructure that is screwed onto the implants.

a natural tooth is that the mobility of the tooth might minimize its load-sharing ability and overload the implant, understimulate the tooth, or cause a breakdown of the intraoral prosthesis. Most complications associated with implant tooth-supported prosthesis arise in the latter half of the first decade leading to long-term complications. Studies confirmed the overall success rates of exclusive implant-supported prostheses and recommended that this be the first approach for treatment.

Summary

- Four basic implant designs—**endosteal, subperiosteal, transosteal,** and **epithelial**.
- Most commonly used implant design—**endosseous implants**.
- **Osseointegration**—implant-to-bone interaction characterized by direct contact between bone and the surface of a functional implant.
- Major difference between implant and natural tooth in the relationship with bone—**periodontal ligament**.
- Parts of a dental implant—**implant fixture, abutment,** and **prosthesis**.
- In the **first-stage surgery**, the implant is placed into the bone through precise drilling.
- **Second-stage surgery** uncovers the osseointegrated implant and exposes to the oral environment.
- **Restorative phase** is the placement of abutments and appropriate fixed or removable prosthesis.
- Protocols for achieving osseointegration are proper aseptic techniques and allowing the bone to heal around the implant for a period of 4–6 months.
- **Implant-retained prosthesis** can be either cement retained or screw retained.
- Methods for surface modifications of metallic implants include passivation, anodization, ion implantation, and texturing.
- Most commonly used titanium products for dental implants are grades 1–4 of commercial pure titanium and titanium alloys like Ti-6Al-4 V and Ti-6Al-7Nb.
- **Bioactive** refers to a variety of inorganic biomaterials that can enhance integration with bone.
- Examples of bioactive materials are calcium phosphates and bioglass.
- Two most commonly used calcium phosphates are hydroxyapatite (HA) and tricalcium phosphate (TCP), they are used

as bone graft materials in granular or block form to serve as a template for the formation of new bone.

- **Mini-implants** are used in orthodontics for appliance anchorage and for overdenture retention in areas where there is minimal bone available or in areas that are narrow.
- The diameter of mini-implants ranges from 1.8 to 2.9 mm.
- The diameter of regular implants ranges from 3.25 to 6 mm.
- **Type I bone** is a homogeneous compact bone.
- **Type II bone** consists of a thick layer of compact bone surrounding a core of dense trabecular bone.
- **Type III bone** is a thin layer of cortical bone surrounding a core of dense trabecular bone.
- **Type IV bone** is composed of a thin layer of cortical bone with a core of low-density trabeculae.
- Frost paradigm correlates microstrain magnitudes with bone conditions of disuse atrophy (less than 500 $\mu\epsilon$), normal function (500–1500 $\mu\epsilon$), and microtrauma (more than 500 $\mu\epsilon$).

Review Questions

1. Write a short note on the historical evolution of dental implants.
2. Classify dental implants.
3. What is osseointegration?
4. Illustrate the different parts of a dental implant.
5. Enumerate the different stages of implant placement.
6. Enumerate the clinical success criteria for implants.
7. What are the different surface treatments done for implants?
8. Which are the commonly used titanium products for implants?
9. Write a short note on "frost paradigm."

Selected Readings

Akagi K.; Okamoto Y.; Matsuura T.; et al. Properties of test metal ceramic titanium alloys. J Prosthet Dent 68 462–467 (1992).

Akca K.; Iplikcioglu H. Finite element stress analysis of the influence of staggered versus straight placement of dental implants. Int J Oral Maxillofac Implants 16 722–730 (2001).

Albrektsson T.; Sennerby L. State of the art in oral implants. J Clin Periodontol 18 474–481 (1991).

Albrektsson T.; Brånemark P.I.; Hansson H.A.; et al. Osseointegrated titanium implants. Requirements for ensuring a long-lasting, direct bone-to-implant anchorage in man. Acta Orthop Scand 52 (2) 155–170 (1981).

Albrektsson T.; Zarb G.; Worthington P.; et al. The long-term efficacy of currently used dental implants: A review and proposed criteria of success. Int J Oral Maxillofac Implants 1 11–25 (1986).

ASTM F 67–00. Standard specification for unalloyed titanium, for surgical implant applications (UNS R 50250, UNS R 50400, UNS R 50550, UNS R 50700). In: Annual Book of ASTM Standards. American Society for Testing and Materials: Philadelphia.

ASTM F 136–98. Wrought titanium–6 aluminum–4 vanadium ELI (extra low interstitial) alloy (UNS R 56401) for surgical implant applications. In: Annual Book of ASTM Standards. American Society for Testing Materials: Philadelphia.

ASTM F 139–00. Standard specification for wrought 18 chromium–14 nickel–2.5 molybdenum stainless steel bar and wire for surgical implants (UNS S 31673). In: Annual Book of ASTM Standards. American Society for Testing Materials: Philadelphia.

Balkin B. Implant dentistry: Historical overview with current perspective. J Dent Educ 52 683–695 (1988).

Baltag I.; Watanabe K.; Kusakari H.; et al. Long-term changes of hydroxyapatite-coated dental implants. J Biomed Mater Res 53 76–85 (2000).

Berman N. Implant technique for full lower denture. Wash Dent J 19 15–17 (1950).

Bosker H.; van Dijk L. The transmandibular implant. Ned Tijdschr Tandheelkd 90 (9) 381–389 (1983).

Bosker H.; van Dijk L. The transmandibular implant: A 12-year-follow-up study. J Oral Maxillofac Surg 47 (5) 442–450 (1989).

Brånemark P.I.; Zarb G.A.; Albrektsson T. Tissue Integrated Prosthesis: Osseointegration in Clinical Dentistry. Quintessence: Chicago.

Brizuela, Aritza, et al. "Influence of the Elastic Modulus on the Osseointegration of Dental Implants." Materials (Basel, Switzerland) vol. 12,6 980. 25 Mar. 2019.

Brunski J.B. Biomechanics of oral implants: Future research directions. J Dent Educ (special issue) 52 755–787 (1988).

Brunski J.B.; Skalak R. Biomechanical considerations in advanced osseointegration surgery: Applications in the maxillofacial region. In: (editors: Worthington P.; Brånemark P.I.) Biomechanical Considerations in Advanced Osseointegration Surgery: Applications in the Maxillofacial Region. Quintessence: Carol Stream, IL, pp. 15–40.

Chang Y.L.; Lew D.; Park J.B.; et al. Biomechanical and morphometric analysis of hydroxyapatite-coated implants with varying crystallinity. J Oral Maxillofac Surg 57 1096–1109 (1999).

Chuang S.K.; Wei L.J.; Douglass C.W.; et al. Risk factors for dental implant failure: A strategy for the analysis of clustered failure-time observations. J Dent Res 81 572–577 (2002).

Cochran D.; Fritz M. Implant therapy I and II. Annals of Perio 1 (1) 707–821 (1996).

In: (editor: Craid R.G.) Restorative Dental Materials. ed 11 Mosby: St. Louis.

Dahl G.S.A. Om mojligheten for inplantation i kaken av metallskelet som bas eller retention for fasta eller avtagbara proteser. Odont T 51 440–446 (1943).

Davies J.E. Mechanisms of endosseous integration. Int J Prosthodont 11 391–401 (1998).

Driskell T.D. History of implants. Calif Dent Assoc J 15 16–25 (1987).

Er N, Alkan A, Ilday S, Bengu E. Improved dental implant drill durability and performance using heat and wear resistant protective coatings. J Oral Implantol. 2018 Jun;44(3):168-175.

Fiorellini J.P.; Chen P.K.; Nevins M.; et al. A retrospective study of dental implants in diabetic patients. Int J Periodont Restor Dent 20 366–373 (2000).

Glossary of Prosthodontic Terms, 7th ed. GPT-7, Mosby, reprinted from. J Prosthet Dent 81 (1) 39–110 (1999).

Gottlander M.; Albrektsson T. Histomorphometric studies of hydroxylapatite-coated and uncoated CP titanium threaded implants in bone. Int J Oral Maxillofac Implants 6 (4) 399–404 (1991).

Gou M, Chen H, Fu M, Wang H. Fracture of zirconia abutments in implant treatments: A systematic review. Implant Dent. 2019 Aug;28 (4):378-387.

Grandi T.; Garuti G.; Guazzi P.; et al. Survival and success rates of immediately and early loaded implants: 12-month results from a multicentric randomized clinical study. J Oral Implantol (April 11, 2011).

Greenfield E.J. Implantation of artificial crown and bridge abutments. Dent Cosmos 55 364 (1913).

Ichikawa T.; Hanawa T.; Ukai H.; et al. Three-dimensional bone response to commercially pure titanium, hydroxyapatite, and calcium-ion-missing titanium in rabbits. Int J Oral Maxillofac Implants 15 231–238 (2000).

Kasemo B.; Lausmaa J. The biomaterial-tissue interface and its analogues in surface science and technology. In: (editor: Davis J.E.) The Bone-Biomaterials Interface. University of Toronto: Toronto, pp. 19–32.
Lacefield W.R. Materials characteristics for uncoated/ceramic-coated implant materials. Adv Dent Res 13 21–26 (1999).
Lautenschlager E.P.; Monaghan P. Titanium and titanium alloys as dental materials. Int Dent J 43 245–253 (1993).
Lee J.J.; Rouhfar; Beirne O.R. Survival of hydroxyapatite-coated implants: A meta-analytic review. J Oral Maxillofac Surg 58 1372–1379 (2000).
Lindh T.; Back T.; Nystromm E.; et al. Implant versus tooth-implant supported prosthesis in the posterior maxilla: A 2-year report. Clin Oral Implants Res 12 441–449 (2001).
Linkow L.I. The bladevent – a new dimension in endosseous implants. Dent Concepts 11 3–13 (1968).
McCracken M. Dental implant material: Commercially pure titanium and titanium alloys. J Prosthodont 8 40–43 (1999).
Meffert R.M. Ceramic-coated implant systems. Adv Dent Res 13 170–172 (1999).
Misch C.M.; Ismail Y.H. Finite element stress analysis of tooth-to-implant fixed partial denture designs. J Prosthodont 2 83–92 (1993).
Misch C.M.; Perel M.L.; Wang H.L.; et al. Implant success, survival and failure: The International Congress of Oral Implantologists (ICOI) Pisa Consensus Conference. Implant Dent 17 (1) 5–15 (2008).
Natiella J.R.; Armitage J.E.; Greene G.W. Jr.; et al. Current evaluation of dental implants. J Am Dent Assoc 84 1358 (1972).
Nikitas Sykaras, Anthony M. Iacopino, Victoria A. Marker, R. Gilbert Triplett, Ronald D. Woody: Implant materials, designs, and surface topographies: Their effect on osseointegration. A literature review. Int J Oral Maxillofac Implants (2000);15:675-690.
Ogiso M.; Yamashita Y.; Matsumoto T. Differences in microstructural characteristics of dense HA and HA coating. J Biomed Mater Res 41 296–303 (1998).
Parr G.R.; Gardner L.K.; Toth R.W. Titanium: The mystery metal of implant dentistry. Dental materials aspect. J Prosthet Dent 54 410–414 (1985).
Prithviraj DR, Deeksha S, Regish KM, Anoop N. A systematic review of zirconia as an implant material. Indian J Dent Res. 2012 Sep-Oct;23(5):643-49.
Rangert B.; Jemt T.; Jörneus L. Forces and moments on Branemark implants. Int J Oral Maxillofac Implants 4 (3) 241–247 (1989).
Rangert B.; Gunne J.; Sullivan D.Y. Mechanical aspects of a Brånemark implant connected to a natural tooth: An in vitro study. Int J Oral Maxillofac Implants 6 177–186 (1991).
Roberts H.D.; Roberts R.A. The ramus endosseous implant. J S Calif Dent Assoc 38 571 (1970).
Rodriguez A.M.; Aquilino S.A.; Lund P.S.; et al. Evaluation of strain at the terminal abutment site of a fixed mandibular implant prosthesis during cantilever loading. J Prosthodont 2 93–102 (1993).
In: (editors: Schnitman P.A.; Shulman L.B.) Dental Implants: Benefits and Risk, An NIH-Harvard Consensus Development Conference. U.S. Department of Health and Human Services: Washington, DC, pp. 1–135.
Schnitman P.A. Implant dentistry: Where are we now? J Am Dent Assoc 124 39–47 (1993).
Schnitman P.A.; Wohrle P.S.; Rubenstein J.E. Immediate fixed interim prostheses supported by two-stage threaded implants: Methodology and results. J Oral Implantol 16 (2) 96–105 (1990).
Shariq Najeeb, Zohaib Khurshid, Jukka Pekka Matinlinna, Fahad Siddiqui, Mohammad Zakaria Nassani, and Kusai Baroudi. Nanomodified peek dental implants: Bioactive composites and surface modification—A review, International Journal of Dentistry Volume 2015, Article ID 381759, 7 pages, http://dx.doi.org/10.1155/2015/381759.
Skalak R. Biomechanical considerations in osseointegrated prostheses. J Prosthet Dent 49 843–849 (1983).
Small I.A.; Chalmers J. Lyons memorial lecture: Metal implants and the mandibular staple bone plate. J Oral Surg 33 (8) 571–585 (1975).
Smith D. Dental implants: Materials and design considerations. Int J Prosthodont 6 106–117 (1993).
Sohn B.S.; Heo S.J.; Koak J.Y.; et al. Strain of implants depending on occlusion types in mandibular implant-supported fixed prostheses. J Adv Prosthodont 3 1–9 (2011).
Steflik D.E.; Corpe R.S.; Young T.R.; et al. The biologic tissue responses to uncoated and coated implanted biomaterials. Adv Dent Res 13 27–33 (1999).
Tonetti M.S. Determination of the success and failure of root-form osseointegrated dental implants. Adv Dent Res 13 173–180 (1999).
Venable C.S.; Stuck W.G.; Beach A. Effects on bone of the presence of metals: Based on electrolysis. Ann of Surg 105 917 (1937).
Vult von Steyern P.; Kokubo Y.; Nilner K. Use of abutment-teeth vs. dental implants to support all-ceramic fixed partial dentures: An in-vitro study on fracture strength. Swed Dent J 29 (2) 53–60 (2005).

PART IV

Fabrication of Prostheses

13

Auxiliary Materials

CHAPTER OUTLINE

KEY TERMS

Base paste (base putty)—The component that forms the main three-dimensional structure of a final impression.

Catalyst paste (catalyst putty)—A component of a polymerization reaction that decreases the energy required for the reaction and usually does not become part of the final product; however, the term *catalyst* has been used for the structural component of dental materials that initiates the polymerization reaction.

Colloid—A solid, liquid, or gaseous substance made up of large molecules or masses of smaller molecules that remain in suspension in a surrounding continuous medium of different matter.

Elastomer—Any of various polymers having the elastic properties of natural rubber.

Gel—A network of fibrils forming a weak, slightly elastic brush heap structure of hydrocolloid; also, the solid network structure of a cross-linked polymer.

Gelation—The process of transforming a hydrocolloid from a sol to a gel.

Imbibition—The displacement of one fluid by another immiscible fluid in a hydrocolloid. In the context of impression materials, imbibition is the uptake by agar or alginate when immersed in water.

Inelastic—Incapable of sustaining significant elastic deformation without fracturing under stress.

Model—A positive full-scale replica of teeth, soft tissues, and restored structures used as a diagnostic aid for the construction of orthodontic and prosthetic appliances; a facsimile used for display purposes.

Shear thinning—The tendency for viscosity to decrease as the shearing rate increases (see *pseudoplasticity* and *thixotropy*).

Static mixing—A technique of transforming two paste-like materials (or fluids) into a homogeneous mixture without mechanical stirring; two streams of material are forced into a mixer cylinder, and the stationary elements in the mixer divide and recombine the feed materials and keep the material streams spiraling through the cylinder simultaneously.

Syneresis—The expression of fluid onto the surface of gel structures.

Thixotropy—The property of certain gels or fluids to become less viscous when sufficient energy in the form of impact force or vibration is applied; at rest, they require a specific duration to return to the previous viscous state. Both pseudoplasticity and thixotropy are shear-thinning processes; the difference is that changes in pseudoplastic viscosity do not exhibit the time-dependency characteristic of thixotropy.

Viscoelastic/viscoelasticity—The ability of a material to strain instantaneously like an elastic solid during rapid stretching or to resist shear flow and to strain linearly over time (like honey) when a stress is applied continuously.

GYPSUM PRODUCTS

Dental plaster (plaster of Paris)—The beta form of calcium sulfate hemihydrate ($CaSO_4 \cdot \frac{1}{2}H_2O$).

Dental stone—The alpha form of calcium sulfate hemihydrate ($CaSO_4 \cdot \frac{1}{2}H_2O$).

Hygroscopic setting expansion—The expansion that occurs when gypsum or a gypsum-bonded investment sets while immersed in water (usually heated to approximately 38°C [100°F]).

Normal setting expansion—The expansion that occurs when gypsum or a gypsum-bonded investment sets in ambient air.

WAXES

Baseplate wax—Dental wax provided in sheet form to establish the initial arch form in the construction of complete dentures.

Bite wax—A wax form used to record the occlusal surfaces of teeth as an aid in establishing maxillomandibular relationships.

Boxing wax—A wax sheet form used as a border at the perimeter of an impression to provide an enclosed boundary for the base of the cast to be made from a poured material such as gypsum or resin.

Corrective wax (dental impression wax)—A thermoplastic wax that is used to make a type of dental impression.

Dental wax—(1) A low-molecular-weight ester of fatty acids derived from natural or synthetic components, such as petroleum derivatives, that soften to a plastic state at a relatively low temperature. (2) A mixture of two or more waxes and additives used as an aid for the production of gypsum casts, the production of nonmetallic denture bases, the registering of jaw relations, and laboratory work.

Flow—Relative ability of wax to plastically deform when heated slightly above body temperature.

Inlay wax—A specialized dental wax that can be applied to dies to form direct or indirect patterns for the lost wax technique, which is used for the casting of metals or hot pressing of ceramics.

Refractory—Capable of sustaining exposure to a high temperature without significant degradation.

Sprue—The mold channel through which molten metal or ceramic flows into a mold cavity.

Sprued wax pattern—A wax form consisting of the prosthesis pattern and the attached sprue network.

Sticky wax—A type of dental wax that exhibits high adhesion to dry, clean surfaces when heated to a plastic condition.

Impression Materials

Making of a **model** or **cast** is an important step in numerous dental procedures. This model or cast is made from an **impression** of the teeth and surrounding soft tissues. Various types of casts and models can be made from gypsum products using an impression mold or negative likeness of a dental structure (Fig. 13.1). The dentist designs and fabricates both removable and fixed prostheses on a gypsum cast. The cast must be an accurate representation of oral structures, which requires an accurate impression.

CRITICAL QUESTION

Which of the seven criteria that ensure accurate impression making are related to the time the impression material is in the mouth? Which one is related primarily to the properties of a **set** impression?

To produce accurate replicas of intraoral and extraoral tissues, the impression materials should have the following properties:

1. sufficient fluidity to adapt to the oral tissues,
2. viscous enough to be held in a tray,

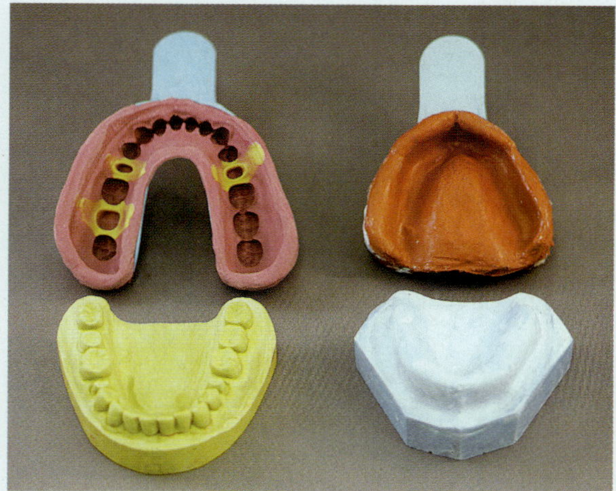

• **Fig. 13.1** Impressions of dentate *(left)* and edentulous arches *(right)* with the resulting respective gypsum casts.

3. able to transform (set) into a rubbery or rigid solid in the mouth in a reasonable time (less than 5 min),
4. resistant to distortion or tearing when removed from the mouth,
5. dimensionally stable long enough to allow one or more casts to be poured,
6. biocompatible, and
7. cost-effective in terms of time as well as the expense of the associated processing equipment.

Environmental conditions and the type of tissue dictate the choice of materials, quality of the impression, and quality of the cast. This chapter discusses the unique properties of currently used impression materials and describes how these characteristics affect the quality of an impression and of the cast made from the impression.

CRITICAL QUESTION

How are dental impression materials classified?

Classification of Impression Materials

Impression materials that are used today can be classified according to the composition, mechanism of setting, mechanical properties, and applications. Table 13.1 shows the classification based on the setting mechanism and mechanical characteristics. The composition of the materials is discussed later.

Setting Mechanism

There are two basic setting mechanisms:

- reversible and
- irreversible.
- *Irreversible* implies that chemical reactions have occurred and that the material cannot revert to the previous state in the dental office. For example, alginate, zinc oxide–eugenol (ZOE) impression paste, impression plaster, and elastomeric impression materials, which set by chemical reactions, are irreversible.
- On the other hand, *reversible materials*, such as agar and impression compound, soften upon heating and solidify slightly above the body temperature without a chemical change.

TABLE 13.1 Classification of Dental Impression Materials

Setting Mechanism	MECHANICAL CHARACTERISTICS	
	Inelastic	Elastic
Chemical reaction (irreversible)	Plaster of Paris Zinc oxide–eugenol	Alginate Polysulfide Polyether Condensation silicone Addition silicone
Thermally induced physical reaction (reversible)	Impression compound	Agar

Mechanical Properties

The set impression materials can be rigid (**inelastic**) or elastic. A set rigid material is resistant to flexure, and when stressed or deformed, it fractures suddenly in a manner similar to that of chalk. ZOE impression paste, impression plaster, and impression compound are inelastic impression materials. The term *elastic* means that the material is flexible and can be deformed and still returns to its original form when unstressed. Examples include agar, alginate, and **elastomers**.

Clinical Application of Impression Materials

Elastic impression materials can be stretched or compressed slightly, and they rebound when the impression is removed from the mouth. They are capable of accurately reproducing both the hard and soft structures of the mouth, including the **undercuts** and interproximal spaces. The extent of the rebound determines the accuracy of the material.

Inelastic impression materials, such as ZOE paste and plaster, are considered ideal for making impressions of edentulous jaw structures or soft tissue because, in the proper consistency, they do not compress the tissue during seating of the impression tray.

Elastomeric Impression Materials

Elastomers comprise a group of synthetic polymer-based impression materials that are chemically cross-linked when set. They can be stretched and yet rapidly recover to their original dimensions, like vulcanized natural rubber when the applied stress is released. Chemically, there are three elastomers based on the backbone of polymer chains: polysulfide, silicone (condensation and addition), and polyether. Representative products are shown in Figure 13.2. In this chapter, they are called elastomeric impression materials.

They are supplied in two components, a **base paste** and a **catalyst paste** (or liquid) that are mixed before making impressions. They are often formulated in several consistencies, including extra low, low, medium, heavy, and putty, in increasing order of filler content. Extra-low and putty forms are available only for condensation and addition silicones. Polysulfide is provided only in light-body and heavy-body consistencies. There is no heavy-body product for condensation silicone. Pigments are added to give each material a distinct color.

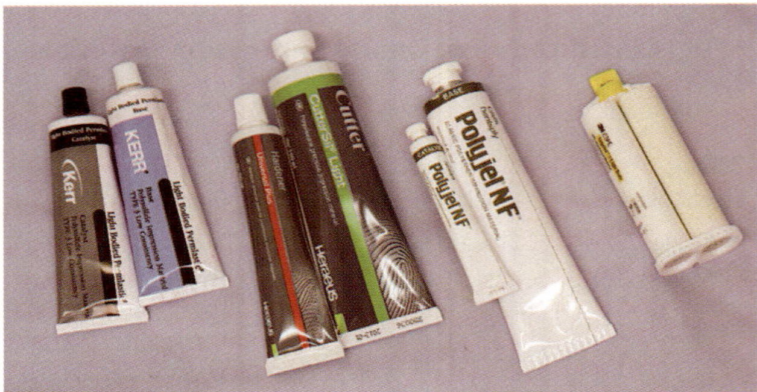

• **Fig. 13.2** Representative commercially available elastomeric impression materials.

Hydrocolloids, which are discussed in later sections, are **elastic impression** materials but they are not categorized as elastomers.

Polysulfide

The base paste consists of:

- A polysulfide polymer that contains a multifunctional mercaptan (-SH) called a polysulfide polymer,
- A suitable filler (such as lithopone or titanium dioxide) to provide the required strength,
- A plasticizer (such as dibutyl phthalate) to confer the appropriate viscosity to the paste, and
- A small quantity of sulfur, approximately 0.5%, as an accelerator.

The catalyst (or accelerator) paste contains lead dioxide, filler, and plasticizer as in the base paste, and oleic or stearic acid as a retarder to control the rate of the setting reaction. Lead dioxide is the component that gives polysulfide impression material its characteristic brown color. The terms *catalyst* and *accelerator* used here and with other impression materials are actually misnomers. *Reactor* is a more appropriate term for the reactions associated with polysulfide and other types of impression materials.

Each paste is supplied in a dispensing tube with appropriately sized nozzle diameters at the tip so that equal lengths of each paste are extruded from each tube to provide the correct ratio of polymer to **cross-linking** agent. Since the composition of the material in the tube is balanced with that of the accelerator, the matched tubes supplied by the manufacturer should always be used.

The reaction starts at the beginning of mixing and reaches its maximum rate soon after spatulation is complete (Fig. 13.3). At this stage, a resilient network starts to form. During the final set,

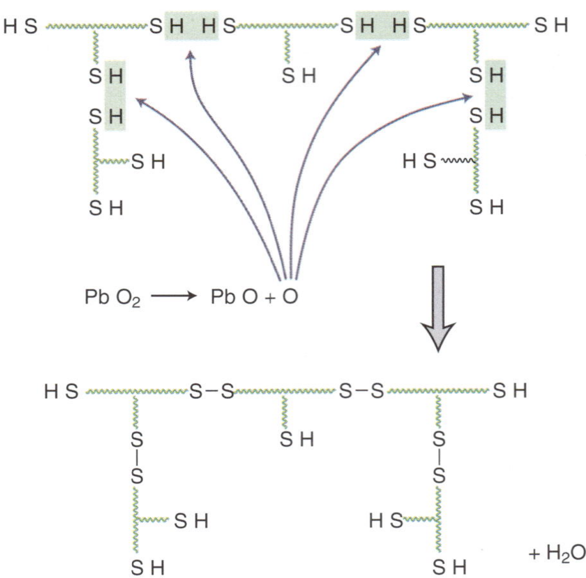

• **Fig. 13.3** Polymerization of polysulfide impression material. SH groups interact with oxygen released from lead dioxide (*left*). Completion of the condensation reaction results in water as a by-product (*right*). Pendant –SH is for cross-linking and terminal –SH is for chain lengthening of the polymer.

a material of adequate elasticity and strength is formed that can be removed past undercuts quite readily. Moisture and temperature have a significant effect on the course of the reaction. In particular, hot and humid conditions will accelerate the setting of polysulfide impression material. The reaction yields water as a by-product. Loss of this small molecule from the set material has a significant effect on the dimensional stability of the impression.

Condensation Silicone

The materials are supplied as a base paste and a low-viscosity liquid catalyst (or paste catalyst), a two-paste system, or a two-putty system. The putty can be used as the tray material in conjunction with a low-viscosity silicone, that is referred to as the putty-wash technique.

The base paste consists of α-ω-hydroxyl-terminated polydimethylsiloxane (Fig. 13.4). The curing of this material involves a reaction of trifunctional and tetrafunctional alkyl silicates in the

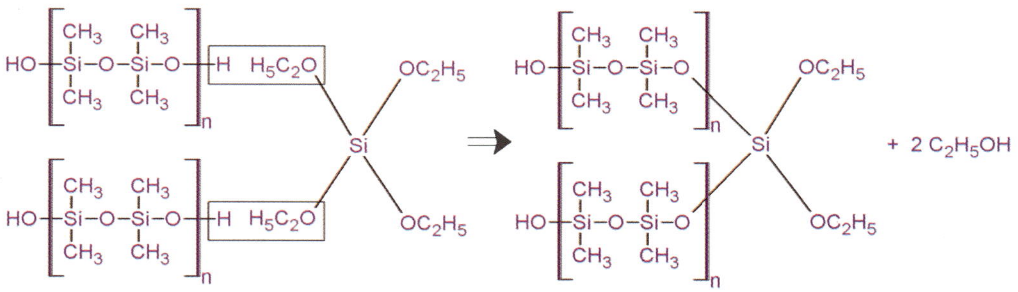

• **Fig. 13.4** Condensation polymerization of α-ω-hydroxyl-terminated poly (dimethylsiloxane) with tetraethyl orthosilicate in the presence of stannous octoate (catalyst). The reaction results in the release of ethanol molecules.

presence of stannous octoate as a catalyst. The material sets by cross-linking between terminal groups of the silicone polymers and the alkyl silicate to form a three-dimensional network (Fig. 13.4). Ethyl alcohol is a by-product of the condensation setting reaction. Its subsequent evaporation accounts for much of the contraction that takes place in the setting impression.

Addition Silicone

This material is often called polyvinyl siloxane (PVS) or vinyl polysiloxane (VPS) impression material. In contrast to the condensation silicone, the addition silicone is based on addition **polymerization** between divinylpolysiloxane and polymethylhydrosiloxane with a platinum salt as the catalyst (Fig. 13.5). The base paste contains polymethylhydrosiloxane, as well as divinylpolysiloxane. The catalyst (or accelerator) paste contains divinylpolysiloxane and a platinum salt. The platinum salt and polymethylhydrosiloxane are separated before mixing. Both pastes contain fillers.

No reaction by-products are formed as long as the correct proportions of divinylpolysiloxane and polymethylhydrosiloxane are used and there are no impurities. However, the residual polymethylhydrosiloxane in the material can lead to a secondary reaction with each other or with moisture, to produce hydrogen gas. Technically, hydrogen gas is a reaction by-product that does not affect the dimensional stability of the impression. Nonetheless, the hydrogen gas evolved can result in pinpoint voids in the gypsum casts poured soon after removal of the impression from the mouth. Manufacturers may add a noble metal, such as palladium, as a scavenger for the released hydrogen gas. The impression should be left overnight if epoxy will be used for pouring models.

One of the disadvantages of the silicone impression materials (including condensation silicones) is their inherent hydrophobic nature. A nonionic surfactant can be added to the paste in the manufacturing process to render a degree of hydrophilicity to the surface of the material. This surfactant migrates toward the surface of the impression material and has its hydrophilic segment oriented toward the surface—a phenomenon that makes the surface more wettable by water. These impression materials still require a dry field for impression making. Pouring the set impression with a gypsum-forming mixture is facilitated because the wet stone has a greater affinity for the hydrophilic surface. The clinical significance of hydrophilic additives is discussed in subsequent sections.

Sulfur contamination from natural latex gloves inhibits the setting of addition silicone. Zinc diethyldithiocarbamate is an accelerator used in the manufacture of the latex gloves. It reacts with the platinum catalyst in the PVS to cause a delay or total inhibition of polymerization. Some vinyl gloves may have the same effect because of the sulfur-containing stabilizer used in the manufacturing process. The contamination is so pervasive that touching the tooth with latex gloves before seating the impression can inhibit the setting of the critical surface next to the tooth. Not all latex gloves will cause an inhibition of set. It has been observed that synthetic latex gloves do not produce this phenomenon, while some natural latex gloves do.

Medium-body addition silicone has also been formulated for making impressions for diagnostic purposes, as a substitute for alginate impression material (discussed later). The advantage of these so-called alginate substitutes is the ability to make multiple, accurate diagnostic casts from one impression. Laboratory studies have reported that they exhibited better detail reproduction and less variability in linear dimensional change than irreversible hydrocolloid.

Polyether

There are two types of polyether impression materials. The first is based on the ring-opening polymerization of aziridine rings,

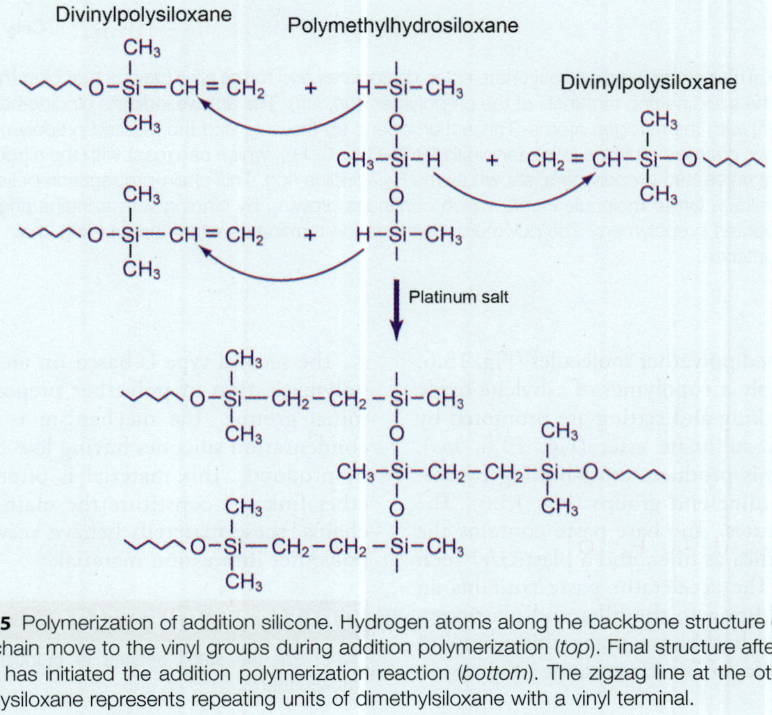

Divinylpolysiloxane

Polymethylhydrosiloxane

Platinum salt

• **Fig. 13.5** Polymerization of addition silicone. Hydrogen atoms along the backbone structure of the vinyl silicone chain move to the vinyl groups during addition polymerization (*top*). Final structure after the platinum salt has initiated the addition polymerization reaction (*bottom*). The zigzag line at the other end of divinylpolysiloxane represents repeating units of dimethylsiloxane with a vinyl terminal.

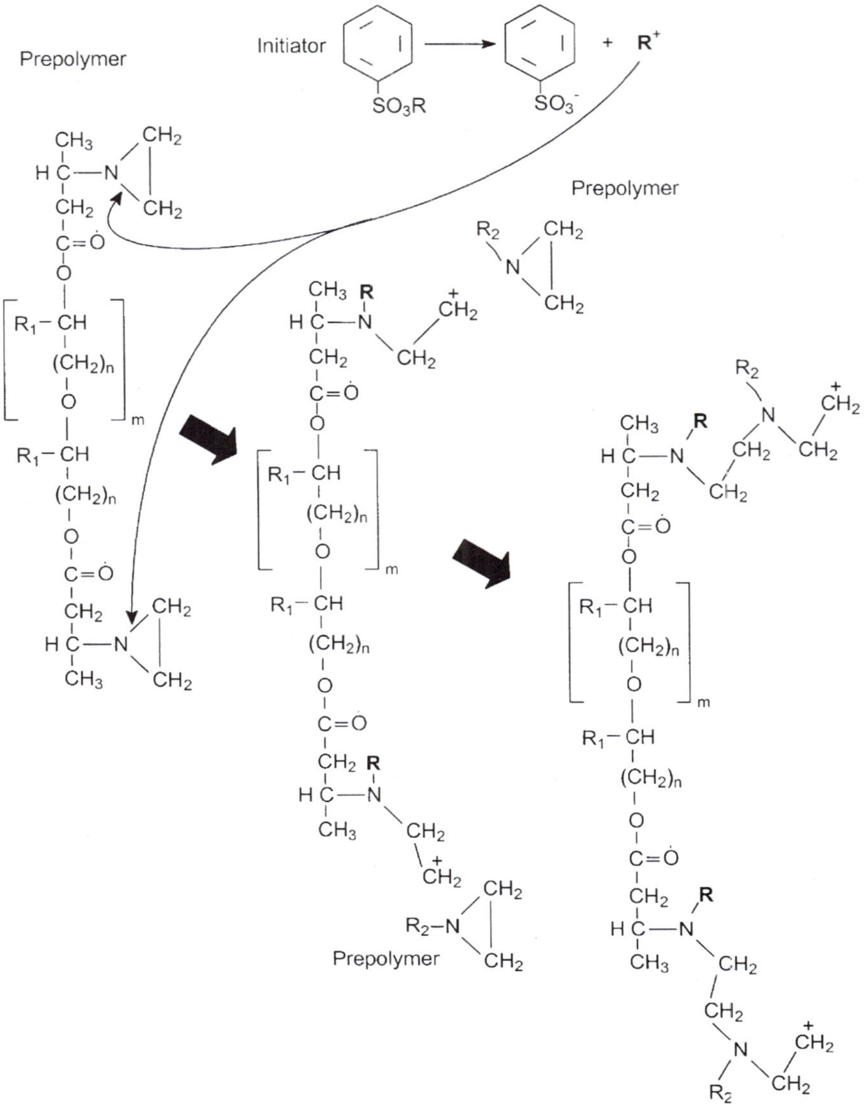

• **Fig. 13.6** The initiator, aromatic sulfonate ester, dissociates and forms alkyl cations that bind the nitrogen atoms of the aziridine ring terminals of the prepolymer (*top, left*). The arrows indicate binding between the cations (R^+) with the nitrogen atoms. This action opens up the ring, and the reacted prepolymer (*center*) now has two charged ethylene imine terminals ($-NR-CH_2-C^+H_2$), which can react with the nitrogen atoms of adjacent unreacted prepolymers, shown as the R_2-aziridine ring. This chain-propagation polymerization reaction yields a larger molecule (*right*), which continues growing by binding with aziridine rings of additional unreacted prepolymers. The polymerization reaction terminates when the growing chain combines with a counterion.

which are at the end of branched polyether molecules (Fig. 13.6, *left*). The main chain is probably a copolymer of ethylene oxide and tetrahydrofuran. Cross-linking and setting are promoted by an **initiator** and an aromatic sulfonate ester (Fig. 13.6, *top*), where R is an alkyl group. This produces cross-linking by cationic polymerization via the imine end groups (Fig. 13.6). The material is supplied as two pastes. The base paste contains the polyether polymer, colloidal silica as filler, and a plasticizer such as glycol ether or phthalate. The accelerator paste contains an alkyl aromatic sulfonate in addition to the filler and plasticizer. The ether-dominated polymer backbones make this group of materials the most hydrophilic of all elastomeric impression materials.

The second type is based on an acid-catalyzed condensation polymerization of polyether prepolymer with alkoxysilane terminal groups. The mechanism is similar to that observed in condensation silicones having low–molecular-weight alcohols as by-products. This material is often called a hybrid. Since the ether linkages constitute the main component of the polymer chains, these materials behave very much like the first type of polyether impression material.

CRITICAL QUESTION

What are the steps needed to produce casts and dies for prosthetic procedures?

Making Impressions With Elastomeric Materials

The use of elastomeric impression material to fabricate gypsum models, casts, and dies involves six major steps:

1. preparing a tray,
2. managing tissue,
3. preparing the material,
4. making an impression,
5. removing the impression, and
6. preparing stone casts and dies.

Impression Trays

Impression trays carry the impression material into the patient's mouth, and the handle of the tray is used to remove the impression. Two types of trays are commonly used: (1) stock trays and (2) custom-made trays. The tray supports the impression material which is generally weak and thereby improves accuracy of the impression.

The use of a custom tray (Fig. 13.7A) is recommended to reduce the quantity of material required to make impressions; thus, any dimensional changes attributed to the materials are minimized. A custom tray allows uniform distribution of impression material between the tray and the object and which also improves accuracy. This is especially true for polysulfide impression material. The use of custom trays for polyether and addition silicone impressions is not critical, since these materials are stiffer and have less polymerization shrinkage than the polysulfide material. In addition, disposable stock trays (Fig. 13.7B) work satisfactorily. Note that the use of less material in a custom tray reduces the compressibility of the impression, which can make removal of the impression tray more difficult. When severe undercuts are present, the use of a custom tray should be avoided. The stock tray should be rigid, thereby minimizing flexure of the tray during impression making. Disposable stock trays are also used to support the putty when the putty-wash technique is used for making impressions. Prior to making an impression, a uniform thickness of tray adhesive is applied on the tray surface, extending over its edge, and it is allowed to dry (through evaporation of solvent). A slightly roughened surface on the tray will increase adhesion. Tray adhesives are not interchangeable among different types of materials.

When the material is used correctly, either custom or stock trays yield clinically acceptable impressions.

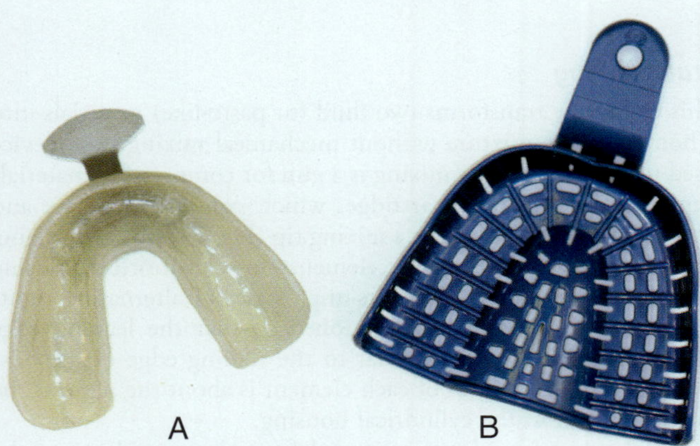

• **Fig. 13.7** Impression trays. Custom tray **(A)** and stock tray **(B)**.

- Impression trays carry the impression material into the patient's mouth.
- The use of a custom tray is recommended to reduce the quantity of material required to make impressions.
- A custom tray allows uniform distribution of impression material between the tray and the object.
- Dimensional changes attributed to the materials are thereby minimized.
- Prior to making an impression, a uniform thickness of tray adhesive is applied on the tray surface, extending over its edge, and it is allowed to dry (through evaporation of solvent).

Tissue Management

The margins of tooth preparations for fixed prostheses often extend to or below the free margin of the gingiva. To ensure access for the tooth preparation and for making the impression, it is necessary to displace the gingival tissues, control gingival hemorrhage, and control sulcular fluids. Among the most popular methods of gingival displacement is the use of gingival retraction cord. An electrosurgical unit or a soft tissue laser can also be used. Newly introduced material in the form of retraction paste like Expasyl (aluminum chloride, kaolin) or Magic Foam Cord (polyvinylsiloxane - addition type) shows better properties and respects periodontium.

The objective of placing a retraction cord is to displace the gingival tissue laterally away from the margin of the preparation. One or two gingival retraction cords are placed under the margin around the tooth for at least 5 min before making impressions. The double-cord technique is used when the margin is very close to the gingival attachment. A fine cord is placed at the base of the crevice to facilitate moisture control, with a larger cord placed on top of the first and near the coronal extent to displace the gingiva laterally. The latter, outermost cord is removed, leaving the fine cord within the crevice while the impression is made. A single cord is sufficient to deflect the soft tissue around the margin when the preparation margin is at or slightly above the gingival crest.

Retraction cords may be impregnated with a hemostatic agent by dipping the cord in a hemostatic solution prior to placement. These agents can have unintended side effects and should be used with caution. For example, epinephrine, which is used widely, is of particular concern in patients with cardiovascular disease. In addition, agents with a low pH can remove the smear layer and superficial dentin apical to the margins of the preparation, possibly leading to postoperative sensitivity of some teeth.

CRITICAL QUESTION

How does **static mixing** achieve a uniform mixture? What is the main difference between static mixing and dynamic mixing?

Manipulation of Impression Materials

Currently, elastomeric impression materials are supplied for three modes of mixing: hand mixing, static mixing, and dynamic mechanical mixing (Fig. 13.8).

Hand Mixing

The user should dispense the same lengths of materials onto a mixing pad or glass slab (Fig. 13.8A). The catalyst paste is first collected on a stainless steel spatula and then spread over the base paste. The mixture is then spread over the mixing pad. The mass is then scraped up with the spatula blade and spread uniformly back and forth on the mixing pad. This process is continued until

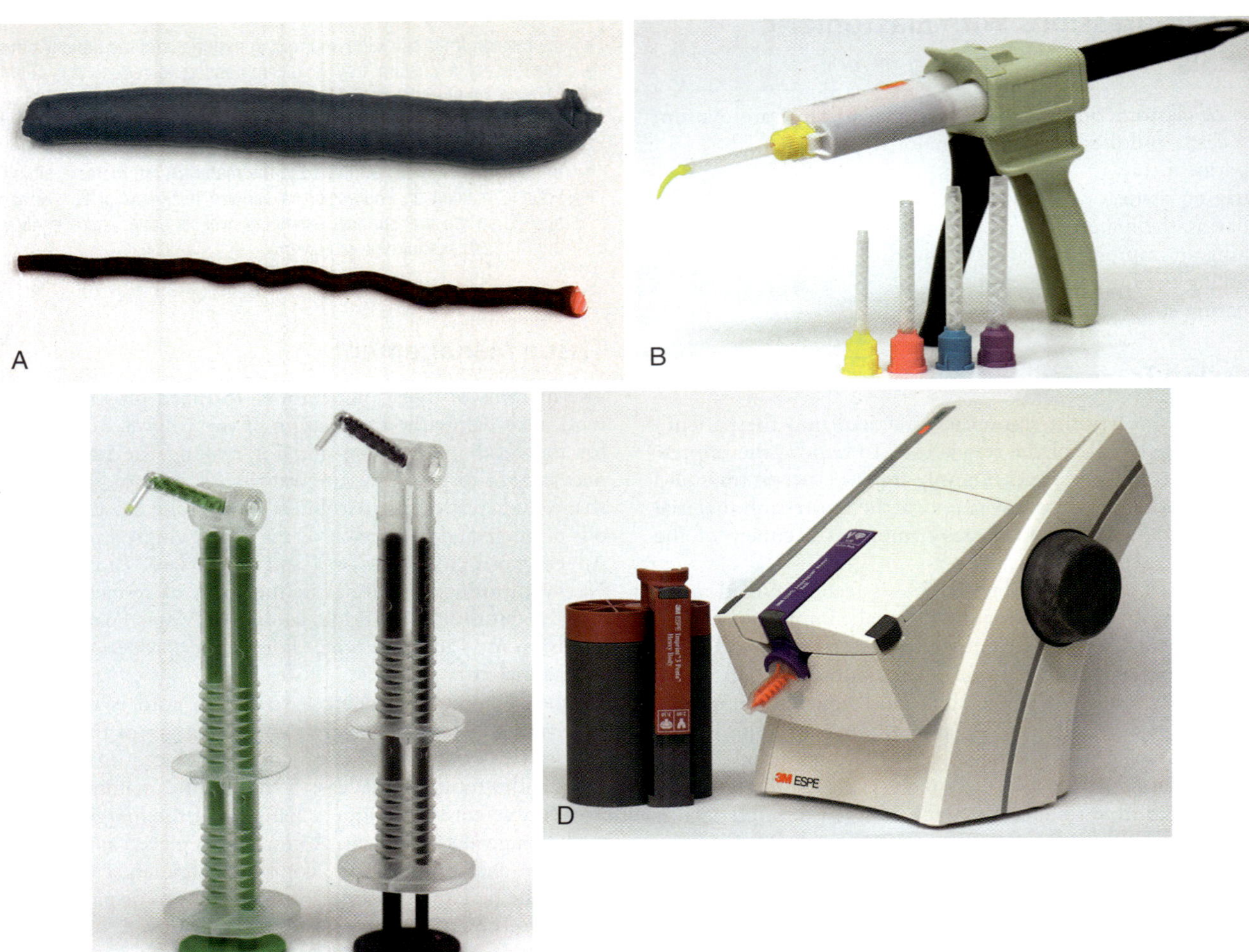

• **Fig. 13.8** Mixing systems. **(A)** Hand mixing. Two equal lengths of the material are dispensed on the mixing pad with the mixing spatula. **(B)** Static mixing. When the trigger is pulled, the plunger is driven forward (*to the left*), so that the base and catalyst pastes are forced from the cartridge into the mixing tip (*extreme left*). The pastes pass through the bore and exit the nozzle as a uniform mixed paste. Four different sizes of mixing tips are shown; the more viscous the material, the larger is the mixing tip that should be used. Syringe tips can be fit to the nozzle to deliver the mixed paste directly to the prepared teeth. **(C)** Static mixing syringe. These syringes fit the cartridge, as the mixing tips shown in **(B)**. The base and catalyst are first injected into the respective barrel. A plunger then forces the material through a smaller static mixing tip. It can deliver the light body material directly onto the abutment(s). **(D)** Dynamic mechanical mixing. The motor-driving mechanism forces the material into the mixing tip and makes the impeller (*insert*) inside the tip rotate. The function of the impeller is only to mix the material.

the mixed paste gets a uniform color, with no streaks of the base or catalyst appearing in the mixture. If one of the components is in liquid form, such as the catalyst for condensation silicones, a length of the base is dispensed from the tube onto a graduated mixing pad and drops of the liquid catalyst corresponding to the length of the base are added. These materials are somewhat difficult to mix because of the difference in the viscosity of the two components.

The two-putty systems available for addition silicone are dispensed by volume using an equal number of scoops of each material. The best mixing technique is to knead the material with one's fingers until a uniform color is obtained. The kneading procedure with the fingers is also applicable with the liquid catalyst of condensation silicone.

Static Mixing

This technique transforms two fluid (or paste-like) materials into a homogeneous mixture without mechanical mixing. The device used to accomplish this mixing is a gun for compressing materials kept in a two-cylinder cartridge, which contains the base and catalyst separately, as well as a mixing tip (Fig. 13.8B). The mixing tip is made of helical mixer elements in a cylindrical housing (Fig. 13.9). The mixer elements are a series of alternating right- and left-turn 180° helixes positioned so that the leading edge of one element is perpendicular to the trailing edge of the next (Fig. 13.9B). The length of each element is about the same as the inner diameter of the cylindrical housing.

The base and catalyst are pressed from the cartridge into the mixing tip as one stream of a two-layer material. The leading edge

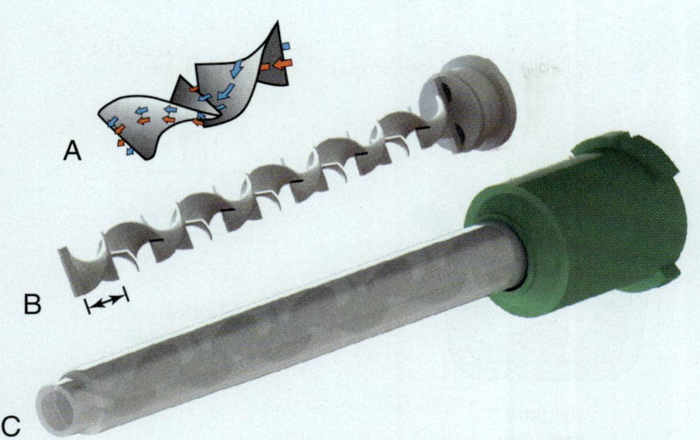

• **Fig. 13.9** Design of a static mixing tip. **(A)** Mechanism of mixing in a two-element model. The two-element model shows that the materials injected into a left-turn helix are immediately split into two streams. Both streams make a 180° counterclockwise turn when they reach the leading edge of the next element, a right-turn helix. Each stream is split as it enters the new element. Two new streams, made of combining two substreams, one from each original stream, now make a 180° clockwise turn when they reach the trailing edge of the element. When there is a third element present, each substream will be split again and the total of substreams will be eight (2^3). **(B)** Mixer elements with 11 helixes. The double-headed arrow delineates the size of one element. The appearance of size difference between neighboring elements is caused by the orientation. **(C)** Mixing tip with encased mixer elements. (Courtesy of K-J. Söderholm.)

of the first element splits the material entering the mixer into two streams. The streams that flow in either side of the helix will make a 180-degree turn (Fig. 13.9A) when they reach the second element. Both streams are split by the leading edge of the second element, and two substreams (one from each original stream) combine into two new streams entering the second element. This process is known as flow division. Assuming that there is no intermixing between the two substreams as they merge, the new stream will have a two-layer structure. After flowing through "n" elements, the number of layers in the stream of material increases to 2^n. The most common mixing tips for impression material mixing have 11 or 12 elements. The stream of material that exits the mixing tip will have a 2048- or 4096-striation structure, which can be treated as a uniformly mixed stream of material. In addition, as the materials make turns along the helix, the rotational circulation causes a radial mixing of the materials. Thus, mixing between substreams occurs before the next flow division that further increases the uniformity of the mixture. Since there is no mechanical mixing, porosity caused by mixing with air is avoided. The mixing tips vary in their diameter, length (number of helical mixer elements), and the size of openings for a specific consistency.

The mixed impression material is injected directly into the adhesive-coated tray or, if the "syringe tip" is in place, onto the prepared teeth. Static mixing provides greater uniformity in proportioning and mixing, yields fewer voids in the mix, and reduces the mixing time. In addition, there are fewer possibilities for contamination of the material. One precaution that should be taken in using these automixing devices is to make sure that the openings of the tubes that dispense the pastes remain unclogged. Problems can be avoided if one expresses a small amount of material from the cartridge before attaching the mixing tip. This type of device has also been adapted to mix and dispense temporary crown and bridge acrylic materials and cements that are used for luting and for producing restorations (Chapter 7).

Dynamic Mechanical Mixing

The device shown in Figure 13.8C uses a motor to drive parallel plungers, forcing the materials into a mixing tip and out into an impression tray or syringe; meanwhile, the motor-driven impeller, which is inside the mixing tip, mixes the materials as they are extruded through the tip. The function of the impeller is only to mix the materials as they are passing through; it does not propel the material. The materials are supplied in collapsible plastic bags housed in a cartridge. The amount of material retained in the mixing tip is slightly greater than that used in static mixing. In using this device, thorough mixing of higher-viscosity materials can be achieved with little effort. Both polyether and addition silicone impression materials of various viscosities are available with this dispensing system.

CRITICAL QUESTION

How does each impression-making technique take advantage of the unique properties of the impression materials?

Making an Impression

Elastomeric impression materials are typically supplied in several viscosities to accommodate different techniques for impression making. Three techniques for making impressions are discussed in this section:

- Multiple-mix technique
- Monophase technique
- Putty-wash technique

Multiple-Mix Technique

A syringe material (light body) and a tray material (heavy body) are used in this technique. Usually, the two groups of materials are mixed simultaneously, each by a different person. With the mechanical devices described earlier, the materials now can be mixed as needed by one individual. The lighter material is injected from the filled syringe or directly from a static mixing gun within and around the tooth preparation. The filled tray is then inserted in the mouth and seated over the syringe material, which has been extruded on hard and/or soft tissue. The tray material will force the syringe material to adapt to the prepared tissues. The two materials should bond together upon setting. If either material has progressed past its working time when the two materials are brought together, the bond between them will be compromised. If a partially set material is seated, it will be compressed elastically. Once removed from the mouth, the impression will "spring back" or relax, and the dies from this impression will be too narrow and too short, as illustrated in Figure 13.10.

In rare cases a clinician may attempt to repair an impression that has small defects or that lacks sufficient detail. This is usually performed by cutting away the interproximal and gingival areas of the impression. Even with proper relief of the initial impression, it will be difficult to reseat the tray precisely. Entrapment of a minute fragment of impression material or debris will eliminate any chance of a successful repair. The impression material's surface must be roughened to ensure that the new material bonds to the set impression. The safest method is to make a new impression when bubbles or similar defects are detected in critical areas.

Monophase Technique

Medium-body polyether and addition silicone are often used for the monophase or single-viscosity technique. The procedure is

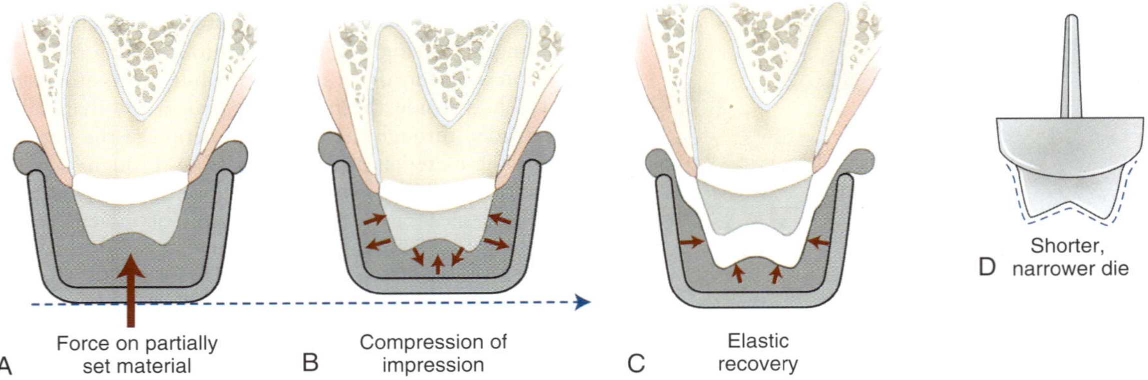

• **Fig. 13.10** Effect of seating tray material that has passed its working time and developed some elasticity. **(A)** Impression tray containing elastomeric impression material is seated too late as elasticity starts to develop. **(B)** Increased seating pressure is applied to overcome the stiffness of impression material. **(C)** Distortion develops during recovery of excessive elastic deformation (spring back). **(D)** The die produced in the inaccurate impression is too narrow and too short.

similar to that of the multiple-mix technique except that only one mixture is made, and part of the material is placed in the tray, and another portion is placed in the syringe for injection in the cavity preparation, prepared teeth, or soft tissue. The success of this technique depends on the pseudoplastic (**shear thinning**) properties of the materials. When a medium-viscosity material is forced through the syringe tip, the viscosity is reduced to allow the material to adapt well to the preparation. Meanwhile, the material in the tray retains its medium viscosity, and, when seated, it can force the syringe material to flow past critical areas of the tooth preparation. Table 13.2 shows the effect of shear rate and elapsed time on some monophase addition silicones.

CRITICAL QUESTION

What are the consequences of placing an impression material in the mouth after the working time has expired?

Putty-Wash Technique

This method was originally developed for condensation silicone to minimize the effect of associated dimensional changes. The thick putty material is placed in a stock tray and a preliminary impression is made. This procedure results in what is essentially an intraoral custom-made tray formed by the putty. Space for the light-body "wash" material is provided either by cutting away some of the "tray" putty or by using a thin polyethylene sheet as a spacer between the putty and the teeth during preliminary impression making. One can also generate the space by vacuum forming a blank plastic sheet on a cast and then make the impression with the putty material. A mixture of the thin-consistency wash material is placed into the putty impression and on the preparation; then the tray is reseated in the mouth to make the final impression.

An alternative approach is to inject the wash material around the preparation and then immediately seat the tray with freshly mixed putty over the wash material. However, this approach risks displacing too much wash material by the putty, so that a critical area of the preparation is reproduced in the putty without the required detail. Occlusal stops should be used in the tray to avoid having the teeth penetrate through the wash or syringe material when the plastic putty mass is being seated.

When the latter technique is used, distortion or incomplete details can result because of excessive pressure applied to the

TABLE 13.2 Viscosity ($\times 10^4$ cp) of Single-Phase Vinyl Polysiloxanes at 37°C

	VISCOSITY AT 1 MIN		VISCOSITY AT 1.5 MIN	
Material	**0.5 rpm**	**2.5 rpm**	**0.5 rpm**	**2.5 rpm**
Baysilex (Miles)	122.1 (2.8)[a]	68.9 (2.5)	211.2 (14.7)	148.8 (1.2)
Green-Mouse (Parkell)	133.7 (8.9)	56.7 (2.9)	247.9 (14.9)	78.0 (2.8)
Hydrosil (Caulk)	194.2 (8.5)	129.4 (4.1)	398.1 (7.8)	153.5[b]
Imprint (3M)	106.5 (12.2)	79.7 (2.2)	245.1 (8.9)	146.2 (5.9)
Omnisil (Coe)	156.8 (11.5)	102.5 (1.9)	347.1 (5.2)	153.5[c]

[a]Numbers within parentheses represent the standard deviation of the mean.
[b]Value at 75 s after mixing.
[c]Value at 77 s after mixing.
From Kim K-N, Craig RG, Koran A: Viscosity of monophase addition silicones as a function of shear rate. *J Prosthet Dent* 67:794, 1992.

setting putty. After being removed from the mouth, the pressure in the impression is released and the putty recovers its "elastic deformation." The distortion produced by the stiff, compressible putty results in a short, narrow die (Fig. 13.10). In addition to excessive pressure, some of the distortion in putty-wash impressions may be attributable to inadequate space for the wash material.

Removal of the Impression

Under no circumstances should the impression be removed until the curing has progressed sufficiently to provide adequate elasticity, so that distortion will not occur. One method for determining the time of removal is to inject some of the syringe material onto a space that is not in the field of operation before inserting the impression tray. This material can be probed with a blunt instrument from time to time; when it is firm and returns completely to its original contour, the impression is sufficiently elastic to be removed. When a multiple-mix technique is used, it is advisable to test both the syringe and the tray materials in this manner. Typically, the impression should be ready for removal within at least 10 min from the time of mixing, allowing 5–8 min for the impression to remain in the mouth. Manufacturers usually provide the optimal time for removal after mixing.

The mechanics of removing the impression involves separation at the impression/tissue interface and stretching of the impression. The first step is to break the physical adhesion between the tissue and the impression; therefore, an impression material, such as polyether, that wets the tissue well will require extra effort to break the seal for the removal. The second step stretches the impression enough to pass under the height of contour of the hard tissue to remove the impression; therefore, using a material of higher rigidity will require a greater force to stretch the impression to facilitate removal. Polysulfide has the lowest viscosity and ranks as one of the least stiff of the elastomeric impression materials of a similar consistency. This flexibility allows the set material to be easily removed from undercut areas and from the mouth with a minimum of stress.

In addition, all elastomeric impression materials are viscoelastic, and it is necessary to use a quick snap to minimize plastic deformation of the impression during the final step of the removal process. The phenomenon of viscoelastic behavior is discussed in subsequent sections.

Preparation of Stone Casts and Dies

The hydrophobic characteristics of silicone impression materials make them suitable for pouring of epoxy resin to produce dies. However, this hydrophobicity makes pouring with gypsum products challenging, as it increases the potential of forming voids in gypsum dies and casts. There are a number of surfactant sprays, also known as debubblizers, which can improve the surface wettability of the silicone impression material for the stone slurry. Only a thin layer of surfactant should be applied to the impression surface. A dilute solution of soap is also an effective surfactant. An alternative to the use of a surfactant is to select a hydrophilized addition silicone (discussed later). Pouring of a stone cast in a polyether or polysulfide impression does not require the aid of a surfactant.

The excellent dimensional stability of addition silicone and polyether impression materials makes it possible to construct two or three casts or dies from these materials. It is also possible to construct successive stone dies or casts from polysulfide impressions when duplicate stone dies are needed. However, each successive die will be less accurate than the first die constructed from the material. The time interval between impression pours should not be greater than 30 min. To minimize tearing and gross distortion after the first pour, the clinician should remove the excess gypsum-forming mass from undercut areas along the periphery of the tray. Be aware that the stiffness of the impression material makes it difficult to remove the stone cast from the impression. A weak stone cast may fracture during removal.

- The hydrophobic characteristics of silicone impression materials make pouring with gypsum products challenging, as it increases the potential of forming voids in gypsum dies and casts.
- There are several surfactant sprays—also known as debubblizers—that can improve the surface wettability of the silicone impression material.

Properties of Elastomeric Impression Materials

The goal of impression making is to produce an accurate impression that can yield a cast or die that reproduces the surface details and precise shape of the original tissue as closely as possible. Meanwhile, the dimensions of the impression should remain stable during the production of dies or casts. In this section, the properties relevant to impression making with elastomers are described.

CRITICAL QUESTION

Why is it not advisable to alter the base/catalyst (accelerator) ratio as a means of controlling working or **setting time**?

Working and Setting Times

Table 13.3 lists working and setting times for the various kinds of elastomeric materials as measured by an oscillating rheometer. The working time, which begins at the start of mixing and ends just before the elastic properties have developed, must be greater than the time required for mixing, filling the syringe and/or tray, injecting the material on tooth preparations, and seating the tray. The setting time is the time that has elapsed from the beginning of mixing until the curing process has advanced sufficiently that the impression can be removed from the mouth with no distortion. However, polymerization may continue for a considerable time after setting. An increase in temperature accelerates the rate of polymerization of all elastomeric impression materials; therefore, the effect of temperature on working and setting time should be taken into consideration.

Working time and setting time decrease as the filler content in the materials increases. Altering the base/catalyst ratio will change the curing rate of these impression materials. Normally, having more base materials in the mixture tends to increase the working and setting times. One should be aware that this is not economical, as a portion of the paste is not used. Moreover, since the accelerator paste contains a retarder as well as a reactor, increasing the base/accelerator ratio may not produce a predictable change in the polymerization rate.

Reproduction of Oral Structure Detail

A surface reproduction test is a requirement of national standards for elastomeric impression materials. There is little doubt that these elastomers can record detail to the finest degree. When

TABLE 13.3 Working and Setting Times of Elastomeric Impression Materials

	MEAN WORKING TIME (MIN)		MEAN SETTING TIME (MIN)	
Impression material	23°C	37°C	23°C	37°C
Polysulfide	6.0	4.3	16.0	12.5
Condensation silicone	3.3	2.5	11.0	8.9
Addition silicone	3.1	1.8	8.9	5.9
Polyether	3.3	2.3	9.0	8.3

From Harcourt JK: A review of modern impression materials. *Aust Dent J* 23:178, 1978.

dental stone is poured on the surface of such test impressions, the finest detail is not always reproduced. The reason for this situation is that the elastomeric impression materials are capable of reproducing detail more accurately than can be transferred from the stone die or cast, which may not be capable of such accuracy.

The clinical significance of the surface reproduction tests is not entirely evident. It is possible that the detail obtained from the elastomeric impression materials under in vitro test conditions might be greater than that obtained in the mouth because of the hydrophobicity exhibited by some of these materials.

CRITICAL QUESTION

Why is rapid seating of an impression tray not advisable for a pseudoplastic impression material?

Rheological Properties

Impression materials are introduced into the mouth as viscous pastes with precisely adjusted flow properties. The viscosity and flow behavior of the unmixed components are also important in regard to the ease of mixing, air entrapment during mixing, and the tendency for the trapped air to escape before the impression is made.

Ideally, the impression material should flow freely and wet the tissue as it is being injected to achieve adaptation, and then resist flow away from the intended surface areas. The same procedure will facilitate spreading of heavy-body material on the impression tray and retain it in the tray. This phenomenon is called shear thinning. Essentially, a stress-thinning material becomes less viscous when stressed as during injection and then recovers its viscosity when it rests on the tissue or in the tray. All elastomeric impression materials exhibit shear-thinning characteristics before setting.

There are two categories of shear-thinning phenomena, **pseudoplasticity** and **thixotropy**, depending on how the material responds to the applied stress and how it behaves at rest. A pseudoplastic material displays decreasing viscosity with increasing shear stress, and recovers its viscosity immediately upon a decrease in shear stress. A thixotropic material does not flow until sufficient energy in the form of an impact force or a vibration force is applied to overcome the yield stress of the material. At rest it takes a specific time to regain its previous viscous state. Drip or run-off tests, which record the quantity of impression material that flows away from the preparation, have been used to demonstrate the phenomenon of thixotropy. Essentially the tests determine whether the impression material at rest continues to flow under the influence of gravity. Manufacturers that emphasize their materials being thixotropic also note that the materials exhibit no slump when injected on a vertical surface. They usually do not mention the duration of time delay. In this context, the phenomenon should be termed extreme shear thinning as the material retains an immobile state at rest but flows freely under stress.

The benefit of thixotropy in impression making has been disputed, since the time duration needed for the impression material to recover the necessary viscosity may be unacceptable. Other reports suggest that a thixotropic material should facilitate handling and make better impressions.

However, the latter does not address the effect of time lag on the impression-making process.

Finally, it is important to note that the shear- thinning property of addition silicone and polyether impression materials enables the clinician to use a monophase impression-making technique to capture the details needed for fixed prostheses to produce an impression that is more stable and resistant to distortion than a light-viscosity material.

CRITICAL QUESTION

How does the viscoelastic property of impression materials dictate the manner in which an impression must be removed from a patient's mouth?

Elasticity and Viscoelasticity

An impression material sustains some deformation as it is removed from the mouth, but it must rebound to its preremoval dimensions. An impression with a sufficiently high elastic limit should not sustain permanent deformation. The elastic properties of these elastomeric impression materials improve with an increase in curing time in the mouth, since the setting time stated by the manufacturer is not always adequate for the development of sufficient elasticity to prevent permanent deformation upon removal of the impression. An extra time of 1 or 2 min before removal may be beneficial.

The relative amount of permanent deformation in compression following strain induced during removal increases in the following order for impression materials: addition silicone, condensation silicone, polyether, and polysulfide. Recovery of elastic deformation following strain is less rapid for the polysulfide material than for the other three types of impression materials.

To understand why impression material may exhibit permanent deformation after being subjected to a compressive force during removal and why recovery of elastic deformation occurs

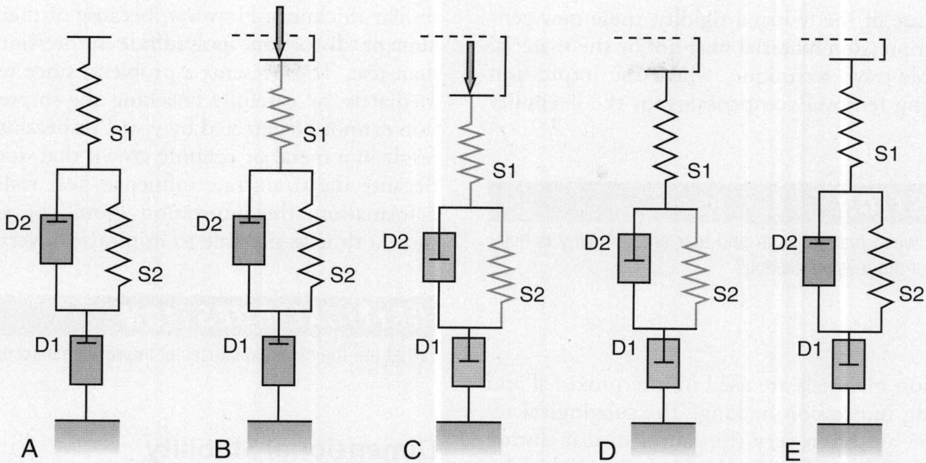

• **Fig. 13.11** A mechanical model showing the response of a viscoelastic material to external loading and unloading. **(A)** Maxwell–Voigt viscoelastic model in a stress-free state. **(B)** During loading, only spring S1 contracts in response to the load. **(C)** When the loading continues, the pistons in dashpot D1 and D2 move proportionally to the duration of loading. Spring S2 contracts along with dashpot D2. No change is expected for spring S1. **(D)** The moment the load is released, spring S1 recovers instantly, whereas the rest of the elements remain unchanged. Spring S2 should also recover instantly but is retarded by the sluggishness of dashpot D2. **(E)** As time passes, spring S2 recovers and extends dashpot D2 slowly to near its original position. Dashpot D1 remains unchanged. The right-hand bracket on the top of each model denotes the degree of deformation.

when an impression material rests on a bench top over time, one must recognize that all elastomeric impression materials are viscoelastic materials. The characteristics of a viscoelastic solid are intermediate between those of an elastic solid and a viscous liquid. An elastic solid can be viewed as a spring (S1 and S2 in Fig. 13.11), which deforms instantly to a certain extent when one applies a specific force. The deformation will be reversed completely when the force is removed. On the other hand, a viscous liquid behaves in a manner similar to that of an oil dashpot (D1 and D2 in Fig. 13.11), which does not respond instantly to any sudden external force but deforms as the load is applied constantly over time. The dashpot continues to deform at a rate proportional to the duration of force application. Compared with the reversible behavior of an elastic solid, the deformation exhibited by the dashpot is permanent. Only a force applied from the opposite direction can restore the dashpot to its original form. The simplest model that demonstrates the viscoelastic behavior is a Maxwell–Voigt model (Fig. 13.11A), which consists of a spring (S1) and a dashpot (D1) in series and a second set (S2 and D2) in parallel.

When a compressive force is applied, S1 responds instantaneously with a definite amount of strain (deformation). At this instant, neither D1 nor D2 responds to the force applied. Meanwhile, S2 cannot respond because the inertia of D2 is preventing S2 from responding (Fig. 13.11B). When the force is maintained on the model, D1 and D2 will begin to move and stop when the force is removed. During this period, S2 moves as much as D2 (Fig. 13.11C). Meanwhile, spring S1 maintains the same magnitude of strain and the amount of movement by D2 is proportional to the duration of force application. When the load is removed, the deformation by spring S1 recovers while the rest remains unchanged (Fig. 13.11D). As time passes, spring S2 slowly overcomes the inertia of dashpot D2 and recovers along with D2 (Fig. 13.11E). This process usually takes time, and the deformation may not recover completely. The deformation of dashpot D1 never recovers.

According to the model, the amount of deformation exhibited by D2 is the permanent deformation observed after removal of the impression. The effort of S2 to recover to its original dimension is equivalent to the elastic recovery of the impression over time. It is apparent from the model that keeping the time of applied force on the impression to a minimum will result in the least amount of permanent deformation. This explains why removal of the impression should be done in a snap, if possible, and a teasing or rocking method should be avoided. However, a slight teasing action will first be required to break the seal between the impression material and the hard and soft tissues.

The PVS impression materials exhibit the most elastic recovery of the currently available materials. Distortion on removal from undercuts is virtually nonexistent because these materials exhibit the lowest permanent distortion after excessive strain in compression. However, the excellent elastic properties present a problem in that the heavy-body putty material begins to acquire elastic properties while it is still in the working-time stage. If the material is at an advanced stage of elasticity and is compressed excessively during the seating of the impression, distortion can occur when the material elastically rebounds (Fig. 13.10).

The stiffness (elastic modulus) of earlier generations of impression materials of similar viscosity was reported to increase in the following order: polysulfide, condensation silicone, addition silicone, and polyether. The difficulty of removing earlier generations of polyether impressions from undercut areas was attributed to their high modulus of elasticity. These materials were so stiff that making impressions of teeth with severe periodontal involvement using polyether carried the risk of tooth extraction. The new generations of polyether impression materials with a stiffness lower than that of hydrophilic PVS were formulated specifically to address concerns about the stiffness of the early materials. Although the new polyether materials are significantly more flexible than that of PVS at the time of removal, their adhesion, which results from the inherent hydrophilicity, can still make the impression removal difficult. Because of the reduced rigidity, these new generations of polyether impression material may not be the material of choice for the "triple-tray" technique, where the impression material's stiffness during removal compensates for the flexibility of the tray.

CRITICAL QUESTION

What is the difference between tear strength and tear energy? Why is tear energy more meaningful for impression making?

Tear Strength

Low-viscosity impression materials are used in interproximal and subgingival areas during impression making. The subgingival regions of the impression are often very thin and can tear during impression removal, leaving a portion embedded within the gingival sulcus (Fig. 13.12). The amount of force needed to tear a specified test specimen divided by the thickness of the specimen is called the tear strength. There is no standard method for testing the tear strength of impression materials, since ISO 4823 (Dentistry—Elastomeric impression materials) does not address such a test method. Figure 13.13 shows two configurations described in a nondental standard (ISO 34-1; Rubber, vulcanized or thermoplastic—Determination of tear strength—Part 1: Trouser, angle and crescent test pieces that have been used by the dental community for testing impression materials).

A tear strength test measures the resistance of an elastomeric material to fracture when subjected to a tensile force acting perpendicular to a surface flaw. The ranking of tear strength from the lowest to highest of the impression materials is as follows: silicones (addition and condensation), polyether, and polysulfide. However, the literature has shown that some polyethers or silicones have higher tear strength than certain polysulfides.

Tear strength is influenced by consistency and the manner of removing the materials. An increased consistency usually increases the tear strength of the material. The addition of a thinning agent to the mixture reduces tear strength slightly but increases flexibility substantially. A quick snap in removing the impression usually increases the tear strength, as the action increases the resistance of the material to deformation (strain).

Polysulfide materials have the highest resistance to tearing. Therefore, thin sections of polysulfide impression material are less likely to tear than polyether or silicone impression materials of a similar thickness. However, because of their susceptibility to permanent distortion, polysulfide impressions may distort rather than tear. This presents a problem, since tearing can be seen immediately by carefully checking the impression, whereas distortion cannot be detected by visual inspection. Thus, distortion can result in a metal or ceramic crown that does not seat completely. Because the strain rate influences tear resistance and permanent deformation, the impression should be strained rapidly for as short a time as possible to minimize adverse effects.

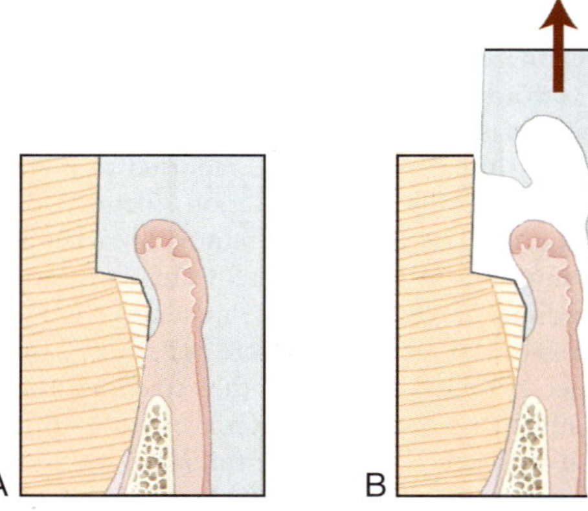

• **Fig. 13.12 (A)** A properly retracted soft tissue will leave a narrow space to be filled by the light-viscosity impression material. **(B)** The impression material has torn during removal.

CRITICAL QUESTION

What are the six main causes of impression inaccuracy?

Dimensional Stability

It is important to distinguish between dimensional accuracy and dimensional stability. The former refers to the lack of dimensional change during curing and shortly after removal from the mouth. The latter refers to the lack of dimensional changes over time. Accuracy is the more important property when impressions are poured up immediately with a die material. This distinction is important because the two do not go hand in hand; materials may be accurate but not stable or inaccurate but stable.

There are six major sources of dimensional change:

1. polymerization shrinkage,
2. loss of a condensation reaction by-product (water or alcohol),
3. thermal contraction from oral temperature to room temperature,
4. absorption of water or disinfectant over a period of time,
5. incomplete recovery of deformation because of viscoelastic behavior, and
6. incomplete recovery because of plastic deformation.

Dimensional changes during curing have been measured directly and indirectly using confined and freestanding specimens of the elastomers in various geometrical shapes. In American National Standards Institute/American Dental Association (ANSI/ADA) Specification No. 19 (ISO 4823), a disk of the impression material is placed on a talc-covered glass plate. At the end of 24 h, the contraction should not exceed 0.5% for type I and III materials, or 1.0% for a type II material. Thus, the measurement includes contraction associated with a thermal change (37–23°C), polymerization shrinkage, and loss of volatile components.

Figure 13.14 shows the mean linear contraction for four elastomers using the method just described. It is evident that all materials change dimensionally over time. The change is greater in magnitude for the polysulfide and condensation silicone materials than for the polyether and addition silicone elastomers. This result is expected because polysulfide and condensation silicone lose polymerization by-products, that is, water and alcohol, respectively.

If maximal accuracy is to be maintained with polysulfide and condensation silicone materials, the slurry mix for a stone die or cast should be poured immediately into the impression after it is removed from the mouth. *Immediately* is defined as within the first 30 min even when the putty-wash technique is used for silicone materials.

The stability of the addition silicone and polyether materials suggests that these impressions do not have to be poured with a gypsum product immediately. In fact, these impressions are often sent to the lab to be poured. It should be noted, however, that some later-generation polyethers are not as dimensionally stable as their predecessors; therefore, immediate pours may be needed.

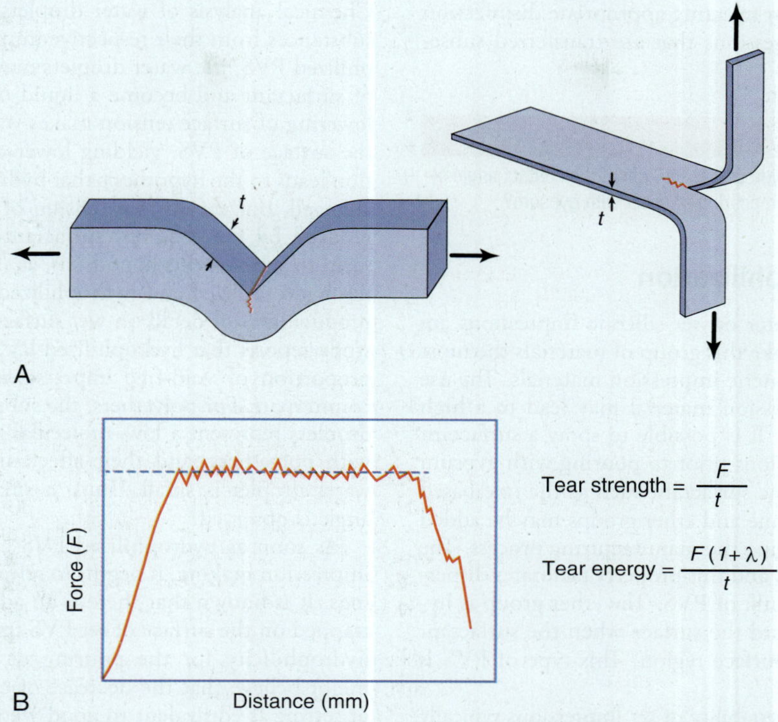

• **Fig. 13.13** **(A)** Two configurations of tear strength test specimens: Die C or right-angle design such as described in the ASTM D624 Plastic Test Standard (*left*) and trouser design configuration (*right*). **(B)** Force–distance curve of a typical tear test and calculation of tear strength and tear energy. The plateau of the curve (*dotted line*) indicates the force (*F*) needed for initiation and propagation of the crack. The thickness of the specimen is *t* and the extension ratio is λ, which equals the extended portion of the specimen length at the end of the test divided by the original length of the specimen.

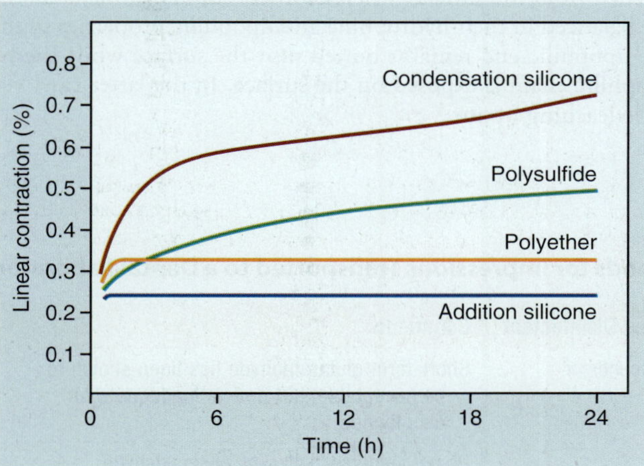

• **Fig. 13.14** Representative linear contraction of four elastomeric impression materials.

Research has shown that a cast produced from an addition silicone impression between 24 h and 1 week is as accurate as a cast made in the first hour assuming that there is no effect associated with the formation of hydrogen bubbles. These materials exhibit the least amount of distortion from the loads imposed on the set material. Thus, multiple pouring of the impressions and removal of the casts will not alter the dimensional stability of the impression even though a substantial force is needed each time a cast is removed from the impression.

One variable that has a negative effect on the polyether impression is the absorption of water or fluids and the simultaneous leaching of the water-soluble plasticizer. Thus, the polyether impression should be stored in a dry (relative humidity below 50%), cool environment to maintain its accuracy and should never be left for protracted periods in disinfecting solutions.

CRITICAL QUESTION

Why are hydrophilic materials potentially more susceptible to distortion during disinfection prior to being poured with a gypsum-forming product?

Disinfection

Condensation silicones, addition silicones, and polysulfides can be disinfected with all Environmental Protection Agency ***(EPA)***-registered disinfectants without the loss of surface quality or accuracy if the disinfection time is short. The impressions should be immersed for the time specified for each disinfectant. After disinfection, the impression should be removed, rinsed, and poured with the gypsum product as soon as possible.

It is important to note that a long immersion time may cause the surfactant in the hydrophilic PVS to leach out and render the impression less hydrophilic. The polyethers are also susceptible to dimensional change if immersed for a long time (more than 10 min) because of their pronounced hydrophilic nature, which tends to promote water absorption from the surroundings.

Table 13.4 shows a guide for selecting appropriate disinfection methods for all types of impressions that are transferred subsequently to a dental laboratory.

CRITICAL QUESTION

How does the surfactant added to hydrophilize PVS affect the contact angle of water droplets during the setting and pouring of casts with gypsum?

Wettability and Hydrophilization

Contact angles of distilled water on set silicone impressions are approximately 100°, which make this group of materials the most hydrophobic among all elastomeric impression materials. The use of a more hydrophobic impression material may lead to a high frequency of voids in the cast. It is possible to spray a surfactant on these hydrophobic impressions prior to pouring with gypsum mixtures. Otherwise a nonionic surfactant such as the one based on a block copolymer of siloxane and ether groups may be added to the bulk of the material during the manufacturing process. The siloxane group is hydrophobic, and this property facilitates dispersion of the surfactant in the bulk of PVS. The ether group is hydrophilic and is oriented toward the surface when the surfactant migrates by diffusion to the surface region. This type of PVS is called a hydrophilized PVS.

In vitro studies of surface wettability of set impressions typically use distilled water as the probing liquid. The results confirm that there is a significant reduction in contact angle of hydrophilized PVS relative to their nonhydrophilized counterparts. Use of an aqueous solution saturated with $CaSO_4$ yields similar results. Examination of stone casts confirms that elastomers, which exhibit the least contact angle with water, also produce stone casts with fewer voids.

The use of optical tensiometry, which analyzes the shape of liquid drops on the surface using a video image, allows observation of contact angles of water droplets on freshly mixed impression materials in real time. Numerous studies have reported a decrease in water contact angles on silicones, hydrophilized PVS, and polyethers over the setting period. This decrease can be as much as 70° for hydrophilized PVS and less for polyether. Chemical analysis of water droplets shows that they all acquire substances from their respective impression materials. For hydrophilized PVS, the water droplets may absorb a sufficient quantity of surfactant and become a liquid of lower surface tension. The lowering of surface tension makes water droplets spread wider on the surface of PVS, yielding lower contact angles. This observation leads to the hypothesis that hydrophilicity of the PVS has not changed, but the surface tension of the probing water has been reduced by the acquired surfactant. Some clinical observations seem to support this hypothesis, as there is no difference between nonhydrophilized and hydrophilized PVS with respect to the reproducibility of detail on wet surfaces. However, another clinical study reports that hydrophilized PVS yields a significantly higher proportion of void-free impressions than its nonhydrophilized counterpart. For polyethers, the substances acquired by the water droplets represent a low–molecular-weight compound associated with polyethers, and their effect on the surface tension of the water droplet is small. Thus, a smaller decrease in the contact angle is observed.

As soon as hydrophilized PVS encounters oral fluids during impression making, it begins to release surfactant to its surroundings. It is known that there is an adequate amount of surfactant trapped on the surface of set PVS impressions, thereby providing hydrophilicity for the pouring of gypsum dies. Whereas one might believe that the decrease of contact angle over the period of setting is equivalent to good wetting of the impression material on moist tooth surfaces, the clinical relevance remains unclear for two reasons. First, the decrease in contact angle may be attributed mainly to the lowering of the surface tension of the water droplets by the surfactant, so the actual improvement in the hydrophilicity of the impression may be much less significant than it appears. Second, there are conflicting clinical observations. This conflict is not surprising when one realizes that some materials contain very hydrophilic surfactants that are readily leached from the surface, whereas others contain surfactants that are balanced in their hydrophilic and lipophilic properties so that the lipophilic end remains buried near the surface while the hydrophilic chain is exposed on the surface. In the latter case, very little leaching occurs.

TABLE 13.4 Guide for the Selection of Appropriate Disinfection Methods for Impressions Transported to a Dental Laboratory

Material	Method	Recommended Disinfectant	Comments
Alginate	Immersion with caution Use only disinfectant for a short-term exposure time (<10 min for alginate)	Chlorine compounds or iodophors	Short-term glutaraldehyde has been shown to be acceptable, but time is inadequate for disinfection
Agar			Do not immerse in alkaline glutaraldehyde
Polysulfide and silicone	Immersion	Glutaraldehydes, chlorine compounds, iodophors, phenolics	Disinfectants requiring more than 30 min exposure time are not recommended
Polyether	Immerse with caution Use disinfectant only for a short exposure time (<10 min)	Chlorine compounds or iodophors	ADA recommends any of the disinfectant classes; however, short-term exposures are essential to avoid distortion
ZOE impression paste	Immersion preferred; spraying can be used for bite registrations	Glutaraldehydes or iodophors	Not compatible with chlorine compounds. Phenolic spray can be used
Impression compound		Iodophors or chlorine compounds	Phenolic spray can be used

CRITICAL QUESTION

How can a torn impression material cause gingival inflammation?

Biocompatibility

The clinical relevance of tests for the assessment of the cytotoxicity of dental materials is widely recognized. Various types of tests are covered in ISO 10993-5, Biological Evaluation of Medical Devices: Tests for In Vitro Cytotoxicity. Comparing the cell cytotoxicity for different impression materials reveals that polysulfide materials result in the lowest cell death count and the set polyether impression material produces the highest cell cytotoxicity scores (Fig. 13.15). Similar results are also observed in multiple exposure tests.

The most likely elastomer-induced biocompatibility problem occurs when a fragment of impression material is trapped in a patient's gingival sulcus. In fact, fragments of impression materials have been found in soft tissues, under the periosteum, in the spongy bone, and in the maxillary sinus. This can also occur in implant dentistry, particularly during second-stage implant surgery or during single-stage surgery. A foreign body of impression material is known to cause a severe gingival inflammation, which may be misdiagnosed as an adverse effect of the tooth preparation or cementation. If evidence of tearing is detected during careful visual inspection of the impression (Fig. 13.12), it is important to examine the gingival sulcus immediately to remove any remnant of the impression or any other foreign body, such as a piece of retraction cord. The radiopacity of polysulfide materials is an advantage in these situations.

Some concerns exist about the hypersensitivity potential of the polyether catalyst system. Contact dermatitis from the polyether, especially as experienced by dental assistants, has been reported. In contrast, no cytotoxic effects have been reported clinically from exposure to polyether components, particularly the imine catalyst.

Shelf Life

Properly compounded impression material does not deteriorate appreciably in the tube or container before the expiration date when it is stored in a dry, cool environment. When one observes clear liquid being expressed along with the material, it is an indication of plasticizer segregation and is indicative of manufacturing error or excessive temperature extremes during storage.

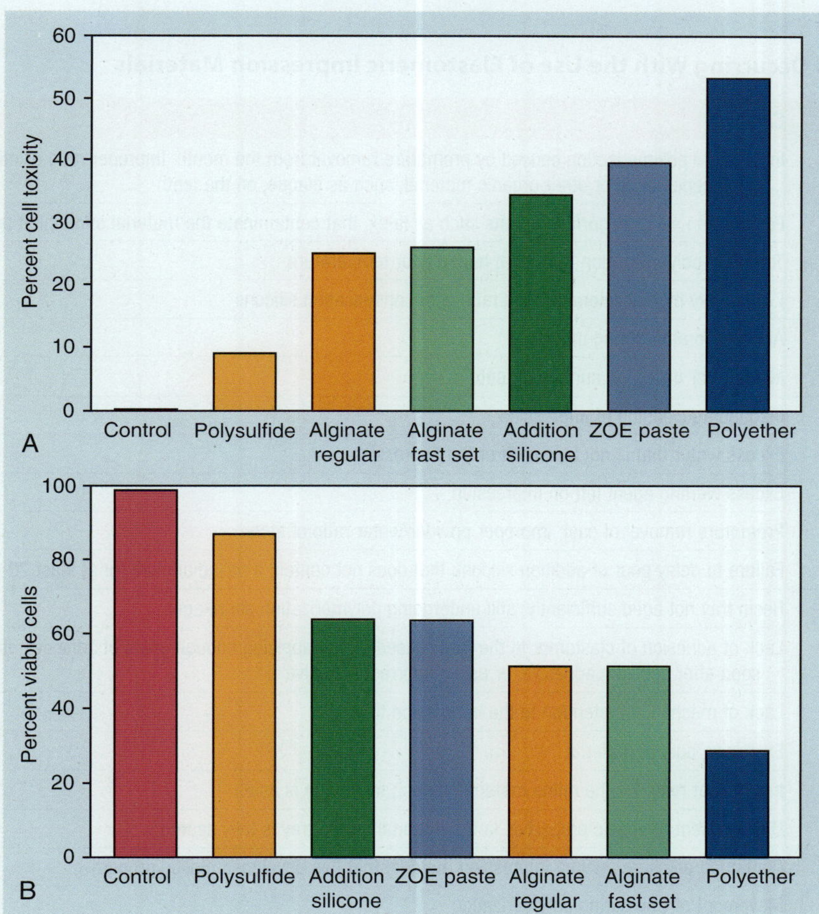

• **Fig. 13.15** Results of a cytotoxicity test of impression materials. **(A)** Graph of cell cytotoxicity shows that, after 3 days of incubation with Vero cells, all of the impression materials were cytotoxic to varying degrees. The relative cytotoxicity of each material is shown relative to the control. **(B)** The graph of cell viability exhibits the relative percent of viable cells after being exposed to the impression materials. (Adapted from Sydiskis RK, Gerhardt DE: Cytotoxicity of impression materials. J Prosthet Dent 69:431, 1993.)

Effect of Mishandling

The failure to produce an accurate epoxy or gypsum die or cast is more likely associated with an error in handling the impression material rather than a deficiency in the material properties. The common failures experienced with impression materials and their causes are summarized in Table 13.5. The comparative properties of elastomeric impression materials are listed in Table 13.6. A summary of the characteristics of the elastomeric impression materials is given in Table 13.7.

CRITICAL QUESTION

What is the difference between a solution and a hydrocolloid?

Hydrocolloids

Colloid is a substance that is microscopically dispersed uniformly throughout another substance. This description appears to be similar to that of a solution. Contrary to the true solutions, which exist as a single phase, a colloidal system consists of two separate phases: the dispersed phase and the dispersion phase. If the dispersion phase of a colloidal system is water, it is called a hydrocolloid. The sizes of the colloid particles range from 1 to 200 nm. In this section the characteristics of the two hydrocolloids for impression making, agar and alginate, are described.

Characteristics of Hydrocolloids

During impression making, the material sets from a flowable state to a solid state. This change of state associated with hydrocolloids is called the sol–gel transformation. A **sol** is a colloidal dispersion of very small particles in a continuous liquid medium and a **gel** is a suspension that behaves like an elastic solid. If a hydrocolloid contains an adequate concentration of the dispersed phase, the sol, under certain conditions, may change to a gel. In the gel state, the dispersed phase forms agglomerates in the form of chains or fibrils, also called **micelles**. The fibrils may branch and intermesh to form a brush heap structure, which can be envisioned as resembling the intermeshing of tree branches or twigs in a brush pile. The dispersion medium is held in the interstices between the fibrils by capillary attraction or adhesion.

Agar (Reversible Hydrocolloid)

The physical change of agar from sol to gel is induced by lowering the temperature. The gel liquefies to a sol when it is heated to a

TABLE 13.5 Common Failures Occurring With the Use of Elastomeric Impression Materials

Type of Failure	Causes
Rough or uneven impression surface	Incomplete polymerization caused by premature removal from the mouth, improper ratio or mixing of components, or presence of oil or other organic material, such as plaque, on the teeth
	For addition silicone, surface agents such as latex, that contaminate the material and inhibit polymerization
	Too rapid polymerization from high humidity or temperature
	Excessively high accelerator/base ratio with condensation silicone
Bubbles	Air incorporated during mixing
Irregularly shaped voids	Moisture or debris on surface of teeth
Rough or chalky stone cast	Inadequate cleaning of impression
	Excess water that is not blown off of the impression
	Excess wetting agent left on impression
	Premature removal of cast; improper powder/water ratio of stone
	Failure to delay pour of addition silicone that does not contain a palladium salt for at least 20 min
Distortion	Resin tray not aged sufficiently; still undergoing polymerization shrinkage
	Lack of adhesion of elastomer to the tray caused by not applying enough coats of adhesive, filling tray with material too soon after applying adhesive, or using incorrect adhesive
	Lack of mechanical retention to the impression tray
	Excessive bulk of material
	Insufficient relief for the reline material (if such technique is used)
	Development of elastic properties in the material before tray is fully seated
	Continued pressure against impression material that has developed elastic properties
	Movement of tray during polymerization
	Premature removal of impression from mouth
	Improper removal of impression from mouth
	Delayed pouring of the polysulfide or condensation silicone impression

TABLE 13.6 **Comparative Properties of Elastomeric Impression Materials**

Property	Polysulfide	Condensation Silicone	Addition Silicone	Polyether
Working time (min)	4–7	2.5–4	2–4	3
Setting time (min)	7–10	6–8	4–6.5	6
Tear strength (N/m)	2500–7000	2300–2600	1500–4300	1800–4800
Percent contraction (at 24 h)	0.40–0.45	0.38–0.60	0.14–0.17	0.19–0.24
Contact angle between set material and water (°)	82	98	98/53[a]	49
Hydrogen gas evolution (Y/N)[b]	N	N	Y[c]	N
Automatic mixing (Y/N)**	N	N	Y	Y
Custom tray (Y/N)[b]	Y	N	N	N
Unpleasant odor (Y/N)[b]	Y	N	N	N
Multiple casts (Y/N)[b]	N	N	Y	Y
Stiffness (value of 1 indicates greatest stiffness)[d]	3	2 (1)	2 (1)	1 (2)
Distortion on removal (value of 1 indicates the greatest and 4 the least potential distortion)	1	2	4	3

[a]The lower contact angle resulted from testing of a hydrophilized PVS.
[b](Y/N) stands for yes or no.
[c]A hydrogen absorber is often included to eliminate hydrogen gas evolution.
[d]The numbers in the parentheses reflect the ranking when soft formulation of polyether impression material is considered.

temperature known as the liquefaction temperature (70–100°C). When the sol is cooled, it becomes a gel at a point known as the **gelation** temperature (between 37°C and 50°C). Thus, it is called a reversible hydrocolloid. The gelation temperature is critical for impression making. If it is too high, the heat from the sol may injure the oral tissues. Conversely, if the gelation temperature is too far below oral temperature, it will be impossible to make the impression because the sol will not convert to a gel.

Composition

Agar, a polysaccharide extracted from certain types of seaweed, is the main active ingredient in the material, while water is the major constituent in the agar impression material (Table 13.8). A small percentage of borax is added to strengthen the gel. Since borax is a potent retarder for the setting of gypsum, an accelerator such as potassium sulfate is added to counteract the effect of borax. Other fillers—such as diatomaceous earth, clay, silica, wax, rubber, and similar inert powders—are used to control strength, viscosity, and rigidity, as previously discussed for elastomeric impression materials. Thymol and glycerin may also be added as a bactericidal agent and plasticizer, respectively. Pigments and flavors are usually included as well. The hydrocolloid is usually supplied in two forms, syringe material and tray material.

CRITICAL QUESTION

What is the purpose of having three water tanks set at three different temperatures in a conditioning unit for agar impression materials?

Making the Agar Impression

This process requires a three-compartment conditioning unit (Fig. 13.16) for the agar tray material that allows liquefaction, storage, and tempering, while the agar syringe material is used only in the liquefaction and storage compartments.

The first step in impression making is to liquefy the hydrocolloid gel in the tube in boiling water at 100°C for a minimum of 10 min. The tube is then placed in a storage bath at 65°C to retain the sol condition until it is needed for impression. For the immediate preparation step, the impression tray is filled with hydrocolloid sol from the tube taken from the storage bath, a gauze pad is placed over the top of the tray material, and the tray is placed in the water-filled tempering compartment (at about 45°C) of the conditioning unit. The tempering time is 3–10 min, just sufficient to ensure that all the material has reached a lower temperature (55°C or less). In any case, the loaded tray should never be left in this bath for more than 10 min as partial gelation can occur, thereby making the material unusable.

Just before tempering the tray material is completed, the syringe material is taken directly from the storage compartment and applied to the prepared teeth. The syringe material is never tempered since it must be maintained in a fluid state to enhance adaptation to the tissues. Normally, the temperature of the syringe material is cooled sufficiently, as it is extruded, so it is comfortable for the patient. The syringe material is first applied to the base of the preparation; then the remainder of the prepared tooth is covered. The tip of the syringe is held close to the tooth, and it remains embedded below the surface of the syringe material to prevent entrapment of air bubbles. The water-soaked outer layer of the hydrocolloid-loaded tray and the gauze covering the tray impression material are removed to ensure firm bonding to the syringe hydrocolloid. The tray is immediately brought into position, seated with light pressure, and held with a very light force. Too much pressure may displace the syringed agar sol from the tooth and distort the impression.

Gelation is accelerated by circulating cool water (approximately 18–21°C) through the tray for 3–5 min. During the gelation process, the tray must be held in the mouth until gelation has proceeded to a point at which the gel strength is sufficient to resist deformation or fracture.

TABLE 13.7 Comparison of characteristics of Elastomers, Agar and Alginate

Generic Type	Advantages	Disadvantages
Polysulfide	Long working time High tear resistance Margins easily seen Moderate cost	Requires custom tray Stretching leads to distortion Compatible with stone Stains clothing Obnoxious odor Pour within 1 h
Condensation silicone (putty wash)	Putty for custom tray Clean and pleasant Good working time Margins easily seen	High polymerization shrinkage Volatile by-product Low tear strength Hydrophobic Pour immediately
Vinyl polysiloxane	One material Putty for custom tray Automix dispense Clean and pleasant Margins easily seen Ideally elastic Pour repeatedly Stable: delay pour	Hydrophobic No flow if sulcus is moist Low tear strength Putty displaces wash Wash has low tear strength Putty too stiff Putty and wash separate Difficult to pour cast
Polyether	Fast setting Clean Automix dispense Least hydrophobic of all elastomers Margins easily seen Good stability Delay pour Shelf life: 2 years	Stiff, high modulus Bitter taste Need to block undercuts Absorbs water Leaches components High cost
Agar	Moist field acceptable Accurate and pleasant Hydrophilic Low cost Long shelf life	Requires special equipment Thermal discomfort Tears easily Pour immediately Difficult to see margins and details
Alginate	Moist field acceptable Clean and pleasant Hydrophilic Low cost Long shelf life	Not accurate/rough Tears easily Pour immediately Can retard setting of gypsum

TABLE 13.8 Composition of Commercial Reversible Hydrocolloid Impression Materials

Component	Function	Composition (%)
Agar	Brush-heap structure	13–17
Borate	Strength	0.2–0.5
Sulfate	Gypsum hardener	1.0–2.0
Wax, hard	Filler	0.5–1.0
Thixotropic materials	Thickener	0.3–0.5
Water	Reaction medium	Balance

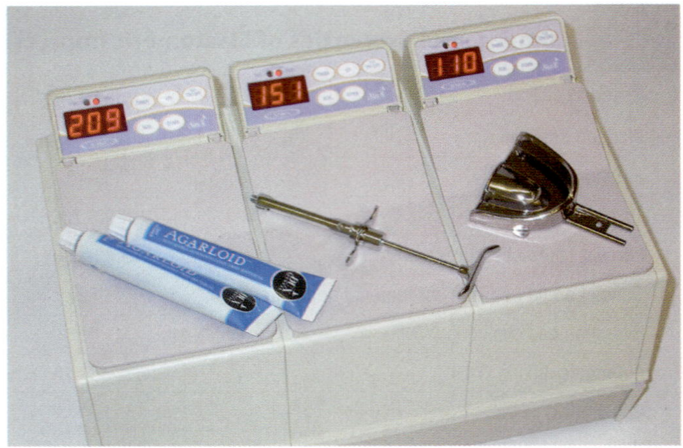

• **Fig. 13.16** Conditioning unit for agar impression materials. The three compartments are used for liquefying the material (*left*), storing after boiling (*middle*), and tempering the tray hydrocolloid (*right*). The number on the display shows the temperature setting in °F. Also shown in the figure are the tray hydrocolloid, a syringe for injecting hydrocolloids, and an impression tray. Note the two tubes are extending out from the handle of the tray for water circulation.

As discussed in the section on elastomeric impression materials, hydrocolloid materials exhibit viscoelastic behavior; therefore, it is necessary to remove the impression with a snap and not to tease it out. Any twisting or flexure should be avoided. Properly done, the resulting impression will accurately reproduce the dimensions and details of hard and soft tissues.

Distortion during Gelation

Some contraction occurs because of the physical change in the hydrocolloid transformation from a sol to a gel. If the material is held rigidly in the tray, the impression material will shrink toward the center of its mass, thereby creating larger dies. Since the sol is a poor thermal conductor, rapid cooling may cause a concentration of stress near the tray where the gelation first takes place. Consequently, water at approximately 20°C is more suitable for cooling the impression than is ice water.

Alginate (Irreversible Hydrocolloid)

The setting of alginate hydrocolloid is a process of cross-linking alginic acids with calcium ions. The alginic acid, which is extracted from certain brown seaweed, is a linear copolymer of β-D-mannuronic acid and α-L-guluronic acid (Fig. 13.17). Mannuronic and guluronic acids are epimers. It is known that the block structure within the alginic acid can vary significantly. Alginates with higher guluronic acid levels normally show a stronger interaction with calcium, and hence, yield greater gel strength. For impression-making purposes, the alginate is richer in mannuronic acid.

Composition

The chief active ingredient in the alginate impression materials is one of the soluble alginates, such as sodium, potassium, or triethanolamine alginate. Table 13.9 shows a formula for the powder component of an alginate impression material. The diatomaceous earth acts as a filler to increase the strength and stiffness of the alginate gel. It also produces a smooth texture and ensures the formation of a firm gel surface that is not tacky. Zinc oxide also acts as filler and has some influence on the physical properties and

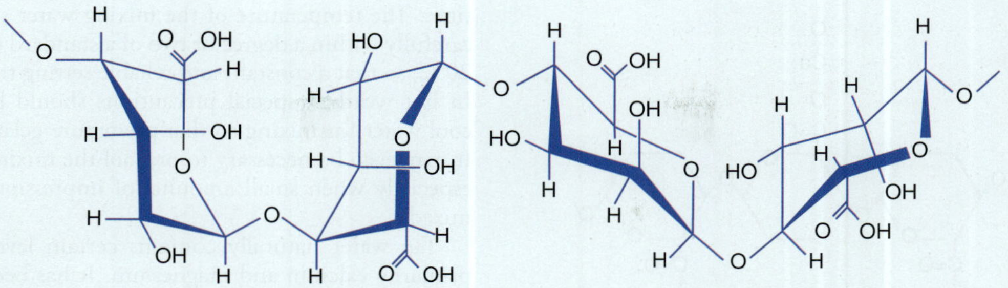

Guluronic Acid

Mannuronic Acid

• **Fig. 13.17** Structural formula of alginic acid. Alginic acid is a linear copolymer with homopolymeric blocks of β-D-mannuronic acid and its epimer α-L-guluronic acid covalently link together in different sequences or blocks.

TABLE 13.9 Powder Composition for an Alginate Impression Material

Component	Function	Weight Percentage
Potassium alginate	Soluble alginate	15
Calcium sulfate	Reactor	16
Zinc oxide	Filler particles	4
Potassium titanium fluoride	Gypsum hardener	3
Diatomaceous earth	Filler particles	60
Sodium phosphate	Retarder	2

setting time of the gel. Calcium sulfate dihydrate is a reactor providing calcium ions that cross-link the alginate sol. A retarder is added to control the setting time. A fluoride, such as potassium titanium fluoride, is added as an accelerator for the setting of the stone to ensure a hard, dense cast surface when the stone is poured in the impression. This fluoride is also called a surface hardener.

When powder in the alginate can is fluffed to break loose the particles, the diatomaceous earth, which is made up of fine porous silica particles, will become airborne when the lid is removed. Long-term exposure through inhalation of these fine silica particles can cause silicosis and pulmonary hypersensitivity. In an effort to reduce the dust encountered after tumbling, manufacturers have introduced a "dustless" alginate in which they have incorporated polyethylene glycol or polypropylene glycol on the alginate powder to agglomerate the particles. This causes the powder to become denser and less able to become airborne. Color indicators have been added in some formulations to reveal the stage of the setting reaction. This is to assist the operator in deciding when to proceed to the next step of impression making.

Two-paste alginate impression materials are also available; these are known as modified alginates. One paste contains a sol of alginate, fillers, retarder, and other ingredients like glycols and dextrose. The other paste consists of gypsum dihydrate, fillers, retarder, glycerol or glycols, gypsum surface modifier, and some silicone oil.

Disinfectant materials like quaternary ammonium compounds, chlorhexidine, bisguanidine compounds were incorporated to make the alginate self-disinfected. Addition of disinfecting agents into alginates eliminates the need for separate disinfection of the impression. Silver nanoparticles within 1 wt% were also tried to get the self-disinfection status for alginate.

CRITICAL QUESTION

How does the retarder optimize the working time of alginate impression material?

Gelation Process

The typical sol–gel reaction can be described simply as a reaction of soluble alginate with calcium ions from calcium sulfate and the formation of an insoluble calcium alginate (Fig. 13.18A). Structurally, calcium ions replace the sodium or potassium ions of two adjacent molecules to produce a cross-linked complex or polymer network (Fig. 13.19). The production of the calcium alginate is so rapid that it does not allow sufficient working time. A water-soluble phosphate salt (e.g., trisodium phosphate) is added to the composition as a retarder to extend the working time. The strategy is that the calcium ions will react preferentially with the phosphate ions in the solution (Fig. 13.18B). Thus, the rapid reaction between calcium ions and the soluble alginate is deferred until phosphate ions from trisodium phosphate are exhausted. The amount of retarder is adjusted to provide the proper setting time.

Controlling Setting Time

A slight modification in the water/powder (W/P) ratio or the mixing time can have marked effects on two important properties of

$$K_{2n} - \text{Alginate} + n\,CaSO_4 \longrightarrow n\,K_2SO_4 + Ca_n - (\text{Alginate})_2 \quad \text{(A)}$$

$$2\,Na_3PO_4 + 3\,CaSO_4 \longrightarrow Ca_3(PO_4)_2 + 3\,Na_2SO_4 \quad \text{(B)}$$

• **Fig. 13.18** **(A)** Setting reaction of alginate. **(B)** Controlling setting time by limiting the availability of calcium ions.

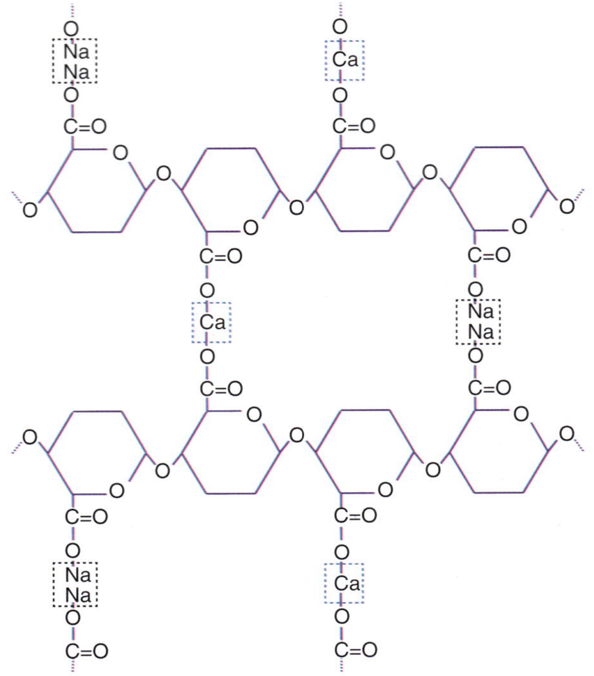

• **Fig. 13.19** Schematic illustration of sodium alginate cross-linked with calcium ions. The base molecules represent the sodium salt of alginic acid, in which hydrogen atoms of carboxyl groups are replaced by sodium atoms. With the exception of polar groups, all side chains have been omitted for simplification.

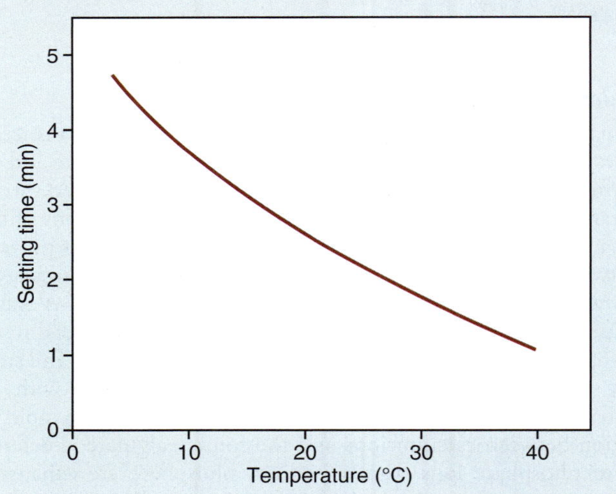

• **Fig. 13.20** Effect of water temperature on the setting time of an alginate impression material.

the gel, tear strength, and elasticity; thus, the setting time is best regulated by the amount of retarder added during the manufacturing process. Usually, the manufacturers make both fast-setting alginate (1.5–3 min) and normal-setting alginate (3–4.5 min) to give clinicians a choice of the materials that best suit their working style.

Clinicians, however, can safely influence the setting time by altering the temperature of the water. It is evident from Figure 13.20 that the higher the temperature, the shorter is the setting time. The temperature of the mixing water should be controlled carefully within a degree or two of a standard temperature, usually 20°C, so that a constant and reliable setting time can be obtained. In hot weather, special precautions should be taken to provide cool water for mixing so that premature gelation does not occur. It may even be necessary to precool the mixing bowl and spatula, especially when small amounts of impression material are to be mixed.

Tap water naturally contains certain levels of metallic ions, primarily calcium and magnesium. It has been shown that compared with distilled water for mixing of alginate impression material, the use of tap water with a high hardness may accelerate the setting of the alginate. If one observes that the setting time has decreased in a new office or clinic location, the effect of the hardness of the tap water on setting time should be considered as a possible cause.

- Tap water naturally contains certain levels of metallic ions, primarily calcium and magnesium.
- Use of tap water with a high hardness may accelerate the setting of the alginate.

CRITICAL QUESTION

Why is it especially important to add water to the rubber mixing bowl before adding the powder when one is mixing a fast-setting alginate impression material?

Preparation of Alginate Impression Materials

A proper mixture of water and powder is essential to obtain a good impression. The measured powder is added slowly to the premeasured water that has already been poured into a clean flexible bowl. The powder is incorporated into the water by carefully mixing with a metal or plastic spatula that is sufficiently flexible to adapt well to the wall of the mixing bowl. If the powder is placed in the mixing bowl first, penetration of the water to the bottom of the bowl is inhibited and a longer mixing time may be required to ensure a homogeneous mix. Care should be taken to avoid incorporating excessive air into the mix. A vigorous stropping motion is best, with the mix being wiped or stropped against the side of the rubber-mixing bowl to express air bubbles. Powder must be incorporated fully in the water.

The mixing time is particularly important; 45 s–1 min is generally sufficient, depending on the brand and type of alginate (fast set or regular set). The instructions on the package should be followed precisely for the mixing time, working time, and setting time for the material one is using. The result should be a smooth, creamy mixture that does not readily drip off the spatula when it is raised from the bowl. Several mechanical mixing devices are available for the alginate materials. They include a rotating mixing bowl, a mechanical mixer with time-control unit, a vacuum mixer for powder/water mixing, and a dynamic mechanical mixer, similar to the one for elastomers (Fig. 13.8D) for two-paste alginate products. Their principal benefits are convenience, speed, and the reduction of human error.

Clean equipment is important because many of the problems and related failures are attributable to dirty or contaminated mixing or handling devices. Contaminants, such as small amounts of gypsum left in the bowl from a previous mix of plaster or stone, can accelerate the set. It is best to use separate bowls for mixing alginate and stone.

Making the Alginate Impression

It is imperative that the impression be retained on the tray so that it can be withdrawn from the perimeter of the teeth. Therefore, a perforated metal tray is preferred. If a plastic tray or a metal rim-lock tray is selected, a thin layer of alginate tray adhesive should be applied and allowed to dry completely before mixing and loading the alginate in the tray. Alginate is a weak material; therefore, a sufficient bulk of material is needed. The thickness of the alginate impression between the tray and the tissues should be at least 3 mm.

As shown in Table 13.10, the compressive strength of alginate doubles during the first 4 min after gelation, but it does not increase appreciably thereafter. Most alginate materials improve in elasticity over time; this minimizes distortion of the material during impression removal, thus permitting superior reproduction of undercut areas. Data clearly indicate that the alginate impression should not be removed from the mouth for at least 3 min after gelation has occurred. It is possible to leave an alginate impression in the mouth too long. With certain alginates, it has been shown that if the impression is held for 6–7 min after gelation rather than 3 min, significant distortion may result.

Since alginate is a viscoelastic material, its tear strength is increased when the impression is removed along a vertical path with a snap. The speed of removal must be a compromise between a rapid movement and a slower rate that is more comfortable for the patient. Usually an alginate impression does not adhere to the oral tissues as with some of the elastomers do, so it is easier to remove the alginate impression rapidly. However, it is always best to avoid torquing or twisting the impression in an effort to remove it quickly. Specifically, the handle should be used minimally during breaking of the air seal ("suction") or removal of the tray from the teeth.

Strength

Manufacturers' directions supplied with the product should be followed in all respects. Any deviation from the instructions can have adverse effects on the gel strength. For example, if too much or too little water is used in mixing, the final gel will be weakened, making it less elastic. Insufficient spatulation results in failure of the ingredients to dissolve sufficiently so that the chemical reactions can proceed uniformly throughout the mass. Overmixing breaks up the formation of the calcium alginate network and reduces its strength.

- Manufacturers' directions supplied with the product should be followed.
- Insufficient spatulation results in failure of the ingredients to dissolve sufficiently so that the chemical reactions can proceed uniformly.

TABLE 13.10 Compressive Strength of an Alginate Gel as a Function of Gelation Time

Time from Gelation (min)	Compressive Strength (kPa)
0	330
4	770
8	810
12	710
16	740

- Overspatulation results in breakup of the calcium alginate network already formed and reduces its strength.
- Alginate impression should not be removed from the mouth for at least 3 min after gelation has occurred.
- Thickness of the alginate impression between the tray and the tissues should be at least 3 mm.

Shelf Life

Two major factors that affect the shelf life of alginate impression materials are storage temperature and moisture contamination from ambient air. The alginate impression powder can be purchased in individually sealed sachets or in bulk form in a can. The individual sachets are preferred since there is less chance for contamination during storage and the correct W/P ratio is ensured. Nevertheless, the bulk form in a can is by far the most popular. If the bulk powder form of alginate is used, the lid should be firmly replaced on the container as soon as possible after dispensing the powder so that moisture contamination is minimized.

An expiration date under a stated condition of storage should be clearly marked by the manufacturer on each packet. It is best not to stock more than a year's supply in the dental office. The material should be stored in a cool, dry environment.

Properties of Hydrocolloid Impression Materials

The quality of a stone cast depends on the properties of the hydrocolloid impressions before pouring and the potential interaction between gypsum and alginate during setting of the gypsum. In this section, details on dimensional stability, gypsum/hydrocolloid interaction, accuracy, disinfection, and effects of mishandling are described.

CRITICAL QUESTION

How can distortion of a hydrocolloid impression be minimized during storage?

Dimensional Stability

Once the hydrocolloid impression is removed from the mouth and exposed to air at room temperature, some shrinkage associated with **syneresis** and evaporation will occur. Conversely, if the impression is immersed in water, swelling caused by **imbibition** can occur. Figure 13.21 shows that the material has shrunk in air and excessive expansion has occurred during subsequent imbibition.

The storage medium, such as 2% potassium sulfate solution, or 100% relative humidity in a storage chamber, is suggested to reduce the dimensional change of agar impressions. Results obtained for impressions made from one agar hydrocolloid product stored in several media are given in Figure 13.22. These results are typical; they indicate that 100% relative humidity is the best storage environment to preserve the normal water content of the impression.

Thermal changes also contribute to dimensional change. With alginates, impressions shrink slightly because of the thermal differential between mouth temperature (37°C) and room temperature (23°C). The agar hydrocolloids experience a temperature shift in the opposite direction, from the chilled water-cooled tray (15°C) to the warmer room temperature. Even this slight change can cause the impression to expand and become less accurate.

If pouring the impression must be delayed, it should be rinsed in tap water, disinfected, wrapped in a surgical paper towel, saturated with water, and placed in a sealed plastic bag or humidor.

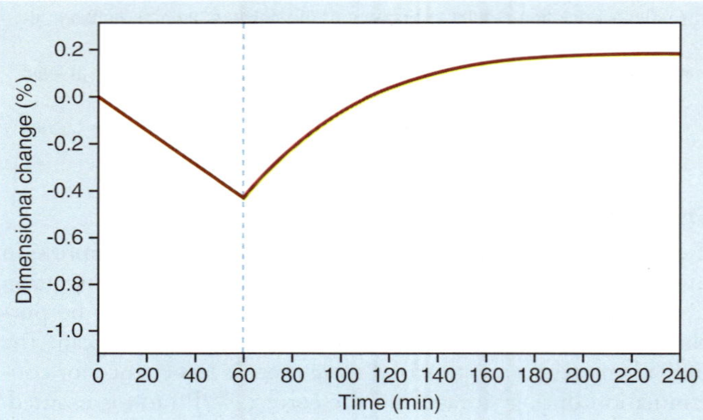

• **Fig. 13.21** Linear contraction of a representative reversible hydrocolloid in air (31%–42% relative humidity) within the initial and subsequent expansions in water. The dashed line indicates the start of water immersion.

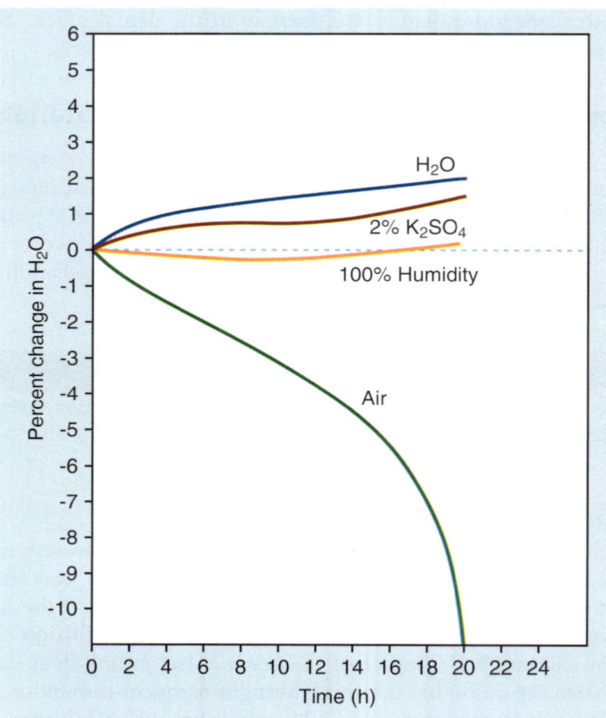

• **Fig. 13.22** Percent change in water content according to weight of an agar impression material in various storage media. At 100% relative humidity, the percent change is minimal.

CRITICAL QUESTION

Why do both agar and alginate include a gypsum hardener and how does it function?

Compatibility With Gypsum

Agar impression material contains borax, which is a known retarder for setting of gypsum products. The gelation process of alginate impressions produces not only insoluble calcium alginate but also sodium sulfate, which is a gypsum-setting accelerator at low concentration, but becomes a retarder at a higher concentration. In addition, polysaccharide also inhibits the setting of gypsum. Because of retardation, the surfaces of the gypsum models prepared from hydrocolloid may be too soft for use as dies or casts.

The deficiency of gypsum setting can be overcome in two ways: (1) by immersing the agar impression in a solution containing a gypsum accelerator, such as 2% potassium sulfate solution, prior to pouring the impression with the gypsum-forming product or (2) by incorporating a gypsum surface hardener in the material, such as the sulfate used in the formulation for agar hydrocolloid (Table 13.8) and the potassium titanium fluoride used in alginate (Table 13.9). The solubility of potassium titanium fluoride is about 1.3 g per 100 mL of water at 20°C. The fluoride on the surface of alginate will form fine calcium fluoride precipitates with the calcium from the gypsum. Fine calcium fluoride particles become nuclei that accelerate the setting of gypsum.

A rough stone surface will result if excess rinsing water has collected on the surface of the impression at the time of pouring the stone mixture. A dried gel surface, on the other hand, will result in its adherence to the surface of the cast, which can result in tearing upon its removal. The surface of the impression should be shiny but with no visible water film or droplets at the time of pouring. After the impression has been filled with stone, somewhat superior stone surfaces may be obtained if the impression is placed in a humidor while the stone hardens.

The stone cast or die should be kept in contact with the impression for a minimum of 30 min, preferably for 60 min, before the cast is separated from the impression. A longer time may be needed for slow-setting gypsum. It is wise to separate the cast from the impression within a reasonable time so that desiccation of the hydrocolloid does not occur, thereby avoiding abrasion of the gypsum cast during its removal.

Digital dental models can be obtained from a CBCT scan of alginate impressions without sending them to a remotely situated laboratory. However, when the impressions are not stored under special conditions, they should be scanned immediately, after the impressions are taken.

CRITICAL QUESTION

What is the optimal method for disinfecting an alginate hydrocolloid impression without causing significant distortion or degradation?

Disinfection

Since the hydrocolloid impression must be poured within a short time after removal from the mouth, the disinfection procedure should be relatively rapid to prevent a dimensional change. The current protocol for disinfecting hydrocolloid impressions recommended by the Centers for Disease Control and Prevention is to use household bleach (1-to-10 dilution), iodophors, or synthetic phenols as disinfectants. After the impression has been rinsed thoroughly, the disinfectant can be sprayed liberally on the exposed surface. The impression is then immediately wrapped in a disinfectant-soaked paper towel and placed in a sealed plastic bag for 10 min. Finally, the wrapped impression is removed from the bag, unwrapped, rinsed, and shaken to remove excess water. The impression is then poured with the stone of choice. An alternative disinfection method is by immersion, but this should not exceed 10 min (Table 13.4).

Accuracy

Agar is among the most accurate of impression materials. Most alginate impressions are not capable of reproducing the finer details observed in impressions with other elastomeric impression materials. Nevertheless, alginate materials are sufficiently accurate that they can be used to make impressions for removable partial dentures.

Effects of Mishandling

Common causes of failures encountered with reversible and irreversible hydrocolloid impression materials are summarized in Table 13.11. See Table 13.7 for a summary of the characteristics of the hydrocolloids.

CRITICAL QUESTION

What is the principle that makes the combined agar–alginate technique effective?

Laminate Technique (Alginate–Agar Method)

A modification of the traditional agar procedure is the combined agar–alginate technique. The agar in the tray is replaced with a mix of chilled alginate that bonds to the agar expressed from a syringe. The alginate gels by a chemical reaction, whereas the agar gels by means of contact with the cool alginate rather than with the water circulating through the tray. Since it is the agar, not the alginate, that contacts the prepared teeth, maximal detail is reproduced. Because only the syringe material needs to be heated, equipment cost is lower and less preparation time is required. Some other benefits of the technique are that agar does not irritate the tissue at the temperature used because the alginate cools the agar to an ideal gelation temperature, agar is more compatible with gypsum model than alginate, less equipment is required, and the time is reduced. The main disadvantages of this technique are as follows: (1) the bond between the agar and the alginate is not always sound; (2) the higher viscosity of the alginate material displaces the agar hydrocolloid during seating; and (3) the dimensional inaccuracy of the alginate hydrocolloid limits its use to single units. To address the bonding issue, ISO 13716 (Dentistry—Reversible-Irreversible Hydrocolloid Impression Material Systems) requires that the bond between the two materials under tensile stress should be in excess of 50 kPa. Nevertheless, this laminate technique is the most cost-effective way of producing an impression with adequate detail.

Duplicating Materials

Both types of hydrocolloids are used in the dental laboratory to duplicate dental casts or models for the construction of prosthetic appliances and orthodontic models. Agar hydrocolloid is more popular in the lab because it can be used many times. In addition, with intermittent stirring, agar hydrocolloid can be kept in a liquid form for 1 or 2 weeks at a constant pouring temperature. These factors make the cost of reversible impression materials quite reasonable.

The hydrocolloid-type duplicating materials have the same composition as the impression materials but their water content is higher. Consequently, the agar or alginate content is lower, which influences their compressive strength and percent permanent set. These property requirements are identified in

TABLE 13.11 Common Causes of Failed Hydrocolloid Impressions

	CAUSES	
Effect	**Agar**	**Alginate**
Grainy material	Inadequate boiling Storage temperature too low Storage time too long	Improper mixing Prolonged mixing Excessive gelation Water/powder ratio too low
Separation of syringe materials	Water-soaked tray material surface not removed material Premature gelation of either material	Not applicable
Tearing	Inadequate bulk Premature removal from mouth Syringe material partially gelled when tray was seated	Inadequate bulk Moisture contamination Premature removal from mouth Prolonged mixing
External bubbles	Gelation of syringe material, preventing flow	Undue gelation preventing flow Air incorporated during mixing
Irregularly shaped voids	Material too cold	Moisture or debris on tissue
Rough or chalky stone model	Inadequate cleansing of impression Excess water or hardening solution left in the impression Premature removal of die Improper manipulation of stone Air drying of the impression before pouring	Inadequate cleaning of impression Excess water left in impression Premature removal of the impression Model left in impression too long Improper manipulation of stone
Distortion	Impression not poured within 30 min Movement of tray during gelation Premature removal from mouth Improper removal from mouth Use of ice water during initial stages of gelation	Impression not poured immediately Movement of tray during gelation Premature removal from mouth Improper removal from mouth

ANSI/ADA Specification No. 20 (ISO 14356; Dentistry—Duplicating Material).

Duplicating silicone – an addition-cured duplicating system is gaining popularity because of greater accuracy and stability. It is easy to manipulate and many numbers of duplicate casts can be prepared from the same mold.

Inelastic Impression Materials

Inelastic impression materials exhibit an insignificant amount of elastic deformation when they are subjected to bending or tensile stresses. In addition, they fracture without exhibiting any plastic deformation if the stress from applied pressure exceeds their tensile, shear, or compressive strength values. These materials include impression plaster, impression compound, and ZOE impression paste. Because of their inability to sustain a substantial amount of elastic deformation without fracture, their use in dental impression making is limited.

Impression Plaster

Impression plaster is a β-calcium sulfate hemihydrate used at a W/P ratio of approximately 0.5–0.6. Its fluidity makes it suitable for making impressions of soft tissues in the uncompressed state, a characteristic of mucostatic impression material. Because of its rigidity, the use of impression plaster has been suggested for making preliminary impressions. This is not currently used in the clinics.

Impression Compound

Impression compound, also called modeling plastic, is a thermoplastic material supplied in the form of sheets and sticks. There are two types of impression compounds available. Type I is a lower-fusing material for making impressions in the oral cavity; it may be supplied in either sheet or stick form (Fig. 13.23). Type II is a higher-fusing material, also called tray compound, used for forming trays to be used in the oral cavity.

An impression of edentulous ridge is obtained with compound. This impression is referred to as the primary impression. It is then used either as a tray to support a thin layer of a second impression material or to prepare a cast for the fabrication of a custom-made tray. Custom tray can be used to make a final impression. This impression is known as the secondary impression. Secondary impressions may also be made with a ZOE wash paste, hydrocolloid, impression plaster, or elastomer. The other common application of compound is for border molding of an acrylic custom tray during fitting of the tray.

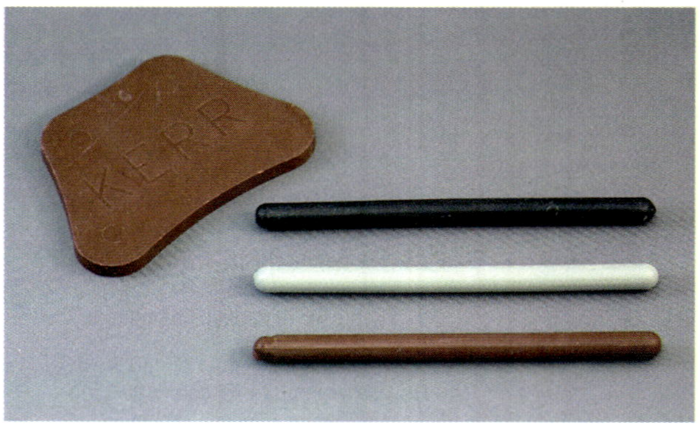

• **Fig. 13.23** Typical type I cake-and-stick configurations of commercial impression compound. The melting temperatures are soft green, 50.0–51.1°C; gray, 53.3–54.4°C; and red, 54.4–55.6°C.

Dimensional Stability

Relaxation of the impression compound can occur in a comparatively short time, especially with an increase in temperature. The result is warping or distortion of the impression. The safest method of minimizing such distortion is to allow thorough cooling of the impression before removal from the mouth and to construct the cast or die as soon as possible after the impression has been obtained—at least within the first hour.

Disinfection

The recommended disinfectant solution for the compound is 2% alkaline glutaraldehyde solution. The impressions should be immersed in this solution for the required time, rinsed, and poured immediately (Table 13.4).

CRITICAL QUESTION

Why does ZOE set faster in a humid environment?

Zinc Oxide–Eugenol (ZOE) Impression Paste

The reaction between zinc oxide and eugenol yields a relatively hard mass that has been involved in a wide range of applications in dentistry, including use as an impression material for edentulous mouths, a surgical dressing, and bite registration paste. The combination of zinc oxide and eugenol is used as temporary filling material, root canal filling material, cementing medium, and temporary relining material for dentures.

Composition and Setting

ZOE impression pastes are dispensed as two separate pastes. A typical formula is shown in Table 13.12. One tube contains zinc oxide and vegetable or mineral oil; the other contains eugenol and rosin. The vegetable or mineral oil acts as a plasticizer and aids in offsetting the action of the eugenol as an irritant.

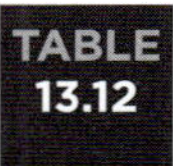

TABLE 13.12 Composition of a Zinc Oxide–Eugenol Impression Paste

Components	Percentage
Tube no. 1 (base)	
Zinc oxide (French processed or USP)	87
Fixed vegetable or mineral oil	13
Tube no. 2 (accelerator)	
Oil of cloves or eugenol	12
Gum or polymerized rosin	50
Filler (silica type)	20
Lanolin	3
Resinous balsam	10
Accelerator solution ($CaCl_2$) and color	5

Oil of cloves, which contains 70%–85% eugenol, is sometimes used because it produces less of a burning sensation when it contacts the patient's soft tissues. The addition of rosin to the paste in the second tube facilitates the speed of the reaction and yields a smoother, more homogeneous product. Canada balsam and Peru balsam are often used to increase flow and improve mixing properties. If the mixed paste is too thin or lacks body before it sets, a filler (such as a wax) or inert powder (such as kaolin, talc, or diatomaceous earth) may be added to one or both of the original pastes.

The setting reaction is ionic in nature and requires an ionic medium in which it can proceed at any desired rate. It is well established that the first reaction is the hydrolysis of zinc oxide to its hydroxide (Fig. 13.24). Some formulations do not contain water in the paste and the setting of the material is retarded until the mixed paste encounters moisture in the patient's mouth. Other anhydrous formulations contain acetic acid or zinc acetate to accelerate the reaction. In any case, water provides additional acceleration. When the two pastes are mixed, the phenol –OH of the eugenol acts as a weak acid and undergoes an acid–base reaction with zinc hydroxide to form a salt, zinc eugenolate (Fig. 13.24). Two further coordinate bonds are formed by donation of pairs of electrons from the methoxy oxygen to zinc. One of the chief disadvantages of the ZOE pastes is the possible stinging or burning sensation caused by the eugenol as it leaches out and contacts soft tissues. Zinc oxide can react with various carboxylic acids and form ZOE-like materials. Orthoethoxybenzoic acid (EBA) is a valuable substitute for eugenol in this regard. Bactericidal agents and other medicaments can be incorporated without interfering with the reaction.

Manipulation

Mixing of the two pastes is accomplished on an oil-impervious paper or glass mixing slab. The proper proportion of the two pastes is generally obtained by squeezing two strips of paste of the same length, one from each tube, onto the mixing slab. A flexible stainless steel spatula is typically used for the mixing procedure. The two strips of contrasting colors are combined with the first stroke of the spatula, and the mixing is continued for approximately 1 min, or as directed by the manufacturer, until a uniform color is achieved.

These materials are classified as a hard paste (type I) or soft paste (type II). The final set should occur within 10 min for a type I paste (hard) and 15 min for a type II paste (soft). When the final set occurs, the impression can be withdrawn from the mouth. The actual time will be shorter when setting occurs in the mouth, since humidity and temperature can accelerate the setting reaction.

The clinician can shorten setting time by adding a small amount of zinc acetate or additional accelerator or a drop of water in the paste before mixing or by extending the mixing time. The use of a cool spatula and mixing slab is also effective in prolonging the setting time.

A paste of a thick consistency or high viscosity can compress the tissues, whereas a thin, fluid material results in an impression that captures a negative replica of the tissues in a relaxed condition with little or no compression. In any event, the impression paste should be homogeneous. Pastes of varying consistencies are commercially available. An advantage of a heavier consistency material is its increased strength.

Dimensional Stability

The dimensional stability of the impression pastes is quite satisfactory. A negligible shrinkage (less than 0.1%) may occur during hardening. No significant dimensional change subsequent to hardening should occur with high-quality commercial products. The impressions can be preserved indefinitely without the change in shape that can result from relaxation or other causes of warping. This condition can be satisfied only if the tray material is dimensionally stable.

Disinfection

The recommended disinfectant solution for ZOE impression paste is 2% alkaline glutaraldehyde solution. The impressions should be immersed in this solution for the required time, rinsed, and poured immediately (Table 13.4).

Other Applications of ZOE Pastes

After a gingivectomy (i.e., the surgical removal of diseased or redundant gingival tissues), a ZOE paste may be placed over the wound to aid in the retention of a medicament and to promote healing. These pastes are generally softer and slower in their setting reaction in comparison with impression pastes. The mixture should be capable of being formed into a rope that is packed into the gingival wounds and the interproximal spaces to provide retention of the dressing. The final product should be strong enough to resist displacement during mastication but not so brittle that it shears readily under localized stresses.

ZOE pastes are also used as bite registration pastes in the construction of complete dentures and fixed or removable dental prostheses. The ZOE impression paste offers almost no resistance to closing of the mandible, thus allowing a more accurate interocclusal relationship record to be formed. Furthermore, the ZOE interocclusal record is more stable than the one made in wax.

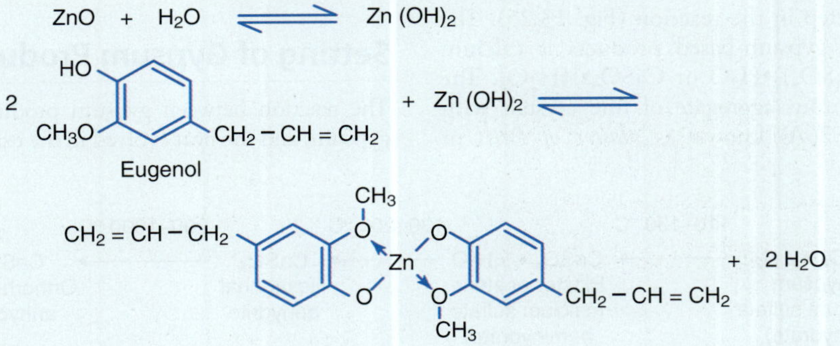

$$ZnO + H_2O \rightleftharpoons Zn(OH)_2$$

2 HO / CH_3O / $CH_2-CH=CH_2$ (Eugenol) + $Zn(OH)_2 \rightleftharpoons$

$CH_2=CH-CH_2$ / CH_3 / O / Zn / O / CH_3 / $CH_2-CH=CH_2$ + $2\,H_2O$

• **Fig. 13.24** Setting reaction of zinc oxide–eugenol. Arrows between zinc and oxygen of methoxy groups indicate coordinate bonds.

Gypsum Products

Gypsum ($CaSO_4{\cdot}2H_2O$; calcium sulfate dihydrate) is a mineral mined in various parts of the world, but it is also produced as a by-product of flue gas desulfurization in some coal-fired electric power plants. Various crystalline forms of gypsum, such as selenite and alabaster, exist in nature. **Gypsum** products are supplied as fine hemihydrate powders that are produced by heating ground gypsum particles. After mixing with water, the mixture reverts back to gypsum. This unique property of gypsum products has led to numerous applications through history. A mixture of plaster (a gypsum product), lime, and water was used in joining the stone blocks of ancient Egypt's pyramids. Gypsum and gypsum products are used today for many applications including building construction, soil conditioning, food additives, pharmaceuticals, medical devices, and dental applications.

The primary applications of gypsum products in dentistry include the production of study models of oral and maxillofacial structures and their use as auxiliary materials for dental laboratory operations involved in the production of dental prostheses. They are also used to make models and casts on which wax models of dental prostheses and restorations are constructed. When a gypsum product is mixed with refractory fillers, such as different crystalline forms of silica, it becomes more heat resistant, which makes it useful to form molds for the casting of dental restorations. This form of material is known as a **gypsum-based investment** and it is discussed in Chapter 14.

Dental cast: a positive life-size reproduction of a part or parts of the oral cavity made from an impression
Die: the positive reproduction of the form of a prepared tooth in any suitable substance
Dental models: three-dimensional replicas of a patient's teeth and parts of oral cavity, used to plan treatment and to observe treatment progress

CRITICAL QUESTION

Calcination is a process of removing the water of crystallization from the dihydrate. What happens if hemihydrate powder is mixed with water?

Production of Gypsum Products

- These materials are produced by calcining calcium sulfate dihydrate (gypsum). Commercially, the gypsum is ground and subjected to temperatures of 110–130°C (230–266°F) in open containers to drive off part of the water of crystallization. This corresponds to the first step in the reaction (Fig. 13.25). The principal constituent of gypsum-based products is calcium sulfate hemihydrate [$(CaSO_4)_2{\cdot}H_2O$ or $CaSO_4{\cdot}\frac{1}{2}H_2O$]. The resulting particle is a fibrous aggregate of fine crystals with capillary pores (Fig. 13.26A) known as *plaster of Paris* or **dental plaster** in dentistry. As the temperature is further raised, it becomes an anhydrite. This process is known as *calcination*.

As shown in Figure 13.1, when gypsum is heated in a closed kettle, vat, or rotary kiln that maintains a wet environment; a crystalline hemihydrate called **dental stone** is produced in the form of rods or prisms (Fig. 13.26B). Because of differences in crystal size, surface area, and degree of lattice perfection, the resulting powders are often referred to as α-hemihydrate for dental stone and β-hemihydrate for plaster of Paris. The β-hemihydrate crystals are characterized by their "sponginess" and irregular shape. In contrast, the α-hemihydrate crystals are denser and have a prismatic shape.

When hemihydrate particles are mixed with water, the reaction in Figure 13.1 is reversed. The α-hemihydrate produces a much stronger and harder dihydrate structure than that resulting from β-hemihydrate. The chief reason for this difference is that the β-hemihydrate crystals are more irregular in shape and porous in character and require more water to wet the powder particles so that they can be stirred and poured. The amount of water required can also be reduced by grinding the hemihydrate particles to eliminate needle-like crystals and to provide better packing characteristics.

It is clear that various gypsum products require different quantities of water. These differences between dental plaster and dental stone are principally due to the shape and compactness of the crystals. These factors are regulated by the manufacturer and they are dependent on the type of process used, dehydration temperatures, particle size of the gypsum calcined, the calcination time, the grinding time for the final product, and the addition of surface-active ingredients to the final product.

If the calcination process occurs under pressure in a 30% calcium chloride solution or in the presence of more than 1% of sodium succinate, the resulting hemihydrate crystals will be shorter and thicker than those produced in a closed container (Fig. 13.26C). Residual calcium chloride or sodium succinate is removed by washing the powder with hot water. This type of gypsum-producing product is called modified α-hemihydrate or **die** stone. These crystals require even less water for mixing.

Water/powder ratio

- For a workable mix of **plaster, 45–50 mL/100 g** (0.45–0.50)
- For a workable mix of **stone, 28–30 mL/100 g** (0.28–0.30)
- For a workable mix of improved **die stone, 19–24 mL/100 g** (0.19–0.24)

CRITICAL QUESTION

Which unique property of hemihydrate and dihydrate makes the dissolution–precipitation theory of gypsum setting possible?

Setting of Gypsum Products

The reaction between gypsum products and water produces solid gypsum, and the heat evolved in the exothermic reaction is equivalent

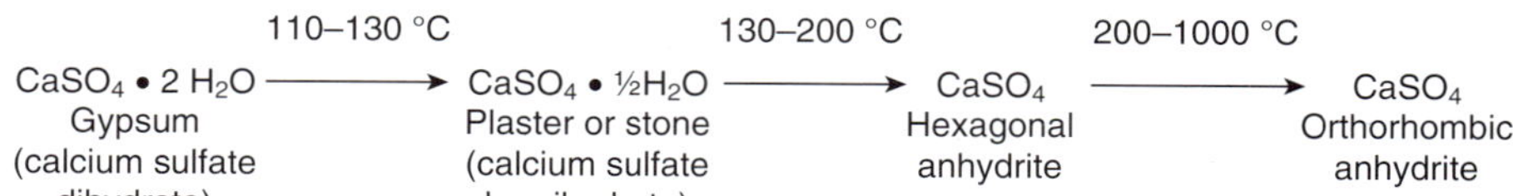

• **Fig. 13.25** Setting reaction of zinc oxide–eugenol. Arrows between zinc and oxygen of methoxy groups indicate coordinate bonds.

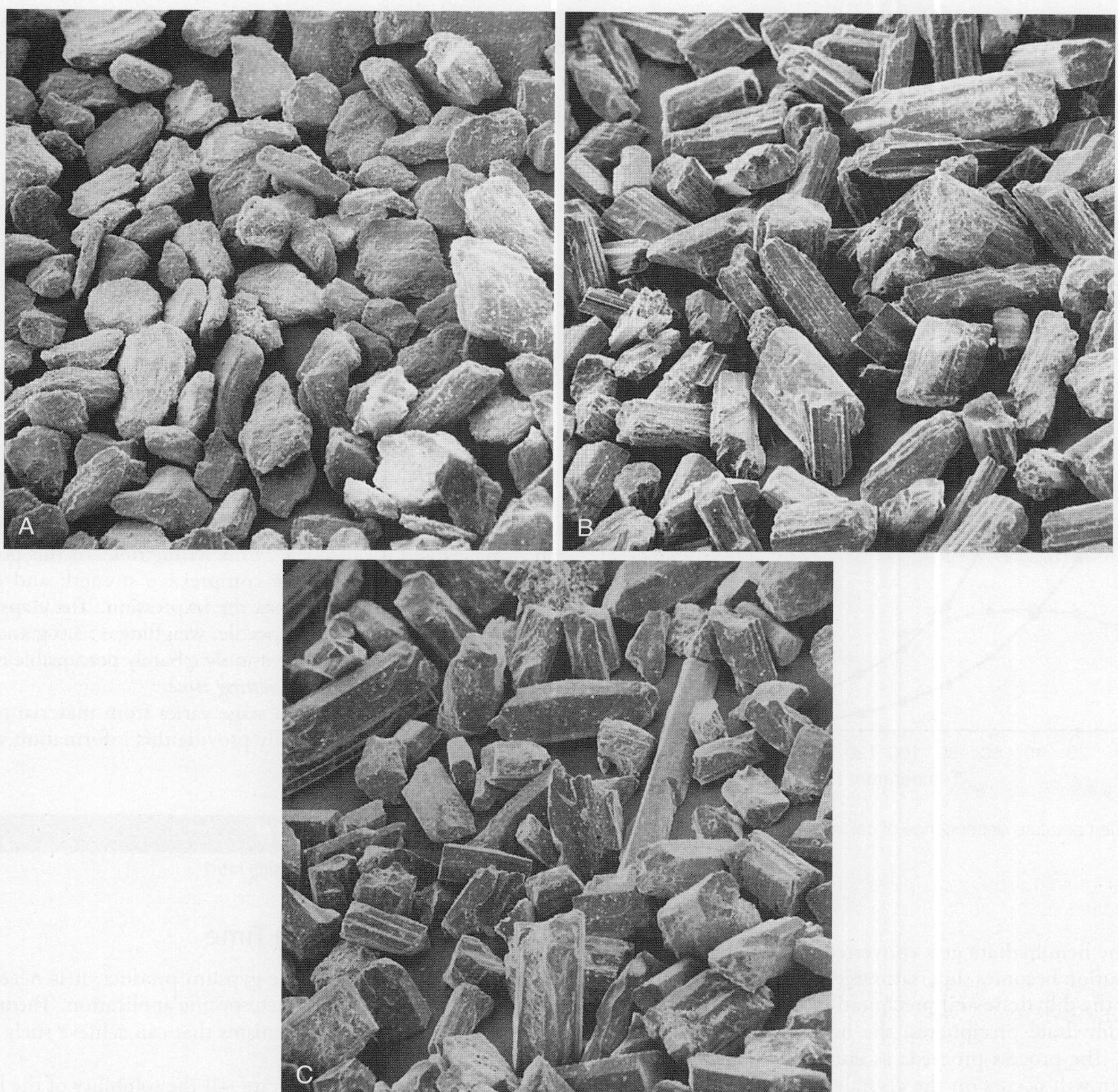

• **Fig. 13.26** Three types of powder particles in gypsum-producing products (×400). **(A)** Plaster of Paris (β-hemihydrate particles); crystals are spongy and irregular in shape. **(B)** Dental stone (α-hemihydrate); crystals are prismatic and more regular in shape than those of plaster. **(C)** Improved stone (modified α-hemihydrate); the cube-shaped particles have a reduced surface area that improves the flow of the mixture.

to the heat used originally for calcination. Set gypsum products probably never attain 100% conversion unless they are exposed to high humidity for a long time. Therefore, there are unreacted hemihydrates remaining in the set materials (Fig. 13.27).

Setting Reactions

There are *three theories* of gypsum setting:

- The colloidal theory proposes that, when mixed with water, hemihydrate enters into the colloidal state through a sol–gel mechanism. In the sol state, hemihydrate particles are hydrated to form dihydrate, thereby entering into an active state. As the measured amount of water is consumed, the mass converts to a solid gel.
- The hydration theory suggests that rehydrated plaster particles unite through hydrogen bonding with sulfate groups to form the set material.
- The most widely accepted mechanism is the dissolution–precipitation theory, which is based on dissolution of the hemihydrate particles in water followed by instant recrystallization to the dihydrate. This reaction has become possible because the *solubility of hemihydrate in water is four times greater than that of the dihydrate* at room temperature (Fig. 13.28). Thus, the setting reactions occur as follows:

1. When the hemihydrate is mixed with water, a suspension is formed that is fluid and workable.
2. The hemihydrate dissolves until it forms a saturated solution of Ca^{2+} and $(SO_4)^{2-}$.

$$\underset{\text{Calcium sulfate hemihydrate}}{(CaSO_4)_2 \bullet H_2O} + 3H_2O \longrightarrow \underset{\text{Calcium sulfate dihydrate}}{2\,CaSO_4 \bullet 2\,H_2O} + \text{unreacted } (CaSO_4)_2 \bullet H_2O + \text{heat}$$

• **Fig. 13.27** Reaction of gypsum-producing products with water.

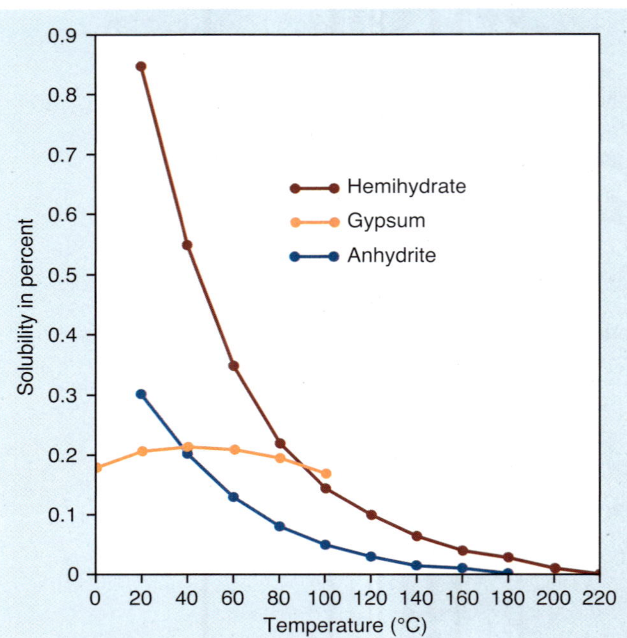

• **Fig. 13.28** Temperature dependence of calcium sulfate solubility in water.

3. When the hemihydrate gets converted to dihydrate, the saturated solution becomes supersaturated with respect to the solubility of the dihydrate and precipitation of dihydrate occurs.
4. As the dihydrate precipitates, the hemihydrate continues to dissolve. The process proceeds as either new crystals form or further growth occurs on the crystals already present until no further dihydrate can precipitate out of solution.

The setting reaction takes time to complete and changes in the mixture begin as soon as the hemihydrate and water are mixed together. X-ray diffraction data for set gypsum products indicate that there is less than 50% dihydrate present in type IV and V stones, about 60% in type II die materials, and over 90% in type I plasters.

CRITICAL QUESTION

How can one determine if the hemihydrate and water mixture has set?

Quantifying Setting Reactions

The hemihydrate and water must be mixed uniformly to ensure a homogeneous reaction through the entire mixture. It must also maintain its workable state as long as possible to facilitate pouring of a **model** or the casting investment. One must also recognize the stage at which the mixture has gained enough strength to resist fracture, which may be caused by the stress produced during removal of the model from the impression.

The time from addition of powder to the water until mixing is completed is called the *mixing time*. Mechanical mixing is usually completed in 20–30 s. Hand spatulation generally requires at least a minute to obtain a smooth mixture. The time from the start of mixing to the point where the consistency is no longer acceptable for the product's intended purpose is the *working time*. Generally, a 3-min working time should allow sufficient time for mixing, pouring an impression and a spare impression, and cleaning the equipment before the gypsum becomes unworkable. As the reaction proceeds, the excess water on the surface is taken up in forming the dihydrate, so that the mix loses its surface gloss and gains strength. When the mix can resist penetration by a Gillmore needle, which has a tip 2.12 mm in diameter and weighs 113.4 g, the time elapsed is called the *initial setting time*. At this point, the mass still has no measurable compressive strength and the cast cannot be safely removed from the impression. The elapsed time at which a heavier Gillmore needle, weighing 453.6 g and with a tip 1.06 mm in diameter, leaves only a barely perceptible mark on the surface is called the *final setting time*.

The elapsed time for each stage varies from material to material. The manufacturers usually provide this information with the product.

CRITICAL QUESTION

How can we control gypsum's setting rate?

Control of the Setting Time

Depending on the use of the gypsum product, it is necessary to control its setting time for each specific application. Theoretically, there are at least three mechanisms that can achieve such control. These include:

1. Solubility of the hemihydrate—If the solubility of the hemihydrate is increased, supersaturation of the dihydrate is achieved faster, which accelerates the rate of dihydrate crystal deposition.
2. Number of nuclei of crystallization—Nucleation is the first step at which Ca^{2+} and SO_4^{2-} in solution start to assemble into clusters on the nanometer scale, becoming stable under the operating conditions. These stable clusters constitute the nuclei. The greater the number of nuclei of crystallization, the faster the dihydrate crystals will form and the sooner the mass will harden. Any pre-existing fine dihydrate particles will also serve as nuclei.
3. Rate of crystal growth—Increasing or decreasing the rate of crystal growth will accelerate or retard the setting time.

In practice, these mechanisms have been incorporated in the formulation of the material by the manufacturer and by manipulation techniques performed by the operator. For example, fine gypsum particle residues from incomplete calcination or addition by the manufacturer will shorten the setting time because of the increase in the number of nuclei. Grinding of hemihydrate particles during manufacturing increases not only the rate of dissolution of the hemihydrate solution but also the number of nuclei. This increase in nuclei density results in a more rapid rate of crystallization.

TABLE 13.13 Effect of Water/Powder Ratio (W/P) and Mixing Time on the Setting Time of Plaster of Paris

W/P Ratio	Mixing Time (min)	Setting Time (min)
0.45	0.5	5.25
0.45	1.0	3.25
0.60	1.0	7.25
0.60	2.0	4.50
0.80	1.0	10.50
0.80	2.0	7.75
0.80	3.0	5.75

From Gibson CS, Johnson RN: Investigation of setting of plaster of Paris. *J Soc Chem Ind* 51:25–38, 1932.

The amounts of water and hemihydrate should be gauged accurately by weight. *The weight (or volume) of the water divided by the weight of the hemihydrate powder is known as the water/powder ratio, which is abbreviated as W/P.* For example, if 100 g of dental stone is mixed with 28 mL of water, the W/P ratio is 0.28. This ratio is an important factor in determining the physical and mechanical properties of the final gypsum product. The use of a higher W/P ratio decreases the number of nuclei per unit volume. Consequently, the setting time is prolonged (Table 13.13). An increase in the W/P ratio also causes a decrease in the strength and a decrease in the setting expansion of the set gypsum products, which will be discussed later.

Some gypsum crystals form immediately when the plaster or stone is brought in contact with the water. As the mixing starts, the formation of these crystals increases. At the same time, the crystals are broken up by the spatulation process, which results in more nuclei of crystallization. Therefore, within practical limits, the longer and the more rapidly the gypsum product is mixed, the shorter is the setting time.

Usually an increase in water temperature leads to an acceleration of a chemical setting reaction. This reaction is more complex for gypsum products. Figure 13.28 shows that the difference in solubility between hemihydrate and gypsum becomes smaller with increasing temperature, and this condition lowers the driving force for forming the dihydrate; it also results in a slower setting reaction. The decreased driving force causes the effect of temperature on the setting time to be erratic and to vary from one material to another. Little change in setting time occurs between 0°C and 50°C. If the temperature of the plaster–water mixture exceeds 50°C, a gradual retardation occurs. As the temperature approaches 100°C, no reaction takes place. This is the reason why very hot water (near the boiling temperature) is used to wash impurities like calcium chloride and sodium succinate from improved stone powder.

CRITICAL QUESTION

What are the recommended methods to accelerate or retard the setting time for a given gypsum-forming product?

Modifiers for Controlling Setting Time

Chemical modifiers have been used extensively to increase or decrease the setting time of gypsum products; they are called *retarders* and *accelerators*, respectively. The manufacturers use both types of compounds to formulate gypsum products with specific setting times.

The chemical that increases the rate of hemihydrate dissolution or precipitation of dihydrate accelerates the setting reaction. The most commonly used accelerator is potassium sulfate, which is particularly effective in concentrations greater than 2%. Slurry water flowing out from a model trimmer contains numerous fine gypsum particles that act as nuclei of crystallization and that can serve as an effective accelerator. It is important that the slurry water be agitated before use to disperse these fine gypsum particles. Increasing the time or speed of mixing can create more nuclei by crushing the developing dihydrate crystals into smaller particles, thereby accelerating the setting of the mix. At a concentration of 2% of the hemihydrate, sodium chloride is an accelerator. Sodium sulfate has its maximum acceleration effect at approximately 3.4%. Several inorganic salts play dual roles in the setting kinetics of dihydrate, which are accelerators at low concentration and retarders at higher concentration. For example, borax, a known retarder for gypsum setting, has been shown also to promote the growth of dihydrate crystals, but only at a concentration lower than 0.2 mM (about 0.08 g/L).

One should recognize that significant acceleration of the reaction time could compromise the optimal flow characteristics of the material. The manufacturer has added accelerators, retarders, and other controlling agents, so it is not wise to add other ingredients that may counteract the effects of components that are already incorporated into the product. Therefore, one should select a product from the manufacturer's catalogue with the specific setting time that the operator needs.

For Faster Setting (Decreased Setting Time)
(a) Long mixing time
(b) Low W/P ratio - a thicker mix
(c) Addition of accelerators. A commonly used **accelerator** is potassium sulfate.

For Slower Setting
(a) Short mixing time
(b) High W/P ratio - a thinner mix
(c) Addition retarders. A commonly used **retarder** is borax.

CRITICAL QUESTION

When a mixture of hemihydrate and water sets, the resulting object is always porous. Why?

Setting Expansion

Regardless of the type of gypsum product selected, an expansion of the mass can be detected during the change from the hemihydrate to the dihydrate. Depending on the composition of the gypsum product, this observed linear expansion may be as low as 0.06% or as high as 0.5%. This phenomenon is contrary to what is expected when hemihydrate reverts to the denser dihydrate form. If equivalent volumes of the hemihydrate, water, and the reaction product (dihydrate) are compared, the volume of the dihydrate formed will be 7.11% less than the equivalent combined volumes of the hemihydrate and water (Fig. 13.29). This represents a 2.37% linear shrinkage of the gypsum object. The phenomenon of *setting expansion* can be explained on the basis of crystallization.

Mechanism of Setting Expansion

The crystallization of dihydrates can be pictured as an outgrowth of crystals from nuclei of crystallization. Crystals growing from the

	$(CaSO_4)_2 \bullet H_2O$ +	$3H_2O$ →	$2\ CaSO_4 \bullet 2\ H_2O$
Molecular mass (g)	290.28	54.05	344.33
Density (g/cm^3)	2.75	1.00	2.32
Equivalent volume (cm^3)	105.56	54.21	148.41

$$\frac{(105.56 + 54.21) - 148.41}{(105.56 + 54.21)} \times 100\% = 7.11\%$$

• **Fig. 13.29** Volume changes from conversion of calcium sulfate hemihydrate to dihydrate.

nuclei can intermesh with and obstruct the growth of adjacent crystals. When the process repeats itself with thousands of the crystals during growth, an outward stress or thrust develops, producing an expansion of the entire mass. Thus, a setting expansion can take place even though the true volume of the crystals alone may be less than calculated. Therefore, the structure immediately after setting is composed of interlocking crystals between which are micropores and pores containing the excess water required for mixing. On drying, the excess water is lost, resulting in a porous structure.

Figure 13.30 shows the dimensional change during setting of a gypsum product. *The mixture exhibits an initial contraction followed by an expansion and smaller contraction.* If the mixture is spread on a glass surface, the distance between any two reference points on the surface of the mixture will not change appreciably during the induction period, the time until the onset of initial setting. It is the adhesion of the mixture to the glass that prevents the expected contraction. In fact, any contraction will appear in the reduction of the height of the mixture on the glass. Only when the crystalline framework is sufficiently rigid (after the initial set) will the force of expansion overcome the adhesion to produce a visible setting expansion.

Therefore, when the technician or dentist produces gypsum models in impression molds, only the setting expansion that occurs after the initial set is of interest. Any contraction that occurs during the induction period does not affect the dimension of the cast relative to the mold because the mixture is still fluid at this stage and the contraction occurs at the free surface, an area that is not in contact with the mold. When enough crystals have formed to produce the outward thrust by impingement, setting expansion follows. The onset of initial setting occurs at approximately the minimal point of the curve, the point at which expansion begins.

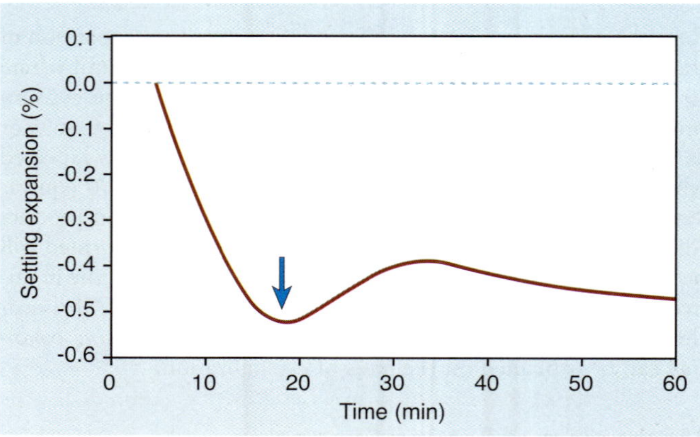

• **Fig. 13.30** Dimensional changes that occur during the setting of a gypsum product. The arrow indicates the initial set at approximately the lowest point of the curve.

Since the contraction prior to initial setting occurs at the free surface, the final dimension of the cast relative to that of the impression mold includes a setting expansion of approximately 0.12%, according to Figure 13.30. Naturally, the quantities of setting expansion vary among different gypsum products.

Control of Setting Expansion

As can be noted from the results presented in Table 13.14, a lower W/P ratio and a longer mixing time will increase the setting expansion. Each of these factors increases the nuclei density. The effect of the W/P ratio on the setting expansion is to be expected on theoretical grounds. At higher W/P ratio, fewer nuclei of crystallization per unit volume are present compared with the greater density of nuclei in thicker mixes. Because it can be assumed that the space between the nuclei is greater in such a case, it follows that there is less growth interaction of the dihydrate crystals and less outward thrust. However, the most effective method by which to control setting expansion is through the addition of chemicals by the manufacturer.

Setting expansion can be controlled by manipulating variables - thicker mix and increased spatulation will cause an increase in setting expansion; a thinner mix and decreased spatulation will cause a decrease in the amount of setting expansion.

CRITICAL QUESTION

Thus far, the setting of plaster or stone has occurred in air. What would happen if the hemihydrate and water mixture were allowed to set under water? Keep in mind that the solubilities of hemihydrate and dihydrate are very low in water, and one should not be concerned that the mixture will dissolve without vigorous stirring.

TABLE 13.14 Effect of Water/Powder Ratio (W/P) and Mixing Time on Setting Expansion of Plaster of Paris

W/P Ratio	Mixing Time (min)	Setting Expansion (%)
0.45	0.6	0.41
0.45	1.0	0.51
0.60	1.0	0.29
0.60	2.0	0.41
0.80	1.0	0.24

From Gibson CS, Johnson RN: J Soc Chem Ind 51:25T, 1932.

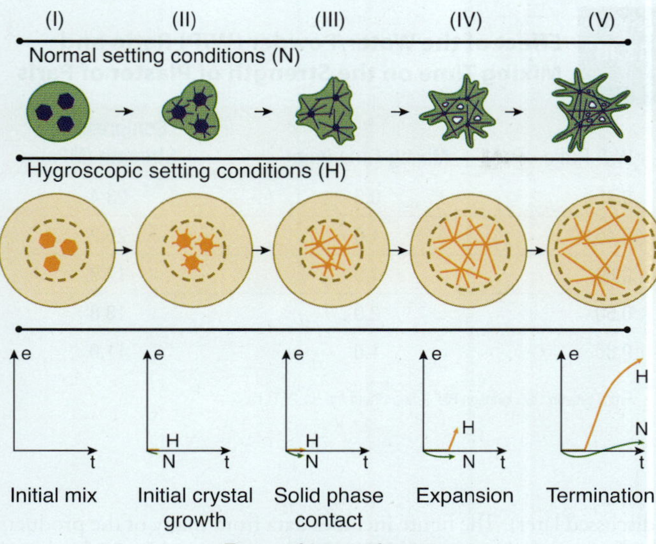

• **Fig. 13.31** Diagrammatic representation of the setting expansion of gypsum products. In the top row, the crystal growth is inhibited by the surface tension of water surrounding the growing crystals. In the middle row, the gypsum mixture (the area surrounded by the dashed circle) is immersed in water during setting (represented by the larger solid circle); the immersion water provides more room for longer crystal growth. The bottom row shows the expansion (e) over time (t) for hygroscopic setting expansion (H) and normal setting expansion (N). (Adapted from Mahler DB, Ady AB: An explanation for the hygroscopic setting expansion of dental gypsum products. J Dent Res 39:378–379, 1960.)

Hygroscopic Setting Expansion

Imagine that the initial mix is represented in the top row of Figure 13.31 (stage I) by the three round particles of hemihydrate surrounded by water. Under normal setting conditions, the crystals of the dihydrate begin to form on the nuclei. The water around the particles is reduced by hydration and these particles are drawn more closely together because surface tension of the water keeps the water surface area at a minimum (stage II). As the crystals of dihydrate grow, they contact each other and the water around the particles again decreases (stage III). Further dihydrate growth consumes more water and should draw the crystals together as before, but the outward thrust of the growing crystals opposes this contraction (stage IV). Eventually, the crystals become intermeshed and entangled (stage V).

Stage I of the middle row (hygroscopic setting conditions) of Figure 13.31 shows an identical mixture of hemihydrate (the area delineated by the dashed circle) under water (the area outside of the dashed circle). The hydration of hemihydrate particles here would proceed as usual. Since they are under water, the water consumed by hydration will be immediately replenished by the immersion water and the distance between the particles would remain the same (stage II). The surface tension of the water will still keep the surface area of the water at a minimum, except that in this case it would be the surface area of the immersion water, which will have no impact on the distance between growing dihydrates. As the dihydrate crystals continue to grow and contact each other, no reduction in the distance between crystals is expected (stage III). This means that the crystals will grow much more freely during the early stages (stage IV), before the intermeshing finally prevents further expansion (stage V). Consequently, the observed setting expansion that occurs when the gypsum product sets under water is greater than that which occurs during setting in air.

To distinguish between the two setting conditions, the setting expansion without water immersion is usually called *normal setting expansion* (N in the bottom row of Figure 13.31), whereas the expansion that occurs under water is known as *hygroscopic setting expansion* (H in the bottom row of Figure 13.31). The **hygroscopic setting expansion** is a physical phenomenon and is not caused by a chemical reaction any more than is the **normal setting expansion**. Therefore, the variables that can cause an increase or decrease in the normal setting expansion will have the same effect on the hygroscopic setting expansion. For example, a reduction in the W/P ratio and increased spatulation will result in a higher hygroscopic expansion.

The hygroscopic expansion obtained during the setting of dental stone or plaster is about twice that of the normal setting expansion. The greater hygroscopic setting expansion of gypsum-bonded casting investments is used in the fabrication of cast gold alloy restorations. Other investment materials that do not use gypsum as binder have also exhibited similar expansion when they set under water. Since warm water (approximately 38°C) is often used as the immersion water for hygroscopic expansion, one theory of hygroscopic expansion suggests that at this higher temperature the wax pattern expands during the setting of the investment material. More discussion on hygroscopic expansion of investment materials is presented in Chapter 14.

Note that *hygroscopy* means the ability of a substance to attract water molecules from the surrounding environment through either absorption or adsorption. The hygroscopic setting expansion described here is not the result of absorption or adsorption. Therefore, the term *hygroscopic setting expansion* of gypsum products is technically incorrect. Nonetheless, this term will be retained in explanations of the setting expansion of gypsum.

> Hygroscopic expansion is approximately twice as great as the normal setting expansion.

> **CRITICAL QUESTION**
>
> How does the presence of water in the pores of set gypsum affect the strength of the gypsum object?

Strength of Set Gypsum Products

The strength of set gypsum products is generally expressed in terms of compressive strength, although diametral tensile strength should also be considered to determine the overall strength characteristics.

Effect of Water Content

As expected from the theory of setting, the strength of plaster or stone increases rapidly as the material hardens after the initial setting time. However, the free water content of the set product definitely affects its strength. For this reason, two strength properties of gypsum are reported:

- *wet strength* (also known as *green strength*), and the
- *dry strength.*

The wet strength is the strength that is determined when water in excess of that required for hydration of the hemihydrate remains in the test specimen. When such excess water is removed by drying,

TABLE 13.15 Effect of Drying on the Strength of Plaster of Paris

Drying Period (h)	Compressive Strength (MPa)	Weight Loss (%)
2	9.6	5.1
4	11.7	11.9
8	11.7	17.4
16	13.0	--
24	23.3	18.0
48	23.3	18.0
72	23.3	--

From Gibson CS, Johnson RN: J Soc Chem Ind 25–38, 1932.

TABLE 13.16 Effect of the Water/Powder (W/P) Ratio and Mixing Time on the Strength of Plaster of Paris

W/P Ratio	Mixing Time (min)	Compressive Strength (MPa)
0.45	0.5	23.4
0.45	1.0	26.2
0.60	1.0	17.9
0.60	2.0	13.8
0.80	1.0	11.0

From Gibson CS, Johnson RN: J Soc Chem Ind 51:25T, 1932.

the strength obtained is the dry strength. The dry strength may be two or more times as high as the wet strength. Consequently, the distinction between the two is of considerable importance.

The effect of drying on the compressive strength of set plaster is shown in Table 13.15. Note the relatively slight gain in strength that occurred after 16 h. Between an 8-h and a 24-h drying period, only 0.6% of the excess water was lost yet the strength doubled. A similar change in surface hardness takes place during the drying process. An explanation of this phenomenon is that as the last trace of water is lost, fine crystals of gypsum precipitate serve as anchors between the larger crystals. Thus, if excess water is reconstituted by immersion or absorption, these small crystals are the first to dissolve and the reinforcing anchors are lost.

Microwave irradiation has been used to speed up the drying of gypsum casts. For example, one study showed that irradiation for 1 min can result in a strength equivalent to that obtained after drying in air for 24 h. Some studies suggest that there is a strengthening effect after casts are dried by microwave irradiation, whereas other studies have shown a slight decrease in strength compared with casts dried in ambient air. In general, microwave irradiation, a timesaving procedure, may be associated with some dimensional changes. The time needed varies with the microwave oven setting and type of cast being dried.

- The dry strength may be two or more times as high as the wet strength.
- Microwave irradiation has been used to speed up the drying of gypsum casts.

Effect of W/P Ratio

As previously noted, the set plaster or stone is porous, and the greater the W/P ratio, the greater the porosity. As might be expected on such a basis, the greater is the W/P ratio, the less is the dry strength of the set material, as shown by the data in Table 13.16, because fewer dihydrate crystals are available per unit volume. Material that is mixed at a high W/P ratio has a diametral tensile strength as high as 25% of the corresponding compressive strength. When materials are mixed at low W/P ratio, the diametral tensile strength is less than 10% of the corresponding compressive strength.

Figure 13.32 is a plot of the strength as a function of the W/P ratio for the five different types of gypsum products used in dentistry (discussed later). The figure includes data from many of the products on the market that meet ANSI/ADA Specification No. 25 for dental gypsum products; the strength ranges represent the wet strength at 1 h. The strength increases as the specimens dry and it can double in a week. Although the W/P ratio varies for the particular brand of plaster or stone, the typical recommended ranges of W/P ratio are shown in Table 13.17 for the five types of gypsum products.

- The strength of set gypsum product depends on the W/P ratio.
- Thicker mixes will increase the strength.
- Thinner mixes will decrease the strength.
- Follow the manufacturer's recommended W/P ratio for optimum strength.
- The strength increases as the specimens dry and it can double in a week.
- Increase in mixing time increases the strength to a limit (1 min).
- Addition of an accelerator or retarder lowers both the wet strength and the dry strength.

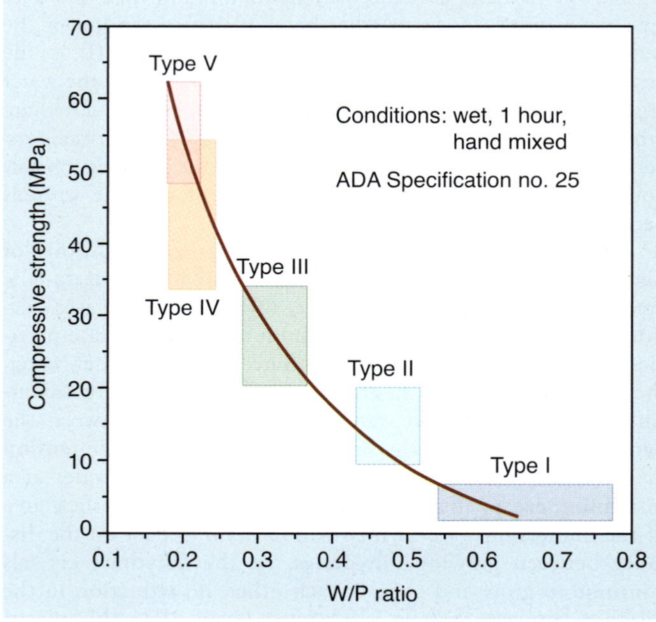

• **Fig. 13.32** Compressive strength as a function of W/P ratio for five types of gypsum products.

TABLE 13.17 **Properties of Five Types of Gypsum Products**[a]

Type	W/P Ratio	Setting Time (min)	2-H SETTING EXPANSION (%)		1-h Compressive Strength[b] (MPa)
			Min	Max	
I. Plaster, impression	0.50–0.75	4 ± 1	0.00	0.15	4.0
II. Plaster, model	0.45–0.50	12 ± 4	0.00	0.30	9.0
III. Dental stone	0.28–0.30	12 ± 4	0.00	0.20	20.7
IV. Dental stone, high strength	0.22–0.24	12 ± 4	0.00	0.10	34.5
V. Dental stone, high strength, high expansion	0.18–0.22	12 ± 4	0.10	0.30	48.3

[a]Properties required of five gypsum products covered by American Dental Association Specification No. 25.
[b]Minimum values.

Effect of Manipulation and Additives

As shown in Table 13.16, the spatulation time also affects the strength of the plaster. In general, an increase in mixing time increases the strength to a limit that is approximately equivalent to that of hand mixing for 1 min. If the mixture is overmixed, the gypsum crystals will be broken up and the final product will hold less crystalline interlocking structure.

The addition of an accelerator or retarder lowers both the wet strength and the dry strength of the gypsum product. Such a decrease in strength can be partially attributed to the salt added as an adulterant and to the reduction in intercrystalline cohesion.

When relatively pure hemihydrate is mixed with minimal amounts of water, the working time is short and the setting expansion unduly high. However, as just noted, dental gypsum products contain additives that reduce the setting expansion, increase the working time, and provide a rapid final set. The addition of more chemicals can upset the delicate balance of these properties. Thus if a change is desired in the setting time, it should be controlled by modest alterations in the W/P ratio and/or the spatulation time.

CRITICAL QUESTION

Which properties are used to classify the various types of gypsum products?

Types of Gypsum Products

ADA Specification No. 25 classifies five types of gypsum products, as shown in Table 13.17, with the property requirement for each type. Some gypsum materials are formulated for special purposes such as for pouring casts or attaching casts to an articulator. The criterion for selecting any particular gypsum product depends on the intended use and the physical properties necessary for that particular use. For example, dental plaster is not suitable for making the die of a prepared tooth because it cannot withstand the laboratory steps viz. waxing up and carving. Die stone is the appropriate choice.

Impression Plaster (Type I)

These impression materials are composed of plaster of Paris (β-hemihydrate; Fig. 13.27A) to which modifiers have been added to regulate the setting time and setting expansion. Impression plaster is rarely used any longer for making dental impressions because it has been replaced by less rigid materials such as the hydrocolloids and elastomers.

Model Plaster (Type II)

This model plaster or laboratory type II plaster is now used principally to fill a flask used in denture fabrication where setting expansion is not critical and the strength is adequate according to the limits cited in the ADA specification or ISO standard. It is usually marketed in the natural white color, to provide contrast with stones, which are generally colored.

Dental Stone (Type III)

With the advent of hydrocolloid impression material and the improved hardness of α-hemihydrate (Fig. 13.27B) made stone dies workable and the fabrication of indirect wax pattern possible.

Type III stone has a minimal 1 h compressive strength of 20.7 MPa (3000 psi), but it does not exceed 34.5 MPa (5000 psi). It is intended for the making of casts to fabricate complete dentures that fit on to soft tissues. For this application, a slight setting expansion of casts that reproduce soft tissues can be tolerated, but not when teeth are involved. Type III stones are preferred for casts used to process dentures because the stone has enough strength for this purpose and the denture can easily be removed after processing.

There are at least two methods for the construction of the cast. One method is to construct a mold by wrapping soft flat wax strips around the impression so that they extend approximately 12 mm beyond the tissue side of the impression. This process is called *boxing*, which forms the base of the cast. The mixture of stone and water is then poured into the impression under vibration. The mixture is allowed to flow slowly in a controlled pathway along the impression so that it forces the air forward as it fills all tooth impressions without entrapment of air bubbles.

Another method is to fill the impression first as described. The remainder of the stone–water mixture is poured on a glass plate. The filled impression is then inverted over a mound of stone, and the base is shaped with the spatula before the stone sets. Such a procedure is not indicated if the impression can easily be deformed or if the stone is “runny.” The cast should not be separated from the impression until it has hardened. The minimal time allowed for setting varies from 45 to 60 min, depending on the rate of setting of the stone or plaster and the type of impression material used.

Dental Stone, High Strength (Type IV)

The principal requisites for a die material are strength, hardness, and minimal setting expansion. To obtain these properties, modified α-hemihydrate (Fig. 13.26C) is used. The cube-shaped particles and the reduced surface area produce such properties without undue thickening of the mix. This material is also called *die stone.*

A hard surface is necessary for die stone because the tooth preparation is covered with wax and carved flush with the margins of the die. A sharp instrument is used for this purpose; therefore, the stone must be resistant to abrasion. It is fortunate that the surface hardness increases more rapidly than the compressive strength because the surface dries more rapidly. This is a real advantage in that the surface resists abrasion, whereas the core of the die is tough and less subject to accidental breakage. The average dry surface hardness of type IV stones is approximately 92 (Rockwell hardness) and that of type III stone is 82. Even though the surface of the type IV stone is harder, care should be taken when the pattern is being carved.

CRITICAL QUESTION

Under what conditions, a type V dental stone is used?

Dental Stone, High Strength, High Expansion (Type V)

This gypsum product exhibits an even higher compressive strength than the type IV dental stone. The improved strength is attained by making it possible to lower the W/P ratio even further than that used for type IV stone. In addition, the setting expansion has been increased from a maximum of 0.10%–0.30% (Table 13.17). The rationale for increasing setting expansion is that certain newer alloys, such as base metal, have a greater casting shrinkage than do the traditional noble metal alloys (Chapter 14). Thus, higher expansion is required in the stone die to aid in compensating for the alloy solidification shrinkage. The use of a type V stone may also be indicated when the expansion achieved during the fabrication of cast crowns is inadequate. One should avoid the use of type V stones for producing dies for inlays and onlays since the higher expansion may lead to an unacceptably tight fit. Additional information on the use of type IV and V stones is provided in the discussion of die materials in Chapter 14.

- Rationale for increasing setting expansion is that certain newer alloys, such as base metal, have a greater casting shrinkage than do the traditional noble metal alloys.
- Higher expansion is required in the stone die to aid in compensating for the alloy solidification shrinkage.

Special Gypsum Products

The orthodontist prefers a white stone or plaster for study models and may even treat the surface with soap to increase their sheen. These products generally have a longer working time, which reduces void formation and facilitates trimming.

The use of an articulator makes it necessary to mount the casts using a gypsum-producing product. These materials are referred to as "mounting" stones or plasters. They are fast setting and have low setting expansion. The mounting plaster has a sufficiently low strength to permit easy trimming and facilitate separating the cast from the articulator mounting plates.

Some products are designed to save time. One type is extremely fast setting and is ready to use in 5 min, but it has little working time. Another product changes color to indicate when it is ready for use. In addition, one specialty product contains a small amount of plastic or resin to reduce brittleness and improve resistance to abrasion during the carving of wax patterns.

Usually, when one feature is improved, another is sacrificed. A faster set is accepted in return for less working time. An improved resistance to carving is accepted in return for more difficult manipulation, decreased detail reproduction, or the need to box the impression because of excessive runniness. Improvements in materials and testing equipment have made it possible to use silicone–stone combinations that can reproduce spaces between lines as fine as 10 μm or less. Current specifications or standards require an accuracy of only 50 μm.

At present many gypsum products are available to suit almost all individual requirements or combinations thereof.

Manipulation of Gypsum Products

So far, we have discussed the types of gypsum products based on their crystal form, their applications, and their setting processes, which may affect the dimensions and strength of the set material. In practice, clinicians and technicians must not only produce a cast using a gypsum-producing material, but they must also store the powder properly and maintain the cast in its best condition for subsequent procedures.

Care of Gypsum Products

The hemihydrate of gypsum absorbs water from the air readily. For example, if the relative humidity of the surroundings exceeds 70%, the plaster absorbs sufficient moisture from the air to start a setting reaction. The first hydration probably produces a few crystals of gypsum on the surface of the exposed hemihydrate crystals. These gypsum crystals can act as nuclei of crystallization and accelerate the setting reaction when they are mixed with water. If the hydration is allowed to continue, this process results in the hemihydrate crystals being completely covered with dihydrate crystals. Under these conditions, the water penetrates the dihydrate coating with difficulty and the setting time is prolonged.

Therefore, it is important that all gypsum products be stored in a dry atmosphere. The best means of storage is to seal the product in a moisture-proof metal container. When gypsum products are stored in closed containers, the setting time is generally retarded only slightly, approximately 1 or 2 min per year. This may be counteracted by a slight increase in the mixing time if necessary.

- It is important that all gypsum products be stored in a dry atmosphere.
- If the relative humidity of the surroundings exceeds 70%, the plaster absorbs sufficient moisture from the air to start a setting reaction.

Proportioning

The recommended W/P ratio should be used. The water and powder should be measured using an accurate graduated cylinder for the water volume and a weighing balance for the weight of powder. The powder should not be measured by volume (using a scoop) as it does not pack uniformly. This characteristic may vary from product to product, and it will pack more densely if the container remains undisturbed. When the container is shaken, the packed particles will be loosened and the volume will increase as a result of air entrapment. Preweighed envelopes are very popular because they promote accuracy, reduce waste, and save time. However, this preweighed, packaged material adds to the cost of producing models and casts.

Mixing and Pouring

If mixing is performed by hand, the bowl should be parabolic in shape, smooth, and resistant to abrasion. The spatula should have a stiff blade and a handle that is convenient to hold. A measured amount of water is placed in the bowl and the weighed powder is sifted into the water as initial hand mixing is performed. The mixture is then vigorously stirred, with periodic wiping of the inside of the bowl with the spatula to ensure wetting of all of the powder and breaking up of any agglomerates or lumps. The mixing should continue until a smooth mix is obtained, usually within a minute. A longer spatulation time drastically reduces the working time, which is of particular importance when pouring models. Entrapment of air in the mix must be avoided, since porosity can lead to weak spots and surface inaccuracies. After mixing, the use of a vibrator of high frequency and low amplitude is helpful in reducing air entrapment.

The preferred method of mixing is to use a mechanical mixer under vacuum. First, the measured water is added to the bowl, followed by gradual addition of the preweighed powder. The powder is incorporated during approximately 15 s of mixing with a hand spatula, followed by 20–30 s of mechanical mixing under vacuum. The strength and hardness obtained from such vacuum mixing usually exceed that obtained by 1 min of hand mixing. Repeatedly adding water and powder by guesswork to achieve the proper consistency should be avoided. This yields a lower strength and may cause distortion.

The mixing bowl with the dental stone mixture is then placed on top of a vibrator to eliminate entrapped air bubbles and the impression tray is held in one hand against the vibrator. The surface of the impression should be free of excess water. With the metal spatula, a small amount of dental stone is added to one open end of the impression (e.g., in the last molar of a full arch impression). The speed of the vibrator should be adjusted high enough to make the stone flow slowly into adjacent spaces. If the speed of vibration is too high, it can generate air bubbles within the stone mixture. The impression may be tilted to control the movement of the stone into the tooth depression. Additional stone is added behind the moving front to promote the flow of stone and to ensure that the previously filled area does not lose much of its volume. Once the tooth depressions are completely filled, larger amounts of dental stone can be added under light vibration to fill the remaining impression up to the mucobuccal fold or rim of the boxed area around the impression tray. The impression is then briefly placed on the vibrator for a few seconds to distribute the stone evenly across the impression.

If the inversion method is used, a mound of stone about 20 mm high is made on a flat surface, such as glass plate, with the remainder of the mixture or with a new mix using a lower W/P ratio. The filled impression, which should exhibit the initial set but not the final set, is then inverted over the mound of stone and the base is shaped with the spatula before the stone sets. The dental stone model should be left undisturbed for 45–60 min until the material has set completely. The dental stone model is now separated from the impression. When tooth preparations are involved, a smaller spatula may be used to deliver a much smaller amount of stone to fill the sites of the preparations and ensure complete filling before the remaining portion of the impression is poured.

For mixing:

- Bowl of parabolic shape.
- Stiff bladed spatula.
- Measured amount of water is placed in the bowl.
- Weighed powder is sifted into the water.
- Mixing to a maximum of 1 min.
- Repeatedly adding water and powder to achieve desired consistency should be avoided. This yields a lower strength and may cause distortion.
- The strength and hardness obtained from vacuum mixing usually exceed that obtained by 1 min of hand mixing.

CRITICAL QUESTION

What storage conditions are necessary to maintain the dimensional accuracy of a gypsum cast?

Care of the Cast

Once the setting reactions in the cast have been completed, its dimensions will be relatively constant under ordinary conditions of room temperature and humidity. However, it is sometimes necessary to soak the gypsum cast in water in preparation for other procedures. When a dry cast is immersed in water, negligible expansion may occur if the water is saturated with calcium sulfate. If the water is not saturated, dissolution of gypsum will occur. For example, a stone cast immersed in a container under running water will lose approximately 0.1% of its linear dimension for every 20 min of immersion. The safest method for soaking the cast is to place it in a water bath with gypsum debris remaining on the bottom of the container to provide a saturated solution of calcium sulfate.

If the storage temperature is raised to between 90°C and 110°C (194–230°F), shrinkage occurs, along with loss of strength as the water of crystallization is removed and the dihydrate reverts to the hemihydrate form. As a rule of thumb, it is not safe to store or heat a stone cast in air at a temperature higher than 55°C (130°F).

CRITICAL QUESTION

What procedure should be followed if it is uncertain whether the impression or the gypsum cast has been disinfected?

Infection Control

Concern over possible cross-contamination of dental office personnel by microorganisms, including hepatitis B virus and human immunodeficiency virus, via dental impressions has prompted study of the effect of spray and immersion-disinfecting techniques on impression materials. The effect of such agents on the surface quality and accuracy of the resulting gypsum casts is an important consideration.

If an impression has not been disinfected or if the laboratory has no assurance that an appropriate disinfection protocol is followed, it will be necessary to disinfect the stone cast. Disinfection solutions can be used that do not adversely affect the quality of the gypsum cast. Alternatively, disinfectants can be incorporated either in the powder or dissolved in the mixing water. Addition of a disinfectant in the gypsum products would undoubtedly have an effect on some of the properties of certain products, such as strength, setting expansion, and setting time. The precise effect depends on the types of gypsum and antimicrobial agents used. Nonetheless, the disinfected stones apparently compare favorably with nondisinfected controls. Ivanovski et al. recommended incorporation of 2% glutaraldehyde which was found to be the most effective disinfectant with the least adverse effects on the physical properties of the set cast.

The same microwave irradiation used in drying gypsum casts has also been evaluated in infection control. One study showed that a 5 min irradiation at 900 W reduced microorganism counts (cfu/mL) with a median log value of six to median counts (cfu/mL) of zero. Data on the effectiveness of microwave irradiation on different microorganism species, based on the power setting, the duration needed, and the influence of prolonged irradiation on the properties of the gypsum cast, are not available.

The widespread availability of a spectrum of disinfected dental stone casts (types II–V) with proven efficacy and unimpaired physical properties will undoubtedly strengthen the barrier system of infection control in the dental laboratory.

CRITICAL QUESTION

A wax pattern of an inlay made using the direct technique may result in a loose-fitting inlay than one made using the indirect technique. Why?

Dental Waxes

Wax has been a valuable commodity for over 2000 years. In ancient times beeswax was used for softening skin, binding together reeds used for flutes, coating and preserving valuable objects, candle production, and making sculptures and statues of highly regarded public figures. Beeswax was derived from secretions that bees use to build honeycombs. Although beeswax is still used today, modern waxes, such as those used to preserve furniture and automobile surfaces and those designed for dental procedures, are made from natural plant and animal sources; some types are derived synthetically from petroleum products and distillates. Synthetic waxes are typically composed of hydrogen, carbon, oxygen, and chlorine. Synthetic waxes are more uniform than natural waxes in their organic structure and more homogeneous in composition.

History of Dental Wax

Carnauba is one of the hardest and most durable waxes. It is derived from the fronds (leaves) of carnauba palm trees and is one of the main components of dental **inlay wax**. Candelilla wax, a major component of some dental waxes, is obtained from Candelilla shrub growing in Costa Rica, Guatemala, Mexico, Nicaragua, Panama, and the southwestern United States. In comparison to plant-derived carnauba and candelilla waxes, animal-derived beeswax, smd mineral-derived paraffin and ceresin waxes, other dental waxes are produced from components of fats, gums, oils, and resins.

Types of Inlay Waxes

The wide variety of dental waxes can be classified into two groups, those used primarily in the clinic and those used in commercial dental laboratories. Clinical products include bite registration wax, disclosing wax (also known as pressure-indicating paste), utility waxes for altering and adapting impression trays, and low-melting type I inlay waxes used in the mouth for direct-waxing processes for pattern production. Laboratory products include **boxing wax**, **baseplate wax**, **sticky wax**, beading wax, utility wax, and hard, medium, and soft type II inlay-type waxes for making patterns on patients' models using the **indirect wax technique**. Type II waxes are required for the lost-wax processing of cast prostheses and frameworks. Each of these waxes has a melting range over which the temperature must be adjusted by means of a burner flame to control the **flow** properties for each specific application.

Dental waxes can also be classified in one of three types:

- pattern wax (inlay, casting, and baseplate types),
- processing wax (boxing, utility, and sticky types), and
- impression wax (bite registration and correction types).

Casting wax is used for partial denture frameworks and other metal frameworks. One of the correction types includes waxes for repairing ceramic margin defects on all-ceramic inlays and crowns.

Inlay waxes are used to prepare patterns. These patterns are reproduced in gold via a casting process and in ceramic by hot isostatic pressing procedures. Inlay wax is sometimes referred to as casting wax, although other types of pattern waxes also fall into this category. Inlay wax must exhibit excellent adaptability to model or die surfaces, and it must be free from distortion, flaking, or chipping during the preparation of patterns. It must also be able to disintegrate, volatilize, and be eliminated completely from an investment mold during the **burnout** or wax elimination procedure. For **direct wax techniques** type I inlay wax must soften at a temperature that is not hazardous to the pulp tissue, and it must harden at a temperature above mouth temperature.

The colors of inlay waxes should contrast with the hues of teeth and dies. Dental waxes are supplied in a variety of colors including blue, green, yellow, red, and ivory. The colors are useful to provide a suitable contrast against a die that is an accurate replica of a prepared tooth or dental arch form. Ivory-colored wax is useful for aesthetic case presentations to patients. If applied as a veneer in a sufficient thickness, its opacity must be sufficient to mask colored die stones.

Inlay waxes may be softened over a flame or in water at 54–60°C to enable their flow in the liquid state and their adaptation to the prepared tooth or die. These waxes are designed to maintain uniform workability over a wide temperature range and to facilitate accurate adaptation to the tooth or die under pressure. Additive layers and corrections may be applied to produce a relatively homogeneous pattern. These fused layers can be carved easily without chipping or flaking. A regular or soft type of wax is typically used for indirect work at room temperature or in cool weather. A harder or medium type with a low flow property is indicated for use in warmer climates.

The first procedure in the casting of an inlay or crown for the lost-wax process is the preparation of a **dental wax** pattern. The cavity is prepared in the tooth and the pattern is carved directly on a die that is a reproduction of the prepared tooth and dental tissues (indirect technique). The direct technique for producing wax inlay patterns within prepared teeth is rarely used because of the wax's sensitivity to changes in pressure, temperature, and heating and cooling rates during manipulation. Because the thermal expansion coefficient of wax is extremely high compared with the values for other dental materials, a wax pattern made in the mouth (direct technique) will shrink appreciably as it is cooled to room temperature. A pattern made by the indirect method may not shrink as much, although the amount depends on whether or not the pattern is allowed to reach room temperature before it is removed from the die. Dipping waxes are used occasionally to facilitate the wax pattern preparation process. This wax is kept molten to provide a station for mass production of patterns.

- The first procedure in the casting of an inlay or crown for the lost-wax process is the preparation of a **dental wax** pattern.
- The wax pattern forms the outline of the mold into which an alloy is cast or a ceramic is hot pressed.

Type I is a *medium wax* employed in direct techniques and type II is a *soft wax* used in the indirect techniques. No matter how a pattern is prepared, it should be an accurate reproduction of the missing tooth structure or part of a prosthesis that is adapted to soft tissues. The wax pattern forms the outline of the mold into which an alloy is cast or a ceramic is hot isostatically pressed (HIP). Consequently, the resulting appliance, device, prosthesis, or framework can be no more accurate than the wax pattern regardless of the care observed in subsequent procedures. Therefore, the pattern should be well adapted to the prepared cavity or replica cavity and properly carved without any significant distortion. Before the adaptation of the wax pattern within a tooth or a die, a separating medium must be used to ensure the complete separation of the wax pattern without distortion. After the pattern is removed from the prepared cavity, it is encased in a gypsum- or phosphate-based material or other type of **refractory** material known as an *investment*. This process is called *investing the pattern*.

After investing anatomically accurate wax or resin patterns of inlays, onlays, crowns, bridges, and frameworks for removable partial dentures, the invested material (wax/resin) must be eliminated completely before molten metal is cast or core ceramic is hot pressed into the mold cavity. Wax patterns are used in the production of several types of complex removable devices or prostheses in addition to single-tooth restorations. However, this chapter is limited primarily to the construction of prostheses employed in operative dentistry and fixed prosthodontics.

Composition of Dental Waxes

The primary components of dental waxes are derived from synthetic waxes and natural waxes (hydrocarbons of the paraffin and the microcrystalline groups, carnauba wax, candelilla wax, and resins). As stated earlier, natural waxes are derived from mineral, vegetable, and animal origins. Synthetic waxes are chemically synthesized from natural wax molecules. Most synthetic waxes are more homogeneous than pure natural waxes. Coloring agents are added for contrast of wax patterns against tooth, die, and model surfaces or to provide an ivory colored or other natural tooth color as demonstration models used for educating patients about treatment options. Some formulations contain a compatible filler to control expansion and shrinkage of the wax product.

Most dental waxes contain 40–60% paraffin by weight, which is derived from high-boiling fractions of petroleum. They are composed mainly of a complex mixture of hydrocarbons of the methane series together with minor amounts of amorphous and microcrystalline phases. The wax can be obtained in a wide range of melting

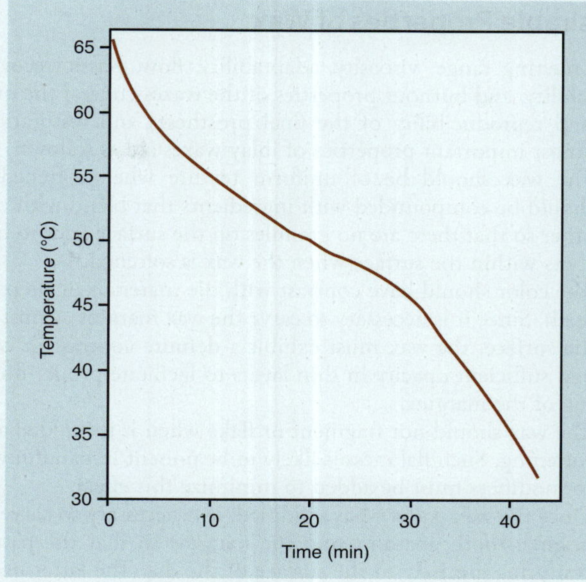

• **Fig. 13.33** Time-temperature cooling curve for type I inlay wax.

or softening temperatures depending on the molecular weight and distribution of the constituents. The melting range can be determined by a temperature versus time cooling curve, as shown in Figure 13.33, for a paraffin-based inlay wax. The temperature–time relationship during cooling indicates the successive solidification of progressively lower–molecular-weight fractions. This condition promotes moldability of the wax below its melting temperature. Paraffin that is used for type I waxes has a higher melting point than the paraffin used for type II waxes. Paraffin wax is likely to flake when it is trimmed, and it does not produce a smooth, glossy surface, which is a desirable requisite for an inlay wax. Thus, other waxes and natural resins must be added as modifying agents.

Gum dammar, or dammar resin, is a natural resin. It is added to the paraffin to improve the smoothness in molding and to render it more resistant to cracking and flaking. It also increases the toughness of the wax and enhances the smoothness and luster of the surface.

Carnauba wax occurs as a fine powder on the leaves of certain tropical palms. This wax is very hard, and it has relatively high melting point and it has an agreeable odor. It is combined with the paraffin to decrease flow at mouth temperature. Carnauba wax contributes greater glossiness to the wax surface than dammar resin.

Candelilla wax can also be added partially or entirely to replace carnauba wax. Candelilla wax provides the same general qualities as carnauba wax but its melting point is lower and it is not as hard as carnauba wax. Ceresin may replace part of the paraffin to modify the toughness and carving characteristics of the wax.

Ceresin is typically a white wax extracted from ozokerite, a waxy mineral mixture of hydrocarbons that is colorless or white when pure, but it has a somewhat unpleasant odor.

Carnauba wax is often replaced in part by certain synthetic waxes that are compatible with paraffin wax. At least two waxes of this type can be used. One is a complex nitrogen derivative of the higher fatty acids and the other contains esters of acids derived from montan wax, a derivative hard wax that is obtained by solvent extraction of certain types of lignite or brown coal. Approximately a third of all montan wax produced is used in automobile polishing pastes.

Desirable Properties of Wax

The melting range, viscosity, adaptability, flow, elastic recovery, carvability, and burnout properties of the waxes control the quality and reproducibility of the final prostheses and restorations. The most important properties of inlay waxes are as follows:

1. The wax should be of uniform texture when softened. It should be compounded with ingredients that blend with each other so that there are no granules on the surface and no hard spots within the surface when the wax is softened.
2. The color should have contrast with die materials or prepared teeth. Since it is necessary to carve the wax margins against the die surface, the wax must exhibit a definite contrast in color and sufficient opacity in thin layers to facilitate proper finishing of the margins.
3. The wax should not fragment or flake when it is molded after softening. Such flakiness is likely to be present in paraffin wax, so modifiers must be added to minimize this effect.
4. Once the wax pattern has solidified, it is necessary to carve the original tooth anatomy and the margins so that the pattern conforms precisely to the surface of the die. The latter procedure sometimes requires that the wax be carved to a very thin layer. The wax must not be pulled away by the carving instrument or chip as it is carved. For lost-wax casting of metals, an investment mold is formed around a wax pattern. After that the wax must be eliminated from the mold. Elimination of the **sprued wax pattern** is usually accomplished by heating the mold to melt and ignite the wax. If the wax leaves a residue or an impervious coating on the walls of the mold, the cast metal inlay may be adversely affected. Consequently, the wax should burn out completely by oxidizing residual carbon to volatile gases. Ideally, when wax melts and is vaporized at 500°C, it should not leave a solid residue that amounts to more than 0.10% of the original weight of the specimen.

Expansion and shrinkage of casting wax are extremely sensitive to temperature. Normally soft wax shrinks more than hard wax. High-shrinkage wax may cause significant pattern distortion when it solidifies. It is necessary to avoid excessive shrinkage and expansion caused by a temperature change. For this reason, organic filler is added to certain wax formulations. Such fillers should be completely miscible with the components of the inlay wax during manufacture, and they should not leave an undesirable residue after burnout.

Flow of Dental Wax

One of the desirable properties of type I inlay wax is that it should exhibit a marked plasticity or flow at a temperature slightly above that of the mouth. The temperatures at which the wax is plastic are indicated by the time–temperature cooling curve for a typical type I wax, as shown in Figure 13.33. The wax begins to harden slowly below 65°C and becomes solid below approximately 48°C, below which it cools rapidly at a constant rate.

Different types of casting waxes exhibit characteristic flow curves as a function of temperature. Each wax exhibits a sharp transition temperature at which it loses its plasticity. Soft wax exhibits a transition point at a lower temperature than hard wax. Inlay waxes do not solidify with a space lattice, as it happens in a metal. Instead, the structure exhibits a combination of crystalline and amorphous structures, with limited short-range order of the molecules. The wax lacks rigidity and may flow under applied pressure even at room temperature.

Requirements for the flow properties of inlay waxes at specific temperatures are summarized in Table 13.18. The flow is measured by subjecting cylindrical specimens to a designated load at the stated temperature and measuring the percentage of reduction in length. The maximum flow permitted for type I waxes at 37°C is 1%. Their low flow at this temperature permits carving and removal of the pattern from the prepared cavity at oral temperature without distortion when a direct technique is employed. In addition, both type I and II waxes at 45°C must have a minimal flow of 70% and a maximum flow of 90%. At this temperature, the wax is inserted into the prepared cavity. If the wax does not have sufficient plasticity, it will not flow into all of the areas in the preparation and reproduce the details.

Thermal Properties of Dental Waxes

Inlay waxes are softened with heat, forced into the prepared tooth cavity in either the tooth or the die, and cooled. The thermal conductivity of the waxes is low (e.g., $k_{paraffin}$ = 0.25 W/mK), and sufficient time must be allowed both to heat them uniformly throughout and to cool them to body or room temperature.

Another thermal characteristic of inlay waxes is their high coefficient of thermal expansion. As shown in Figure 13.34, the wax may expand as much as 0.7% with an increase in temperature of 20°C or contract as much as 0.35% when it is cooled from 37°C to 25°C. The average linear thermal expansion coefficient over this temperature range is 350×10^{-6}/K, with values ranging from 217 to 512×10^{-6}/K.

A comparison of the thermal expansion coefficients of dental materials given in the chapters on physical properties and ceramics indicates that inlay wax expands and contracts thermally more per degree temperature change than any other dental material. This property is less significant when the wax is used in the indirect technique because the pattern is not subjected to a change from mouth to room temperature.

The thermal dimensional change may be affected by the previous treatment of the wax. Curve A in Figure 13.34 represents the thermal expansion of inlay wax as a function of temperature. The expansion rate increases abruptly above approximately 35°C. The temperature at which a change in expansion rate occurs is known as the *glass transition temperature*. Some constituents of the wax probably change in their crystalline form at this temperature, and the wax is more plastic at higher temperatures. Not all waxes

TABLE 13.18 Requirements for Inlay Wax Flow (%)

Type of Wax	T = 30 °C Maximum	T = 37 °C Maximum	T = 40 °C Minimum	T = 40 °C Maximum	T = 45 °C Minimum	T = 45 °C Maximum
I	—	1	—	20	70	90
II	1	—	50	—	70	90

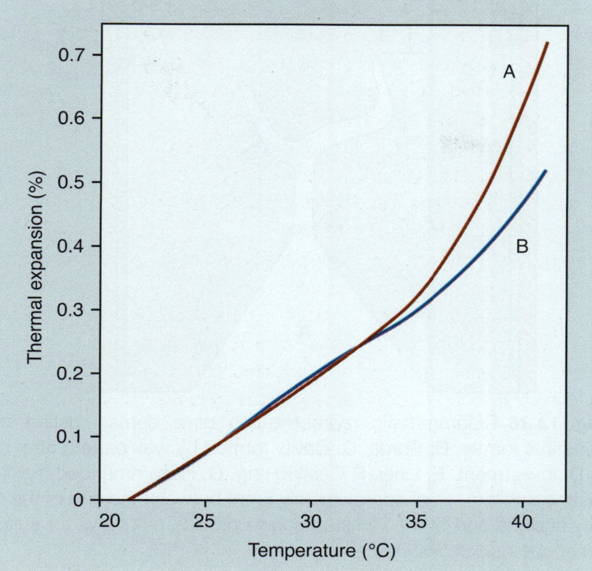

• **Fig. 13.34** Thermal expansion of inlay wax. Curve A represents the thermal expansion when the wax was held under pressure while it was cooling from the liquid state. When the same wax was allowed to cool without pressure and again heated, the behavior shown by curve B occurs.

exhibit transition temperatures. The transition point shown in Figure 13.34 appears to be characteristic of an inlay wax with a high paraffin wax content. If the wax is allowed to cool without being placed under pressure, the transition temperature region is neither as pronounced when it is reheated, nor there is much change in the thermal expansion coefficient, as shown in curve B of Figure 13.34.

- The temperature at which a change in expansion rate occurs in waxes is known as the *glass transition temperature.*
- Some constituents of the wax probably change in their crystalline form at this temperature, and the wax is more plastic at higher temperatures.

Manipulation of Inlay Wax

The higher flow of softer waxes produces larger cast metal or HIP ceramic prostheses than harder waxes because the soft waxes expand more as the investment heats up during setting. Waxes oxidize on heating, and on prolonged heating some waxes evaporate, so that the storage container for melted wax will be coated by gummy deposits. Therefore, care should be exercised to use the lowest temperature possible and to clean the wax pot and replace the wax periodically.

To manipulate inlay wax, dry heat is preferred to the use of a water bath. The latter can result in the inclusion of droplets of water, which can splatter on flaming, smear the wax surface during polishing, and distort the pattern during temperature changes. To avoid distortion during removal of the pattern, it should be penetrated slightly with an explorer point and carefully removed from the cavity. A mesial-occlusal-distal pattern can best be removed by inserting a staple-like wire within the surface so that each prong is positioned above the proximal wall areas of the pattern. It should be removed with dental floss looped through the staple and withdrawn in a direction parallel to the axial walls and with minimum distortion. After removal, touching the pattern with the fingers should be avoided as much as possible to prevent any temperature changes and distortion.

To fabricate indirect patterns, the die should be lubricated, preferably with a lubricant containing a wetting agent. Any excess must be avoided because it will prevent intimate adaptation to the die. The melted wax may be added in layers with a spatula or a waxing instrument. The prepared cavity should be overfilled, and the wax then carved to the proper contour. When the margins are being carved, care should be taken to avoid abrading any surface of the stone die. A silk or other fine cloth may be used for a final polishing of the pattern, rubbing toward the margins. Theoretically, applying pressure is undesirable, as shown by change in shape of the stick of wax in Figure 13.35. However, some clinicians prefer to apply finger pressure as the wax is cooling to help fill the cavity and prevent distortion during cooling. The fingers also accelerate the cooling rate. Although temperature changes should be avoided, some technicians prefer to repeatedly remelt small areas along the margins and examine them under a low-power microscope. Regardless of the method chosen, the most practical method for avoiding any

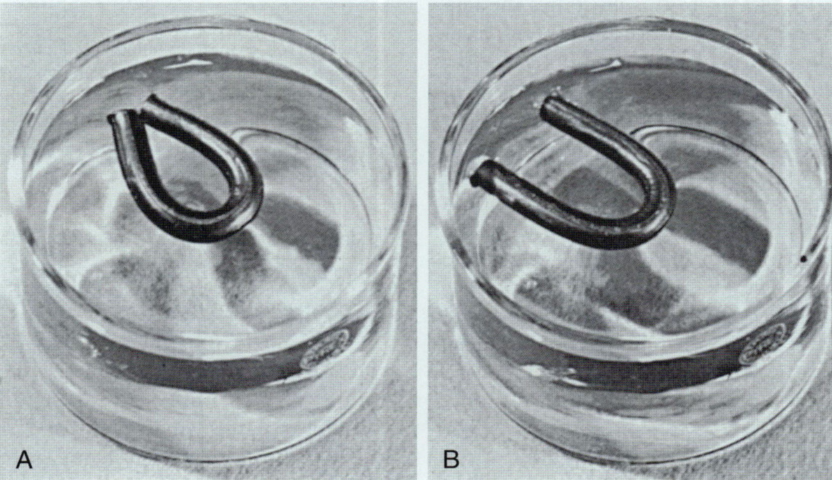

• **Fig. 13.35 A,** A stick of inlay wax is bent into the shape of a horseshoe and floated on water at room temperature. **B,** After 24 hours the same stick of wax tends to relax and distortion occurs.

possible delayed distortion is to invest the pattern immediately after removal from the mouth or die, as noted earlier. Once the investment hardens (sets), no distortion of the pattern will occur.

- The higher flow of softer waxes produces larger cast metal or HIP ceramic prostheses.
- To manipulate inlay wax, dry heat is preferred.
- To fabricate indirect patterns, the die should be lubricated.
- Delayed distortion of the wax pattern can be avoided by investing the pattern immediately after removal from the die.

CRITICAL QUESTION

How can one best minimize potential distortion effects associated with **elastic memory** and temperature changes?

Wax Distortion

Distortion of wax patterns is the most serious problem one can experience in forming and removing the pattern from a tooth or die. Distortion of a wax pattern results from occluded air in the pattern, physical deformation (during molding, carving, or removal), release of stresses "trapped" during previous cooling, excessive storage time, and extreme temperature changes during storage. A newly made wax pattern tends to change its shape and size over time. Upon cooling it contracts and, after attaining equilibrium, reaches a state of dimensional stability. It is important that the wax pattern be retained on the die for several hours to avoid distortion and ensure that equilibrium conditions are established.

Like other thermoplastics, waxes tend to return partially to their original shape after manipulation. This is known as *elastic memory*. To demonstrate this effect, a stick of inlay wax can be softened over a Bunsen burner, bent into a horseshoe shape, and chilled in this position. If it is then floated in room temperature water for a number of hours, the horseshoe will open, as shown in Figure 13.35A and B. This is more critical for inlay waxes because the metal or hot-pressed ceramic restorations made from the wax must fit onto unyielding hard tooth tissue.

The elastic memory of waxes is further illustrated during measurement of the thermal expansion of a wax held under pressure during cooling. The expansion increases above the glass transition temperature more than when it is cooled without pressure, as shown in curve B of Figure 13.34. Again, this illustrates the tendency of wax to return to its normal undisturbed state. In recalling Figure 13.35A, when the wax is bent into a horseshoe, the inner molecules are under compression, and the outer ones are in tension. Once the stresses are gradually relieved at room temperature, the wax tends to recover its elastic strain.

The components of a casting ring with a wax pattern surrounded by casting investment are shown in Figure 13.36. A sprued wax pattern is shown in the center of the investment ring. Examples of properly sprued wax patterns for a single crown and for a three-unit bridge are shown in Figure 13.37. Note the spherical reservoir that is attached to the single-crown pattern. The purpose of the reservoir is to maintain a molten pool of metal to ensure complete filling of the crown area of the mold cavity. For the bridge pattern on the right side of Figure 13.37, a runner bar is used as a reservoir.

Storage of a wax pattern for too long can lead to a distortion of its form because of stress relaxation effects. A casting will fit most accurately when the pattern is invested immediately after its removal from the preparation.

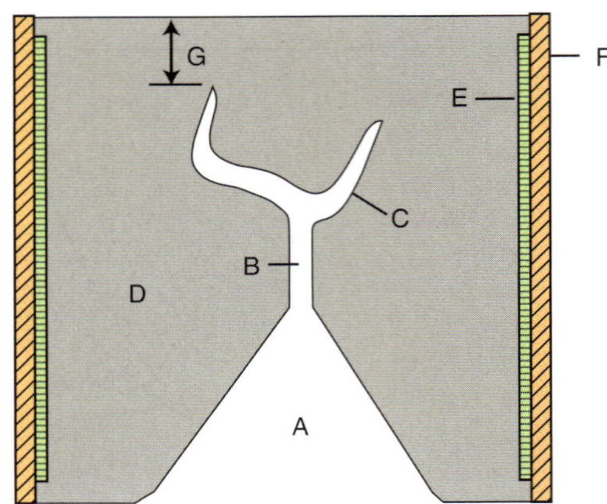

• **Fig. 13.36** Diagrammatic representation of a dental casting mold: **A**, Crucible former. **B**, Sprue. **C**, Cavity formed by wax pattern after burnout. **D**, Investment. **E**, Liner. **F**, Casting ring. **G**, Recommended maximum investment thickness of approximately 6mm between the end of the mold cavity and the end of the invested ring to provide pathways for sufficient gas escape during casting

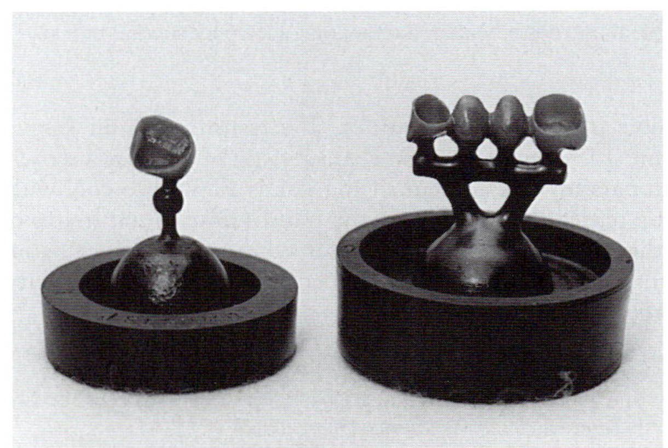

• **Fig. 13.37** Primary sprue oriented directly toward the wax pattern *(left)*. Note the spherical reservoir on the vertical sprue. Indirect sprue design showing a horizontal reservoir runner bar that is positioned near the heat center of the invested ring *(right)*.

- Reservoir is a small amount of additional wax which is added to the sprue former near the junction of wax pattern.
- It prevents localized shrinkage porosity as the alloy in this part solidifies last after the solidification of metal in mold.

CRITICAL QUESTION

Under what conditions should medium and hard waxes be used?

Specialty Waxes

A pattern made of hard wax is less sensitive to temperature conditions than one made of soft wax. The exothermic heat generated during the setting of an investment affects the pattern selectively. A soft wax pattern may result in a slightly larger and relatively rougher casting than a hard wax pattern. This tendency of softer inlay waxes to expand during setting in a hygroscopic bath at 37.8°C (100°F) may contribute to the phenomenon of **hygroscopic expansion**.

Other types of waxes are employed for different purposes than those described for the inlay waxes. The composition of each type is adjusted for the particular requirements. One of the most common is baseplate wax.

Baseplate wax is used to establish the initial arch form in the construction of complete dentures. Supplied in 1–2-mm thick red or pink sheets, the wax is approximately 75% paraffin or ceresin with additions of beeswax and other resins or waxes. Harder the wax, the less is the flow at a given temperature. The difference in flow of the three types may be advantageous for a particular application. There are three types of waxes according to the flow and each one is indicated for a particular purpose.

- Type I, a soft wax, is used for building veneers.
- Type II, a medium wax, is designed for patterns to be placed in the mouth in normal climatic conditions.
- Type III, a hard wax, is used for trial fitting in the mouth in tropical climates.

Because residual stress is present within the wax from contouring and manipulating the wax, the finished denture pattern should be flasked as soon as possible after completion of all adjustments and manipulations.

The *impression waxes*, also referred to as ***bite waxes*** or ***corrective waxes***, tend to distort if they are withdrawn from undercut areas. Thus, they are limited to use in edentulous sites of the mouth or in occlusal surface areas. Although corrective waxes are relatively soft at mouth temperature, they have sufficient body to register the detail of soft tissues, and they are rigid at room temperature.

Other types of dental waxes include *sticky wax*, yellow- or orange-colored stick wax, which is tacky when melted but firm and brittle when cooled. Sticky waxes are used to temporarily fasten gypsum model components, join and temporarily stabilize the components of a bridge before soldering, or attach pieces of a broken denture prior to a repair.

Boxing wax is another useful material for enclosing an impression before plaster or stone cast is poured. Typically provided in pink-colored flat sheets, this wax is relatively soft and pliable and can easily be pressed to the desired contour around the perimeter of an impression and self-sealed at the overlapped area with firm pressure.

Carving wax and *presentation wax* are used for demonstration purposes. Such waxes contain synthetic and polymeric materials with additives such as fillers and coloring agents.

Summary

- **Irreversible impression material** means that chemical reactions have occurred and the material cannot revert to the previous state, for example, alginate, zinc oxide–eugenol (ZOE) impression paste, impression plaster, and elastomeric impression materials.
- Reversible impression materials soften upon heating and solidify slightly above body temperature with no chemical change taking place, for example, agar and impression compound.
- **Elastomeric impression materials** (rubber base) are polysulfide, silicone (condensation and addition), and polyether.
- Different consistencies (viscosity) of elastomeric impression materials—extra low, low, medium, heavy, and putty, in increasing order of filler content.
- Three modes of mixing elastomers are hand mixing, static mixing (using a gun), and dynamic mechanical mixing.
- **Putty-wash technique:** Putty can be used as the tray material in conjunction with a low-viscosity silicone as a wash impression.
- **Multiple-mix technique:** A syringe material (light body) and a tray material (heavy body) are used in this technique. Both materials are mixed simultaneously, each by a different person. The lighter material is injected from the filled syringe or directly from a static mixing gun within and around the tooth preparation. The filled tray is then inserted in the mouth and seated over the syringe material, which has been extruded on hard and/or soft tissue.
- **Monophase technique:** The procedure is similar to that of the multiple-mix technique except that only one mixture is made, and part of the material is placed in the tray, and another portion is placed in the syringe for injection in the cavity preparation, prepared teeth, or soft tissue.
- **Addition silicone** is also called polyvinyl siloxane (PVS) or vinyl polysiloxane (VPS) impression material.
- Sulfur contamination from natural latex gloves inhibits the setting of addition silicone.
- Tear strength of elastomers in the ascending order: **Polysulfide $<$ polyether $<$ silicone.**
- Dimensional stability of elastomers in the ascending order: **Polysulfide $<$ condensation $<$ polyether $<$ addition**.
- Biocompatibility of impression materials in the ascending order: **Polyether $<$ alginate $<$ silicones $<$ ZOE $<$ polysulfides.**
- Reversible hydrocolloid is otherwise known as agar.
- Irreversible hydrocolloid is otherwise known as alginate.
- The agar gel liquefies to a sol when it is heated to a temperature known as the ***liquefaction temperature*** (70–100°C). When the sol is cooled, it becomes a gel at a point known as the ***gelation temperature*** (between 37°C and 50°C).
- **Laminate technique,** also called alginate–agar method, alginate is used as a tray material while agar is expressed from a syringe.
- **Duplicating materials**—both types of hydrocolloids are used in the dental laboratory to duplicate dental casts or models. The hydrocolloid-type duplicating materials have the same composition as the impression materials but their water content is higher.
- **Impression plaster** is a β-calcium sulfate hemihydrate used at a water/powder ratio of approximately 0.5–0.6. It was once used to make wash impressions of edentulous ridges in combination with impression compound. Because of its rigidity, the use of impression plaster has been suggested for making splinting transfer coping utilized to produce long-span implant-supported prostheses.
- **Impression compound** also called modeling plastic, is a thermoplastic material. Type I impression compound is a lower-fusing material for making impressions in the oral cavity; it may be supplied in either sheet or stick form. Type II is a higher-fusing material, also called tray compound, used for forming trays to be used in the oral cavity.
- An impression of soft tissue obtained with tray compound is referred to as the primary impression. It is then used as a tray to support a thin layer of a second impression material, which is to be placed against the tissues. This impression is known as the **secondary impression** or a **wash impression.**
- Secondary impressions may also be made with a ZOE wash paste, hydrocolloid, impression plaster, or light body elastomer.

- Zinc oxide–eugenol (ZOE) is used as an impression material for edentulous mouths, a surgical dressing, bite registration paste, temporary filling material, root canal filling material, cementing medium, and temporary relining material for dentures.

Gypsum Products

- **Gypsum products** are supplied as fine powder of hemihydrate of calcium sulfate and that is produced by heating ground gypsum (dihydrate of calcium sulfate) particles.
- **ADA Specification No. 25** classifies five types of gypsum products: Impression plaster (type I); model plaster (type II); dental stone (type III); dental stone, high strength (type IV); dental stone, high strength, high expansion (type V).
- The primary applications of gypsum products in dentistry include the production of study models of oral and maxillofacial structures and their use as auxiliary materials for dental laboratory operations involved in the production of dental prostheses.
- The most widely accepted setting mechanism of gypsum is the **dissolution–precipitation theory,** which is based on dissolution of the hemihydrate particles in water followed by instant recrystallization to dihydrate.
- **Water/powder (W/P) ratio** is an important factor in determining the physical and mechanical properties of the final gypsum product.
- **Chemical modifiers** have been used extensively to increase or decrease the setting time of gypsum products. They are called *retarders* and *accelerators*, respectively.
- Depending on the composition of the gypsum product, the observed linear expansion may be as low as 0.06% or as high as 0.5%.
- Lower W/P ratio and a longer mixing time will increase the setting expansion.
- The **setting expansion** is usually called *normal setting expansion* whereas the expansion that occurs under water is known as *hygroscopic setting expansion.*
- Two strength properties of gypsum are reported—the *wet strength* also known as *green strength* and the *dry strength.*
- The effect of disinfecting agents on the surface quality and accuracy of the resulting gypsum casts is an important consideration.

Waxes

- **Synthetic waxes** are typically composed of hydrogen, carbon, oxygen, and chlorine.
- Paraffin wax flakes when it is trimmed, and does not produce a smooth, glossy surface.
- Gum dammar added to paraffin improves the smoothness and renders it more resistant to cracking and flaking.
- Carnauba wax when combined with paraffin wax decreases its flow at mouth temperature.
- Candelilla wax can also be used instead of carnauba wax.
- **Type I inlay wax** has a maximum flow of 1% at 37°C, this permits carving and removal of the pattern without distortion.
- Both **type I and II** inlay waxes must have a minimal flow of 70% and a maximum flow of 90% at 45°C.
- Distortion of a wax pattern occurs due to release of stresses trapped during previous cooling.

Review Questions

1. List the ideal properties of an impression material.
2. Classify impression materials. Enumerate the different elastomeric impression materials and write a detailed note on addition silicones.
3. Write a note on tissue management prior to impression making.
4. Enumerate and briefly describe different techniques used for impression making with elastomeric impression materials.
5. Classify hydrocolloid impression materials. Describe alginate impression material in detail.
6. Write a short note on compatibility of hydrocolloids with gypsum.
7. What is laminate technique in impression making?
8. Enumerate the different uses of zinc oxide–eugenol in dentistry.

Gypsum Products

1. Discuss types of gypsum products and their properties.
2. Describe the setting reaction of dental stone.
3. Explain the mechanism of setting expansion in dental stone.
4. Give a brief note on the composition and properties of die stones.

Waxes

1. Describe composition, properties, manipulation, and uses of inlay casting wax.
2. Classify waxes. Discuss in detail impression waxes.
3. Write a short note on causes of wax distortion.
4. Discuss briefly sticky wax.
5. Discuss in brief composition of dental waxes.
6. Write briefly on the desirable properties of dental waxes.

Selected Readings

Alaghari S, Velagala S, Alla RK, Ramaraju AV. Advances in alginate impression materials: a review. Int J Dent Mater 2019;1(2): 55–59.

Balkenhol M.S.; Haunschild S.; Lochnit G.; et al. Surfactant release from hydrophilized vinylpolysiloxanes. J Dent Res 88 668–672 (2009); Water droplets placed on the hydrophilized VPS absorbed surfactant from the VPS reduced the surface tension of the water droplet. It resulted in lower contact angle over time; surface properties of the VPS did not change.

Barnes H.A. Thixotropy—a review. J Non-Newtonian Fluid Mech 70 1–33 (1997); This review article describes in detail the thixotropic phenomenon with examples of thixotropic systems.

Blatz M.B.; Sadan A.; Burgess J.O.; et al. Selected characteristics of a new polyvinyl siloxane impression material: a randomized clinical trial. Quintessence Int 36 97–104 (2005); Hydrophilized PVS impression material provided a significantly higher proportion of impressions free of bubbles and voids than the nonhydrophilized PVS.

Boening K.W.; Walter M.H.; Schuette U. Clinical significance of surface activation of silicone impression materials. J Dent 26 447–452 (1998); This study shows no significant correlation between sulcus reproduction and free surface energy or between quality ranking and free surface energy.

Bradna P.; Cerna D. Impact of water quality on setting of irreversible hydrocolloid impression materials. J Prosthet Dent 96 443–448 (2006); The use of tap water with high water hardness accelerated setting of alginate impression as opposed to the use of distilled water.

Chai J.; Pang I.-C. A study of the "thixotropic" property of elastomeric impression materials. Int J Prosthodont 7 155–158 (1994); The study shows shear thinning does not have a lasting effect on the viscosity of vinyl polysiloxane, polyether, or polysulfide.

Chen S.Y.; Liang W.M.; Chen F.N. Factors affecting the accuracy of elastomeric impression materials. J Dent 32 603–609 (2004); This study evaluates the effects of storage times and the proportion of inorganic filler on the accuracy and stability of elastomeric impression materials.

Craig R.G. Review of dental impression materials. Adv Dent Res 2 51–64 (1988); This article reviews published works from 1975 to 1986. Advances during the period included disinfection solutions, the agar/alginate technique, dustless alginate, new formulations of polyether and PVS, elimination of hydrogen gas from PVS, the static mixing of PVS, and hydrophilization of PVS.

Davis B.A.; Powers J.M. Effect of immersion disinfection on properties of impression materials. J Prosthodont 3 31–34 (1994); Two 30-min cycles of disinfection in 2% acid-potentiated glutaraldehyde reduced wettability but had little effect on the dimensional change of addition silicones and polyethers.

Grundke K.; Michel S.; Knispel G.; et al. Wettability of silicone and polyether impression materials: characterization by surface tension and contact angle measurements. Colloids and Surfaces A: Physicochem Eng Aspects 317 598–609 (2008); The decrease of the water contact angle was directly related to the decrease in the liquid surface tension of the water droplet during spreading. The migration of the surfactant to the outermost surface was increasingly hindered with the progression of the polymerization and cross-linking process.

Hosseinpour D.; Berg J.C. The dynamic interaction of water with four dental impression materials during cure. J Prosthodont 18 292–300 (2009); All materials investigated in the fresh, uncured state showed qualitative decomposition, such as formation of a crater and a scum of material at its surface, from interaction with probing water. These effects diminished with curing time until, beyond a critical value, no effects were evident. The initial hydrophilicity was highest for polyether. Beyond the critical curing time, different degrees of hydrophilicity were observed, with Aquasil showing the lowest final contact angle.

Kim K.-N.; Craig R.G.; Koran A. Viscosity of monophase addition silicones as a function of shear rate. J Prosthet Dent 67 794–798 (1992); All products showed a 6- to 10-fold decrease in viscosity with an increasing shear rate (shear thinning).

Klooster J.; Logan G.I.; Tjan A.H.L. Effects of strain rate on the behavior of elastomeric impressions. J Prosthet Dent 66 292–298 (1991); This study reported that (1) polysulfide exhibited the greatest deformation with the lowest tensile strengths; (2) higher strain rates yielded higher tensile strength; and (3) polysulfides showed the greatest elongation at rupture, with the highest values for higher strain rates.

Lim K.-C.; Chong Y.-H.; Soh G. Effect of operator variability on void formation in impressions made with an automixed addition silicone. Aust Dent J 37 35–38 (1992); Automixing produced substantially fewer voids than hand mixing. There was a significant difference in the number of voids in the impressions made by the two operators.

Lu H.; Nguyen B.; Powers J.M. Mechanical properties of 3 hydrophilic addition silicone and polyether elastomeric impression materials. J Prosthet Dent 92 151–154 (2004); The study shows that a new "soft" polyether impression materials had higher strain in compression and lower tensile strength compared to new "hydrophilic" addition silicone materials.

Michael N. Mandikos, Polyvinyl siloxane impression materials: An update on clinical use, Australian Dental Journal 1998;43:(6):428–34.

Martinez J.E.; Combe E.C.; Pesun I.J. Rheological properties of vinyl polysiloxane impression pastes. Dent Mater 17 471–476 (2001); Both PVS materials investigated in the study exhibited thixotropic properties.

McCabe J.F.; Carrick T.E. Recording surface detail on moist surfaces with elastomeric impression materials. Eur J Prosthodont Restor Dent 14 42–46 (2006); It was concluded that the more hydrophilic nature of the polyether and hybrid materials enabled them to record more accurate impressions of moist surfaces, particularly in areas of difficult access such as deep grooves.

McCormick J.T.; Antony S.J.; Dial M.L.; et al. Wettability of elastomeric impression materials: effect of selected surfactants. Int J Prosthodont 2 413–420 (1989); There are two distinct groups of impression materials classified by surface wettability: agar, alginate, and polyether are hydrophilic, while polysulfide and silicone (not hydrophilized) are more hydrophobic.

Norling B.K.; Reisbick M.H. The effect of nonionic surfactants on bubble entrapment in elastomeric impression materials. J Prosthet Dent 42 342–347 (1979); The incorporation of nonionic surfactants into silicone and polysulfide elastomers increases their wettability by gypsum products and results in fewer bubbles in poured casts.

Phatale S, Marawar P P, Byakod G, Lagdive SB, Kalburge JV. Effect of retraction materials on gingival health: a histopathological study. J Indian Soc Periodontol 2010;14:35-9.

Pratten D.H.; Novetsky M. Detail reproduction of soft tissue: a comparison of impression materials. J Prosthet Dent 65 188–191 (1991); Polyether and hydrophilized addition silicone were judged best in detail reproduction and ZOE and polysulfide low-viscosity materials were judged worst in this regard. Voids were minimized with low-viscosity polysulfide and ZOE relative to addition silicones.

Rupp F.D.; Axmann D.; Jacobi A.; et al. Hydrophilicity of elastomeric non-aqueous impression materials during setting. Dent Mater 21 94–102 (2005); Real time observation shows that contact angle on nonaqueous elastomeric impression material decreases rapidly during setting. The rate of reduction is faster with hydrophilized PVS.

Salem N.S.; Combe E.C.; Watts D.C. Mechanical properties of elastomeric impression materials. J Oral Rehab 15 125–132 (1988); This study investigated four elastomeric impression materials. The polysulfide had the greatest resistance to tearing but the elastic modulus and tensile strength were less than that of the other three materials.

Sydiskis R.K.; Gerhardt D.E. Cytotoxicity of impression materials. J Prosthet Dent 69 431–435 (1993); Comparison of cell cytotoxicity and cell viability for seven types of impression materials showed that polyether exhibited the most adverse effects in both categories.

Tingting Jianga, Sang-Mi Leea, Yanan Houa, Xin Changc, Hyeon-Shik Hwang. Evaluation of digital dental models obtained from dental cone-beam computed tomography scan of alginate impressions: The Korean J. of Orthodontics; kjod.(2016).46.3:129–136.

Takahashi H.; Finger W.J. Dentin surface reproduction with hydrophilic and hydrophobic impression materials. Dent Mater 7 197–201 (1991); No difference was found in the detail reproduction of the dentin surface by either type of PVS. It was concluded that the surface tension of PVS before complete setting is lower than that of the dentin surface; therefore PVS, regardless of hydrophobicity, will spread on wet dentin.

von Berg G.B. Accuracy of polyether vs plaster impressions for long-span implant supported prostheses. MSc Thesis. University of the Witwatersrand: Johannesburg; This study shows that for polyether impressions, the use of plaster resulted in smaller interabutment error but with less predictable variance in dimensions.

Wassell R.W.; Ibbetson R.J. The accuracy of polyvinyl siloxane impressions made with standard and reinforced stock trays. J Prosthet Dent 645 748–757 (1992); Using stock trays, the heavy-body/light-body combination was superior to the putty-wash impression made with the addition silicone.

Webber R.L.; Ryge G. The determination of tear energy of extensible materials of dental interest. J Biomed Mater Res 2 281–296 (1968); An equation was used that takes dimensional change of the test specimen into consideration in calculating tear energy.

Gypsum Products

Bailey J.H.; Donovan T.E.; Preston J.D. The dimensional accuracy of improved dental stone, silver-plated, and epoxy resin die materials.

J Prosthet Dent 59 307–310 (1988); Silver-plated and epoxy resin die systems were found to be acceptable alternatives to the improved dental stones.

Berg E.; Nielsen O.; Skaug N. High-level microwave disinfection of dental gypsum casts. Int J Prosthodont 18 (6) 520–525 (2005); Microwave treatment was capable of eliminating microorganisms on gypsum casts, whereas casts poured from disinfected alginate impressions were not free of microorganisms.

Brukl C.E.; McConnell R.M.; Norling B.K.; et al. Influence of gauging water composition on dental stone expansion and setting time. J Prosthet Dent 51 218–223 (1984); This study investigated the influence of water purity on the setting of dental stones. It confirmed that a slurry of fine gypsum particles was the most effective accelerator but showed that solutions of supernatant had no significant influence on the setting of dental stones.

Chan T.K.C.; Darvell B.W. Effect of storage conditions on calcium sulphate hemihydrate-containing products. Dent Mater 17 134–141 (2001); This article shows that at a relative humidity less than 70%, it would take in excess of 1000 h of exposure before reaction within the gypsum products began. There is no evidence to suggest that there is a safe humidity level for exposure.

Dilts W.E.; Duncanson M.G. Jr.; Collard E.W. Comparative stability of cast mounting materials. J Okla Dent Assoc 68 11–13 (1978); Certain properties of mounting gypsum products are cited, particularly their low-setting expansion.

Ivanovski S.; Savage N.W.; Brockhurst P.J.; et al. Disinfection of dental stone casts: antimicrobial effects and physical property alterations. Dent Mater 11 19–23 (1995); This article shows that the incorporation of disinfectant in mixing water affected the setting time, setting expansion, compressive strength, and detail reproduction; it delayed expansion of the stone, but the changes observed were within the specification limit. Casts poured from contaminated alginate impression showed antimicrobial effects depending on the disinfectant used.

Jørgensen K.D. Studies on the setting of plaster of Paris. Odontol Tidskr 61 304–346 (1953); The porosity of set gypsum was calculated as a function of W/P ratio. The higher the ratio, the greater the porosity.

Kuntze R.A. The Chemistry and Technology of Gypsum. American Society for Testing and Materials: Philadelphia; This is an excellent reference on the basic chemistry and technological aspects of gypsum.

Lautenschlager E.P.; Harcourt J.K.; Ploszaj L.C. Setting reactions of gypsum materials investigated by x-ray diffraction. J Dent Res 48 43–48 (1969); This article demonstrates the conversion of the hemihydrate to the dihydrate of calcium sulfate.

Lewry A.J.; Williamson J. The setting of gypsum plaster. J Mater Sci 29 5279–5284 (1994); The article describes the reaction occurring in three steps: dissolution, nucleation and precipitation, as well as completion associated with depletion of reactants.

Lucas M.G.; Arioli-Filho J.N.; Nogueira S.S.; et al. Effect of incorporation of disinfectant solutions on setting time, linear dimensional stability, and detail reproduction in dental stone casts. J Prosthodont 18 521–526 (2009); This article shows that addition of sodium hypochlorite significantly altered, adversely, all of the evaluated properties. However, the addition of glutaraldehyde and chlorhexidine did not make any significant changes in the evaluated properties.

Mahler D.B.; Ady A.B. Explanation for the hygroscopic setting expansion of dental gypsum products. J Dent Res 39 578–589 (1960); This is a classic study that best defines the mechanics of hygroscopic expansion.

Saso Ivanovski S, Savage N W, Brockhurst P J, Bird P S. Disinfection of dental stone casts: antimicrobial effects and physical property alterations. Dent Mater 11:19–23, January, 1995.

Yap A.U.; Yap S.H.; Teo J.C.; et al. Microwave drying of high strength dental stone: effects on dimensional accuracy. Oper Dent 28 193–199 (2003); This study shows that there was no significant difference in percentage weight loss from specimens that were either air dried for 24 h or microwaved at each time interval. Significant differences in dimensional change were observed between specimens microwaved at higher energy levels with shorter duration and those air-dried for 24 h.

Waxes

Baum L.; Phillips R.W.; Lund M.R. Textbook of Operative Dentistry. ed 2 Saunders: Philadelphia; Techniques for manipulating wax and forming the pattern are described.

Craig R.G.; Eick J.D.; Peyton F.A. Strength properties of waxes at various temperatures and their practical application. J Dent Res 46 300 (1967); Properties of waxes are controlled by the composition and melting range of certain components.

Ito M.; Kuroiwa A.; Nagasawa S.; et al. Effect of wax melting range and investment liquid concentration on the accuracy of a three-quarter crown casting. J Prosthet Dent 87 56–57 (2002); The relationship between wax characteristics and the casting accuracy of a three-quarter crown was investigated using four different wax materials: paraffin 135 with a softening temperature of 37.5°C (P38), paraffin 1080 with a softening temperature of 63.5°C, one with a softening temperature of 41.5°C, and a hard wax with a softening temperature of 51°C. Two mixtures of phosphate-bonded investment were prepared, one with 100% special liquid and another with 75% special liquid plus 25% distilled water. P38 demonstrated the best results. Casting shrinkage was smaller with the use of 100% special liquid. Casting shrinkage was affected by the type of wax used and was sensitive to the site at which dimensional measurements were made. The casting shrinkage increased when waxes with a higher softening temperature were used.

Ito M.; Yamagishi T.; Oshida Y.; et al. Effect of selected physical properties of waxes on investments and casting shrinkage. J Prosthet Dent 75 (2) 211–216 (1996); This study evaluated the relationship between flow characteristics, bending strength, and softening temperature of paraffin and dental inlay waxes to casting shrinkage when patterns were invested with a phosphate-bonded investment. Casting shrinkage decreased as the flow of the wax pattern increased. If a low-flow wax or thick pattern is used, the size of the casting ring should be increased.

Jorgensen K.D.; Ono T. Distortion of wax crowns. Scand J Dent Res 92 (3) 253–256 (1984); Distortion of wax crowns is sufficient to reduce the fit of the final restoration to a degree that is clinically unacceptable. This study suggests that wax pattern distortion may be minimized only by use of a pattern/die investing technique.

Kotsiomiti E.; McCabe J.F. Experimental wax mixtures for dental use. J Oral Rehabil 24 (7) 517–521 (1997).

Kotsiomiti E.; McCabe J.F. Stability of dental waxes following repeated heatings. J Oral Rehabil 22 (2) 135–143 (1995); The flow and strength properties of dental waxes were examined following excessive and repeated heatings. Reductions in flow and elastic modulus were observed in some cases after the heating temperature had been increased to 300°C. Repeated exposure of dental waxes to temperatures higher than 200°C may affect the composition and properties, resulting in inferior materials.

McMillan L.C.; Darvell B.W. Rheology of dental waxes. Dent Mater 16 (5) 337–350 (2000); The rheological properties of waxes were evaluated using a modified Stokes' falling ball method. Waxes were shown to be pseudoplastic and did not display a yield point. The pseudoplasticity followed a power law whose exponent was temperature dependent in a complex manner. A standardized viscosity number was defined to characterize the flow behavior of dental waxes. The reciprocal of the pseudoplasticity parameter provides a similarly convenient measure of the stress sensitivity of the wax.

Saso Ivanovski S, Savage N W, Brockhurst P J, Bird P S. Disinfection of dental stone casts: antimicrobial effects and physical property alterations. Dent Mater 11:19–23, January, 1995.

Steinbock A.F. An overview of dental waxes. Dental Lab News (1989). July, p. 50; An excellent review of the various types of waxes, their composition, and their properties.

14

Casting Investments and Casting Procedures

CHAPTER OUTLINE

KEY TERMS

Burnout—Process of heating an invested mold to eliminate the embedded wax or plastic pattern.

Casting—(1) The process by which a wax pattern is converted to a metallic replica of a prepared tooth restoration. (2) A dental restoration formed by the solidification of a molten metal in a mold.

Divesting—Process of removing investment from a cast metal or hot-pressed ceramic.

Hygroscopic expansion—Amount of setting expansion that occurs when a gypsum-bonded casting investment is immersed in 38°C water during setting. (see Chapter 13, Auxiliary Materials, for more information on this process.)

Refractory—Capable of sustaining exposure to a high temperature without significant degradation.

Sprue—The mold channel through which molten metal or ceramic flows into a mold cavity.

Sprued wax pattern—A wax form consisting of the prosthesis pattern and the attached ingate or sprue network.

The lost-wax method has been used to fabricate prostheses made of metal, ceramic, and polymers. Although the principle of the process is the same for all three classes of materials, there are distinct differences unique to each material. Fabrication of ceramic- and polymer-based prostheses was presented in Chapters 10 and 11, respectively. This chapter will focus on the metals only.

The process requires a die that duplicates the oral tissue needing a replacement or prosthesis. A wax pattern (Fig. 14.1) of the prosthesis is built on the laboratory indirect die by carving wax to the exact dimension. The wax pattern is then removed from the die and placed in a casting ring to be filled with investment materials. After the investment sets, the casting ring is heated to melt and burn out the wax. The investment material in the casting ring is now a negative of the final prosthesis. The negative mold is then filled with molten metal or ceramic. After the metal cools, the investment is fragmented and removed, leaving the prosthesis. This is a very brief description of the process. In practice, there are many fine details. The focus of this chapter is first to prepare a die suitable for fabricating the wax pattern. The wax pattern is then fixed in a casting ring with cylindrical segments known as an *ingate* or *sprue* for the flow of molten metal or ceramic to fill the mold cavity, made by investing in a refractory material (Fig. 14.2). The molten metal or ceramic is introduced to the empty space with pressure. Finally, there is a discussion of casting defects.

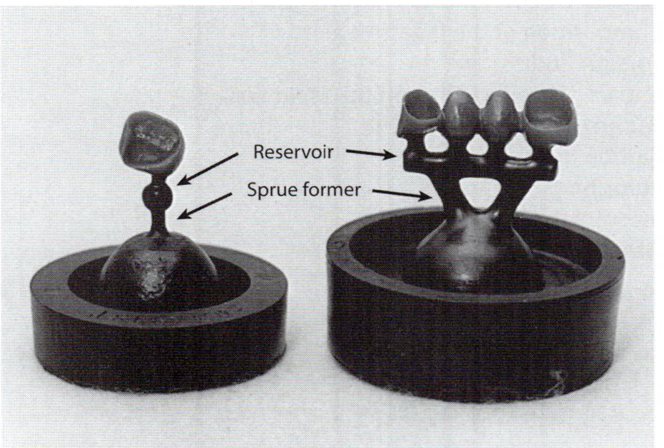

• **Fig. 14.1** Primary sprue oriented directly toward the wax pattern (*left*). Note the spherical reservoir on the vertical sprue. Indirect sprue design showing a horizontal reservoir runner bar that is positioned near the heat center of the invested ring (*right*).

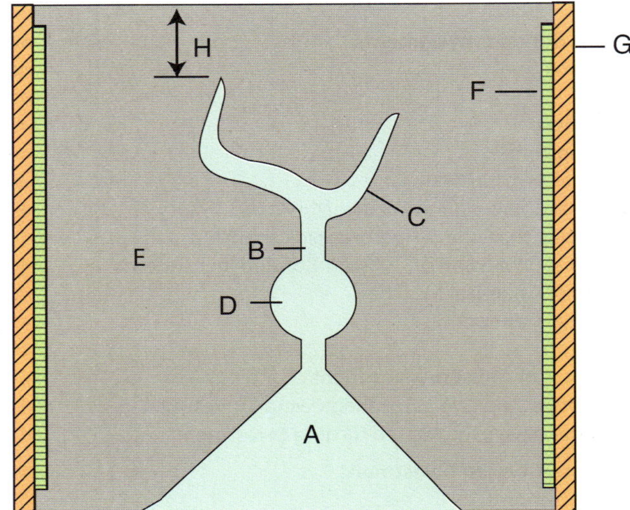

• **Fig. 14.2** Diagrammatic representation of a dental casting mold. **(A)** Crucible former. **(B)** Sprue. **(C)** Cavity formed by wax pattern after burnout. **(D)** Reservoir. **(E)** Investment. **(F)** Liner. **(G)** Casting ring. **(H)** Recommended maximum investment thickness of approximately 6 mm between the end of the mold cavity and the end of the invested ring to provide pathways for sufficient gas escape during casting.

CRITICAL QUESTION

Why should gypsum-bonded investment not be heated above 700°C?

Gypsum-Bonded Investments

The most common method used to form metal inlays, onlays, crowns, bridges, and other metal frameworks is to cast molten alloys by centrifugal force, under pressure, or under vacuum and pressure into a mold cavity. The material used for the mold must be sufficiently refractory and thermally stable that it can withstand exposure to the high temperatures of molten metal as the metal solidifies and cools to room temperature. In addition, the mold or investment material must not interact chemically with the metal surface, and it must be easy to remove from the metal casting.

Refractories are materials that are resistant to high temperature.

The mold cavity is produced by eliminating a wax or resin pattern by heating the mold to a specific temperature and for a specific time. This is called the *burnout process*. To provide a pathway to the mold cavity for molten metal, the wax or resin pattern must have one or more cylindrical wax segments attached at the desired point(s) of metal entry; this arrangement is termed as *sprued wax pattern*. A **sprue** is the channel in a refractory investment mold through which molten metal flows. After the wax pattern has been made, on a replica die of the tooth, a sprue former base is attached to the sprued wax pattern, a ring is pressed into the sprue former base, and an investment slurry is vibrated into the ring to embed the wax pattern. Examples of sprued wax patterns on a sprue former base are shown in Figure 14.1. The investment material is mixed in the same manner as plaster or dental stone, poured around the pattern, and allowed to set. After the investment hardens, the sprue former base is removed. The wax pattern inside the investment is eliminated by heating, thereby forming the mold. The molten metal is then forced through the sprue or ingate created by the sprue former into the mold cavity. The remainder of this chapter deals with refractory investments and casting methods used for the fabrication of small dental crown and bridge prostheses either by casting metal or by hot-pressing ceramic.

Generally, two types of investments—gypsum bonded and phosphate bonded—are employed, depending on the melting range of the alloy to be cast. The gypsum-based materials are traditionally used for conventional casting of gold alloy inlays, onlays, crowns, and larger fixed dental prostheses (FDPs). Phosphate-based investments are designed primarily for base metal alloys which are used to produce copings or frameworks for metal–ceramic prostheses. It can also be used for pressable ceramics. A third type is the ethyl silicate–bonded investment, which is used principally for the casting of removable partial dentures made from base metals (cobalt-based and nickel-based alloys). Commercially pure titanium and titanium alloys require a special investment (zirconia and alumina based) as well as a controlled atmosphere to achieve satisfactory castings.

The type of investment used depends on whether the appliance to be fabricated is fixed or removable and on the method of obtaining the expansion required to compensate for the contraction of the molten alloy during solidification. Type I investments are those employed for the casting of inlays or crowns when the compensation for alloy casting shrinkage is accomplished principally by thermal expansion of the investment. Type II investments are also used for casting inlays, onlays, or crowns, but the major mode of compensation for alloy shrinkage during solidification is by hygroscopic expansion achieved by immersing the invested ring in a warm water bath. Burnout of the wax pattern is performed at a lower temperature than that used for the high-heat burnout technique. Type III investments are used rarely in the construction of partial dentures because they are designed for casting gold alloys. This chapter focuses primarily on type I and type II investments.

Composition

The ingredients of dental inlay investments employed with conventional gold casting alloys are α-hemihydrate of gypsum, and quartz, or cristobalite, which are forms of silica. Most investments contain the α-hemihydrate of gypsum because of its greater strength. This gypsum product serves as a binder for the other ingredients and to provide rigidity. The strength of the investment is dependent on the amount of binder used. The investment powder may contain 25–45% of calcium sulfate hemihydrate. The remainder consists of silica allotropes and controlling chemicals.

The α-hemihydrate form of gypsum is generally the binder for investments used in casting gold-containing alloys with melting ranges below 1000°C. When this material is heated at temperatures sufficiently high to completely dehydrate the investment and to ensure complete castings, it shrinks considerably and occasionally fractures.

The thermal expansion curves for the three common forms of gypsum products are shown in Figure 14.3. All forms shrink considerably after dehydration between 200°C and 400°C. A slight expansion takes place between 400°C and approximately 700°C, and a large contraction then occurs. This latter shrinkage is most likely caused by decomposition and the release of sulfur dioxide. This decomposition not only causes shrinkage but also contaminates the castings with the sulfides of the nonnoble alloying elements, such as silver and copper. Thus, it is imperative that gypsum investments not be heated above 700°C. However, for gypsum products containing carbon, the maximum temperature is 650°C. In this way proper fit and uncontaminated alloys are obtained.

Usually castings made from *pure gypsum* ($CaSO_4 \cdot 2H_2O$) molds are extremely undersized. The α-hemihydrate product, which requires less mixing water and shrinks less, is the optimal choice as a binder.

Silica

The wax pattern is usually eliminated from the mold by heat. During heating, the investment is expected to expand thermally to compensate partially or totally for the casting shrinkage of the

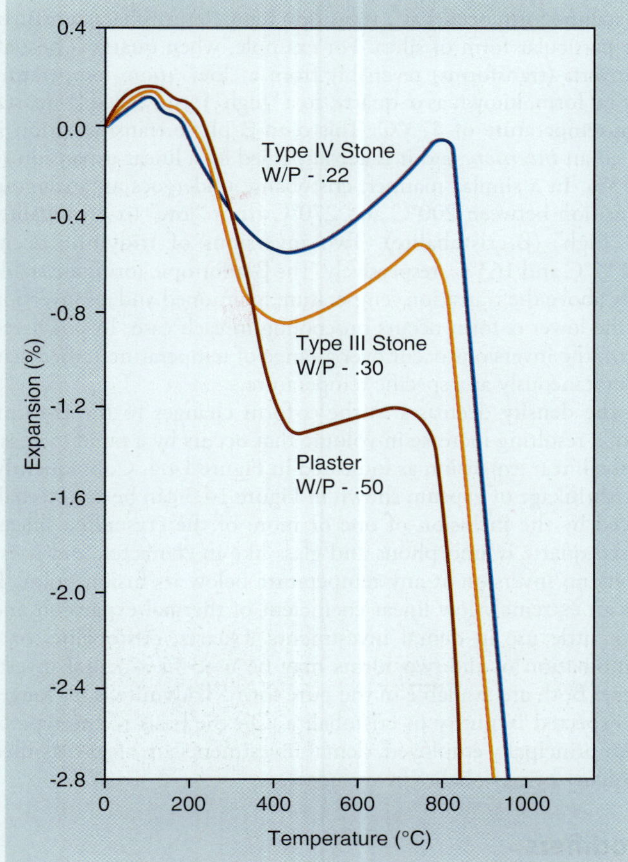

• **Fig. 14.3** Dimensional change of three forms of gypsum when heated. (Courtesy of R Neiman, Whip-Mix Corporation, Louisville, KY.)

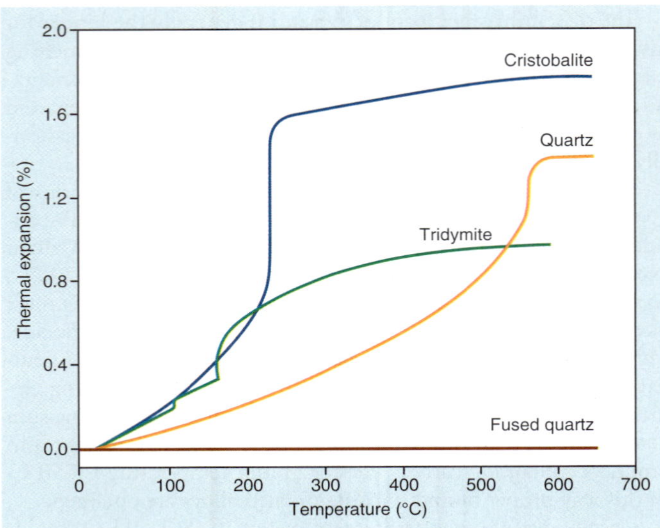

• **Fig. 14.4** Thermal expansion of four forms of silica. (Courtesy of R Neiman, Whip-Mix Corporation, Louisville, KY.)

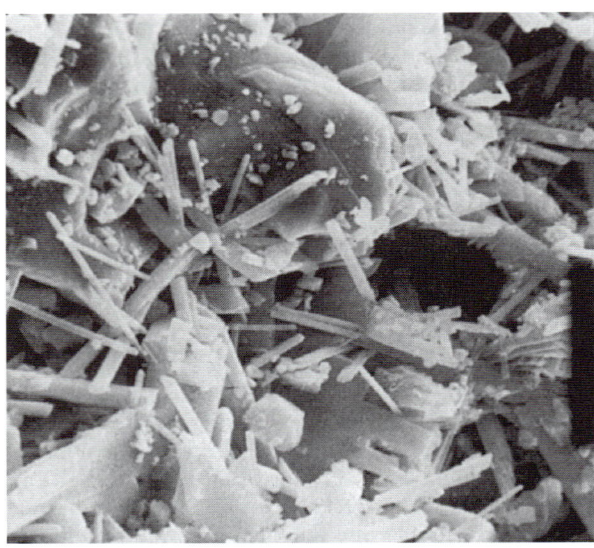

• **Fig. 14.5** Microstructure of the surface of a set cristobalite investment. The large irregular particles are silica and the rod-like particles are cristobalite (×3000). (Courtesy of R Earnshaw.)

solidifying alloy. As shown in Figure 14.1, gypsum shrinks considerably when it is heated. If the proper forms of silica are incorporated in the investment, this contraction during heating can be eliminated and changed to expansion. Silica exists in at least four allotropic forms: quartz, tridymite, cristobalite, and fused quartz. Quartz and cristobalite forms are of particular dental interest.

When quartz, tridymite, or cristobalite is heated, a change in crystalline form occurs at a transition temperature characteristic of the particular form of silica. For example, when quartz is heated, it inverts (transforms) reversibly from a "low" room-temperature crystal form, known as α-quartz, to a "high" form, called β-quartz, at a temperature of 573°C. This α-to-β phase transformation is called an *inversion,* and it is accompanied by a linear expansion of 0.45%. In a similar manner, cristobalite undergoes an analogous transition between 200°C and 270°C from "low" (α-cristobalite) to "high" (β-cristobalite). Two inversions of tridymite occur at 117°C and 163°C, respectively. The β-allotropic forms are stable only above the transition temperature mentioned and an inversion to the lower α-form occurs on cooling in each case. In powdered form, the inversions occur over a range of temperature rather than instantaneously at a specific temperature.

The density decreases as the α-form changes to the β-form, with a resulting increase in volume that occurs by a rapid increase in the linear expansion as indicated in Figure 14.4. Consequently, the shrinkage of gypsum shown in Figure 14.3 can be counterbalanced by the inclusion of one or more of the crystalline silicas. Fused quartz is amorphous and glass like in character, and it exhibits no inversion at any temperature below its fusion point. It has an extremely low linear coefficient of thermal expansion and is of little use in dental investments. Quartz, cristobalite, or a combination of the two forms may be used in a dental investment. Both are available in the pure form. Tridymite is no longer an expected impurity in cristobalite. On the basis of the type of silica principally employed, dental investments are often classified as quartz or cristobalite investments.

Modifiers

In addition to silica, certain modifying agents, coloring matter, and reducing agents, such as carbon and powdered copper, are present. The reducing agents are used in some investments to provide a nonoxidizing atmosphere in the mold when a gold alloy is cast.

Unlike the dental stones, a setting expansion is usually desirable to assist in compensating for the contraction of the alloy. Some of the added modifiers—such as alkali-earth and transition metal chlorides, boric acid, and sodium chloride—not only regulate the setting expansion and the setting time but also prevent most of the shrinkage of gypsum when it is heated above 300°C. In some instances, the modifiers are needed to regulate the setting time and setting expansion, as described for the dental stones. The microstructure of a set gypsum-bonded investment can be seen in Figure 14.5.

Setting Time

The setting time of an investment can be measured in the same manner as plaster. Furthermore, it can be controlled in the same manner. The setting time for dental inlay casting investment should not be less than 5 or more than 25 minutes. Usually, the modern inlay investments set initially in 9–18 minutes. Sufficient time should be allowed for mixing and investing the pattern before the investment sets.

Normal Setting Expansion

A mixture of silica and calcinated gypsum powder (calcium sulfate hemihydrate, $CaSO_4 \cdot \frac{1}{2}H_2O$) results in setting expansion greater than that of the gypsum product used alone. The silica particles probably interfere with the intermeshing and interlocking of the crystals as they form. Thus, the thrust of the crystals is outward during growth, and they increase expansion. Generally, the resulting setting expansion in such a case is high. Type I investments should exhibit a maximum setting expansion in air of 0.6%. The purpose of the setting expansion is to aid in enlarging the mold to compensate partially for the casting shrinkage of the alloy. Typically, the setting expansion of these investments is approximately 0.4%. This expansion is controlled by retarders and accelerators.

Variables other than the exothermic heat of reaction also influence the effective setting expansion. As the investment sets and setting expansion occurs, it eventually gains sufficient strength to produce a dimensional change in the wax pattern and mold cavity. The inner core of the investment adjacent to a mesial-occlusal-distal (MOD) wax pattern can actually force the proximal walls outward to a certain extent. If the pattern has a thin wall, the effective setting expansion is somewhat greater than that of a pattern with thicker walls because the investment can move the thinner wall more readily. Also, softer the wax, the greater is the effective setting expansion, because the softer wax is more readily moved by the expanding investment. If a wax softer than a type II inlay wax is used, the setting expansion may cause an excessive distortion of the pattern.

Hygroscopic Setting Expansion

The theory of hygroscopic setting expansion was previously described in connection with the setting of dental plaster and stone. Hygroscopic setting expansion, is greater in magnitude than normal setting expansion and differs from normal setting expansion. It occurs when the gypsum product is allowed to set in contact with heated water.

Hygroscopic setting expansion was first discovered in connection with an investigation of the dimensional changes of a dental investment during setting. As illustrated in Figure 14.6, the hygroscopic setting expansion may be six or more times greater than the normal setting expansion of a dental investment. In fact, it may be as high as 5 linear percent. The hygroscopic setting expansion is one of the methods for expanding the casting mold to compensate for the casting shrinkage of gold alloys.

Commercial investments exhibit different amounts of hygroscopic expansion. Although all investments appear to be subject to hygroscopic expansion, the expansion in some instances is not as great as in others. For this reason, certain investments are specially formulated to provide a substantial hygroscopic expansion when the investment is permitted to set in contact with water. Type II investments should exhibit a minimum setting expansion in water of 1.2%. The maximum expansion permitted is 2.2%. As

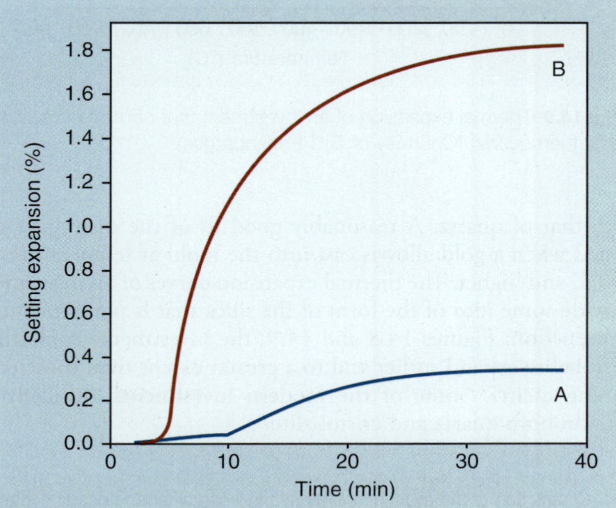

• **Fig. 14.6** Setting expansion and hygroscopic expansion of a gypsum-bonded investment. **(A)** Normal setting expansion of dental investment. **(B)** Hygroscopic setting expansion. The investment was immersed in water 5 minutes after the beginning of mixing; the water/powder ratio was 0.30.

discussed in the following sections, a number of factors are important in the control of hygroscopic expansion.

Variables That Affect Hygroscopic Expansion

The magnitude of the hygroscopic setting expansion of a dental investment is generally proportional to the silica content of the investment, other factors being equal. The finer the particle size of the silica, the greater is the hygroscopic expansion. In general, α-hemihydrate is apt to produce a greater hygroscopic expansion in the presence of silica than with the β-hemihydrate alone, particularly when the expansion is unrestricted.

A dental investment should have enough hemihydrate binder with the silica to provide sufficient strength after hygroscopic expansion; otherwise, shrinkage occurs during the subsequent drying of the set investment. At least 15% of binder is necessary to prevent drying shrinkage.

With most investments, the hygroscopic expansion is decreased when the mixing time is reduced. This factor is also important in the control of the effective setting expansion.

The older the investment, the lower is its hygroscopic expansion. Hence, it is desirable to limit the quantity of investment purchased at one time. The greatest amount of hygroscopic setting expansion is observed if the immersion takes place before the initial set. If the duration of immersion of the investment in the water bath, crosses the initial setting time of the investment, the lower is the hygroscopic expansion.

Both the normal and hygroscopic setting expansions are confronted by opposing forces, such as those exerted by the walls of the container in which the investment is poured or by the walls of the wax pattern. However, the confining effect on hygroscopic expansion is more pronounced than the similar effect on the normal setting expansion. Therefore, the effective hygroscopic setting expansion is likely to be less, relative to the expected expansion compared with the normal setting expansion.

When the dimensional change in the wax pattern is measured after investing, the increase in the effective setting expansion during immersion of investment in a 37.7°C (100°F) water bath is apparently not due to hygroscopic expansion alone. Rather, it may be caused mainly by heating and expansion of the wax pattern and softening of the pattern at the water temperature, permitting an increase in effective setting expansion. The latter results from a combination of thermal expansion of the wax pattern plus the softened condition of the wax, reducing its confining effect on the expansion of the setting investment. This is substantiated by the fact that immersion in water at room temperature (rather than 37.7°C) reduces the effective expansion.

The magnitude of the hygroscopic setting expansion can be controlled by the quantity of water added to the setting investment. It has been proved that the magnitude of the hygroscopic expansion is proportional to the quantity of water added during the setting period. Beyond which no further expansion is evident regardless of the amount of water added.

The effect of some of the factors previously discussed (W/P ratio, mixing, and shelf life) on the maximal hygroscopic setting expansion is illustrated in Figure 14.6 relative to the amount of water added. As shown in Figure 14.6, the magnitude of the hygroscopic setting expansion below the maximal expansion value is dependent only on the quantity of water added (independent of the W/P ratio), the amount of mixing, and the age or shelf life of the investment. This finding is the basis for the mold expansion technique.

Hygroscopic setting expansion is a continuation of ordinary setting expansion because the immersion water replaces the water

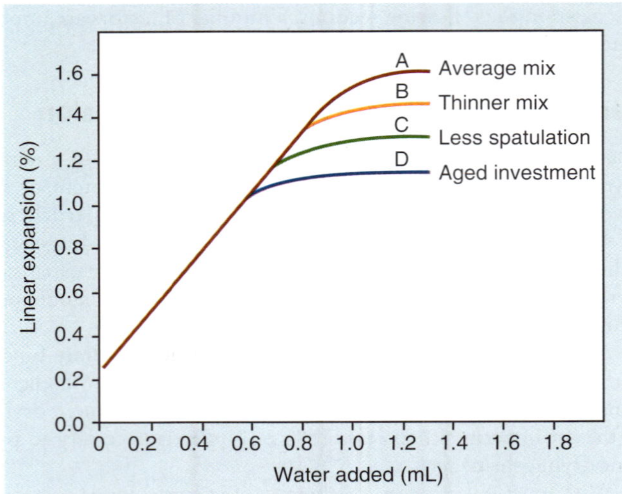

• **Fig. 14.7** Relationship of the linear hygroscopic setting expansion and the amount of water added as influenced by certain manipulative factors. (Data from Asgar K, Mahler DB, Peyton FA: Hygroscopic technique for inlay casting using controlled water additions. *J Prosthet Dent* 5:711, 1955.)

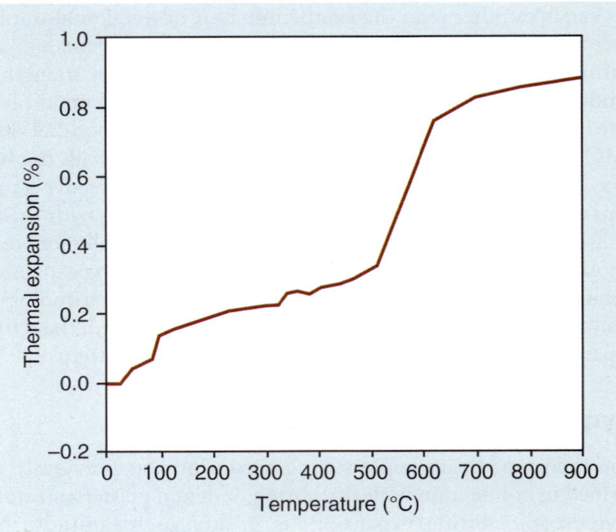

• **Fig. 14.8** Thermal expansion of an investment that contains 25% plaster of Paris and 75% quartz. (Courtesy of G C Paffenbarger.)

of hydration, thus preventing confinement of the growing crystals by the surface tension of the excess water. Because of the dilution effect of the quartz particles, the hygroscopic setting expansion in these investments is greater than that of the gypsum binder when used alone. This effect is the same as previously described for normal setting expansion. This phenomenon is purely physical. Investments with binders other than hemihydrates also exhibit a similar expansion when they are allowed to set under water. Expansion can be detected when water is poured into a vessel containing only small smooth quartz particles. The water is drawn between the particles by capillary action, thereby causing the particles to separate, creating an expansion. The effect is not permanent after the water is evaporated unless a binder is present.

Greater the quantity of silica or the inert filler, more rapidly the added water can diffuse through the setting material and greater is the expansion. The role of manipulation technique on hygroscopic expansion is given in Figure 14.7.

Thermal Expansion of Gypsum-Bonded Investments

To achieve sufficient expansion of gypsum-bonded investment, the silica must be increased to counterbalance the contraction of the gypsum during heating. However, when the quartz content of the investment is increased to 60%, with the balance being the calcium sulfate hemihydrate binder, the initial contraction of the gypsum is not eliminated. The contraction of the gypsum is entirely balanced when the quartz content is increased to 75% (Fig. 14.8). If sufficient setting expansion is present, a casting made at 700°C would probably have a fit on the die reasonably well. The thermal expansion curves of quartz investments are influenced by the particle size of the quartz, the type of gypsum binder, and the resultant W/P ratio necessary to provide a workable mix.

The effect of cristobalite compared with that of quartz is demonstrated in Figure 14.9. Because of the much greater expansion that occurs during the inversion of cristobalite, the normal contraction of the gypsum during heating is readily eliminated. Furthermore, the expansion occurs at a lower temperature because of the lower inversion temperature of the cristobalite in comparison with that of quartz. A reasonably good fit of the castings is obtained when a gold alloy is cast into the mold at temperatures of 500°C and higher. The thermal expansion curves of an investment provide some idea of the form of the silica that is present. As can be seen from Figures 14.8 and 14.9, the investments containing cristobalite expand earlier and to a greater extent than those containing quartz. Some of the modern investments are likely to contain both quartz and cristobalite.

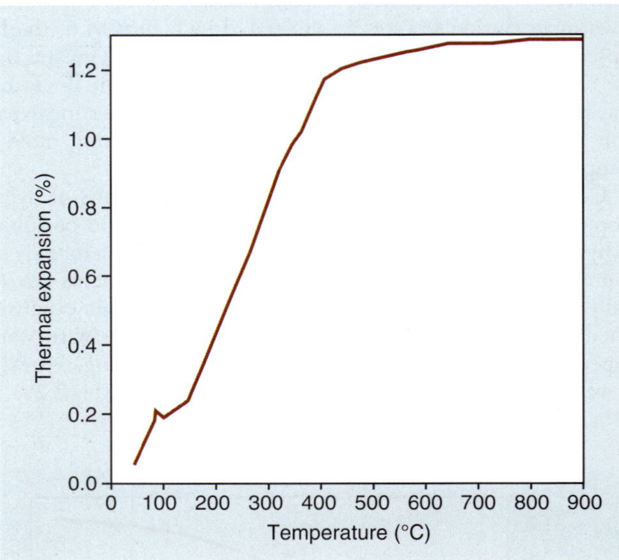

• **Fig. 14.9** Thermal expansion of an investment that contains cristobalite rather than quartz. (Courtesy of G C Paffenbarger.)

- Contraction of the gypsum is entirely balanced when the quartz content is 75%. Casting is made at 700°C.
- Cristobalite balances contraction of the gypsum at a lower temperature of 500°C.
- Modern investments contain both quartz and cristobalite.

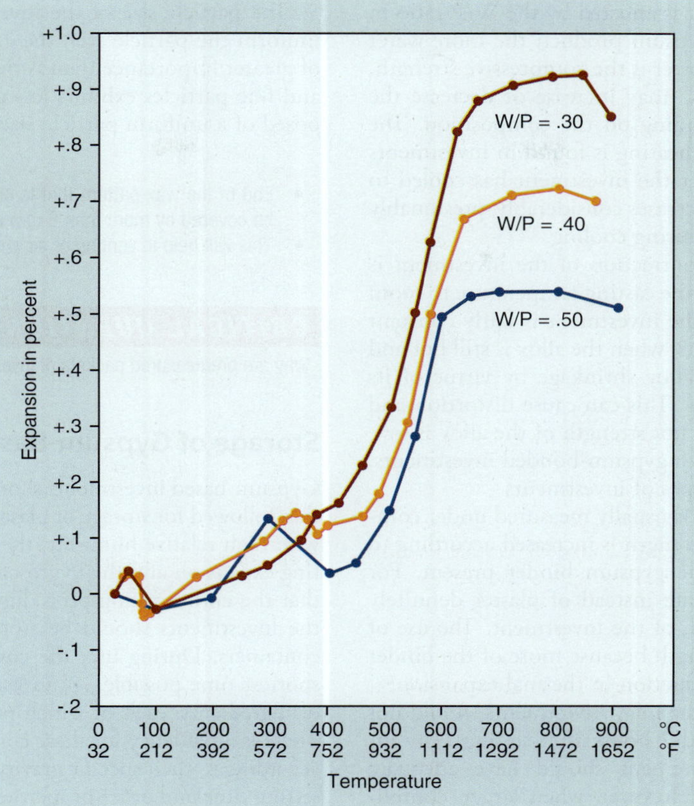

• **Fig. 14.10** Effect of water/powder ratio on the thermal expansion of an investment containing 20% plaster of Paris and 80% quartz. (Courtesy of G C Paffenbarger.)

The desired magnitude of the thermal expansion of a dental investment depends on its use. If the hygroscopic expansion is to be used to compensate for the contraction of the gold alloy, as for the type II investments, thermal expansion should be between 0% and 0.6% at 500°C. However, for type I investments, which rely principally on thermal expansion for compensation, the thermal expansion should not be less than 1% or greater than 1.6%.

The magnitude of thermal expansion is related to the amount of solids present. Therefore, it is apparent that the more water used in mixing the investment, the less is the thermal expansion that is produced during subsequent heating. This effect is demonstrated by the curves shown in Figure 14.10. Although the variations in the W/P ratio shown are rather extreme, the curves indicate that it is imperative to measure the water and powder accurately if the proper compensation is to be achieved.

Effect of Chemical Modifiers

Disadvantage of an investment, that contains sufficient silica to prevent contraction during heating, is related to the weakening effect of the silica in such quantities and which is likely to be too great. Addition of small quantities of sodium, potassium, or lithium chlorides to the investment, eliminates the contraction caused by the gypsum and increases the expansion without the need for an excessive amount of silica.

Boric acid has a similar effect. It also hardens the set investment. However, it apparently disintegrates during the heating of the investment and a roughened surface on the casting may result. Silicas do not prevent gypsum shrinkage but counterbalance it, whereas chlorides actually reduce gypsum shrinkage below temperatures of approximately 700°C.

Thermal Contraction

When an investment is cooled from 700°C, its contraction curve follows the expansion curve during the inversion of the β-quartz or β-cristobalite to its stable α-form at room temperature. Actually, the investment contracts to less than its original dimension. This contraction below the original dimension is unrelated to any property of the silica; it occurs because of the shrinkage of gypsum when it is first heated.

As the investment is reheated, it expands thermally to the same peak value reached when it was first heated. However, in practice the investment should not be heated a second time because internal cracks can develop.

Strength

The fracture resistance of the investment must be adequate to prevent cracking, bulk fracture, or chipping of the mold during heating and casting of gold alloys. Although a certain minimal strength is necessary to prevent fracture of the investment mold during casting, the compressive strength should not be unduly high. It has been found that all castings for the standardized MOD die used by the National Institute of Standards and Technology showed a constant pattern of distortion. The distortion apparently results from a directional restraint by the investment to the thermal contraction of the alloy casting as it cools to room temperature.

The strength of the investment is affected by the W/P ratio in the same manner as any other gypsum product; the more water that is employed in mixing, the lower is the compressive strength. Heating the investment to 700°C may increase or decrease the strength as much as 65%, depending on the composition. The greatest reduction in strength on heating is found in investments containing sodium chloride. After the investment has cooled to room temperature, its strength decreases considerably, presumably because of fine cracks that form during cooling.

Although the total thermal contraction of the investment is similar to that of gold alloys from the casting temperature to room temperature, the contraction of the investment is fairly constant until it cools to below 550°C. Thus, when the alloy is still hot and weak, the investment can resist alloy shrinkage by virtue of its strength and constant dimensions. This can cause distortion and even fracture of the casting if the hot strength of the alloy is low. Although this is rarely a factor with gypsum-bonded investments, it can be important with other types of investments.

The strength of an investment is usually measured under compressive stress. The compressive strength is increased according to the quantity and the type of the gypsum binder present. For example, the use of α-hemihydrate instead of plaster definitely increases the compressive strength of the investment. The use of chemical modifiers increases strength because more of the binder can be used without a marked reduction in thermal expansion.

The compressive strength for the inlay investments should not be less than 2.4 MPa when tested 2 hours after setting. Any investment that meets this requirement should have adequate strength for casting of an inlay. However, when larger, complicated castings are made, greater strength is necessary, as required for type III partial denture investments.

Fineness of Gypsum Investment

The fineness of the investment may affect its setting time, the surface roughness of the casting, and other properties. A fine silica results in a higher hygroscopic expansion than does a coarser silica. A fine particle size is preferable to a coarse one because the finer the investment, the smaller the surface irregularities on the casting.

CRITICAL QUESTION

What are the two measures that may be taken to minimize porosity in dental castings?

Porosity of the Gypsum-Based Casting Investment

As the molten metal enters the mold under pressure during casting, the trapped air must be forced out ahead of the inflowing metal. If the air is not completely eliminated, a back pressure builds up to prevent the molten alloy from completely filling the mold. The simplest method for venting the mold is through the pores of the investment. Thus, it is important that the end of the wax pattern that is nearest to the end of the investment ring should not be covered by more than 6 mm of investment, to allow sufficient interconnectivity of the porous network for escape of gas from the mold cavity during filling of the mold with molten metal.

In general, the more gypsum crystals that are present in the set investment, the less is its porosity. Thus, the lower the amount of calcium sulfate hemihydrate and the more gauging water used in mixing the investment, the more porous it will be.

The particle size of the investment is also a factor. The more uniform the particle size, the greater is its porosity. This factor is of greater importance than is the particle size. A mixture of coarse and fine particles exhibits less porosity than an investment composed of a uniform particle size.

- End of the wax pattern that is nearest to the end of the ring should not be covered by more than 6 mm of investment.
- This will help in venting of air ahead of the entry of molten metal.

CRITICAL QUESTION

Why are premeasured packets of investments sometimes more cost-effective?

Storage of Gypsum-Based Casting Investment

Gypsum-based investments should be stored in the same manner as that followed for storage of plaster or dental stone. In storage rooms with high relative humidity, the setting time may change. The setting expansion and the hygroscopic expansion may be altered such that the entire casting procedure may be adversely affected. Thus, the investments should be stored in airtight and moisture-proof containers. During use, the containers should be opened for the shortest time possible. All investments are composed of a number of ingredients, each of which possesses a different specific gravity. There is a tendency for these components to separate as they settle, according to their specific gravity. This separation may influence the setting time and other properties of the investment. Because of this settling and the danger of accidental moisture contamination, it is advisable to purchase prepackaged investments in relatively small quantities. If investments are needed on an infrequent basis, prepackaged products are more cost-effective because less waste is likely, especially in storage areas with relatively high humidity.

The investment supplied in bulk packages should be weighed and the water should be measured according to the proportion of the investment mix. In this manner one can control the setting or the thermal expansion in relation to the compensation needed for the casting shrinkage and other important properties. One need only measure the gauging water.

Manufacturers also supply preweighed packets of investment powder. However, one should be aware of slight variations in the weight of premeasured packets of powder. The quality control of investment products is related not only to the homogeneity of particulate components but also to variations in the weight of powder in the packets. Products with weight variations of 2% or less between packets in a box of preweighed investment powder packets represent excellent quality control. Weight variations of 5% or more among packets may have serious consequences in terms of the flow characteristics of the investment slurry, setting time, setting expansion, and fracture resistance.

Phosphate-Bonded Investment

Rapid growth in the use of metal–ceramic and hot-pressed ceramic prostheses has resulted in the increased use of phosphate-bonded or silicate-bonded investments. Although these investments are more difficult to remove from castings than are gypsum-based investments, this problem has been reduced recently, and the phosphate-bonded investments now produce satisfactory results with conventional gold alloys.

Phosphate-bonded investments are becoming more widely used than gypsum-bonded investments. The tremendous increase in the use of metal–ceramic prostheses necessitates the use of higher melting gold alloys that do not cast well into gypsum investments. Likewise, with the recent increase in the cost of the noble metals and silver (starting in 2010), there will likely be a recurrent trend toward the use of the less expensive base metal alloys, most of which require phosphate investments. Commercially pure titanium and titanium alloys require specially formulated investments to minimize the interaction of the molten metal with the investment.

Composition

Like gypsum-based investments, phosphate-based investments contain refractory fillers and a binder. The silica filler, typically 80% by weight, is in the form of cristobalite, quartz, or a mixture of the two forms. The purpose of the filler is to provide thermal shock resistance (refractoriness) and a high thermal expansion. The particle size varies from a submicron level to that of fine sand. The sandy feel of the investment does not necessarily relate to casting smoothness or affect the ease of removing the casting from the investment.

The binder consists of magnesium oxide (basic) and a phosphate that is acidic in nature. Originally phosphoric acid was used, but monoammonium phosphate has replaced it because it can be incorporated into the investment powder.

Because several of the newer gold-containing alloys and other alloys used for metal–ceramic restorations have higher melting temperature ranges than traditional gold alloys, it usually follows that their contraction during solidification is also greater. This necessitates a greater expansion of the investment. In this regard, colloidal silica suspensions in place of water are beneficial for mixing the phosphate investments.

Because colloidal silica liquid suspensions can freeze and become unusable, these suspensions and their investment powders should be stored in a frost-free environment. Some suspensions are available as freeze-stable products. Although they freeze solid at low temperatures, they become useful again after they have been thawed out and shaken. Some phosphate investments are made to be used with water for the casting of alloys. In addition, for predominantly base metal alloys, a 33% dilution of the colloidal silica is required.

Carbon is often added to the powder to produce clean castings and facilitate the **divesting** of the casting from the investment mold. This addition is appropriate when the casting alloy is gold, but there is disagreement regarding the effects of carbon in phosphate investments used for casting silver–palladium alloys, palladium–silver alloys, or base metal alloys. It is believed that carbon can embrittle the alloys, even though the investment is heated to temperatures that burn out the carbon. Some evidence indicates that palladium reacts with carbon at temperatures above 1504°C. Thus, if the casting temperature of an alloy with high palladium content exceeds this critical point, a phosphate investment without carbon should be used. Also, a carbon crucible should not be employed for melting the alloy. Generally, even gold alloys used with porcelain should not be premelted or fluxed on charcoal blocks because trace elements that provide high strength may be removed or are reduced below the desired level.

Setting Reaction

The chemical reaction for the phosphate-based binder system that causes the investment to set and harden is described in the following.

(1)

$$NH_4H_2PO_4 + MgO + 5H_2O \rightarrow NH_4MgPO_4 + 6H_2O$$

For example, in some products the magnesium ammonium phosphate formed is polymeric. Although the stoichiometry (*Stoichiometry is the quantitative description of the proportions by moles of the substances in a chemical reaction.*) suggests the use of equal quantities or equal molecules of magnesia and monoammonium phosphate, an excess of magnesia is usually present, and some of it is never fully reacted. The product formed is the predominantly colloidal multimolecular $(NH_4MgPO_4{\cdot}6H_2O)_n$ aggregate around excess MgO and fillers. On heating, the binder of the set investment undergoes thermal reactions as suggested by the following sequence:

(2)

$MgO + NH_4H_2PO_4 + H_2O$

↓ Room temperature

$(NH_4MgPO_4 + 6H_2O)_n$
MgO
$NH_4H_2PO_4$
H_2O

Colloidal-type particles

↓ Prolonged set at 25 °C/ Dehydration at 50 °C

$(NH_4MgPO_4 + 6H_2O)_n$

↓ Dehydrated at 160 °C

$(NH_4MgPO_4 + H_2O)_n$

↓ Heated from 300 to 650 °C

$(Mg_2P_2O_7)_n$

↓ Noncrystalline polymeric phase

$Mg_2P_2O_7$

↓ Heated above 1040 °C

$Mg_3(P_2O_4)_2$

The resulting reaction products of phosphate-bonded investments are crystalline $Mg_2P_2O_7$, excess MgO, and essentially unchanged quartz, cristobalite, or both. In addition, $Mg_3(P_2O_4)_2$ may be formed if the investment is grossly overheated or if the molten metal contacts the mold cavity surfaces.

Setting and Thermal Expansion of Phosphate-Bonded Investment

In theory, the setting reaction should result in shrinkage, as is also expected for gypsum-based investments. However, a slight expansion actually occurs, which can be increased considerably by using a colloidal silica solution (sometimes called a special liquid) instead of water. This solution allows phosphate investments to expand considerably rather than shrink according to predictions. Figure 14.11 shows the effect of the concentration of colloidal silica in aqueous suspension on increasing the setting and thermal expansion.

Shown in Figure 14.12 is the thermal expansion of a typical phosphate investment mixed with water as compared with the same investment mixed with its accompanying special liquid. When phosphate investments are mixed with water, they shrink over the same temperature range as gypsum-bonded investments (200–400°C). This contraction is practically eliminated when a colloidal silica solution replaces water. Some users of phosphate-bonded investment prefer to decrease expansion by increasing the L/P ratio rather than by decreasing the concentration of the special liquid, or they may use a combination of these methods.

The early thermal shrinkage of phosphate investments is associated with decomposition of the binder, magnesium ammonium phosphate, and is accompanied by evolution of ammonia, which

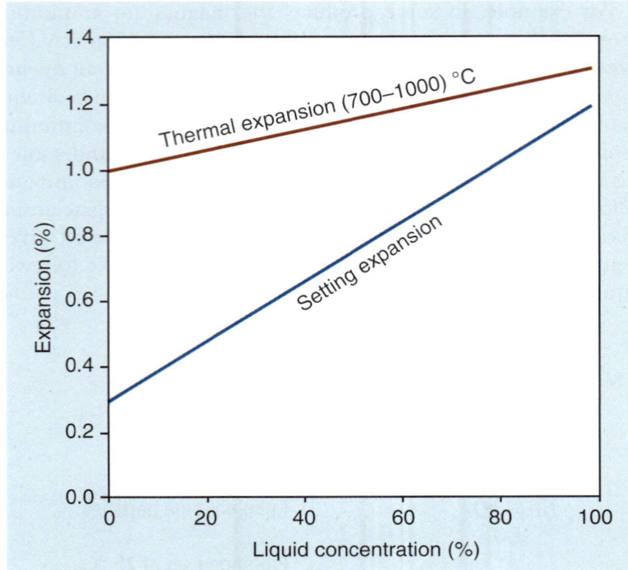

• **Fig. 14.11** Influence of liquid concentration on the setting and thermal expansion of a phosphate-bonded investment. (Courtesy of R Neiman, Whip-Mix Corporation, Louisville, KY.)

is readily apparent by its odor. For gypsum investments the shrinkage is caused by the transformation of calcium sulfate from the hexagonal to the rhombic form. However, some of the shrinkage is masked because of the expansion of the refractory filler, especially for cristobalite.

Working and Setting Time

Unlike gypsum investments, phosphate investments are markedly affected by temperature. The warmer the mix, the faster it sets. The setting reaction itself gives off heat, and this further accelerates the rate of setting. Increased mixing time and mixing efficiency, as determined by the type of mixer and speed of mixing, result in a faster set and a greater rise in temperature. In general, the more efficient the mixing, the better is the smoothness and accuracy of the casting. The ideal technique is to mix as long as possible yet have just enough time for investing. Mechanical mixing under vacuum is preferred.

A third variable that has a considerable effect on the working and setting time is the L/P ratio, which often varies considerably depending on user preference. An increase in the L/P ratio increases the working time, which can be very short (2 minutes or less) when the investment is mixed at the manufacturer's recommended L/P ratio at high speed (1750 rpm) for the recommended time. Prolonged working time occurs at higher laboratory temperatures and also when the liquid has not been chilled.

Surface Quality of Cast Metals

In the past, detail reproduction and surface smoothness of a metal–ceramic gold alloy restoration cast in a phosphate-bonded investment were considered inferior to those characteristics of a conventional gold alloy that had been cast in a gypsum-bonded investment. However, increasing the ratio of special liquid to water used for the mix markedly enhances casting surface smoothness, but it can lead to oversized extracoronal castings. Improvement in the technique and also in the investment composition now make it possible to fabricate castings having few surface imperfections when phosphate-bonded investment is used with either a low-fusing gold alloy, a high-fusing gold alloy, or a base metal alloy. Phosphate-bonded investments now approach the surface quality or fineness of the gypsum investments. However, their ability to improve the smoothness is dependent on the alloy and casting procedure employed.

Ethyl Silicate–bonded Investment

The use of ethyl silicate–bonded investments has declined because of the more complex and time-consuming procedures involved with their use; however, they are still used in the

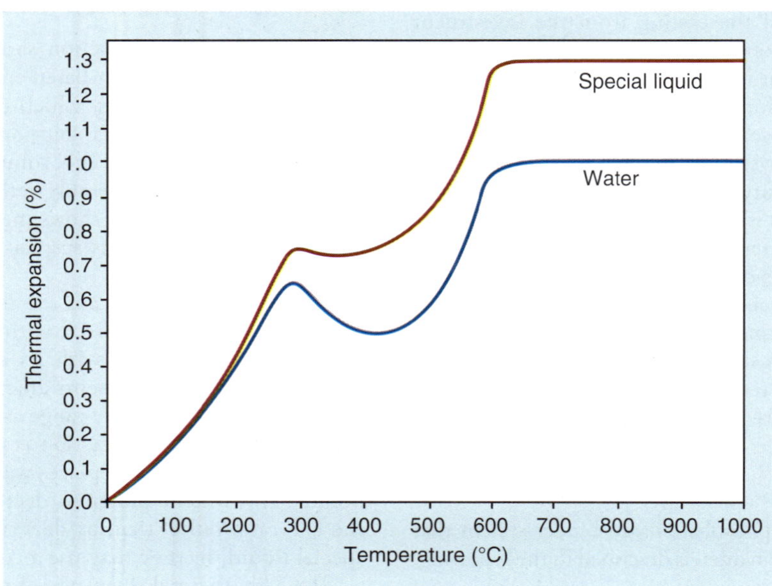

• **Fig. 14.12** Thermal expansion of a phosphate-bonded investment mixed with water as compared with the special liquid. (Courtesy of R Neiman, Whip-Mix Corporation, Louisville, KY.)

construction of high-fusing base metal partial denture alloys. In this case, the binder is a silica gel that reverts to silica (cristobalite) on heating. Several methods may be used to produce the silica or silicic acid gel binders. When the pH of sodium silicate is lowered, by the addition of an acid or an acid salt, a bonding silicic acid gel forms. The addition of magnesium oxide strengthens the gel. An aqueous suspension of colloidal silica can also be converted to a gel by the addition of an accelerator, such as ammonium chloride.

Another system for binder formation is based on ethyl silicate. A colloidal silicic acid is first formed by hydrolyzing ethyl silicate in the presence of hydrochloric acid, ethyl alcohol, and water. In its simplest form, the reaction can be expressed follows:

$$Si(OC_2H_5)_4 + 4H2O \rightarrow Si(OH)_4 + 4C_2H_5OH \quad (3)$$

Since an ethyl silicate polymer is used, a colloidal sol of polysilicic acids is expected instead of the simpler silicic acid sol shown in the reaction. The sol is then mixed with quartz or cristobalite, to which is added a small amount of finely powdered magnesium oxide to render the mixture alkaline. A coherent gel of polysilicic acid then forms, accompanied by a setting shrinkage. This soft gel is dried at a temperature below 168°C. During the drying process, the gel loses alcohol and water to form a concentrated, hard gel. As might be expected, a volumetric contraction accompanies the drying, which reduces the size of the mold. This contraction is known as green shrinkage, which is additive to the setting shrinkage.

Gelation is likely to be slow and time-consuming. A faster method for the production of the silica gel can be used. Certain types of amines can be added to the solution of ethyl silicate so that hydrolysis and gelation occur simultaneously. The mold enlargement before casting must compensate not only for the casting shrinkage of the metal but also for the green shrinkage and the setting shrinkage of the investment.

CRITICAL QUESTION

Why is the marginal fit of cast crowns on a prepared tooth essential to the long-term clinical success of metal prostheses?

Clinical Evaluation of Casting Fit

Dental castings can be produced in any size (from a denture base to the smallest inlay). The procedures employed for the construction of small restorations, such as inlays, onlays, crowns, and endodontic posts, are the primary topic of this chapter. The fundamental principles are the same, regardless of the size of the casting, and the techniques differ only in sprue design, type of investment, and method of melting the alloy.

The casting process is designed to provide a metallic duplication of missing tooth structure with as much accuracy as possible. The tolerance limits for the fit and marginal adaptation of a cast restoration are not known. In a clinical study, 10 experienced dentists were asked to evaluate the marginal adaptation of a group of inlays, using an explorer and radiographs. After the cemented restorations were graded, they were microscopically measured at the marginal openings of various areas. For "acceptable" restorations, the mean opening was 21 μm at the occlusal surface and 74 μm at the gingival region, which is not as accessible visually. There was little agreement among these 10 dentists on the acceptability of the marginal openings when evaluated by either explorers or radiographs.

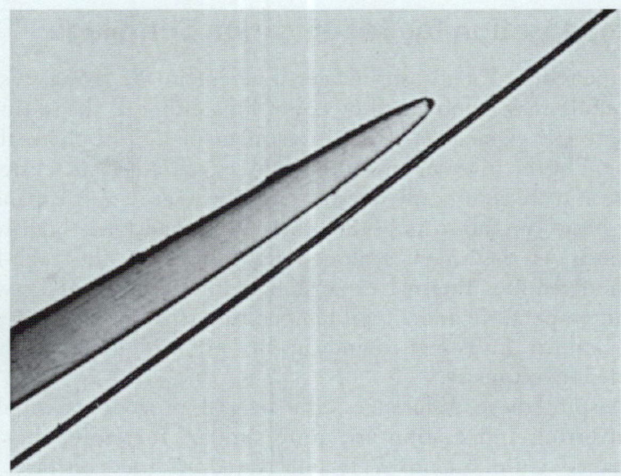

• **Fig. 14.13** Longitudinal section of an unused explorer tip (*top*) and a 60 μm hair (×25). (From McLean JW, Van Fraunhofer JA: The estimation of cement film thickness by an in vivo technique. *Br Dent J* 131:107, 1971.)

The difficulty in detecting small discrepancies at the margins of cemented restorations is associated with the use of explorers that have a relatively large radius of curvature at the tip compared with the width of margin gaps that are being evaluated. As shown in Figure 14.13, the tip of this unused explorer may not "catch" a 60 μm margin gap, whose width is the diameter of a human hair, as it traverses along a path perpendicular to the gap. If this explorer tip substantially penetrates into a gap during probing, the fit of a crown, inlay, or onlay will not be clinically acceptable. The illustration poses the question of how readily a hairline gap can be detected by running an explorer over the margins of the restoration, especially in interdental areas that must often be probed at a small angle to the surface. It is obvious that the accuracy of the inlay or crown should be greater than what can be detected by the eye or by the conventional methods of clinical testing. At the margins of the cemented restoration, a thin line of cement is always present, even though it may not be readily visible. With the exception of resin-based luting materials, the present dental cements are somewhat soluble and can deteriorate in the oral cavity. Thus, the less accurate the casting fit and the greater the amount of cement exposed, the more likely it is that the cement will degrade. Certainly a high degree of accuracy in marginal adaptation of 25 μm or less cannot be guaranteed for all cast restorations. It stands to reason that the more accurate the fit of the casting, the less the likelihood of leakage, plaque accumulation on the cement, and secondary caries.

- For "acceptable" restorations, the mean opening is 21 μm at the occlusal surface and 74 μm at the gingival region.

Assuming that the wax pattern is satisfactory, the procedure then becomes a matter of enlarging the mold uniformly and sufficiently to compensate for the casting shrinkage of the alloy. Theoretically, if the shrinkage of the wax and the alloy is known, the mold can be expanded enough to compensate for such shrinkage. The overall dimensional accuracy possible with current techniques has not been clearly defined. Thus, neither the allowable tolerance of accuracy in the fit of the casting nor that obtainable during the casting procedure is known. In the final analysis, the casting procedure is partly empirical and previous experience is very beneficial.

Compensation for Solidification Shrinkage

Compensation for the shrinkages inherent in the dental casting procedure may be obtained by controlling either (l) the setting or hygroscopic expansion of the investment or (2) the thermal expansion of the investment. Both of these techniques are currently in use and are commonly referred to as the hygroscopic expansion (low-heat) method and the thermal expansion (high-heat) method. As their names alone might indicate, the high-heat method requires thermal expansion of the investment between room temperature and a high temperature (650–700°C) for gypsum-bonded investments and up to 1050°C for phosphate-bonded investments.

Despite these differences, the overall procedures involved in investing and casting are quite similar; therefore, they are described simultaneously. If not stated to the contrary, the reader can assume that the procedures mentioned are common to both the high-heat and the low-heat techniques. For best results, the manufacturer's recommendations for the specific alloy used should be followed.

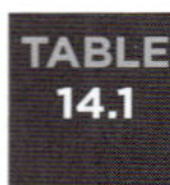

Dimensional Change in Dies Made From a Silicone Impression Compared With a Standardized Die

	DIMENSIONAL CHANGE (%)	
Die Material	**Occlusal**	**Cervical**
Type IV die stone	0.06	0.00
Type IV stone plus hardener A	0.16	0.08
Type IV stone plus hardener B	0.10	0.10
Silica-filled epoxy resin	−0.15	−0.26
Aluminum-filled epoxy resin	−0.14	−0.19
Electroformed silver	−0.10	−0.20

Reproduced with permission from Toreskog S, Phillips RW, Schnell RJ: *J Prosthet Dent* 16: 119, 1966.

Ringless Casting System

A ringless system provides maximum expansion of investment. This system, called the Power Cast Ringless System (Whip-Mix Corporation, Louisville, KY), consists of three sizes of rings and formers, preformed wax sprues and shapes, investment powder, and a special investment liquid. The tapered plastic rings allow for removal of the investment mold after the material has set. This system is suited for the casting of alloys that require greater mold expansion than traditional gold-based alloys.

CRITICAL QUESTION

What methods can be used to increase the abrasion resistance of master dies?

Preparation of the Master Die

The most commonly used die materials are type IV (dental stone, high-strength) and type V (dental stone, high-strength, high-expansion) improved stones. These materials are relatively inexpensive, easy to use, and generally compatible with all impression materials. Type IV stones should have a setting expansion of 0.1% or less, whereas the harder type V stones may expand as much as 0.3%. This greater expansion is useful in compensating for the relatively large solidification shrinkage of base metal alloys.

The chief disadvantage of the type IV gypsum die is its susceptibility to abrasion during carving of the wax pattern. Gypsum dies are sometimes modified to (1) make them more abrasion resistant, (2) change the dimensions of the dies, (3) increase the refractoriness of the dies, or (4) produce a combination of these effects. Several means are used to increase the abrasion resistance, including silver plating, coating the surface with cyanoacrylate adhesive, and adding a die hardener to the gypsum. However, each of these methods can also increase the die dimensions slightly, thus reducing accuracy (Table 14.1).

Methods of Altering Die Dimensions

Additional accelerator (potassium sulfate) and retarder (borax) can be added to the gauging water to reduce the setting expansion of the type IV die stone to less than 0.1% and, therefore, to reduce the diameter of the die. To produce relief space for cement, clinicians commonly use a die spacer that is coated on a stone die. The most common die spacers are resins. Although proprietary paint-on liquids are sold for this purpose, model paint, colored nail polish, and thermoplastic polymers dissolved in volatile solvents are also used. Such spacers are applied in several coats, 0.5 mm short of the preparation finish line to provide relief for the cement luting agent and ensure complete seating of an otherwise precisely fitting casting or coping.

- Die Spacer is a colored, paint-on material applied to dies that adds a desired dimension to the surface of the die to function as a "spacer."
- The extra thickness created by the Die Spacer results in additional space between the finished restoration and the natural tooth surface to accommodate the cement used for luting.

Die Stone/Investment Combination

Another technique employs a die material and the investing medium with a comparable composition. One of the commercial gypsum-bonded materials (Divestment, Whip-Mix Corporation, Louisville, KY) is mixed with a colloidal silica liquid. The die is made from this mix, and the wax pattern is constructed on it. Then the entire assembly (die and pattern) is invested in a mixture of the investment and water, thereby eliminating the possibility of distortion of the pattern on removal from the die or during the setting of the investment. When it is heated to 677°C, the setting expansion of the material is 0.9% and the thermal expansion is 0.6%. Because this type of investment is a gypsum-bonded material, it is not recommended for high-fusing alloys used for metal–ceramic restorations. However, it is a highly accurate technique for use with conventional gold alloys, especially those selected for extracoronal preparations.

A phosphate-bonded investment is used in the same manner as gypsum-based material, and it is suitable for use with high-fusing alloys. Phosphate-bonded die investment materials formulated for use in making ceramic prostheses can also be used when casting high-fusing alloys.

Other Die Materials

Nongypsum die materials are also available, such as acrylic, polyester, and epoxy resins. These materials are limited in their compatibility with impression materials, which would ordinarily be nonaqueous elastomers rather than hydrocolloid or compound. Compatibility is specific and applicable only to the particular brand rather than to chemical types of impression materials. Moreover, in the case of filled autopolymerizing acrylic resins, the curing contraction is excessive (0.6 linear percent for one material). Therefore, acrylic resin cannot be used when an accurate die is required. The same is true for polyester resin materials.

Various epoxy die materials are reliable with respect to the 0.1–0.2% dimensional change on polymerization (Table 14.1). Even though epoxy dies are generally undersized in comparison with the prepared tooth, especially in the axial direction, they are used successfully by some commercial dental laboratories, presumably because of their superior abrasion resistance.

A cast crown that is fabricated on a slightly undersized resin die may not seat completely on the tooth compared with one made on a slightly large stone die.

The high-strength stones (types IV and V) appear to be the most successful die materials available. With care, abrasion during carving of the wax pattern can be avoided. However, in the construction of a metal–ceramic crown that is made with a metal foil coping (such as Captek), the metal is burnished on the die. This process requires the application of high localized pressure to adapt the metal foil intimately on the die surface. Gypsum dies may be readily damaged, so a less brittle material, such as resin or metal, is sometimes preferred.

Recently several gypsum die stones have been compounded with resins to provide the advantages of both materials. These modified die stones maintain the low expansion of stone, but they also have the increased toughness and resistance to carving imparted by the resins.

- The high-strength stones (types IV and V) are the most successful die materials.

CRITICAL QUESTION

Why is the term "silver-plated die" technically incorrect?

Electroformed Dies

Metal dies produced from electroplated impression material have moderately high strength, adequate hardness, and excellent abrasion resistance. Detail reproduction of a line 4 μm or less in width is readily attainable on the resulting metal-covered die when a nonaqueous elastomeric impression material is used.

Copper-plated compound dies first became popular in the early 1930s, and silver-plated dies became more popular in later years. Several modifications of the fabrication technique are used, but the following description is typical.

The first step in the procedure is to treat the surface of the impression material so that it conducts electricity. This process is referred to as metallizing. In this process, a thin layer of metal, such as silver powder, is deposited on the surface of the impression material. This metal layer determines to a large extent the surface character of the finished die. Various metallizing agents are available, including bronzing powder and aqueous suspensions of silver powder and powdered graphite. These agents can be deposited on the surface of the impression with a camel-hair brush.

The electroplating bath itself is primarily a solution of silver cyanide. Care must be taken to avoid the addition of acids to the cyanide solution, which can cause the release of cyanide vapor, a "death chamber" gas. Chemical deposition of silver from a silver nitrate solution can be used if greater surface detail reproduction is desired. In the silver-plating process, the greater the concentration of silver in the bath, the faster the silver is deposited. The acid content increases the throwing power, a term that refers to the penetration of current into a concave structure, such as an impression for a full crown. Impressions of teeth generally have walls with significant depth relative to the location of the occlusal area. Therefore, a considerable amount of throwing power is desirable. An electrical contact is made with the metallized surface of the impression, which is the cathode in the electroplating bath. A plate of silver is used as the anode. A direct current is applied for approximately 10 hours.

Hydrocolloid impressions are extremely difficult to electroplate, and the process is not feasible for dental use. Electroformed dies made from polysulfide rubber impressions are clinically acceptable when a silver cyanide bath is used, although they are generally slightly less accurate than a properly constructed stone die.

Polysulfide rubber impressions are cleaned thoroughly and dried. They are then metallized with a fine silver powder. Although other metallizing agents can be used, the silver powder results in a superior surface on the electroformed die. An anode of pure silver, at least twice the size of the area to be plated, is employed, and the electroplating is carried out as before for approximately 10 hours, using 5–10 mA/cm^2 of cathode surface.

An impression that contains the electroformed die surface is then filled with dental stone. When the stone hardens, it is mechanically locked into the rough interior of the electroformed metal shell. The impression material is then removed to provide a die with greater surface hardness and resistance to abrasion than one of gypsum. The model and die are prepared in the normal manner, and the margins of the die are trimmed with a finishing disk. It should be clear to the reader that the terms "electroplated die" and "silver-plated die" are technically incorrect because it is the impression material surface that receives the electrodeposited metal.

- Electroplated die is obtained by depositing a layer of pure metal (copper/silver) on the impression and is supported with type IV stone or resin.

CRITICAL QUESTION

What casting deficiencies may result when (1) the sprue former is too small in diameter, (2) the sprue former is attached without flaring to thinner areas, (3) the sprues are oriented toward thin areas of a wax pattern, or (4) the sprues are of inadequate length to position the wax pattern within 6 mm of the end of the invested ring?

Variables and Principles of Optimal Sprue Design

The purpose of a sprue former, or sprue pin, is to provide a channel through which molten alloy can reach the mold in an invested ring after the wax has been eliminated. With large restorations or prostheses, such as removable partial denture frameworks and FDPs, the sprue formers are made of wax.

The diameter and length of the sprue former (also referred to simply as the sprue) depend to a large extent on the type and size of the pattern, the type of casting machine to be used, and the dimensions of the flask or ring in which the casting will be made. Prefabricated sprue formers are available in a wide range of gauges or diameters (Table 14.2).

Wax Pattern Removal

The sprue former should be attached to the wax pattern with the pattern on the master die provided that the pattern can be removed directly in line with its path of withdrawal from the die. Any motion that might distort the wax pattern should be avoided during removal. The gauge selection and design for the sprue former are often empirical, but optimal performance during the casting process is based on the following five general principles.

Sprue Diameter

Select a sprue former with a diameter that is approximately the same size as the thickest area of the wax pattern. If the pattern is small, the sprue former must also be small, because attaching a large sprue former to a thin, delicate pattern could cause distortion. On the other hand, if the sprue former's diameter is too small, this area will solidify before the casting itself and localized shrinkage porosity ("suck-back" porosity) may develop. As shown in Figure 14.1, reservoir sprues are used to help overcome this problem.

Sprue Position

The position of the sprue former attachment is often a matter of individual judgment and intuition, based on the shape and form of the wax pattern. Some clinicians prefer placement at the occlusal surface, whereas others choose sites such as a proximal wall or just below a nonfunctional cusp to minimize subsequent grinding of occlusal anatomy and contact areas. As indicated earlier, the ideal area for the sprue former is the point of greatest bulk in the pattern to avoid distorting thin areas of wax during attachment to the pattern and permit complete flow of the alloy into the mold cavity.

Sprue Attachment

The sprue former connection to the wax pattern is generally flared for high-density gold alloys but often restricted for lower-density alloys. Flaring of the sprue former may act in much the same way as a reservoir, facilitating the entry of the fluid alloy into the pattern area. If possible, the sprue former should be attached to the portions of the pattern with the largest cross-sectional areas. It is best for the molten alloy to flow from a thick section to surrounding thin areas (e.g., the margins) rather than the reverse. This design minimizes the risk of turbulence. Also, the orientation of the sprue former should minimize the risk for metal flow onto flat areas of the investment or onto small areas such as line angles.

The sprue former should be long enough to position the pattern properly in the casting ring within 6 mm of the trailing end (see Fig. 14.2) and yet short enough so that the molten alloy does not solidify before it fills the mold. The type of sprue former selected influences the burnout technique used. Wax sprue formers are more common than plastic. It is advisable to use a two-stage burnout technique whenever plastic sprue formers or patterns are involved to ensure complete carbon elimination because plastic sprues soften at temperatures above the melting point of inlay waxes. Patterns may be sprued either directly or indirectly. For direct spruing, the sprue former provides a direct connection between the pattern area and the sprue base or crucible former area (see Fig. 14.2). With indirect spruing, a connector or reservoir bar is positioned between the pattern and the crucible former (see Fig. 14.2). It is common to use indirect spruing for multiple single units and fixed partial dentures, although several single units can be sprued with multiple direct sprue formers.

A reservoir should be added to a sprue network to prevent localized shrinkage porosity (Fig. 14.14). When the molten alloy fills the heated casting ring, the pattern area should solidify first and the reservoir last. Because of its large mass of alloy and position in the heat center of the ring, the reservoir remains molten to furnish liquid alloy into the mold as it solidifies. Assuming that the reservoir bar is larger in volume than that of the patterns, and that the sprue formers attached to those patterns were of the correct diameter and placed in the appropriate position, the resulting solidification shrinkage occurs in the reservoir bar and not in the prosthesis.

TABLE 14.2 Wire Gauge Versus Diameter

AWG Gauge	Conductor Diameter (mm)
0000	11.68400
000	10.40384
00	9.26592
0	8.25246
1	7.34822
2	6.54304
3	5.82676
4	5.18922
5	4.62026
6	4.11480
7	3.66522
8	3.26390
9	2.90576
10	2.58826
11	2.30378
12	2.05232
13	1.82880
14	1.62814
15	1.45034
16	1.29032
17	1.15062
18	1.02362
19	0.91186
20	0.81280
21	0.72390
22	0.64516
23	0.57404
24	0.51054
25	0.45466

(Adapted from Engineering ToolBox, (2004). Wire Gauge Converter - AWG versus square mm. [online] Available at: https://www.engineeringtoolbox.com/awg-wire-gauge-d_731.html)

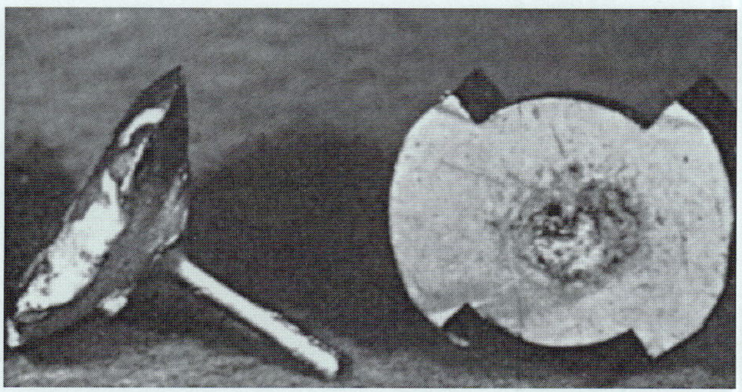

• **Fig. 14.14** Localized shrinkage caused by using a sprue of improper diameter.

Sprue Direction

The sprue former should be directed away from any thin or delicate parts of the pattern because the molten metal may abrade or fracture investment in this area and result in a casting failure. The sprue former should not be attached to a broad flat surface at a right angle. Such an orientation leads to turbulence within the mold cavity and severe porosity in this region (Fig. 14.15A). When this same pattern is sprued at a 45° angle to the proximal area, a satisfactory casting is obtained (Fig. 14.15B).

Sprue Length

The length of the sprue former depends on the length of the casting ring. If the sprue is too short, the wax pattern may be so far removed from the end of the casting ring that gases cannot be adequately vented to permit the molten alloy to fill the ring completely. When these gases are not completely eliminated, porosity may result. Therefore, the sprue length should be adjusted so that the top of the wax pattern is within 6 mm of the open end of the ring for gypsum-bonded investments (Fig. 14.16). With the higher-strength phosphate-bonded investments, it may be possible to position the wax pattern within 3–4 mm of the top of the investment. For reproducibility of casting accuracy, the pattern should be placed as close as possible to the center of the ring. However, the position of the wax pattern for vacuum pressure casting may be different.

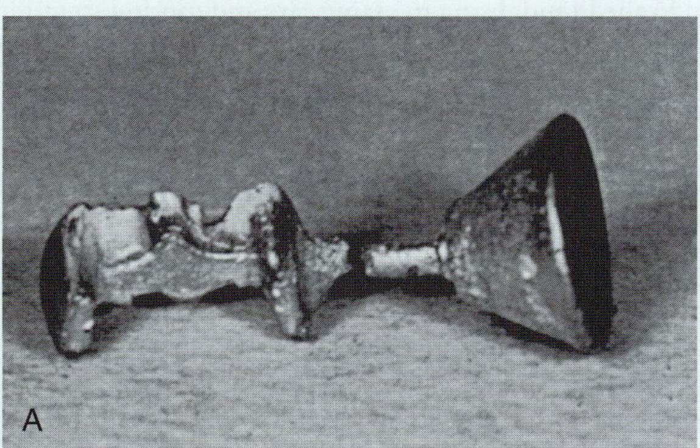

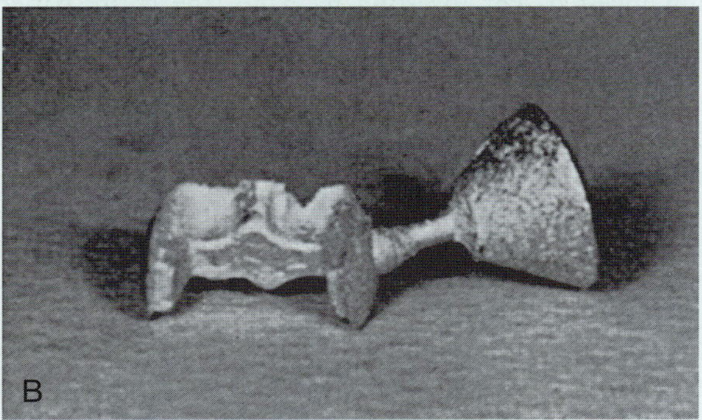

• **Fig. 14.15** **(A)** Detached sprue indicates severe porosity at the point of attachment because of turbulence caused by an improper sprue angle. **(B)** Sound casting results with sprue at approximately 45° to the proximal wall.

- Sprue diameter: Select a sprue former with a diameter that is approximately the same size as the thickest area of the wax pattern.
- Sprue position: The ideal area for the sprue former is the point of greatest bulk in the pattern.
- Sprue length: Should be long enough to position the pattern in the casting ring within 6 mm of the trailing end.
- A reservoir should be added to a sprue network.
- The sprue former should not be attached to a broad flat surface at a right angle.

CRITICAL QUESTION

How does nonuniform investment expansion occur? How can excessive longitudinal expansion be minimized?

Casting Ring Liner

With the use of solid metal rings or casting flasks, provision must be made to permit investment expansion. The mold may actually become smaller rather than larger because of the reverse pressure resulting from the confinement of the setting expansion. This effect can be overcome by using a split ring or flexible rubber ring that permits the setting expansion of the investment.

However, the most commonly used technique to provide investment expansion is to line the inner walls of the ring with a ring liner. Traditionally, asbestos was the material of choice, but it can no longer be used because its carcinogenic potential makes it a biohazard. Two types of nonasbestos ring liner materials have been produced: an aluminosilicate ceramic liner and a cellulose (paper) liner.

To ensure uniform expansion, the clinician or technician cuts the liner to fit the inside diameter of the casting ring with no overlap. The dry liner is tacked in position with sticky wax, and it is then used either dry or wet. With a wet liner technique, the lined ring is immersed in water for a time, and the excess water is shaken away. Squeezing the liner should be avoided, because this leads to variable amounts of water removal and nonuniform expansion. Although a ceramic liner may not absorb water like a cellulose liner, its network of fibers can retain water on the surface.

The liner affords greater normal setting expansion in the investment and the absorbed water causes a semihygroscopic expansion as it is drawn into the investment during setting, as shown for gypsum investments in Figure 14.6. The use of one liner (C) increases the normal setting expansion compared with no liner. Using a thicker liner material or two layers of liner (D) provides even greater semihygroscopic expansion and also affords a more unrestricted normal setting expansion of the investment. As shown in Figure 14.17, two layers of liner can be used to increase the expansion slightly compared with that obtained from one liner. In any case, the thickness of the liner should not be less than approximately 1 mm.

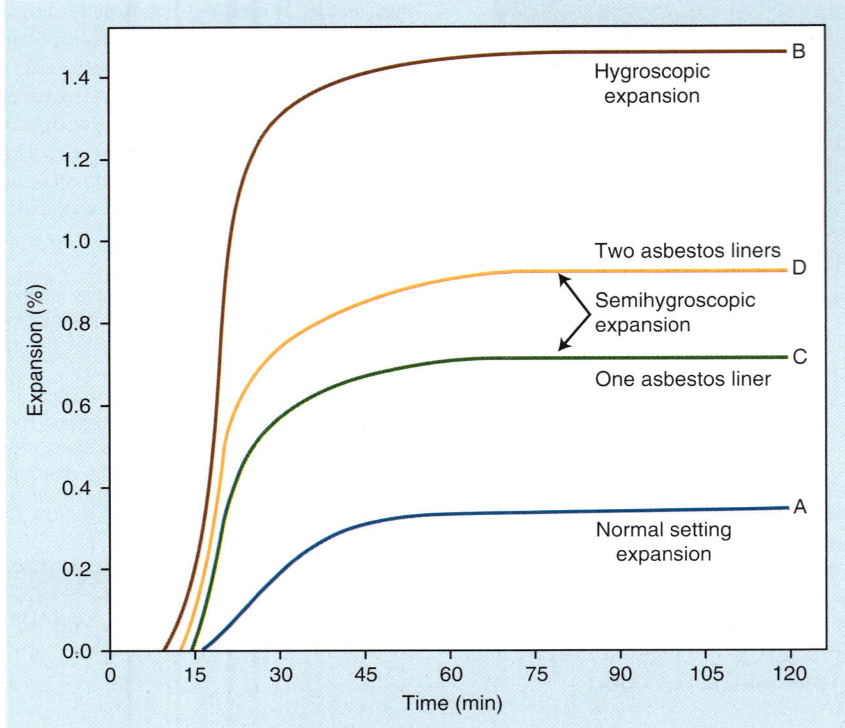

• **Fig. 14.16** **(A)** Normal setting. **(B)** Hygroscopic expansion of an investment compared with somewhat restricted expansion that occurs in an inlay ring containing **(C)** one liner and **(D)** two liners. (Courtesy of R Neiman, Whip-Mix Corporation, Louisville, KY.)

Because cellulose liners are paper products, they are burned away during the burnout procedure and a technique must be found to secure the investment in the ring. However, the desired length (height) of the liner remains a matter of controversy. If the length (height) of the liner is somewhat shorter than that of the ring itself, the investment will be confined at one or both ends of the ring. The longitudinal setting and hygroscopic expansion are thereby restricted as compared with an arrangement where the liner is flush with the ends of the ring.

The expansion of the investment is always greater in the unrestricted longitudinal direction than in the radial direction—that is, toward the ring. Therefore, it is desirable to reduce the expansion in the longitudinal direction. Placing the liner somewhat short (3.25 mm) of the ends of the ring tends to produce a more uniform expansion; thus, there is less chance for distortion of the wax pattern and the mold.

Investing Procedure

The wax pattern should be cleaned of any debris, grease, or oils. A commercial wax pattern cleaner (Debubblizer—detergent emulsions) or a diluted synthetic detergent may be used. Any excess liquid is shaken off, and the pattern is left to air-dry while the investment is being prepared. The thin film of cleanser left on the pattern reduces the surface tension of the wax and permits better "wetting" of the investment to ensure complete coverage of the intricate portions of the pattern.

While the wax pattern cleaner is air-drying, the appropriate amount of distilled water (gypsum investments) or colloidal silica special liquid (phosphate investments) is dispensed. The liquid is added to a clean dry mixing bowl, and the powder is gradually added to the liquid, using the same care and caution to minimize air entrapment as was discussed for the mixing of dental stones. Mixing is performed gently until all the powder has been wet; otherwise, the unmixed powder may inadvertently be pushed out of the bowl. Although hand-mixing is an option, it is far more common to mix all casting investments mechanically under vacuum.

Vacuum Mixing

Mechanical mixing under vacuum removes air bubbles created during mixing and evacuates any potentially harmful gases produced by the chemical reaction of the high-heat investments. Once mixing is complete, the pattern may be hand invested or vacuum invested. For investing by hand, the entire pattern is painted (inside and out) with a thin layer of investment. The casting ring is positioned on the crucible former, and the remainder of the investment is vibrated slowly into the ring. With vacuum investing, the same equipment used to mix the investment is employed to invest the pattern under vacuum.

As noted, the amount of porosity in the investment is reduced by vacuum investing. As a result, the texture of the cast surface is somewhat smoother with better detail reproduction. The tensile strength of vacuum-mixed investment is also increased. In one study, it was found that 95% of vacuum-invested castings were free of nodules, whereas only 17% of castings made in hand-invested molds were entirely free of defects. Freedom of any surface imperfections is highly important, because even a small nodule on a casting may damage a fragile enamel margin when the casting is evaluated for fit in the prepared cavity. The finished casting should always be checked under magnification for such defects before fitting it on the die.

Air bubbles that remain in the mix, even with vacuum mixing, can be entrapped on flat or concave surfaces that are not oriented suitably for air evacuation. Tilting the ring slightly aids in releasing these bubbles so that they can rise to the surface. Excessive vibration should be avoided because it can cause solids in the investment to settle and may lead to free-water accumulation adjacent to the wax pattern, resulting in surface roughness. Excessive vibration can also dislodge small patterns from the sprue former (Fig. 14.15), resulting in a miscast. 50–100 Hz is considered as optimum vibration frequency to be used in investing.

If the hygroscopic technique is employed, the filled casting ring is immediately placed in a 37°C water bath with the crucible former's side down. For the thermal expansion or high-heat technique, the invested ring is allowed to bench set undisturbed for the time recommended by the manufacturer.

Compensation for Shrinkage

Occasionally it may be desirable to alter the mold dimensions of a full cast crown compared with a small inlay. A number of factors influence mold size. As previously discussed, two liners allow for greater setting and thermal expansion than does a single liner. Also the setting, hygroscopic, and thermal expansions of investments can be controlled to a certain extent by varying the L/P ratio of the investment. The lower the L/P ratio, the greater the potential for investment expansion. Conversely, thinner mixes reduce the expansion. With some investments, however, the effect of minor adjustments to the L/P ratio is insignificant.

There is a limit to how much the L/P ratio can be altered. If the mix is too thick, it cannot be applied to the pattern without a likelihood of distorting the pattern and producing air voids during investing. On the other hand, if the mixture is too thin, a rough surface may result on the casting.

Another possible problem is too much expansion of the mold when the thermal expansion technique is used with a cristobalite investment. A thermal expansion of 1.3% may take place. If an effective setting expansion of 0.3%–0.4% is added to such a thermal expansion, a total linear expansion as high as 1.7% may be obtained, higher than the average casting shrinkage of a gold alloy. As a result, a cast crown may be too large.

In addition to controlling the hygroscopic expansion by the L/P ratio, the clinician can regulate expansion by reducing the time of immersion of the setting investment or by controlling the amount of water to be added during the setting process. The longer the delay before the investment is immersed in the water bath, the less is the amount of hygroscopic expansion that can occur.

Controlled Water-Added Technique

The linear hygroscopic expansion increases directly with the amount of water added until maximum expansion is attained. The compositions of investments used with the water-added hygroscopic casting technique ensure maximal expansion during immersion in water. The amount of hygroscopic expansion needed for compensation is then obtained by adding only enough water to provide the desired expansion.

A soft, flexible rubber ring is used instead of the usual asbestos-lined metal ring. The pattern is invested as usual. A specified amount of water is then added on top of the investment in the rubber ring, and the investment is allowed to set, usually at room temperature. The controlled water-added technique is rarely used, however, because the hygroscopic expansion method described earlier provides adequate expansion in most cases.

Casting Procedure

Once the investment has set for an appropriate period—approximately 1 hour for most gypsum- and phosphate-bonded investments—it is ready for burnout. The procedures for the two types of investments are similar, so the following discussion focuses on gypsum investments. The crucible former and any metal sprue formers are carefully removed. Any debris from the ingate area (funneled opening at the end of the ring) is cleaned with a brush. If the burnout procedure does not immediately follow the investing procedure, the invested ring is placed in a humidor at 100% humidity. Preferably, the investment should not be allowed to dry out. Rehydration of a set investment that has been stored for an extended period may not replenish all of the lost water.

Wax Elimination and Heating

The invested rings are placed in a room-temperature furnace and heated to the prescribed maximum temperature. For gypsum-bonded investments, this temperature can be either 500°C for the hygroscopic technique or 700°C for the thermal expansion technique. With phosphate-bonded investments, the maximum temperature setting may range from 700°C to 1030°C, depending on the type of alloy selected. The temperature setting is more critical with gypsum-bonded investments than for the phosphate type because the gypsum investments are more prone to investment decomposition. During burnout, some of the melted wax is absorbed by the investment and residual carbon produced by ignition of the liquid wax becomes trapped in the porous investment. It is also advisable to begin the burnout procedure while the mold is still wet. Water trapped in the pores of the investment reduces the absorption of wax, and as the water vaporizes, it flushes wax from the mold. This process is facilitated by placing the ring with the sprue hole down over a slot in a ceramic tray in the burnout furnace. When the high-heat technique is used, the mold temperature generates enough heat to convert carbon to either carbon monoxide or carbon dioxide. These gases can then escape through the pores in the heated investment.

Hygroscopic Low-Heat Technique

Hygroscopic expansion of gypsum-bonded investments was described earlier in this chapter. This technique (Fig. 14.16) obtains its compensation expansion from three sources: (1) the 37°C water bath expands the wax pattern, (2) the warm water entering the investment mold from the top adds some hygroscopic expansion, and (3) the thermal expansion at 500°C provides the needed thermal expansion. The low-heat technique offers the advantages of less investment degradation, a cooler surface for smoother castings, and the convenience of placing the molds directly in the 500°C furnace. The last benefit makes it possible to keep one or more furnaces at the burnout temperature so that molds may be put in as they are ready. This is particularly useful in large laboratories where molds are ready for burnout at various times. Care must nevertheless be taken to allow sufficient burnout time because the wax is more slowly oxidized (eliminated) at the low temperature.

The molds should remain in the furnace for at least 60 minutes, and they may be held up to 5 hours longer with little damage. Since the temperature of the furnace gets lowered each time a mold is placed, extra time should be allowed to ensure complete wax elimination when molds are placed at intervals. Even though the mold is usually held at this temperature for 60–90 minutes, sufficient residual fine carbon may be retained to reduce the venting of the mold. Because of this potential for reduced venting, back-pressure porosity is a greater hazard in the low-heat technique than in the high-heat technique, since the investments generally employed with the low-heat technique may be denser.

The standardized hygroscopic technique was developed for alloys with a high gold content; the newer noble alloys may require slightly more expansion. This added expansion may be obtained by making one or more of the following changes:

1. Increasing the water bath temperature to 40°C
2. Using two layers of liner
3. Increasing the burnout temperature to a range of 600–650°C

High-Heat Thermal Expansion Technique

This approach depends almost entirely on using a high-heat burnout to obtain the required expansion while at the same time eliminating the wax pattern. Additional expansion results from the slight heating of gypsum investments on setting, thus expanding the wax pattern, and the water entering the investment from the wet liner adds a small amount of hygroscopic expansion to the normal setting expansion.

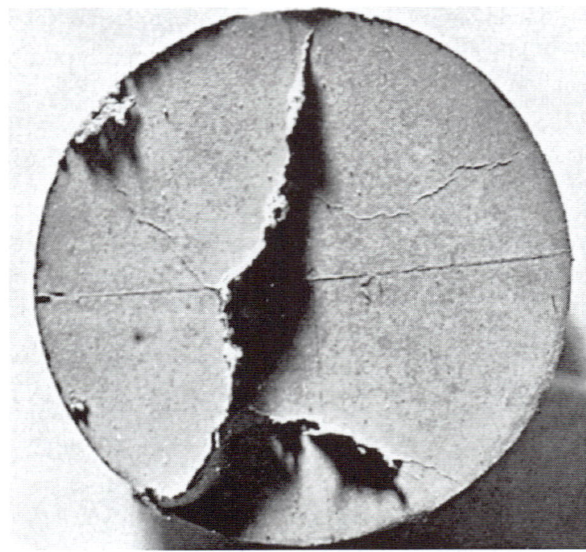

• **Fig. 14.17** Fins on the surface of a casting that formed as a result of cracks in the investment before casting of the metal.

Casting Metal in Gypsum Investments

These casting investments are relatively fragile and require the use of a metal ring for protection during heating. The molds are usually placed in a furnace at room temperature, slowly heated to 650–700°C in 60 minutes, and held for 15–30 minutes at the higher temperature.

The rate of heating has some influence on the smoothness and, in some instances, the overall dimensions of the investment. Initially the rapid heating can generate steam, which can cause flaking of the mold walls. Too many patterns in the same plane within the investment often cause separation of a whole section of investment because the expanding wax creates excessive pressure.

Too rapid a heating rate may also cause cracking of the investment. In such a case, the outside layer of the investment expands much more than the central sections. Consequently, the outside layer starts to expand thermally, resulting in compressive stress in the outside layer, which counteracts tensile stresses in the middle regions of the mold. Such a stress distribution causes radial cracks in the brittle investment. These cracks, in turn, produce a casting with fins or spines similar to those shown in Figure 14.17. This condition is likely to be present with a cristobalite investment. Low inversion temperature of the cristobalite and the rapid rate of expansion during the inversion make it important to heat the investment slowly.

Breakdown of the dental investment and the resulting contamination and brittleness of the gold alloy casting probably occur more frequently than is generally understood. The mechanism of investment decomposition and alloy contamination is related to a chemical reaction between the residual carbon and calcium sulfate binder. Calcium sulfate per se does not decompose unless it is heated above 1000°C. However, the reduction of calcium sulfate by carbon takes place rapidly above 700°C in accordance with the following reactions:

(4)

$$CaSO_4 + 4C \rightarrow CaS + 4CO$$
$$3CaSO_4 + CaS \rightarrow 4CaO + 4SO_2$$

This reaction takes place whenever gypsum investments are heated above 700°C in the presence of carbon. The sulfur dioxide as a product of this reaction contaminates gold castings and makes them extremely brittle. This fact emphasizes the need for completely eliminating the wax and avoiding burnout temperatures above 700°C, particularly if the investment contains carbon. Furthermore, sulfur gases are generated by the gypsum investment when it is heated above 700°C.

After the casting temperature has been reached, the casting should be made immediately. Maintaining a high temperature for a considerable length of time may result in sulfur contamination of the casting and also in a rough surface on the casting because of the disintegration of the investment. To avoid this problem, some technicians use furnaces with heating elements on all four sides, thereby reducing the burnout time.

Despite all these precautions and reasons for using a slow burnout technique, the desire for rapid results has led to improved investment formulations. A few gypsum investments, some with a considerable amount of cristobalite, are now offered to be used with a much more rapid burnout procedure. Some suggest placing the mold in a furnace at 315°C for 30 minutes and following this with very rapid heating to the final burnout temperature. In addition, a few investments may be placed directly into a furnace at the final burnout temperature, held for 30 minutes, and cast. Because of the furnace design, the proximity of the mold to the heating element, and the availability of air in the muffle may affect size and smoothness.

Casting in Phosphate Investments

Many of the earlier statements about gypsum investments also apply to phosphate investments. There are several differences, however, because the setting mechanism and reactions on heating are quite different.

Phosphate investments obtain their expansion from the following sources:

1. Expansion of the wax pattern—this is considerable because the setting reaction raises the mold temperature substantially.
2. Setting expansion—this is usually higher than in gypsum investments, especially because special liquids are used to increase such expansion.

3. Thermal expansion—this is greater when taken to temperatures higher than those used for gypsum-bonded investments.

A total expansion of 2% or more is required for alloys used to produce metal–ceramic prostheses, since these gold-based, palladium-based, and base metal alloys have higher melting and solidification temperatures.

Although phosphate investments are usually much harder and stronger than gypsum investments, they are nevertheless quite brittle and are subject to the same unequal expansion of adjacent sections as phase changes occur during heating.

The usual burnout temperatures for phosphate-bonded investments range from 750°C to 1030°C. The highest temperatures are required for base metal alloys. The heating rate is usually slow up to 315°C and is quite rapid thereafter, reaching completion after a hold at the upper temperature for 30 minutes. Most burnout furnaces are capable of being programmed for heating rates and holding times.

Time Allowable for Casting

The investment contracts thermally as it cools. When the thermal expansion or high-heat technique is used, the investment loses heat after the heated ring is removed from the furnace and the mold contracts. Because of the liner and the low thermal conductivity of the investment, a short time can elapse without much appreciable effect. Under average conditions of casting, approximately 1 minute can pass without a noticeable loss in dimension.

In the low-heat casting technique, the temperature gradient between the investment mold and the room is not as great as that employed with the high-heat technique. Also, the thermal expansion of the investment is not as important to the shrinkage compensation. However, the burnout temperature lies on a fairly steep portion of the thermal expansion curve rather than on a plateau portion, as in the high-heat technique. Therefore, in the low-heat casting technique, the alloy should also be cast soon after removal of the ring from the oven; otherwise, a significant variation from the desired casting dimensions may occur.

Casting Machines

Alloys are melted in one of the four following ways, depending on the available types of casting machines:

1. The alloy is melted in a separate crucible by a torch flame and cast into the mold by centrifugal force (Fig. 14.18).
2. The alloy is melted electrically by a resistance heating or induction furnace and then cast into the mold centrifugally by motor or spring action. A representative casting machine of this type is shown in Figure 14.19.
3. The alloy is melted by induction heating and then cast into the mold centrifugally by motor or spring action. A representative casting machine of this type is shown in Figure 14.20.
4. The alloy is vacuum arc melted and cast by pressure in an argon atmosphere.

In addition to these melting methods, the molten metal may be cast by air pressure, vacuum, or both. The general procedure for each is described in the following sections, with certain advantages and disadvantages cited. However, it is important to follow the manufacturer's directions precisely for any of these devices.

Torch Melting/Centrifugal Casting Machine

The casting machine spring is first wound two to five turns (depending on the particular machine and the speed of casting rotation desired). The alloy is melted by a torch flame (Fig. 14.21) in a glazed ceramic crucible attached to the "broken arm" of the casting machine. The torch flame is generated from a gas mixture of propane and air, natural gas and air, acetylene and air, or acetylene and oxygen. The broken arm feature accelerates the initial rotational speed of the crucible and casting ring, thus increasing the linear speed of the liquid casting alloy as it moves into and through the mold. Once the metal has reached the casting temperature and the heated casting ring is in position, the machine is released and the spring triggers the rotational motion.

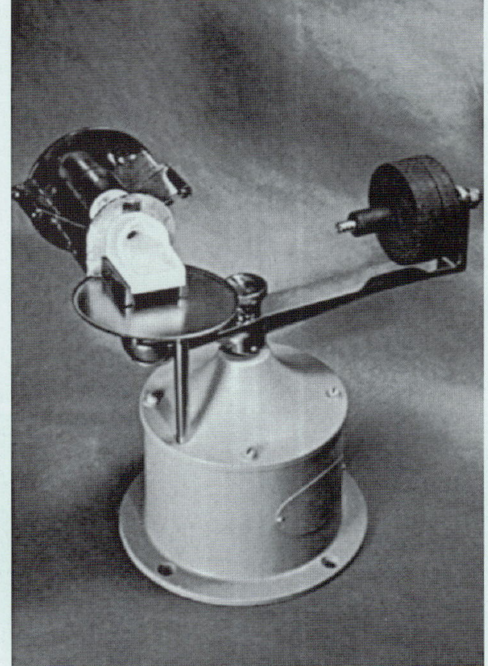

• **Fig. 14.18** Centrifugal casting machine, spring wound.

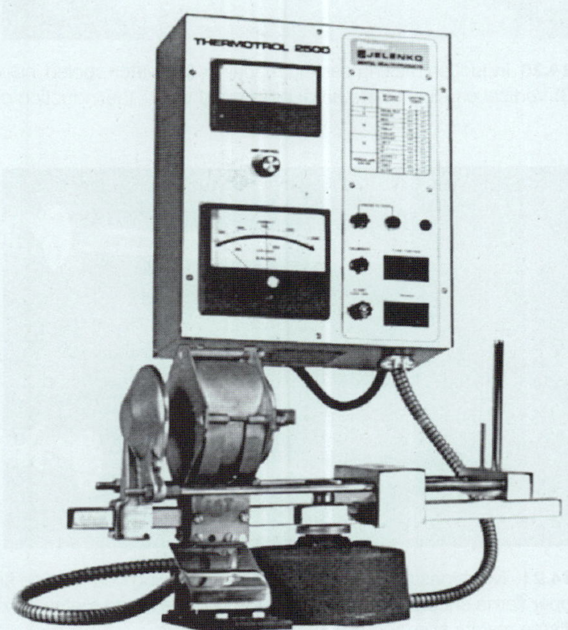

• **Fig. 14.19** Spring-wound casting machine with electrical resistance melting furnace.

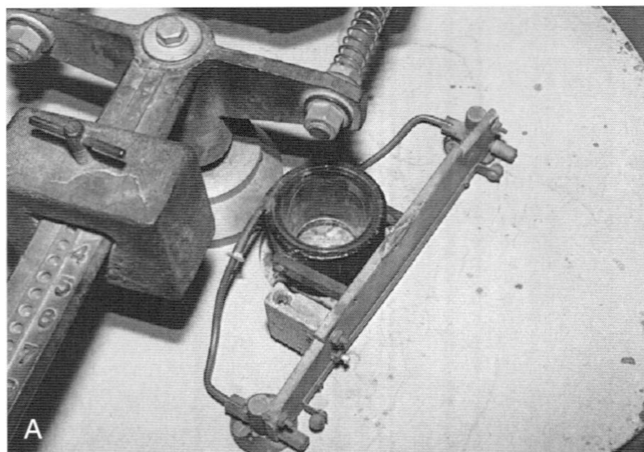

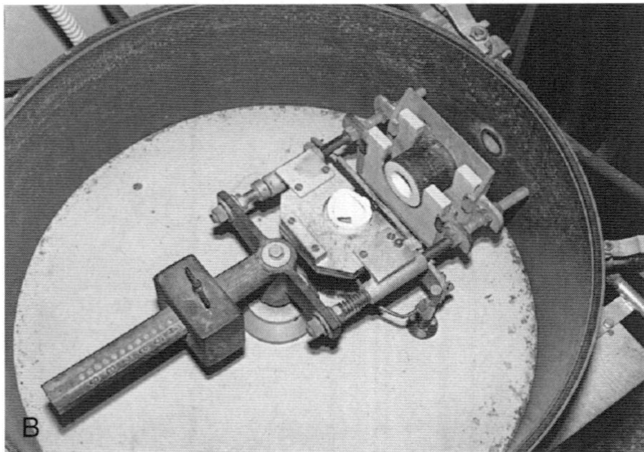

• **Fig. 14.20** Induction melting casting machine. **(A)** Water-cooled induction coil. **(B)** Vertical crucible (*white area*) positioned within the induction coil.

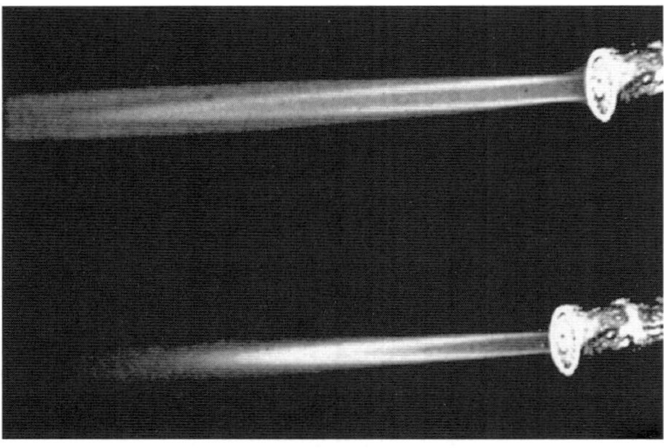

• **Fig. 14.21** Two types of nonluminous flames showing combustion areas. The upper flame should be employed for fusing the noble metal alloy. The lower flame results from too much air in the mixture.

Electrical Resistance–Heated Casting Machine

In this device, current is passed through a resistance heating conductor, and automatic melting of the alloy occurs in a graphite or ceramic crucible. This is an advantage, especially for alloys such as those used for metal–ceramic prostheses, which are alloyed with base metals in trace amounts that tend to oxidize on overheating. Another advantage is that the crucible in the furnace is located flush against the casting ring. Therefore, the alloy button remains molten slightly longer, again ensuring that solidification progresses completely from the tip of the casting to the button surface. A carbon crucible should not be used in the melting of high-palladium alloys, palladium–silver alloys, nickel–chromium alloys, or cobalt–chromium base metal alloys. An example of the electrical resistance casting machine is shown in Figure 14.19.

Induction Melting Machine

With this unit, the alloy is melted by an induction field that develops within a crucible surrounded by water-cooled metal tubing (see Fig. 14.20). The electric induction furnace is a transformer in which an alternating current flow through the primary winding coil and generates a variable magnetic field in the location of the alloy to be melted in a crucible. Once the alloy reaches the casting temperature in air or in vacuum, it is forced into the mold by centrifugal force, air pressure, or vacuum. The device has become popular in the casting of jewelry, but it has not been used as much as the other two techniques for noble alloy castings. It is more commonly used for melting base metal alloys.

There is little practical difference in the properties or accuracy of castings made with any of the three types of casting machines. The choice is a matter of access to specialized equipment and personal preference.

Direct-Current Arc Melting Machine

The direct-current arc is produced between two electrodes: the alloy and the water-cooled tungsten electrode. The temperature within the arc exceeds 4000°C and the alloy melts very quickly. This method poses a high risk of overheating the alloy, and damage may result after only a few seconds of prolonged heating.

Vacuum- or Pressure-Assisted Casting Machine

For this method, the molten alloy is heated to the casting temperature, drawn into the evacuated mold by gravity or vacuum, and subjected to additional pressure to force the alloy into the mold. For titanium and titanium alloys, vacuum arc heated argon pressure casting machines are required.

Casting Crucibles

Generally, four types of casting crucibles are available: clay, carbon, quartz, and zirconia–alumina. Clay crucibles are appropriate for many of the crown and bridge alloys, such as the high-noble and noble types. Carbon crucibles can be used not only for high-noble crown and bridge alloys but also for the higher-fusing gold-based metal–ceramic alloys.

Crucibles made from alumina, quartz, or silica are recommended for high-fusing alloys of any type. These are especially suited for alloys that have a high melting temperature or those that are sensitive to carbon contamination. Crown and bridge alloys with high palladium content—such as palladium–silver alloys for metal–ceramic copings and any of the nickel-based or cobalt-based alloys—are included in this category.

Torch Melting of Noble Metal Alloy

This type of alloy is best melted by placing it on the inner sidewall of the crucible. Thus, the operator can better observe the progress of the melting and there is a better opportunity for any gases in the flame to be reflected from the surface of the alloy rather than being absorbed.

The fuel used in most instances is a mixture of natural or artificial gas and air, although oxygen–air and acetylene can also be used. The temperature of the gas–air flame is greatly influenced by the nature of the gas and the proportions of gas and air in the mixture. Considerable care should be taken to obtain a nonluminous brush flame with the different combustion zones clearly differentiated. Two types of flames can be obtained with a casting torch, as shown in Figure 14.21. The air supply for the lower flame (Fig. 14.22) is excessive, so that incomplete combustion and a lower temperature will result. This type of flame is likely to be favored by the beginner because the roaring sound that accompanies this flame adjustment "sounds" hot. The upper brush flame indicates the proper adjustment for maximal efficiency and temperature.

With a little practice, the clinician can readily detect whether the proper zone of the flame is in contact with the metal by observing the condition of the alloy surface. When the reducing zone is in contact, the surface of the gold alloy is bright and mirror like, as indicated in Figure 14.22. When the oxidizing portion of the flame is in contact with the alloy, a dull film of "dross" develops over the surface, as seen in Figure 14.22B. Although care should be taken not to overheat the alloy, there is generally more likelihood of underheating when the gas–air flame is used. The alloy first appears to be spongy and then small globules of fused alloy appear. The molten alloy soon assumes a spheroidal shape, as indicated in Figure 14.22A. At the proper casting temperature, the molten alloy is light orange and tends to spin or follow the flame when the latter is moved slightly. At this point, the alloy should be approximately 38–66°C above its liquidus temperature.

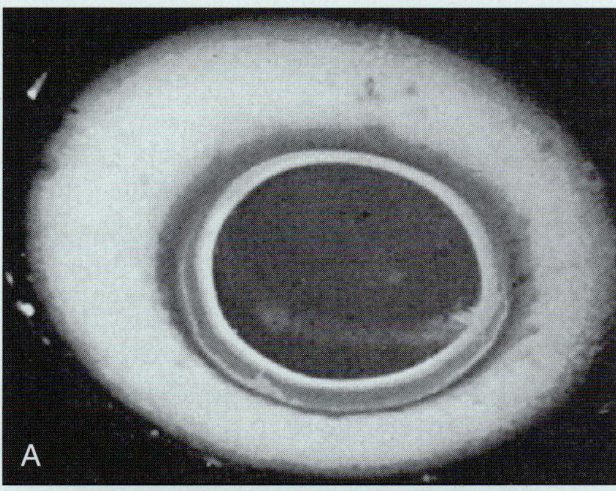

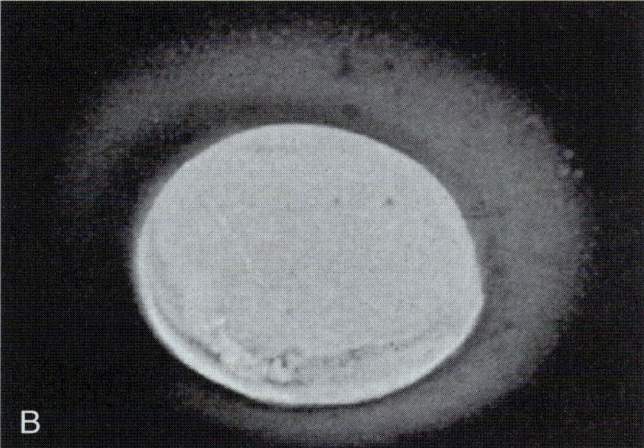

• **Fig. 14.22** **(A)** Mirror-like surface of the metal indicates proper fusion. **(B)** Cloudy surface indicates surface oxidation by improper positioning of the torch flame.

The casting should be made immediately when the proper temperature is reached. As previously discussed, various devices are also available for melting the alloy electrically.

Cleaning the Casting

When a type III or IV gold alloy has been cast and it has solidified, the ring should be quenched in water as soon as the button exhibits a dull-red glow. Two advantages are gained in quenching: (1) the noble metal alloy is left in an annealed condition for burnishing, polishing, and similar procedures and (2) when the water contacts the hot investment, a violent reaction ensues, resulting in a soft, granular investment that is easily removed.

Often the surface of the casting appears dark because of oxides and tarnish. Such a surface film can be removed by a process known as pickling, which consists of heating the discolored casting in an acid. One of the best pickling solutions for gypsum-bonded investments is a 50% hydrochloric acid (HCl) solution. The HCl aids in the removal of any residual investment, as well as of the oxide coating. The disadvantage of HCl is that the fumes from the acid are likely to corrode laboratory metal furnishings. In addition, these fumes are a health hazard and should be vented via a fume hood. However, the pickling process can be performed ultrasonically while the prosthesis is sealed in a Teflon container. A solution of sulfuric acid (H_2SO_4) may also be more advantageous in this respect. Ultrasonic devices are useful for cleaning the casting, as are commercial pickling solutions made of acid salts. Abrasive blasting devices are also useful for cleaning the surface of castings.

The best method for pickling is to place the casting in a test tube or dish and to pour the acid over it. It may be necessary to heat the acid, but boiling should be avoided because of the considerable amount of acid fumes involved. After pickling, the acid is poured off and the casting is removed. The pickling solution should be renewed frequently, because it is likely to become contaminated after reusing the solution several times.

In no case should the casting be held with steel tongs so that both the casting and the tongs come into contact with the pickling solution, because this may contaminate the casting. The pickling solution usually contains small amounts of copper dissolved from previous castings. When the steel tongs contact this electrolyte, a small galvanic cell is created and copper is deposited on the casting at the point where the tongs grip it. This copper deposition extends into the alloy and is a future source for discoloration in the area.

If gold-based and palladium-based metal–ceramic alloys and base metal alloys are bench cooled to room temperature before the casting is removed from the investment, these alloys are generally not pickled.

- Pickling is the immersion of metals in an acid solution for the purpose of removing surface fire scale and oxides caused by heating, annealing, casting, soldering, etc.
- For gypsum-bonded investment, pickling is done with hydrochloric acid/sulfuric acid.

Melting of Base Metals

Although torch melting can be used in some cases, most base metals of Ni–Cr, Ni–Cr–Be, Co–Cr, Co–Ni–Cr, commercially pure Ti, and Ti–Al–V require special melting equipment, such as induction melting machines, vacuum melting devices, or arc melting units. The procedures required are designed to minimize the risk for excessive oxidation or an interaction of the molten alloys with the recommended casting investments. It is beyond the scope of this book to discuss these methods; the reader is referred to specialized instruction manuals developed by the manufacturers of these products.

Technical Considerations for Phosphate-Bonded Investment

The procedure for investing a wax pattern in a phosphate-bonded investment is essentially the same as that for a gypsum-bonded investment. As previously mentioned, the working time can vary depending on the L/P ratio, special liquid concentration, temperature, mixing time, mixing rate, and operator skill and experience.

As with any investment that has a high thermal expansion, especially when marked changes in expansion or contraction occur, it is necessary to use a slow heating rate during burnout to prevent possible cracking or spalling. Some furnaces provide slow rates of heating. For those that do not, it is advisable to use a two-stage burnout, holding at 200–300°C for at least 30 minutes before completing the burnout. Recommendations for the rate of heating vary, so it is wise to follow the instructions for the specific investment used.

Although phosphate investments appear strong, they are still susceptible to a number of disrupting influences during burnout. When the wax softens, it expands much more than does the investment. When investing, it is desirable to leave 3–6 mm of investment around each pattern and to stagger the patterns if several are placed in the same ring. A number of patterns positioned along a plane can exert tremendous pressure and fracture almost any investment, but particularly the phosphate-bonded materials. The rapid expansion of cristobalite investment at approximately 300°C requires slow heating to prevent fracture. After the temperature reaches 400°C, the rate of heating can be safely increased. After burnout, usually at a final temperature of 700–1030°C depending on the alloy melting range, the casting is made. The permeability of the phosphate investment is low compared with that of a gypsum-bonded investment. Therefore, the required casting pressure should be greater than that for a gypsum mold.

- It is desirable to leave 3–6 mm of investment around each pattern.
- Stagger the patterns if several patterns are placed in the same ring.

Recovery and cleaning of the casting are more difficult when a phosphate-bonded investment is used because such materials do not contain the soft gypsum products. Also, the particles usually include large grains of quartz. In some instances, such as with gold-containing alloys, the investment adheres rather tenaciously, usually requiring cleaning in an ultrasonic device. Neither the phosphate binder nor the silica refractory is soluble in HCl or H_2SO_4. Old hydrofluoric acid (HF) dissolves the silica refractory quite well without damage to a gold-based or a palladium–silver alloy, but this acid must be used carefully with other alloys. In fact, even dilute HF should not be used unless the necessary neutralizing solutions are immediately at hand and the clinician is familiar with the correct handling techniques. However, once tissue injury has occurred, it cannot be reversed with such solutions. Alternative commercially available solutions can be used with greater safety.

- HF differs from other acids because it readily penetrates the skin and dissociates into fluoride ions, causing destruction of deep tissue layers, including bone.
- Ensure that calcium gluconate antidote is on hand before handling HF.
- Neutralize small spills by covering with magnesium sulfate (dry).
- Wash the spill site with a sodium bicarbonate solution.

Base metal alloys require a light sandblasting, usually with fine alumina. Chromium-based partial dentures are usually sandblasted to remove the investment. Acid should not be used for cleaning base metal alloys.

The selection of the appropriate phosphate-bonded investment must be made on the basis of the composition of the alloy to be used. Carbon-containing investments are well suited for gold-based crown and bridge casting alloys and metal–ceramic alloys. However, if the alloy is carbon sensitive (such as in silver–palladium, high palladium, palladium–silver, nickel–chromium–beryllium, nickel–chromium, and cobalt–chromium alloys), a noncarbon investment should be used.

Causes of Defective Castings

An unsuccessful casting results in considerable trouble and loss of time. In almost all instances, defects in castings can be avoided by strict observance of procedures governed by certain fundamental rules and principles. Seldom is a defect in a casting attributable to factors other than the carelessness or ignorance of the operator. With present techniques, casting failures should be the exception, not the rule.

Defects in castings can be classified under four headings:

1. Distortion
2. Surface roughness and irregularities
3. Porosity (Fig. 14.23)
4. Incomplete or missing detail

The porosity in the pontic area of Figure 14.23 was caused by the retention of heat by the pontic because of its bulk and because it was located in the heat center of the ring. This problem can be solved simply by attaching one or more small-gauge sprues (e.g., 18 gauge) at the surface most distant from the main

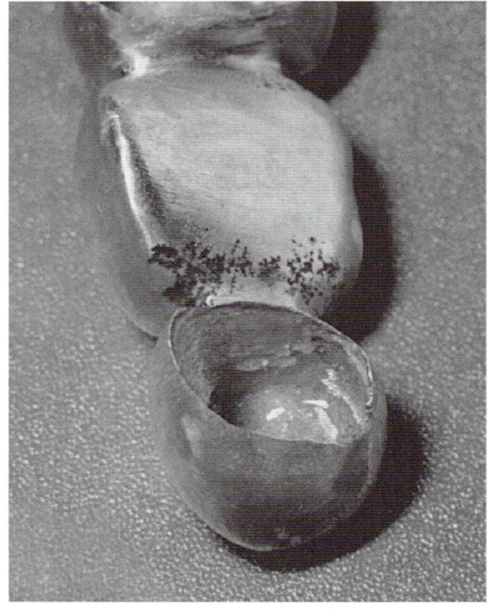

• **Fig. 14.23** Localized shrinkage porosity in pontic of three-unit bridge caused by delayed solidification and lack of a chill-set sprue.

sprue attachment and extending the sprue(s) laterally within 5 mm of the edge of the ring. These small chill-set sprues ensure that solidification begins within the sprues, and they act as cooling pins to carry heat away from the pontic. Other types of casting porosities are described in a later section.

Distortion

Any marked distortion of the casting is probably related to a distortion of the wax pattern, as described in the section on inlay wax. This type of distortion can be minimized or prevented by proper manipulation of the wax and handling of the pattern.

Unquestionably some distortion of the wax pattern occurs as the investment hardens around it. The setting and hygroscopic expansions of the investment may produce a nonuniform expansion of the walls of the pattern. This type of distortion occurs in part from the nonuniform outward movement of the proximal walls. The gingival margins are forced apart by the mold expansion, whereas the solid occlusal bar of wax resists expansion during the early stages of setting. The configuration of the pattern, the type of wax, and the thickness influence the distortion that occurs, as has been discussed. For example, distortion increases as the thickness of the pattern decreases. As would be expected, the lower is the setting expansion of the investment, the less low is distortion. Generally, this is not a serious problem, but it accounts for some of the unexplained inaccuracies that may occur in small castings.

Surface Roughness, Irregularities, and Discoloration

The surface of a dental casting should be an accurate reproduction of the surface of the wax pattern from which it is made. Excessive roughness or irregularities on the outer surface of the casting necessitate additional finishing and polishing, whereas irregularities on the cavity surface prevent proper seating of an otherwise accurate casting.

Surface roughness should not be confused with surface irregularities. Surface roughness is defined as relatively finely spaced surface imperfections whose height, width, and direction establish the predominant surface pattern. Surface irregularities are isolated imperfections, such as nodules, that are not characteristic of the entire surface area.

Even under optimal conditions, the surface roughness of the dental casting is invariably somewhat greater than that of the wax pattern from which it is made. The difference is probably related to the particle size of the investment and its ability to reproduce the wax pattern in microscopic detail. With proper manipulative techniques, the normal increased roughness in the casting should not be a major factor in dimensional accuracy. However, improper technique can lead to a marked increase in surface roughness as well as to the formation of surface irregularities.

Air Voids

Small nodules on a casting are caused by air bubbles that become attached to the pattern during or subsequent to the investing procedure. Such nodules can sometimes be removed if they are not in a critical area. However, for nodules on margins or on internal surfaces, removal of these irregularities might alter the fit of the casting. As previously noted, the best method to avoid air bubbles is to use the vacuum investing technique.

If a manual method is used, various precautions can be taken to eliminate air from the investment mix before the investing. As previously outlined, a mechanical mixer with vibration both before and after mixing should be used routinely. A wetting agent may be helpful in preventing the collection of air bubbles on the surface of the pattern, but it is by no means a certain remedy. As previously discussed, it is important that the wetting agent be applied in a thin layer. It is best to air-dry the wetting agent, because any excess liquid dilutes the investment, possibly producing surface irregularities on the casting.

Water Films

Wax is repellent to water; if the investment becomes separated from the wax pattern in some manner, a water film may form irregularly over the surface. Occasionally this type of surface irregularity appears as minute ridges or veins. If the pattern is slightly moved, jarred, or vibrated after investing or if the painting procedure does not result in intimate contact of the investment with the pattern, such a condition may result. A wetting agent is useful for the prevention of such irregularities. Too high an L/P ratio may also produce these surface irregularities.

Liquid/Powder Ratio (L/P)

The amount of water and investment should be measured accurately. The higher the L/P ratio, the rougher the casting. However, if too little water is used, the investment may be unmanageably thick, so that it cannot be properly applied to the pattern. In vacuum investing, the air may not be sufficiently removed. In either instance, a rough surface on the casting may result.

Composition of the Investment

The ratio of the binder mass to that of the quartz influences the surface texture of the casting. In addition, a coarse silica causes surface roughness.

Foreign Bodies

When foreign substances get into the mold a surface roughness may be produced. For example, a rough crucible former with investment clinging to it may roughen the investment on its removal so that bits of investment are carried into the mold with the molten alloy. Carelessness in the removal of the sprue former may also be a cause.

Usually, contamination results not only in surface roughness but also in incomplete areas or surface voids. Any casting that shows sharp, well-defined deficiencies indicates the presence of some foreign particles in the mold, such as pieces of investment and bits of carbon from a flux. Bright-appearing concavities may be the result of flux being carried into the mold with the metal.

Surface discoloration and roughness can result from sulfur contamination. An example of this effect may be seen in Figure 14.24, either from investment breakdown at elevated temperatures or from a high sulfur content of the torch flame. The interaction of the molten alloy with sulfur produces a black or gray layer on the surface of gold alloys that is brittle and does not clean readily during pickling.

Impact of Molten Alloy on the Mold Wall

The direction of the sprue former should be such that the molten gold alloy does not impact a weak portion of the mold surface. Occasionally, the molten alloy may fracture or abrade the mold

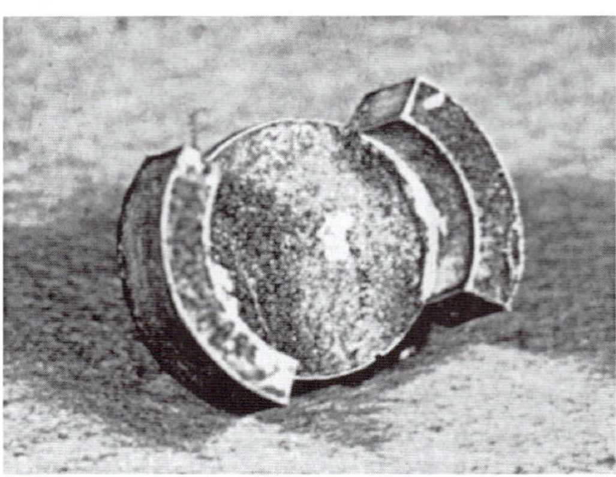

• **Fig. 14.24** A black-coated noble metal alloy casting resulting from sulfur contamination or oxidation during melting of the alloy.

surface on impact, regardless of its bulk. It is unfortunate that sometimes the abraded area is smooth, so that it cannot be detected on the surface of the casting. Such a depression in the mold is reflected as a raised area on the casting, often too slight to be noticed yet sufficiently large to prevent complete seating of the casting. This type of surface roughness or irregularity can be avoided by proper spruing so as to prevent the direct impact of the molten metal at an angle of 90° to the investment surface. A glancing impact is likely to be less damaging, and at the same time an undesirable turbulence is avoided.

Pattern Position

If several patterns are invested in the same ring, they should not be placed too close together. Likewise, positioning too many patterns in the same plane in the mold should be avoided. The expansion of wax is much greater than that of the investment, and this may cause breakdown or cracking of the investment if the spacing between patterns is less than 3 mm.

Carbon Inclusions

Carbon from a crucible, an improperly adjusted torch, or a carbon-containing investment, can be absorbed by the alloy during casting. These particles may lead to the formation of carbides or even create visible carbon inclusions.

CRITICAL QUESTION

How can the risk for porosity and incomplete castings be minimized?

Porosity

Cast metal prostheses such as inlays, onlays, crowns, and bridges represent the most durable and long-lasting materials and devices used for dental restorations. They are quite costly, so dental patients expect a high degree of precision and quality in their manufacture. In this regard, extreme care should be taken to prevent the casting defects already mentioned. In addition, care should also be taken to avoid producing one of the most common types of defects, that is, casting porosity.

Where is porosity most likely to occur? It may occur both within the interior region of a casting and in the external surface. The latter effect results in surface roughness, but it is also a manifestation of internal porosity. Not only does the internal porosity weaken the casting, but it also extends to the surface, which may also cause discoloration. If severe, it can cause plaque accumulation at the tooth–restoration interface, and secondary caries or periodontal disease may result within the adjacent tooth structure. Although porosity in a casting cannot be prevented entirely, it can be minimized by the use of proper techniques.

Porosities in noble metal alloy castings are classified in the following. Illustrations of some of these defects are also noted.

I. Solidification defects
   A. Localized shrinkage porosity (Fig. 14.23)
   B. Microporosity (Fig. 14.23A)
   C. Suck-back porosity (Fig. 14.26)
II. Trapped gases
   A. Pinhole porosity (Fig. 14.25A)
   B. Gas inclusions
   C. Subsurface porosity (Fig. 14.25B)
   D. Back pressure porosity (Fig. 14.27)

Localized shrinkage is generally caused by premature termination of the flow of molten metal during solidification. The linear contraction of noble metal alloys from a liquid state to a solid state is at least 1.25%. Therefore, continual feeding of molten metal through the sprue must occur to make up for the shrinkage of metal volume during solidification. If the sprue freezes in its cross-section before this flow is completed to the casting proper, a localized shrinkage void will occur in the last portion of the casting that solidifies. Four types of porosities are shown in Figure 14.25A and B: (a) localized shrinkage porosity, (b) microporosity, (c) pinhole

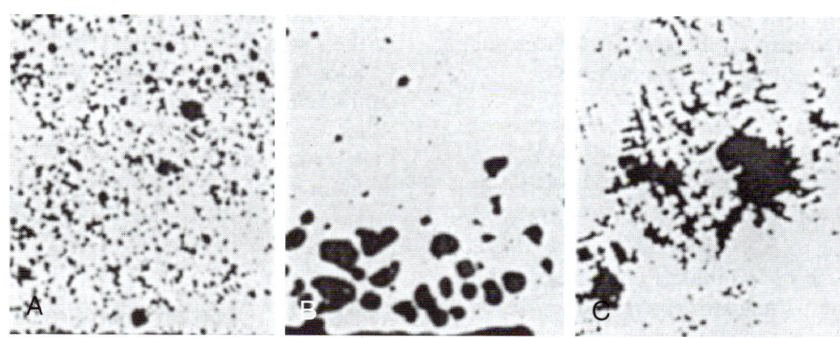

• **Fig. 14.25** **(A)** Microporosity, pinhole porosity, and gas inclusions. Microporosity voids are irregular in shape, whereas the two other types tend to be spherical; the largest spherical voids are gas inclusions. **(B)** Subsurface porosity. **(C)** Localized shrinkage porosity. (Courtesy of G Ryge.)

porosity, and (d) subsurface porosity. Localized shrinkage porosity is shown in Figure 14.25C. Localized shrinkage generally occurs near the sprue–casting junction, but it may occur anywhere between dendrites, as shown in Figure 14.25C, where the last part of the casting to solidify was between the dendrite branches as they developed.

Microporosity also occurs from solidification shrinkage, but it is generally present in fine-grain alloy castings when the solidification is too rapid for the microvoids to segregate to the liquid pool. This premature solidification causes the formation of small, irregular voids. Such phenomena can occur from rapid solidification if the mold or casting temperature is too low. Unfortunately, this type of defect is not detectable unless the casting is sectioned. In any case, it is generally not a serious defect. Oxygen is dissolved by some of the metals, such as silver, in the alloy while they are in the molten state. During solidification, the gas is expelled to form blebs and pores in the metal. As was pointed out earlier, this type of porosity may be attributed to abuse of the metal. Castings that are severely contaminated with gases are usually black when they are removed from the investment and do not clean easily on pickling (see Fig. 14.24). The porosity that extends to the surface is usually in the form of small pinpoint holes (see Fig. 14.25A). When the surface is polished, other pinholes appear.

Both pinhole and gas inclusion porosities are related to the entrapment of gas during solidification. Both are characterized by a spherical contour but are decidedly different in size. The gas inclusion porosities are usually much larger than pinhole porosity, as indicated in Figure 14.25A. Many metals dissolve or occlude gases while they are molten. For example, both copper and silver dissolve oxygen in large amounts in the liquid state. Molten platinum and palladium have a strong affinity for hydrogen as well as oxygen. On solidification, the absorbed gases are expelled and pinhole porosity results. The larger voids (Fig. 14.25A) may also result from the same cause, but it is more logical to assume that such voids are caused by gas that is mechanically trapped by the molten metal in the mold or by gas that is incorporated during the casting procedure.

Larger spherical porosities can be caused by gas occluded from a poorly adjusted torch flame or by use of the mixing or oxidizing zones of the flame rather than the reducing zone (Fig. 14.25A). If the alloy has been used before, these types of porosities can be minimized by premelting the gold alloy on a graphite crucible or a graphite block and correctly adjusting and positioning the torch flame during melting.

Subsurface porosity occurs on occasion, as shown in Figure 14.25B. At other times it may be particularly evident. The reasons for such voids are not well understood. They may be caused by the simultaneous nucleation of solid grains and gas bubbles at the first moment that the alloy freezes at the mold walls. As has been explained, this type of porosity can be diminished by controlling the rate at which the molten metal enters the mold.

As described previously in this chapter, suck-back porosity, another type of localized shrinkage porosity, may also occur externally, usually in the interior of a crown near the area of the sprue, if a hot spot has been created by the hot metal impinging from the sprue channel on a point of the mold wall. This hot spot causes the local region to freeze last and results in what is called suck-back porosity, as shown in Figure 14.26 (left). Suck-back porosity often occurs at an occlusoaxial line angle or incisoaxial line angle that is not well rounded. The entering metal impinges onto the mold surface at this point and creates a higher localized mold temperature in this region, known as a hot spot. A hot spot may retain a localized pool of molten metal after other areas of the casting have solidified. This, in turn, creates a shrinkage void or suck-back porosity. This type of porosity defect can be eliminated by flaring the point of sprue attachment and reducing the mold-melt temperature differential—that is, lowering the casting temperature by about 30°C. Such a result is shown on the right side of Figure 14.26.

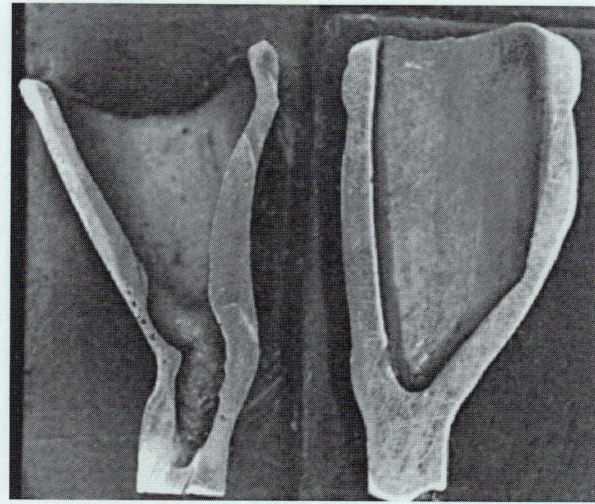

• **Fig. 14.26** Examples of suck-back porosity. The coping on the left was cast at 1370°C. The coping on the right side was cast at 1340°C. (Courtesy of J Nielsen.)

Entrapped air bubbles on the inner surface of the casting, are sometimes referred to as back-pressure porosity, can produce large concave depressions such as those seen in Figure 14.27. This is caused by the inability of the air in the mold to escape through the pores in the investment or by the pressure gradient that displaces the air pocket toward the end of the investment via the molten sprue and button. The entrapped air voids are frequently found in a "pocket" at the cavity surface of a crown or mesio-occlusal-distal casting. Occasionally it is found even on the outside surface of the casting when the casting temperature or mold temperature is so low that solidification occurs before the entrapped air can escape. The incidence of entrapped air can be increased by use of the dense modern investments, by an increase in mold density produced by vacuum investing, and by the tendency for the mold to clog with residual carbon when the low-heat technique is used. Each of these factors tends to slow the venting of gases from the mold during casting.

All castings probably contain a certain amount of porosity, as exemplified by the photomicrographs shown in Figure 14.28. This porosity should be kept to a minimum because it may adversely affect the physical properties of the casting. Proper burnout, an adequate mold and casting temperature, a sufficiently high casting pressure, and proper L/P ratio can minimize or eliminate entrapped air porosity. It is a good practice to make sure that the thickness of investment between the tip of the pattern and the end of the ring is not greater than 6 mm.

- Localized shrinkage is generally caused by premature termination of the flow of molten metal during solidification.
- Microporosity also occurs from solidification shrinkage, when the solidification is too rapid.
- Both pinhole and gas inclusion porosities are related to the entrapment of gas during solidification. Many metals dissolve or occlude gases while they are molten.

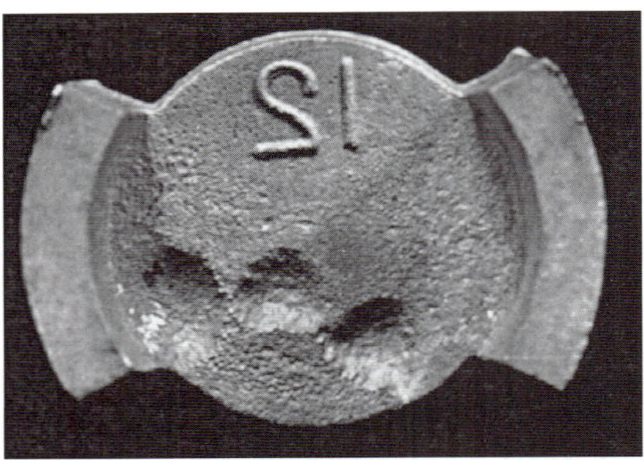

• **Fig. 14.27** Surface irregularity on the cavity side of a casting caused by back-pressure porosity.

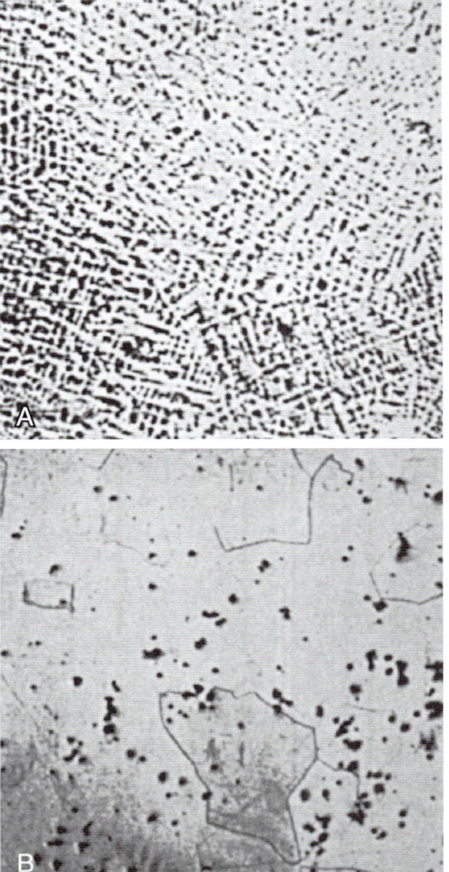

• **Fig. 14.28** **(A)** Grain structure of an as-cast type III noble metal alloy. **(B)** Same alloy after a homogenization heat treatment at 725°C for 70 minutes. Pinhole porosity is visible. (Courtesy of B Hedegard.)

- Subsurface porosity may be caused by the simultaneous nucleation of solid grains and gas bubbles at the first moment that the alloy freezes at the mold walls.
- If a hot spot is created by the hot metal impinging from the sprue channel, the local region freezes last and results in what is called suck-back porosity.
- Entrapped air bubbles on the inner surface of the casting, are sometimes referred to as back-pressure porosity and can produce large concave depressions.

Incomplete Casting

Occasionally only a partially complete casting or perhaps no casting at all is found. The obvious cause is that the molten alloy has been prevented in some manner from completely filling the mold. At least two factors that may inhibit the ingress of the liquefied alloy are insufficient venting of the mold and high viscosity of the fused metal.

The first consideration, insufficient venting, is directly related to the back pressure exerted by the air in the mold. If the air cannot be vented quickly, the molten alloy does not fill the mold before it solidifies. In such a case, the magnitude of the casting pressure should be suspected. If insufficient casting pressure is used, the back pressure cannot be overcome. Furthermore, the pressure should be applied for at least 4 seconds. The mold is filled and the alloy solidified in 1 second or less, yet it is quite soft during the early stages. Therefore, the pressure should be maintained for a few seconds beyond this point. An example of an incomplete casting that is caused by insufficient casting pressure is shown in Figure 14.29. These failures are usually exemplified by rounded, incomplete margins.

A second common cause of an incomplete casting is incomplete elimination of wax residues from the mold. If too many products of combustion remain in the mold, the pores in the investment may become filled, so that the air cannot be vented completely. If moisture or particles of wax remain, the contact of the molten alloy with these foreign substances produces an explosion that may lead to sufficient back pressure to prevent the mold from being filled. An example of a casting failure caused by incomplete wax elimination can be seen in Figures 14.30 and 14.31. Although the rounded margins in Figure 14.31 are similar to those of the

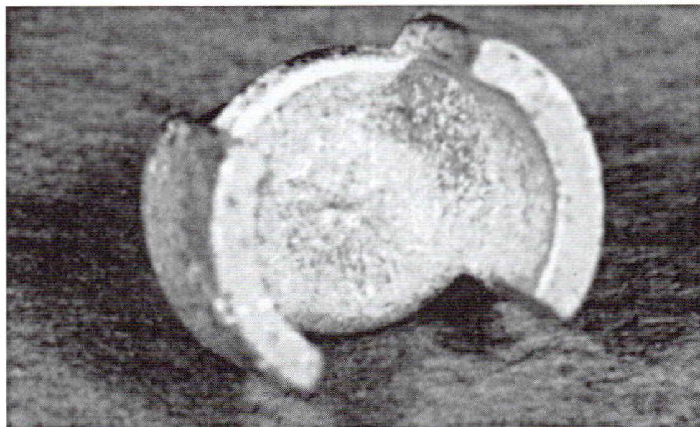

• **Fig. 14.29** Rounded, incomplete margins are evidence of insufficient casting pressure.

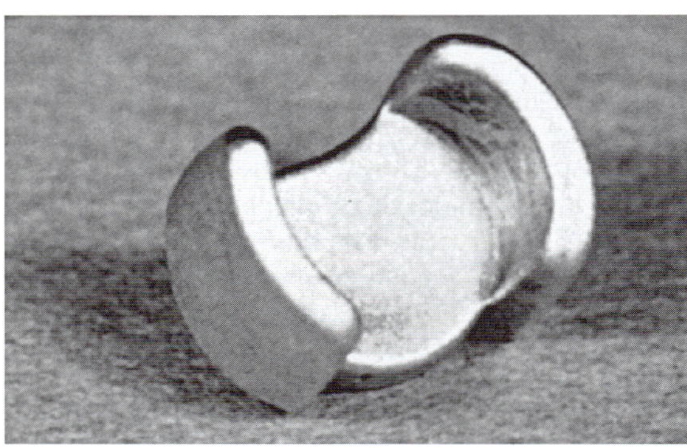

• **Fig. 14.30** Incomplete casting resulting from incomplete wax elimination is characterized by rounded margins and shiny appearance.

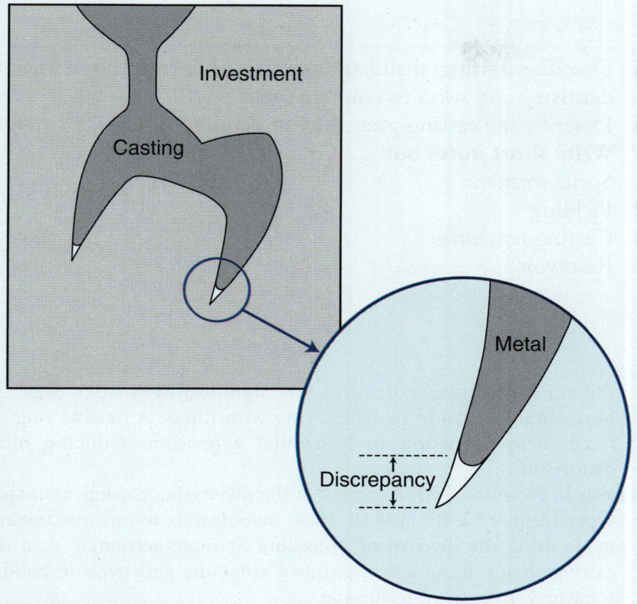

• **Fig. 14.31** Schematic illustration of an incomplete casting.

incomplete casting in Figure 14.29, they are quite shiny rather than dull. This shiny condition of the metal is caused by the strong reducing atmosphere created by carbon monoxide left by the residual wax.

Casting alloys probably exhibit varying viscosities in the molten state, depending on composition and temperature. Since both the surface tension and the viscosity of a molten alloy increase with a decrease in temperature, incomplete casting results from high viscosity of the molten metal and that is attributed to insufficient heating. The temperature of the alloy should be raised higher than its liquidus temperature so that its viscosity and surface tension are decreased so that it does not solidify prematurely as it enters the mold. Such premature solidification may account for the greater susceptibility of the white gold alloys to porosity because their liquidus temperatures are higher. Thus, white gold alloys are more difficult to melt with a gas–air torch flame.

Other Causes

Certain surface discolorations and roughness may not be evident when the casting is completed but may appear during service. For example, various gold alloys—such as solders, bits of wire, and mixtures of different casting alloys—should never be melted together and reused. The resulting mixture would not possess the proper physical properties and might form a eutectic phase with low corrosion resistance. Discoloration and corrosion can also occur.

An often overlooked source of discoloration is the surface contamination of a gold alloy restoration by mercury. Mercury penetrates rapidly into the alloy and causes a marked loss in ductility and a greater susceptibility to corrosion. Thus, it is not a good practice to place a new amalgam restoration adjacent to a high-noble alloy restoration. In addition, these dissimilar metals form a galvanic cell that can lead to breakdown of the anode (amalgam) relative to the cathode (noble alloy).

Summary

- The channel in the investment mold through which molten metal flows is the sprue.
- The **gypsum-based investments** are traditionally used for conventional casting of gold alloys.
- **Phosphate-based investments** are used to produce copings or frameworks for metal–ceramic prostheses and base metal alloys.
- The **ethyl silicate–bonded investment** is principally used for the casting of removable partial dentures made from base metals.
- Commercially pure titanium and titanium alloys require a special investment as well as a controlled atmosphere to achieve satisfactory castings.
- The **α-hemihydrate form** of gypsum is generally used as the binder in gypsum-bonded investments.
- When gypsum-bonded investments are heated over 700°C, it decomposes to release sulfur dioxide which contaminates the casting.
- If **hygroscopic setting expansion** is employed, the filled casting ring is immediately placed in a 37°C water bath with the crucible former down.
- The compressive strength for the inlay investments should not be less than 2.4 MPa when tested 2 hours after setting.
- The silica filler used in the investments provides resistance to thermal shock, that is, refractoriness and a high thermal expansion.
- The use of colloidal silica instead of water practically eliminates the contraction of phosphate-bonded investments while heating.
- The **casting shrinkage** can be compensated by controlling the setting or hygroscopic expansion of the investment or the thermal expansion of the investment.
- The **ringless casting system** is suited for the casting of alloys that require greater mold expansion than the gold-based alloys.
- The selected sprue former should have a diameter that is approximately the same size as the thickest area of the wax pattern.
- A reservoir should be added to a sprue network to prevent localized shrinkage porosity.
- If the **sprue former** is attached at right angle to a broad flat surface, turbulence is formed within the mold cavity leading to severe porosity.
- The aluminosilicate ceramic liner and the cellulose liner have replaced the carcinogenic asbestos liners.
- The gypsum-bonded investments are best pickled with a warm 50% HCl solution.
- Only **sandblasting** and not acid should be used to clean base metal alloys.

Review Questions

1. Describe the types of casting defects, and the reasons and methods to avoid them.
2. What are the different types of ring liners and their mechanism of expansion?
3. Classify investments and write in detail about the composition and function of each component of a gypsum-bonded investment material.
4. What are the causes of wax pattern distortion and describe the methods of prevention?
5. Describe casting shrinkage of various metal alloys used in dentistry and ways to counter them.
6. Describe the casting procedure in detail for a Co–Cr crown.

Write short notes on:

1. Sprue formers
2. Pickling
3. Casting machines
4. Reservoir

Selected Readings

Christensen G.J. Marginal fit of gold inlay castings. J Prosthet Dent 16 297–305 (1966); In this laboratory study, 10 dentists accepted cemented gold inlays with a mean occlusal margin opening of 21 μm (range of 2–51 μm), a mean proximal margin opening of 26 μm (range of 9–34 μm), and a gingival margin opening of 74 μm (range of 34–119 μm). Explorer examination of visually accessible areas was superior to either explorer or radiographic examination of visually inaccessible areas.

Cooney J.P.; Caputo A.A. Type III gold alloy complete crowns cast in a phosphate-bonded investment. J Prosthet Dent 46 414–419 (1981); Marginal fit was superior for castings made in phosphate-bonded investment; surface roughness was less when cast in the gypsum-bonded investment.

Dootz E.R.; Asgar K. Solidification patterns of single crowns and three-unit bridge castings. Quint Dent Technol 10 299–305 (1986); Solidification rates and patterns differed for type III gold alloy and a palladium-silver alloy. The gold alloy solidified in a random pattern, whereas the palladium-silver metal-ceramic alloy solidified in a unidirectional manner.

Eames W.B.; O'Neal S.J.; Monteiro J.; et al. Techniques to improve the seating of castings. J Am Dent Assoc 96 432–437 (1978); Die spacing was the most suitable method to compensate for casting variables and to ensure improved marginal adaptation while also increasing retention by 25%.

Earnshaw R. The effect of casting ring liners on the potential expansion of a gypsum-bonded investment. J Dent Res 67 1366–1370 (1988); Total expansion, setting expansion, and thermal expansion of the investment setting against a smooth dry surface was 1.7%; against a dry ceramic liner, 1.6%–1.7%; and against wet cellulose or wet asbestos, 2.2–2.3%. The ceramic liner can be used wet if it is treated with a surfactant instead of water.

Finger W. Effect of the setting expansion of dental stone upon the die precision. Scand J Dent Res 88 159–160 (1980); The addition of potassium sulfate and borax to type IV gypsums reduced setting expansion without affecting the physical properties.

Finger W.; Ohsawa M. Accuracy of cast restorations produced by a refractory die-investing technique. J Prosthet Dent 52 800–803 (1984); By minimizing distortion of the wax pattern, the refractory die-investing procedure can produce consistently accurate cast gold alloy restorations.

Jorgensen K.D.; Okamoto A. Restraining factors affecting setting expansion of phosphate-bonded investments. Scand J Dent Res 94 178–181 (1986); The authors suggest that setting expansion is a highly unreliable means to compensate partially for the thermal contraction of casting alloys.

Jorgensen K.D.; Ono T. Distortion of wax crowns. Scand J Dent Res 92 (3) 253–256 (1984); Distortion of wax crowns is sufficient to reduce the fit of the final restoration to a degree that is clinically unacceptable. This study suggests that wax pattern distortion may be minimized only by use of a pattern/die investing technique.

Junner R.E.; Stevens L. Anisotropic setting expansion of phosphate-bonded investment. Aust Dent J 31 434–439 (1986); In this study the vertical setting expansion was significantly greater than the horizontal expansion in a rigid ring with liners. A flexible ring offered little restriction to horizontal expansion, reducing mold distortion.

Kaplan J.; Newman S.M. Accuracy of the divestment casting technique. Oper Dent 8 82–87 (1983); These investigators found that castings made using the divestment procedure fit more accurately than did castings made using a conventional stone-die and gypsum-bonded refractory investment technique.

Kotsiomiti E.; McCabe J.F. Experimental wax mixtures for dental use. J Oral Rehabil 24 (7) 517–521 (1997).

Kotsiomiti E.; McCabe J.F. Stability of dental waxes following repeated heatings. J Oral Rehabil 22 (2) 135–143 (1995); The flow and strength properties of dental waxes were examined following excessive and repeated heatings. Reductions in flow and elastic modulus were observed in some cases after the heating temperature had been increased to 300°C. Repeated exposure of dental waxes to temperatures higher than 200°C may affect the composition and properties, resulting in inferior materials.

Lautenschlager E.P.; Harcourt J.K.; Ploszaj L.C. Setting reaction of gypsum materials investigated by X-ray diffraction. J Dent Res 48 43–48 (1969); An early study of the conversion from calcium sulfate hemihydrate to calcium sulfate dihydrate.

Mackert J.R. Jr. An expert system for analysis of casting failures. Int J Prosthodont 1 268–280 (1988); An expert system was proposed for the diagnosis of common lost-wax casting problems, based on an interactive consultation session at a PC station, during which the user answered questions about defective castings. The computer responded with conclusions on the most likely cause of each problem.

Mahler D.B.; Ady A.B. An explanation for the hygroscopic setting expansion of dental gypsum products. J Dent Res 39 578 (1960); A classic publication on the theory of hygroscopic setting expansion. An excellent reference for those interested in the mechanics of this phenomenon.

Martin K.H. An investigation of the effect of the water/powder ratio on the accuracy of the fit of gold alloy castings. Aust Dent J 1 202 (1956); Use of the correct water/powder ratio with a gypsum investment is essential to obtain a good fit of castings, especially when the low-heat technique is used.

Matsuya S.; Yamane M. Decomposition of gypsum-bonded investments. J Dent Res 60 1418–1423 (1981); At 900°C, decomposition of gypsum-bonded investments occurred, leading to the formation of $CaSiO_3$ and Ca_2SiO_4.

Mueller H.J.; Reyes W.; McGill S. Surfactant-containing phosphate investment. Dent Mater 2 42–44 (1986); The addition of surfactants in a phosphate-bonded casting investment can increase the hygroscopic setting expansion. The surfactant also makes the unset investment more viscous and reduces the compressive strength.

Naylor W.P.; Moore B.K.; Phillips R.W. A topographical assessment of casting ring liners using scanning electron microscopy (SEM). Quint Dent Technol 11 413–420 (1987); Three types of nonasbestos ring liners exist: ceramic, cellulose, and a ceramic-cellulose combination. A liner containing an aluminosilicate component has the potential to produce respirable-size ceramic particles.

Neiman R.; Sarma A.C. Setting and thermal reactions of phosphate investments. J Dent Res 59 (9) 1478–1485 (1980); The setting reactions and thermal degradation of phosphate binders were interpreted from DTA and X-ray diffraction data. The authors concluded that setting took place through the complex formation of $(NH_4MgPO_4{\cdot}6H_2O)n$, excess reactants, and water and that dehydration and thermal reactions led to a sequence of reactions resulting in the formation of $(NH_4MgPO_4{\cdot}H_2O)$, $(Mg_2P_2O_7)n$, $Mg_2P_2O_7$, and $Mg_3(PO_4)_2$.

Nielsen J.P. Pressure distribution in centrifugal dental casting. J Dent Res 57 261–269 (1978); This article discusses the factors contributing to the pressure gradient that develops along the length of a casting in a centrifugal casting machine.

Nielsen J.P.; Ollerman R. Suck-back porosity. Quint Dent Technol 1 61–65 (1976); Using a gold-palladium-silver alloy with different sprue former lengths, diameters, and angles of attachment, lower casting temperature and flaring of the sprue former reduced suck-back porosity. The authors postulated that a "hot spot" is created in the mold that causes this type of porosity.

Nomura G.T.; Reisbick M.H.; Preston J.D. An investigation of epoxy resin dies. J Prosthet Dent 44 45–50 (1980); In a comparison of three epoxy die materials with a type IV stone, full crown epoxy dies were undersized, MOD onlay resin dies were accurate, and detail reproduction was found to be comparable to the type IV gypsum. However, only one epoxy material had a hardness approaching that of the dental stone.

Santos J.F.; Ballester R.Y. Delayed hygroscopic expansion of phosphate-bonded investments. Dent Mater 3 165–167 (1987); Delayed hygroscopic expansion occurs when the investment is immersed in water after setting. Increased time of immersion and an increase in the special liquid concentration increased the hygroscopic setting expansion.

Stevens L. The effect of early heating on the expansion of a phosphate-bonded investment. Aust Dent J 28 366–369 (1983); The thermal expansion of a phosphate-bonded investment decreased as heating was delayed from 1 to 6 hours after mixing. The setting expansion increased as the special liquid replaced water for mixing.

Taggart W.H. A new and accurate method of making gold inlays. Dent Cosmos 49 1117 (1907); The dental "lost wax" process was developed by Taggartopening up the opportunity to cast accurate restorations in an investment mold.

Vaidyanathan T.K.; Schulman A.; Nielsen J.P.; et al. Correlation between macroscopic porosity location and liquid metal pressure in centrifugal casting technique. J Dent Res 60 59–66 (1981); Radiographic analysis of uniform cylindrical castings revealed that the porosity is dependent on the location at which the sprue is attached to the casting. The location of the macroscopic porosity, at portions of the casting close to the free surface of the button, is dependent on the pressure gradient and therefore different heat transfer rates in different portions of the casting.

Verrett R.G.; Duke E.S. The effect of sprue attachment design on castability and porosity. J Prosthet Dent 61 418–424 (1989); Flared and straight sprue attachments optimized castability and minimized porosity.

Zeltser C.; Lewinstein I.; Grajower R. Fit of crown wax patterns after removal from the die. J Prosthet Dent 53 (3) 344–346 (1985); The effects of loading wax patterns before investment was determined. Repetitive loading revealed that the plastic deformation in wax was less after the second loading than after the first cycle for a specific load.

15

Digital Technology in Dentistry

CHAPTER OUTLINE

KEY TERMS

Additive manufacturing (AM)—A process of constructing objects where material is incrementally added according to a computer-aided design (CAD) file; also known as *three-dimensional (3-D) printing.*

Augmented reality (AR)—A form of virtual reality in which interacting with the real world is through simulation.

Computer-aided design (CAD)—A computer technology that designs an object and creates a computer file for manufacture of the design.

Computer-aided manufacturing (or milling) (CAM)—The use of software and computer-controlled machinery to automate a manufacturing process.

Cone beam computed tomography (CBCT)—An X-ray three-dimensional (3-D) imaging technology in which the radiation is divergent and forms a cone.

Digital—An electronic technology that records or stores information in the form of binary digits (i.e., 1 and 0) or technology characterized by electronic and computerized devices (e.g., digital images).

Digital impression—A virtual scan (digital model) of a patient's dentition and other structures that is generated with laser or other optical scanning devices and converted into a digital format.

Prototyping—The creation, modification, and optimization of two-dimensional or three-dimensional models of objects, which may be the final desired object or an interim object for examination of fit.

Virtual reality (VR)—A computer-generated simulation that allows for interactive experiences.

We are living in a digital world. The evidence is everywhere: Websites, buying and selling online, smartphones, digital televisions, video streaming, eBooks, digital music, geolocation, social media, computers, printers, ATMs, digital cameras, clocks, robotics, drones and guided missiles, banking and finances, and driverless cars. Digital technology is a broad-based term which connotes computer-based products and solutions. Technically digital technology may refer to using new algorithms, which means a set of instructions designed to perform a specific task or applications to solve a problem. There seems to be a growing concern that if we are not going digital, being digital, or dreaming digital, then we are relegating ourselves to be museum pieces. The word digital started out in the mid-17th century, evolving from digits. In the initial stages, it was fingers and later it changed to numerical digits. In the early 20th century, it was radio and recording technologies and in the 1950s world of computers opened up.

Digital dentistry has dawned to dentistry with three main foci:

1. Computer-aided design/Computer-aided manufacturing (CAD/CAM)

   CAD/CAM dentistry is employed to improve the design and creation of dental restorations including removable and fixed prosthesis.
2. Imaging (digital radiography)

   Dentists use digital dental radiographs (digital X-rays) to detect, diagnose, treat, and monitor oral conditions and diseases. Digital radiography is a type of X-ray imaging that uses digital X-ray sensors to replace traditional X-ray film, producing enhanced computer images of teeth and other oral structures and conditions.

3. Practice/patient management systems

Practice management system is a type of healthcare software that captures patient demographics, schedules appointments, initiates, interacts with insurance companies, and tracks billing and generates reports. Along with this it can produce electronic patient records, a digital version of patient-centered clinically oriented information and mining data for research.

CRITICAL QUESTIONS

What is prototyping?

What are subtractive and additive processes, and what are their relative advantages and disadvantages?

Prototyping Tools

CAD technology is based on using computer software and systems to assist in the creation, modification, analysis, and optimization of two-dimensional (2-D) or three-dimensional (3-D) models of objects. Any computer program that includes computer graphics and engineering functions for manipulation can be classified as CAD software. CAM in dentistry is the construction of a restorative device using the output from the CAD software. CAM may be additive (buildup of a material) or subtractive (removal of material from a larger starting piece).

CAD/CAM

In 1985, Dentsply Sirona introduced the first intraoral scanner, chairside economical restoration of esthetic ceramics (CEREC) as an exciting alternative to conventional impression making. This marked the dawn of digital dentistry. Intraoral scanners precisely recorded the 3-D geometry of an object and subsequently allowed this to be used to produce customized dental restorations. The intraoral scanner uses structured light which falls on an object to be scanned by a handheld device. Images of the object are then captured by image sensors of the scanner, to be processed by a software. This results in the production of a 3-D surface model. The most widely used output file is the stereolithography/standard tessellation language (STL).

Two types of scanners are popularly used in dentistry—intraoral and extraoral. Real-time scanning produces digital images of single or multiple teeth, complete arches, opposing arches, occlusion, and surrounding soft tissues. Patients appreciate digital impressions because of the comfort and dentists accept it because of the avoidance of space-demanding plaster casts which are replaced by easily archived digital files. Scanners have become so sophisticated that they weigh between 70 and 500 g only and are wireless in connection. Current studies suggest that digital impressions produce crowns as or more accurate than conventional impressions. Conventional impressions still appear to be the best solution currently for long-span restorations, such as fixed full arches on natural teeth and implants. Laboratory-based scanners—optical or mechanical—are capable of scanning either stone casts or impressions and have proved to be highly accurate. Currently available options for integrating CAD/CAM based systems is provided in Box 15.1.

• BOX 15.1 Flowchart on Available CAD/CAM Technique Options

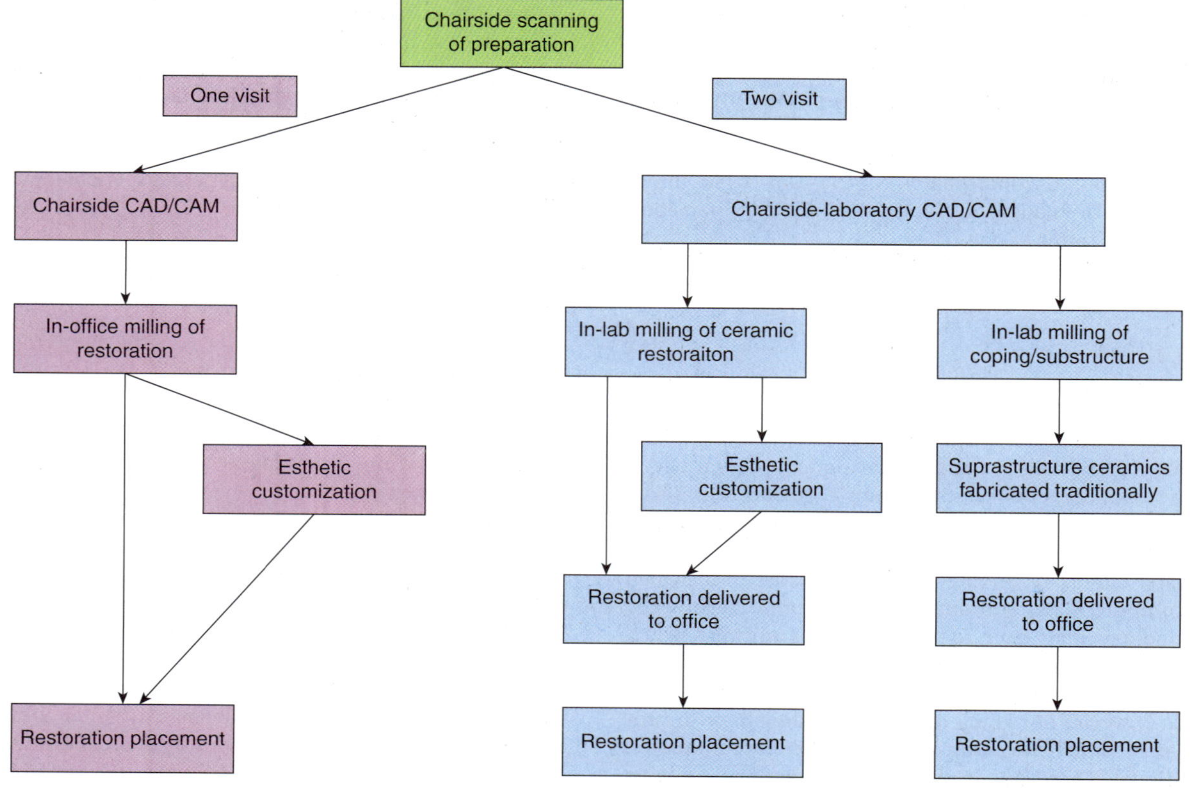

From 1. Corrales E, editor Innovation in Dentistry : CAD / CAM Restorative Procedures 2008.

Digital planning, designing, and manufacturing technologies have become the common standard in dental laboratory technology. Digital tooth design and treatment planning have changed the laboratory processes fundamentally. Digital wax-ups allow the use of scanned files of natural teeth and smiles and hence achieve superior ability to mimic nature. Combined with current face-scanning technologies, artificial intelligence (AI) and machine learning tools may allow automated generation of individual digital smile designs and treatment plans in the near future.

Presently used CAD/CAM technologies with the assistance of machines, and other tools, the dentists experience virtually no limit to the type of dental restoration that can be fabricated, from single-unit inlays, onlays, crowns, veneers, implant abutments and restorations to fixed and removable dental prostheses for partially and completely edentulous patients. Though the prominent method of fabrication is subtractive through milling processes, additive technologies such as 3-D printing are becoming increasingly popular and are already in use for printing models, impression trays, night guards, surgical guides, orthodontic aligners, dentures, provisionals, crowns and other devices using a range of materials from plastics to metals. The most unique factor in additive technology is the flexibility of design. No longer is the solid block in the milling machine, the starting point of fabrication of the prosthesis. Instead products are created layer-by-layer even with high degree of geometric complexity.

Despite the documented advantages, CAD/CAM technology has not yet been fully embraced by the dental profession. The main reasons are the high initial and maintenance cost, a steep learning curve, and the need to change procedures that practitioners have learned in the dental colleges and are comfortable with.

CRITICAL QUESTION

Which dental applications can be used with CAD/CAM technology?

Indications for CAD/CAM

Many indications and materials are available for chairside CAD/CAM restorations, as shown in the list that follows. Each type of material offers unique features for its indications. The CAD/CAM system represents the process by which these materials are fabricated, and the clinical outcome of the restoration is determined by the restorative material.

- Ceramic-, metal-, and resin-based crowns and bridges
- Copings and frameworks for metal–ceramic prostheses
- Full and partial dentures
- Inlays, onlays, partial crowns, and provisionals
- Implant abutments and crowns, including screw-retained crowns
- Orthodontic printed models and clear appliances
- Maryland bridges and veneers

Subtractive Manufacturing—CAM Milling Machines

CAD/CAM crown fabrication is a state-of-the-art technique for certain crown materials. With CAD/CAM technology in a dental office, a patient may receive a crown with the same-day delivery and reduced chairside adjustments. Representative CAD/CAM systems are offered by Dentsply Sirona (CEREC) and Planmeca USA (Emerald). This group of equipment can be used to fabricate ceramic and composite inlays, onlays, crowns, and veneers from an optical impression of the prepared tooth made from a digital impression. The restoration is designed using the system's software and milled from a solid block of ceramic or composite using diamond and carbide burs. Restorations and prostheses may be prepared in a single appointment, which eliminates the impression material, preparation of a model, preparation of a provisional restoration, and laboratory fabrication of the final restoration or prosthesis.

CAD/CAM Systems

Today's dental CAD/CAM systems can be divided into four groups.

1. The first group is the chairside systems, such as CEREC from Dentsply Sirona and Emerald from Planmeca USA. The Primescan (Dentsply Sirona) uses blue light-emitting diode (LED) light and smart pixel sensor video imaging for 24 frames per second and processes more than 1 million 3-D data points per second. The Emerald uses a multicolor laser-based system.
2. The second group is the commercial laboratory systems. For these systems, the dentist should send physical impressions, master models, or raw scans to the laboratory of choice for the fabrication of the final prosthesis.

   The chairside system usually operates on a closed architecture format, which requires the scan to be used only within the manufacturer's proprietary CAD/CAM workflow, and this system uses its own specific file format for CAD/CAM functions. The laboratory system uses an open architecture format that allows a variety of file formats, such as STL, OBJ - Object (Relocatable Object module), and PLY - Polygon (Polygon file format). The STL is the most popular file format in the field. The scan data can be easily exported as an STL file format compared with other file formats.
3. The third group is stand-alone digital impression systems. This type of system is based on an open architecture format and takes only intraoral or extraoral scans. The raw file format is electronically transferred to a designated commercial laboratory for the fabrication of the final prosthesis. The Medit i500 (Medit Corp) works based on 3-D video technology. The TRIOS 3 (3Shape) uses fast confocal microscopy optical scanning technology. The iTero (Align Technology) uses laser light beams based on parallel confocal microscope technology. The True Definition Scanner (Midmark) uses structured pulsating blue light with active wavefront sampling 3-D video technology. The CS 3600 (Carestream Dental) uses LED light with active-speed 3-D video technology.
4. The fourth group is hybrid systems; these are a kind of mix-and-match system based on an open architecture format. A hybrid system allows communication between products of many different manufacturers, such as intraoral and extraoral scanners, CAD units, and CAM units. The dentist and laboratory can choose their preferred scanners, CAD/CAM software, computer hardware, 3-D printers, and milling machines from a variety of vendors.

The common disadvantages of the laboratory, digital impression, and hybrid systems are the need for multiple clinical appointments, the making of physical impressions, the fabrication of provisionals, the increased total costs of fabrication, and the delayed delivery time compared with the chairside systems.

CAD/CAM Materials

All classes of dental materials, including ceramics, polymers, and metals, can be processed with CAD/CAM systems. In this chapter, ceramics are discussed, which is the most widely used material, among others.

The CAD/CAM ceramics can be categorized into three main groups, mainly by the glass content, and subgroups by the type of material, as follows:

- Aesthetic ceramics with high glass content
  - *Aluminosilicate* (feldspathic or synthetic)—This material is a mixture of high-melting glasses, nepheline, and albite, such as the Mark II (VITA North America).
  - *Lucite* (40%–50%) containing glass—The typical material of this group is IPS e.max (Ivoclar Vivadent).
- Structural ceramics with low glass content
  - *Lithia disilicate and zirconia-reinforced lithia silicate*—This material group includes e.max CAD (Ivoclar Vivadent), Suprinity (VITA North America), and Celtra Duo (Dentsply Sirona).
  - *Alumina, spinel, and alumina/zirconia*—This material group comprises In-Ceram Alumina, In-Ceram Spinel, and In-Ceram Zirconia (VITA North America).
- Structural ceramics without glass content
  - *Polycrystalline alumina* (with 3 wt% Mg for grain growth control)—This material group includes VITA All-Cubes (VITA North America).
  - *Polycrystalline zirconia* (with 3–5 wt% of Y for transformation toughening)—This material group includes VITA YZ HT (VITA North America), CEREC Zirconia Blocks (Dentsply Sirona), IPS e.max ZirCAD LT (Ivoclar Vivadent), and KATANA Zirconia Blocks (Kuraray America).

All materials presented here can be processed by either a chairside or a laboratory milling machine. The commercial labs use disks for bulk production of multiple units, and chairside milling units work with individual blocks. The manufacturers produce only feldspathic (aluminosilicate) blocks for chairside milling. Thus, there are no laboratory-milled feldspathic CAD/CAM prostheses.

CAD/CAM Case

The advantage of the chairside CAD/CAM systems is that the dentist can create any preparation design to preserve tooth structure as long as enough enamel structure remains for desirable adhesion between the ceramic and the enamel. Because one-visit CAD/CAM dentistry does not require provisional restorations and temporary cement, contamination of the prepared tooth structure is minimized, and the dentist can gain strong bonding for optimal results.

The following clinical case demonstrates a CAD/CAM chairside partial coverage (inlay or onlay) crown. The occlusal surface of an existing composite resin restoration shows the existence of a large marginal gap but without radiographic evidence of recurrent caries. After the old composite resin restoration was removed, lesions of recurrent caries were revealed. The tooth was prepared to receive a ceramic onlay. Once the cavity preparation was completed (Fig. 15.1A), the intraoral scans of the prepared tooth were made (Fig. 15.1B). Scans of the unprepared teeth of the opposing arch and the buccal bite registration were also taken (not shown). The next step includes the occlusal relation adjustment (Fig. 15.1C) and the design of the prosthesis (Fig. 15.1D). The final preview of the milling process prior to the actual manufacturing process is shown in Figure 15.1E. The CAD/CAM restorations were then tried and inserted with dual-cure resin cement. The final occlusal photo (Fig. 15.1F) shows a well-integrated aesthetic ceramic restoration.

Additive Manufacturing—3-D Printing

Additive manufacturing (AM) or 3-D printing includes processes in which material is incrementally joined or solidified under computer control to create an object. The object is formed layer-by-layer, such as fusing of particles or curing of light-sensitive

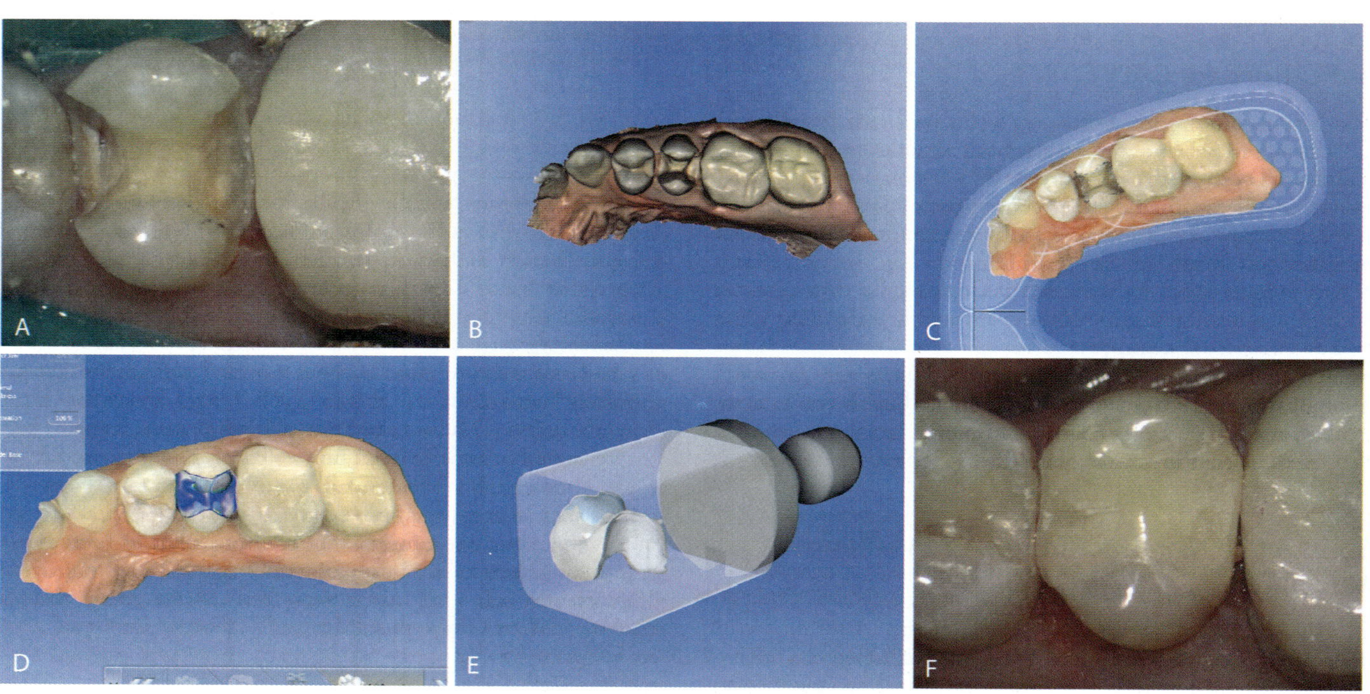

• **Fig. 15.1** Computer-aided design/computer-aided manufacturing (CAD/CAM) processing of an onlay. **(A)** Tooth preparation. **(B)** Intraoral scan of the preparation. **(C)** Occlusal relation adjustment step. **(D)** Virtual restoration editing step. **(E)** Final milling preview. **(F)** Postoperative photo.

polymers. A key advantage of 3-D printing is the ability to produce very complex geometries of restorations designed from intraoral impressions.

Desktop 3-D printers use dental resins for the fabrication of temporary prosthetics, surgical guides, orthodontic models, retainers, and aligners. Various dental resins for printing applications may be chosen for any of the desired characteristics, such as transparency for optical clarity, translucency for esthetics, flexibility for patient comfort, or high-impact resins that resist wear and fracture. The most common applications are transparent aligners and night guards. Aligners serve as alternatives to braces and have become especially popular because of their invisibility. This technology may also be used for printing diagnostic casts (Fig. 15.2). Oral surgery guides from 3-D printing offer the required precision to verify proper implant positioning where bone is present (Fig. 15.3A), adequate bone reduction for bone recontouring (Fig. 15.3B), and precise drill positions (Fig. 15.3C), to name a few. These guides also facilitate immediate placement and loading of implants where a provisional restoration can be printed prior to the surgery (Figs 15.4 and 15.5). A printable material with contact bactericidal activity is also possible, which may lead to crowns, retainers, aligners, and implants that are resilient to degradation under oral conditions, with longer clinical lifetimes.

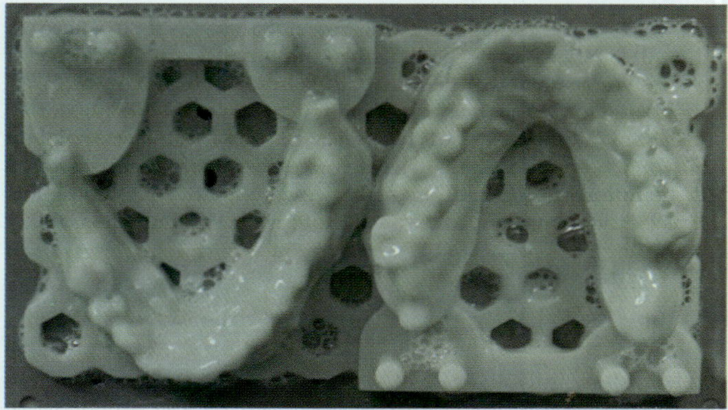

• **Fig. 15.2** Three-dimensional (3-D) printed model of diagnostic casts. (Courtesy Dr Luiz Gonzaga.)

Current Additive Manufacturing Technologies

Currently, 3-D printing includes stereolithography (SLA), fused deposition modeling (FDM), selective laser melting (SLM), and direct metal laser sintering (DMLS). The most commonly used 3-D printing process (46% as of 2018) is FDM, a material extrusion technique. All 3-D printing requires a CAD file for execution of the manufacturing.

Stereolithography

For this CAM method, thin layers of a photocurable resin are cured to create the computer-designed geometry. Liquid resin is photopolymerized by using small-spot-size LEDs or laser radiation to locally cure the liquid resin. As the liquid resin cures on the surface, the platform holding the object is gradually lowered in the pool of liquid, allowing liquid resin to flow to the area to be cured. The resin objects shown in Figures 15.2–15.5 were all made by SLA.

SLA printers achieve the most accurate results because of the precision of the layers this type of printer creates. The thickness of the printed layers can be controlled by adaptive slicing. If the surface has been designed with a high curvature, for example, thinner layers will be applied than would be the case for a low-curvature surface. Adaptive slicing yields a better surface quality than uniform slicing, which minimizes variations in the cusp height across the layers.

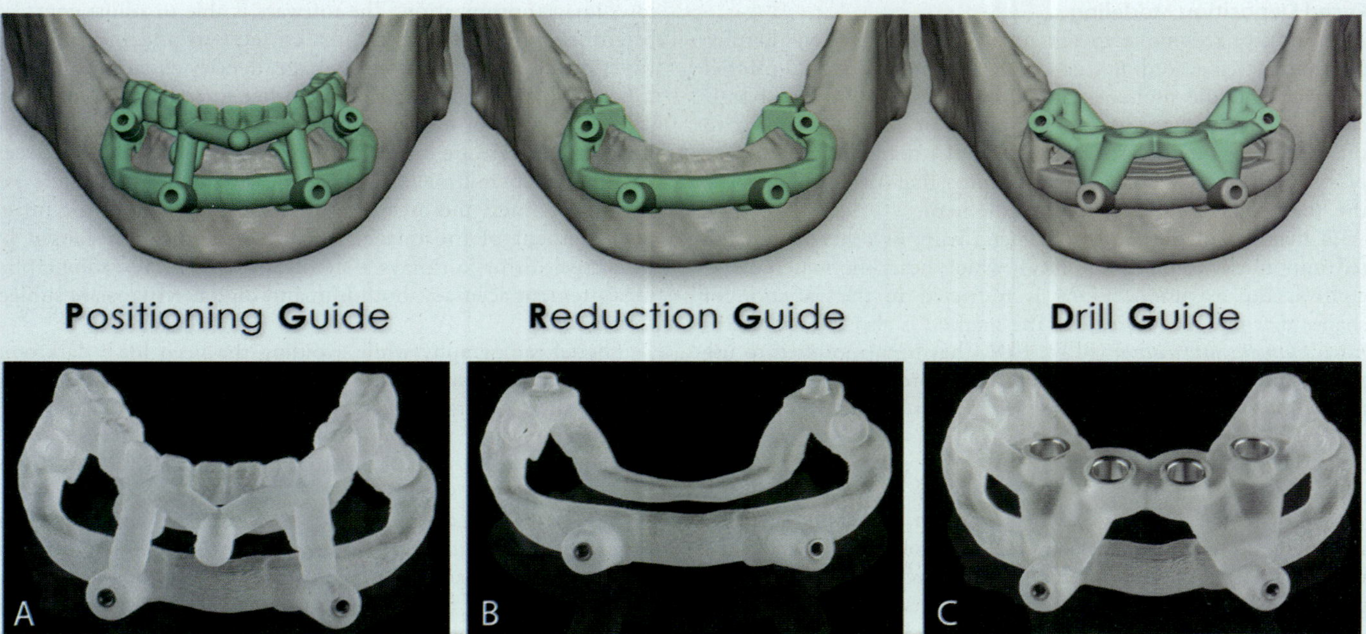

• **Fig. 15.3** **(A)** Computer-aided design/computer-aided manufacturing (CAD/CAM) image of a positioning guide for implant placement (*top*), final processed three-dimensional (3-D) printed guide (*bottom*). **(B)** CAD/CAM image of bone reduction guide (*top*), final 3-D printed guide (*bottom*). **(C)** CAD/CAM image of drill positioning guide (*top*), final 3-D printed guide (*bottom*). (Courtesy Dr Luiz Gonzaga.)

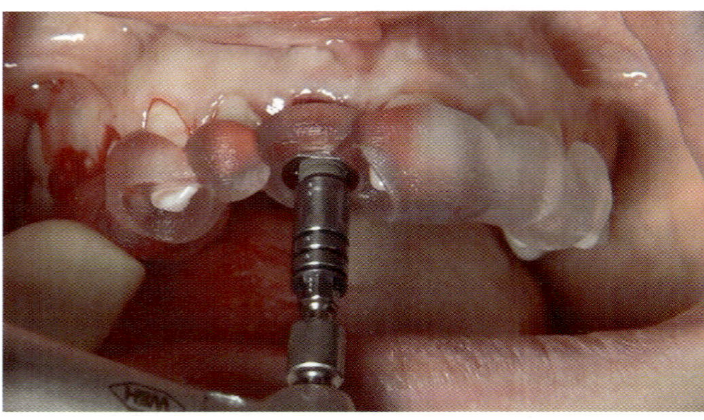

• **Fig. 15.4** Surgical placement of anterior implant using a three-dimensional (3-D) surgical guide. (Courtesy Dr Luiz Gonzaga.)

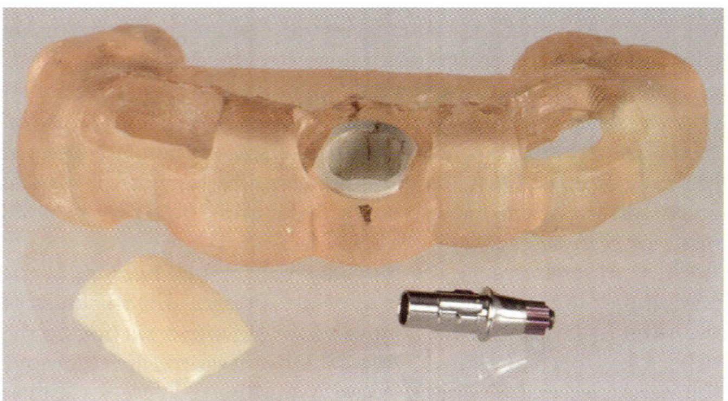

• **Fig. 15.5** Because of the accuracy of this technology, a provisional restoration can be printed to fit exactly where the implant was placed and be loaded immediately. (Courtesy Dr Luiz Gonzaga.)

Fused Deposition Modeling

This additive technique incrementally deposits molten thermoplastic material according to a CAD file. The item is 3-D printed by layer, and the molten material becomes a solid object as it cools. FDM printing uses an additive layer approach similar to that in SLA but uses plastic filaments rather than liquid resin. The plastic filament is fed through an extruder that melts and deposits the material layer-by-layer to form the item.

A filament of thermoplastic, metal wire, or other material is fed into an extrusion nozzle head, which heats the material and controls the extrusion. FDM is restricted in the variation of shapes that may be fabricated. The method is also known also as *fused filament fabrication* (FFF). FDM has been modified to use pellets directly instead of filament. This process is called *fused particle fabrication* (FPF) or *fused granular fabrication* (FGF).

Selective Laser Melting

This AM technique uses a high-power laser to melt and fuse a variety of metal and alloy powders together. The 2-D layers are incrementally melted and assembled to form a 3-D object. SLM is also known as *DMLS* or *laser powder bed fusion* (LPBF). The term *DMLS* is misleading in that the object is melted during production, a variation of liquid-phase sintering.

Materials for Additive Manufacturing

All classes of materials discussed in Chapter 2 are currently used to fabricate objects by AM technology, but these materials need to be in a flowable state or powder for processing. For polymeric objects, photocuring liquid monomers have been used with SLA, and thermoplastic pellets or wires are used with FDM. Postcuring of objects made of SLA is often needed. For metal objects, metal powder form made by atomization is the most popular feedstock that is selectively melted by laser. Even though not all ceramics include or form a liquid phase as with resins and metals, sintering of ceramic particles by selective laser is possible. However, these ceramic parts have a rough and porous surface and are suitable as tissue-engineering scaffolds. To improve the densification of ceramic objects, a photocuring liquid filled with a high amount of ceramic fillers is cured with SLA, and the resulting green body is heat treated in a furnace to burn off resin residue and densify the desired ceramic structure.

The mechanical properties of 3-D printed parts limit the potential of large-scale printing. Therefore, an optimized pattern of 3-D printing is important to control flaw sensitivity. Also, changes in the printing environment have an influence on the quality of the finished products. AM is capable of fabricating parts of various sizes, from the microscale to macroscale. However, the precision of the printed parts is dependent on the accuracy of the method employed and the scale of printing. For instance, microscale 3-D printing poses challenges with the resolution, surface finish, and layer bonding, which sometimes require postprocessing techniques such as sintering.

Digital Imaging

The value of digital radiography in dental diagnosis is well established, especially during operative procedures. Advantages of digital radiography are: reduction in radiation dose to the patient; patient education; image optimization and computer-aided feature extraction, workflow improvement; avoidance of darkroom and chemical processing; environmental waste reduction; improved electronic communications and image archiving.

The software that accompanies most of the direct sensors allows image optimization. The software is able to adjust contrast, brightness, and perform gamma corrections and measurement functions. Creating an inverse image, density equalization, magnification, and image rotation are other standard imaging tools. The three types of measurement generally available with digital imaging software are linear measurement—the distance between two points in millimeters; angle measurement—the angle between two lines; and area measurement—the area of the image or a segment of the image. Because magnification caused by projective distortion plays a significant role in all radiographic measurement accuracy, both film and digital systems are subject to error.

Digital radiography while avoiding the need for a darkroom and its space, it eliminates the cost of stocking film and chemicals. Film packets generate lead waste and film processors use large amounts of water, creating further environment impact. X-ray developer and fixer contain hazardous chemicals which must not be poured into the sewer system.

The last two decades have witnessed extensive development in diagnostic dental imaging. In spite of the compelling research interest in cone beam computed tomography (CBCT), magnetic resonance imaging (MRI) has also shown significant potential to clarify relevant clinical questions. However intraoral radiographs remain the most common imaging method of dental practice. The shift from analog to digital imaging was the earliest revolution in modern dental and maxillofacial radiology, bringing many advantages to the clinical work flow.

Cone Beam Computed Tomography

CBCT systems are a variation of traditional computed tomography (CT) systems. The CBCT systems used by dental professionals rotate around the patient, capturing data using a cone-shaped X-ray beam.

Cone beam imaging technology is commonly referred to as CBCT. The terminology "cone beam" refers to the conical shape of the beam that scans the patient in a circular path around the vertical axis of the head. First introduced toward the end of the millennium, CBCT heralded a new dental technology for the 21st century. Initially its practical applications were limited to implant dentistry and orthognathic/orthodontic patient care. CBCT scanners use comparably less sophisticated hardware and software than CT scanners, resulting in simpler, more compact and less expensive machines, but produce comparable, or better images of the *hard* tissue structures of the jaws and skull. These advantages make CBCT technology particularly well suited to hard tissue imaging and dentistry. CBCT applications that are helpful in a multitude of dental disciplines. These applications include, but are not limited to, dentoalveolar abnormality, vertical root fractures, jaw tumors, prosthodontic evaluations, and advances in orthodontic/orthognathic and implant patient evaluations. CBCT scan data can bridge with CAD/CAM image files for the fabrication of various dental restorations. This facilitates implant and prosthodontic rehabilitation by synchronous planning and subsequently milling coronal restorations for teeth and root form implants. New requirements for improved diagnostic techniques will keep the CBCT technology alive with more sophistication.

Optically Based Caries Diagnosis

Caries causes demineralization of enamel and dentin. Demineralized areas have greater porosity than the surrounding tissue, which changes the optical properties of the mineral tissue. This change in optical properties is used to locate caries. Quantitative light induced fluorescence (QLF) is such a nondestructive diagnostic method for the assessment of early caries lesions. Teeth fluoresce because of the presence of minerals in the enamel and dentin. When a tooth becomes carious, the fluorescence of the carious lesion decreases. The fluorescence image of enamel with incipient lesions can be digitized, and then the loss of fluorescence at the lesion site can be quantified in comparison to the fluorescence of sound enamel. The QLF image provides a measure of the extent and severity of the lesion. Changes in fluorescence and lesion area can be followed over time to measure lesion development before intervention. QLF has been successfully applied to smooth surfaces and occlusal surfaces but not interproximal lesions.

The new QLF-D BiLuminator allows ordinary white light images to be collected simultaneously with fluorescent images. The images aid in direct visual assessment and highlight features such as leaking restoration margins with secondary caries, occlusal and interproximal caries, sealant integrity, cariogenic activity under sealants, and the presence of calculus and gingivitis. Other recently introduced fluorescent detection systems include the CamX Spectra Caries Detection System (Air Techniques, Melville, NY) and the SoproLIFE Dental Caries Detection System (Acton North America, Mount Laurel, NJ).

Practice Management Systems

Along with patient care, the present day dental practice involves the following practice management systems: accessing and searching patient-related records, designating the roles of staff, evaluating the productivity of staff members, and tracking patient visits including their electronic health records. Practice management system guides dentists and their office personnel to manage the day to day and real-time tasks of patient care.

Present day dentists are guided not only by the knowledge and skills they acquired from the dental colleges but also through a greater extent by evidence-based dentistry (EBD). Research-based decision-making is gaining priority in dental practice. Dental practice management systems give easy and reliable access to scientific literature which provides useful data, reviews, and reliable analysis. Dentists with updated knowledge will perform better in comparison to fellow professionals.

Dental practices are no more handled by a single person and most of the practices involve multiple specialists and scheduling appointments manually is almost impossible. Dentists will find it difficult to manage both dentistry and office work together. The reception staff consistently coordinates with the dentist to know the phases of treatment and schedule upcoming activities. Fortunately, dental practitioners can achieve efficiency with the help of technology. Oral health providers equipped with the right tools can save time and can provide hassle-free services. The role of dental practice software becomes very crucial in mitigating the issues related to time management and scheduling. Dental practice software can improve the productivity and clinical efficiency while simultaneously streamlining the day-to-day operations.

Dental practice software should have the following features:

- *Scheduling*—Dental practice software should have an in-built digital calendar to record all visits, appointments, timing of treatment plan and any other important event to attend. This helps the dentist to visualize free slots and occupied slots so that they can manage their present and future commitments.
- *Electronic health record*—This is a collection of patient's data that includes the demographic status, contact information, treatment information, medical records and lab reports. Dental practice software helps dentists to store, organize, and provide easy access in the database.
- *Dental charting*—This is a process of listing and organizing information about teeth in a graphical manner. Dentist can note down missing teeth, bleeding teeth, impacted teeth, cavities, etc. and makes an appropriate chart. This can be done easily with the help of a dental charting tool of dental practice software.
- *Reports and analytics*—This feature provides dental practitioners with reports and analytics to better judge the clinical profile as well as business growth. It can generate reports in the graph and chart format.
- *Patient communication*—The software sends email reminders, alerts, and SMS regarding upcoming appointments to the patients. It can send reminders for due payments also.
- *Management of reception*—This feature of the software helps in managing the reception area. The first interaction of the patient with staff becomes systematic and efficient even before meeting the dentist. Time management especially of the waiting patients can be made smoothly with the software.
- *Billing*—This feature of dental practice software allows the dentist to define the billing methods. It covers payment methods such as card, cheque, cash, payment wallets, online payment, etc. This also helps dentists to keep accurate records of their dental-based finances.

Dental practice software makes the life of both dentists and patients easy.

Artificial Intelligence (AI)

AI refers to the simulation of human intelligence in machines that are programmed to think like humans and mimic their actions. The term may also be applied to any machine that exhibits traits associated with a human mind such as learning and problem solving.

The term AI first appeared in a proposal for a "2 month, 10 man study of artificial intelligence" submitted on August 31, 1955 by John McCarthy of Dartmouth College, Marvin Minsky of Harvard University, Nathaniel Rochester of IBM, and Claude Shannon of Bell Telephone Laboratories. The workshop, which took place a year later, in July and August 1956, is generally considered as the official birthdate of AI. Two years later McCarthy developed the most popular programming language "Lisp" in AI research. In 1959 Arthur Samuel coined the term "machine learning," in an article entitled "Some Studies in Machine Learning Using the Game of Checkers."

Machine learning is a subset of AI that uses techniques (such as deep learning) that enable machines to use experience to improve at tasks. Deep learning is a subset of machine learning that is based on artificial neural networks. The *learning process* is *deep* because the structure of artificial neural networks consists of multiple input, output, and hidden layers. Each layer contains units that transform the input data into information that the next layer can use for a certain predictive task. Thanks to this structure, a machine can learn through its own data processing.

Deep learning technology is used in image analysis technology. Deep learning has been used not only in face detection, but also in dental radiology. AI has been used to improve image interpretation in dental radiology. AI programs "learn" to analyze the digital image. Digital radiographs can be calculated using the algorithms to detect caries. The experienced clinician who has superior clinical acumen and the expert software engineer utilizing the training set—the information used to *train* a machine learning—teach the AI, the required skill of caries diagnosis. Subsequently clinicians and engineers will verify the precision of the skill of AI. The accuracy is rated between 80% and 90%.

In 3-D radiographs, such as tomography scans, the annotation of anatomical landmarks and segmentation of bone and teeth structures are achieved by AI. Annotation provides the initial set up for training a machine learning model with what it needs to understand and how to discriminate against various inputs to come up with accurate outputs.

Through AI, from a CBCT a panoramic and lateral cephalometric view can be generated. Nerve recognition and pathology identification are also possible and it happens automatically. The software used for this purpose has the potential for self-improvement and hence it is called intelligent.

Another area in which AI is gaining popularity is in intraoral scanning. In the fabrication of fixed prosthesis, after tooth preparation intraoral scanning is employed. If the margin is visible, an accurate scanning will automatically mark the margins on the tooth preparations. The scans can now advance to the stage of digital designing and subsequent milling. Single crown fabrication is almost fully automated in the advanced laboratories.

Digital smile designing (DSD) technique. DSD is a technical tool which is used to design and modify the smile of patients digitally and help them to visualize it before undergoing the treatment by creating and presenting a digital mockup of their new smile. It helps in visual communication and involvement of the patients in their own smile design process, thus ensuring predictable treatment outcome and increasing case acceptance. Once the required patient data (photographs) are uploaded, the AI engine searches and proposes well-suited morphology of teeth and alignment. Clinician has the freedom to modify the proposed smile design and the STL file for creation of mock-up model, preparation guide, or surgical guide.

The use of AI for assisting in orthodontic treatment planning has been a reality for some time. AI assists in decision-making and helps orthodontists to choose the best way to move, a tooth or group of teeth. This is useful because orthodontics performed in a totally traditional way require high manual skill and AI helps those who have limitations in the skills especially during the initial phases of professional life. More than one Aligner Company claims to use AI algorithms to optimize orthodontic planning, thereby saving the time of orthodontists in this process. While accepting the fact that AI assists in treatment planning, we should recognize that it completely ignores the existence of oral diseases, does not fully integrate facial analysis in its algorithms, and is unable to consider the impact of functional problems in treatments.

AI can diagnose and predict periodontally compromised teeth with the radiographs and convolutional neural networks (CNNs) were used. Using deep learning algorithms, the diagnostic accuracy rates were 81.0% and 76.7% in premolars and molars, respectively. The accuracy of predicting extractions was 82.8% and 73.4% in premolars and molars, respectively. AI is rated equivalent to a good clinician in diagnosing periodontally compromised teeth.

CAD/CAM technology which has become popular with removable and fixed prosthesis has the support of AI especially in the decision-making process. Deciding on the selection of implant systems based on evidence has strengthened the armamentarium of practicing dentist. Integrating radiographs with implant software has become very popular these days. Very soon AI will automatically merge CBCT scan and intraoral scan, design the restoration, and suggest the correct implant with the proper design in the ideal position based on tissue thickness, emergence profile, bone type, and the patient's medical history. Soon the dentist will be witnessing with mixed feelings, the robot placing the implant.

In future AI will analyze patient history and will evaluate the treatment plan cross-checking the investigation reports. While giving the diagnostic support, AI can suggest treatment based on documented evidence which will be updated in real time from a scientific database. Teaching institutions and students will be benefitted from enormous data. Evaluation and assessment process can become unbiased when AI starts assessing. However, clinician should exercise caution before switching over to AI-supported clinical techniques. May be AI will suggest when to have a complete conversion because it can also learn like human beings.

- In future, AI will analyze patient history and will evaluate the treatment plan cross-checking the investigation reports.

Robotics

History of robots can be traced to Leonardo da Vinci who created many human-inspired, robot-like sketches, designs, and models in early CE 1500. Word robot has a Czech origin meaning worker or servant. The word robot first appeared in print in 1920 in a play entitled "Rossum's Universal Robots" authored by Karl Kapek, a Czechoslovakian playwright. Isaac Asimov coined and popularized the term robotics through many science fiction novels. He has gone beyond fiction and formulated three laws of robotics:

- A robot may not injure a human being or through inaction, allow a human being to come to harm.

- A robot must obey the orders given to it by human beings except when such orders would conflict with the First Law.
- A robot must protect its own existence as long as such protection does not conflict with the First or Second Laws.

These laws are considered valid even in the present day world.

Robot is an electromechanical device with multiple degrees of freedom (DOF) (movements) and that is programmable to accomplish a variety of tasks. May be it appears strange but it is difficult to define a "robot" precisely. However, there are some essential characteristics that a robot must have.

- **Ability to sense**—A robot should be able to sense its surroundings just like the human beings through different types of sensors: light sensors (eyes), sonar sensors (ears), chemical sensors (nose), touch and pressure sensors (hands), and taste sensors (tongue). Sensors will give robot, the awareness of its environment.
- **Ability to move**—A robot should be able to move around its environment. Whether rolling on wheels, walking on legs, or propelling by thrusters a robot should have the ability to move. To be considered as a robot either it should move in whole or in parts.
- **Energy**—A robot has energy requirements for its working. A robot can be solar powered, electrically powered, or battery powered. The way the robot gets its energy will depend on the job specification of the robot.
- **Intelligence**—A robot needs some intelligence and it is obtained through the programs it receives. The robot should have built-in facility to receive the programs.

Robots can replace humans and human activities in many fields. A wide range of devices are produced by robotics: from autonomous vacuum cleaners to military drones to entire factory production lines. Robots use technology to increase the quality and safety of a variety of tasks based on control, feedback, and processing. Because of their ability to do precise work without exhaustion it has made its way into dentistry as well.

Robots can replace humans and human activities in many fields.

Robot Patients

For giving clinical training and to develop clinical skills for dental students and dentists, patient robots have been designed to simulate real-life treatment scenarios. Robot can perform a variety of patient gestures and reactions such as blinking, sneezing, coughing, rolling of eyes, shaking the head, moving tongue, and even get fatigue for mouth opening for too long. It can simulate gag reflex, making it no different from an actual patient. Robot is also equipped with voice recognition and it allows the training dentist to carry out some basic conversation with the robot during the exam or procedure.

Endodontic Micro Robot

Endodontic therapy, also called root canal treatment, is an advanced clinical procedure performed to remove damaged tissue from the inner canal of a tooth and seal the canal to prevent the tooth from being a source of infection. A typical procedure includes access opening, root canal preparation, and root canal filling. The treatment process is time-consuming and prone to human error. The outcome relies on the clinician's master skills that can be gained only through years of training and practice. The success rate is 60–65% by general dentists and 90% by specialists. In order to improve the quality and reliability of endodontic therapy, endodontic micro robot is used.

The automated treatment using micro endodontic robot prevents problems identified with conventional techniques and provides safe, accurate, and reliable root canal treatment for patients. With on-line monitoring and intelligent control, the robot will perform the automatic probing, drilling, cleaning, and filling of root canal. The computer-aided method of root canal treatment deals with tool positioning and movement control for automated endodontic therapy.

Nano Robots

Dental nano robots can be used in different areas with improved effectiveness.

Nano robots can be used to induce anesthesia. A colloidal suspension containing millions of active, analgesic, micron-sized robots will be instilled on to the gum and the robots will respond to the input supplied by the dentist. Nano robots will then shut down all sensations by establishing control over nerve-impulse traffic in any tooth that requires treatment. After the treatment, the nano robots restore sensation, providing the patient with anxiety-free needleless comfort. The anesthesia is fast acting and reversible, with no side effects or complications associated with it.

Orthodontic nano robots are expected to manipulate the periodontal tissues, allowing rapid and painless tooth movements including rotating and vertical repositioning within minutes to hours. This is in contrast to the conventional techniques which are time-consuming.

Dentinal hypersensitivity may be caused by changes in pressure transmitted hydrodynamically to the pulp. Etiology is related to the finding that hypersensitive teeth have eight times higher surface density of dentinal tubules and the tubules have diameters twice as large as that of nonsensitive teeth. Nano robots can identify teeth with hypersensitivity and selectively seal the dentinal tubules with desensitizing agents. This would offer immediate and long-lasting relief to the patient as compared to conventional methods.

Nanorobotic dentifrice (dentifrobots): A subocclusal-dwelling nanorobotic dentifrice delivered by mouthwash or toothpaste can patrol supragingival and subgingival surfaces at least once a day, metabolizing trapped organic matter into harmless and odorless vapors and performing continuous calculus debridement. These invisibly small (1–10 μm) dentifrobots, perhaps numbering 10^3–10^5 nanodevices per oral cavity and crawling at 1–10 μm/s. These devices would safely deactivate themselves if swallowed.

Robot-assisted surgery originates from the pioneering work done at the National Aeronautics and Space Administration (NASA). In the 1980s, NASA developed a remotely controlled robotic system to operate on astronauts in space, as well as on soldiers on the battlefield.

A robotic system provides advanced maneuverability for the surgeon and an improved working space for the entire surgical team. The system consists of a master–slave setup—surgeon console (master unit) and robotic arms (slave unit). By the turn of the 21st century, the system could function even in transcontinental destinations. Advancing frontiers of robotic surgery have successfully included dental implant placement.

Robotic implant surgery: Surgical guide template is always considered as a reliable strategy to assist in diagnosis and facilitate proper positioning of implants according to the design of prosthesis. However, the physical position of a surgeon is often constrained due to the limitation of patient's mouth opening and poor accessibility of the location of the missing teeth. Though the strategy is clinically acceptable, the possibility of human error cannot be ruled out. Robotic surgery has the advantage of precision, greater efficiency, increased stability, and more flexibility for assisting dental implant osteotomy and implantation.

In 2017, World's first commercial dental robotic system, YOMI (Neosis, Miami, FL, USA), was developed. The guidance system, termed haptic robotic technology, directed surgeons during the drilling process based on the desired preoperative trajectory. It eliminates the need of a surgical guide but maintains accuracy, ensures full visualization of the operating site, and prevents drill deviation and over drilling past preplanned depths to avoid critical anatomy like nerves and sinus space.

Robots are generally defined as computer-controlled devices with five or six DOF (movements) that can execute complex movements with high accuracy. Remarkable progress has been achieved in automatic robotic systems. However, robotic application capable of determining implant insertion torque is not developed yet. Despite limitations and initial developmental difficulties, the future of robotic implant surgery seems to be bright. It appears to flourish when the systems improve concomitant with the reduction in cost.

Tooth-Arrangement Robot

A number of robot systems have been developed. CRS robot—this is a single manipulator robot system which can be used for the fabrication system having six DOF (movements). This consists of the following components: CRS robot, electromagnetic gripper, computer, a central control system with tooth-arrangement and robot control software for tooth arrangement, motion planning and control, denture base, light source device, and light-sensitive glue.

84DOF multimanipulator tooth-arrangement robot has 14 independent manipulators, a dental arch generator with five point control. Manipulators positioned in a dental arch form can move along its own trail to satisfy the requirements of the position of each tooth. The dental arch matches the one of the patients.

Another robot has a 3-D Cartesian structure. A Cartesian coordinate robot (also called linear robot) is primarily an industrial robot with three principal axes of control which are linear. They move in a straight line and are at right angles to each other. The three sliding joints correspond to movement of the wrist up-down, in-out, and back-forth.

Orthodontics Archwire Bending Robot

A robotic bending apparatus for automatically bending orthodontic archwires into a particular shape. The bending apparatus comprises a robot mounted to a base. A first gripping tool has a structure for holding the archwire and is either be fixed with respect to the base or may be incorporated into a moveable arm. The second gripping tool is mounted to the end of a moveable six-axis robot arm. Three axes are translational and the other three rotational. Another Cartesian type archwire bending robot mechanism is composed of a base, a rotary feed, supporting structure for archwire, bending die, and archwire bending mechanism.

Virtual Reality and Augmented Reality

Recent times have ushered in a lot of computer-based technologies to dentistry such as virtual reality (VR) and augmented reality (AR).

VR can be described as the combination of multiple technologies allowing users to interact with virtual entities in real time. The two main features of VR are immersion and interaction. Immersion refers to the sense of presence in a virtual environment, while interaction refers to the user's power of modification. AR is a type of technology in which an environment is enhanced through the process of superimposing computer-generated virtual content over real structure enhancing the sensory perception of reality.

Use of AR has been well recognized in industry, sightseeing, marketing, entertainment, architecture, education, and medicine. Surgeons were the first to adopt AR in their respective fields, for example, neurosurgery, urology, spine surgery, laparoscopic surgery, endoscopic surgery, hepatobiliary and pancreatic surgery, and cancer surgery. In dentistry, AR technology can be successfully utilized to enhance diagnosis, treatment, and education outcomes.

AR and maxillofacial and implant surgery: Oral and maxillofacial regions contain many surgically and anatomically important structures, including nerves and vessels. The intricate anatomy of the craniofacial structures necessitates precise presurgical planning. AR technology is well suited for this purpose and also fits the currently favored minimally invasive philosophy.

Based on AR principles, the real operative site of a patient is provided with graphic information that was extracted and modified from a data source. Previously acquired diagnostic images such as radiographs, CT scans, MRI scans, and angiography can also be good sources of additionally integrated AR information.

In contrast to conventional image-guided surgery, where a surgeon must look away from the operative field to view the informative data, AR guidance systems provide real-time intraoperative information with real surgical fields. In AR the virtual image is superimposed onto the real environment, forming the "integrated image." AR provides the possibility of keeping 3-D images on the patient's body rather than a separate screen and surgeon gets more clarity.

A dental implant positioning system with a superimposed graphic suggestion on the patient was introduced as early as 1995. Teleplanning and surgical navigation of implant placement can also be achieved using AR systems. The AR surgical navigation systems for implant placement use retinal imaging display rather than watching the monitor because looking away from the restricted oral surgical site during the operation will have dangerous consequences. Surgical template if integrated with the AR system can significantly reduce deviations in the placement of implants. However, experienced professionals feel that the accuracy of AR systems still needs to be improved. AR system can make dental implantology treatment cost-effective because of its ability to reduce time and additional expenditure.

Orthodontics and endodontics: Guided bracket placement can be done using a light-weight AR system. This is considered as a practical and feasible system. In endodontics, application of AR technology helps in real-time detection of root canal orifices.

Dental education: AR provides new educational opportunities by blending digital elements with a real learning environment. Traditional anatomy teaching using atlas and cadaver is time-consuming and laborious. AR can make it possible to visualize internal structures and integrate digital ultrasound.

Virtual tooth models are developed that indicate enamel, dentine, and pulp. Augmented video and audio rendering are also used to help dental students learn the tooth preparation techniques. Traditional and AR-supported teaching when compared exhibited equal effectiveness but virtual teaching involves more man power and infrastructure.

With varied use of simulators, AR technology has proved its suitability in dental education especially in anatomy, surgery, and restorative dentistry. With other state-of-the-art technologies, such as haptics and robotics, AR applications in dentistry are expected to become more prevalent in the near future.

Summary

Digital dentistry has dawned to dentistry with three main foci:

- Computer-aided design/computer-aided manufacturing (CAD/CAM)
- Digital Imaging (digital radiography)
- Practice/patient management systems

CAD/CAM

Two types of scanners are popularly used in dentistry—intraoral and extraoral. Real-time scanning produces digital images of single or multiple teeth, complete arches, opposing arches, occlusion, and surrounding soft tissues.

Digital planning, designing, and manufacturing technologies have become the common standard in dental laboratory technology.

Presently used CAD/CAM technologies with the assistance of machines, and other tools, the dentists experience virtually no limit to the type of dental restoration that can be fabricated.

Though the prominent method of fabrication is subtractive through milling processes, additive technologies such as three-dimensional (3D) printing are becoming increasingly popular.

Indications:

- Ceramic-, metal-, and resin-based crowns and bridges
- Copings and frameworks for metal–ceramic prostheses
- Full and partial dentures
- Inlays, onlays, partial crowns, and provisionals
- Implant abutments and crowns, including screw-retained crowns
- Orthodontic printed models and clear appliances
- Maryland bridges and veneers

Digital Imaging

The value of digital radiography in dental diagnosis is well established, especially during operative procedures. The software is able to adjust contrast, brightness, and perform gamma corrections and measurement functions.

Cone beam computed tomography systems (CBCT) are a variation of traditional computed tomography (CT) systems. The CBCT systems used by dental professionals rotate around the patient, capturing data using a cone-shaped X-ray beam.

CBCT scan data can bridge with CAD/CAM image files for the fabrication of various dental restorations.

Practice Management Systems

Along with patient care, the present day dental practice involves the following practice management systems: accessing and searching patient-related records, designating the roles of staff, evaluating the productivity of staff members, and tracking patient visits including their electronic health records.

Present day dentists are guided not only by the knowledge and skills they acquired from the dental colleges but also through a greater extent by evidence-based dentistry (EBD). Research-based decision-making is gaining priority in dental practice.

Artificial Intelligence

- Artificial intelligence (AI) refers to the simulation of human intelligence in machines that are programmed to think like humans and mimic their actions.
- The term may also be applied to any machine that exhibits traits associated with a human mind such as learning and problem solving.
- Another area in which AI is gaining popularity is in intraoral scanning. In the fabrication of fixed prosthesis, after tooth preparation intraoral scanning is employed.
- AI assists in decision-making and helps orthodontists to choose the best way to move, a tooth or group of teeth.

Robotics

- Robot is an electromechanical device with multiple degrees of freedom (movements) and that is programmable to accomplish a variety of tasks.
- *Robot patients:* For giving clinical training and to develop clinical skills for dental students and dentists.
- *Endodontic micro robot:* The automated treatment using micro endodontic robot prevents problems identified with conventional techniques and provides safe, accurate, and reliable root canal treatment for patients.
- *Nano robots:* Can be used to induce anesthesia.
- *Robotic implant surgery:* Robotic surgery has the advantage of precision, greater efficiency, increased stability, and more flexibility for assisting dental implant osteotomy and implantation.

Virtual Reality and Augmented Reality

Virtual reality (VR) can be described as the combination of multiple technologies allowing users to interact with virtual entities in real time. Augmented reality (AR) is a type of technology in which an environment is enhanced through the process of superimposing computer-generated virtual content over real structure enhancing the sensory perception of reality.

Suggested Readings

Ahrberg D, Lauer HC, Ahrberg M, et al.: Evaluation of fit and efficiency of CAD/CAM fabricated all-ceramic restorations based on direct and indirect digitalization: A double-blinded, randomized clinical trial. *Clin Oral Investig* 20: 291, 2016. DOI:10.1007/s00784-015-1504-6.

Dutã M, Amariei CI, Bogdan CM, et al.: An overview of virtual and augmented reality in dental education. *Oral Health Dent Manag* 10: 42–48, 2011.

Haag M, Igel C, Fischer MR: Digital teaching and digital medicine: A national initiative is needed. *GMS J Med Educ* 35:Doc43, 2018.

Jung EH, Lee ES, Jung HI, et al.: Development of a fluorescence-image scoring system for assessing noncavitated occlusal caries. *Photodiagn Photodyn* 21:36–42, 2018.

Ngo TD, Kashani A, Imbalzano G, et al.: Additive manufacturing (3D printing): A review of materials, methods, applications and challenges. *Compos Part B-Eng* 143:172–196, 2018.

Oberoi G, Nitsch S, Edelmayer M, et al.: 3D Printing-encompassing the facets of dentistry. *Front Bioeng Biotechnol* 6: 172(1–13), 2018.

Park S, Kim S, Lee H, et al.: Comparison of fluorescence parameters between three generations of QLF devices for detecting enamel caries *in vitro* and on smooth surfaces. *Photodiagn Photodyn* 25:142–147, 2019.

Tofail SAM, Koumoulos EP, Bandyopadhyay A, et al.: **Additive manufacturing: Scientific and technological challenges, market uptake and opportunities.** *Mater Today* 21:22–37, 2018.

van der Veen M, de Josselin de Jong E: Application of quantitative light-induced fluorescence for assessing early caries lesions: In Faller RV (editor): Assessment of Oral Health. Monogr Oral Sci., Basel, Karger, 2000, vol 17, pp. 144–162.

Yue J, Zhao P, Gerasimov JY, et al.: 3D-Printable antimicrobial composite resins. *Adv Funct Mater* 25: 6756–6767, 2015.

Digital Dentistry

Gutmann J L. The evolution of America's scientific advancements in dentistry in the past 150 years, JADA 2009;140(9 suppl):8S–15S

Markus B. Blatz, Julian Conejo. The current state of chair side digital dentistry and materials, Dent Clin N Am 63 (2019) 175–197, https://doi.org/10.1016/j.cden.2018.11.002

Rekow E D. Digital dentistry: The new state of the art — Is it disruptive or destructive? Dent Mater (2019), https://doi.org/10.1016/j.dental.2019.08.103

Tehran Peffley-Routt. The advantage of digital dentistry, https://www.researchgate.net/publication/324603548

Al-Mussawi, Farid. Computer-based technologies in dentistry: Types and applications,

Journal of Dentistry, Tehran University of Medical Sciences, Tehran, Iran (2016); Vol. 13, No. 3)

CBCT

Abramovitch K, Rice D D. Basic principles of cone beam computed tomography

Dent Clin N Am 58 (2014) 463–484, http://dx.doi.org/10.1016/j.cden.2014.03.002

Dawood A, Patel S, Brown J. Cone beam CT in dental practice, bdj. 2009; 207: 23–28, DOI: 10.1038/sj. bdj.2009.560

AI

Yo-wei Chen, Kyle Stanley, Wael Att. Artificial intelligence in dentistry: Current applications and future perspectives, Quintessence International | volume 51 • number 3 • March 2020, 248–257

Zeba Jafria, Nafis Ahmadb, Madhuri Sawaia, Nishat Sultana, Ashu Bhardwaja

Digital smile design-An innovative tool in aesthetic dentistry, Journal of Oral Biology and Craniofacial Research 10 (2020) 194–198

F. Schwendicke, W. Samek, and J. Krois. Artificial intelligence in dentistry:

Chances and challenges, Journal of Dental Research, 2020, Vol. 99(7) 769–774, DOI: 10.1177/0022034520915714

Virtual Reality/Augmented Reality

Ta-Ko Huang, Chi-Hsun Yang, Yu-Hsin Hsieh, Jen-Chyan Wang, Chun-Cheng Hung. Augmented reality (AR) and virtual reality (VR) applied in dentistry, Kaohsiung Journal of Medical Sciences (2018) 34: 243–248

Ming Zhu1, Fei Liu1, Gang Chai1, Jun J. Pan, Taoran Jiang, Li Lin, Yu Xin, Yan Zhang, Qingfeng Li. A novel augmented reality system for displaying inferior alveolar nerve bundles in maxillofacial surgery, Scientific Reports (2017) 7:42365 | DOI: 10.1038/srep42365, www.nature.com/scientificreports

Ho-Beom Kwon, Young-Seok Park, Jung-Suk Han (2018): Augmented reality in dentistry: A current perspective, Acta Odontologica Scandinavica, DOI:10.1080/00016357.2018.1441437www.nature.com/scientificreports

T. Jodaa, G.O. Galluccib, D. Wismeijerc, N.U. Zitzmanna. Augmented and virtual reality in dental medicine: A systematic review, Computers in Biology and Medicine (2019) 108:93–100

Robotics

Yiqun Wu, Feng Wang, Shengchi Fan, James Kwok-Fai Chow. Robotics in dental implantology, Oral Maxillofacial Surg Clin N Am 31 (2019) 513–518, https://doi.org/10.1016/j.coms.2019.03.013

Jin-gang Jiang, Yong-de Zhang, Chun-ge Wei, Tian-hua He, Yi Liu. A review on robot in prosthodontics and orthodontics, Hindawi Publishing Corporation, Advances in Mechanical Engineering, Article ID 198748 (2014)

Intraoral Scanners

Francesco Mangano, Andrea Gandolfi, Giuseppe Luongo, Silvia Logozzo. Intraoral scanners in dentistry: A review of the current literature, BMC Oral Health (2017) 17:149, DOI 10.1186/s12903-017-0442-x

16

Materials and Processes for Cutting, Grinding, Finishing, and Polishing

CHAPTER OUTLINE

KEY TERMS

Abrasive—A product that has a hard phase as an essential constituent that provides many individual particles with sharp cutting edges.

Air–particle abrasion—The process of material removal by way of air pressure–propelled abrasive particles. Typical applications are surface cleaning, cavity preparation, and surface preparation for bonding. The process is also known as *erosion* in the field of tribology.

Bonded abrasive—An abrasive instrument containing a phase that holds abrasive particles in a more or less tight grip with spaces in between that allow air or liquids to pass. The strength of bonding in a product varies based on its intended use. Strong bonding is required for work on hard materials. Breaking away of grains from the bond of an abrasive is desirable as they become dull. Bond materials include organic (resin or rubber), vitrified (glass or glass–ceramic), and metal.

Buffing—Polishing with a soft absorbent material such as cloth or leather, typically in combination with a medium containing very fine abrasive particles.

Bulk reduction and contouring—An early process that precedes finishing and polishing, whereby excess restorative material is removed to develop the anatomical form of the final restoration.

Cutting—Reduction of a material by use of an edged instrument, such as a bladed dental bur, or a bonded abrasive disk or wheel; implies material removal by a slicing action.

Dressing—The use of a variety of tools to remove any debris that may be clogging the spaces between abrasive particles on a bonded abrasive instrument to expose fresh abrasive and restore grinding efficiency. Diamond-coated tools or bonded abrasive stones of aluminum oxide or silicon carbide are the most common devices used for dressing grinding wheels.

Erosion—A process of material removal achieved by (1) air pressure–propelled abrasives *(air–particle abrasion)*, (2) pressurized liquid abrasive mixtures *(slurry erosion)*, or (3) chemical dissolution using strong acids or alkali (*chemical erosion* or *acid etching*).

Finishing—The process of removing surface defects or scratches created during the contouring process through the use of cutting or grinding instruments or both.

Grinding—A machining process that uses coated or bonded abrasive wheels or points to turn against the surface of a material workpiece in order to reduce the surface. Ground surfaces typically display linear scratch marks where abrasive particles have ground material away.

Polish, polishing—A process that uses very fine abrasives to bring a material surface to a highly developed, finished, or refined state. A minimal amount of material is removed from the workpiece to generate a smooth, glossy appearance. The force per unit area for polishing is the lightest of all processes that use abrasives.

True/truing—A process of correcting the concentricity and shape of a grinding wheel; truing keeps the grinding wheel rotating concentrically with the spindle axis of the motor or handpiece head without vibration or wobble.

A Brief History of Abrasives

Abrasive processes have been used since prehistoric times. Hunting and gathering instruments were shaped and sharpened by chipping and abrading one surface against another over 10,000 years ago to produce sharp edges on hard natural materials. Spear points, arrowheads, scraper tools, and hoes were made by chipping, **grinding**, and honing the surfaces and edges of relatively hard rock-like materials. Sandstone was used to produce smoother surfaces on the Egyptian pyramids.

Grinding wheels of a primitive type were created over 4000 years ago by taking a cylindrical stone with an **abrasive** surface and spinning it against metals and ceramics to adjust their shapes, reduce rough areas, and produce smoother surfaces. These processes were refined over subsequent millennia to produce, by the Middle Ages, metal daggers, swords, spears, and shields of relatively high quality. The Chinese introduced the first coated abrasives in the 13th century by embedding seashell fragments in natural gums that were spread on a parchment backing.

In the early 1900s, abrasive technology advanced further through the development and use of alumina grains, diamond particles, and silicon carbide grit. New products in the form of powders, slurries, particle-embedded disks and wheels, and burs of different types soon emerged for use in dentistry. The further refinement of dental handpieces, air or abrasive technology, and methods of bonding abrasives to various binders has led to major processing breakthroughs that have rapidly advanced the quality of treatment in the current era of restorative dentistry, particularly with adhesive and esthetic dentistry.

CRITICAL QUESTION

What are the main benefits of finishing and polishing the surfaces of restorative materials? What are the goals of finishing and polishing?

Finished and polished restorations provide four benefits of dental care:

- Better gingival health
- Chewing efficiency
- Patient comfort
- Esthetics

Additional benefits of finishing and polishing include:

- Surface changes greater than 1 μm can also lead to increased bacterial adhesion as well as surface staining. A well-contoured and polished restoration promotes gingival health by resisting the accumulation of food debris and pathogenic bacteria. This is accomplished through a reduction in total surface area and reduced roughness of the restoration surface. Smoother surfaces have less retention areas and are easier to maintain in a hygienic state when preventive oral home care is practiced because dental floss and the toothbrush bristles can gain more complete access to all surfaces and marginal areas.
- Tarnish and corrosion activity of some metallic materials can be significantly reduced if the entire metal restoration is highly polished.
- Oral function is enhanced with a well-polished restoration because food glides more freely over occlusal and embrasure surfaces during mastication.
- Smooth restoration surfaces minimize wear rates on opposing and adjacent teeth. This is particularly true for restorative materials such as ceramics, which contain phases that are harder than tooth enamel and dentin.
- Rough material surfaces lead to the development of high, two-body contact stresses that can cause the loss of functional and stabilizing contacts between teeth or a reduction in the vertical dimension of occlusion. Rough surfaces on ceramics also act as stress concentration points.
- Finishing and polishing these surfaces can improve the strength of the restoration, especially in areas that are under tension, such as the perimeter of ceramic–ceramic crowns where unsupported areas of veneering ceramic are present.
- Finally, esthetic demands may require the dentist to finish and polish highly visible surfaces of restorations differently from those that are not accessible. Although a mirror-like polish is preferred for previously mentioned reasons, this type of surface may not be esthetically compatible with adjacent teeth in highly visible areas, such as the facial surfaces of maxillary anterior teeth. Fortunately, these surfaces are not subject to high contact stresses and they are easily accessible for cleaning. Subtle anatomic features and textures may be added to these areas without affecting oral health or function.

In summary, the goals of finishing and polishing procedures are

1. To obtain the desired anatomy
2. Proper occlusion
3. Reduction of roughness and the depth of gouges and scratches produced by the contouring and finishing instruments

The instruments available for finishing and polishing restorations include fluted carbide burs, diamond burs, stones, coated abrasive disks and strips, polishing pastes, and soft and hard polymeric cups, points, and wheels impregnated with specific types and sizes of abrasive particles.

The polished surface should be smooth enough to be well tolerated by oral soft tissues and to resist bacterial adhesion and excessive plaque accumulation. When plaque deposits exist on restorative material surfaces, they should be easily removable by brushing and flossing.

Applications of Abrasives in Dentistry

The intraoral surfaces of virtually every direct and indirect restoration must be contoured by grinding, **finishing**, and **polishing** procedures. The goal of these procedures is to produce the smoothest surface possible in a limited time. A single type of abrasive cannot be used effectively for all types of dental materials. Different abrasives are used for the three major classes of materials: ceramics, metals, and resin-based composites.

Why are abrasives different?

- The abrasive instruments used for metals must be able to remove metal particles quickly and efficiently without generating excessive heat or becoming clogged with debris.
- Flexible disks used for resin composites can be used for metals, they are incapable of removing large amounts of metal quickly.
- Likewise, although diamond burs have been developed for grinding and finishing zirconia frameworks, specialized Zir-Cut (Axis/SybronEndo, Coppell, Texas) coarse blue wheels with embedded diamond particles may be more effective because they may not wear out as fast as diamond burs and they can remove relatively large amounts of zirconia from framework surfaces rather efficiently.

It is essential to have suitable finishing and polishing instruments for the respective dental materials.

Form of polishing instruments

The form of polishing instruments also affects the rate of material removal and the surface finish. Some common examples include:

1. **Disks:** Regular and extrathin Sof-Lex (3M ESPE St. Paul, MN) **contouring** and polishing disks are useful for finishing and polishing resin-based materials. They are provided in the stiff and flexible disk forms to allow either light or heavy pressure to be applied, depending on the amount of composite that needs to be removed. The polymer backing allows the disks to be used either in the dry or wet condition.

   The regular Sof-Lex disks are available in four grades of abrasiveness:
   - Coarse (black)
   - Medium (dark blue)
   - Fine (medium blue)
   - Superfine (light blue)

   The extrathin disks and gapped strips are also provided in these four abrasive grades, but their colors are different. A word of caution is important here. The abrasive disks and strips of other manufacturers may not follow the same convention for Sof-Lex disks (i.e., darker colors corresponding to coarser abrasives and lighter colors to finer abrasives).
2. **Cups, cones and wheels:**

   The Astropol finishing and polishing system (Ivoclar Vivadent, Amherst, NY) is a comprehensive finishing and polishing set that consists of four differently shaped polishers in three grit sizes for interdental and occlusal applications.

   The shapes include:
   - Small flame
   - Large flame
   - Cup
   - Disk forms

   The grit sizes are designated as
   1. Finish (Astropol F for the removal of excess material and prepolishing)
   2. Polish (Astropol P, for polishing of restorations: especially those made from microfilled composite materials)
   3. High-gloss polish (Astropol HP, that is best suited for hybrid composites)

Usually a combination of shapes, grits, or materials is required to achieve the final polish. Newer systems are evolving which involve fewer steps to achieve an acceptable result.

Benefits of Finishing and Polishing Restorative Materials

Principles of Cutting, Grinding, Finishing, and Polishing

Particles of a substrate material (workpiece) are removed by the action of a harder material that makes frictional contact with the substrate. This contact must generate sufficient tensile and shear stresses to break atomic bonds and release particles from the substrate. With rotary instrumentation, the blades of a carbide bur or the tips of abrasive particles transfer the force to the substrate. These tensile and shear stresses are induced in both the substrate and the rotary instrument. The instrument will fail to cut, grind, or polish if the stress that develops in any part of the cutting or grinding surface exceeds the strength of the instrument blade edges or particle bond strength to the binder compared with the strength of the substrate (workpiece). As a result, blade edges will become dull, and abrasive particles will fracture or tear away from their binder.

Subtle differences distinguish the cutting, grinding, and polishing processes.

- A **cutting** operation usually involves the use of a bladed instrument or any other instrument in a blade-like fashion. Substrates may be divided into large separate segments, or they may sustain deep notches and grooves by the cutting operation. High-speed tungsten carbide burs have numerous regularly arranged blades that remove small pieces or segments of the substrate as the bur rotates. As shown in Figure 16.1A, the unidirectional cutting pattern reflects the action of the regularly arranged blades on a tungsten carbide bur. The pattern produced by a diamond bur is shown in Figure 16.1B. The surface of a coarse diamond bur is shown in Figure 16.1C. When 30-fluted finishing burs have been used on a surface, the regular pattern of the cutting blades is discernible only if the surface is magnified for inspection. On the other hand, a separating wheel is an example of an instrument that can be used in a blade-like fashion. A separating wheel does not contain individual blades, but its thin blade design allows it to be used in a rotating fashion to grind through cast metal sprues and die stone materials.
- A **grinding** operation removes small particles of a substrate through the action of bonded or coated abrasive instruments. Grinding instruments contain many randomly arranged abrasive particles. Each particle may contain several sharp points that run along the substrate surface and remove particles of

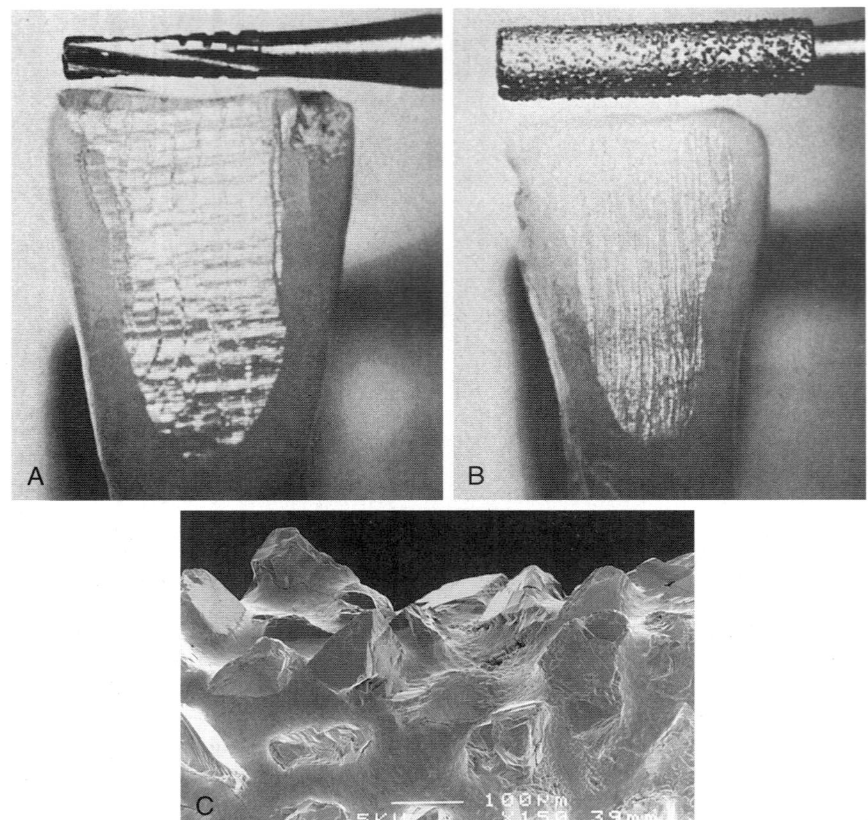

• **Fig. 16.1** **(A)** Tooth cut by a carbide bur. Note the regular pattern of removal of tooth structure, which corresponds to the regular arrangement of blades on the bur. **(B)** Tooth ground by a diamond bur. Note the multiple scratches formed by the random arrangement of abrasive particles on the diamond bur. **(C)** Magnified image of the bonded diamond particles on a coarse diamond bur (×150).

material. For example, a diamond-coated rotary instrument may contain many sharp diamond particles (see Fig. 16.1C) that pass over a tooth during each revolution of the instrument. Because these particles are randomly arranged, many unidirectional scratches are produced within the material surface, as illustrated in Figure 16.1B, which shows a tooth surface ground by a diamond bur. Cutting and grinding are both considered predominantly unidirectional in their action. This means that a cut or ground surface exhibits cuts and scratches oriented in one predominant direction.

Different types of burs have unique effects on surfaces. In general, a carbide bur with more blades will produce a smoother surface than a carbide bur containing fewer blades. For example, a 16-fluted carbide bur produces a smoother finish than an 8-fluted carbide bur, but the latter removes material more rapidly. Similarly, the coarsest diamond bur removes material more quickly but leaves a rougher surface. (See Fig. 16.2 for scanning electron microscopy [SEM] images of carbide and diamond burs.)

Bulk Reduction Process

Bulk reduction can be achieved through the use of instruments such as diamond burs, tungsten carbide burs, steel burs, abrasive wheels, and separating disks. Whereas diamond burs and abrasive wheels provide this action by grinding, steel and carbide burs remove materials through a cutting action of the hard blades. Abrasive-coated disks are popular instruments for bulk reduction of resin-based composite restorations. For bulk reduction of composites, the clinician should choose 8- to 12-fluted carbide burs or abrasives with a particle size of 100 μm or larger and sufficient hardness (9–10 Mohs hardness). SEM images of the surface finishes produced on a resin-based composite by a coarse diamond, a 12-fluted carbide bur, a 16-fluted carbide bur, and two types of finishing or polishing systems are shown in Figure 16.3. For bulk reduction of ceramics and metals, the user should follow the manufacturers' instructions to minimize the time required. In some cases, instruments used in the dental lab may be different from those used chairside, so the abrasiveness of an unknown instrument should be tested on a scrap piece of the material that will be used for a specific task.

Contouring

Even though contouring can be achieved during the bulk reduction process, in some cases, it requires finer cutting instruments or abrasives to provide better control of contouring and surface details. At the end of this process, the desired anatomy and margins should be established. The smoothness of the surface at this stage depends on the instrument used and may require extra steps to establish a smoother surface. Usually 12- to 16-fluted carbide burs or abrasives ranging in size from 30 to 100 μm provide a fine contouring action.

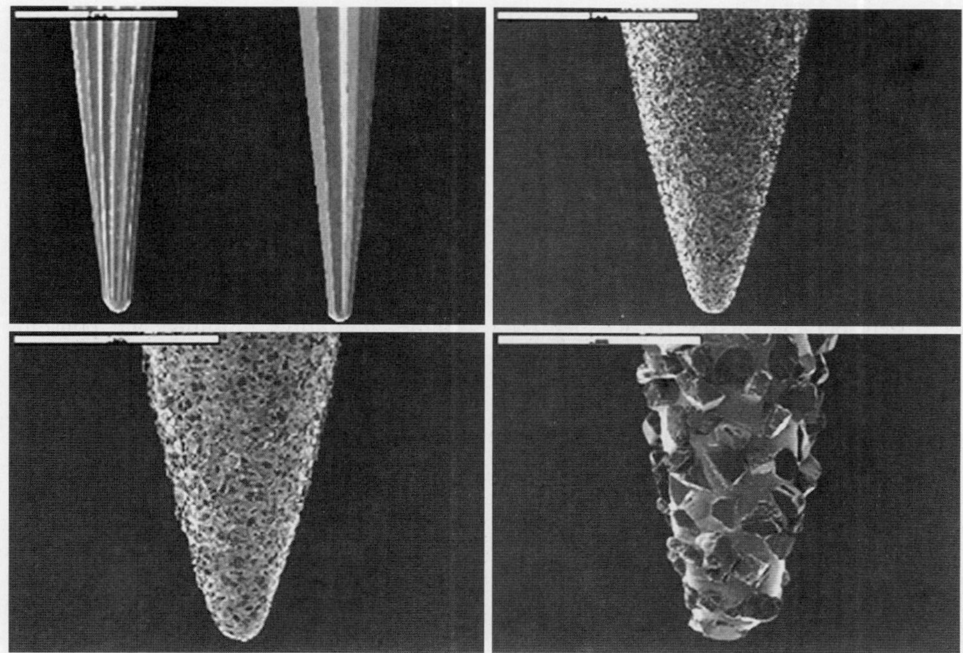

• **Fig. 16.2** Scanning electron microscopy (SEM) images. *Upper left*, 16-fluted (*left*) and 8-fluted (*right*) tungsten carbide finishing burs. *Upper right*, fine diamond bur. *Bottom left*, medium-grit diamond bur. *Bottom right*, coarse-grit diamond bur.

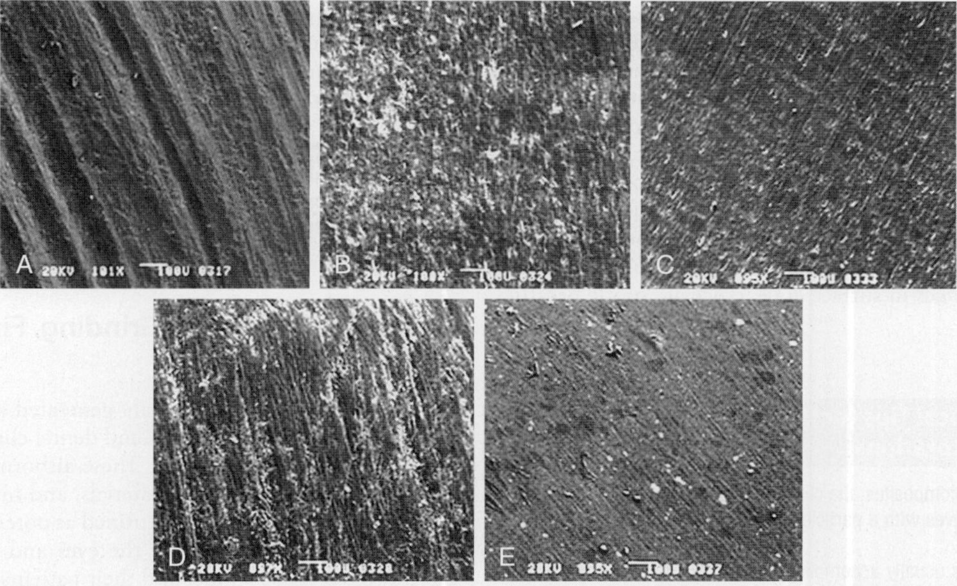

• **Fig. 16.3** Scanning electron microscopy (SEM) images of the surface of a resin-based composite after the grinding, finishing, and polishing processes using five instruments. **(A)** A coarse diamond. **(B)** A 12-flute carbide bur. **(C)** A 16-flute carbide bur. **(D)** An abrasive-impregnated finishing disk. **(E)** An abrasive-impregnated polishing disk.

Finishing

In general, finishing and polishing processes require a stepwise approach, introducing finer scratches to the surface of the substrate to methodically remove deeper scratches. This process may require several steps to reach the desired surface smoothness. Surface imperfections can be an integral part of the internal structure, or they can be created by the instruments that are used for gross removal because of the size of the abrasives or the flute geometry. Finishing provides a relatively blemish-free smooth surface. The finishing action is usually accomplished using 18- to 30-fluted carbide burs, fine and superfine diamond burs, or abrasives that are between 8 and 20 μm in size.

Polishing

The purpose of polishing is to provide an enamel-like luster to the restoration. Smaller particles provide smoother and shinier surfaces. The speed of achieving a luster, however, depends on the hardness and size of the abrasive particles and the method of abrasion (e.g., two-body abrasion or three-body abrasion). Ideally, abrasive particles in the range of particle sizes up to 20 μm provide luster at a low magnification. At the end of this process, there should be no visible scratches. However, there will always be scratches that are detectable at higher magnification. The surface must be cleaned between steps because abrasive particles left on the surface from the previous step can cause deep scratches.

Polishing procedures, the most refined of the finishing processes, remove the finest surface particles. Each type of polishing abrasive acts on an extremely thin region of the substrate surface. Polishing progresses from the finest abrasive that can remove scratches from the previous grinding procedure and is completed when the desired level of surface smoothness is achieved. Each step is followed by the use of progressively finer polishing media until no further improvement in surface finish is observed. The final stage produces scratches so fine that they are not visible unless greatly magnified. Polishing should be terminated when no further change in surface luster or glossiness occurs during the application of the finest abrasive that is used for that application. Further attempts to improve the surface appearance may actually degrade the surface by generating heat and by smearing dislodged material across the surface (Box 16.1).

Examples of polishing instruments are rubber abrasive points, fine particle disks and strips, and fine particle polishing pastes. Polishing pastes are applied with soft felt points, muslin (woven cotton fabric) wheels, prophylaxis rubber cups, or **buffing** wheels. A nonabrasive material should be used as an applicator while using polishing pastes. Felt, leather, rubber, and synthetic foam are popular applicator materials for buffing. A common feature of some of these materials is their porous texture, which allows fine abrasive particles to be retained during the buffing procedure.

Polishing is considered multidirectional, which means that the final surface scratches are oriented in many directions. Some examples of ground and polished surfaces are shown in Figure 16.3. Note that the differences in surface appearance are subtle because of the transitional nature of the grinding and polishing processes. If there were larger differences in the size of particles removed, the surface change would be more easily detected.

Heat generation during the cutting, contouring, finishing, and polishing processes of direct restorations is a major concern. To avoid adverse effects to the pulp, the clinician must cool the surface with a lubricant, such as an air–water spray, and avoid continuous contact of high-speed rotary instruments with the substrate. Intermittent contact during operation is necessary not only to cool the surface but also to remove debris formed between the substrate and the instrument. The effectiveness and the speed of the contouring, finishing, and polishing procedures will be greatly improved by the removal of debris.

• BOX 16.1 Clinical Tips for Polishing Composite Restorations

- For bulk reduction of composites, the clinician should choose 8- to 12-fluted carbide burs or abrasives with a particle size of 100 μm or larger and sufficient hardness.
- The finishing action is usually accomplished using 18- to 30-fluted carbide burs, fine and superfine diamond burs, or abrasives that are between 8 and 20 μm in size.
- When a handpiece and bur are translated in a direction opposite to the rotational direction of the bur at the surface being abraded, a smoother grinding action is achieved.
- Polish with fine and extrafine polishing paste (aluminum oxide or diamond); extrafine abrasive-coated disks; silicon carbide–impregnated brushes; or diamond-impregnated rubber polishing disks, cups, or points.
- Diamond abrasive pastes are used in a relatively dry condition. The instruments that apply the paste to the material surface are equally important. These include ribbed prophy cups (the ribbed type or the more flexible nonribbed type), brushes, and felt wheels.

Abrasive-Impregnated Brushes and Felt Devices

Abrasive-impregnated, latch-type polishing brushes come in several shapes (pointed, cup shaped), with a variety of polymer "bristles" impregnated with silicon carbide or aluminum oxide. The brushes can reach into the grooves, fissures, and interproximal areas of ceramic and resin composite restorations that are not easy to reach with other finishing or polishing devices without unintended removal of anatomic grooves, fissures, and contours.

Liquid Polish

Low-viscosity fluid resins are being used as liquid polishers and surface sealants that provide a gloss over composite resin restorations. These liquid polishers or surface sealants also aid in creating a marginal seal, and they have the ability to fill microgaps. Liquid polishers reduce microleakage at composite margins and have been found to be effective in helping prevent stain penetration and discoloration of composite resins, which results in greater shade stability.

CRITICAL QUESTION

What precautions should be taken to minimize the generation of aerosols? What precautions should be taken to minimize exposure to and inhalation of aerosols?

Biological Hazards of Grinding, Finishing, and Polishing Processes

Dispersions of solid particles are generated and released into the breathing space of laboratories and dental clinics whenever finishing operations are performed. These airborne particles may contain tooth structure, dental materials, and microorganisms.

Such aerosols have been identified as potential sources of infectious and chronic diseases of the eyes and lungs and present a hazard to dental personnel and their patients. Silicosis, also called *grinders disease*, is a major illness caused by inhalation of aerosol particles released from any of a number of silica-based materials that are used in the processing and finishing of dental restorations. Silicosis is a fibrotic pulmonary disease that severely debilitates the lungs and doubles the risk for lung cancer. The risk for silicosis is substantial, because 95% of generated aerosol particles are smaller than 5 μm in diameter and can readily reach the pulmonary alveoli during normal respiration. Additionally, 75% of airborne particles are potentially contaminated with infectious microorganisms. Furthermore, aerosols can remain airborne for more than 24 hours before settling and are, therefore, capable of cross-contaminating other areas of the treatment facility.

Aerosols produced during finishing procedures may be controlled in three ways:

- First, they may be controlled at the source through the use of adequate infection control procedures, water spray, and high-volume suction.
- Second, personal protective equipment (PPE) such as safety glasses and disposable face masks can protect the eyes and respiratory tract from aerosols. Masks should be chosen to provide the best filtration along with ease of breathing for the wearer.
- Third, the entire facility should have an adequate ventilation system that efficiently removes any residual particulates from the air. Many systems are also capable of controlling chemical contaminants such as mercury vapor from amalgam scrap and monomer vapor from acrylic resin.

CRITICAL QUESTION

How can the amount of lubricant either increase or decrease cutting efficiency?

Abrasion and Erosion

Abrasion

Wear is a material removal process that can occur whenever surfaces slide against each other. The process of finishing a restoration involves abrasive wear through the use of hard particles. In dentistry, the outermost particles or surface material of an abrading instrument is referred to as the *abrasive*. The material being finished is called the *substrate*. In the case of a diamond bur abrading a tooth surface, as illustrated in Figure 16.4, the diamond particles bonded to the bur represent the abrasive, and the tooth is the substrate. Also, note that the bur in the high-speed handpiece rotates in a clockwise direction as observed from the head of the handpiece.

The rotational direction of a rotary abrasive instrument is an important factor in controlling the instrument's action on the substrate's surface. When a handpiece and bur are translated in a direction opposite to the rotational direction of the bur at the surface being abraded, a smoother grinding action is achieved. However, when the handpiece and bur are translated in the same direction as the rotational direction of the bur at the surface, the bur tends to "run away" from the substrate, thereby producing a more uncontrolled grinding action and a rougher surface.

Abrasion is further divided into the processes of two-body and three-body wear. *Two-body abrasion* occurs when abrasive particles are firmly bonded to the surface of the abrasive instrument and no other abrasive particles are used. A diamond bur abrading a tooth represents an example of two-body wear. *Three-body abrasion* occurs when abrasive particles are free to translate and rotate between two surfaces. An example of three-body abrasion involves the use of nonbonded abrasives such as those in dental prophylaxis pastes. These nonbonded abrasives are placed in a rubber cup, which is rotated against a tooth or material surface. These two processes are not mutually exclusive. Diamond particles may debond from a diamond bur and cause three-body wear. Likewise, some abrasive particles in the abrasive paste can become trapped in the surface of a rubber cup and cause two-body wear. Lubricants are often used to minimize the risk of these unintentional shifts from two-body to three-body wear, and vice versa. Thus, the efficiency of cutting and grinding will be improved with the use of lubricants such as water, glycerin, or silicone. Intraorally, a water-soluble lubricant is preferred. Excessive amounts of lubricant may reduce the cutting efficiency by reducing the contact

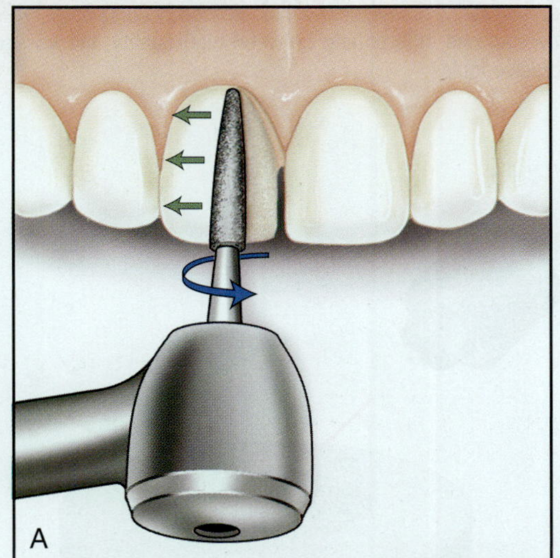

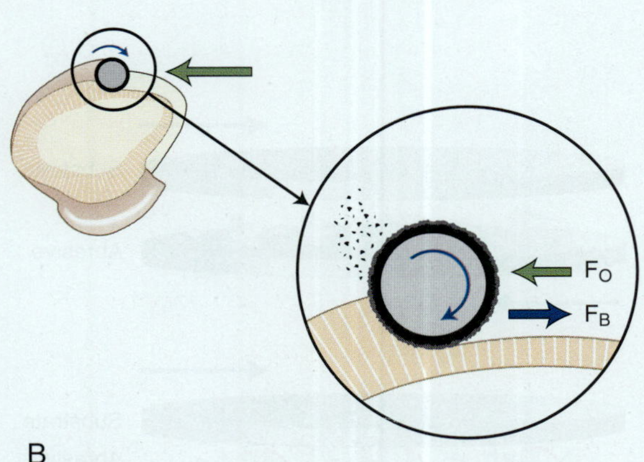

• **Fig. 16.4** The mechanics of high-speed rotary instrumentation. **(A)** The blue circular arrow indicates that the high-speed diamond bur rotates in a clockwise direction when viewed from the head of the handpiece. The green arrows indicate the direction that the instrument should be drawn to counteract the rotational force of the bur and achieve the most rapid abrasive action of the bur. **(B)** Incisal view of the forces generated during high-speed rotary tooth preparation. As the bur rotates in a clockwise direction, it generates a rotational force at the tooth surface, F_B (*large blue arrow* that represents schematically the force of tooth structure against the bur). The operator of the instrument must generate an opposing force, F_o (*green arrow*), which will exceed the rotational force of the bur, F_B, and carry the instrument against the tooth surface where the surface will be abraded.

between the substrate and the abrasive. Too little lubricant results in increased heat generation and reduced cutting efficiency.

Erosion

Erosive wear is caused by hard particles impacting a substrate surface, carried by either a stream of liquid or a stream of air, as occurs in sandblasting a surface. Figure 16.5 illustrates schematically the processes of two-body abrasion, three-body abrasion, and hard particle erosion. Most dental laboratories have air-driven grit-blasting units that employ hard particle erosion to remove surface material. A distinction must be made between this type of erosion and chemical erosion, which involves chemicals such as acids and alkalis instead of hard particles to remove substrate material. Chemical erosion, more commonly called *acid etching* in dentistry, is not used as a method of finishing dental materials. It is used primarily to prepare tooth surfaces to enhance bonding or coating.

Hardness of Abrasives

As stated previously, the inherent strength of cutting blades or abrasive particles on a dental instrument must be great enough to remove particles of substrate material without becoming dull or fracturing too rapidly. The durability of an abrasive is related to the hardness of its particles or surface material. Hardness is a surface measurement of the resistance of one material to be plastically deformed by indenting or scratching another material. The first ranking of hardness was published in 1820 by Friedrich Mohs, a German mineralogist. He ranked 10 minerals by their relative scratch resistance in relation to one another. The least scratch-resistant mineral, talc, received a score of 1 and the most scratch-resistant mineral, diamond, received a score of 10.

Knoop and Vickers hardness tests are based on indentation methods that quantify the hardness of materials. The tip of a Knoop diamond indenter has an elongated pyramidal shape, whereas the Vickers diamond indenter has an equilateral pyramidal design. Both tests involve the application of the indenter to a test surface under a known load (usually 100 Newtons, or 100 N). The depth of surface penetration is reported as hardness in units of force per unit area. Although a number of other factors affect a material's abrasiveness, the farther apart a substrate and an abrasive are in hardness, the more efficient is the abrasion process. On the basis of a comparison of hardness values for several dental materials listed in Table 16.1, it is expected that silicon carbide and diamond abrasives will abrade dental porcelain more readily compared with garnet, even though the abrasive particles for all three materials have very sharp edge characteristics.

CRITICAL QUESTION

Why is it sometimes inappropriate to select the hardest abrasive to reduce the time required for finishing and polishing a prosthesis?

Abrasive Instrument Design

Abrasive Grits

Abrasive grits are derived from materials that have been crushed and passed through a series of mesh screens (sieves) to obtain different particle size ranges. Table 16.2 lists grit and particle sizes for commonly used dental abrasives. Dental abrasive grits are classified as coarse, medium coarse, medium, fine, and superfine, according to particle size. Experience generally indicates which grades of an abrasive give the best results in finishing a given material. Keep in mind that the rate of material removal is not the only important factor. The surface finish obtained with each abrasive is just as important. If too hard an abrasive is used or if the grain size is too coarse for use on a given material, deep scratches result in the substrate that cannot be removed easily in subsequent finishing operations. Additionally, if an abrasive does not have the proper particle shape or does not break down in a manner that creates or exposes new sharp-edged particles, it will tend to gouge the substrate.

CRITICAL QUESTION

How can one differentiate between high-quality and low-quality bonded abrasive tools?

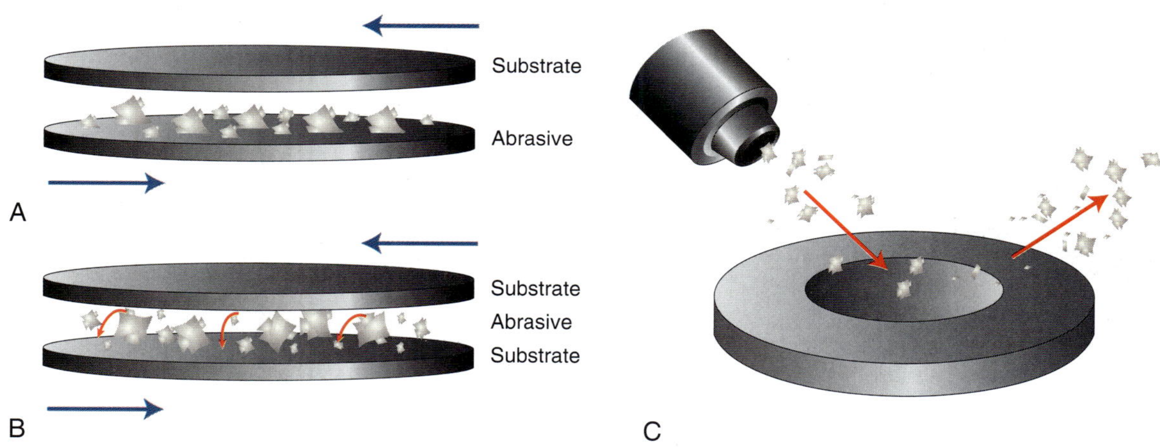

• **Fig. 16.5** Illustrations of two-body abrasion, three-body abrasion, and hard-particle erosion. **(A)** Two-body abrasion occurs when abrasive particles are tightly bonded to the abrasive instrument that is removing material from the substrate surface. **(B)** Three-body abrasion occurs when abrasive particles are free to translate and rotate between two surfaces. **(C)** Hard-particle abrasion (also called "air abrasion") is produced when abrasive particles are propelled against a substrate by air pressure.

TABLE 16.1 **Hardness Values of Dental Materials, Tooth Structure, and Abrasives**

Material	Mohs Hardness	Knoop Hardness (kg/mm^2)	Vickers Hardness (kg/mm^2)
Talc	1	—	—
Gypsum	2	—	12
Denture base resin	2–3	20	—
Cementum	—	40	—
Calcite	3	135	—
Metal-reinforced glass ionomer		14–24	40
Dentin	3–4	70	57–60
Type III gold alloy	3	—	122–180 (softened)/155–250 (hardened)
Type IV gold alloy	4	220	150–194 (softened)/248–280 (hardened)
Amalgam	4–5	90	120 (Ag_2Hg_3 phase)
Enamel (apatite)	5	340–431	294–408
Rouge	5–6	—	—
Glass (glass–ceramics)	5–6	360	—
Microfilled composite	5–7	30	37–160
Hybrid composite	5–7	55	61–159
Titanium (Ti)	—	—	210
Ti–6Al–4V	—	—	320
Nickel–chromium (Ni–Cr) alloy (as cast)	—	153–328	200–395
Cobalt–chromium (Co–Cr) alloy (as cast)	—	—	280–380
Layered gold alloy (for porcelain fused to metal [PFM])	—	—	35
Pressed lithia disilicate core	—	—	640
Tripoli	6	—	—
Pumice	6–7	460–560	—
Porcelain	6–7	560	430
Tin oxide	6–7	—	—
Sand	7	—	—
Cuttle	7	800	—
Quartz	7	820	—
Zirconium silicate	7.5	—	—
Garnet	8–9	1350	—
Emery	7–9	2000	—
Corundum	9	2000	—
Aluminum oxide	9	2100	1200
Tungsten carbide	9.8	1900	—
Silicon carbide	9–10	2500	—
Diamond	10	7000–10,000	—

Bonded Abrasives

Bonded abrasives consist of abrasive particles incorporated through a binder to form grinding tools such as points, wheels, separating disks, coated thin disks, and a wide variety of other abrasive shapes. Particles are bonded by four general methods: (1) sintering, (2) vitreous bonding (glass or ceramic), (3) resinous bonding (usually phenolic resin), and (4) rubber bonding (latex-based or silicone-based rubber). Because most of the rubber wheels, cups, and points contain latex, a known allergen, all residues must be removed from polished surfaces.

TABLE 16.2 Abrasive Particle Sizes[a]

Grit/Mesh (USA)	Aluminum Oxide, Silicon Carbide, and Garnet (μm)	Grade[b]	Coated Disk Diamond (μm)	Abrasive Descriptions for Diamond Burs and Diamond Polishing Paste
120	142	Coarse	142	Supercoarse–coarse
150	122		122	Coarse–regular
180	70–86		86	Coarse–regular
240	54–63		60	Fine
320	29–32	Medium	52	Fine
400	20–23		40	Fine–superfine–coarse finishing
600	12–17	Fine	14	Superfine–medium finishing
800	9–12		8	Ultrafine–fine finishing
1200	2–5	Superfine	6	Milling pastes
1500	1–2		4	Polishing pastes (2–5 μm)
2000	1		2	Polishing pastes (2–5 μm)

[a]Average particle sizes. Grades vary among manufacturers.
[b]Four grades used for a popular brand for aluminum oxide–coated disks. Silicon carbide (SiC) and garnet may vary among manufacturers.

Abrasive disks are used for bulk reduction, contouring, finishing, and polishing of restoration surfaces. Most types of disks are coated with aluminum oxide abrasive. Abrasive strips with either a plastic or metal backing are also available to smooth and polish the proximal surfaces of all direct and indirect bonded restorations. Metal strips are usually limited to situations in which very tight proximal contacts are involved. They are particularly useful for ceramic restorations but are also used for resin composites and amalgams. However, care must be taken to avoid lacerating the gingival tissues. Metal-backed strips are more costly, but they can be autoclaved and used several times if they are not damaged. Plastic-backed strips are used primarily for resin composites, compomers, hybrid ionomers, and resin cements.

Sintered abrasives are the strongest type because the abrasive particles are fused together. Vitreous-bonded abrasives are mixed with a glassy or ceramic matrix material, cold pressed to the instrument shape, and fired to fuse the binder. Resin-bonded abrasives are cold pressed or hot pressed and then heated to cure the resin. Hot pressing yields an abrasive binder with extremely low porosity. Rubber-bonded abrasives are made in a manner similar to that for resin-bonded abrasives.

The type of bonding method employed for the abrasive greatly affects the grinding behavior of the tool on the substrate. Bonded abrasives that tend to disintegrate rapidly against a substrate are too weak and result in increased abrasive costs because of the reduced instrument life. Those that tend to degrade too slowly get clogged with grinding debris, which results in loss of abrasive efficiency, increased heat generation, and increased finishing time. An ideal binder holds the abrasive particles in the tool long enough to cut, grind, or polish the substrate, and yet it releases the particles either before cutting efficiency is lost or before heat buildup causes thermal damage to the substrate. Binders are specially formulated for substrate-specific applications. Several examples of bonded abrasives are shown in Figure 16.6.

CRITICAL QUESTION

What are the purposes of truing a grinding instrument?

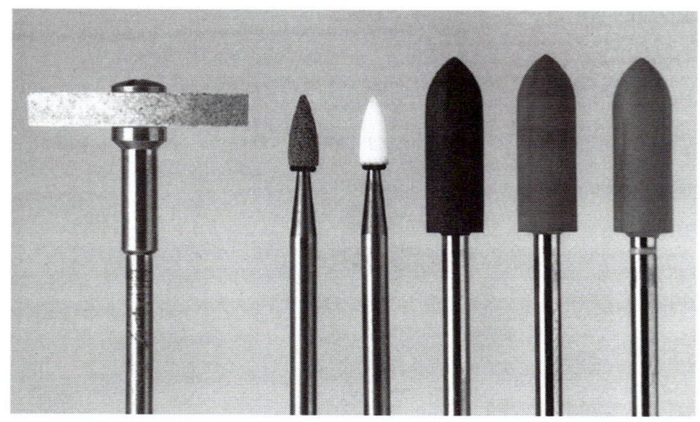

• **Fig. 16.6** Typical bonded abrasive instruments used in the dental laboratory include vitreous-bonded abrasive wheels and points (*three instruments on left*) and rubber-bonded abrasive bullets (*three instruments on right*).

A bonded abrasive instrument should always be trued and dressed before use. *Truing* is a procedure by which the abrasive instrument is run against a harder abrasive block until the abrasive instrument rotates in the handpiece without eccentricity or runout when placed on the substrate. The *dressing* procedure, like truing, is used to shape the instrument, but it accomplishes two different purposes as well. First, the dressing procedure reduces the instrument to its correct working size and shape. Second, it is used to remove clogged debris from the abrasive instrument to restore grinding efficiency during the finishing operation. The clogging of the abrasive instrument with debris is called *abrasive blinding*. Abrasive blinding occurs when the debris generated from grinding or polishing occludes the small spaces between the abrasive particles on the tool and reduces the depth that particles can penetrate into the substrate. As a result, abrasive efficiency is lost and greater heat is generated. A blinded abrasive appears to have a coating of the substrate material on its surface. Frequent dressing of the abrasive instrument during the finishing operation on a truing instrument, as illustrated in Figure 16.7, maintains the efficiency of the abrasive in removing the substrate material.

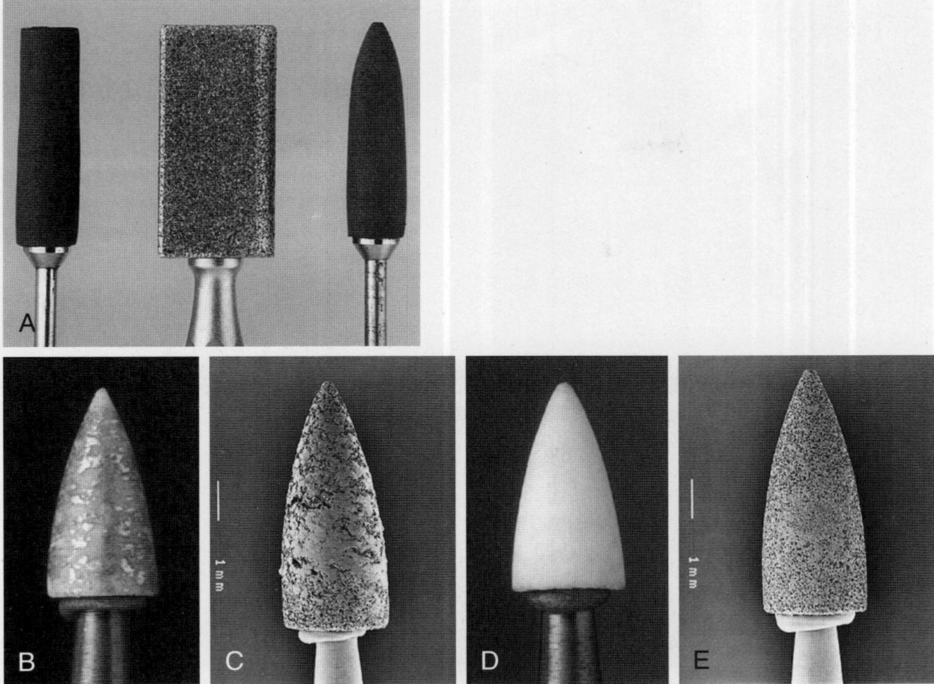

• **Fig. 16.7** A dressing tool is used to true, shape, and clean bonded abrasive instruments both before and during the finishing procedure. **(A)** A rubber-bonded abrasive cylinder (*left*) shows irregular external contours, which will cause it to run eccentrically. The cylinder is first trued against a diamond-coated abrasive dressing tool (*center*) to make it rotate around the central axis of the instrument. Once trued, the abrasive is further dressed to a desired working shape (*right*). **(B)** Instruments that are blinded with debris lose their cutting efficiency and generate more heat during operation. Note the coating of debris on the abrasive surface. **(C)** A scanning electron micrograph of the same instrument reveals the significant amount of debris that is clogging the instrument surface. **(D)** Frequent dressing of the abrasive on the dressing tool shown in the first photograph removes accumulated debris and restores cutting efficiency. **(E)** A scanning electron micrograph of the blinded abrasive after dressing reveals that the debris has been removed and the abrasive surface restored.

Binders for diamond abrasives are manufactured specifically to resist abrasive particle loss rather than to degrade at a certain point and release particles. One reason for this is that diamond is the hardest material known—so hard that diamond abrasive particles do not lose their cutting efficiency against substrates and, therefore there is no need for new abrasive particles to be exposed during the grinding process. Another reason is that diamond grits are expensive and must be used in limited quantities for instrument manufacture. Special bonding processes have been designed to allow for extended instrument life by keeping the abrasive particles firmly bound to the instrument shank with maximum particle exposure.

Diamond particles are bonded to metal wheels and bur blanks with special heat-resistant resins such as polyimides. The supercoarse through fine grades are then plated with a refractory metal film such as nickel. The nickel plating provides improved particle retention and acts as a heat sink during grinding. Titanium nitride coatings are used as an additional layer on some of the recent diamond abrasive instruments to further extend their longevity. Finishing diamonds used for resin-based composites contain diamond particles 40 μm or less in diameter, and many are not nickel plated. Therefore, they are highly susceptible to debonding and should always be used with light force and copious water spray to ensure retention of the very fine diamond particles. Diamond burs should always be used in the presence of water spray and at rotational speeds of less than 50,000 revolutions per minute (rpm).

Diamond instruments are preshaped and trued; they are not treated like other bonded abrasives. Diamond cleaning stones are used on the supercoarse through fine grades to remove debris buildup and to maintain grinding efficiency. An example of a diamond cleaning stone is shown in Figure 16.8. Cleaning stones should not be used on finishing diamonds because their bonded particles are quickly removed. Manufacturers provide special operating and cleaning instructions for these instruments.

Coated Abrasive Disks and Strips

Coated abrasives are fabricated by securing abrasive particles to a flexible backing material (heavyweight paper, metal, or Mylar) with a suitable adhesive material. These abrasives typically are supplied as disks and finishing strips. Disks are available in different diameters and with thin and very thin backing thicknesses. A further designation is made in regard to whether or not the disk or strip is moisture resistant. It is advantageous to use abrasive disks or strips with moisture-resistant backings because their stiffness is not reduced by water degradation. Furthermore, moisture acts as a lubricant to improve cutting efficiency. Examples of coated abrasives are shown in Figure 16.9.

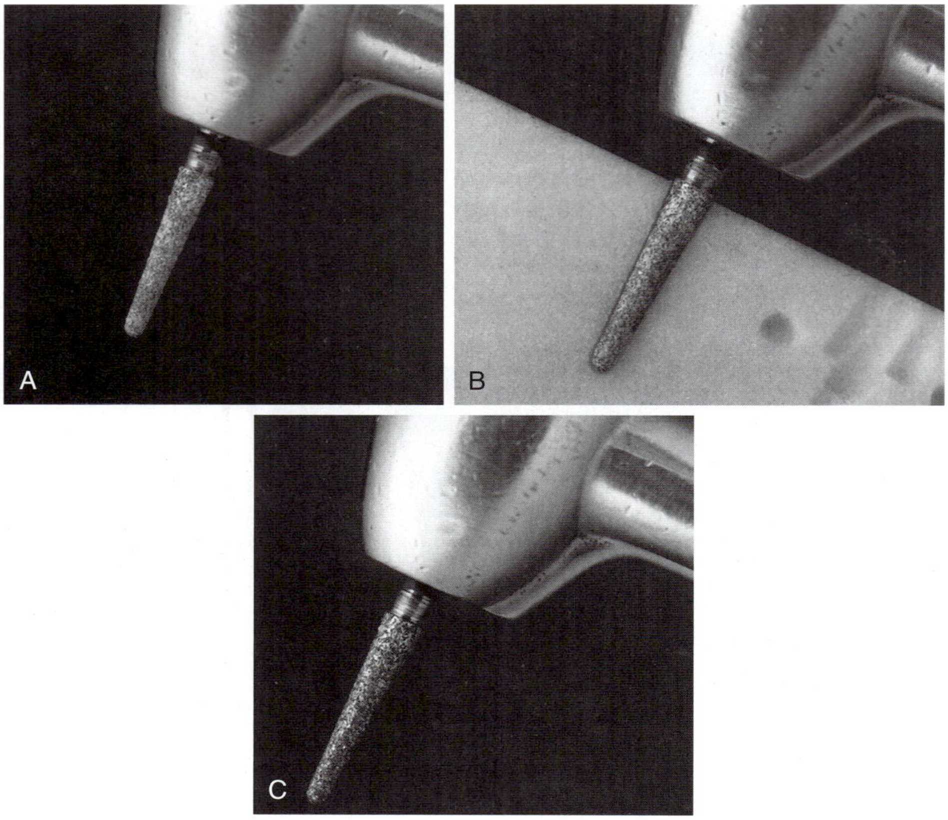

• **Fig. 16.8** A diamond cleaning stone is used to remove debris from diamond instruments. **(A)** Diamond bur in high-speed rotary handpiece before cleaning. Note the accumulated debris. **(B)** The bur is cleaned by running it against the moistened diamond cleaning stone for 2–4 seconds. **(C)** The cleaned diamond bur has no debris remaining between the diamond abrasive particles.

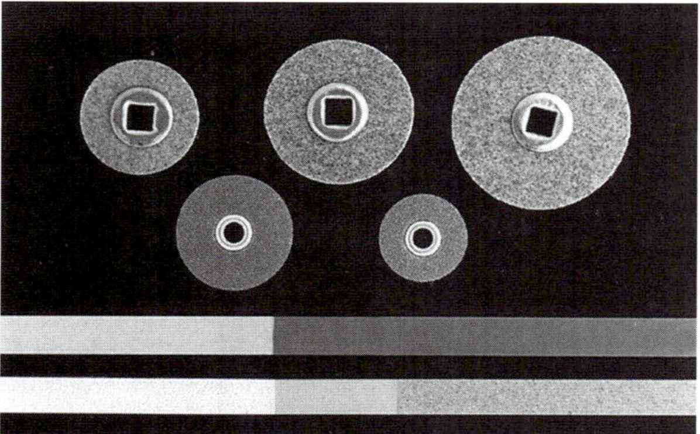

• **Fig. 16.9** Coated abrasive disks and strips. Disks are available in several sizes and with both paper and moisture-resistant backings. Paper-backed disks are represented by the top row of disks; moisture-resistant Mylar-backed disks are shown in the second row. Mylar-backed abrasive strips may be coated with two different grades of abrasive. The coatings are separated in the center of the strip by an uncoated area, which allows the strip to be passed between teeth.

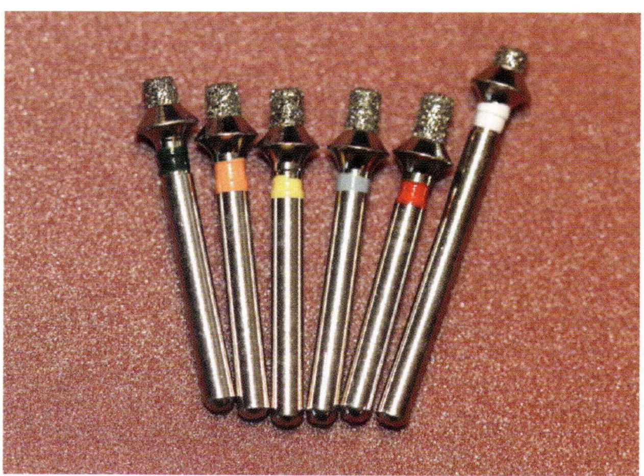

• **Fig. 16.10** Specialized diamond burs for occlusal reduction of tooth surfaces. The color-coded bands refer to the depth of the cutting portion. The depths are as follows: 1.0 mm (white), 1.5 mm (green), 1.8 mm (orange), 2.0 mm (yellow), 2.2 mm (blue), and 2.4 mm (red).

Different manufacturers use various coding conventions to allow the user to differentiate between coarse, medium, and fine abrasive grits. This situation was explained earlier for Sof-Lex disks. Examples of different types of abrasive instruments and abrasive grades are shown in Figures 16.10–16.15.

Nonbonded Abrasives

Polishing pastes are considered nonbonded abrasives and are primarily used for final polishing. They must be applied to the substrate with a nonabrasive device such as synthetic foam, rubber, felt, or chamois cloth. The abrasive particles are dispersed in a

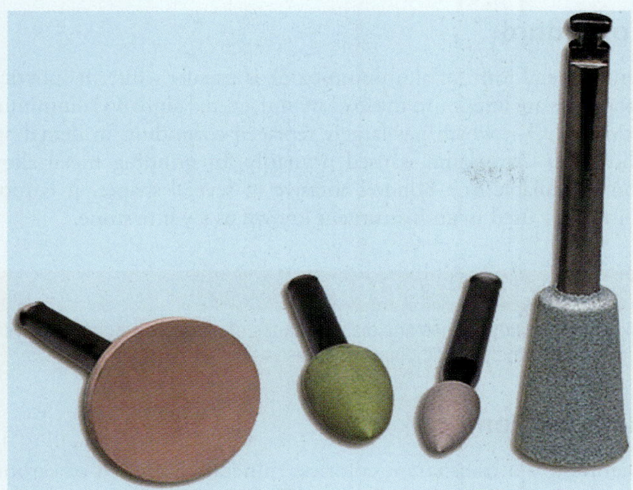

• **Fig. 16.11** Astropol (Ivoclar Vivadent) polishing kit with wheel, point, and cup shapes.

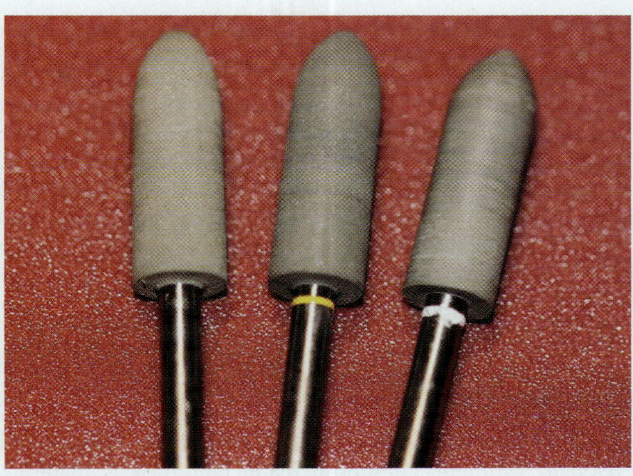

• **Fig. 16.13** Rubberized abrasive points with color-coded bands or no band to indicate relative levels of abrasiveness. Because of variability in color coding, the websites of the manufacturer or supplier should be referred to for the color codes and indications for use.

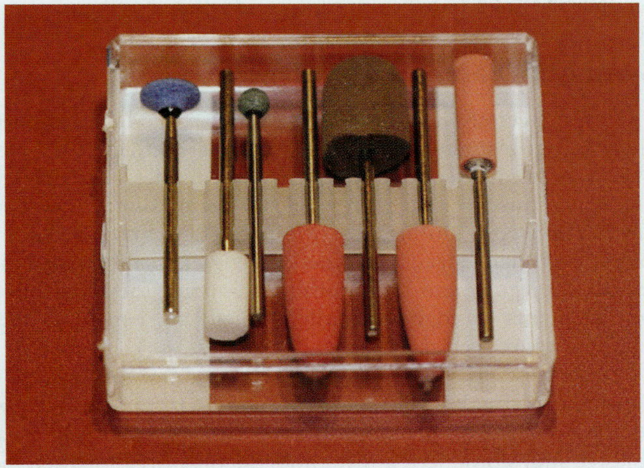

• **Fig. 16.12** Kit for laboratory grinding and finishing of metals. Typically, green mounted stones contain silicon carbide and are useful for shaping, adjusting, finishing, and fine grinding of high-noble and noble cast alloys. The blue, brown, and white mounted stones are useful for noble and base metal alloys that are used for metal–ceramic prostheses. The pink mounted points and cylinder are used for hard metals such as cobalt–chromium alloys. The user should check whether these devices are intended for benchtop lathes or for handpieces.

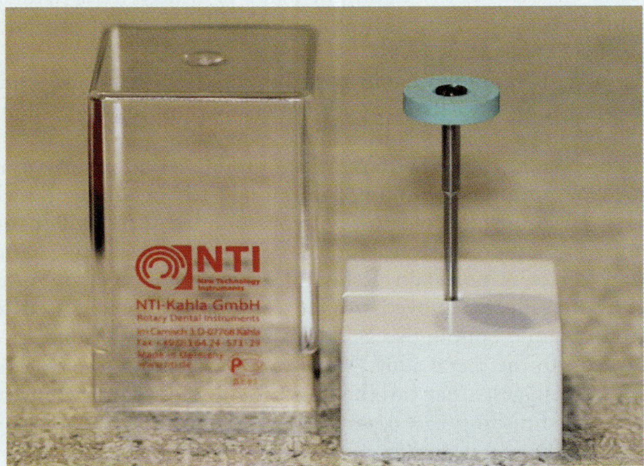

• **Fig. 16.14** Abrasive wheel for grinding zirconia and other ceramics.

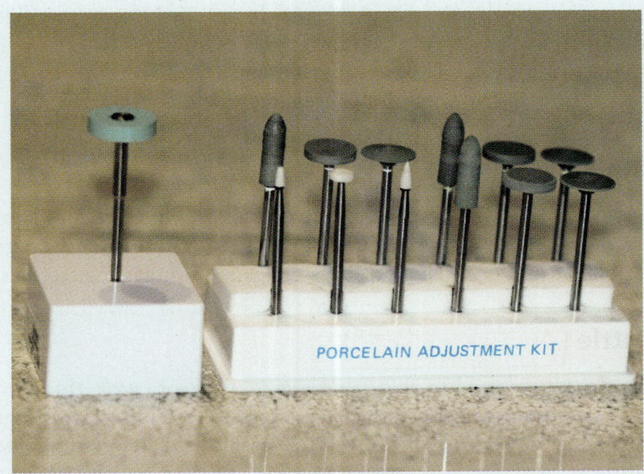

• **Fig. 16.15** Porcelain finishing kit. Note the yellow and white bands on the mandrels (shanks) to distinguish the levels of abrasiveness.

water-soluble medium such as glycerin for dental applications. Aluminum oxide and diamond are the most popular nonbonded abrasives.

Abrasive Motion

The motion of abrasive instruments is classified as rotary, planar, or reciprocal. In general, burs act in a rotary motion and disks in a planar motion, and reciprocating handpieces provide a cyclic motion and are reciprocal in relationship to their direction of motion. Different sizes of abrasives can be incorporated with each motion. Reciprocating handpieces especially provide the benefit of accessing interproximal and subgingival areas to remove overhangs, finish subgingival margins without creating ditches, and create embrasures.

Types of Abrasives

Many types of abrasive materials are available, but only those commonly used in dentistry are discussed in this section. Natural abrasives include Arkansas stone, chalk, corundum, diamond, emery, garnet, pumice, quartz, sand, tripoli, and zirconium silicate. Cuttle and kieselguhr are derived from the remnants of living organisms. Manufactured abrasives are synthesized materials, which are generally preferred because of their more predictable physical properties. Silicon carbide, aluminum oxide, synthetic diamond, rouge, and tin oxide are examples of manufactured abrasives.

Aluminum Oxide

Fused aluminum oxide was the second synthetic abrasive to be developed. Synthetic aluminum oxide (alumina) is made as a white powder and can be somewhat harder than corundum (natural alumina) because of its purity. However, corundum has a Mohs hardness of approximately 9 (on a scale of 1–10). Alumina can be processed with different properties by slight alteration of the reactants in the manufacturing process. Several grain sizes of alumina are available, and alumina has largely replaced emery for several abrasive uses. Aluminum oxide is widely used to make bonded abrasives, coated abrasives, and air-propelled grit abrasives for dental applications.

Sintered aluminum oxide is used to make white stones, which are popular for adjusting dental enamel and finishing metal alloys, resin-based composites, and ceramic materials.

Pink and ruby variations of aluminum oxide abrasives are made by adding chromium compounds to the original melt. These variations are sold in a vitreous-bonded form as noncontaminating mounted stones for the preparation of metal–ceramic alloys to receive porcelain. Remnants of these abrasives and other debris should be removed from the surface of metals used for metal–ceramic bonding so as not to prevent optimal bonding of porcelain to the metal alloy. A review by Yamamoto (see Selected Reading) suggests that carbide burs are the most effective instruments for finishing this type of alloy because they do not contaminate the metal surface with entrapped abrasive particles.

Arkansas Stone

This abrasive material is a semitranslucent light-gray siliceous sedimentary rock mined in Arkansas. It contains microcrystalline quartz and is dense, hard, and uniformly textured. Small pieces of this mineral are attached to metal shanks and trued to various shapes for fine grinding of tooth enamel and metal alloys.

Chalk

One of the mineral forms of calcite is chalk, a white abrasive composed of calcium carbonate. Chalk is used as a mild abrasive paste to polish tooth enamel, gold foil, amalgam, and plastic materials.

Cuttle

Commonly referred to as *cuttlefish*, *cuttlebone*, or *cuttle*, this abrasive is a white calcareous powder made from the pulverized internal shell of a Mediterranean marine mollusk of the genus *Sepia*. Cuttle is available as a coated abrasive and is useful for delicate abrasion operations such as the polishing of metal margins and dental amalgam restorations.

Corundum

This mineral form of aluminum oxide is usually white. Its physical properties are inferior to those of manufactured alpha (α) aluminum oxide (Al_2O_3), which has largely replaced corundum in dental applications. Corundum is used primarily for grinding metal alloys and is available as a bonded abrasive in several shapes. It is most commonly used in an instrument known as a white stone.

CRITICAL QUESTION

What are the advantages and disadvantages of natural diamond abrasives compared with synthetic diamond abrasives?

Natural Diamond

Diamond is a transparent colorless mineral composed of carbon. It is the hardest known substance. Diamond is called a *superabrasive* because of its ability to abrade any other known substance. Diamond abrasives are supplied in several forms, including bonded abrasive rotary instruments, flexible metal-backed abrasive strips, and diamond polishing pastes. They are mostly used on ceramic and resin-based composite materials.

Synthetic Diamond Abrasives

The advantages of synthetic diamonds over natural diamonds include their consistent size and shape as well as their lower cost. The shape of the diamond determines the binder needed for its use, which can be either resin or metal. Resin-bonded diamonds have sharp edges. During use, the sharp edges break down and expose new sharp edges and corners. However, metal-bonded diamonds are regular and more consistent in size. They function as cutting points or edges primarily through the benefit of their hardness rather than their shape.

Larger synthetic diamond particles appear greenish because of the chemical reaction with nickel during the manufacturing process. Manufactured diamond is used almost exclusively as an abrasive and is produced at five times the quantity of natural diamond abrasive. This abrasive is used in the manufacture of diamond saws, wheels, and burs. Blocks with embedded diamond particles are used to true other types of bonded abrasives. Diamond polishing pastes are also produced from particles smaller than 5 μm in diameter. Synthetic diamond abrasives are used primarily on tooth structure, ceramic materials, and resin-based composite materials.

Emery

This abrasive is a grayish-black corundum prepared in a fine grain form. Emery is used predominantly in coated abrasive disks and is available in a variety of grit sizes. It may be used for finishing metal alloys or acrylic resin materials.

Garnet

The term *garnet* includes a number of different minerals that possess similar physical properties and crystalline forms. These minerals are the silicates of aluminum, cobalt, iron, magnesium, and manganese. The garnet abrasive used in dentistry is usually dark red. Garnet is extremely hard and, when fractured during the grinding operation, it forms sharp, chisel-shaped plates, making it a highly effective abrasive. Garnet is available on coated disks and arbor bands. It is used in grinding metal alloys and acrylic resin materials.

Kieselguhr

This material is composed of the siliceous remains of minute aquatic plants known as *diatoms*. The coarser form of kieselguhr is called *diatomaceous earth* and is used as a filler in many dental materials such as the hydrocolloid impression materials. Kieselguhr is an excellent mild abrasive; however, the risk of respiratory silicosis caused by chronic exposure to airborne particles of this material is significant, so appropriate precautions should always be taken.

Pumice

Volcanic activity produces this light-gray highly siliceous material. It is used mainly in grit form but can be found in some rubber-bonded abrasives. Both pumice forms are used on acrylic resin materials. Flour of pumice, an extremely fine grained volcanic rock derivative from Italy, is used in polishing tooth enamel, direct-filling gold, dental amalgam, and acrylic resins.

Quartz

The most commonly used form of silica (SiO_2) is quartz, a very hard (Mohs hardness of 7), colorless, and transparent mineral. It is the most abundant and widespread of minerals. Quartz crystalline particles are pulverized to form sharp, angular particles that are useful in making coated abrasive disks. Quartz abrasives are used primarily to finish metal alloys, and they may also be used to grind dental enamel.

Sand

This abrasive is a mixture of small mineral particles predominantly composed of silica. These particles represent a mixture of colors, making sand abrasives distinct in appearance. Sand particles have a rounded to angular shape. They are applied under air pressure, through a process called *sandblasting*, to remove refractory investment materials from base metal alloy castings. They are also coated onto paper disks for grinding metal alloys and acrylic resin materials.

Tripoli

This abrasive is derived from a lightweight, friable siliceous sedimentary rock. Tripoli can be white, gray, pink, red, or yellow. The gray and red types are most frequently used in dentistry. The rock is ground into very fine particles and formed with soft binders into bars of polishing compound. Tripoli is used for polishing metal alloys and some acrylic resin materials.

Rouge

Iron oxide is the fine red abrasive component of rouge. Like tripoli, rouge is blended with various soft binders into a cake form. It is used to polish high-noble metal alloys such as yellow gold alloys.

Silicon Carbide

This extremely hard abrasive was the first of the synthetic abrasives to be produced. Green and blue–black types of silicon carbides are produced; both types have equivalent physical properties. The green form is often preferred because substrates are more visible against the green color. Silicon carbide is extremely hard and brittle. The particles are sharp, and they break to form new sharp particles. This results in highly efficient cutting of a wide variety of materials, including metal alloys, ceramics, and acrylic resin materials. Silicon carbide is available as an abrasive in coated disks and as vitreous- and rubber-bonded instruments.

Tin Oxide

This extremely fine abrasive material is used extensively as a polishing agent for polishing teeth and metallic restorations such as dental amalgams in the mouth. It is mixed with water, alcohol, or glycerin to form a mildly abrasive paste.

Zirconium Silicate

Zircon or zirconium silicate ($ZrSiO_4$) is supplied as an off-white mineral. It is ground to various particle sizes and used to make coated abrasive disks and strips. It is frequently used as a component of dental prophylaxis pastes.

Zirconium oxide: This abrasive is tougher than aluminum oxide and usually used as a mixture with aluminum oxide primarily in elastic or rubber-like finishing and polishing rotary-shaped instruments.

Abrasive Pastes

The most commonly used abrasive pastes contain either aluminum oxide (alumina) or diamond particles. Alumina pastes should be used with a rotary instrument and increasing amounts of water as the polishing process proceeds from the use of coarser to finer abrasive particles. Diamond abrasive pastes are used in a relatively dry condition. The instruments that apply the paste to the material surface are equally important. These include ribbed prophy cups (the ribbed type or the more flexible nonribbed type), brushes, and felt wheels. Abrasive pastes have several disadvantages: First, they are relatively thick and cannot gain access to embrasures. Second, the pastes tend to splatter when they spin off of the instruments at excessive rotational speeds or if they become wet. Third, heat is generated when insufficient coolant is used or when continuous polishing pressure is applied without allowing coolant to reach the surface.

CRITICAL QUESTION

Which procedure will ensure that progressively finer abrasives completely remove scratches made by previous coarse abrasives?

Finishing and Polishing Procedures

Resin-Based Composite Restorations

Dental composites are among the most difficult types of materials to predictably finish and polish to a high luster because they contain a relatively soft resin matrix and hard filler particles in their structures. Each resin composite brand contains a different microstructure. Therefore, there are varying methods for finishing and polishing different composites and different time requirements for achieving a desirable luster (Fig. 16.16). Additionally, the maintenance of the luster over time can vary considerably because of the microstructural differences (Fig. 16.17). This means that there

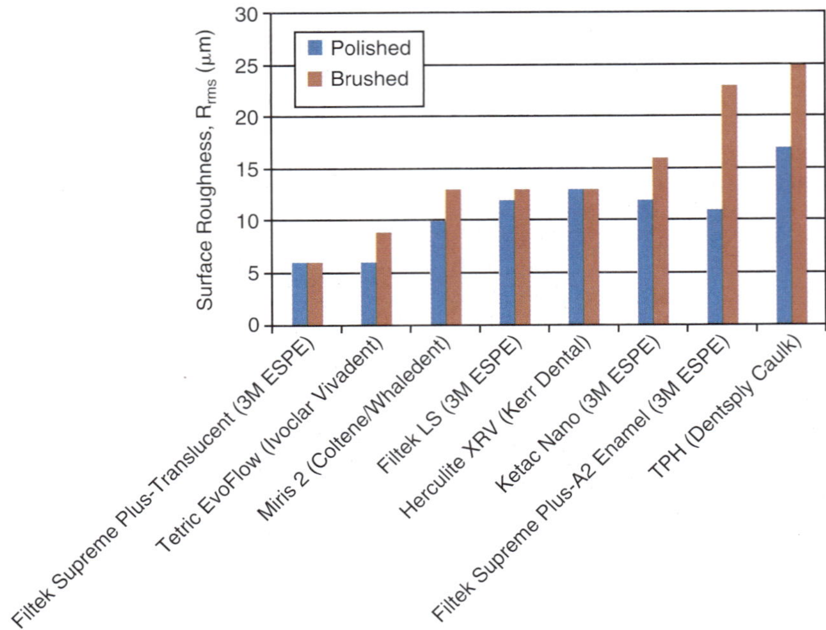

• **Fig. 16.16** Influence of toothbrushing on surface roughness of various direct restorative materials. (Courtesy of Dr J-H Phark.)

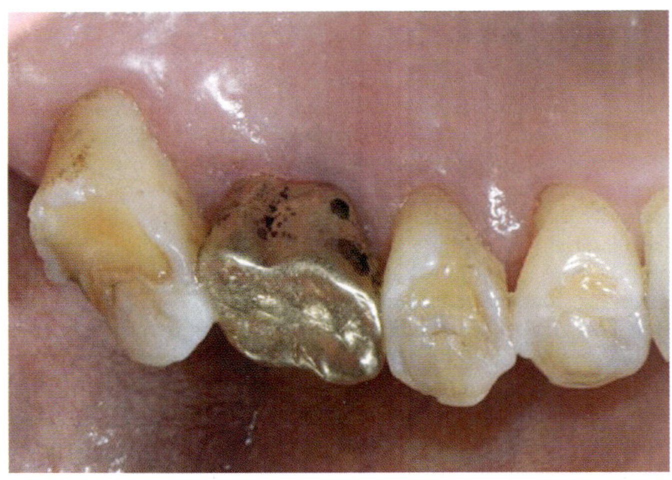

• **Fig. 16.17** Maintenance of gloss for different resin composites subjected to toothbrush abrasion.

must be selective grinding associated with the soft material and the harder particles, a situation that is especially apparent with hybrid composites. In addition, the final finish of a composite restoration depends on the fillers and resin matrix, the preparation design, curing effectiveness, and postcuring time required for the material to achieve its final properties. For some composite materials, a delay of 10 minutes or more is recommended after curing to allow complete polymerization to occur.

Exposed filler particles create peaks and valleys that prevent the surface from acquiring a high luster. During each stage of finishing and polishing, the operator should proceed in one direction only. Then, after the use of the next abrasive in the sequence, polishing should continue in a direction perpendicular to the previous one. This process ensures that scratches become more visible and that the effectiveness of scratch removal can be assessed more rapidly. The recommended abrasives and polishing instruments should be used in the proper sequence, and intermediate abrasive steps should never be skipped. For example, following a coarse abrasive disk with a fine abrasive rather than a medium-grit abrasive would leave some of the scratches produced by the coarse abrasive. The operator can choose to use one system from start to finish (such as abrasive-coated or flexible abrasive-impregnated rubber disks) or combine different systems based on preference and the location of the restoration (such as impregnated disks for anterior or a brush for posterior sites).

The material's intrinsic factors, such as resin monomer type and concentration of filler particles, are important for the clinical performance of restorative materials. It is important for manufacturers to inform clinicians about the specific finishing and polishing systems for their materials depending on the composition, filler size, type and loading, and hardness.

Recently some manufacturers have introduced spirals that are made with either aluminum oxide or diamond particles impregnated in a thermoplastic elastomer (Fig. 16.18) (Sof-Lex Spirals, 3M). The universal shape allows for usage on all tooth surfaces and reduces the need for different shaped tools (e.g., points, cups, disks, and brushes), which are designed for specific shapes and contours.

The claimed advantages include:

- Adapts to all tooth surfaces
- Works from any angle
- Effective for anterior and posterior restorations
- Helps create natural gloss in two steps

These can be used with direct and indirect restorations and work with a variety of materials including, composite restorations, resin-modified glass ionomers, bisacrylic temporary materials, CAD/CAM restorative materials like zirconia, and precious and semiprecious metals. Another advantage of these spirals is that they can be sterilized and reused making them cost-effective.

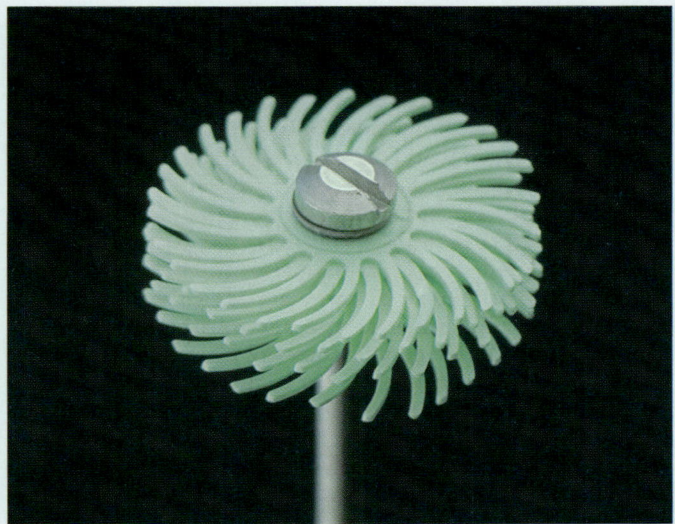

• **Fig. 16.18** Spiral wheel polishers are designed for maximal flexibility of use on most areas of a restoration. These polishers have a polyamide rubber construction and are available in different diameters with several types and grits of embedded abrasive. Laboratory and clinic polishers are available for use on denture acrylics, composites, ceramics, and precious metals. (Courtesy Dr Farzan Pouranfar.)

Additionally, multiple polishing pastes are available some of which contain diamond as the polishing agent. These could be used with a buff or goats hair brush to get the final luster (Box 16.2).

The finishing and polishing technique consists of these essential steps:

- First, contour the restoration either with 12-fluted carbide burs, 30–100 μm diamond burs, or coarse abrasive-coated disks, depending on the dentist's preference.
- Next, finish with 16- to 30-fluted carbide burs, fine and extrafine diamond burs, white stones (aluminum oxide), white Arkansas stones, or medium and fine abrasive-coated disks.
- Interproximal finishing and polishing are accomplished with gapped finishing and polishing strips covered with aluminum oxide abrasive particles, or with metal strips covered with submicron diamond particles.
- Finally, polish with fine and extrafine polishing paste (aluminum oxide or diamond); extrafine abrasive-coated disks; silicon carbide–impregnated brushes; or diamond-impregnated rubber polishing disks, cups, or points or spirals. Most finishing and polishing systems, whether impregnated or coated with abrasive, are available in a variety of color-coded kits. Manufacturers' instructions for their use must be followed to obtain the optimal outcome.

Shown in Figure 16.19 are two clinical photographs of a class II composite restoration made of Tetric EvoCeram (Ivoclar Vivadent) resin-based composite after polishing (top left) and after 12 months of clinical service (top right). The bottom center image represents a laser-scanned image resulting from the superposition of the second surface scan over the one made at baseline. The red areas represent the loss of composite or tooth enamel during the 12-month period. The maximum wear depths at two of the sites were 160 and 190 μm. Well finished and polished restoration however large can survive for long periods with proper maintenance (Fig. 16.20A and B).

• BOX 16.2 Clinical Steps for Polishing Anterior Composite Restorations

1. Check the shape of the tooth by observing the angle lines, which create a reflective zone between the line angles and the shadow area, which lies outside the angle lines and is rounded. This correction of angle lines and flat area is made with medium grain disks or with fine grained diamond tips.
2. Then the contour of the incisal embrasures must be done. This contour may range from straight or curved. The outline of the embrasures is usually made with abrasive disks.
3. To finalize the details of shape, medium or fine grain diamond drills are used.
4. Interproximal polishing should be done with interproximal strips. Cervical excess can be removed with a #12 surgical blade.
5. After the details of shape and contour, pass a rubber or a rubber disk on the composite resin to smoothen the entire surface.
6. Create the vertical macrotexture. These vertical grooves are usually more open in incisal and will narrow toward the cervical giving the "V" shape to this depression.
7. The horizontal macrotexture is more evident in the cervical third and in the transition with the middle third of the tooth. This procedure is usually done with fine grain spherical diamond drills in low rotation.
8. Smoothen the macrotexture using rubber cups or cones.
9. Create vertical and horizontal microtexture as required using a very thin tipped diamond. The position of the tip relative to the vestibular surface of the restoration should be about 45°, using a very gentle pressure and always in the same direction.
10. Smoothen the surface using 3 m Sof-Lex spirals to create a shine on the restoration. In low gloss scenarios this would be the final step.
11. To finish the finishing and polishing process and give to the composite resin a natural appearance of enamel gloss, it is recommended to use a low-grade (less than 0.5 μm) diamond pastes or aluminum oxide pastes. These pastes should be applied with a felt disk or a soft-brushed brush.
12. These steps described earlier can be performed with water or without water. The advantage of not using water is to have a better visibility of the details. In this case, plenty of water should be used between each step to cool the tooth and clean all debris created by the instruments.

Dental Amalgam

Burnishing prior to carving provides the removal of the excess mercury and improves marginal adaptation, and burnishing after carving improves smoothness. However, burnishing alone will not provide a completely scratch- and retention-free surface for amalgam restorations. Slow-speed handpieces should be used for finishing and polishing amalgam restorations. In the past, a recommendation was made to wait 24 hours before polishing the amalgam restorations to allow amalgam to set completely. However, if the restoration's surface is finished initially with a very fine prophylaxis paste applied with a cotton pellet or a nonribbed rubber prophy cup rotated at slow speed and light pressure, a smooth, velvety finish is achieved that will acquire a luster as it is abraded normally in the mouth. Spherical amalgams set faster and can be finished and polished sooner.

If amalgam has hardened to an advanced stage in which the abrasion by a fine prophylaxis paste is no longer effective, the following procedure may be used at the next dental appointment: (1) Contour with slow-speed green stones or diamond burs or brown and green rubber points. (2) Apply a mixture of fine pumice and water or alcohol with a rotary brush or felt wheel to polish the surface (Fig. 16.20C).

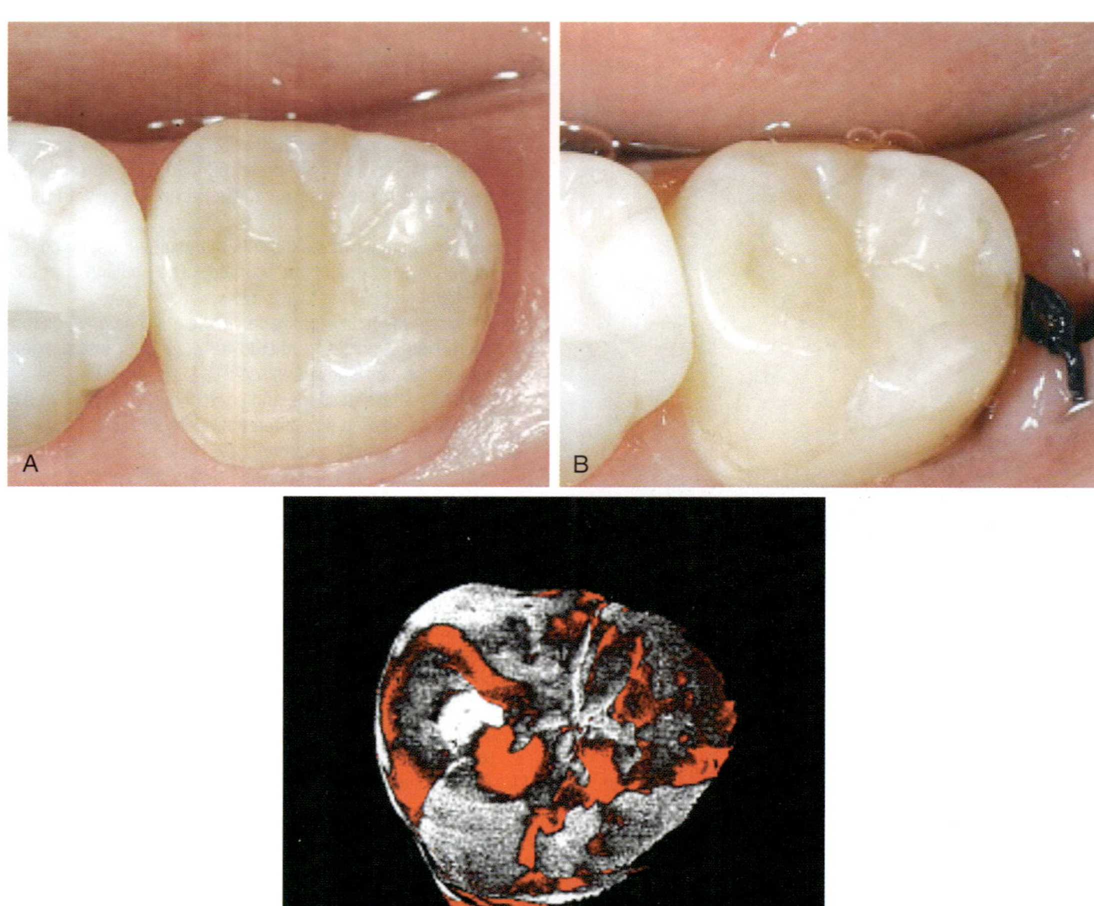

• **Fig. 16.19** Class II composite restoration made of Tetric EvoCeram (Ivoclar Vivadent) resin-based composite. **(A)** Baseline view of occlusal and buccal surfaces after polishing. **(B)** View of occlusal and buccal surfaces after 12 months. The material loss (red areas) between these surfaces **(C)** is revealed by superposing the two scanned images. The red areas indicate the loss of enamel or composite. Two areas with maximum wear depths of 160 and 190 μm that were measured via laser scanning, were not detectable by visual examination. (Photos provided courtesy of Dr Siegward Heintze.)

Gold Alloy

Pure gold is a very soft and ductile metal. Therefore, it requires a different approach from that used for many other metals used in dentistry. Slow-speed handpieces should be used for finishing and polishing gold alloys. This technique consists of the following steps: (1) contour with carbide burs, green stones (silicon carbide), or heatless stones; (2) finish with pink stones (aluminum oxide) or medium-grade abrasive-impregnated rubber wheels and points (brown and green); (3) apply fine abrasive-impregnated rubber wheels, cups, and points; and, if necessary, (4) apply tripoli or rouge with rag or leather wheels.

CRITICAL QUESTION

What are the differences between finishing and polishing a ceramic restoration extraorally and intraorally?

Ceramic Restorations

The ideal surface for ceramic restorations is a polished and glazed one. However, the production of a **glaze ceramic** through a **natural glaze** or **overglaze** process will not necessarily yield a smooth surface if the initial ceramic surface has significant roughness. The smoothest surfaces can be achieved extraorally before a prosthesis is cemented. In the mouth, minor roughness can be successfully polished without compromising the surface quality. In addition, polishing can improve the strength within the surface region of a ceramic prosthesis because it removes pores, microcracks, and other microscopic flaws. In addition (Fig. 16.21A and B), there is a strong correlation between the surface roughness and the color change of ceramics. Adequate cooling is important when ceramic restorations are finished and polished in vivo (Figs 16.22 and 16.23, Box 16.3). The use of an air–water spray device and maintaining intermittent contact between the restoration and the rotary instrument are critical during the operation.

Different ceramic materials need different polishing systems to achieve smooth finish. Continuous contact between the restoration and the rotary instrument should be avoided. A heatless stone (silicon carbide) provides heat reduction and can be used as an alternative. Several kits are available for finishing and polishing ceramic restorations (Figs 16.22 and 16.23). Manufacturers' instructions should be followed when these systems

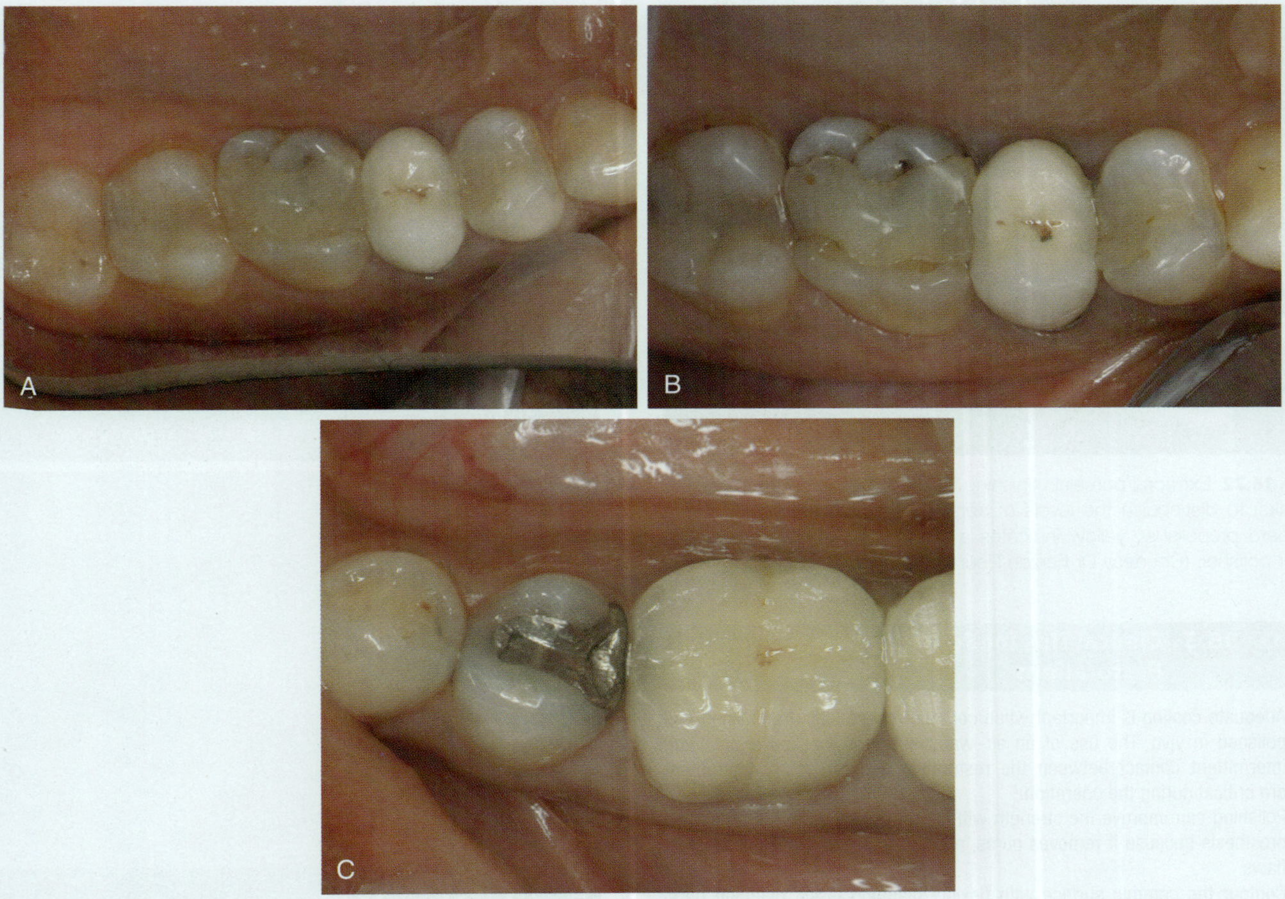

• **Fig. 16.20** **(A)** Large MOD restoration on 16 five years after placement. **(B)** MOD on 26 at 12 years. Disto-occlusal restoration on 14 is 14 years old. **(C)** Finished and polished amalgam restoration after 15 years of clinical service.

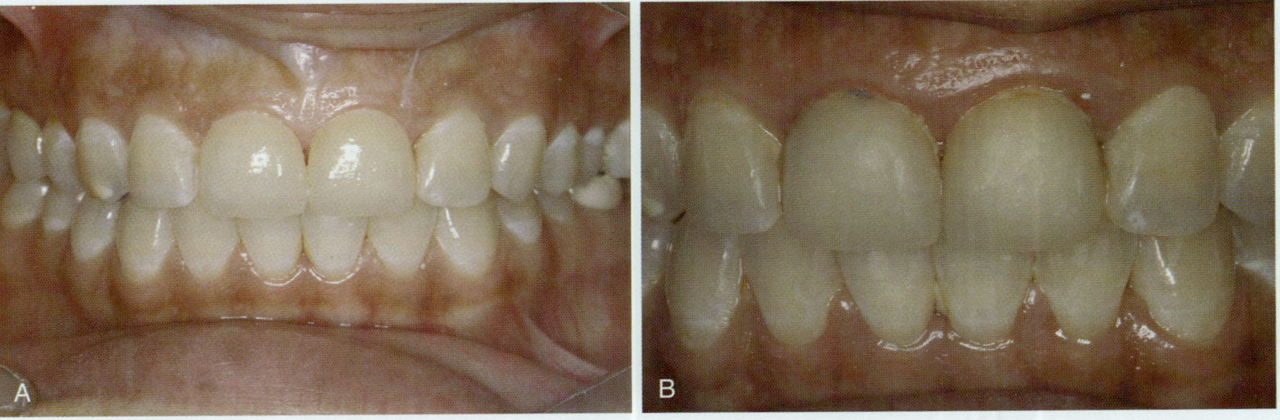

• **Fig. 16.21** **(A** and **B)** Left image shows anterior ceramic veneers immediately after placement. Right image shows same veneers after 7 years of clinical service with dicoloration and margin deterioration.

are used. Depending on the dentist's preference, a general technique is as follows:

1. Contour the ceramic surface with flexible diamond disks, diamond burs, heatless or polymer stones, or green stones (silicon carbide).
2. Finish with white stones or abrasive-impregnated rubber disks, cups, and points. This process may require two or three steps, depending on the system used.
3. Polish with fine abrasive-impregnated rubber disks, cups, and points or, if necessary, use a diamond paste applied with a brush or felt wheel.
4. Apply an overglaze layer or natural glaze on the ceramic, if necessary. For intraoral polishing, use an intermittent application of rotating instruments with a copious amount of water as a coolant.

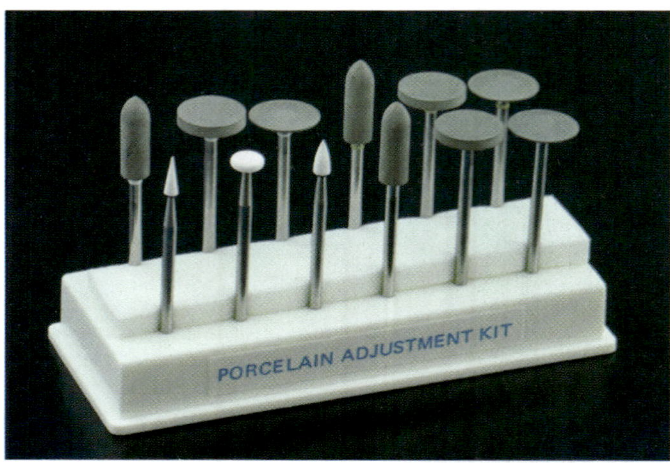

• **Fig. 16.22** Extraoral porcelain finishing kit. Note bands on the mandrels (shanks) to distinguish the levels of abrasiveness. No band indicates a standard prepolisher, yellow indicates a polisher, and white indicates a super polisher. (Courtesy Dr Farzan Pouranfar.)

• BOX 16.3 Clinical Tips for Polishing Ceramic Restorations

- Adequate cooling is important when ceramic restorations are finished and polished in vivo. The use of an air–water spray device and maintaining intermittent contact between the restoration and the rotary instrument are critical during the operation.
- Polishing can improve the strength within the surface region of a ceramic prosthesis because it removes pores, microcracks, and other microscopic flaws.
- Contour the ceramic surface with flexible diamond disks, diamond burs, heatless or polymer stones, or green stones (silicon carbide).
- Finish with white stones or abrasive-impregnated rubber disks, cups, and points. This process may require two or three steps, depending on the system used.
- Polish with fine abrasive-impregnated rubber disks, cups, and points or, if necessary, use a diamond paste applied with a brush or felt wheel.
- Apply an overglaze layer or natural glaze on the ceramic, if necessary. For intraoral polishing, use an intermittent application of rotating instruments with a copious amount of water as a coolant.

Monolithic zirconia is commonly used today to eliminate the chipping fractures of veneers that have been reported for several types of ceramic–ceramic systems based on an yttria-stabilized tetragonal zirconia particle (Y-TZP) system. Depending on the particle-size distribution of the zirconia and the amount of surface grinding required to adjust occlusion, the surface may be very difficult to grind and polish. Therefore, intraoral finishing and polishing may take significant chair time (Fig. 16.24).

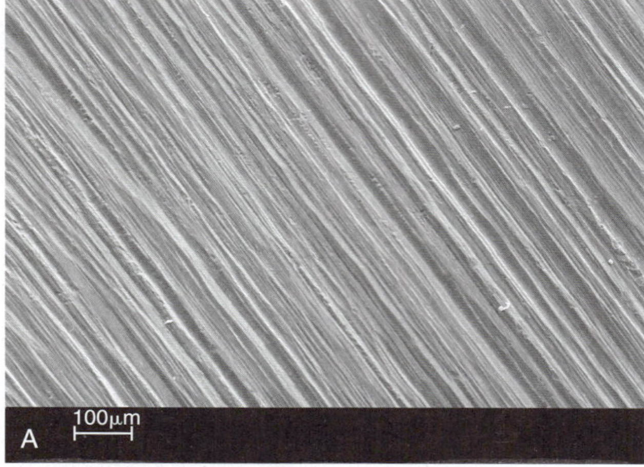

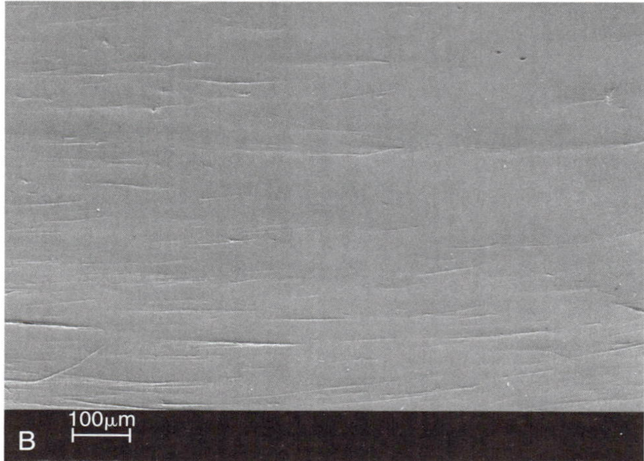

• **Fig. 16.24** **(A)** Zirconia surface finished with a fine diamond bur. **(B)** Zirconia surface polished using the Dialite/Diashine system. (Courtesy of Dr Siegward Heintze.)

For those providing chairside CAD-CAM zirconia restorations, carefully contouring and polishing milled zirconia restorations in their presintered state are recommended so that the sintered restorations have a near-perfect surface upon removal from the sintering furnace. This approach greatly reduces or eliminates the need for postsintering finishing and polishing. Figure 16.25 shows that milling markings will persist after sintering if not removed. In addition to time savings, there are two additional advantages to this approach: avoiding the risk of weakening the restoration from the conversion of the tetragonal zirconia phase to the monoclinic phase caused by grinding and eliminating the risk of creating a displeasing pearl-like surface appearance to the restoration from polishing.

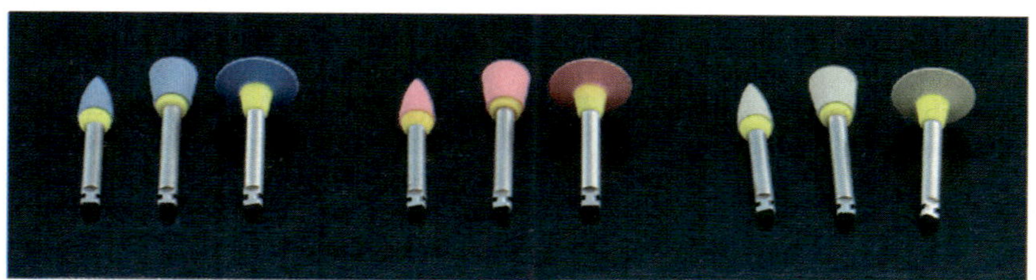

• **Fig. 16.23** Intraoral ceramic polishers for laminate veneer (Dialite intraoral polishers; Brasseler USA). Abrasive levels are blue (coarse), pink (medium), and gray (fine). (Courtesy Dr Farzan Pouranfar.)

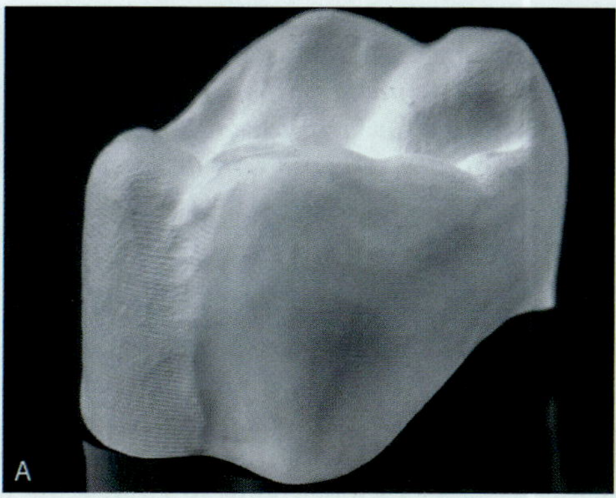

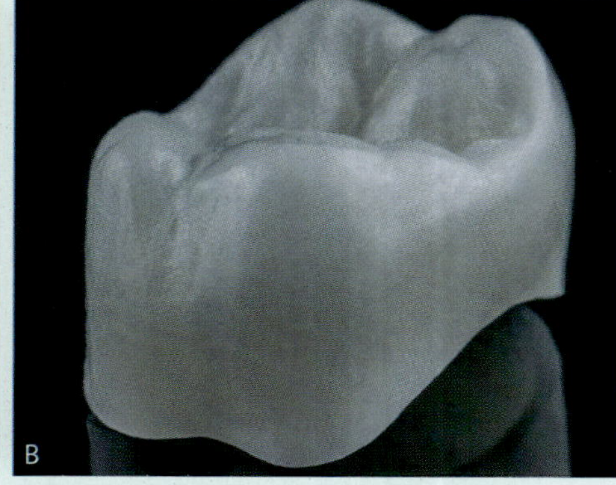

• **Fig. 16.25** Effect of sintering on milled and partially prepolished zirconia crown. **(A)** Presintered zirconia crown showing as-milled surface *(left)* and prepolished surface *(right)*. **(B)** Same restoration after fully sintering. Note difference in smoothness and that sintering does not remove milling striations. (Courtesy Dr Troy Decker.)

As mentioned previously, leaving rough contact surfaces on zirconia restorations is not recommended. This may result in a relatively rough surface, which may cause severe wear of opposing enamel or restorative material surfaces. A glaze layer may also wear rapidly, exposing the rough-milled surface of the zirconia (Figs 16.26 and 16.27).

New translucent monolithic zirconia has been developed to merge strength with improved tooth color matching. Unfortunately, the changes required to increase the translucency, also lead to a decrease in strength. The higher susceptibility to surface damage, as a result of increasing dopant concentration, may render polishing of ground, translucent zirconia more complicated compared to the conventional 3Y-TZP counterparts.

It is recommended that if occlusal adjustment is needed after delivery, the restoration should ideally be polished with a diamond-impregnated silicone polishing instrument (Fig. 16.28).

This should be followed by polishing paste which contains up to 20% diamond particles with a grain size of 2–4 μm and a maximum rotational speed of 15,000 rpm. This would also add to the overall luster and appearance of the restoration.

For occlusal adjustment, the use of a special diamond instrument with diamond grit (e.g., ZR grinder, Komet, Gebr. Brasseler; or K-Diamonds, Edenta) under water cooling has been recommended since they deliver greater performance and durability.

Monolithic translucent zirconia can also be adjusted using surface staining or a glaze spray. More esthetic results might be achieved by coloring presintered zirconia with an infiltration technique. Here, noncolored presintered zirconia is immersed in a colored liquid or the color is applied on the material using a brush. Fischer et al. (2013) introduced a multicolor concept for translucent zirconia. This method is especially useful when occlusal adjustment is anticipated and translucency of the monolithic material compromises the esthetic results.

It should also be considered that any coloring process may affect the physical and visual aspect of dental zirconia. It has been shown that coloring liquid had no effect on translucency of partially stabilized translucent zirconia, while it decreased the translucency of fully stabilized translucent zirconia types.

It has been suggested that 15,000 rpm is the optimum speed which produces the best polish.

Glaze ceramic layers over rough zirconia will eventually wear and expose the rough-milled surface of the zirconia (Fig. 16.26), which can cause greater wear on opposing enamel surfaces (Fig. 16.27). Lawson et al. demonstrated the advantages

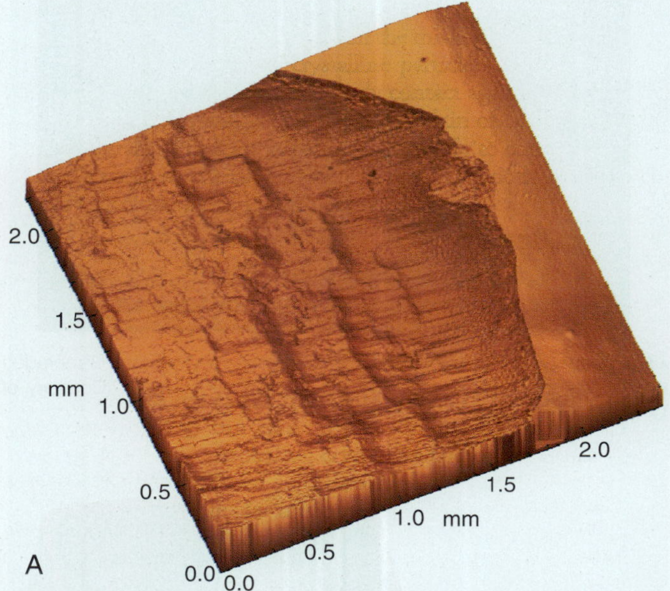

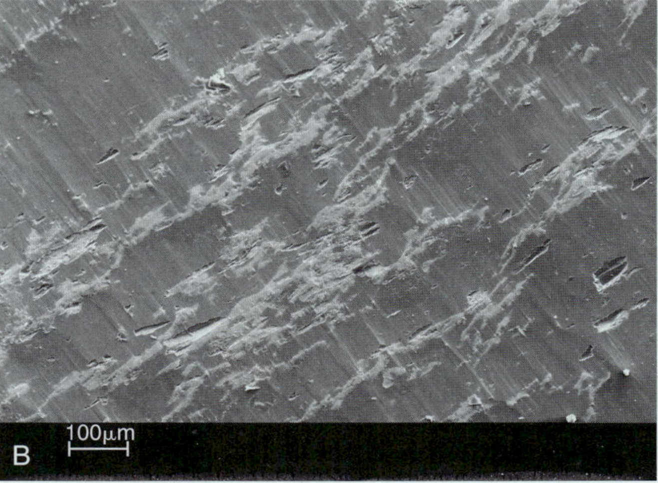

• **Fig. 16.26** Wear facet of a milled and glazed ceramic after wear simulation. Three-dimensional image generated with FRT MicroProf sensor **(A)** and a scanning electron micrograph **(B)** (×100 magnification). (Courtesy of Dr Siegward Heintze.)

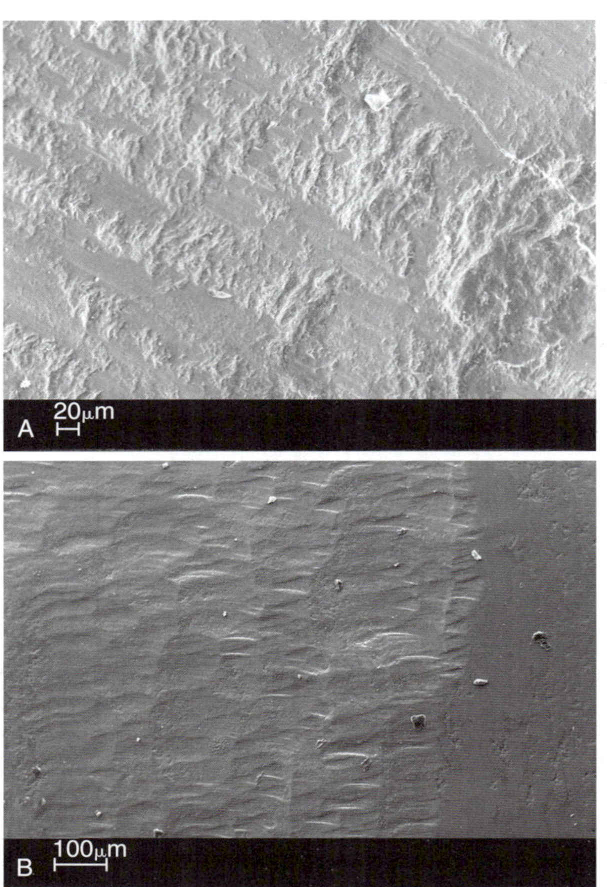

• **Fig. 16.27** Scanning electron micrograph images of enamel stylus abraded by glazed crowns **(A)** and by optimally polished crowns **(B)**. (Courtesy of Dr Siegward Heintze.)

of placing polished zirconia and lithia disilicate in opposing contact with natural enamel.

By and large polished zirconia causes the least amount of enamel wear, glazed zirconia the most, and polished then reglazed zirconia will be intermediate.

Acrylic Resins for Denture Bases and Veneers

Resins are relatively soft materials. To avoid overheating, a large amount of pumice slurry should be applied to the surface. Intermittent contact with the substrate also helps to avoid overheating. The following technique is recommended:

1. Contour with tungsten carbide burs and sandpaper
2. Use a rubber point to remove the scratches
3. Apply pumice with a rag wheel, felt wheel, bristle brush, or prophy cup, depending on the size of the area that needs to be polished
4. Apply tripoli or a mixture of chalk and alcohol with a rag wheel

Air–Particle Abrasion Technology

As an alternative to the use of rotary instrument cutting, air–particle abrasive systems can deliver a fine, precisely controlled high-pressure stream of 25–30 μm aluminum oxide particles to remove enamel, dentin, and restorative materials. Because air–particle abrasion generates minimal heat and vibration, there is relatively little potential for tooth chipping or microfracturing. These systems have been used for the following applications: tooth preparation, removal of defective resin-based composite restorations, endodontic access through porcelain crowns, a minimal preparation to repair crown margins, tunnel preparations, superficial removal of stains, cleaning of tooth surfaces before adhesive bonding, and roughening of internal surfaces of

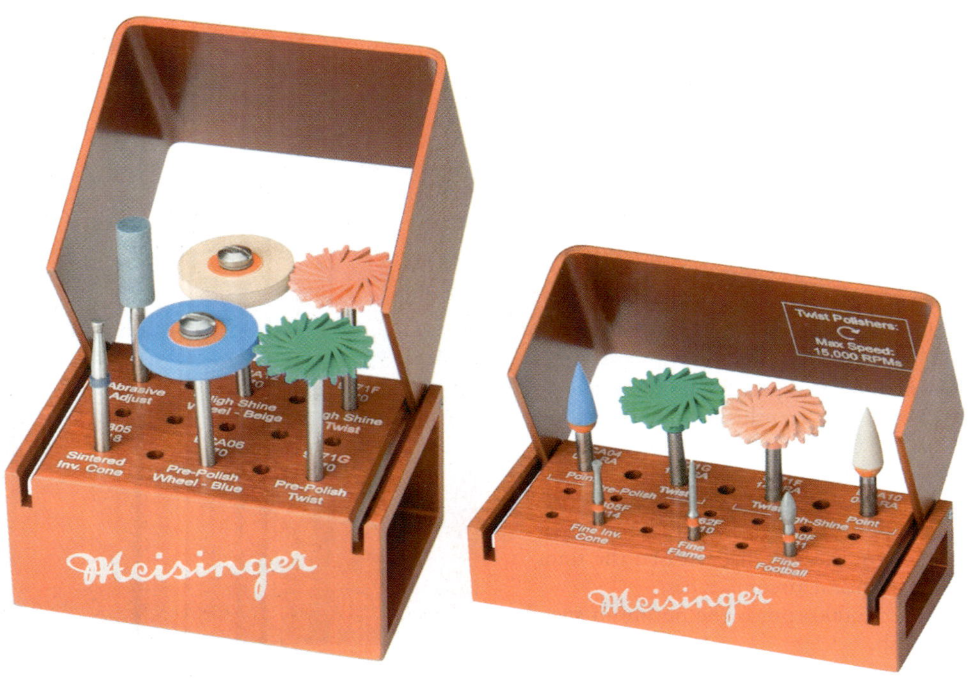

• **Fig. 16.28** Typical finishing and polishing kits for zirconia ceramics: extraoral kit for laboratory use (*left*) and intraoral kit for chairside use (*right*). Note that the extraoral kits for laboratory kits contain abrasives that will allow for heavier adjustments. (Courtesy Meisinger USA.)

indirect porcelains or composite restorations before adhesive bonding.

Prophylaxis Paste Selection for Dental Hygiene Procedures

It should be noted that, depending on the particle size of the abrasive and its composition, the abrasiveness of the prophy pastes may have adverse effects on exposed cementum and dentin surfaces as well as esthetic restorative materials. Table 16.3 shows the mean roughness values obtained on glazed ceramic surfaces after three rounds of 10-second application of various prophy pastes by the same operator. Only one of the pastes (Proxyt Fine) did not alter the surface smoothness significantly. Similarly, another study revealed the effect of the same prophy pastes on the gloss reduction of a polished resin composite (Table 16.4).

Dentifrices

Tooth cleaning substances such as dentifrices are available as toothpastes, gels, and powders. Dentifrices have three important functions: (1) their abrasive and detergent actions provide more efficient removal of debris, plaque, and stained pellicle compared with use of a toothbrush alone; (2) they polish teeth to provide increased light reflectance and superior esthetic appearance, and the high polish, as an added benefit, enables teeth to resist the accumulation of microorganisms and stains better than rougher surfaces could; and (3) they act as vehicles for the delivery of therapeutic agents with known benefits—for example, fluorides, tartar control agents, desensitizing agents, and remineralizing agents.

Fluorides improve resistance to caries and may, under a proper oral hygiene regimen, enhance the remineralization of tooth surfaces with incipient noncavitated enamel lesions, thereby hardening the surface. Tartar control agents such as potassium and sodium pyrophosphates can reduce the rate at which new calculus deposits form supragingivally. Desensitizing agents with proven clinical efficacy are strontium chloride and potassium nitrate. The therapeutic benefits of other additives such as peroxides and bicarbonates are under investigation. The products advertised as "whitening toothpastes" may contain an abrasive agent alone or both a chemical agent and an abrasive agent. The former type of additive acts through a surface stain removal mechanism, whereas the latter additives act through a combined mechanism of abrasion and bleaching.

TABLE 16.3 Effect of Prophylaxis Pastes on Glazed Ceramic Surface Roughness

Product	Surface Roughness
Proxyt coarse (Ivoclar Vivadent, Amherst, NY)	0.183 ± 0.08
Proxyt fine (Ivoclar Vivadent, Amherst, NY)	0.066 ± 0.03
Nupro coarse (Dentsply International, York, PA)	0.209 ± 0.11
Nupro fine (Dentsply International, York, PA)	0.188 ± 0.07
Control (glazed surface)	0.061 ± 0.03

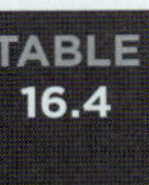

TABLE 16.4 Effect of Prophy Pastes on Polished Composite Surface Gloss Reduction, Measured by Gloss Units, After a 60-Second Application

Product	Mean GU ± SD
Nupro coarse	−40.86 ± 4.22[a]
Nupro fine	−40.57 ± 5.64[a]
Proxyt coarse	−41.61 ± 3.32[a]
Proxyt fine	−16.24 ± 3.34[b]

The difference between mean values of groups represented by the same superscripts is not statistically significant.

Dentifrice Composition

Typical components of some dentifrices are listed in Table 16.5. The abrasive concentrations in paste and gel dentifrices are 50%–75% lower than those of powder dentifrices. Therefore, powders should be used more sparingly and with greater caution by patients (especially where cementum and dentin are exposed) to avoid excessive dentinal abrasion and pulpal sensitivity.

Dentifrice Abrasiveness

The ideal toothpaste should provide the greatest possible cleaning action on tooth surfaces with the lowest possible abrasion rate. Dentifrices do not have to be highly abrasive to clean teeth effectively. This is fortunate because exposed root surface cementum and dentin, respectively, are abraded at rates of 35 and 25 times the rate of enamel. Standardized laboratory tests have been developed to measure the cleaning ability and abrasiveness of dentifrices. Only the abrasiveness test is discussed in this section.

Currently, the preferred means of evaluating dentifrice abrasiveness is to employ irradiated dentin specimens and brush them for several minutes with test and reference dentifrices. An abrasiveness ratio is then calculated by comparing the amounts of radioactive phosphorus (P^{32}) released by each dentifrice, and this value is multiplied by 1000. A dentifrice must obtain an abrasiveness score of 200–250 or less to satisfy the abrasiveness test requirements proposed by the American Dental Association (ADA) and the International Organization for Standardization (ISO). This means that a test dentifrice must abrade dentin at 20%–25% of the rate of the reference standard to be considered safe for normal usage. A problem with this laboratory test is that it does not account for all variables that would affect abrasiveness under in vivo conditions. Some of the factors affecting dentifrice abrasiveness are listed in Box 16.4.

Another problem is that not all dentifrices respond in a similar manner under this test. For example, dentifrices that contain sodium bicarbonate yield poor test results because the particles dissolve completely approximately 1 minute into the 8-minute test. This illustrates that it is very difficult or impossible to use a laboratory test to predict the in vivo abrasiveness of various dentifrices. Patients should experience similar amounts of relative wear from the various dentifrices as those found in laboratory tests. The majority of modern dentifrices are not exceedingly abrasive. In fact, one published document has rated four dozen dentifrices with regard to cleaning ability and abrasiveness. The products are ranked as high, moderate, or low in abrasiveness. It

TABLE 16.5 Typical Dentifrice Components[a]

Component	Composition (wt%) Pastes and Gels	Composition (wt%) Powders	Materials	Purpose
Abrasive	20–55	90–98	Calcium carbonate, dibasic calcium phosphate dihydrate, hydrated alumina, hydrated silica, sodium bicarbonate, mixtures of listed abrasives	Removes plaque or stain, polishes tooth surface
Detergent	1–2	1–6	Sodium lauryl sulfate	Aids in debris removal
Colorants	1–2	1–2	Food colorants	Are used for appearance
Flavoring	1–2	1–2	Oils of spearmint, peppermint, wintergreen, or cinnamon	Provides flavor
Humectant	20–35	0	Sorbitol, glycerine	Maintains moisture content
Water	15–25	0	Deionized water	Acts as suspension agent
Binder	3	0	Carrageenan	As thickener, prevents liquid–solid separation
Fluoride	0–1	0	Sodium monofluorophosphate, sodium fluoride, stannous fluoride	Prevents dental caries
Tartar control agents	0–1	0	Disodium pyrophosphate, tetrasodium pyrophosphate, tetrapotassium pyrophosphate	Inhibits formation of calculus above the gingival margin
Desensitization agents	0–5	0	Potassium nitrate, strontium chloride	Promotes occlusion of dentinal tubules

[a]Some compositional information provided by Dr George Stookey.

• BOX 16.4 Factors Affecting Dentifrice Abrasiveness

Extraoral Factors

- Abrasive particle type, size, and quantity in dentifrice
- Amount of dentifrice used
- Toothbrush type
- Toothbrushing method and force applied during brushing
- Toothbrushing frequency and duration
- Patient's coordination and mental status

Intraoral Factors

- Saliva consistency and quantity (normal variations)
- Xerostomia induced by drugs, salivary gland pathology, and radiation therapy
- Presence, quantity, and quality of existing dental deposits (pellicle, plaque, calculus)
- Exposure of dental root surfaces
- Presence of restorative materials, dental prostheses, and orthodontic appliances

is highly probable that most of the evaluated products meet the American National Standards Institute (ANSI)/ADA and ISO test requirements. Thus, these rankings should be considered a guide to products that do not exceed a maximum acceptable (safe) abrasiveness value.

Toothbrushes

The bristle stiffness of toothbrushes alone has been shown to have no effect on the abrasion of hard dental tissues. However, when a dentifrice is used, there is evidence that more flexible toothbrush bristles bend more readily and bring more abrasive particles into contact with tooth structure, albeit with relatively light forces. This interaction should produce more effective abrasion and cleaning action on the areas that the bristles can reach. Battery-powered toothbrushing devices provide a variety of cleansing actions that are claimed to improve tooth-cleaning actions even further than those achieved by manual toothbrushes.

Summary

- **Finished and polished restorations** provide four benefits of dental care:
  - Better gingival health
  - Chewing efficiency
  - Patient comfort
  - Esthetics
- **Principles of cutting, grinding, finishing, and polishing**
  - Particles of a substrate material (workpiece) are removed by the action of a harder material that makes frictional contact with the substrate.
  - A cutting operation usually involves the use of a bladed instrument or any other instrument in a blade-like fashion.
  - A grinding operation removes small particles of a substrate through the action of bonded or coated abrasive instruments. Grinding instruments contain many randomly arranged abrasive particles.
  - In general, a carbide bur with more blades will produce a smoother surface than a carbide bur containing fewer blades.
  - The coarsest diamond bur removes material more quickly but leaves a rougher surface.
- **Bulk reduction process**
  Bulk reduction can be achieved through the use of instruments such as diamond burs, tungsten carbide burs, steel burs, abrasive wheels, and separating disks.
- **Contouring**
  At the end of this process, the desired anatomy and margins should be established.
- **Finishing**
  Finishing provides a relatively blemish-free smooth surface. The finishing action is usually accomplished using 18- to 30-fluted carbide burs.

- **Polishing**
  - The purpose of polishing is to provide an enamel-like luster to the restoration.
  - Examples of polishing instruments are rubber abrasive points, fine-particle disks and strips, and fine-particle polishing pastes.
- **Abrasion and erosion**
- **Abrasion**
  - *Wear* is a material removal process that can occur whenever surfaces slide against each other.
  - In dentistry, the outermost particles or surface material of an abrading instrument is referred to as the *abrasive.*
  - The material being finished is called the *substrate.*
  - *Two-body abrasion* occurs when abrasive particles are firmly bonded to the surface of the abrasive instrument and no other abrasive particles are used.
  - *Three-body abrasion* occurs when abrasive particles are free to translate and rotate between two surfaces.
- **Erosion**
  Erosive wear is caused by hard particles impacting a substrate surface, carried by either a stream of liquid or a stream of air, as occurs in sandblasting a surface.
- **Hardness of abrasives**
  - Hardness is a surface measurement of the resistance of one material to be plastically deformed by indenting or scratching another material.
  - The first ranking of hardness was published in 1820 by Friedrich Mohs, a German mineralogist.
  - Knoop and Vickers hardness tests are based on indentation methods that quantify the hardness of materials.
- **Abrasive instrument design**
- **Abrasive grits**
  - Abrasive grits are derived from materials that have been crushed and passed through a series of mesh screens (sieves) to obtain different particle size ranges.
  - Dental abrasive grits are classified as coarse, medium coarse, medium, fine, and superfine, according to particle size.
- **Bonded abrasives**
  - Bonded abrasives consist of abrasive particles incorporated through a binder to form grinding tools such as points, wheels, separating disks, coated thin disks.
  - Abrasive disks are used for bulk reduction, contouring, finishing, and polishing of restoration surfaces.
  - Metal strips are usually limited to situations in which very tight proximal contacts are involved.
  - *Truing* is a procedure by which the abrasive instrument is run against a harder abrasive block until the abrasive instrument rotates in the handpiece without eccentricity or runout when placed on the substrate.
  - The *dressing* procedure, like truing, is used to shape the instrument, but it accomplishes two different purposes as well.
- **Coated abrasive disks and strips**
  Coated abrasives are fabricated by securing abrasive particles to a flexible backing material (heavyweight paper, metal, or Mylar) with a suitable adhesive material. These abrasives typically are supplied as disks and finishing strips.
- **Nonbonded abrasives**
  Polishing pastes are considered nonbonded abrasives and are primarily used for final polishing. The abrasive particles are dispersed in a water-soluble medium such as glycerin for dental applications. Aluminum oxide and diamond are the most popular nonbonded abrasives.
- **Abrasive motion**
  The motion of abrasive instruments is classified as rotary, planar, or reciprocal.
- **Types of abrasives**
  - Natural abrasives include Arkansas stone, chalk, corundum, diamond, emery, garnet, pumice, quartz, sand, tripoli, and zirconium silicate. Cuttle and kieselguhr are derived from the remnants of living organisms.
  - Manufactured abrasives are synthesized materials, which are generally preferred because of their more predictable physical properties. Silicon carbide, aluminum oxide, synthetic diamond, rouge, and tin oxide are examples of manufactured abrasives.
- **Abrasive pastes**
  The most commonly used abrasive pastes contain either aluminum oxide (alumina) or diamond particles. Alumina pastes should be used with a rotary instrument and increasing amounts of water as the polishing process proceeds from the use of coarser to finer abrasive particles.
- **Finishing and polishing procedures**
- **Resin-based composite restorations**
  - First, contour the restoration either with 12-fluted carbide burs, 30–100 μm diamond burs, or coarse abrasive-coated disks, depending on the dentist's preference.
  - Next, finish with 16- to 30-fluted carbide burs, fine and extrafine diamond burs, white stones (aluminum oxide), white Arkansas stones, or medium and fine abrasive-coated disks.
  - Finally, polish with fine and extrafine polishing paste (aluminum oxide or diamond); extrafine abrasive-coated disks; silicon carbide-impregnated brushes; or diamond-impregnated rubber polishing disks, cups, or points.
- **Dental amalgam**
  - Contour with slow-speed green stones or diamond burs or brown and green rubber points.
  - Apply a mixture of fine pumice and water or alcohol with a rotary brush or felt wheel to polish the surface.
- **Gold alloy**
  - Contour with carbide burs, green stones (silicon carbide), or heatless stones.
  - Finish with pink stones (aluminum oxide) or medium-grade abrasive-impregnated rubber wheels and points (brown and green).
  - Apply fine abrasive-impregnated rubber wheels, cups, and points; and, if necessary apply tripoli or rouge with rag or leather wheels.
- **Ceramic restorations**
  - Contour the ceramic surface with flexible diamond disks, diamond burs, heatless or polymer stones, or green stones (silicon carbide).
  - Finish with white stones or abrasive-impregnated rubber disks, cups, and points. This process may require two or three steps, depending on the system used.
  - Polish with fine abrasive-impregnated rubber disks, cups, and points or, if necessary, use a diamond paste applied with a brush or felt wheel.
  - Apply an overglaze layer or natural glaze on the ceramic.
  - If necessary, for intraoral polishing, use an intermittent application of rotating instruments with a copious amount of water as a coolant.
  - Leaving rough contact surfaces on zirconia restorations is not recommended. This may result in a relatively rough surface, which may cause severe wear of opposing enamel or restorative material surfaces.
  - By and large polished zirconia causes the least amount of enamel wear, glazed zirconia the most, and polished then reglazed zirconia will be intermediate.

Review Questions

1. Discuss in detail the different types of abrasives used in dentistry.
2. Discuss in detail abrasive and polishing agents.
3. Discuss in brief bonded abrasives.
4. Discuss in detail rotary cutting instruments.
5. Discuss in brief design of a dental bur.
6. Discuss in brief Beilby layer.
7. Describe the action of abrasives and state the requirements of abrasive materials.
8. Write a short note on polishing of gold alloys and role of rouge.
9. Discuss in brief dentifrices.
10. Discuss in brief role of pumice in dentistry.
11. Discuss in brief diamond abrasives.
12. Discuss in brief polishing agents for cast restorations.
13. Discuss in detail materials used and technique for polishing composite restorations.
14. Discuss in detail factors affecting final polish of ceramic restorations and techniques for achieving the same.
15. Discuss in brief technique for polishing dental amalgam.
16. Discuss in brief technique for polishing ceramic restorations.
17. Enumerate the steps involved in finishing and polishing precious metal restorations.
18. Enumerate various abrasives used in dentistry and elaborate on diamond abrasives.
19. Discuss the difference between abrasion and cutting and its effect on surface finish.
20. Discuss in brief basic concepts of finishing and polishing.

Selected Readings

Carr M.P.; Mitchell J.C.; Seghi R.R.; et al. The effect of air polishing on contemporary esthetic restorative materials. Gen Dent 50 (3) 238–241 (2002); This article describes the effects of air polishing on different dental materials.

Consumer Reports: Toothpastes. September: 602–606, 1992; This study evaluated 48 toothpastes in independent laboratories for abrasiveness and cleaning effectiveness. All toothpastes were subsequently ranked for these criteria.

Cooley R.L. Aerosol hazards. In: (editors: Goldman H.S.; Hartman K.S.; Messite J.) Occupational Hazards in Dentistry. Yearbook Medical: Chicago, pp. 21–33; Sources of dental aerosols, their hazards, and preventive measures are presented.

Dorfer C.E.; Hefferren J.; Gonzales-Cabezas C.; et al. Methods to determine dentifrice abrasiveness. Summary proceedings of a workshop in Frankfurt, Germany. J Clin Dent 21 (Suppl) (2010).

Fairhust C.W.; Lockwood P.E.; Ringle R.D.; et al. The effect of glaze on porcelain strength. Dent Mater 8 203–207 (1992).

Fruits T.J.; Miranda F.J.; Coury T.L. Effects of equivalent grit sizes utilizing different polishing motions on selected restorative materials. Quintessence Int 27 (4) 279–285 (1996).

Hefferren J.J. Laboratory method for assessment of dentifrice abrasivity. J Dent Res 55 563 (1976); This reference describes the dentifrice abrasiveness test.

Hutchings I.M. Tribology: Friction and Wear of Engineering Materials. CRC Press: Boca Raton, FL; This publication thoroughly describes the scientific basis of friction, wear, and lubrication.

Jones C.S.; Billington R.W.; Pearson G.J. The in vivo perception of roughness of restorations. Brit Dent 196 42–45 (2004); The tactile ability of the tongue to discern very small changes in surface roughness intraorally is suggested in this study.

Jefferies S.R. Abrasive finishing and polishing in restorative dentistry: A state-of-the-art review. Dent Clin North Am. 51 (2) 379–397 (2007 Apr).

In: (editors: Kroschwitz J.I.; Howe-Grant M.) ed 4 Kirk-Othmer Encyclopedia of Chemical Technology. Vol 1 Wiley: New York, pp. 17–37; This encyclopedia presents a thorough review of specific abrasives, their physical properties, and their methods of manufacture.

Moda MD, Godas AG de L, Fernandes JC, Suzuki TYU, Guedes APA, Briso ALF, et al. Comparison of different polishing methods on the surface roughness of microhybrid, microfill, and nanofill composite resins. J Invest Clin Dent. 2017 Apr 10;9(1):173–9.

Mackert J.R. Side effects of dental ceramics. Adv Dent Res 6 90–93 (1992); This article presents information on silicosis and the potential hazards of porcelain dust generation during grinding procedures.

Nakazato T.; Takahashi H.; Yamamoto M.; et al. Effects of polishing on cyclic fatigue strength of CAD/CAM ceramics. Dent Mater J 18 (4) 395–402 (1999).

Phark J.-H.; Huh I.; Botta A.C.; Duarte S.; et al. Influence of tooth brushing on surface roughness of restorative materials. J Dent Res 89 (Special Issue A) 1052 (2010).

Powers J.M.; Bayne S.C. Friction and wear of dental materials. In: (editor: Henry S.D.) Friction Lubrication and Wear Technology, ASM Handbook. Vol 18 American Society of Metals International: Materials Park, OH, pp. 665–681; This article, a compilation of information from more than 200 sources, presents a review of friction and wear as they relate to human dental tissues and restorative materials.

Proxyt Scientific Documentation, Ivoclar Vivadent. http://www.ivoclarvivadent.us/en-us/download-center/scientific-documentation/#P; This document outlines the principles of professional prophylaxis, including the properties of prophy pastes and their effects on dental tissues and various restorative surfaces.

Ratterman E.; Cassidy R. Abrasives. In: (editors: Lampman S.R.; Woods M.; Zorc T.P.) Engineered Materials Handbook. Ceramics and Glasses. Vol 4 ASM International: Materials Park, OH, pp. 329–335; A system for selecting abrasives for glasses and ceramics based on a comparison of physical properties is presented. Mechanical property tables are presented for several materials.

Stookey G.K.; Burkhard T.A.; Schemehorn B.R. In vitro removal of stain with dentifrices. J Dent Res 61 1236 (1982); The method used to measure the cleaning effectiveness of a dentifrice is presented.

Williamson R.T.; Kovarik R.E.; Mitchell R.J. Effects of grinding, polishing, and over glazing on the flexure strength of a high-leucite feldspathic porcelain. Int J Prosthodont 9 (1) 30–37 (1996).

Yamamoto M. Metal-Ceramics. Quintessence: Chicago; This volume discusses the preparation of metal–ceramic alloys for porcelain application, including several excellent photographs.

Safoura Ghodsi ZJ. A review on translucent zirconia. European Journal of Prosthodontics and Restorative Dentistry. 2018 May 22;26:62–74; This article reviews the translucent zirconia and influence of polishing procedures on the same.

Rinke S and Fischer C. Range of indications for translucent zirconia modifications: Clinical and technical aspects. Quintessence Int 2013; 44:557-566.

Yazici A.R.; Antonson D.; et al. Effect of prophylactic pastes on composite surface gloss. J Dent Res 90 (Special Issue A) 3046 (2011); This abstract outlines the study showing the effect of different prophylactic pastes on the gloss of resin composite.

PART V

Clinical Aspects of Dental Restorations

17 Biocompatibility

CHAPTER OUTLINE

KEY TERMS

The descriptions of key terms are derived from the scientific literature, US agencies, or the International Organization for Standardization (ISO), and the terms are grouped by general terms, biological or clinical effects, and limit values.

GENERAL

Adverse reaction—Any unintended, unexpected, and harmful response of an individual to a (dental) treatment or biomaterial.

Bioactive materials—Biomaterials that, in addition to their primary function (e.g., to restore dental hard tissues), actively stimulate a specific positive tissue response or control their microbiologic environment.

Biocompatibility—The ability of a biomaterial to perform its desired function with respect to a medical (or dental) therapy, without eliciting any undesirable local, allergic, or systemic effects in the recipient or beneficiary of that therapy but generating the most appropriate beneficial cellular or tissue response in that specific situation and optimizing the clinically relevant performance of that therapy.

Biointegration—The process of forming an interface between bone or other living tissue and an implanted material with no intervening space. Biocompatibility is a prerequisite for biointegration.

Osseointegration—The process of forming a direct structural and functional interface between live bone and an artificial implant surface without any intervening fibrous connective tissue. Biocompatibility is a prerequisite for osseointegration.

Risk—Combination of the probability of harm to health occurring as a result of adverse reactions associated with a biomaterial interaction and the severity of that harm.

Safety—The absence (freedom) from unacceptable risks in the context of the intended use.

Xenoestrogen—A chemical that is not indigenous to the body but acts in a manner similar to that of estrogen.

BIOLOGICAL OR CLINICAL EFFECTS

Allergy—A clinical hypersensitivity reaction initiated by specific immunological mechanisms.

Carcinogenicity—Malignant tumor formation caused by an exposure to a chemical or biomaterial.

Cytotoxicity—Cell death or impairment of cell metabolism caused by an exposure to a chemical or biomaterial.

Estrogenicity—Body reaction in a manner similar to that of estrogen, the female sex hormone, from exposure to a chemical or biomaterial.

Genotoxicity—A change of the DNA or of chromosomes caused by an exposure to a chemical or biomaterial.

Hypersensitivity—The objectively reproducible symptoms or signs initiated by an exposure to a defined stimulus at a dose tolerated by normal persons.

Mutagenicity—A change of the DNA or of chromosomes, which is transferred to the next cell generation, caused by an exposure to a chemical or biomaterial.

Sensitization—The process by which antibodies are produced, which react specifically to the causative foreign substance.

Toxicity—The relative ability (dose-related effect) of a substance or a material to cause injury to biological tissues, ranging from improper biochemical function, organ damage, and cell destruction to death. Depending on the duration of exposure period, the terms *acute toxicity* ($\leq$24 hours), *subacute toxicity* ($>$24 hours but $\leq$30 days), and *chronic toxicity* ($>$30 days) are used.

LIMIT VALUES

Lethal dose fifty (LD50)—The calculated dose of a substance that is expected to cause the death of 50% of the entire population of a biological collective, such as specific experimental animals or cells.

No-observed-adverse-effect level (NOAEL)—The highest tested dose of a substance that has been reported to have no harmful (adverse) health effects on people, animals, or cells.

This chapter describes the conceptual aspects of **biocompatibility** with specific emphasis on the solid and liquid materials of greatest relevance to dentistry. Details on test methods for biocompatibility and the monitoring of inorganic and organic species are not included because these tests are not the responsibility of practicing dentists. Many excellent textbooks and reference sources are available that describe these test methods in great detail.

Placement of a material in the body creates an interface that must exhibit both biological and structural stability during the lifetime of the implanted device. These interfaces are dynamic, and their transitional functionality is dependent on the quality of the junction and the biocompatibility of the material. The dynamics of the interfacial interaction affect the material's biocompatibility and its acceptance by the body, which depend on the shape, size, and location of the material, its physical properties, its composition, and the stresses that develop during function.

CRITICAL QUESTION

There are many types of tests for biocompatibility. Which tests can provide conclusive evidence to identify the specific cause of an allergic or **toxic** response to a restorative material?

Three major factors are linked to the success of dental materials:

1. Material properties
2. The design of the dental device
3. The biocompatibility of component materials

The biocompatibility of dental restorative materials is evaluated using compositional analysis, surface degradation tests, cell culture tests, clinical testing in humans, and animal model tests. The biocompatibility of a material depends on several factors:

1. The chemical nature of its components
2. The physical nature of the components
3. The types and locations of patient tissues that will be exposed to the device
4. The duration of the exposure
5. The surface characteristics of the material
6. The amount and nature of substances eluted from the material

The primary purpose of biocompatibility tests is to protect dental patients who will be treated with the materials and the office staff and lab technicians who will be handling these materials. Since no dental biomaterial is absolutely free from the potential risk of **adverse reactions**, the testing of biocompatibility is related to risk assessment. Thus, the challenge for the users of dental biomaterials is to select those products for which the known benefits far outweigh the known risks. Specific tests have been developed to screen restorative and implant materials for their biocompatibility. For materials, models have been developed to analyze the uptake, distribution, biotransformation, and excretion of metal ions or metal complexes in the body.

CRITICAL QUESTION

Which five adverse reactions are *not* types of allergic reactions?

A *critical adverse effect* is the first event that is observed at the lowest exposure level. The location of this effect is called the *critical tissue*, or *critical organ*, and the concentration of a substance that produces this effect is the *critical concentration*. A metal such as mercury can be exposed to tissues as a solid binary phase (Ag_2Hg_3), as dissolved ions in saliva, and as atoms in the vapor form. For this metal, one must be concerned about exposure levels, absorbed dose, body burden, and critical target tissue concentrations. Shown schematically in Figure 17.1 are the critical tissue and organ sites that can be affected by exposure to dental restorative materials and auxiliary materials used to make impressions and models. Material components can be released during melting and casting of metals, fabrication of prostheses, grinding and polishing procedures, adhesive bonding, or cementing to prepared teeth. Exposure by deposition and possibly by local uptake occurs when any one of the four types of epithelial surfaces—oral tissue, gastrointestinal tract tissue, respiratory tract tissue, and skin—makes contact with one of these metal forms.

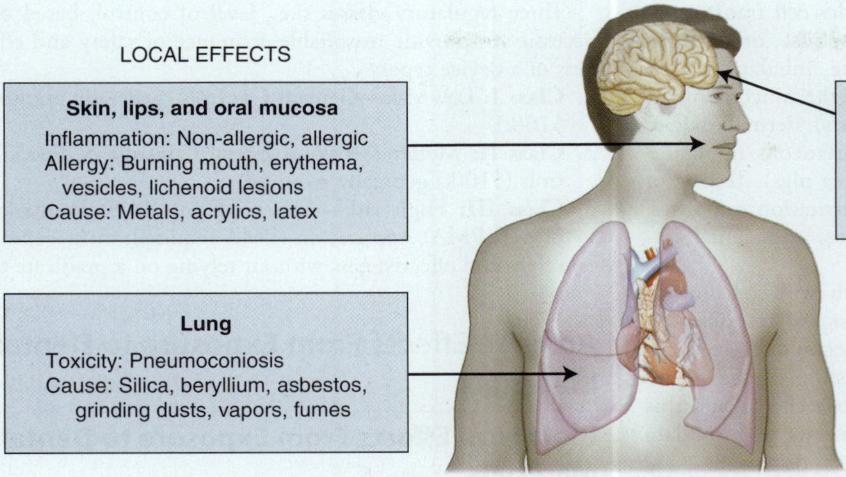

LOCAL EFFECTS

Skin, lips, and oral mucosa
Inflammation: Non-allergic, allergic
Allergy: Burning mouth, erythema, vesicles, lichenoid lesions
Cause: Metals, acrylics, latex

Lung
Toxicity: Pneumoconiosis
Cause: Silica, beryllium, asbestos, grinding dusts, vapors, fumes

SYSTEMIC EFFECTS

Brain and nervous system
Toxicity: Neurobehavioral effects, multiple sclerosis, Alzheimer's, Parkinson's disease, epilepsy
Cause: Unknown

• **Fig. 17.1** Schematic illustration of critical tissues and organs that may be susceptible to the adverse effects of dental materials.

Determining the biocompatibility of dental materials is an extremely complex task that requires consideration of cell biology, patient risk factors, clinical experience, and materials science. This chapter discusses the types of biological responses that materials may cause, types of tests used to characterize biocompatibility, and anatomical aspects of the oral cavity (OC) that influence biological responses to materials. Finally, recommendations are proposed on how clinical judgments should be made in assessing the biological safety of restorative materials.

Adverse reactions to dental restorative materials and auxiliary materials include one or more of the following effects:

- Allergic reaction
- Chemical burn
- Pulp irritation
- Pulp damage
- Thermal injury
- Tissue irritation
- Toxic reaction

The specific causes of these effects are difficult to diagnose because of the multifactorial nature of dental treatment and the subjective nature of patients' complaints or descriptions of their symptoms. Furthermore, there are no perfect tests for the confirmation or validation of diagnoses. A patch test with dental test substances administered by an allergist may provide additional evidence of a potential **allergy** to one of the components of the material. Yet, the results of such testing are not 100% conclusive. There are no direct tests for the diagnosis of **toxicity** reactions. Specific tests such as urinary mercury concentration can help clinicians complement their differential diagnoses. Toxicity diagnoses are also based on the signs and symptoms presented by the patient and by a review of the history of possible exposures to a suspected toxin.

Traditionally, we have accepted the view that toxicity is dose dependent and allergy is dose independent. However, there is considerable uncertainty about which types of exposures lead to the **sensitization** of individuals to substances or ions released from dental restorative materials and auxiliary dental materials. We must rely on the signs and symptoms expressed by our patients and the visual signs observed during clinical exams. In certain cases, allergy tests may have to be performed by an allergist or dermatologist (if appropriate) to assist in the diagnostic process. Specific dental test substances have been established for this purpose, and the treating dentist may have to make additional suggestions to the allergist for tests of other dental substances that are of potential significance in each case (Gawkrodger, 2005; Khamaysi et al 2006).

This chapter is not intended to offer a course on biocompatibility test methods or theory. It is an overview of biocompatibility concepts, terminology, outcome data from national registries of adverse effects, and principles of established test methods. This overview is designed to provide a brief review of established concepts to assist dentists and other health care professionals in the conservative selection and use of dental restoratives and auxiliary materials. It also provides the essential background information and statistics on adverse events that may be needed to draft evidence-based statements on the positive and negative aspects of biomaterials and to ensure that optimal informed consent procedures on material use are employed.

Historical Perspective

CRITICAL QUESTION

How do national and international governments protect dentists and their patients against the use of unsafe or bioincompatible dental products?

Tests for the safety of restorative dental materials must ensure that a candidate material is nontoxic and unlikely to cause adverse immunological effects. Evaluations of toxicity are designed to identify adverse health events caused by physical agents, chemical agents, or both. Paracelsus (1493−1541) correctly proposed that only the dose of a substance differentiates a toxic agent from a remedy (Siddiqui et al 2003). No pharmacological agent is free of potential toxic effects, and no drug is free from the possibility of causing an adverse event in certain individuals. No test can produce results that can guarantee that a substance will not cause adverse effects in all individuals who are treated with the substance. The allowable percentage of adverse effects in a population is based on the risks to the health and life expectancy of the individuals who will be exposed to the product under the indicated conditions and the corresponding exposure doses for its components.

Biological testing of materials has evolved significantly over the past 50 years. Since the 1980s, testing has focused on primary tests for cytotoxicity, hemolysis, Styles cell transformation, the Ames test, the dominant lethal response, oral **LD**50, intraperitoneal (IP) LD50, and the acute inhalation test. Secondary tests are also used. These include the mucous membrane irritation test (in hamsters cheek pouches), dermal toxicity from repeated exposures, responses to subcutaneous implantation (e.g., in rats), and sensitization (of guinea pigs). Testing of dental materials also includes tests for pulp irritation responses, pulp capping effects, endodontic applications, and dental implant performance.

As cell culture techniques evolve, research will continue to focus on mechanisms that control the biological responses to materials. Molecular biology and imaging techniques have recently been introduced. Biocompatibility testing in the future may lead to more reliable predictions of adverse effects, and this knowledge of biological properties may allow us to formulate materials that provide specific, desired biological responses.

Influence of the American Dental Association

Methods and standards for testing the safety and effectiveness of dental materials have evolved slowly during the 20th century. In 1930, the American Dental Association (ADA) formed a Council on Dental Therapeutics to oversee the evaluation of dental products. Also in 1930, the Council established the ADA's Seal of Acceptance program to promote the safety and effectiveness of dental products. However, in 2005, the ADA decided to phase out the Seal of Acceptance program for professional products. Instead, a decision was made to publish a product evaluation newsletter for ADA member dentists that focused on a specific category of professional products in each article. This newsletter, called the *Professional Product Review*, was initiated in July 2006 and the final phase-out of the ADA seal for professional products occurred on December 31, 2007. One of the major accomplishments of the ADA was the development and acceptance of ANSI/ADA Specification No. 41. Recommended Standard Practices for Biological Evaluation of Dental Materials. This specification represented great progress toward the establishment of biological tests for dental materials.

Requirements of the US Food and Drug Administration

The Dental Products Panel of the US Food and Drug Administration (FDA) Medical Devices Advisory Committee reviews and evaluates data concerning the safety, effectiveness, and regulation of products for use in dentistry, and bone physiology relative to the oral−maxillofacial complex and makes appropriate recommendations to the FDA Commissioner.

In 1938, the US Federal Food, Drug, and Cosmetic Act (FFDCA) authorized the FDA to oversee the safety of foods, drugs, and cosmetics. This act required evidence of drug safety before pharmaceutical products could be distributed to the public. More recently, in 1976, Medical Device Amendments (MDA) to the FFDCA included regulation of medical devices, including dental devices, for the first time. The MDA of 1976 required that FDA classifies all medical devices into one of three classes, according to risk, class I, class II, and class III. Dental devices, which are not specifically exempted, are required to be cleared by FDA prior to distribution into interstate commerce. Currently, the Dental Devices Branch of the Center for Devices and Radiological Health regulates premarket clearance of dental devices.

Three regulatory classes (i.e., level of control, based on risk; necessity to provide reasonable assurance of safety and effectiveness of a device type):
1. **Class I:** Low risk—General Controls (generally exempt from 510(k))
2. **Class II:** Moderate risk—General Controls & Special Controls (510(k) generally required)
3. **Class III:** High risk—General Controls & Premarket Approval (PMA) Application (PMA required; must demonstrate safety and effectiveness without relying on a predicate device)

Adverse Effects From Exposure to Dental Materials

Biological Effects From Exposure to Dental Materials

There are five main pathways through which harmful substances can enter the body:
1. Absorption through skin/mucosa/dentin and eye contact
2. Leakage through the tooth apex
3. Direct contact with bone (implants)
4. Inhalation
5. Ingestion

Systemic Effects of Materials

Systemic effects from dental materials are a function of the distribution of substances released from dental materials in the body. Their migration to other sites of the body can occur by diffusion through tissues or by flow through lymphatic channels or blood vessels.

The ultimate systemic response depends on six key variables:
1. Site of exposure
2. The intrinsic (i.e., molecular) toxicity
3. The effective concentration of the substance at the site of action
4. The time of exposure
5. The excretion rate of the substance
6. The target organ (site of action): When substances are excreted slowly, their critical concentrations are reached more rapidly than are those concentrations of substances that are excreted quickly

CRITICAL QUESTION

Why might the local response and systemic response to a dental material differ? Which factors come into play to explain these differences?

Local and Systemic Effects of Materials

Any biomaterial that is placed adjacent to a natural tissue in the body can induce local or systemic biological effects. These effects are controlled by the substances that are released from the material and the biological responses to those substances. The nature, severity, and location of these effects are determined by the distribution of released substances. For dental materials, local effects might occur in the pulp tissue, in the periodontium (PD), at the root apex, or in nearby oral tissues such as the buccal mucosa or tongue (Fig. 17.2). The arrows in this figure indicate the pathways that foreign substances from a restorative material, if present, take into the oral environment, the tissue space next to the

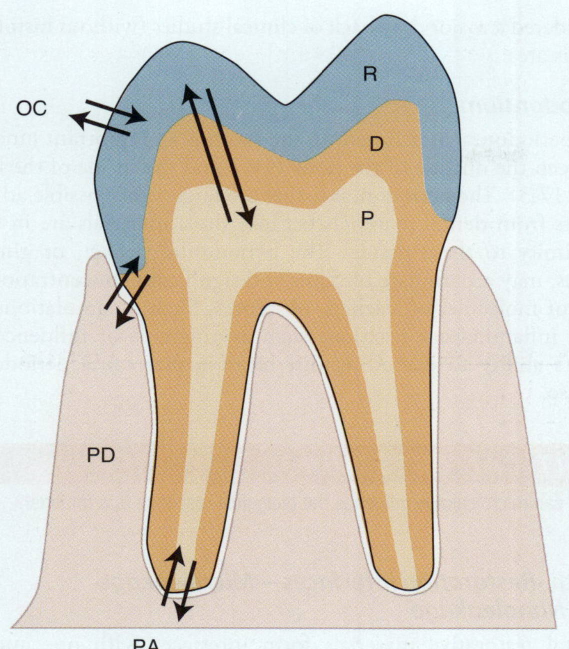

• **Fig. 17.2** Schematic illustration of pathways that leached ions or substances may follow during in vivo degradation of a dental restoration *(R)* into the oral cavity *(OC)*, dentin *(D)*, the pulp chamber and the pulp tissue *(P)*, the periodontium *(PD)*, and periapical tissue and bone *(PA)*.

PD, the pulp chamber (P), or the periapical region (PA). The periodontal ligament is also an important tissue, since it is located in proximity to the pocket or attachment area, which is often a site for accumulation of biofilms and ions, atoms, or molecules of substances released from the cervical region of dental restorations that can extend into this area. Such accumulations can be metabolized, which could then change their biological properties. These local effects are a function of (1) the ability of substances to be distributed to these sites, (2) their concentrations, and (3) exposure times, which may range from seconds to years.

CMR Effects

The term *CMR effects* refers to carcinogenicity, mutagenicity, and reproductive toxicity. Any adverse effect on the DNA of an organism caused by a chemical or a material is termed **genotoxicity**. If the adverse effect is transferred to the next (heritable) generation of cells, the effect is called **mutagenicity**. Thus, genotoxicity can be regarded as the first and necessary step for mutagenicity. Genotoxic reactions occur when a physical or chemical agent changes the genetic material of an organism. Mutations are common occurrences in the DNA of all humans, and they may result from many factors, such as radiation, genotoxic chemicals, and genetic errors in the DNA replication process. Several metal ions, such as beryllium, copper, and nickel, are known mutagens. Some components in root canal sealers and resin-based materials have exhibited mutagenic potential in vitro. Mutagenicity does not have the same consequences as carcinogenicity, and many mutations are repaired. Others are irrelevant or insignificant, or the affected cell undergoes apoptosis, preventing the transfer of the DNA damage to the next cell generation. No dental material has ever been shown to be carcinogenic in dental patients. Reproductive toxicity plays virtually no role in dental materials but has to be considered during preclinical risk assessments performed by the manufacturer.

Estrogenicity

Estrogenicity is the ability of a chemical to act as the hormone estrogen does in the body. If these chemicals are not indigenous to the body, the substances are called xenoestrogens. In 1996 Olea et al. claimed that dental sealants released estrogenic substances in sufficient quantities to warrant concern. The compound of concern is called *bisphenol-A (BPA),* which is a precursor of the bisphenol-A glycidyl dimethacrylate (*bis*-GMA) monomer widely used in the formulation of dental composites and sealants and a building block of plastics like the polycarbonates used in some orthodontic brackets. BPA is a known xenoestrogen. The fear is that the release of these substances from dental materials will compound exposure to other (nondental) sources of endocrine disruptors, which in turn may lead to (claimed!) diseases such as type II diabetes, obesity, premature puberty, and even (breast) cancer, albeit such claims are highly controversial. The amounts of BPA released from dental resin composites are very low. Therefore, the estrogenicity of dental composites has also been questioned, particularly for use in children. For more details, see the discussion on resin-based composites.

Local Effects of Materials

The arrows in Figure 17.2 indicate the pathways that foreign substances from a restorative material can take leading into the OC, the tissue space next to the PD, the pulp chamber (P), or the PA region. Local effects that occur on nearby oral tissues such as the buccal mucosa, the PD, or tongue are generally apparent to visual inspection. Local effects also occur, often hidden from our eyesight, including in the pulp tissue, tooth–restoration interfaces, and bone–implant interfaces.

Pulp Tissue

Postoperative discomfort/sensitivity or pain, which may occur shortly after the treatment with dental restorative materials, may result from several factors, including thermal trauma, chemical injury, microleakage, and allergy. The perception of this postoperative sensitivity is generally believed to be related to the movement of extracellular fluid in the dentinal tubules and the influence of this fluid movement on the odontoblastic processes, as proposed in the so-called *hydrodynamic theory* of postoperative sensitivity. As a result of this movement, cell receptors on the surface of the odontoblast processes are stimulated, and the odontoblasts transfer this signal to afferent nerves, which are closely associated with the odontoblast layer. Therefore, sealing the dentinal tubules during the restorative procedure is clinically important to prevent or reduce intratubular fluid movement and thus postoperative sensitivity.

Pulp damage (inflammation) caused by a restorative material may very often occur without any clinical symptoms at the beginning and is only detected histologically. The intratubular fluid becomes the medium for the diffusion of foreign substances into the pulp chamber. However, the thickness of the remaining dentin between the material and the pulp chamber can slow down the process, and dentinal sclerosis under a carious lesion will further decrease the dentin permeability. Furthermore, dentin may act as a buffer for acidic substances like self-etch adhesives. Therefore, dentin can be regarded as a partial barrier. A major problem in the diagnosis of potential pulp damage caused by a restoration is the fact that there is virtually no correlation between the histologically documented damage to the pulp and clinical symptoms. This is

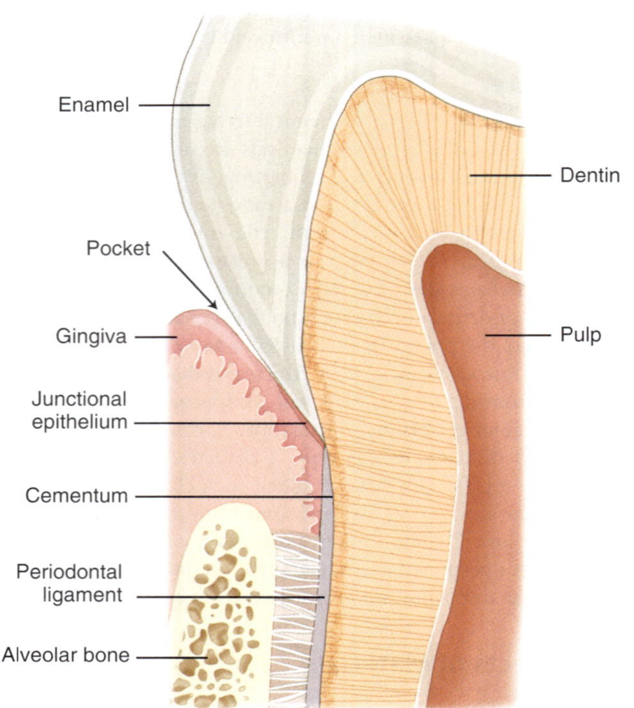

• **Fig. 17.3** Schematic illustration of the periodontal attachment area. The gingiva is attached to the tooth's cementum surface just below the enamel with a specialized epithelium, which is called the *junctional epithelium.* The periodontal "pocket" is formed from the gingival tissue extension above the junctional epithelium. Cementum covers the dentin, starting at the enamel–dentin junction. Below the gingiva, alveolar bone attaches to cementum through a tissue called the *periodontal ligament.* This ligament is not present when implants are osseointegrated with bone.

considered a major drawback of clinical studies (without histology) in this area.

Periodontium

The periodontal attachment to the tooth is an important junction between the outside of the body (OC) and the inside of the body (Fig. 17.3). The periodontal tissues are targets for possible adverse effects from dental materials because these materials are in close proximity to these tissues. The periodontal pocket, or gingival sulcus, may accumulate biofilms and significant concentrations of ions or molecules of leached substances. Such accumulations can elicit inflammatory reactions such as gingivitis or influence the body's ability to defend against bacteria that cause periodontal disease.

CRITICAL QUESTION

How can microleakage influence the biological response to a material?

Tooth–Restoration Interfaces—Microleakage and Nanoleakage

Dental restorative materials form interfaces with one another (adhesives with resin composites or cements with dental alloys) and with the dental hard tissues. The tooth–restoration interface is critical for the transfer of leached substances into dentinal fluid. As shown in Figure 17.4, debonding of the adhesive layer from the dentin, as a result of, for example, polymerization stress, can lead to fluid ingress along gaps, which leads to so-called microleakage, or the diffusion of bacteria and fluids into this gap. The microscopic gap and the microleakage may lead to several undesirable events. Bacteria may migrate into this gap and may even form a thin biofilm, which then initiates an inflammation of the pulp tissue. The gap also promotes material breakdown and

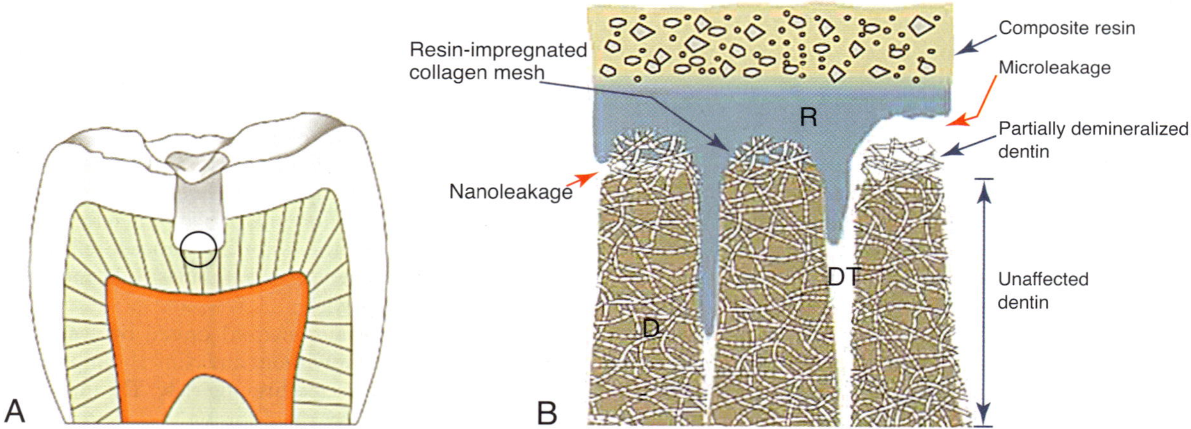

• **Fig. 17.4** Concepts of microleakage and nanoleakage. **(A)** Cross-section of class I composite restoration. **(B)** Diagram illustrating the interphase of bonding resins *(R)* to dentin *(D).* The dentin has been acid etched in preparation for the application of the resin adhesive, which leaves the collagenous matrix of the dentin exposed (demineralized dentin). If the resin does not completely penetrate the collagen network *(left),* then a small space of communication exists between the tubules *(DT)* and the collagen network *(red arrow, left).* This situation allows for nanoleakage. On the other hand, if the resin fails to penetrate the collagen network at all, or debonds from it, then the space is much larger *(red arrow, right).* This situation allows for microleakage. In the ideal situation *(center),* the resin penetrates the collagen network all the way to the mineralized dentin.

secondary caries along the unsupported margin. This breakdown increases the gap width, which allows larger particles and molecules to progress toward the pulp chamber. The presence of this gap also causes marginal staining and compromised esthetics that may lead to restoration replacement.

If the resin from dental adhesives penetrates the collagen network of the acid-treated dentin but does not penetrate the network completely, then a much smaller gap (less than 0.1 μm in most cases) may develop between the mineralized matrix of dentin and the collagen–resin hybrid layer (Fig. 17.4). This much smaller gap may lead to nanoleakage, which probably does not permit bacteria penetration but allows fluid exchange that may degrade the resin or the collagen network and subsequently reduce the longevity of the dentin–resin bond.

Micromechanical interlocking occurs between the bonding of resins from dental adhesives to enamel. Enamel does not contain collagens, and the bond to resin is based on the interlocking of the resin with the etched enamel surface and potentially on chemical bonding between the resin and the enamel apatite (for 10-methacryloyloxydecyl dihydrogen phosphate–based adhesives). Therefore, nanoleakage is not known to occur between restorations and enamel.

Bone–Implant Interface

The success of endosseous dental implants depends on the stability of the implant, which is determined by the biomechanical properties of the bone–implant interface. The initial stability is gained from introducing the implant into a prepared cavity slightly smaller than the size of implant, which allows the implants to be threaded into bone. The final stability is achieved by the ingrowth and integration of new bone onto the implant surface through the process of **osseointegration**. Materials that allow osseointegration have very low degradation rates, and they tend to form biocompatible surface oxides that enhance bony approximation. The general process of **biointegration** involves the adaptation of bone or other tissue to the implanted material without any intervening space along the tissue–material interface. The majority of current dental implants are made of commercially pure titanium (CPTi) or titanium alloy (Chapter 12).

Inflammatory and Allergic Reactions

Different types of biological responses to substances can occur in humans. These include inflammatory, allergic, toxic, and mutagenic reactions. However, not all of these have been documented for dental material exposures. The inflammatory response involves the activation of the host's immune system to ward off some challenge or threat. Inflammation may result from trauma (excessive force, laceration, and abrasion), allergy, or toxicity. Histologically, the inflammatory response is characterized by edema of the tissue caused initially by an infiltration of inflammatory cells such as neutrophils and, later in the chronic stage, to the action of monocytes and lymphocytic cells. The relationship of dental materials to inflammatory reactions is important because of chronic inflammatory responses such as pulp inflammation and periodontal disease. As indicated previously, teeth with cervical restoration margins can release ions or other substances into the gingival sulcus, and adverse reactions can affect the periodontal attachment and the periodontal ligament.

An allergic reaction occurs when the body recognizes a substance, molecule, or ion as foreign, and the human immune system can react quickly, as during an anaphylactic reaction or slowly in delayed contact dermatitis. These reactions are insensitive to the amount of the allergen that is available or released.

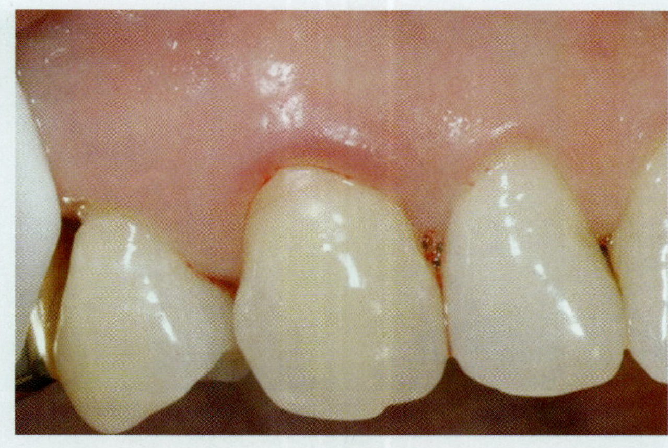

• **Fig. 17.5** Inflammatory response or possible allergic reaction adjacent to a class V resin-based composite. However, no patch test was performed to confirm this response. (Courtesy of Dr Hyun-Ju Chung.)

An allergic reaction induces an inflammatory response that cannot easily be distinguished from reactions caused by a nonallergic inflammatory process or by low-grade toxicity. However, by observing the signs of the effect or the absence of the signs in other locations and by the process of elimination, some reasonably logical inferences may be drawn. In some cases, observation for 2 weeks or more, when possible, can lead to a resolution of the response because the effect was caused either by trauma, another noninflammatory process, or a self-limiting allergic condition. Examples of inflammatory reactions that may be caused by allergens leached as ions from metals or other substances released by dental materials are shown in Figures 17.5–17.11. Figure 17.6 illustrates three potential sites for allergic reactions to nickel-containing metals: (1) a watchband buckle; (2) bilateral, fixed metal–ceramic prostheses with copings and framework made from nickel alloy (crown on left and three-unit FDP on right); and (3) a severe reaction of lips to nickel-containing wire. Figure 17.7D illustrates positive responses to patch test substances on a patient's back. In addition, bilateral lichenoid mucositis lesions which will be discussed later, are shown in Figure 17.12 on the buccal mucosa adjacent to gold alloy crowns.

Some materials, such as latex, can cause allergy directly by activating antibodies to the material. These are classified as type I, II, or III reactions, according to the Gell and Coombs classification of immune responses (Gell & Coombs, 1963; Rajan, 2003). These reactions occur quickly and are modulated by antibody-producing eosinophils, mast cells, or B lymphocytes. In comparison, metal ions must first interact with a host molecule to produce a delayed type IV **hypersensitivity** reaction, which is modulated by monocytes and T cells. This type is often associated with contact dermatitis.

- A type I reaction (mediated by IgE or IgG4) is an immediate atopic reaction (based on a genetic predisposition to the development of immediate hypersensitivity reactions to a common environmental antigen) or anaphylactic reaction when an antigen interacts with mast cells or basophils. *Atopy* refers to a personal tendency, familial tendency, or both occurring in childhood or adolescence whereby one becomes sensitized and produces immunoglobulin E (IgE) antibodies in response to normal exposures to allergens, usually proteins. As a result, these individuals develop symptoms such as asthma, rhinoconjunctivitis, or eczema.

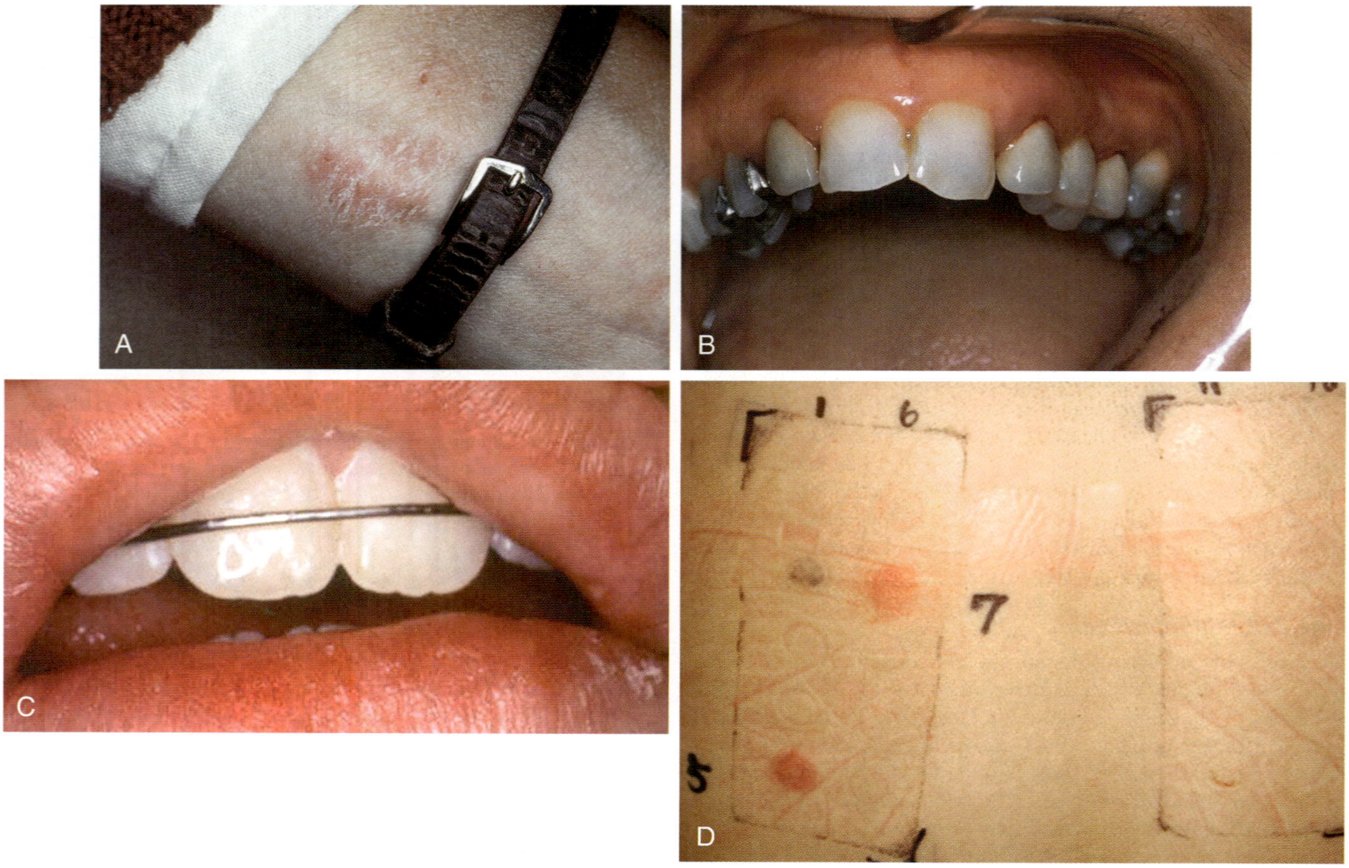

• **Fig. 17.6 (A)** Possible allergic reaction to nickel alloy in watchband buckle. **(B)** Bilateral erythema in a female patient that may have been associated with allergic reactions to nickel in a recently cemented metal–ceramic crown (*left side of photo*) and in two metal–ceramic crowns (*right side of photo*) of a three-unit fixed dental prosthesis. **(C)** Severe allergic reaction in the lips of a patient who was exposed to a nickel-containing orthodontic wire. **(D)** Positive responses to patch tests on a patient's back. (C, Courtesy of Dr Donald Cohen; D, Courtesy of Dr Young Ho Won.)

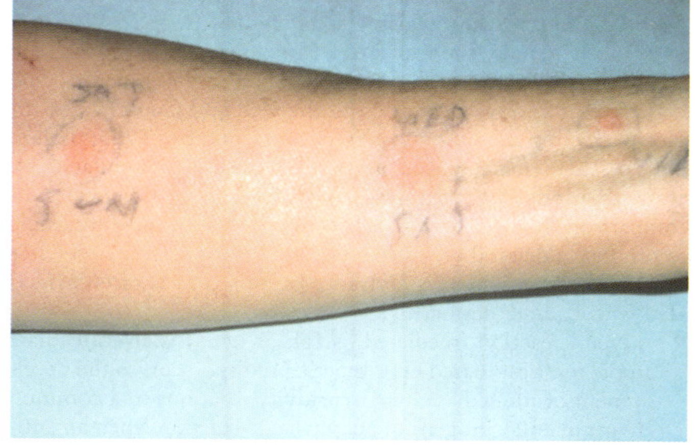

• **Fig. 17.7** Photo of a patient's arm after she tested herself with metal disks made of a nickel–chromium (Ni–Cr) alloy. Note that the patient has noted the period during which the disks were taped to her arm prior to examination of the sites in a dental clinic. This type of test is not standardized, and the test results should not be used to confirm or reject the diagnosis of a suspected allergy to nickel or any of the other alloy components.

- A type II response is a cytotoxic hypersensitivity reaction.
- Type III is an immune complex hypersensitivity reaction.
- Type IV is a delayed or cell-mediated hypersensitivity.
- Type V is a stimulating antibody reaction, which is rare and sometimes classified as a subcategory of type II (Rajan, 2002).

CRITICAL QUESTION

How does the corrosion of metals contribute to their biocompatibility?

Precursors to Adverse Effects of Dental Materials

Each biomaterial can degrade and release components under certain environmental and physical conditions.

Metals can degrade by wear, dissolution, or corrosion. The difference between dissolution and corrosion is primarily related to the difference between chemical concentration gradients and electrical current gradients. A metal restoration can release metal ions as a result of chemical reactions, electrochemical forces, or mechanical forces (such as during abrasion). For some materials, such as ceramics and resin-based composites, cyclical stresses contribute to the breakdown of the material and release of components. Thus, the biocompatibility of the material is controlled by

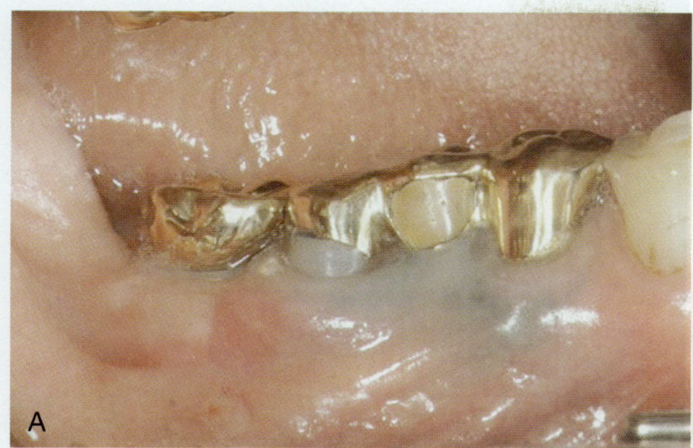

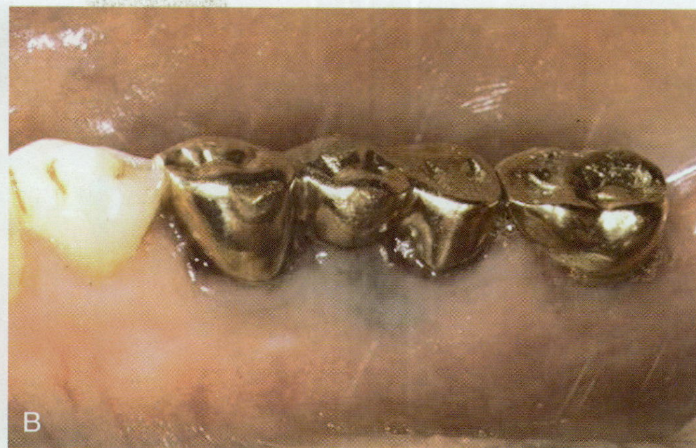

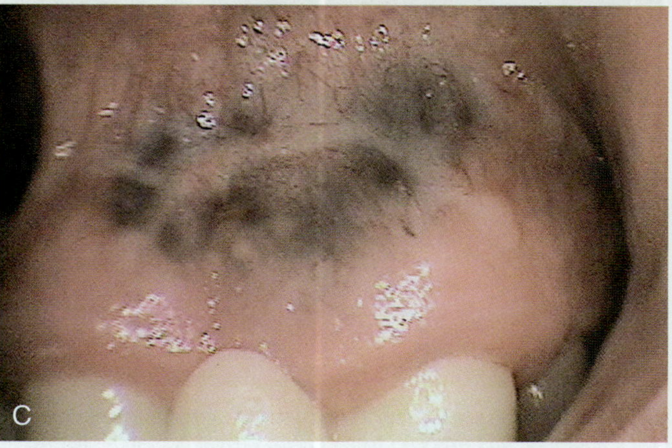

• **Fig. 17.8** Large blue-colored areas, typically referred to as an amalgam tattoo, which is a benign area of discolored membrane in the mouth. These examples are not associated with allergic reactions to mercury or any other metallic elements in the amalgam fillings. The discoloration is caused by small amalgam granules that have fallen into open wounds created during the condensation and carving of amalgam fillings in prepared teeth **(A and B)** or retrograde fillings in root apices **(C)**. (Upper two photos courtesy of Dr Hyun-Ju Chung.)

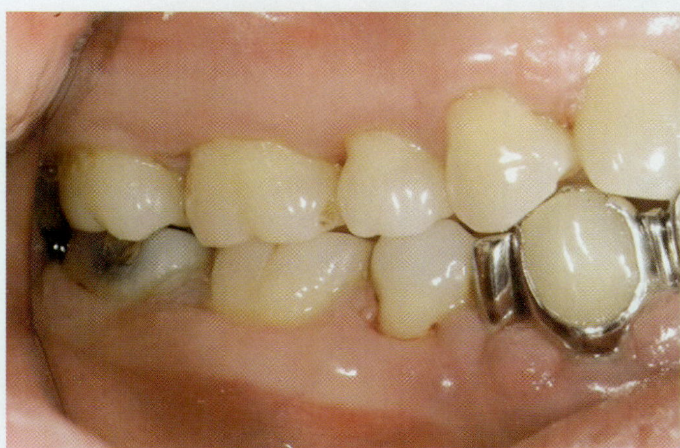

• **Fig. 17.9** Inflammatory response adjacent to a crown (*lower right*) made from a metal coping. No definitive diagnosis can be made of a potential allergy to one of the component metals without testing the individual to a battery of dental patch test substances. Thorough dental and medical histories are also required for the evaluation of this condition. (Courtesy of Dr Hyun-Ju Chung.)

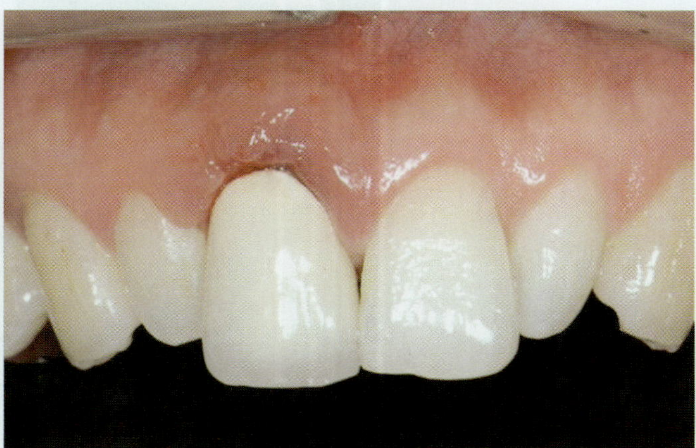

• **Fig. 17.10** Inflammation adjacent to the metal margin of a metal–ceramic crown. A potential allergy to one of the metal components should be explored, since such tissue response to leached metal ions is one of the most prevalent adverse effects reported by national adverse effect registries. Furthermore, gingival reactions to metal oxides that were produced during the firing process for metal–ceramic crowns have also been proposed. (Schmalz, Langer, and Schweikl. J Dent Res 77:1772-1778, 1998; Schmalz and Garhammer, Dent Mater 18:396-406, 2002; courtesy of Dr Hyun-Ju Chung.)

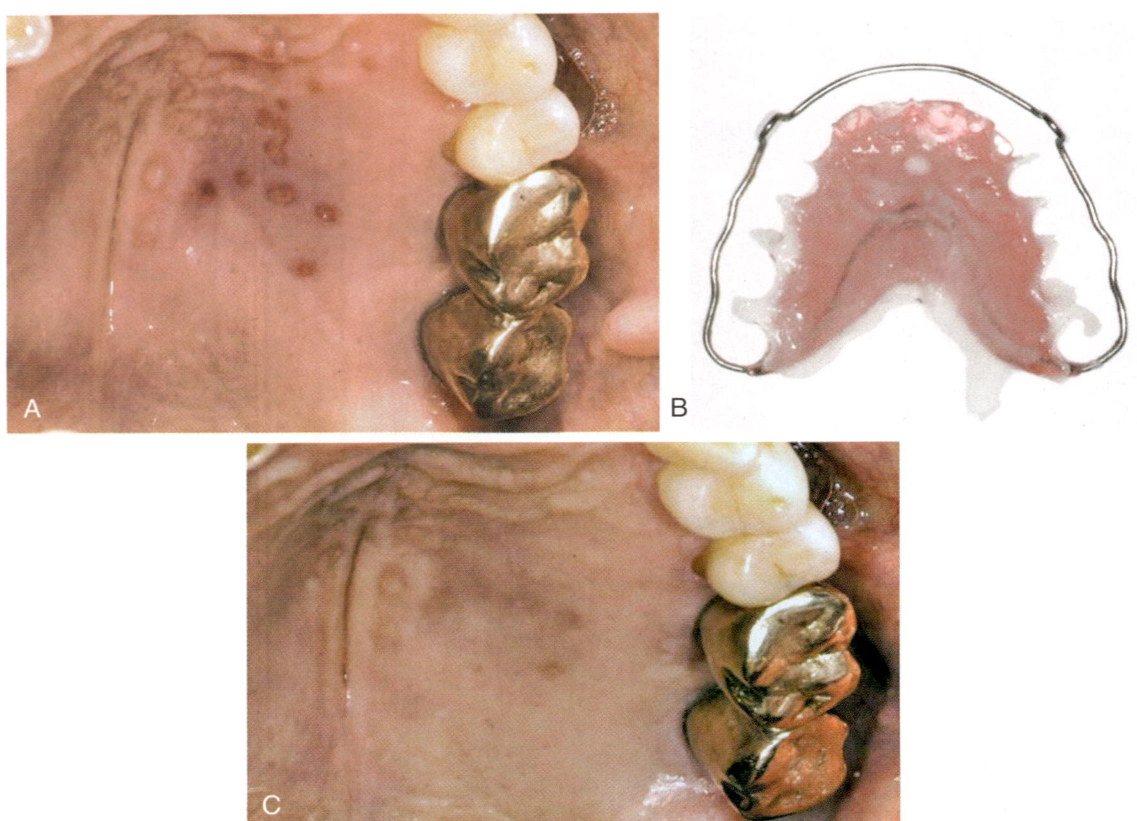

• **Fig. 17.11** Erythematous reaction sites. Patch testing was not performed to confirm a suspected allergic response. **(A)** Palatal area that was exposed to an acrylic palatal appliance. **(B)** Acrylic appliance with embedded wire. **(C)** Initial healing of palatal tissue shown in A within 2–3 days after removal of the palatal appliance. (Courtesy of Dr Byung-Gook Kim.)

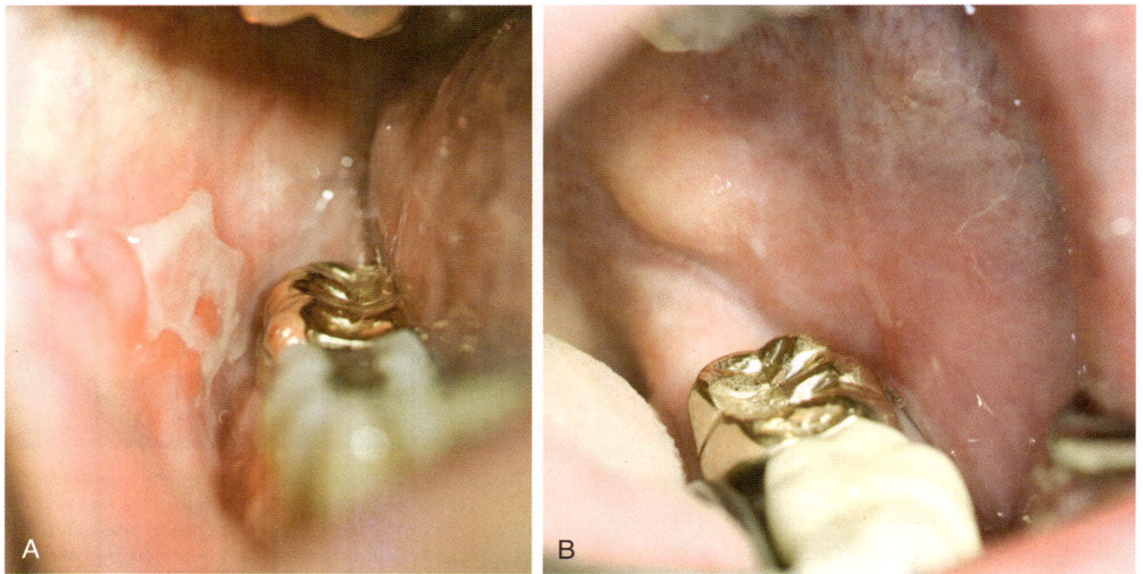

• **Fig. 17.12** Bilateral lichenoid lesions that are associated with gold alloy crowns. **(A)** Lichenoid mucositis lesion (*white area*) in tissue adjacent to a gold alloy crown. **(B)** Lichenoid mucositis lesion in vestibular tissue next to gold alloy crown on opposite side of the arch. Patch testing of the patient was not performed. (Courtesy of Dr Donald Cohen.)

the degradation process. The biological response to a corrosion process depends on the composition of the material, the amount of the offending species released over time, the shape of the prosthesis, and its location on or within tissues.

Corrosion is not determined only by a metal's composition but also by the environment in contact with the metal. For example, acidic substances such as citrus juices or regurgitated hydrochloric acid alter the surfaces of ceramics. High pH environments may also increase the dissolution of some glass-phase ceramics. The environment–metal interface creates the conditions for corrosion. This interface is active and dynamic, the material breakdown products affect the body, and the body's environment affects the material's surface structure.

In addition to the degradation process, the biocompatibility of a material is also affected by its surface characteristics. Material surfaces are often different in composition from those of the interior structures of metals and resin-based composites.

Another factor that increases the potential for the release of potential allergens, mutagens, or toxins is the surface roughness of a restoration or prosthesis. For metals, a rough surface promotes corrosion, which increases the release of ions that may lead to adverse effects. Several types of beverages have caused degradation of two types of dental ceramics. Plaque accumulation also increases on roughened surfaces, and this may contribute to periodontal disease or caries.

Unfinished surfaces of resin-based composites and pit-and-fissure sealants have an oxygen-inhibited outer layer that may be more susceptible to leaching impurities such as BPA. Some studies indicate that leaching of BPA decreases over a relatively short period, and the results suggest that the toxicity risk is extremely low. However, the concentration of BPA is dependent on the quality standards that the manufacturer follows relative to allowable impurity levels.

CRITICAL QUESTION

Is it possible for a material to have no obvious biological effects by itself but still alter body functions?

Products that pass the primary tests, such as the toxicity test, then progress to secondary and usage tests (Fig. 17.13). Today, the choice of the test method is based on risk assessment, which is also divided into separate stages of analysis. Details on such testing are provided in relevant ISO standards such as ISO 14971. This risk assessment is the basis for deciding whether new tests are necessary or not, or whether data from the scientific literature are sufficient. If they are necessary, cell culture tests are regarded as the first choice combined with animal tests for sensitization. Subsequently, risk assessment continues and decisions are made on whether or not further tests (e.g., animal tests or human clinical tests) are needed. Clinical tests in some countries are mandatory for materials that are considered to be of high risk. The final decision for market clearance is then made by an interchange between manufacturers and a third party such as a governmental agency or a private organization to which this authority has been granted by a government agency. Our profession seems to be overly complacent in its acceptance of new materials without demanding proof of their safety and efficacy. When a new product is introduced on the dental market, the advertisements tend to promote the clinical performance but rarely summarize the biocompatibility tests and results of these tests compared with results from control materials.

Dentists must rely on the appropriate test methods that are required in standards and in legal regulations and assume that

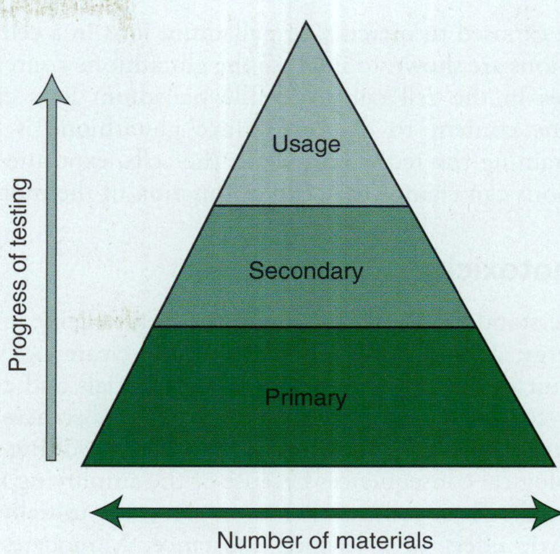

• **Fig. 17.13** Classical progression of biocompatibility tests for evaluating a group of new dental materials. All of the products are screened initially using primary tests. Those that have favorable test results are then subjected to secondary tests. Finally, the best materials of the initial group are subjected to clinically relevant usage tests prior to decisions on whether or not they will be used for clinical trials in humans. (Courtesy of J Wataha.)

sufficient evidence of safety has been established for dental devices once they have been cleared for market use.

Since toxicity is dose dependent, it is obvious that materials that release too much of a substance can cause overt toxicity. The terms and definitions given previously indicate that there are different dose thresholds for various levels and probabilities of risk. Figure 17.14 shows a plot of cellular glutathione from monocytes

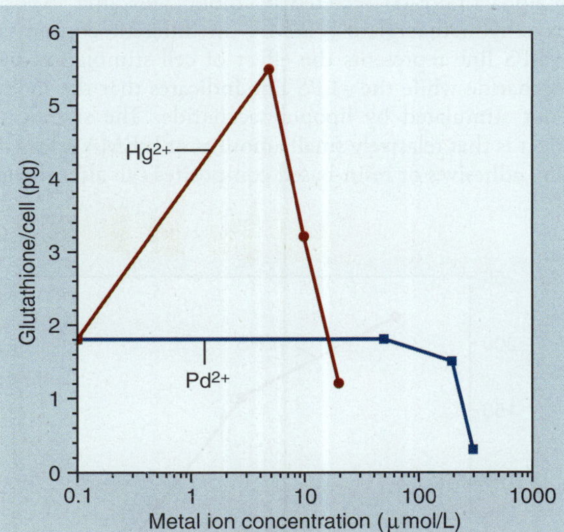

• **Fig. 17.14** Response of monocytes in a cell culture after a 24-hour exposure to mercury ions (Hg^{2+}) or palladium ions (Pd^{2+}). Mercury ions produced a spike in glutathione at an ion concentration of about 8 μmol/L and a subsequent decrease as mercury became toxic to the cells. In contrast, during exposure to palladium ions, the glutathione content did not decrease significantly until the palladium ion concentration increased to between 200 and 300 μmol/L, which is far below the ion concentrations required to induce toxicity in these cells. Because both types of metal ions alter the chemical defense (glutathione production) against oxidative stress at subtoxic ion levels, these processes are believed to affect the immunotoxicity of these metals. (Courtesy of J Wataha.)

that were exposed to mercury or palladium ions in a cell culture. Mercury ions are shown to increase the glutathione content of the monocytes in the cell culture, while palladium ions cause the glutathione content to decrease. Since glutathione is essential for maintaining the redox balance in the cells, exposure to these metallic ions can change the cellular function of the monocytes.

Immunotoxicity

Our understanding of the differences between toxicity, inflammation, allergy, and mutagenicity has become clearer as we learn more about the interactions between biomaterials and cells. The principal concept of immunotoxicity is that substances leached from materials can alter immune system cells, resulting in enormous biological consequences because of the amplifying nature of immune cells. These cellular alterations can occur initially because of the toxic effect of a leached substance. Monocytes control chronic inflammatory and immune responses, and they also secrete many substances that alter the actions of other cells. Thus, if substances leached from a biomaterial change the monocyte's ability to secrete these substances, the biological response can be greatly influenced and this may greatly impair cellular defense mechanisms against bacteria (Schmalz et al., 2011).

As stated earlier, cell function can either increase or decrease as a result of immunotoxic effects. As shown in Figure 17.14, mercury ions are known to increase the glutathione content of human monocytes in cell culture, whereas palladium ions decrease the cells' glutathione content. Glutathione is important in maintaining oxidative stress in cells, and any change in its concentration can alter cell function. Higher concentrations of mercury can also decrease glutathione as the ion concentration becomes more toxic.

Figure 17.15 shows a graph of the amount of tumor necrosis factor alpha (TNF-α) secreted by monocytes after exposure to hydroxyethylmethacrylate (HEMA) in different concentrations. The +LPS line represents the effect of cell stimulation by lipopolysaccharide while the –LPS line indicates that the monocytes were not stimulated by lipopolysaccharide. The significance of this effect is that relatively small amounts of HEMA released from bonding adhesives or resin-based composites can alter the normal functions of monocytes, thereby contributing to the potential immunotoxicity of some resin-based products.

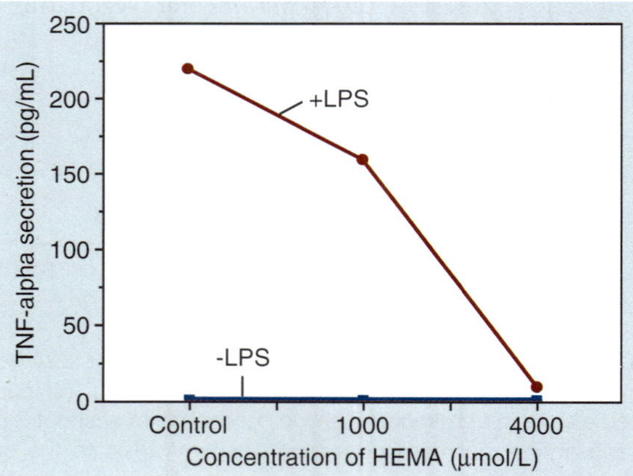

• **Fig. 17.15** Reduction in secretion of tumor necrosis factor alpha (TNF-α) by monocytes after exposure to different concentrations of hydroxyethylmethacrylate (HEMA). The TNF-α secretion shown on the y-axis is plotted against HEMA concentration on the x-axis for cells that were either stimulated by lipopolysaccharide (+LPS) or not stimulated by lipopolysaccharide (−LPS). (Courtesy of J Wataha.)

Pulpal and Periodontal Effects

The postoperative discomfort or pain caused by treatment with dental materials may result from any of several factors, including thermal trauma, chemical injury, microleakage, and allergy. The hydrodynamic theory of pulp pain is related to the movement of dentinal fluid and its influence on the odontoblastic processes. It is well known that dentin permeability increases substantially in areas closer to the pulp chamber. Thus, the damaging effect of a material, if such an effect occurs, is strongly influenced by the remaining thickness of dentin between the material and the pulp chamber. This outward fluid pressure from the pulp chamber toward the enamel is not sufficient to eliminate the inward diffusion of bacteria, bacterial products, or material components into the pulp. A major problem in the diagnosis or potential pulp damage caused by a material or substance is the fact that there is virtually no correlation between the histologically documented damage to the pulp and clinical symptoms. This is considered as a major drawback of clinical studies in this area.

Because the cervical margins of many dental restorations are near the periodontal attachment area, the biocompatibility of these materials may influence the body's ability to defend against bacteria that cause periodontal disease. Further, the periodontal pocket, or gingival sulcus, may accumulate significant concentrations of leached substances that do not accumulate to these levels in other areas. In addition to the accumulation of leached or dissolved substances in subgingival areas, substances that are leached from root canal filling materials may accumulate next to the apical foramen. Substances that accumulate in these areas can lead to inflammatory reactions, allergic reactions, periodontal pathology, and PA lesions.

CRITICAL QUESTION

How can microleakage influence the biological response to a material?

Interfaces With Dental Materials

Tooth-supported dental restorations consist of one or more prepared teeth, a monolayer or multilayer restorative material, and auxiliary dental biomaterials such as dental adhesives, cements, and sealing agents. Although several interfaces may be present in these restorations, the dentin−cement or dentin−resin interfaces are the most important in transition areas for transfer of leached substances into dentinal fluid. Dental cements such as zinc phosphate, glass ionomer, zinc polycarboxylate, and zinc oxide−eugenol do not require etching of dentin to be used as luting agents. In contrast, adhesive-bonded, resin-based cements may require acid etching of dentin to remove the smear layer and to expose the collagen mesh that allows infiltration of the bonding resin. This resin layer acts as a partial barrier to the transport of elements, ions, or substances that are released from a variety of restorative materials.

If the resin material does not penetrate the collagenous network or debonds from it as the resin shrinks during polymerization, a microscopic gap will form between the resin and dentin. This shrinkage may also occur with enamel. Although this gap is only a few microns wide, it is wide enough to permit bacteria to penetrate this interfacial space, since the average size of a *Streptococcus* bacterium is only about 1 μm in diameter. The dentin−resin interface occurs when the clinician attempts to bond resin-based restorative materials to dentin. The interface actually forms between the resin and the collagen network. Thus, the integrity of the resin–collagen interface will control the potential pulp-damaging effect of these restorations.

As shown in Figure 17.4, incomplete bonding or resin penetration into the collagen mesh of acid-etched dentin can lead to fluid ingress along gaps wider than 1 μm, which is referred to as *microleakage*. The microscopic gap for the so-called microleakage process may lead to several undesirable events. The bacteria that migrate to the pulp may initiate an infection of pulp tissue. The gap also promotes material breakdown along the unsupported margin. This breakdown increases the gap width, which allows larger particles and molecules to progress toward the pulp chamber. It also causes marginal staining and compromised esthetics that may lead to premature replacement. One in vitro study revealed less leakage for amalgam restorations compared with resin-bonded composites (Őzer et al., 2002).

If the resin penetrates the collagen network of dentin but does not penetrate it completely, then a much smaller gap (less than 0.1 μm in most cases) will exist between the mineralized matrix of dentin and the collagen–resin hybrid layer (see Figure 17.4). This much smaller gap has been claimed to allow nanoleakage, which probably does not allow bacteria or bacterial products to penetrate the marginal gaps of the restoration and the pulp. However, fluid exchange most likely occurs, and this may degrade the resin or the collagen network that is incompletely embedded with the resin, thereby reducing the longevity of the dentin–resin bond.

Nanoleakage is not known to occur between restorations and enamel because enamel contains virtually no organic mass and therefore has no collagenous matrix into which a resin may penetrate. Although it is unclear whether leakage toward or into the dental pulp chamber is a major factor in the biological response to dental materials, one must be aware of potential immune responses in the pulp and PA tissues that may occur independently of leakage phenomena.

Mercury and Amalgam

The controversy over the biocompatibility of amalgam has waxed and waned several times in the 170-plus year history of its dental use in the United States. Most of the controversy stems from the known toxicity of mercury and the question of whether mercury from amalgam restorations has toxic effects. Mercury occurs in four forms: as the metal (Hg^0), as an inorganic ion (Hg^{2+}), as a component of the silver–mercury phase, or in one of several organic forms such as methyl or ethyl mercury. Metallic mercury gains access to the body via the skin or as a vapor through the lungs. Ingested metallic mercury is poorly absorbed from the gut (0.01%), so the primary portal into the body is through inhalation of mercury vapor.

Absorption of specific metals through the oral mucosa, gastrointestinal tract, or respiratory tract can vary considerably for different chemical forms of a metal. Excretion may occur through exhaled vapor or through urine, feces, or skin. For example, mercury vapor is readily absorbed after inhalation. Dissolved mercury can be transported through blood and distributed to the brain and other organs and excreted by exhalation and in urine. Elemental mercury is transported to blood cells and tissues, where it is oxidized rapidly to mercuric mercury (Hg^{2+}).

The most common forms of mercury that occur naturally in the environment are metallic mercury, inorganic salts, mercuric sulfide (HgS), mercuric chloride ($HgCl_2$), and methyl mercury (CH_3Hg^+). Mercury forms numerous compounds, assuming +1 valence in mercurous compounds and +2 valence in mercuric compounds. The transformative ability of mercury can be either helpful or harmful. Microorganisms and various natural processes can convert metallic mercury to inorganic mercury compounds, inorganic mercury compounds to organic mercury compounds, and organic to inorganic compounds. Methyl mercury is the most common form that is transformed by natural processes; it is a more toxic form than ethyl mercury ($C_2H_5Hg^+$) or elemental mercury. Methyl mercury is a major safety concern because it bioaccumulates through the food chain; its pharmacokinetic half-life is longer (1.5–3 months) than that of ethyl mercury (less than 1 week). Moreover, it is accumulated in the body rather than being excreted in the gut, as occurs with ethyl mercury. In air, the concentrations of mercury range from about 0.01 to 0.02 μg/m³.

Mercury accumulates in the kidneys. In the brain, metallic mercury can be converted to an inorganic form that is retained in the brain. Elemental mercury and mercury vapor have a half-life of 1–3 months. Mercury leaves the body by excretion through urine and feces.

Exposure to high levels of mercury can injure the brain, kidneys, and the developing fetus. The nervous system is sensitive to all forms of mercury, although the brain is most sensitive to metallic mercury and methyl mercury. Chronic mercury toxicity may be manifested as tremors; memory loss; and changes in personality, vision, and hearing. Children and fetuses are most sensitive to the effects of mercury on the nervous system. Selenium, an essential element, is claimed to be protective against the toxic effects of mercury.

For air in the workplace, the Occupational Safety and Health Administration has set a permissible exposure limit (PEL) for mercury vapor in air of 0.1 mg/m³.

The United Nations Environment Programme (UNEP) has organized global meetings through the UNEP Global Mercury Partnership to protect human health and the global environment from the release of mercury and its compounds by minimizing and, where feasible, ultimately eliminating global, anthropogenic mercury releases to air, water, and land. Since 2001 the Governing Council/Global Ministerial Environment Forum of UNEP has discussed the need to protect human health and the environment from the releases of mercury and its compounds. By the end of 2011, three sessions of the Intergovernmental Negotiating Committee (INC) organized by UNEP had been held to prepare a Global Legally Binding Instrument on Mercury: INC1 (June 7–11, 2010, Stockholm, Sweden), INC2 (January 24–28, 2011, Chiba, Japan), and INC3 (October 31–November 4, 2011, Nairobi, Kenya). Although no globally binding document on controlling mercury in dental amalgam and other mercury-containing products had been approved, a proposal for a "phase-down" of dental amalgam was supported combined with a need for research on more durable alternatives to dental amalgam and a renewed emphasis on prevention of caries and the associated need to reduce the need for restorations throughout the world.

Several studies have shown that amalgams release sufficient vapor to cause absorption of between 1 and 3 μg/day of mercury, depending on the number and size of amalgam restorations present (Langworth et al., 1988; Berglund, 1990; Mackert & Berglund, 1997; Ekstrand et al., 1998). The inhaled mercury gains access to the bloodstream via the alveoli of the lungs. From the blood, mercury is distributed throughout the body, with a preference for fat and nerve tissues. Mercury is also ingested as particles produced by wear, and about 45 μg/day of mercury may reach the gut either as the amalgam form or as dissolved and released Hg^{2+} ions. The absorption of ionic mercury is also poor (approximately 1%–7%). Mercury trapped in amalgam particles is also poorly resorbed. Methyl mercury is not produced from amalgams but is generally a product of bacteria or other biological systems acting on metallic mercury. Methyl mercury is the most toxic form of mercury and is also very efficiently absorbed from the gut (90–95%). Methyl mercury is absorbed mainly from the diet, particularly from fish (especially shark, swordfish, and tuna), which contribute a significant portion.

Concerns about mercury stem from its toxicity and its relatively long half-life in the body. The toxicity of mercury is well known; the symptoms depend somewhat on the form. Acute symptoms are neurologically based or kidney based, ranging from paresthesia (at 500 μg/kg or above) to ataxia (at 1000 μg/kg or above), joint pain (at 2000 μg/kg or above), and death (at 4000 μg/kg or above). The lowest known level for any observable toxic effect is 3 μg/kg. This level translates to about 30 μg of mercury per gram of creatinine clearance in the urine. At chronic exposure levels, the symptoms are more subtle and include weakness, fatigue, anorexia, weight loss, insomnia, irritability, shyness, dizziness, and tremors in the extremities or the eyelids. Although amalgams do not release anywhere near toxic levels of mercury, the long half-life of mercury in the body raises concerns among some individuals. The half-life ranges from 20 to 90 days, depending on the form, with methyl mercury exhibiting the longest half-life and inorganic forms the shortest. Numerous tests for the body burden of mercury have been developed, including those based on the analysis of blood, urine, and hair. Of these test parameters, measurement of mercury in the urine after 24 hours may be the best long-term indicator of the total metallic mercury body burden, normalized to grams of creatinine clearance from the kidneys.

Humans are exposed to mercury from a variety of sources in addition to dental amalgams. There are extremely sensitive methods for detecting mercury in parts per trillion; these methods have made it possible to analyze the sources of mercury exposure for humans. Estimates of intake levels from air (in micrograms per day) are 0.12 for Hg^0, 0.04 for Hg^{2+}, and 0.03 for methyl mercury. Water probably contributes about 0.05 μg/day and food about 20.0 μg/day in the form of Hg^{2+}. Depending on one's diet, the consumption of fish contributes about 0.9 μg/day of Hg^0 and 3.8 μg/day of methyl mercury. These values place the 1–3 μg/day of absorbed Hg^0 vapor from amalgams in perspective. Thus, the intake of mercury is a complex issue with many sources and forms of exposure. Furthermore, there is considerable variability from individual to individual depending on diet, environment, and dental status. Despite the confirmed exposure of humans to these low levels of mercury, the biological effects of these levels are insignificant.

Numerous studies have attempted to determine whether mercury exposure from dental restorations or other sources contributes to any documentable health problem. Several studies have estimated the number of amalgam surfaces needed to expose an individual to mercury concentrations with a minimum observable effect (slightly impaired psychomotor performance, detectable tremor, and impaired nerve conduction velocity). Estimates are that several hundred amalgam surfaces would be necessary to achieve these levels. Even if all 32 teeth were restored on all surfaces with amalgam, the total number of surfaces (counting incisal edges) would be only 160. Other studies have measured renal function in patients in whom all of the amalgam was removed at the same time (the worst possible case). Despite markedly elevated blood, plasma, and urine levels of mercury, no renal impairment was noted. Still other studies have attempted to look at blood cell types and cell numbers in dentists, who are presumably exposed to higher levels of mercury because of their daily occupational exposure. No effects of mercury have been noted. Other studies for neurological symptoms in children populations occupationally exposed have shown no effects (Bellinger et al., 2006, 2007; DeRouen et al., 2002, 2006). In summary, there are simply no data to show that mercury released from dental amalgam is harmful to the general population.

Methacrylates and Resin-Based Composites

The best screening substance for methacrylate allergy caused by dental material products is HEMA. This result confirms previous findings (Goon et al., 2006), which revealed that HEMA alone picked up 96.7% of the patients with methacrylate allergy and 100% of the dental personnel with methacrylate allergy.

The frequency of positive responses to the common allergen test substances was reported as follows: gold sodium thiosulfate, 14.0%; nickel sulfate, 13.2%; mercury, 9.9%; palladium chloride, 7.4%; cobalt chloride, 5.0%; and HEMA 5.8% (Goon et al., 2006).

Estrogenicity

In 1996, a research group claimed that dental sealants released estrogenic substances in sufficient quantities to warrant concern (Olea et al., 1996). Since then, the **estrogenicity** of dental composites has also been questioned, particularly for use in children. Estrogenicity is the ability of a chemical to act as the hormone estrogen does in the body. If these chemicals are not indigenous to the body, the substance is called a **xenoestrogen**. The occurrence of xenoestrogens in the environment has been a concern for many years. Environmentalists fear that these substances will alter reproductive cycles and developmental processes in wildlife, and there is evidence to support these concerns with regard to humans. The concern about estrogens in dentistry centers around a chemical called *BPA*, which is a synthetic starting point for bis-GMA composites in dentistry as well as many other plastics. The fear is that the release of these substances might alter normal cellular development or cell maintenance if BPA has estrogenic effects, even at the impurity levels that may be encountered in practice. It is generally accepted that BPA is released from bis-DMA, which is also used in dental products. However, if bis-DMA is used, the amount released after placement of a restorative filling is too small to be of concern. However, to overcome any concerns, products free of bis-DMA can be used.

There is fairly convincing evidence that BPA and BPA dimethacrylate may act on the estrogenic receptors in cells. Thus, these chemicals are probably xenoestrogens. One test commonly used to assess xenoestrogenic activity is the *E-screen assay*. This in vitro test relies on the growth response of breast cancer cells, which are sensitive to potential estrogenic compounds.

Although the estrogenicity of BPA has been confirmed, there is little evidence that dental composites have estrogenic effects in vitro or in vivo. The original report of estrogenic effects in 1996 appears to have been overstated because several errors in the method and interpretation have subsequently been reported in the literature. Studies have shown only trace amounts of BPA in dental composites, and attempts at eluting BPA from polymerized composites have yielded either low or undetectable amounts. Coupled with the relative insensitivity of BPA as an estrogen and the likely dilution of any released BPA, the risks of estrogenic effects in vivo appear low. No studies have convincingly shown evidence of these effects from dental resin–containing materials.

Other Biological Considerations for Resins

The explosion in the use of resin-based composites for restorative work has raised questions about the biological safety of these materials. The primary risk of these materials appears to be allergy related, and the risk is highest for dental personnel because of frequent exposure to nonpolymerized materials. Allergy to other types of dental materials such as latex gloves and monomeric substances also represents the greatest risks of an adverse biological effect for dental office staff. The allergenicity of methylmethacrylate is well documented, and the use of gloves is not effective in preventing contact because most resin monomers pass easily through gloves. Also, allergic reactions to other methacrylates have been reported. The allergic reactions occur primarily as contact dermatitis, with the resins acting as haptens via delayed hypersensitivity (type IV) mechanisms.

Resins also have significant toxic effects, which are clearly demonstrated through the use of in vitro tests. The results of these tests are often comparable with, and sometimes worse than, the effects resulting from the use of metals. There is ample evidence that resins release nonpolymerized components into biological environments, although the release in vivo of specific substances is not well documented for either resins or metals. Resin components have also been shown to traverse dentin, and newer techniques that advocate direct pulp capping with resins expose pulp directly to these materials.

Titanium and Titanium Alloys

In vitro evaluation of titanium biocompatibility, percentage attachment efficiency, and proliferation of human fetal fibroblasts and human gingival fibroblasts reveals that a surface layer of titanium oxide (Ti_2O_3) has the ability to coexist with living tissues and organisms. Based on these studies one can conclude that titanium is relatively nontoxic, noninjurious, and not physiologically reactive. Titanium has a light weight, high strength, and excellent durability when exposed to chemical agents. However, it is susceptible to attack by acidic fluoride products.

Base Metal and Noble Metal Alloys

Predominantly base metal alloys are classified by the ADA as those containing less than 25% by weight of noble metals (gold, platinum, palladium, rhodium, ruthenium, iridium, and osmium). Noble alloys are classified as those that contain between 25% and 60% of these noble metal elements. High-noble (HN) metal alloys are classified by the ADA as those containing at least 40% gold and 60% of noble metal elements. Stainless steel (Fe–C–Ni–Cr), cobalt–chromium (Co–Cr), nickel–chromium (Ni–Cr), and cobalt–nickel–chromium (Co–Ni–Cr), classified as base metal alloys, and CPTi are used most often for removable fixed restorations and orthodontic appliances. Some evidence suggests that metal appliances can lead to gingivitis or periodontitis. The severity of these adverse effects varies as a function of atomic or molecular characteristics (Schmalz & Garhammer, 2002). Metallic components and microparticles from cast metal restorations have been found in contiguous plaque and gingival tissues. Although high-gold-content noble alloys are more resistant to corrosion than other alloys, most local adverse effects seem to occur when noble and base alloys are used together.

Metal ions can be leached from cast metal restorations or wrought appliances into the OC. Since HN and noble (N) alloys are corrosion resistant, one might expect a negligible level of leaching. However, allegations of adverse effects caused by leaching of palladium have raised concerns on the biocompatibility of these alloys (Wataha & Hanks, 1996). Biocompatibility studies have revealed that the strongest responses were derived from the Ni–Cr alloy and the weakest response was from the 22k gold alloy. The high-gold alloy and the high-palladium group showed reactions similar to those of the 22k gold alloy. However, the low-gold alloy and the Pd–Ag alloys ranked between the base metal alloy and the precious metal alloys.

Metallic ions released through corrosion processes are responsible for much of the metal−protein or metal−cell interaction behavior of dental metals and alloys. However, the surface structure of the metal, its composition, and its electrochemical properties also contribute to local interactions. Increased plaque accumulation can cause adverse inflammatory reactions in the adjacent soft tissues. Ions released from the superficial layers of cast alloys may be quite cytotoxic.

No correlation has been found between the noble metal content of alloys and the severity of corrosion. However, some base metals, such as nickel–chromium–beryllium (Ni–Cr–Be) alloys, exhibit increased corrosion in low-pH environments. Also, microscopic particles can be abraded from metallic restorations during wear processes. In sufficient quantities, metal ions such as copper, nickel, and beryllium can be released and subsequently induce inflammation of the adjacent periodontal tissues and the oral mucosa.

No evidence exists to prove that dental metallic materials are mutagenic, genotoxic, or carcinogenic. Although in vitro evidence suggests that the immune response can be altered by various metal ions, their role in oral inflammatory diseases such as gingivitis and periodontitis is unknown. Allergic reactions to metallic dental restorations have been described earlier. Nickel is known to be highly allergenic, especially in females. It has been reported that 34%–65% of patients who are allergic to nickel are also allergic to palladium. Further, palladium allergy seems to occur when individuals have been sensitized to nickel.

Nickel and Beryllium

Of many metals used in dentistry, nickel is a common chemical element in many base metal dental alloys, such as those used for crowns, fixed dental prostheses, removable partial dentures, and some orthodontic appliances. Nickel is also used in many types of endodontic files, although the duration of exposure through the use of files is far shorter. The use of nickel-based alloys for fixed prosthodontics in the United States has increased dramatically over the past 30 years and its use currently represents somewhere between 30% and 50% of the market. The use of nickel in dental alloys has been controversial for many years because of the allergenic potential of nickel ions and nickel compounds.

Nickel is the most allergenic metal known, with an incidence of allergic reactions between 10% and 20%. Reactions to nickel are more common among women, presumably because of the chronic exposure to nickel through jewelry, although the incidence among men is increasing. Reactions to nickel-containing dental alloys are well documented, and these can be quite severe in sensitized individuals. These reactions are probably under-reported because they are often subtle and can resemble periodontal inflammation (see Fig. 17.6A and B) or the erythema that results from excessive pressure on the palatal mucosa by metal frameworks. These reactions may also occur only outside the mouth.

Not all individuals with nickel allergy will react to intraoral nickel, and it is currently not possible to predict which individuals will react. Because the frequency of nickel allergy is high, it is possible that individuals will become sensitized to nickel after placement of nickel-containing alloys in the mouth.

The mechanisms of the high allergy frequency to nickel are not known, but there is probably a genetic component. Nickel has other adverse biological effects in addition to allergy. Nickel ions (Ni^{2+}) are a documented mutagen in humans, but there is no evidence that nickel ions cause any carcinogenic response intraorally. Nickel ions, along with cobalt and mercury, have also been shown to be nonspecific inducers of inflammatory reactions. It is well known that nickel-based alloys can exhibit significant corrosion and release of nickel ions in a low-pH environment. Beryllium-free Ni–Cr alloys are more corrosion resistant than beryllium-containing alloys. Base metal alloys containing both beryllium and nickel exhibit high beryllium release rates, which may pose a health risk.

In vitro environments do not necessarily simulate in vivo conditions. Many biological factors—including the biofilm characteristics, organic acid composition, and types of enzymes produced by oral microorganisms or those present in food—may contribute to alloy corrosion in vivo. Interactions between metallic restorations and patient factors such as consumption frequency of acidic foods and beverages and composition of saliva, can significantly affect intraoral corrosion. Corrosion may also be accelerated by phagocytotic cells such as human neutrophils (Yang et al., 1992). This has been demonstrated in clinical observations of removable partial denture frameworks made of titanium.

Wear can also accelerate the corrosion processes in vivo because of the local breakdown of the passivation layer (Khan et al., 1999). The dual action of corrosion and wear may accelerate breakdown in the oral environment.

In one study (Reuling et al., 1990), the corrosion rates of two Ni–Cr alloys with nearly identical compositions were significantly different. These results confirm that the release of metal ions from the alloys is not necessarily proportional to the nominal alloy composition (Wataha et al., 1991). On the basis of these studies, it is clear that the release of metal ions cannot be predicted from the nobility or the overall composition of cast alloys. Each product must be evaluated individually for its corrosion behavior and the release of metal ions in specific corrosive environments.

Although no general correlation has been demonstrated between alloy composition and cytocompatibility, severely cytotoxic alloys generally have contained higher amounts of nickel than biocompatible products.

Although beryllium is known to be highly toxic, it is used in some Ni–Cr alloys in concentrations of 1%–2% by weight (approximately 5.5%–11% atomic content) to increase the castability of these alloys and lower their melting range. It also tends to form thin adherent oxides that are required to promote atomic bonding of porcelain. The use of beryllium in dental alloys is controversial because of its biological effects. First, beryllium is a documented carcinogen in either the metallic (Be^0) or ionic (Be^{2+}) state, although there are no studies showing that dental alloys containing beryllium cause cancer in humans. Any reaction is most probably mediated by beryllium released from the alloys, and although such release has been documented intraorally and in vitro, it is not as prominent as for nickel. Acidic environments enhance beryllium release from Ni–Cr alloys.

Furthermore, beryllium-containing particles that are inhaled and reach the alveoli of the lungs may cause a chronic inflammatory condition called berylliosis. In this condition, the alveoli of the lung are engorged with lymphocytes and macrophages. T cells in susceptible individuals proliferate locally in the lung tissue, presumably in a delayed hypersensitivity reaction to the beryllium metal. Berylliosis occurs only in individuals with a hypersensitivity to beryllium and may occur from inhalation of beryllium dusts (from grinding or polishing alloys), salts, or fumes such as those encountered in casting beryllium-containing alloys. Thus, dental lab technicians would presumably be at the highest risk of adverse effects from exposure to beryllium dusts and vapors.

Cytotoxicity of Metals and Dental Casting Alloys

Cytotoxicity is often reported by an IC_{50} value, which is the inhibitory concentration (IC) that causes a 50% reduction in cell growth. A study of 43 metal salts, using the colony formation method and two types of cells (fibroblasts and osteoblast-like cells), revealed that IC_{50} depends on the types of metallic elements, their chemical states, and their elemental concentrations (Yamamoto et al., 1998). The IC_{50} for the salts with the highest toxicity (greater than 10^{-5} mol/L) were $CdCl_2$, VCl_3, $AgNO_3$, $HgCl_2$, $SbCl_3$, $BeSO_4$, and $InCl_3$. Their IC_{50}s differed by four orders of magnitude from the IC_{50} of the lowest-toxicity salt. The relatively high-toxicity salts—HgCl, $Ti(NO_3)_3$, $TiNO_3$, $GaCl_3$, $CuCl_2$, $MnCl_2$, $CoCl_2$, $ZnCl_2$, $NiCl_2$, $SnCl_2$, $IrCl_4$, CuCl, $RhCl_3$, $Pb(NO_3)_2$, $Cr(NO_3)_3$, and $Bi(NO_3)_3$—had IC_{50}s below 10^{-4} mol/L for each cell line (Arvidson et al., 1987).

Another study reported the metabolic as well as the morphological response of cultured human gingival fibroblasts to salt solutions of beryllium (Be^{2+}), chromium (Cr^{6+} and Cr^{3+}), nickel (Ni^{2+}), and molybdenum (Mo^{6+}) ions that may be released from dental alloys (Messer et al., 1999). The evaluation parameters included viability, lysosomal activity, oxygen consumption, membrane integrity, DNA synthesis, ribonucleic acid (RNA) synthesis, protein synthesis, intracellular adenosine triphosphate (ATP) levels, and glucose-6-phosphate dehydrogenase activity. Whereas Ni^{2+} ion solutions altered metabolic functions at concentrations of 3–30 parts per million (ppm) compared with Cr^{3+} and Mo^{6+} at concentrations of 10 and 100 ppm, Cr^{6+} and Be^{2+} were the most toxic ions, which caused cellular alterations at concentrations of 0.04–12 ppm. Heavy metal ions such as Ni^{2+} and Co^{2+}, released from an implanted alloy by corrosion, can be distributed systemically by proteins, such as albumin. Cast CPTi has been found to be highly biocompatible (Berstein et al., 1992; Wang & Li, 1998). Further, it was observed that the corrosion resistance of a noble or base metal alloy does not permit one to draw conclusions as to its biocompatibility. It was also found that solid specimens of gold-based solders combined with a substrate alloy were very often less cytotoxic than the solders alone. Only three solder-substrate alloy combinations revealed more pronounced toxic reactions than the single solders (Wataha et al., 1995).

Various studies have shown that copper is more toxic than gold, palladium, and titanium. However, this result may be misleading since copper is more susceptible to corrosion. Thus, analyses of cytotoxicity test results should also consider the relative corrosion rates of specific elements in various solutions including artificial saliva.

In addition to the nature and quantity of released cations, surface topography of a cast metallic structure may be an important factor for biocompatibility. Thus, released metal ions as well as surface topography may contribute to local adverse effects in the gingiva and PD adjacent to cast restorations.

Dental Ceramics

Dental materials are exposed to a wide range of solids and liquids with a range of pH values and temperatures in the oral environment.

Therefore, excellent chemical durability is an important prerequisite in selecting ceramics as well as other restorative dental materials. Overall, the risk of surface degradation is low, and feldspathic ceramics have been used as clinical veneers for many years without significant biocompatibility issues.

Ceramic materials are known for their high levels of biocompatibility. Metal oxides such as Al_2O_3, BaO, CaO, K_2O, Li_2O, Na_2O, ZnO, and ZrO_2 are components of either dental core ceramics or dental veneering (layering) ceramics, and silicone dioxide (SiO_2) is the principal matrix phase component of all veneering ceramics. These oxides and related compounds in dental ceramics exhibit minimal dissolution in normal oral fluids and beverages. However, highly acidic environments can increase the release rates of certain metal and silicone ions. For example, acidulated phosphate fluoride (APF) is known to corrode the surfaces of veneering porcelains as well as glaze and stain ceramics. This is an extreme case, which suggests that APF should not be used in patients who have ceramic or metal−ceramic restorations.

Zirconia Biocompatibility

Yttria-stabilized zirconia (Y-TZP) has a material density of greater than 6.0 g/cm^3 and a maximum operating temperature of 2000°C. This material has the highest flexural strength (900 MPa) of the zirconia materials. Its flexural strength can increase to 1400 MPa when it is processed by hot isostatic pressing (HIP). The hardness of Y-TZP is 13–13.5 GPa. Its fracture toughness is 8 MPa·m$^{1/2}$, and its coefficient of thermal expansion (CTE) is relatively low (10.2×10^{-6}/K). The excellent mechanical properties of this material are a result of a very small grain size, extremely low porosity, and transformation toughening.

The biocompatibility of zirconia has been evaluated extensively. No local or systemic cytotoxic effects or adverse reactions have been traced to zirconia. The bone response of zirconia in vivo and the inflammation adjacent to zirconia have been shown to be satisfactory. Furthermore, bacteria and pathogen seem to adhere to zirconia to the same extent as to other materials.

Sensitization to and Irritation by Ceramics

Several investigators have demonstrated that, unlike other dental materials, most dental ceramics do not induce an adverse effect when they contact the oral mucous membrane. Others have shown that glazed ceramics, which have been used in implant trials, caused very mild inflammatory reactions. These glazed ceramics were less irritating than resin-based composite or gold.

Thus, compared with other dental materials, ceramic has no or very limited potential to induce irritation or sensitizing reactions. Since this evidence shows that ceramic materials do not cause direct irritation to cells of the mucous membrane, one can conclude that minor observed irritations may be attributed to mechanical irritation, for example, from roughened surfaces.

Radioactivity

Naturally occurring radioactivity has been detected in certain dental ceramics. Veronese et al. (2006) reported that the dose rates from natural radionuclides in feldspathic porcelains and glass ceramics were about 10 times higher than the background value, whereas resin-based composites and alumina-based ceramics exhibited negligible beta dose rates, which were similar to those from natural teeth.

Latex

Both patients and office staff are exposed to latex from many sources, including toy balloons, condoms, swim goggles, dishwashing gloves, hairnet elastics, clothing elastics, footwear, cervical diaphragms, and hot water bottles. Of particular interest in dentistry is the use of latex gloves and latex rubber dams, which expose both patients and dental personnel to this potential allergen. In the early 1980s, when HIV infection became a major safety issue, dental personnel began to routinely wear gloves to reduce the risk of transmission. Since that time, the incidence of latex hypersensitivity reactions has increased enormously. In 1991, the FDA estimated that about 6%–7% of surgical personnel may be allergic to latex. Surveys of dental professionals have shown that 42% have adverse reactions to occupational materials, most of which were related to dermatoses of the hands and fingers. Adverse reactions to latex gloves have been reported in 3.7% of adult patients and 5.7% of pediatric patients.

Natural latex products are made from a white milky sap harvested from a tree growing in tropical regions. Ammonia is added to the sap to preserve it, but at the same time, the ammonia hydrolyzes and degrades the sap proteins to produce allergens. Vulcanization is the process by which liquid latex is hardened into rubber through the use of sulfur compounds and heat. These chemicals may be allergenic themselves and are often present to some degree in the final product. The manufacturing process leaches the allergens by soaking the rubber products in hot water. The leaching water is changed repeatedly to decrease the concentration of the allergens, but leaching brings other allergens to the surface and unfortunately places the highest concentrations near the skin of the wearer. Thus, the allergenicity of a given batch of latex will be dependent on how the latex was collected, preserved, and processed. Synthetic latex is also available, but it produces the same problems except that naturally occurring proteins and their degradation products are not present.

CRITICAL QUESTION

What evidence or documentation can you provide to dental patients to assure them that amalgam is a safe material for dental restorations?

Adverse Effects Data From National Registries

Reporting systems for monitoring intraoral reactions to dental materials complement traditional biocompatibility evaluations of dental materials products. Because of the overwhelming number of dental biomaterials that have been developed in recent years, it is essential that such reporting systems be established to assist dental practitioners in their optimal selection and use.

From 1993 to 2011, three countries had established registries for spontaneous reporting of adverse effects that result from the use of dental materials. In 1993, a national reporting system was established in Norway, funded by the Ministry of Health and Social Affairs. Similar reporting registries were established in Sweden in 1996 and in the United Kingdom in 1999.

Although some countries have established systems for submitting adverse effects reports, only a few of these are sufficiently comprehensive to encourage periodic reviews of the data and publication of the results. Reports from these programs are described below.

Some Scandinavian studies (Jacobsen & Hensten-Pettersen, 1989, 1993; Kallus & Mjör, 1991) revealed that adverse effects on personnel associated with exposure to dental materials were extremely rare. The incidence of these reactions ranges from 0.038% (1 in 2600) to 0.143% (1 in 700).

One study (Vamnes et al., 2004) investigated the relationship between patient complaints and objective clinical findings based on 899 adverse effects reports that had been submitted between 1993 and 1999 to the Dental Biomaterials Adverse Reaction Unit (DBARU) at the University of Bergen in Norway. The reports submitted by dentists and physicians were based on subjective symptoms, objective findings, or both. Reported reactions were compared with clinical findings obtained after dental and medical examinations at the DBARU. These examinations involved patients who had reported reactions primarily to amalgam fillings (84%) and metals in fixed dental prostheses (11%). Reactions to resins, cements, removable denture materials, and endodontic materials were also reported but at a much lower frequency (2%–4%). In 80 of the patients, the examinations revealed edema, lichenoid reactions, ulcers, vesicles, erythema, and atrophy. For 35 of these patients, the intraoral findings from examinations at the DBARU were similar to those in the dentists' reports. For another 45 patients, objective intraoral signs of reactions that had not been reported were found upon examination. Patients with suspected adverse reactions have reported anxiety, burning sensation, concentration difficulty, depression, dry mouth, disturbance of taste, pain in muscles and joints, dizziness, fatigue, headache, memory problems, and restlessness. Many patients reported subjective symptoms without any observed objective signs of adverse effects or reactions.

Another DBARU report was based on 296 patients, 70% of them were women between 40 and 49 years of age, who were referred primarily for effects attributed to dental amalgam (85%) and metals in crowns and bridges (11%). Nearly all of the patients (96%) reported general subjective symptoms of muscle and joint pain, fatigue, and memory problems. Complaints involving the orofacial tissues (lips, face, and temporomandibular joint) and intraoral symptoms were also reported. The investigators could not identify a specific cause-and-effect relationship between the dental biomaterials in question and the patients' general symptoms.

A study of a preliminary survey (Scott et al., 2004) by the UK Adverse Reactions Reporting Project (ARRP) was designed to measure the severity of adverse reactions to dental materials in the United Kingdom. The reporting forms distributed to dental professionals were modified versions of the forms used by adverse reaction units in Bergen, Norway, and Umeå, Sweden. The ARRP received 1075 complete reports of adverse reactions observed or experienced by dental staff and patients. Most of the patient-related adverse reactions (16.3%) were associated with metals (n = 175). These metal exposure effects were mainly lichenoid reactions associated with amalgam restorations (n = 124, or 70.9%). Dental technicians reported acrylic resin as the cause of hand dermatitis in 61.1% (44 out of a total 72) of the reported cases. Dental surgery staff reported gloves as the cause of hand dermatitis in 75.0% of cases (398 out of a total 531). These results indicate that dental staff members are at risk mostly from an adverse reaction to latex gloves, whereas most patients are at risk for reactions associated with metals. For dental technicians, the greatest danger of an adverse reaction was from acrylic resins. The Swedish National Register of Side Effects (SNRSE) was established in 1996. It was set up in collaboration with Medical Odontological faculty of the University of Umeå, Sweden. This reporting registry is similar to the one that has been in use since 1993 at the University of Bergen, Norway, and the Swedish unit has collaborated with the Norwegian unit.

One study revealed the types and duration of side effects to resin-based dental materials based on 618 reports (456 on patients and 162 on dental practitioners) from 1996 to 1999 that had been submitted to the SNRSE (Tillberg et al., 2009). The link between the material and the reaction was assessed as *probable*, *possible*, *uncertain*, or *unclassifiable*, depending on the probability of the relationship and the quality of information submitted by the observer. The inclusion criteria for the patients to be accepted into the study were (1) reactions thought to be caused by direct resin-based restorations; (2) reactions that the expert group of the SNRSE had assessed to be *probable* or *possible*; and (3) reactions occurring during the years 1996–1999. Fifteen percent of the patients made complaints related to treatment with composite and bonding materials. The majority of complaints were based on intraoral effects or a combination of intraoral and extraoral effects that occurred within 24 hours after treatment. The most common adverse effects were related to skin, oral ulcers, and burning mouth complaints. These effects disappeared in 50% of the patients in less than a week. The investigators concluded that immediate reactions to resin-based materials were more common than delayed allergic reactions and the mechanism responsible for the immediate reactions was probably nonallergic in most cases.

Dental materials are among the most widely used synthetic biomaterials to be placed in the human body. They are classified as medical devices according to the European Medical Devices Directive (EMDD). According to the EMDD, reports of serious or life-threatening reactions should be sent to the manufacturers of the products and not necessarily to a neutral oversight organization.

In the United States, the 1976 MDA, which became effective in 1984, require device manufacturers to report deaths, serious injuries, and malfunctions to the US FDA. The FDA receives adverse event reports on devices as either individual reports or summary reports. Individual reports include voluntary reports submitted by health care providers and consumers through MedWatch (http://www.fda.gov/Safety/MedWatch/default.htm), the safety information and adverse event reporting program of the FDA. Mandatory reports are submitted by manufacturers and user facilities. Fuller and Parmentier (2001) reported that 28,555 reports on dental devices were submitted to the FDA over a 35-month period between 1996 and 1999. Injuries represented 64.4% of the reports, 90% of which were associated with endosseous implants. Malfunction of dental devices accounted for 34.8% of these reports. Only two deaths were reported (0.007%) during this period.

Allergic Reactions

The previous reviews of reports from three national registries of adverse events reveal that most of the effects were associated with metals. Furthermore, patch tests for potential allergies to dental materials also suggest that the most likely allergens were components of cast dental alloys (Ditrichova et al., 2007). In this study, patch tests were performed on 25 subjects with lichenoid lesions located on the buccal mucosa, tongue, and lips. Two sets of allergens, the "European Standard" and "Dental Screening" (Chemotechnique Diagnostics, Sweden) were used, supplemented with pulverized amalgam, iridium, indium, menthol, sorbic acid, and platinum.

Tests were performed in accordance with International Contact Dermatitis Research Group guidelines. A total of 15 patients (60% overall) exhibited sensitization to one or more allergens, with a total of 31 positive reactions. The greatest frequency of positives was associated with dental metals (27 positive reactions). The order of tested metals according to frequency of positive reactions was mercury (24%), amalgam (24%), nickel (16%), palladium (16%), cobalt (12%), gold (8%), chromium (4%), and indium (4%). The correspondence of the material's presence in the mouth to the positive test result was 44%. However, susceptibility to allergic reactions varies considerably from one metal to another. Some estimates indicate that 15% of the population is sensitized to nickel, whereas only 4.2% (Valentine-Thon et al., 2006) of the population is sensitized to titanium.

No standard patch test for Ti has so far been adopted, and positive reactions to Ti have only rarely been demonstrated with skin testing. Patch testing in general has been validated only for the epidermal antigen contact test, which may itself induce sensitization of naive T lymphocytes, and is relevant primarily for detecting dermal effects of hypersensitivity (contact dermatitis). *In vitro* testing with the lymphocyte transformation test (LTT) on the other hand, can detect both dermally and nondermally sensitizing allergens (e.g., beryllium). A version of LTT called memory lymphocyte immunostimulation assay (MELISA®) was selected for investigating hypersensitivity to Ti. Müller and Valentine-Thon (2006) demonstrated that titanium can induce clinically relevant hypersensitivity in a subgroup of patients chronically exposed via dental or endoprosthetic implants.

Palladium-based alloys have been associated with stomatitis and oral lichenoid reactions, and palladium allergy seems to occur mainly in patients who have been sensitized to nickel. Except for titanium, many casting metal elements, including nickel, palladium, cobalt, gold, and chromium, have the potential to induce adverse reactions in hypersensitive patients. Individuals who are allergic to a metal are likely to exhibit allergic contact dermatitis as well as lichenoid lesions. Based on one study of 25 patients with lichenoid lesions, positive responses to standard patch tests were found for amalgam (25%), nickel (16%), palladium (16%), cobalt (1%), gold (8%), chromium (4%), and indium (4%). In another study of patients who exhibited patch test reactions to mercury compounds, partial or complete replacement of amalgam fillings led to a significant improvement in nearly all patients (Laeijendecker et al., 2004).

In 1996, the Finnish Contact Dermatitis Group patch tested more than 4000 patients (2300–2600 of the patients for most allergens) with a dental screening series (Kanerva et al., 1996, 2001). The irritant reactions were scored as "irritant" or "doubtful," and allergic responses were scored as +, ++, or +++, respectively. A reaction index was calculated, on the irritancy of the patch test substances. The most frequent allergic patch test reactions were induced by nickel (14.6%), ammoniated mercury (13%), mercury (10.3%), gold (7.7%), benzoic acid (4.3%), palladium (4.2%), cobalt (4.1%), and 2-hydroxyethylmethacrylate (HEMA) (2.8%).

Nickel is one of the metals most likely to initiate such reactions. Individuals who wear jewelry are also more susceptible because of the common addition of nickel as an alloying element. Men who have body piercings and metallic decorations are susceptible to metal allergies (Ehrlich et al., 2001). This study supported the theory of coreactivity of nickel and cobalt but not for nickel and palladium.

Other high-risk situations for metal allergies are exposures to soil, saltwater, cement, leather, antiperspirants, belt buckles, metal denture frameworks, pins, bra strap attachments, and zippers. However, one investigator (Hensten-Pettersen, 1992) concluded that even though base metal alloys were alleged to be a major concern to the dental profession, relatively few case reports have substantiated this concern. In fact, allergy to gold-based dental restorations has been more commonly reported. He hypothesized that tolerance induction may be a possible benefit of the use of intraorally placed alloys. In nonsensitized individuals, oral antigenic contacts to nickel and chromium may induce tolerance rather than sensitization.

Few studies have classified the clinical manifestations of contact allergic dermatitis from exposure to specific allergens in the dental series for contact dermatitis. The results from one study (Khamaysi et al., 2006) indicate that the most frequent oral manifestations were cheilitis and perioral dermatitis (25.6%), burning mouth (15.7%), lichenoid lesions (14.0%), and orofacial granulomatosis (10.7%). A total of 14.9% of the patients were dental personnel, each of whom suffered from hand dermatitis. The most common allergens were gold sodium thiosulfate (14.0%), nickel sulfate (13.2%), mercury (9.9%), palladium chloride (7.4%), cobalt chloride (5.0%), and HEMA (5.8%). Positive reactions to metals were frequent in all the clinical variants, and no specific association between a specific clinical presentation and a particular allergen was found. An allergy to mercury does not seem to contribute to the pathogenesis of oral lichenoid reactions. One should note that oral lichen planus lesions are more generalized and that oral lichen planus–like (lichenoid) lesions occur primarily/only at the contact area with the causative material, although such a reaction can also be caused by chronic mechanical trauma.

A 2009 study (Raap et al., 2009) explored the relationship between positive patch test reactions to metal alloys used in dentistry or their salts and clinical symptoms. This study comprised 206 patients who underwent patch testing with dental metals because of suspected contact allergy. Twenty-eight patients (13.5%) had positive patch test reactions to dental metals. The majority of positive patch test reactions occurred for gold sodium thiosulfate, palladium chloride, and nickel sulfate, followed by amalgam, ammoniated mercury, and cobalt chloride and amalgam metals (copper, tin, and zinc), and ammonium tetrachloroplatinate (n = 1). Only 7% of the patients had a clinically relevant contact allergy on the oral mucosa (3.5% with lichen planus and 3.5% with stomatitis). The conclusions of the study were that contact allergies to dental metals are infrequent and that the most frequent contact allergens were gold sodium thiosulfate and palladium chloride.

Hosoki et al. (2009) revealed that allergies to metals in some patients were manifested not only as lichen planus and contact dermatitis responses but also as psoriasis-like reactions (pustulosis palmaris et plantaris), which may occur on hands, feet, or the entire body. Patch testing of 78.8% females and 21.2% males indicated that 68.8% of the patients had one or more positive patch test reactions. The most common allergens were nickel (25.0%), palladium (24.4%), chromium (16.7%), cobalt (15.9%), and tin (12.5%). Pustulosis palmaris et plantaris reactions are considered a subcategory of psoriasis and affect the palms of the hands and the soles of the feet. These effects can be very painful and may make it difficult to perform manual tasks or to walk. Thus, treatment of these patients is critically important to relieve their suffering.

If a patient is allergic to a metal or other material, an allergic response to it on first contact and allergy symptoms will appear within 10 days. After sensitization to the particular substance, even brief contact with that allergen may cause the allergic contact dermatitis to reappear within 24–48 hours (Website, Asthma and Allergy Foundation of America: http://www.aafa.org/display.cfm?id=9&sub=23&cont=329). One of the most common signs is a change in the color of the skin, which usually appears on the spot that was in contact with the metal. Other areas can exhibit signs after the initial reaction has occurred. The general signs of contact allergies include (1) reddish, itchy, swollen skin; (2) vesicles; (3) scaly areas; (4) darkening of affected tissue; (5) leathery skin; and (6) cracked skin. The best "cures" for these reactions are avoidance of the suspected metals, use of nonmetallic jewelry, use of hypoallergenic jewelry such as that containing titanium, or a high gold content (e.g., 18 karat or more).

A study of 139 published cases of allergic reactions to dental metallic restorations showed that these patients suffered from local irritations primarily in the form of gingivitis and stomatitis (Hildebrand et al., 1989). Only 23.7% of 139 persons revealed general reactions. When the restorations were removed, 82.7% of the patients recovered from the allergic reactions. Analysis of these data demonstrates that local allergic reactions to metals may often be underdiagnosed as inflammatory reactions.

In other studies, lichenoid reactions, swelling, and pain in oral soft tissues and lips have been observed. In several patients, gold ions caused an allergic contact gingivostomatitis, which was similar in appearance to erosive lichen planus (Izumi, 1982; Laeijendecker & van Joost, 1994). Many of these patients had a history of reactions to gold jewelry.

Observations in another study, Vamnes et al. (2004) revealed that patch testing with substances in dental materials produced 23% positive responses to gold sodium thiosulfate, 28% to nickel sulfate, 14% to cobalt chloride, 9% to palladium chloride, 6% to mercury, and 8% to components of resin-based materials (18 substances).

Exposure of patients to dental materials and other products can elicit signs or symptoms such as burning, tingling, cheilitis, oral lichenoid lesions, and swelling of the face, lips, tongue, palate, and buccal mucosa. The main cause of immediate-type allergic reactions was latex. Adverse reactions following the use of local anesthetics occurred in less than 5% of cases, and immediate-type allergic reactions to these agents were rare.

Marcusson et al. (1998) evaluated the relationship between the test results of metal allergies for 397 patients who claimed to have experienced a variety of subjective symptoms related to dental restorative materials and the corresponding allergies of eczematous patients. The difference between the frequencies of metal allergy in the dental group was statistically significant or close to significance for nickel sulfate, potassium dichromate, cobalt chloride, palladium chloride, and gold sodium thiosulfate. These findings suggest that the dental patient group represents a subgroup with a high frequency of metal allergies.

Based on a retrospective study of patch tests (Finn Chambers on Scanpor Tape applied to the upper back) from a medical center in Israel from 2000 to 2004, the extent and severity of adverse reactions to dental materials were evaluated to determine the frequency of allergens of the dental series associated with contact dermatitis and to identify the relationship between the allergens of dental relevance and clinical manifestations (Khamaysi et al., 2006). Between 2000 and 2004, 121 patients aged 20–80 years were patch tested and evaluated. Examinations revealed that the most frequent oral manifestations were cheilitis and perioral dermatitis (25.6%), burning mouth (15.7%), lichenoid reaction (14.0%), and orofacial granulomatosis (10.7%). Dental personnel, representing 18 (14.9%) of the 121 patients, all suffered from hand dermatitis.

It has been observed that patients with a previous history of positive skin reactions to nickel did not develop local or systemic adverse effects in response to a nickel-containing alloy. No association between patients' orofacial complaints and patch test results was found (Yontchev et al., 1986).

The components of dental allergy tests have included both noble metal and base metal elements. One group has proposed an allergy test for metal ions released from dental restorations, including the following elements/ions: Au^{3+}, Pd^{2+}, Zn^{2+}, Mo^{6+}, Sn^{2+}, Ga^{3+}, Co^{2+}, Cr^{3+}, Cr^{6+}, Ni^{2+}, Fe^{2+}, Fe^{3+}, and Si^{4+} (van Loon et al., 1986).

A study of 60 persons documented that nickel has the highest allergenic potency, followed by chromium, cobalt, silver, copper, palladium, platinum, and gold (Kansu & Aydin, 1996). Allergic reactions to 49 selected casting alloys, CPTi, and amalgam were investigated in an epidemiological study population of 763 patients. Most frequently, nickel, cobalt, and silver caused allergic irritations. In addition, a surprisingly high incidence of positive dermal reactions to titanium (4.2%) has been reported (Valentine-Thon et al., 2006). This result indicates that titanium should also be considered in the diagnosis of allergic reactions to metallic dental restorations.

Metals of the platinum group exhibit a considerable allergenic potency. In particular, allergic reactions to palladium—including contact dermatitis, intraoral contact mucositis, and lichenoid reactions—have been reported. However, Wataha and Hanks (1996) concluded that palladium does not pose an increased risk to the health of patients because of the limited dissolution rate of palladium from these alloys. However, one should note that palladium in cast metals may react differently in single phase compared with multiphase dental alloys that tend to be less corrosion resistant. The corrosion products of these multiphase alloys may affect the allergenicity as well as the cytotoxicity of palladium-based alloys differently compared with single-phase alloys. The presence of gold alloy restorations significantly increases the prevalence of gold sensitivity. A total of 136 asymptomatic patients were patch tested for gold sensitivity. Of 136 patients tested, 33.8% of those with gold restorations had positive skin reactions, whereas only 10.8% of the patients without gold restorations exhibited positive reactions (Schaffron et al., 1999).

CRITICAL QUESTION

When a dentist decides to place an implant or to restore a tooth, which potential adverse effects can be caused solely by the material used?

Toxicity

Toxicologists are trained to analyze the biochemical and molecular mechanisms that produce adverse effects through foreign substances such as restorative materials and auxiliary dental products. Paracelsus (1493−1541), who is sometimes referred to as the first modern medical scientist or as the father of toxicology, stated in German, *"Alle Ding' sind Gift, und nichts ohn' Gift; allein die Dosis macht, daß ein Ding kein Gift ist."* This is translated as, "All things are poison, and nothing is without poison; only the dose permits something not to be poisonous." Alternative translations of the latter phrase are: "The right dose differentiates a poison from a remedy," and "The dose makes the poison."

Toxicity Tests

These tests are designed with the following elements: (1) a test organism such as cells and selected strains of bacteria through higher-order plants and animals, (2) a specific response or biological endpoint, (3) an exposure or test period, and (4) a dose or a dose curve. The test design should be a good human model—that is, an objective response that can be reproduced with comparable results—and the test time should be of reasonable length.

Dose–Response Relationships

Toxicity tests exhibit a dose–response relationship when there is a consistent mathematical relationship between the proportion of individuals responding and a given dose for a given exposure period. For example, the number of mortalities increases with an increase in the dose of chemicals given to a group of organisms. Since toxicity is dose dependent, the effect of a specific dose of a therapeutic substance may be toxic, nontoxic, or beneficial. The quantity of a substance (in milligrams) ingested by test animals is often expressed as a ratio of milligrams per kilogram of body weight (mg/kg).

The species of test organisms differ in how they respond to specific chemicals. The same species of an organism may show variations in response to a given dose. Typically, this intraspecies variation follows a normal distribution when one plots the number of responding organisms against the response for a given dose. A dose can be described either as a lethal dose (LD) in a test when the response is death or an effective dose (ED), for which the response is another observable outcome. A dose–response plot allows us to identify the doses that affect a percentage of the exposed population. For example, LD50 is the dose that kills 50% of the test organisms.

Significance of Dose–Response Relationships

By comparing the LD50 of chemicals in animals we can rate the relative **acute toxicity** of each chemical. For example, DDT (LD50 for rats = 113 mg/kg), an insecticide, is considered more toxic than ethyl alcohol (LD50 for rats = 1400 mg/kg). By multiplying this LD50 dose (mg/kg) by 70 kg (the average weight of a human) and assuming that humans are as sensitive as the species that were exposed to the test substance, we can estimate the LD50 for humans of average size. However, the LD50 serves only as a rough estimate of one aspect of the toxic potential of a substance.

Shortcomings of Dose–Response Data

Before using the LD50 dose–response data to assess the overall toxicity of a compound, one should note that an LD50 dose is a single value on a plotted graph and does not identify the time dependency of the dose–effect relationship. Second, the LD50 is a measure of acute toxicity, not chronic effects. A complete battery of toxicity tests includes analyses of subacute toxicity, chronic toxicity, carcinogenicity, and reproductive toxicity. Thus, the LD50 dose should be used with extreme caution.

Exposure Pathways for Toxins in Humans

The three main pathways through which harmful substances are likely to enter the body are (1) absorption through skin and eye contact, (2) inhalation, and (3) ingestion. Skin acts as a barrier against the entry of foreign substances into the body. If this protective barrier is broken by abrasions or lacerations, toxic chemicals can penetrate the barrier and migrate into the body. In addition, exposure to some organic solvents can increase the permeability of skin to substances that would ordinarily be able to penetrate the surface. Furthermore, skin has a large surface area, which facilitates contact by toxic substances.

The fastest way for toxic substances to enter the body is through inhalation (see Fig. 17.1). Inhaled vapors or particulate matter can make immediate contact with respiratory tissues and soon thereafter with the bloodstream. Once a substance has entered the bloodstream, it is transported rapidly throughout the body.

Based on the patch testing of dental personnel who were referred as patients to the Department of Occupational and Environmental Dermatology, Stockholm, hand eczema was diagnosed in 63% of 174 cases, 67% being classified as irritant contact dermatitis and 33% as allergy-induced contact dermatitis (Wrangsjo et al., 2001). Further diagnoses included other eczemas, urticaria, rosacea, psoriasis, tinea pedis, bullous pemphigoid, and no skin disease. A total of 59% of the participants had positive reactions to substances in the standard series and 40% to substances exclusive of the dental series. Of the 22% patients who had positive reactions to methacrylates, the majority reacted to several test preparations. Reactions to HEMA, EGDMA (ethyleneglycol dimethacrylate), and MMA (methylmethacrylate) were most frequent, and 37% were positive only to methacrylates; the remaining 15 also had reactions to allergens in the standard series; 95% of these had hand eczema and 5% had facial eczema. The most frequent allergens besides methacrylates were nickel, cobalt, palladium, fragrance mix, colophonium, and thiuram mix. Allergy to natural rubber latex was diagnosed in 14 of 137 (10%) subjects. In summary, irritant hand dermatitis was the dominant diagnosis. Contact allergy to methacrylate was seen in 22% of the patch-tested patients.

Ingestion of potentially harmful substances by lab technicians and dental staff is not as great a concern as is exposure through skin and lungs. Compared with penetration of skin, ingestion opportunities are limited because there are very few dental substances that can be swallowed.

Reactions to Toxic Agents

There are several adverse reactions that can be caused by exposure to biomaterial substances and processes. These include reactions to the following:

1. Systemic toxins such as chemical agents, which can act on target organs or organ systems.
2. Asphyxiants, which deprive the tissues of oxygen (anoxia).
3. Irritants, which cause inflammation of tissues by direct contact.
4. Allergic sensitizers, which activate the production of antibodies—which, in turn, react with the antigen to make it a latent complex (when the body becomes exposed one or more times to the sensitized agent, the concentration of antibodies increases until an antigen–antibody reaction, or allergic reaction, results in one or more symptoms).
5. Carcinogens, which are substances known to cause cancer in an organism.
6. Reproductive toxins, such as mutagens or teratogens.

Toxic chemicals, such as those that may be handled by dentists and lab technicians, can cause a localized or systemic reaction by contacting the skin or tissue directly by ingestion in liquid or solid form or by inhalation as dusts, particles, mists, fumes, or other types of vapors. In addition to reacting to chemical carcinogens, patients may also be affected by physical carcinogens, such as ionizing radiation. Further discussion of the nature of carcinogens or reproductive system toxins is beyond the scope of this book.

Genotoxicity, Mutagenicity, and Carcinogenicity

Genotoxicity refers to any adverse effect on the DNA of an organism. If the adverse effect is transferred to the next (heritable) generation of cells, the effect is called mutagenicity. Mutagenic reactions occur when a physical or chemical agent changes the genetic material of an organism, usually deoxyribonucleic acid (DNA) permanently, thereby increasing the frequency of mutations above the normal background level. Mutations may be caused directly, through interactions between a substance and DNA, or indirectly, by altering cellular processes that control DNA integrity. Mutations are common occurrences in the DNA of all humans and they may result from many factors such as radiation, chemicals, and genetic errors in the DNA replication process. Several metal ions from dental materials—such as beryllium, copper, and nickel—are known mutagens, and some components of other materials such as root canal sealers have also been shown to be mutagenic. Resin-based materials have also been identified as having some mutagenic potential. However, it must be emphasized that mutagenicity does not have the same consequences as carcinogenicity, or the ability to form tumors. In fact, many mutations are repaired and others are irrelevant or insignificant. Equally important is the fact that the material and nature of an exposure can control the mutagenic or carcinogenic response. No dental material has ever been shown to be carcinogenic in dental patients.

Much effort has been devoted to validating the potential of certain metals, monomers, and other dental substances to impair the local and systemic immune responses of dental patients with cast metallic restorations. Why is our interest in immunological effects so high? The adverse effects of dental material substances generally are limited to local tissue reactions, and toxic effects from typical concentrations of metal ions, monomers, and other substances have not been proven. However, if any impairment of the autoimmune system was traced to an interaction with dental materials, the impact on the practice of dentistry and on the quality of life of our patients could be enormous. Gender may play a significant role in this scenario. Both the innate and adaptive immune responses of females are somewhat more robust than those of males. Females are somewhat more susceptible to autoimmune disorders such as systemic lupus erythematosus, rheumatoid arthritis, and multiple sclerosis.

Since these gender differences are largely attributed to estrogen levels, any interaction of the body with biomaterial substances that affect the production of estrogen or its associated enzymes or that attack native cells as if they were foreign bodies may play a major role in causing these severe systemic diseases. Thus, research must continue to screen material components for their ability to induce autoimmune disturbances. Such research may focus on cytokines (the molecules that carry signals between the immune system cells), apoptosis (a measure of the relative ability of the immune system to eliminate cells that die normally), and B cells (which are unique white blood cells that are important for fighting off bacteria). Too little or excessive estrogen production may lead to insufficient B cells or the inability to support their survival longer than is desirable.

The induction of immune mediators by metallic materials has been investigated using lymphocyte cell lines. Expressions of the inflammatory mediator interleukin 2 (IL-2) and the immune effector IgG by T and B cells were found after incubation with three copper-based casting alloys. The production of these immune mediators was altered by released cations (Bumgardner et al., 1993). Lipopolysaccharide (LPS)–stimulated osteoblast-like cells increased IL-1a and TNF-α after the cells were incubated with cobalt, chromium, and titanium. This study showed that metal ions disrupted cytokine release, osteoblast function, and the synthesis of type I collagen.

Cytokines can be released from unstimulated and stimulated peripheral blood mononuclear cells after incubation with chromium ions. In addition, chromium cations can reduce cell viability, DNA synthesis, secretion of IL-6, and expression of soluble IL-2 receptor. These results suggest that chromium may suppress the immune system (Donati et al., 1998).

Several metal ions (Ag, Au, Cu, Hg, Ni, Pd, Pt, and Zn) have induced the secretion of proteins from macrophages (Wataha et al., 1995). Subtoxic concentrations of a nickel solution also induced an increase of IL-1a and TNF-α secretion from unstimulated and LPS-stimulated THP-1 monocytes (macrophages) (Wataha & Hanks, 1996). In most cases, carcinogenic metal ions are not mutagenic in bacterial test assays. Alteration of DNA repair processes and carcinogenic effects have been reported for Cd^{2+}, Ni^{2+}, and Co^{2+} (Hartwig, 1995). Nickel has exhibited a relatively weak mutagenic activity.

There is evidence that metallic components derived from cast dental prostheses can modulate the expression of various immunological factors. An increased expression of cytokines after LPS stimulation by various cell types indicates that bacterial toxins and cations released by corrosion may collectively cause inflammatory effects related to oral mucositis, gingivitis, periodontitis, and alveolar bone resorption.

Genotoxic effects have been reported for beryllium and gallium salts (Kuroda et al., 1991). Occupational data indicate that beryllium may increase the risk of lung cancer and other tumors in humans (Aller, 1990; Ashby et al., 1990; Hayes, 1997). No genotoxic effects were found for orthodontic appliances (wires, brackets, extension screws) fabricated with base metal alloys and CPTi (Assad et al., 1998; Tomakidi, 2000; Wever et al., 1997). No genotoxic effects were found for several titanium-containing alloys, CPTi, and one Ni–Cr−based alloy (Wang & Li, 1998). There is some evidence, which suggests that nickel, cobalt, chromium, and beryllium tend to increase cancer risk in humans. However, there is no validated evidence to prove that dental casting alloys are genotoxic or carcinogenic.

CRITICAL QUESTION

Which risks are associated with handling of base metal alloys? Which dental personnel are most likely to exhibit adverse effects to dental materials?

Occupational Hazards for Dental Personnel

Dental technicians seem to have an increased risk for occupational diseases during the fabrication of dental metallic restorations. Technicians are exposed to significantly more platinum, palladium, and gold than do road construction workers or high school graduates. This confirms that laboratory technicians work in areas of high occupational metal exposure. Inhalation and aspiration of various dust and toxic vapors, which are generated during the heating and melting of certain alloys, may irritate the respiratory and gastrointestinal systems of these technicians.

Pneumoconiosis is a severe fibrotic lung disease that can be caused by **chronic exposure** to inorganic dust. The fabrication of base metal prostheses can significantly increase the incidence of pneumoconiosis among dental technicians working in laboratories with insufficient dust-handling facilities. A clinical screening of dental technicians in Crete revealed a 9.8% prevalence of pneumoconiosis. Previous epidemiological studies have documented a prevalence of this lung disease in approximately 15.4% of technicians after 20 years or more of exposure. The prevalence in the general population is less than 1%.

Exposure to dust from Co–Cr, Co–Cr–Mo, and Ni–Cr–Be alloys was identified as a possible reason for pneumoconiosis in dental technicians. The risks of benign pneumoconiosis induced by hard metals are well documented. Malignant pneumoconiosis is caused by dust from crystalline silica, asbestos, or beryllium. Silicosis is the most common occupational disease among dental technicians, whereas the risk for berylliosis is not well documented.

There is no evidence proving that metallic restorations threaten the health of dental personnel other than technicians. Because of the increased risk for pneumoconiosis, the installation of dust exhaust collectors in dental laboratories is highly recommended.

There is no evidence to suggest that metallic dental restorations increase mutagenic and carcinogenic risks in humans. Except for laboratory technicians, there is also no indication that metallic dental materials are an occupational hazard for dental personnel. The laboratory technicians have a higher risk for fibrotic lung diseases caused by dust from metals and abrasives, but only if there is insufficient exhaust ventilation in dental laboratories. Adverse occupational reactions are common and dental staff exhibits various forms of hand or facial dermatitis as well as respiratory disease. Contact-type reactions seem to occur most often because of exposure to acrylates, formaldehyde, fragrances, latex, and rubber additives. Latex allergies are well recognized because dental office staff seems to be most susceptible to this type of allergen.

Irritation problems are more likely to cause hand dermatitis in dental personnel compared with dermatitis caused by contact allergy. Patch testing of patients is recommended for those who exhibit contact-type allergy and blood tests for those who have experienced immediate-type allergic reactions possibly related to dental treatments or materials. Testing of dental personnel is also indicated for individuals who exhibit hand or facial dermatitis or respiratory distress as a result of their exposure to work materials (restorative materials and auxiliary materials) and their work environment (dusts, fumes, and vapors). Such individuals should be referred to medical specialists for proper testing, diagnosis, and treatment (if indicated).

Hydrofluoric Acid

Etching of glass-phase ceramics and glass ceramics by hydrofluoric acid (HF) has been performed occasionally to promote bonding of these ceramics to resin-based composites. This etching process has been performed both in the lab and in the mouth. Since HF is an extremely corrosive acid, it is significantly more hazardous than many of the other acids used in dental labs and offices. Technicians and dentists should be well informed on the risks of exposure to HF and methods that are effective in dealing with accidental HF exposures.

Exposure of Skin, Mucosa, and Eyes to Hydrofluoric Acid

HF is corrosive and readily destroys tissue. Exposure of the eyes to HF may result in blindness or permanent eye damage. HF readily penetrates human skin, allowing it to destroy soft tissues and to decalcify bone. Chemical burns from HF are typically very painful and slow to heal. Skin exposure to high concentrations of HF (≥50%) immediately causes significant and painful destruction of tissue. In addition to the chemical burns induced by exposure to skin or other tissues, systemic fluoride poisoning can also occur. A significant concern over the use and possible exposure of tissue to relatively low concentrations of HF is that the pain or burning sensations may not be experienced until several hours after exposure. Because of this delayed effect of HF to produce severe tissue damage possibly without pain, all tissues that have been exposed to HF should receive immediate first aid care, medical evaluation, and follow-up evaluations even if the injury appears insignificant and no pain is experienced.

Inhalation of Hydrofluoric Acid Vapor

Inhaled HF vapor can damage the lungs. Delayed effects may not be apparent for hours after the initial exposure. The US Occupational Safety and Health Administration (a division of the US Department of Labor) has set a limit for exposure to individuals for airborne concentrations to an average of 3 ppm HF over an 8-hour workday. Long-term or chronic exposure to HF can result in *fluorosis*, a syndrome characterized by weight loss, bone embrittlement, anemia, and general ill health.

Ventilation During Use of Hydrofluoric Acid

To minimize inhalation of HF vapor, gels and liquids should be used with adequate ventilation. Concentrations greater than 5% should be handled inside a chemical fume hood.

Eye and Skin Exposure to Hydrofluoric Acid

When eyes have been exposed to HF, they should immediately be irrigated at an eyewash station for at least 15 minutes with large volumes of water while the eyelids are held apart and away from the eyeballs. Calcium gluconate gel must not be applied to the eyes. In all cases of where the eyes have been exposed to acids, immediate medical attention should be sought.

Skin Exposure to Hydrofluoric Acid

If small areas of the hand or forearm have been contaminated, these areas must immediately be washed in a sink. If calcium gluconate gel is readily available, rinsing should be limited to 5 minutes so that application of the gel can be quickly initiated so as to limit the migration of fluoride ions. The calcium gluconate gel should be reapplied to the affected areas every 15 minutes. If calcium gluconate gel is not available, the affected areas should be rinsed for at least 15 minutes. Contaminated clothing must be removed and placed in a hood or plastic bag. Prompt medical attention should be sought in all instances of skin exposure to HF.

Neutralization of Hydrofluoric Acid by Calcium Gluconate Gel

Available as a commercial product, this gel is a topical antidote for HF residue on exposed skin. It combines with HF to form insoluble calcium fluoride, thereby preventing the extraction of calcium from tissues and bones. Calcium gluconate has a limited shelf life and should be refrigerated and replaced with a fresh supply after its expiration. Disposable gloves should be used in applying calcium gluconate gel to the skin.

Hazards Associated With Other Fluorine Compounds

Other chemicals containing fluorine—such as ammonium fluoride, ammonium bifluoride, and sodium fluoride—may react with acid or water to produce HF. One should review the Material Safety Data Sheets (MSDSs) of all fluoride compounds to learn the safety precautions that are recommended to reduce the risk of HF exposure.

CRITICAL QUESTION

Which factors influence the conditions for a biocompatibility test?

Biocompatibility Tests

Test Requirements

The specific use of a material in the body has a direct bearing on the biological response it produces. There are some major requirements of any test for biocompatibility. Three of the most significant ones are that:

1. The test should be performed under conditions that simulate the actual use of the material in the body.
2. The test conditions should reflect the effects of the material's time in the body on the biological response.
3. The stresses induced in the material under its intended function should be considered in the interpretation of the biological response.

The test conditions should reflect whether or not the material will (1) contact soft tissue or mineralized tissue; (2) be external to the oral epithelium; (3) serve as an endosseous implant; (4) be exposed directly to bone, tissue fluid, blood, and saliva; and (5) be separated by some barrier such as dentin between the material and living cells. Special attention must be paid to materials that communicate through the epithelium or lie completely beneath the epithelium.

Short-term exposures such as those of impression materials or temporary cements are used only for a few minutes to a few weeks in the mouth. Their biological responses are likely to differ from those that occur after 10 years of exposure. The short-term responses are likely to be allergic reactions, but they are unlikely to be toxic or mutagenic effects. In general, the most demanding tests are designed to evaluate materials that are expected to remain present for the longest times.

The induced stresses may be physical, chemical, or thermal in nature. Thus, biomaterials that flex, deform plastically, leak, or fracture easily in the oral environment may cause adverse effects, including discomfort, sensitivity, restoration failure, postoperative pain, and pulp trauma related to filling removal, tooth preparation, and replacement of the restorative material.

CRITICAL QUESTION

Is there one best test to measure biocompatibility?

Advantages and Disadvantages of Biocompatibility Tests

Three types of tests are used to analyze the biocompatibility of dental materials:

1. An in vitro test
2. An animal test
3. A usage test performed clinically in animals or humans

Each of these tests has advantages and disadvantages, and each type is used to evaluate a material before it can be sold to dental practitioners. No single test can accurately estimate the biological response to a material. In addition, there is no clear consensus on the optimal combinations of tests that must be performed for each type of material.

For in vitro tests, the candidate material or an extract of the material is placed in direct or indirect contact with some biological system outside of an organism. Direct contact exposes a material or an extract of a material directly to the biological environment, whereas indirect contact involves a barrier such as agar, a membrane filter, or dentin. In vitro tests can be conducted in cell culture dishes, test tubes, or other containers. Biological systems may consist of mammalian cells, cellular organelles, tissues, bacteria, or certain enzymes. These tests can be used to measure cell growth, cellular function, and the integrity of a cell's genetic material.

In vitro tests are relatively fast and inexpensive and they can be standardized relatively easily. Also, in vitro tests can be controlled very well to provide highly reliable data and reproducible measurements. Perhaps the greatest disadvantage of in vitro tests is their limited relevance to clinical practice. For example, a test that measures cytotoxicity using osteoblast cell cultures may be somewhat irrelevant if the material never contacts osteoblasts in vivo. The in vitro tests lack the ability to simulate complex interactions that exist in an organism between and among the immune, inflammatory, and circulatory systems. In vitro tests can be used to check if a substance eluted from the test material has the general potential to be harmful to cells.

Animal tests involve the placement of a material in an organism. Test animals include baboons, cats, dogs, ferrets, guinea pigs, hamsters, mice, monkeys, pigs, rats, and sheep. Animal tests differ from vitro tests in that an intact animal is used rather than cells or tissues from an animal. In some animal tests, the test materials are not applied as in the patient, for example, when restorative materials are implanted subcutaneously in rats. In this case a more nonspecific toxic response is evaluated. In other animal tests, the materials are ground and fed to the animals (e.g., rats) in so-called acute or chronic toxicity tests; this process simulates the oral uptake of the materials, although oral ingestion in such quantities is not realistic. Therefore, these tests are becoming discontinued. In other animal tests, for example, those involving guinea pigs, the ability of a substance from a material to sensitize and then elicit an allergic reaction is evaluated. These test methods have provided reliable data that can be extrapolated to humans. Many other animal-based test methods are described in the literature for testing certain material properties, for example, mutagenicity or carcinogenicity, but they are seldom used for testing dental materials. In contrast, tests are applied in the test animal as they are in the patient, for example, a restorative material in class V cavity preparations is placed in monkey teeth. However, such usage tests can also be performed in humans, for example, in teeth that are scheduled for extraction because of orthodontic reasons.

Thus, the advantage of animal tests lies in their ability to permit an intact biological system to respond to or interact with a candidate material. The material can thereby interact with many complex biological systems to obtain a biological response. The disadvantages of animal tests are their high cost, control difficulty, and the length of time that may be required to obtain a measurable response. These tests are criticized by animal rights activists and other individuals because of concerns regarding the ethical treatment of test animals. Finally, the relevance of animal tests in simulating human responses is often challenged. In spite of these disadvantages, animal tests are essential for evaluating new materials prior to their clinical use.

Usage tests are the most clinically relevant tests. They are performed either in animals or humans. Such a test requires that the material be placed in a clinically relevant environment similar to that to which the material would be exposed in clinical practice. When a usage test is performed in humans, it is called a *clinical trial*. The choice of animals for a usage test is more limited than that for other animal tests because of the size or anatomy of a given animal species. Consequently, usage tests tend to involve larger animals with anatomy similar to that of humans. The ultimate relevance of a usage test depends on the extent to which the test simulates the clinical use of the product.

It is tempting to consider a usage test involving humans as the best test method. However, even human clinical trials have some limitations. Very often no histology is performed, and from clinical symptoms alone, no evaluation of the real damage, for example, of the pulp after placement of a restorative material, is possible. Furthermore, teeth that are scheduled for extraction because of orthodontic reasons are normally obtained from young patients. These teeth may have open apices, which may react differently from teeth of older patients with narrow apical openings and with potentially previous damage from caries.

Usage tests have several disadvantages, including their design complexity, difficulty to control experimentally, and interpretation challenges. These tests are also extremely costly. If humans are used in a clinical trial, approval for the proposed usage tests must be obtained from an institutional review board. A test for the long-term performance of a material may take 5 years or more, which adds considerably to the typically high cost of using human subjects. Finally, human usage tests may involve legal and confidentiality issues that do not occur for animal and in vitro tests.

CRITICAL QUESTION

If you were presented with a new material, never before used in a human being, how would you decide if it was safe as a dental restorative material?

How Tests Are Used Collectively to Measure Biocompatibility

Advertisements for new restorative materials rarely provide comprehensive information on the biocompatibility tests that were performed to judge the safety of the products. This situation exists for several reasons. First, the dental profession has not observed many severe toxic reactions or anaphylactic reactions that are of life-threatening proportions. Second, dentists are often more concerned with potential clinical performance and simplicity of technique than with poorly defined side effects. Third, the profession is well aware that there is no single simple test that unequivocally establishes biocompatibility of products on a quantitative basis. Finally, the profession seems to operate on the assumption that most if not all of the potential adverse effects can be corrected simply by removing the suspected material.

Dental health professionals are well aware of the fact that no single test is sufficient to evaluate the biocompatibility of a new material. Rather, in vitro, animal, and usage tests can collectively classify a material's general safety for clinical use. However, the role of each of these basic tests in the overall evaluation process is unclear. Three test phases have been distinguished in the testing of a new biomaterial: primary, secondary, and usage tests (see Fig. 17.13). Primary tests are performed initially for screening a new material; these tests are usually in vitro in nature and may include cytotoxicity and mutagenicity tests. Primary tests can also include animal tests to measure systemic toxicity. Secondary tests are usually conducted in animals to observe outcomes such as the immune response, dermal irritation, chronic toxicity, or response upon implantation.

The test of a new material represents a relatively linear progression from primary to secondary to usage tests (see Fig. 17.14). Initially, primary tests are performed, and materials that pass these tests then undergo secondary tests. Similarly, materials that pass the secondary tests are subjected to usage tests.

In the late 1970s and early 1980s, research was performed to compare in vitro animal tests, and usage tests for materials employed clinically in dentistry for many years. These studies revealed that in vitro and animal tests do not necessarily predict the results of usage tests or successful clinical experience with the material. So how is a dental practitioner to decide whether a material is sufficiently safe or not? The manufacturer must perform the required tests, which ensure that its products are safe, that is, free from unacceptable risks of the probability and severity of harmful effects. Thus, the primary responsibility falls on the producer although the dentist must be familiar with the potential adverse effects of restorative materials.

One of the criteria for selecting a material is the time the product has been used in service without any reports of adverse events. Where are adverse events recorded and how can these reports be accessed? The answer to this question was given in an earlier section on adverse event registries in several countries. A search of the websites in Norway, Sweden, and the United Kingdom would allow a clinician to review reports on existing materials to determine the types of adverse effects that were most likely for specific types of materials. Next, a search of the PubMed or Web of Science literature with key words or MeSH terms, which can be identified by librarians, if necessary, should be performed to identify if any reports of the specific product have been recorded. Finally, a request should be made to national agencies in the dentist's home country to determine whether any adverse events reports have been made. As one might expect, unless catastrophic failures have occurred soon after the product's introduction, the shorter the time that the product has been in existence, the smaller is the number of adverse effects reports that will be found.

A major concern on regarding in vitro test data used to select a material is the relatively poor correlation among these tests. However, when tests are performed under simulated clinical conditions, more reasonable correlations are found.

Biocompatibility Standards

The first biocompatibility test standard, Document No. 41 for Recommended Standard Practices for Biological Evaluation of Dental Materials was formalized by the passage of the Medical Device Bill in 1976. The FDA classifies dental materials as *devices*. This classification requires less stringent testing than is required for drugs, which must pass performance tests for safety and efficacy. Dental devices need to meet only safety test requirements.

An update to ADA Document No. 41 for the biological testing of dental materials was published in 1982 to include tests for mutagenicity. The initial tests require in vitro assays for cytotoxicity, red blood cell membrane lysis, mutagenesis, carcinogenesis, and animal tests for systemic toxicity (by oral ingestion). Secondary evaluations include animal tests for inflammatory or immune responses, and usage tests include tests for pulp and bone response. Based on a thorough risk assessment according to relevant ISO standards and an evaluation of the existing literature, the manufacturers have the responsibility of selecting the appropriate and necessary biological tests for their products. Finally, the manufacturer is fully responsible legally for any adverse effects arising from the use of the products, which may have been prevented by performing state-of-the-art tests.

ISO Standard 10993

To evaluate the biocompatibility of a medical device (which includes dental materials) prior to testing in a clinical study, a series of standards were developed. Unlike ADA/ANSI Document No. 41, ISO 10993 is not restricted to dental materials. In 2010, ISO Standard 10993 consisted of 20 parts, each addressing a different area of biological testing. The standard identifies initial tests for cytotoxicity, sensitization, systemic toxicity, and supplementary tests for chronic toxicity, carcinogenicity, and biodegradation. The initial tests may be either in vitro or animal tests, whereas the supplementary tests are performed on animals or humans. The document provides suggestions for test selection based on how long the material will be present; whether it will contact the body surface, blood, or bone; and if it will communicate externally once it is placed internally. For dentistry, ISO 7405 is also relevant. It describes the tests that are specific for dental materials or for which ample evidence exists for the materials. For example, all usage tests are described in ISO 7405 as well as cell culture tests that are specially designed for restorative materials such as the dentin barrier test.

Because of the multifactorial nature of biocompatibility, standardization is essential for the unbiased comparison of results from different studies, but they have some significant disadvantages. Many standards cannot keep pace with the development of new scientific technology. In addition, standards are developed based on agreements and compromises among manufacturers, academicians, and the lay public. Thus, they tend to be developed quite slowly. Standards are also arbitrary in nature because proposed thresholds for acceptability and criteria for determining unacceptable performance are rarely accepted universally. However, in spite of these limitations, standards for biological testing are necessary to ensure the biological safety of medical and dental products.

Material Safety Data Sheets

Each dental product is supplied with an *MSDS*, also known as a *Product Safety Data Sheet*, or a COSHH data sheet in the United Kingdom. This is a report on the properties of a particular substance, for example, melting point, boiling point, and flash point. This report is intended for occupational settings and is essential for workers and emergency personnel because it describes procedures for handling or working with the material safely. In addition to physical data, it identifies toxicity risks, health effects, first aid procedures, reactivity, storage and disposal conditions, and, where applicable, procedures for firefighting, the types of protective equipment that should be used and procedures that must be followed for accidental releases and handling of spills.

Potentially harmful substances must be properly labeled to minimize the risk of injuries to personnel and others who may come in contact with the material or substance, risks to the health of individuals, and risks of environmental exposure. Labels may include hazard symbols, for example, the European Union label, with a black diagonal cross on an orange background.

Labeling on packages or delivery devices that contain potentially hazardous substances exhibits symbols indicating the types of hazards that may be encountered. The color-coded markings fall into one of four categories: (1) *blue* for the level of health hazard, (2) *red* for flammability, (3) *yellow* for (chemical) reactivity, and (4) *white* for unique hazards. Each of the health, flammability, and reactivity categories is rated on a scale from 0 (no hazard or normal substance) to 4 (severe risk). An example of such a label is shown in Figure 17.16.

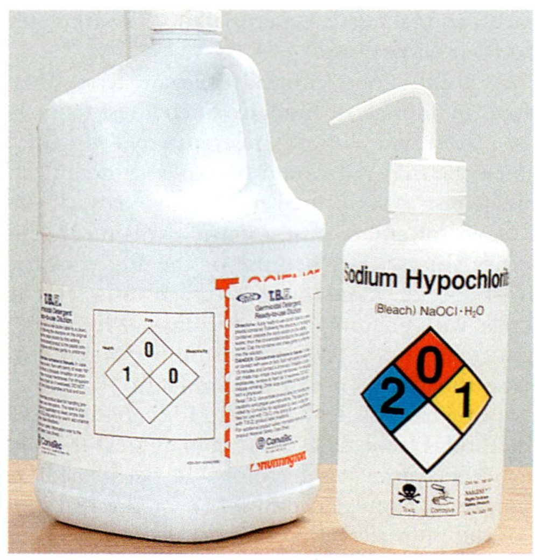

• Fig. 17.16 Labeling on a liquid dispenser that indicates the color-coded hazard levels in each of four categories. (From Sorrentino SA, Remmert LN: Mosby's Textbook for Nursing Assistants, 8th ed. St. Louis, 2012, Mosby.)

CRITICAL QUESTION

What information is required to judge the safety of metallic, resin composite, and ceramic products?

Clinical Guidelines for Selecting Biocompatible Materials

Clinicians need to evaluate claims of the biological safety of new materials made by the manufacturers. With knowledge of biocompatibility issues, clinicians can make rational judgments about biological safety. Several critical steps described here will ensure an informed decision.

Define the Intended Use and Indications for Restorative Materials

As discussed previously, the intended use of a material plays a crucial role in the material's biocompatibility. Clinicians should inquire when the material is proposed for a new indication and if the material has been tested in the proposed use. If the material is used in a new way or new environment, more caution is advised. To minimize the risk of litigation resulting from unexpected adverse events, the lab technician and dentist must adhere to the instructions for use and use the material as indicated by the manufacturers. For other applications, such as off-label use, the practitioner is fully liable for any adverse effects that may occur. Furthermore, many dental materials are supplied by the manufacturer as a semifinal product, and the dentist finalizes the product through other processes, such as light curing a resin composite. Correct handling according to the instructions for use is essential for acceptable biocompatibility.

Identify the Main Components of the Material

The principal components of materials are listed in the SDS, but this list is not always complete, and elemental concentrations are not included. This is especially relevant for potential allergens, where even small amounts in the material may cause adverse reactions. Studies have shown repeatedly that a small change in the composition or processing of a material can cause a significant change in the material's biocompatibility. In case of doubt, clinicians should ask the manufacturer for specific information. They also should request written information from the lab technicians certifying that the materials used are the ones the clinician has prescribed and that all instructions for use of the manufacturer have been followed. Generally, caution is advised in applying previous biological data and processing principles to new situations.

CRITICAL QUESTION

A sales representative introduces a new restorative material in your office or at a trade show. What do you need to know from him or her about the material's biocompatibility tests?

Evaluate the Safety and Performance of Dental Materials

In vitro or animal tests are sometimes difficult to relate to clinical applications. However, there are instances when clinicians do not have sufficient data from clinical trials to make an informed decision, so they must rely on in vitro or animal tests. Clinicians should not simply accept nondescript statements, such as "The material has been subjected to biocompatibility tests, and no adverse effects were observed," but should ask for the type of tests used. If clinical trial results are available, inquiring if the conditions and duration of the test are relevant for the practice is important.

The quality and relevance of usage test data depend on the fidelity of reproducing the clinical use. If animal or in vitro test results are the only ones available, then clinicians should question the design of these tests and the methods employed, making sure that testing conditions were as relevant as possible, including multiple types of tests performed under different clinically relevant conditions. A well-controlled comparison with existing similar types of materials is always preferable to an isolated test on one material. The known potential or claimed adverse effects of dental materials, such as those summarized in Table 17.1, should be investigated periodically to ensure that patients will be presented with accurate information related to the benefits and risks of proposed treatments.

CRITICAL QUESTION

Based on the effect of substances eluted from dental materials on the immune system, who is responsible for deciding which materials are biologically safe for use—the patient, the dentist, the manufacturer, or the FDA?

TABLE 17.1 Potential and Claimed Adverse Effects and Drawbacks of Dental Restorative Materials

Restorative Material	Potential Adverse Effects
Dental amalgam	Contact dermatitis or sensitization/allergic reactions to metal elements Localized lichenoid lesions Postoperative sensitivity Thermal sensitivity of pulp Symptoms of mercury toxicity, especially neurotoxicity Environmental concerns
Dental adhesives/ resin composites	Contact dermatitis or sensitization/allergic reactions to methacrylates Localized lichenoid lesions Estrogenic effects of bisphenol A Postoperative sensitivity from polymerization stresses and marginal gaps Pulp damage in deep cavities/pulp exposure Cytotoxicity or genotoxic effects
Dental alloys	Contact dermatitis or sensitization/allergic reactions to metals, especially nickel, cobalt, and beryllium Localized lichenoid lesions Thermal sensitivity of pulp Systemic effects of leached metal ions
Conventional glass ionomer cements	Postoperative pain (luting materials) Pulp damage when placed on exposed pulp
Resin modified glass-ionomer cements	Contact dermatitis or sensitization/allergic reaction to methacrylates Localized lichenoid lesion Postoperative sensitivity from polymerization stresses and marginal gaps Pulp damage in deep cavities/pulp exposure Cytotoxicity or genotoxic effects Systemic effects of other free monomers or leached substances
Dental ceramic	Respiratory effects from silica dust, excessive wear of antagonist tooth structure Radioactivity Toxicity of hydrofluoric acid

Risks Versus Benefits of Dental Materials

The risk of using Ni–Cr alloy for crowns and bridges is the potential of releasing cations as a result of corrosion, especially at low pH values. These ions may be distributed in the OC and may enter the systemic circulatory system. The benefit of using an Ni–Cr alloy over an HN alloy is the low cost and higher elastic modulus of the Ni–Cr alloy. In the case of *bis*-GMA–based resin, one of the potential adverse effects is the release of BPA. However, the quantity of BPA released is extremely small, and the sealing of pits and fissures in enamel surfaces is a highly effective means for preventing caries lesions or lesion progression in these sites. Both examples depict the process of comparing the risks and benefits of a material.

Anamnesis (Patient's Account of Medical History)

Dental practitioners cannot simply follow a "cookbook" approach to select restorative materials for their patients. Instead, they must use their best clinical judgment based on scientific evidence and personal experience with the material and, more importantly, statements from patients, their physicians, and their previous dentists to ensure that all possible risks are minimized. For example, local and systemic allergic reactions to many alloys have been observed, with nickel being the most frequent allergenic element. Questioning the patient, parent, or caregiver about existing allergies would quickly eliminate certain alloys from consideration. Also, severe renal disease with impaired renal clearing function is a contraindication for amalgam use. Information provided by the patient should be documented and regularly updated.

Treatment Planning

There is considerable variability in the treatment-planning process. The benefits and risks stated to patients by their practitioners are also likely to vary significantly from practice to practice. Obviously, some of the decisions will be based on accepting greater risks for the predicted benefits, whereas others will be based on a very conservative philosophy, which suggests that the risks of adverse effects should be exceptionally low. In some of these cases, when considerable risks exist, no treatment may be the best choice. For example, if some patients claim that they are allergic to several types of potential allergens, including metals, cosmetics, and foodstuffs, extreme caution is indicated to minimize related items. However, if the restorative treatment is essential to restore occlusion and function, these risks may be accepted, although informed consent procedures must still be satisfied before treatment begins. Once the practitioner makes a treatment decision, the patient should be informed of the benefits and risks of the proposed treatment and of any alternative treatments. Then, for medical and legal requirements to be satisfied, the patient must give his or her consent for the proposed treatment.

Risk Communication

Patients may ask the dentist before the treatment if the materials selected are safe. From a patient's viewpoint, safety often means that nothing bad will ever happen. However, this is not always possible. One may ask the patients about their hobbies or favorite sports and then inquire about the potential risks these activities may carry. The patients may soon realize that there is always a chance for adverse events to happen.

The clinician can refer to the fact that the probability of adverse effects from dental materials is generally low (0.3%). In contrast, the rate of adverse reactions toward cosmetic products has been reported as 12%. This means that the probability for an adverse reaction from contact with dental materials is about 40 times less than that with cosmetics if generally accepted good practice for patient treatment is followed. Finally, the risk should be "individualized," meaning the clinician should explain to the patient the specific situation in the patient's case, such as allergies, cavity sizes, or the situation of the dentition in general. This specific and unique expertise enables the clinician to put Internet-derived information into clinical perspective for individual patients.

Summary

- The biocompatibility of dental restorative materials is evaluated using compositional analysis, surface degradation tests, cell culture tests, clinical testing in humans, and animal model tests. The biocompatibility of a material depends on several factors:
  - The chemical nature of its components
  - The physical nature of the components
  - The types and locations of patient tissues that will be exposed to the device
  - The duration of the exposure
  - The surface characteristics of the material
  - The amount and nature of substances eluted from the material
- Adverse reactions to dental restorative materials and auxiliary materials include one or more of the following effects:
  - Allergic reaction
  - Chemical burn
  - Pulp irritation
  - Pulp damage
  - Thermal injury
  - Tissue irritation
  - Toxic reaction
- **Local and systemic effects of materials**
  Their routes of entry into the body include the following sources:
  - Ingestion and absorption
  - Inhalation of vapor
  - Leakage through the tooth apex
  - Absorption through the oral mucosa
- **Inflammatory and allergic reactions**
  - The inflammatory response involves the activation of the host's immune system to ward off some challenge or threat.
  - An allergic reaction occurs when the body recognizes a substance, molecule, or ion as foreign, and the human immune system can react quickly, as during an anaphylactic reaction or slowly in delayed contact dermatitis.
- **Immunotoxicity**
  The principal concept of immunotoxicity is that substances leached from materials can alter immune system cells, resulting in enormous biological consequences because of the amplifying nature of immune cells.
- **Mercury and amalgam**
  - Most of the controversy over amalgam stems from the known toxicity of mercury and the question of whether mercury from amalgam restorations has toxic effects.
  - For air in the workplace, the Occupational Safety and Health Administration has set a permissible exposure limit (PEL) for mercury vapor in air of 0.1 mg/m^3.
  - Concerns about mercury stem from its toxicity and its relatively long half-life in the body. Acute symptoms are neurologically based or kidney based, ranging from paresthesia to ataxia, joint pain, and death.
- **Methacrylates and resin-based composites**
  The best screening substance for methacrylate allergy caused by dental material products is HEMA.
- **Estrogenicity**
  Estrogenicity is the ability of a chemical to act as the hormone estrogen does in the body. If these chemicals are not indigenous to the body, the substance is called a **xenoestrogen**. The concern about estrogens in dentistry centers on a chemical called *bisphenol A* (*BPA*), which is a synthetic starting point for bis-GMA (bisphenol-A-glycidyldimethacrylate) composites in dentistry as well as many other plastics.
- **Titanium and titanium alloys**
  Titanium is relatively nontoxic, noninjurious, and not physiologically reactive.

- **Base metal and noble metal alloys**
  Metal ions can be leached from cast metal restorations or wrought appliances into the oral cavity. Metallic ions released through corrosion processes are responsible for much of the metal−protein or metal−cell interaction behavior of dental metals and alloys. No evidence exists to prove that dental metallic materials are mutagenic, genotoxic, or carcinogenic.
- **Nickel and beryllium**
  - Nickel is the most allergenic metal known, with an incidence of allergic reactions between 10% and 20%.
  - The mechanisms of the high allergy frequency to nickel are not known, but there is probably a genetic component.
  - The use of beryllium in dental alloys is controversial because of its biological effects. Furthermore, beryllium-containing particles that are inhaled and reach the alveoli of the lungs may cause a chronic inflammatory condition called beryIliosis.
- **Dental ceramics**
  Ceramic materials are known for their high levels of biocompatibility.
- **Latex**
  Of particular interest in dentistry is the use of latex gloves and latex rubber dams, which expose both patients and dental personnel to this potential allergen. Adverse reactions to latex gloves have been reported in 3.7% of adult patients and 5.7% of pediatric patients.
- **Allergic reactions**
  - Patch tests for potential allergies to dental materials also suggest that the most likely allergens were components of cast dental alloys.
  - Exposure of patients to dental materials and other products can elicit signs or symptoms such as burning, tingling, cheilitis, oral lichenoid lesions, and swelling of the face, lips, tongue, palate, and buccal mucosa.
- **Toxicity tests**
  These tests are designed with the following elements:
  - A test organism such as cells and selected strains of bacteria through higher-order plants and animals.
  - A specific response or biological endpoint.
  - An exposure or test period.
  - A dose or a dose curve.
- **Dose–response relationships**
  Toxicity tests exhibit a dose−response relationship when there is a consistent mathematical relationship between the proportion of individuals responding and a given dose for a given exposure period.
- **Reactions to toxic agents**
  There are several adverse reactions that can be caused by exposure to biomaterial substances and processes. These include reactions to the following:
  - Systemic toxins such as chemical agents, which can act on target organs or organ systems.
  - Asphyxiants, which deprive the tissues of oxygen (anoxia).
  - Irritants, which cause inflammation of tissues by direct contact.
  - Allergic sensitizers, which activate the production of antibodies—which, in turn, react with the antigen to make it a latent complex (when the body becomes exposed one or more times to the sensitized agent, the concentration of antibodies increases until an antigen–antibody reaction, or allergic reaction, results in one or more symptoms).
  - Carcinogens, which are substances known to cause cancer in an organism.
  - Reproductive toxins, such as mutagens or teratogens.
- **Genotoxicity, mutagenicity, and carcinogenicity**
  - Genotoxicity refers to any adverse effect on the DNA of an organism.
  - If the adverse effect is transferred to the next (heritable) generation of cells, the effect is called mutagenicity.
  - Carcinogenicity refers to the ability or tendency to produce tumors.
- **Occupational hazards for dental personnel**
  - The fabrication of base metal prostheses can significantly increase the incidence of pneumoconiosis among dental technicians working in laboratories with insufficient dust-handling facilities.
  - Contact-type reactions seem to occur most often because of exposure to acrylates, formaldehyde, fragrances, latex, and rubber additives.
  - Latex allergies are well recognized because dental office staff seems to be most susceptible to this type of allergen.
- **Biocompatibility tests**
  Three types of tests are used to analyze the biocompatibility of dental materials:
  - An in vitro test.
  - An animal test: *Animal tests* involve the placement of a material in an organism.
  - A usage test performed clinically in animals or humans. *Usage tests* are the most clinically relevant tests.

Review Questions

1. Define biocompatibility. Discuss the various tests used for determining biocompatibility of dental materials.
2. Discuss biocompatibility of dental materials. Add a note on pulp capping.
3. Discuss in brief toxicity tests.
4. Discuss the hazards and side effects of beryllium and nickel in dental alloys.
5. Discuss in detail mercury toxicity and its management.
6. Discuss biologic effects of restorative materials on the pulp.
7. Discuss in detail advantages and disadvantages of biocompatibility tests.
8. Discuss in detail occupational hazards for dental professionals.
9. Write a brief note on latex allergy.
10. Discuss in brief cytotoxicity.
11. Discuss in brief mutagenicity and carcinogenicity.
12. Discuss in brief factors influencing biocompatibility of dental materials.
13. Discuss in detail local and systemic effects of dental materials.
14. Discuss in brief allergic reactions.
15. Discuss in detail allergic and inflammatory reactions.
16. Classify allergic reactions to restorative materials.
17. Discuss in brief in vitro testing.
18. Discuss in brief estrogenicity.
19. Tissue reactions related to alloys used in dentistry.
20. Write a short note on reaction to toxic agents.

Acknowledgments

The contributions of Dr John Wataha to the previous version of this chapter in the 11th edition are greatly appreciated. His conceptual descriptions and images developed for Figures 7.2, 7.3, and 7.12–7.15 are of special value to the 12th edition. Dr Yeong-Joon Park provided helpful suggestions and several images. The input of Michael E Adjodha, Dental Devices Branch, Center for Devices and Radiological Health, US Food and Drug Administration, is also greatly appreciated. Dr Donald Cohen provided clinical images of lichenoid lesions. The artistic suggestions of Dr Inchan Ko and Miss Jihae Ahn are also appreciated.

Suggested Readings

This comprehensive list of biocompatibility references supplements the key references cited in the chapter.

Aberer W.; Holub H.; Strohal R.; et al. Palladium in dental alloys—the dermatologists' responsibility to warn? Contact Dermat 28 163–165 (1993).

Aller A.J. The clinical significance of beryllium. J Trace Elem Electrolytes Health Dis 4 1–6 (1990).

Arenholt-Bindslev D. Environmental aspects of dental filling materials. European J Oral Sci. 106 713–720 (1998).

Arikan A.; Kulak Y. A study of chromium, nickel and cobalt hypersensitivity. J Marmara Univ Dent Fac 1 223–229 (1992).

Arvidson K.; Cottler-Fox M.; Hammarlund E.; et al. Cytotoxic effects of cobalt-chromium alloys on fibroblasts derived from human gingiva. Scand J Dent Res 95 356–363 (1987).

Ashby J.; Ishidate M. Jr.; Stoner G.D.; et al. Studies on the genotoxicity of beryllium sulphate in vitro and in vivo. Mutat Res 240 217–225 (1990).

Assad M.; Yahia L.H.; Rivard C.H.; et al. In vitro biocompatibility assessment of a nickel-titanium alloy using electron microscopy in situ end-labeling (EM-ISEL). J Biomed Mater Res 41 154–161 (1998).

Bellinger D.C.; Trachtenberg F.; Barregard L.; et al. Neuropsychological and renal effects of dental amalgam in children: A randomized clinical trial. JAMA 295 1775–1783 (2006).

Bellinger D.C.; Daniel D.; Trachtenberg F.; et al. Dental amalgam restorations and children's neuropsychological function: The New England Children's Amalgam Trial. Environ Health Perspect 115 440–446 (2007).

Bergenholtz G. Evidence for bacterial causation of adverse pulpal responses in resin-based dental restorations. Crit Rev Oral Biol Med 11 467–480 (2000).

Berglund A.; Pohl L.; Olsson S.; et al. Determination of the rate of release of intra-oral mercury vapor from amalgam. J Dent Res 67 (9) 1235–1242 (1988).

Berglund A. Estimation by a 24-hour study of the daily dose of intra-oral mercury vapor inhaled after release from dental amalgam. J Dent Res 69 (10) 1646–1651 (1990).

Berstein A.; Bernauer I.; Marx R.; et al. Human cell culture studies with dental metallic materials. Biomaterials 13 98–100 (1992).

Bumgardner G.L.; Mauer S.M.; Ascher N.L.; et al. Long-term outcome of renal transplantation in patients with systemic lupus erythematosus. Transplant Proc 21 2031–2032 (1989).

Bumgardner J.D.; Lucas L.C.; Alverson M.W. Jr.; et al. Effects of copper-based dental casting alloys on two lymphocyte cell lines and the secretion of interleukin 2 and IgG. Dent Mater 9 85–90 (1993).

Bumgardner J.D.; Doeller J.; Lucas L.C. Effect of nickel-based dental casting alloys on fibroblast metabolism and ultrastructural organization. J Biomed Mater Res 29 611–617 (1995).

Bumgardner J.D.; Lucas L.C. Cellular response to metallic ions released from nickel-chromium dental alloys. J Dent Res 74 1521–1527 (1995).

Bumgardner J.D.; Johansson B.I. Effects of titanium-dental restorative alloy galvanic couples on cultured cells. J Biomed Mater Res 43 184–191 (1998).

Camargo S.E.; Camargo C.H.; Hiller K.A.; et al. Cytotoxicity and genotoxicity of pulp capping materials in two cell lines. Int Endod J 42 227–237 (2009).

Choudat D. Occupational lung diseases among dental technicians. Tuberc Lung Dis 75 99–104 (1994).

Craig R.G.; Hanks C.T. Cytotoxicity of experimental casting alloys evaluated by cell culture tests. J Dent Res 69 1539–1542 (1990).

Deichmann W.B.; Henschler D.; Holmsted B.; et al. What is there that is not poison? A study of the Third Defense by Paracelsus. Arch Toxicol 58 207–213 (1986).

Demirci M.; Hiller K.A.; Bosl C.; et al. The induction of oxidative stress, cytotoxicity, and genotoxicity by dental adhesives. Dent Mater 24 362–371 (2008).

DeRouen T.A.; Leroux B.G.; Martin M.D.; et al. Issues in design and analysis of a randomized clinical trial to assess the safety of dental amalgam restorations in children. Control Clin Trials 23 301–320 (2002).

DeRouen T.A.; Martin M.D.; Leroux B.G.; et al. Neurobehavioral effects of dental amalgam in children: A randomized clinical trial. JAMA 295 1784–1792 (2006).

Ditrichova D.; Kapralova S.; Tichy M.; et al. Oral lichenoid lesions and allergy to dental materials. Biomed Pap Med Fac Univ Palacky Olomouc Czech Repub 151 333–339 (2007).

Dodes J.E. The amalgam controversy-An evidence-based analysis. J Am Dent Assoc 132 (3) 348–356 (2001).

Donati M.E.; Savarino L.; Granchi D.; et al. The effects of metal corrosion debris on immune system cells. Chir Organ Mov 83 387–393 (1998).

Durner J.; Spahl W.; Zaspel J.; et al. Eluted substances from unpolymerized and polymerized dental restorative materials and their Nernst partition coefficient. Dent Mater 26 91–99 (2010).

Durner J.; Kreppel H.; Zaspel J.; et al. The toxicokinetics and distribution of 2-hydroxyethyl methacrylate in mice. Biomaterials 30 2066–2071 (2009).

Eckhardt A.; Gerstmayr N.; Hiller K.A.; et al. TEGDMA-induced oxidative DNA damage and activation of ATM and MAP kinases. Biomaterials 30 2006–2014 (2009).

Eckhardt A.; Muller P.; Hiller K.A.; et al. Influence of TEGDMA on the mammalian cell cycle in comparison with chemotherapeutic agents. Dent Mater 26 232–241 (2010).

Ehrlich A.; Kucenic M.; Belsito D.V. Role of body piercing in the induction of metal allergies. Am J Contact Derm 12 151–155 (2001).

Ekstrand J.; Bjorkman L.; Edlund C.; et al. Toxicological aspects on the release and systemic uptake of mercury from dental amalgam. Eur J Oral Sci 106 678–686 (1998).

Ersev H.; Schmalz G.; Bayirli G.; et al. Cytotoxic and mutagenic potencies of various root canal filling materials in eukaryotic and prokaryotic cells in vitro. J Endod 25 359–363 (1999).

Froudarakis M.E.; Voloudaki A.; Bouros D.; et al. Pneumoconiosis among Cretan dental technicians. Respiration 66 338–342 (1999).

Galler K.M.; Schweikl H.; Hiller K.A.; et al. TEGDMA reduces mineralization in dental pulp cells. J Dent Res 90 257–262 (2011).

Gawkrodger D.J. Investigation of reactions to dental materials. Br J Dermatol 153 479–485 (2005).

In: (editors: Gell P.G.H.; Coombs R.R.A.) Clinical Aspects of Immunology. ed 1 Blackwell: Oxford, England.

Goon A.T.; Isaksson M.; Zimerson E.; et al. Contact allergy to (meth) acrylates in the dental series in southern Sweden: Simultaneous positive patch test reaction patterns and possible screening allergens. Contact Dermatitis 55 219–226 (2006).

Hartwig A. Current aspects in metal genotoxicity. Biometals 8 3–11 (1995).

Hayes R.B. The carcinogenicity of metals in humans. Cancer Causes Control 8 371–385 (1997).

Heintze U.; Edwardsson S.; Derand T.; et al. Methylation of mercury from dental amalgam and mercuric chloride by oral streptococci in vitro. Scand J Dent Res 91 (2) 150–152 (1983).

Hensten-Pettersen A. Casting alloys: Side-effects. Adv Dent Res 6 38–43 (1992).

Hildebrand H.F.; Veron C.; Martin P. Non-precious metal dental alloys and allergy [translation]. J Biol Buccale 17 227–243 (1989).

Hosoki M.; Bando E.; Asaoka K.; et al. Assessment of allergic hypersensitivity to dental materials. Biomed Mater Eng 19 53–61 (2009).

Izumi A.K. Allergic contact gingivostomatitis due to gold. Arch Dermatol Res 272 387–391 (1982).

Jacobsen N.; Hensten-Pettersen A. Occupational health problems and adverse patient reactions in orthodontics. Eur J Orthod 11 254–264 (1989).

Jacobsen N.; Pettersen A.H. Self-reported occupation-related health complaints among dental laboratory technicians. Quintessence Int 24 409–415 (1993).

Johansson B.I.; Bergman B. Corrosion of titanium and amalgam couples: Effect of fluoride, area size, surface preparation and fabrication procedures. Dent Mater 11 41–46 (1995).

Johansson S.G.; Bieber T.; Dahl R.; et al. Revised nomenclature for allergy for global use: Report of the Nomenclature Review Committee of the World Allergy Organization, October 2003. J Allergy Clin Immunol 113 832–836 (2004).

Junpoom P.; Kukiattrakoon B.; Hengtrakool C. Surface characteristic changes of dental ceramics after cyclic immersion in acidic agents and titratable acidity. Eur J Prosthodont Restor Dent 18 177–184 (2010).

Kallus T.; Hensten-Pettersen A.; Mjör I.A. Tissue response to allergenic leachables from dental materials. J Biomed Mater Res 17 741–755 (1983).

Kallus T.; Mjör I.A. Incidence of adverse effects of dental materials. Scand J Dent Res 99 236–240 (1991).

Kanerva L.; Kerosuo H.; Kullaa A.; et al. Allergic patch test reactions to palladium chloride in school children. Contact Dermatitis 34 39–42 (1996).

Kanerva L.; Rantanen T.; Aalto-Korte K.; et al. A multicenter study of patch test reactions with dental screening series. Am J Contact Derm 12 83–87 (2001).

Kansu G.; Aydin A.K. Evaluation of the biocompatibility of various dental alloys: Part 2-Allergenical potentials. Eur J Prosthodont Restor Dent 4 (4) 155–161 (1996).

Khamaysi Z.; Bergman R.; Weltfriend S. Positive patch test reactions to allergens of the dental series and the relation to the clinical presentations. Contact Dermatitis 55 216–218 (2006).

Khan M.A.; Williams R.L.; Williams D.F. The corrosion behaviour of Ti-6Al-4V, Ti-6Al-7Nb and Ti-13Nb-13Zr in protein solutions. Biomaterials 20 631–637 (1999).

Krifka S.; Petzel C.; Hiller K.A.; et al. Resin monomer-induced differential activation of MAP kinases and apoptosis in mouse macrophages and human pulp cells. Biomaterials 31 2964–2975 (2010).

Krifka S.; Seidenader C.; Hiller K.A.; et al. Oxidative stress and cytotoxicity generated by dental composites in human pulp cells. Clin Oral Invest 16 (1) 215–224 (2012).

Krifka S.; Petzel C.; Bolay C.; et al. Activation of stress-regulated transcription factors by triethylene glycol dimethacrylate monomer. Biomaterials 32 1787–1795 (2011).

Kulak Y.; Arikan A. Effect of dental base metal alloys on IgE levels and some blood parameters. J Oral Rehabil 24 749–754 (1997).

Kuroda K.; Endo G.; Okamoto A.; et al. Genotoxicity of beryllium, gallium and antimony in short-term assays. Mutat Res 264 163–170 (1991).

Laeijendecker R.; van Joost T. Oral manifestations of gold allergy. J Am Acad Dermatol 30 205–209 (1994).

Laeijendecker R.; Dekker S.K.; Burger P.M.; et al. Oral lichen planus and allergy to dental amalgam restorations. Arch Dermatol 140 1434–1438 (2004).

Langworth S.; Kohlbeck K.G.; Akesson A. Mercury exposure from dental restorations, II: release and absorption. Swed Dent J 12 (1-2) 71–72 (1988).

Lee J.Y.; Yoo J.M.; Cho B.K.; et al. Contact dermatitis in Korean dental technicians. Contact Dermatitis 45 13–16 (2001).

Leyhausen G.; Abtahi M.; Karbakhsch M.; et al. Biocompatibility of various light-curing and one conventional glass-ionomer cement. Biomaterials 19 559–564 (1998).

Lygre G.B.; Gjerdet N.R.; Gronningsaeter A.G.; et al. Reporting on adverse reactions to dental materials—intraoral observations at a clinical follow-up. Community Dent Oral Epidemiol 31 200–206 (2003).

Mackert J.R. Jr. Factors affecting estimation of dental amalgam mercury exposure from measurements of mercury vapor levels in intraoral and expired air. J Dent Res 66 (12) 1775–1780 (1987).

Mackert J.R. Jr.; Leffell M.S.; Wagner D.A.; et al. Lymphocyte levels in subjects with and without amalgam restorations. J Am Dent Assoc 122 (3) 49–53 (1991).

Mackert J.R. Jr.; Berglund A. Mercury exposure from dental amalgam restorations: Absorbed dose and the potential for adverse health effects. Crit Rev Oral Biol Med 8 (4) 410–436 (1997).

Mackert J.R. Jr. Side-effects of dental ceramics. Adv Dent Res 6 90–93 (1992).

Marcusson J.A. Contact allergies to nickel sulfate, gold sodium thiosulfate and palladium chloride in patients claiming side-effects from dental alloy components. Contact Dermatitis 34 320–323 (1996).

Marcusson J.A.; Cederbrant K.; Heilborn J. Indium and iridium allergy in patients exposed to dental alloys. Contact Dermatitis 38 297–298 (1998).

Messer R.L.; Bishop S.; Lucas L.C. Effects of metallic ion toxicity on human gingival fibroblasts morphology. Biomaterials 20 1647–1657 (1999).

Mjör I.A.; Hensten-Pettersen A.; Skogedal O. Biologic evaluation of filling materials. A comparison of results using cell culture techniques, implantation tests and pulp studies. Int Dent J 27 124–129 (1977).

Müller K.; Valentine-Thon E. Hypersensitivity to titanium: Clinical and laboratory evidence. Neuroendocrinology Letters 27 (suppl 1) 31–35 (2006).

Nayebzadeh A.; Dufresne A. Evaluation of exposure to methyl methacrylate among dental laboratory technicians. Am Ind Hyg Assoc J 60 625–628 (1999).

Nayebzadeh A.; Dufresne A.; Harvie S.; et al. Mineralogy of lung tissue in dental laboratory technicians' pneumoconiosis. Am Ind Hyg Assoc J 60 349–353 (1999).

Olea N.; Pulgar R.; Pérez P.; et al. Estrogenicity of resin-based composites and sealants used in dentistry. Environ Health Perspect 104 (3) 298–305 (1996).

Olsson S.; Berglund A.; Pohl L.; et al. Model of mercury vapor transport from amalgam restorations in the oral cavity. J Dent Res 68 (3) 504–508 (1989).

Ozer F.; Unlu N.; Ozturk B.; et al. Amalgam repair: Evaluation of bond strength and microleakage. Oper Dent 27 199–203 (2002).

Raap U.; Stiesch M.; Reh H.; et al. Investigation of contact allergy to dental metals in 206 patients. Contact Dermatitis 60 339–343 (2009).

Rajan A. The Gell-Coombs classification of hypersensitivity reactions: A re-interpretation. Trends Immunol 24 (7) 376–379 (2003).

Reuling N.; Wisser W.; Jung A.; et al. Release and detection of dental corrosion products in vivo: Development of an experimental model in rabbits. J Biomed Mater Res 24 979–991 (1990).

Rom W.N.; Lockey J.E.; Lee J.S.; et al. Pneumoconiosis and exposures of dental laboratory technicians. Am J Public Health 74 1252–1257 (1984).

Schaffran R.M.; Storrs F.J.; Schalock P. Prevalence of gold sensitivity in asymptomatic individuals with gold dental restorations. Am J Contact Derm 10 201–206 (1999).

Schmalz G. Concepts in biocompatibility testing of dental restorative materials. Clin Oral Invest 1 154–162 (1997).

Schmalz G.; Garhammer P. Biological interactions of dental cast alloys with oral tissues. Dent Mater 18 396–406 (2002).

In: (editors: Schmalz G.; Arenhold-Bindslev D.) Biocompatibility of Dental Material (G Schmalz and D Arenhold-Bindslev). Springer-Verlag: Berlin-Heidlberg, p. 329; This book presents a comprehensive science-based overview of biocompatibility aspects of dental materials. Concepts of biocompatibility assessment are also presented on most material types used in clinical practice.

Schmalz G.; Schuster U.; Schweikl H. Influence of metals on IL-6 release in vitro. Biomaterials 19 1689–1694 (1998).

Schmalz G.; Garhammer P. Biological interactions of dental cast alloys with oral tissues. Dent Mater 18 396–406 (2002).

Schmalz G.; Langer H.; Schweikl H. Cytotoxicity of dental alloy extracts and corresponding metal salt solutions. J Dent Res 77 1772–1778 (1998).

Schmalz G.; Preiss A.; Arenholt-Bindslev D. Bisphenol-A content of resin monomers and related degradation products. Clin Oral Investig 3 (3) 114–119 (1999).

Schmalz G. The biocompatibility of non-amalgam dental filling materials. Eur J Oral Sci 106 696–706 (1998).

Schmalz G.; Arenholt-Bindslev D. Biocompatibility of Dental Materials. In: (editors: Schmalz G.; Arenholt-Bindslev D.) Springer-Verlag: Berlin, Heidlberg, Germany.

Schmalz G.; Krifka S.; Schweikl H. Toll-like receptors, LPS, and dental monomers. Adv Dent Res 23 302–306 (2011).

Schuurs A.H.B. Reproductive toxicity of occupational mercury. A review of the literature. J Den 27 249–256 (1999).

Schweikl H.; Schmalz G.; Bey B. Mutagenicity of dentin bonding agents. J Biomed Mater Res 28 1061–1067 (1994).

Schweikl H.; Schmalz G.; Gottke C. Mutagenic activity of various dentine bonding agents. Biomaterials 17 1451–1456 (1996).

Schweikl H.; Schmalz G. Toxicity parameters for cytotoxicity testing of dental materials in two different mammalian cell lines. Eur J Oral Sci 104 292–299 (1996).

Schweikl H.; Schmalz G. Glutaraldehyde-containing dentin bonding agents are mutagens in mammalian cells in vitro. J Biomed Mater Res 36 284–288 (1997).

Schweikl H.; Schmalz G.; Rackebrandt K. The mutagenic activity of unpolymerized resin monomers in *Salmonella typhimurium* and V79 cells. Mutat Res 415 119–130 (1998).

Schweikl H.; Schmalz G.; Federlin M. Mutagenicity of the root canal sealer AHPlus in the Ames test. Clin Oral Invest 2 125–129 (1998).

Schweikl H.; Schmalz G. Triethylene glycol dimethacrylate induces large deletions in the hprt gene of V79 cells. Mutat Res 438 71–78 (1999).

Schweikl H.; Schmalz G.; Spruss T. The induction of micronuclei in vitro by unpolymerized resin monomers. J Dent Res 80 1615–1620 (2001).

Schweikl H.; Schmalz G.; Weinmann W. Mutagenic activity of structurally related oxiranes and siloranes in Salmonella typhimurium. Mutat Res 521 19–27 (2002).

Schweikl H.; Hiller K.A.; Bolay C.; et al. Cytotoxic and mutagenic effects of dental composite materials. Biomaterials 26 1713–1719 (2005).

Schweikl H.; Altmannberger I.; Hanser N.; et al. The effect of triethylene glycol dimethacrylate on the cell cycle of mammalian cells. Biomaterials 26 4111–4118 (2005).

Schweikl H.; Spagnuolo G.; Schmalz G. Genetic and cellular toxicology of dental resin monomers. J Dent Res 85 870–877 (2006).

Schweikl H.; Hartmann A.; Hiller K.A.; et al. Inhibition of TEGDMA and HEMA-induced genotoxicity and cell cycle arrest by N-acetylcysteine. Dent Mater 23 688–695 (2007).

Schweikl H.; Muller R.; Englert C.; et al. Proliferation of osteoblasts and fibroblasts on model surfaces of varying roughness and surface chemistry. J Mater Sci Mater Med 18 1895–1905 (2007).

Scott A.; Egner W.; Gawkrodger D.J.; et al. The national survey of adverse reactions to dental materials in the UK: A preliminary study by the UK Adverse Reactions Reporting Project. Br Dent J 196 471–477 (2004). discussion 465.

Selden A.I.; Persson B.; Bornberger-Dankvardt S.I.; et al. Exposure to cobalt chromium dust and lung disorders in dental technicians. Thorax 50 769–772 (1995).

Siddiqui M.A.; Mehta N.J.; Khan I.A. Paracelsus: The Hippocrates of the Renaissance. J Med Biogr 11 78–80 (2003).

Spagnuolo G.; D'Anto V.; Cosentino C.; et al. Effect of N-acetyl-L-cysteine on ROS production and cell death caused by HEMA in human primary gingival fibroblasts. Biomaterials 27 1803–1809 (2006).

Spagnuolo G.; D'Anto V.; Valletta R.; et al. Effect of 2-hydroxyethyl methacrylate on human pulp cell survival pathways ERK and AKT. J Endod 34 684–688 (2008).

Tillberg A.; Stenberg B.; Berglund A. Reactions to resin-based dental materials in patients—type, time to onset, duration, and consequence of the reaction. Contact Dermatitis 61 313–319 (2009).

Tomakidi P.; Koke U.; Kern R.; et al. Assessment of acute cyto- and genotoxicity of corrosion eluates obtained from orthodontic materials using monolayer cultures of immortalized human gingival keratinocytes. J Orofac Orthop 61 2–19 (2000).

Traisnel M.; le Maguer D.; Hildebrand H.F.; et al. Corrosion of surgical implants. Clin Mater 5 309–318 (1990).

Valentine-Thon E.; Müller K.; Guzzi G.; et al. LTT-MELISA® is clinically relevant for detecting and monitoring metal sensitivity. Neuroendocrinology Letters 27 17–24 (2006).

Vamnes J.S.; Morken T.; Helland S.; et al. Dental gold alloys and contact hypersensitivity. Contact Dermatitis 42 128–133 (2000).

Vamnes J.S.; Lygre G.B.; Gronningsaeter A.G.; et al. Four years of clinical experience with an adverse reaction unit for dental biomaterials. Community Dent Oral Epidemiol 32 150–157 (2004).

van Loon L.A.; van Elsas P.W.; van Joost T.; et al. Test battery for metal allergy in dentistry. Contact Dermatitis 14 158–161 (1986).

Wang R.R.; Li Y. In vitro evaluation of biocompatibility of experimental titanium alloys for dental restorations. J Prosthet Dent 80 495–500 (1998).

Wataha J.C. Predicting clinical biological responses to dental materials. Dent Mater 28 23–40 (2012); This article describes methods and measures that are used to predict clinical biological responses to dental materials. Emphasis is placed on the global nature and universal importance of issues associated with the assessment of the biological safety of these materials. The importance of the active interface between biomaterials and biological systems is highlighted including concepts of interactions at the interface, the dynamic nature of the interface, the function of the type of tissue where the interface is created, the foreign body nature of biomaterials, and the potential to customize interactions at the material–tissue interface.

Wataha J.C.; Craig R.G.; Hanks C.T. The release of elements of dental casting alloys into cell-culture medium. J Dent Res 70 1014–1018 (1991).

Wataha J.C.; Hanks C.T.; Sun Z. In vitro reaction of macrophages to metal ions from dental biomaterials. Dent Mater 11 239–245 (1995).

Wataha J.C.; Hanks C.T. Biological effects of palladium and risk of using palladium in dental casting alloys. J Oral Rehabil 23 309–320 (1996).

Waxman S.G. The molecular pathophysiology of pain: Abnormal expression of sodium channel genes and its contributions to hyperexcitability of primary sensory neurons. Pain Suppl 6 S133–S140 (1999).

Waxman S.G.; Dib-Hajj S.; Cummins T.R.; et al. Sodium channels and pain. Proc Natl Acad Sci USA 96 7635–7639 (1999).

Wever D.J.; Veldhuizen A.G.; Sanders M.M.; et al. Cytotoxic, allergic and genotoxic activity of a nickel-titanium alloy. Biomaterials 18 1115–1120 (1997).

Wrangsjo K.; Swartling C.; Meding B. Occupational dermatitis in dental personnel: Contact dermatitis with special reference to (meth)acrylates in 174 patients. Contact Dermatitis 45 158–163 (2001).

Yamamoto A.; Honma R.; Sumita M. Cytotoxicity evaluation of 43 metal salts using murine fibroblasts and osteoblastic cells. J Biomed Mater Res 39 331–340 (1998).

Yang J.; Shanbhag A.; Lilien J.; et al. Human neutrophil response to short-term exposure to F-75 cobalt-based alloy. J Biomed Mater Res 26 1217–1230 (1992).

18

Clinical Research on Restorations

CHAPTER OUTLINE

KEY TERMS

Case–control studies—Type of study that examines two groups at a point in time, usually groups with and without disease or intervention, and makes inferences from these.

Evidence-based dentistry—An approach to oral health care that requires the judicious integration of systematic assessments of clinically relevant scientific evidence, relating to the patient's oral and medical condition and history, with the dentist's clinical expertise and the patient's treatment needs and preferences.

Fractography—The study of fractured surfaces of materials.

Prospective analysis study—Type of study that plans interventions, examines the results of these interventions over a period of time, and makes conclusions.

Randomized controlled clinical trial—A prospective study that randomizes participants and employs a control group.

Retrospective study—Type of study that examines past occurrences and interventions and deducts results and conclusions.

One of the most difficult areas in dental materials research is the ability to predict their clinical performance through in vitro testing methodologies. The oral environment is almost impossible to simulate in a laboratory setting because of the many variables that need to be introduced, such as occlusal forces, the pH of the surrounding environment, diet, the buffering capacity of saliva, and muscle and soft tissue cleansing action. As such, most in vitro testing methodologies evaluate how a material responds to a specific testing condition, and the experimental data are used to differentiate between materials. The true test for a restorative dental material is clinical performance, which includes longevity and predictability of use. In recent years, there has been a push from the medical community to implement evidence-based dentistry (EBD) in dental education and practice.

What Is Evidence-Based Dentistry?

EBD is defined as an approach to oral health care that requires the judicious integration of systematic assessments of clinically relevant scientific evidence, relating to the patient's oral and medical condition and history, with the dentist's clinical expertise and the patient's treatment needs and preferences. Three main areas in evidence-based dental care are relevant scientific evidence, patient needs and preference, and dentists' clinical expertise. Since the patient needs/preferences and clinical expertise are subjective, relevant scientific evidence is of critical importance. The types of evidence were ranked, with laboratory or standardized testing as being the lowest tier of evidence, followed by in vivo observations in the form of clinical studies and case studies. The highest form of evidence is the controlled, randomized clinical trial, where clinical interventions are allocated by chance and evaluated based on performance. The randomization eliminates the effect of multiple patient variables, which can skew (a bias toward one particular group or subject) results.

CRITICAL QUESTION

Why are clinical trials essential in testing the performance of dental biomaterials?

Level of Evidence in Evidence-Based Dentistry

Among the available hierarchy of evidence, systematic reviews and meta-analyses of randomized controlled clinical trials (RCTs) take the top position and contribute to the highest level of evidence, followed by RCTs and cohort studies. These are followed by case–control studies, cross-over studies, cross-sectional studies, case studies, and case reports. Finally, there are animal research and in vitro laboratory testing. At each level of evidence, there is a body of knowledge, but not all levels are equally useful for making patient care decisions. As we progress up the pyramid, the number of studies and, correspondingly, the amount of available literature decreases while at the same time, their relevance to answering clinical questions increases.

From a dental material point of view, we will discuss the evidence in three categories: in vitro testing, observational studies, and randomized control clinical studies.

In Vitro Testing

Although necessary, these standardized tests often evaluate a limited number of variables in one test condition and are not representative of the true oral environment. The International Organization for Standardization (ISO) is an independent, nongovernmental international organization that develops specifications for products and services to ensure quality, safety, and efficiency. The ISO/Technical Committee 106 (TC 106) was specifically designed to develop standards for dental materials testing. Unfortunately, dental manufacturers' adherence to ISO standards is desirable but not required. Additionally, most of these in vitro tests cannot be correlated with what occurs in the oral environment. For example, the ISO standard for wear of enamel and a dental material is measured using a pin-on-disk system. The setup is that one material is in the form of a disk or a pin and the opposing material (preferably enamel) is on the other end. Both materials are rotating in a circular motion on a flat plane. The reality is that teeth are not flat, and the temporomandibular joint functions on an arch and then a slide to produce a complex movement along cuspal inclines and fossae. So, the wear of a dental material as measured by these standards cannot reasonably be correlated with clinical performance.

Another example is the test for the chemical durability of ceramic materials, which is conducted by immersing the ceramic in a pH 2.4 buffer solution at 80°C for 16 hours. This scenario does not represent the oral environment in that the diet of each individual exposes the material to a myriad of pH changes. In addition, the buffering capacity of saliva continually strives to neutralize this environment to pH 7.4, so there is a constant fluctuation of pH in the oral cavity. A recent in vitro study introduced the concept of pH cycling, where ceramic disks were exposed to a sequence of pH 2, 7, and 10 over a period of 30 days at 80°C. This study demonstrated that the surface degradation and material loss were significantly greater during the pH-cycling testing methodology than the constant immersion currently being employed as a standard test. There are two different dissolution mechanisms involved that work synergistically when the pH is cycled. In an acidic solution, an ionic exchange mechanism occurs where the network modifiers (Al, Ca, K, Zn) are exchanged for the ions in solution. This leaves a weakened corrosive layer on the surface. In a basic solution, a total dissolution process occurs where the Si–O bonds are cleaved, and the surface layer is corroded. In a constant immersion environment, a steady state is reached where no further corrosion occurs. However, in a pH-cycled environment, alternating between acid and base, the basic solution will attack not only the Si–O bonds but also the corroded layer produced by immersion in an acidic environment. Thus, there is a constant dissolution process that is corroding the surface of ceramic. Although the pH cycling test represents extremes in the oral environment, this method suggests that the current standard of constant immersion could be underestimating the potential for surface degradation of materials in the mouth. Therefore in vitro testing is ranked as the lowest form of evidence by EBD standards.

CRITICAL QUESTION

What is the best type of clinical study and why?

Observational Studies

In vivo observations are the second tier of dental evidence as classified by EBD. These types of studies include retrospective studies, prospective studies, case–control studies, and cohort studies. The dental literature is replete with observational studies that examine the performance of dental materials over a predetermined time.

Retrospective Studies

Retrospective studies look back in time for applied interventions and examine the outcome in the present time. For example, a retrospective analysis can be performed on the longevity of the types of post and core materials by performing a chart review, categorizing the types of materials used, and evaluating the duration these post and cores were in service intraorally. The advantages of these studies are that data are readily available to be analyzed, and they are relatively inexpensive to execute. The disadvantages include no standardization of placement of these materials because there are multiple operators involved, records may be incomplete, and the presence of multiple variables is very difficult to ascertain. Statistically, there is a higher chance of error with these types of studies, resulting from confounding variables and bias.

Case–Control Studies

Case–control studies are also observational studies and are generally retrospective. These studies have an outcome status and an exposure status that are not determined by the investigator. This type of study will generally examine two groups, one with and one without the outcome, to determine whether there is an exposure and try to infer causation. An example of this could be the neurological effects of dental amalgam where investigators identify groups with an outcome (neurological defects) and an exposure status (presence of amalgam in their mouths) and try to find an association. As with retrospective studies, these are relatively inexpensive, although they provide less evidence for causation.

Prospective Studies

Prospective studies can be observational or controlled and randomized, and they are planned longitudinal experiments—for example, a study comparing the wear of enamel against metal–ceramic crowns and all-ceramic crowns. These two groups (or cohorts) can be followed over a specified period of time to determine which material is more wear friendly to enamel. These studies are more expensive because they have to be planned, and participants must be followed for long periods of time.

Randomized Controlled Clinical Trials

RCTs are considered the gold standard of evidence-based sciences. These studies randomize the allocation of participants into groups to minimize bias and confounding variables and are controlled, meaning there is the presence of a control group where participants receive no treatment or the current standard of treatment. These studies are prospective and longitudinal, which is one of the reasons they are not very common because they are expensive and logistically very difficult to conduct. An example of an RCT is comparing the survival of metal–ceramic crowns and ceramic–ceramic crowns in three-unit fixed dental prosthesis. The metal–ceramic material serves as the control or the standard of care. The objective is to determine whether there are advantages to the new material over the old material and whether these outweigh the disadvantages.

Evidence Syntheses: Systematic Reviews and Meta-analysis

Most experts consider well done systematic reviews, with or without meta-analysis, to provide the best evidence for all question types. The major advantage of systematic reviews is that they are based on the findings of multiple studies that were identified in comprehensive, systematic literature searches.

The position of systematic reviews at the top of the evidence hierarchy is not absolute, however:

- You must appraise a systematic review's methodological rigor and the strength of its findings before applying those findings to patient care.
- Systematic reviews often take months to years to conduct. Make sure that the findings of a systematic review have not been superseded by newer evidence.
- A large, well-conducted randomized controlled trial may provide more compelling evidence than a systematic review of small, underpowered trials.

Systematic Reviews Versus Narrative Reviews

It is important to understand the difference between systematic reviews (with or without meta-analysis) and narrative reviews.

Systematic reviews seek to answer a specific and clearly formulated question by using rigorous, explicit protocols to identify, select, and appraise relevant research studies; and to collect and analyze data from the selected studies. To minimize bias, systematic reviews include or exclude evidence on the basis of explicit quality criteria. They may incorporate meta-analysis.

Narrative reviews, often just called Reviews, articles may be ***evidence based***, but they are not evidence. Rather than answering a specific clinical question, they provide an overview of the research landscape on a given topic. They usually lack systematic search protocols or explicit criteria for selecting and appraising evidence.

CRITICAL QUESTION

What are the factors that would limit interventions applied in a clinical study?

Clinical Analysis of Survival and Acceptability

As mentioned earlier, the best form of evidence is clinical performance studies, either as observational studies or randomized and controlled interventional studies. Because human experiments are well controlled and regulated by ethical boards, intervention has to fall within a reasonable benefit-to-risk ratio. In other words, the risks for conducting the study should not outweigh the benefits, and no harm should be promoted in the experiment. For this reason, clinical studies are limited to mostly observation of occurrences. For example, a crack cannot purposely be introduced into a ceramic crown and cemented onto a patient's mouth to enable observation of the phenomena of progression of slow crack growth in vivo. Similarly, a biopsy of a healthy peri-implant site cannot be performed for the sole purpose of being able to compare bacterial flora to a diseased peri-implant site. This section will describe several in vivo measurements that are currently being employed to assess the clinical performance of dental materials. First is a description of how restorations are being assessed after periodic performance intraorally. Second are two methods of measuring and quantifying wear in vivo. Third is a forensic assessment of clinical fractures through fractographic analysis.

CRITICAL QUESTION

What is the rationale for calibrating evaluators in a clinical study, and why is there a need for dual evaluation?

Clinical Assessment of Restorations

Perhaps the oldest and most important clinical assessment tool is the rating scale published by Cvar and Ryge in 1971 in the US Public Health Service Guidelines (USPHS; Box 18.1). The original

• BOX 18.1 Original Cvar and Ryge Criteria Used to Evaluate Restorations

Color Match

Oscar (O)	Anterior restoration, invisible without a mirror
Alfa (A)	Posterior restoration, matching the adjacent tooth in color, shade, and translucency
Bravo (B)	Posterior restoration; the mismatch in color, shade, and translucency between the restoration and the adjacent tooth within normal range
Charlie (C)	Posterior restoration; the mismatch in color, shade, and translucency between the restoration and the adjacent tooth outside normal range

Cavosurface Marginal Discoloration

Alfa (A)	No discoloration anywhere on the margin between the restoration and the tooth
Bravo (B)	Discoloration present but does not penetrate along the margin toward the pulp
Charlie (C)	Discoloration present and penetrates along the margin toward the pulp

Anatomical Form

Alfa (A)	Restoration continuous with existing anatomical form
Bravo (B)	Restoration undercontoured, i.e., discontinuous with existing anatomical form but dentin/base not exposed
Charlie (C)	Restoration undercontoured, i.e., discontinuous with existing anatomical form and dentin/base exposed

Marginal Adaption

Alfa (A)	No visible evidence of a crevice along the margin into which an explorer penetrates
Bravo (B)	Visible evidence of a crevice along the margin into which an explorer penetrates but dentin/base not exposed
Charlie (C)	Visible crevice along the margin with exposed dentin/base; the restoration is not mobile, fractured, or missing in part of the tooth
Delta (D)	Restoration mobile, fractured, or missing in part of the tooth

Caries

Alfa (A)	Caries absent along the restoration margin
Bravo (B)	Caries present along the restoration margin

parameters used for evaluating dental restorations were color match, marginal discoloration, marginal integrity, anatomical form, and the presence of dental caries. The parameters were graded alfa (A), bravo (B) and charlie (C). These rankings were created to differentiate restorations that were within the range of excellent, acceptable, needing future replacement to prevent damage, and needing immediate replacement. The key to the success of this grading scale is the systematic calibration of the reviewers to ensure that (1) the evaluators are familiar with the grading scale, (2) they possess the visual discrimination for assessment, and (3) they maintain consistency in grading longitudinal studies. Another requirement is the implementation of dual evaluators and a process by which they can resolve differences in grading. The original study noted that the accuracy of a trained and calibrated evaluator is about 85%. The inclusion of a second trained and calibrated evaluator increases the accuracy of the rating to 98%. One aspect of this study that was never really implemented is the universal collection of photographs and study models to enable calibration across clinical studies. With time, modified versions of the clinical assessment tool have come to include additional parameters, such as occlusion, postoperative sensitivity, fracture, retention, and others, depending on the needs of the study and the restoration being evaluated. Perhaps the biggest obstacle to clinical studies is cost, which largely explains why most studies have no controls and only one evaluator.

In 2007, the Fédération Dentaire Internationale (FDI) released its own version of the clinical assessment of restorations. The FDI subdivided the different parameters according to esthetic, functional, and biological groups (Box 18.2) for a total of 16 parameters in all. The grading scale was expanded to include clinically excellent, clinically good, clinically satisfactory, clinically unsatisfactory, and clinically poor. To facilitate calibration between multiple sites, the FDI also posted an online calibration guide, but this, of course, is no replacement for the hands-on clinical calibration that occurs. As with the USPHS scale, investigators are able to tailor the criteria based on their studies and needs.

• BOX 18.2 Fédération Dentaire Internationale (FDI) Revised Criteria for Evaluating Clinical Restorations

Esthetic Criteria

Surface luster
Staining: (a) surface and (b) margin
Color match and translucency
Esthetic anatomical form

Functional Criteria

Fracture of material and retention
Marginal adaptation
Occlusal contour and wear
Approximal anatomical form: (a) contact point and (b) contour
Radiographic examination, where applicable
Patient's view

Biological Criteria

Postoperative sensitivity and tooth vitality
Recurrence of caries, erosion, abfraction
Tooth integrity
Periodontal response
Adjacent mucosa
Oral and general health

For all three groups, the following gradings are used for evaluation:
Clinically excellent/very good
Clinically good
Clinically sufficient/satisfactory
Clinically unsatisfactory
Clinically poor

CRITICAL QUESTION

What qualities of wear are desirable in a dental material?

Wear Analysis

One of the most important criteria for dental materials is durability and compatibility with existing structures. These two parameters are clearly measured through wear analysis, in that these materials must be durable enough to withstand occlusal forces by not wearing away and at the same time exhibiting comparable wear of opposing enamel. Wear of restorative material surfaces can cause damage to the existing structures. A worn surface usually translates into a roughened surface, which can encourage plaque accumulation, caries formation, and wear of the opposing tooth surface. Consequently, worn surfaces can result in a decrease in the occlusal vertical dimension, which could then lead to occlusal trauma, periodontal disease, and temporomandibular joint dysfunction. As mentioned earlier, the standard test for wear is not representative of occlusal function. Several wear machines or chewing simulators were developed that introduced varying load, vertical and horizontal movement, and thermocycling. However, none of these chewing simulators was found to correlate well with clinical scenarios. Therefore, the best measure is to determine the wear of enamel and dental materials in a clinical setting. There are two ways to quantify clinical wear: indirect and direct.

Indirect Method

The indirect method is the most commonly used method for measuring clinical wear. The method is indirect because replicas are made using an elastomeric impression of the area of interest (dental material and/or opposing tooth enamel), and stone models are made where the measurements are conducted. The measuring devices are diverse and can include laser scanners, microcomputed tomography (micro-CT), or surface profilometers.

A laser scanner produces a three-dimensional (3-D) image through the movement of an object (in this case, a tooth replica) under the projection of a laser beam. The reflection of the cross-section profile of the object is detected by sensors, which produce an image consisting of "point clouds." Each point represents *x*-, *y*-, and *z*-coordinates on the scanned surface. Each profile can then be combined and transformed into high-resolution images through advanced software that allows for comparison and measurement. The edge effect is an error or artifact that is produced when the laser beam hits a sharp edge or the bottom of a groove, producing overshot reflections. Laser beam measurements are also affected by surface reflections of the material being scanned, so stone or elastomeric impression materials are used as replicates to minimize these reflections.

Laser scanners can either have red or blue laser beams. Higher wavelength beams (red beams) have lower resolution, more diffraction, and less intensity compared with the blue laser beams. Depending on the nature of the material being scanned, the laser can penetrate through the material to cause a diffusion on the surface, which can result in a loss of focus on the surface being measured and sends inaccurate readings back to the detector, which in turn leads to invalid measurements.

When measuring the clinical wear of a dental material, a baseline impression and a replica model of the teeth involved in the measurement are first made. Depending on the study protocol, an impression and replica are once again produced during the designated follow-up time, either in months or years. The wear that occurred between baseline and the period of interest is measured using specialized scanners with software that can superimpose images by using known landmarks and calculating volume loss and maximum wear depth. Figure 18.1 demonstrates teeth-opposing ceramic crowns that were monitored for 10 months. Baseline and period replicas are shown on the left, with yellow arrows pointing to areas that are worn. A laser scanner device was used to superimpose the two replicas. The image on the right demonstrates red areas that highlight the areas on the teeth where wear occurred. The maximum wear or the maximum wear depth value is perhaps more important than calculating the volume loss of a material. Volumetric wear can occur over a large surface area and therefore not be detrimental to the integrity of the tooth or the restoration if the depth is shallow and remains superficial. However, maximum wear indicates maximum depth, which can prove to be more damaging. For example, when calculating the wear of enamel, if volume loss is large but occurs over a wide area, the wear can be limited to enamel. However, if the maximum wear refers to depth and the value is large, then there is a possibility of wear through the dentin. There are several laser scanners available on the market that are used for quantifying wear. Unfortunately, the validity of these measurements is rarely verified with calibrated instruments such as micro-CT or a profilometer. As mentioned earlier, there are errors that can be produced from the laser-scanning process. Figure 18.2 demonstrates the discrepancies between a laser scanner and surface profilometer in measuring the depth profile of indentations produced by different grit diamond burs on a ceramic surface to simulate wear. This in vitro study evaluated the validity of a red laser scanner in measuring depth and volume against a surface profilometer, in addition to the effect of bur grit on these measurements. Gross over and underestimations of depth and volume wear measurements were observed with the laser scanner compared with the surface profilometer. These errors probably resulted from a combination of the edge effect mentioned previously, the nature of the material being scanned, and the high wavelength of the beams. Nonetheless, although laser scanners are a convenient tool for measuring clinical wear, the users have to be judicious in determining the accuracy and the validity of the wear measurements.

Micro-CT can also be used to measure clinical wear using the indirect method. Micro-CT uses X-rays to see through an object slice by slice. These two-dimensional (2-D) images are then rendered through a software program to produce a 3-D model of the object or analyzed in cross-sections. For the purpose of wear analysis, wear can be quantified through analysis of the replicas. Figure 18.3 demonstrates the mesial and occlusal views of a dentoform tooth that has been placed in a chewing simulator to receive random wear at multiple sites. The micro-CT was used to scan the tooth before and after wear occurred, and the results are shown in Figure 18.3, where the colored areas refer to the areas of wear, which are quantified according to the grid shown on the side.

Surface profilometry can also be used for quantitative wear evaluation using the indirect technique. The contact profilometer has a stylus that traverses the surface of the object being measured, whereas the noncontact profilometer uses a laser beam or white

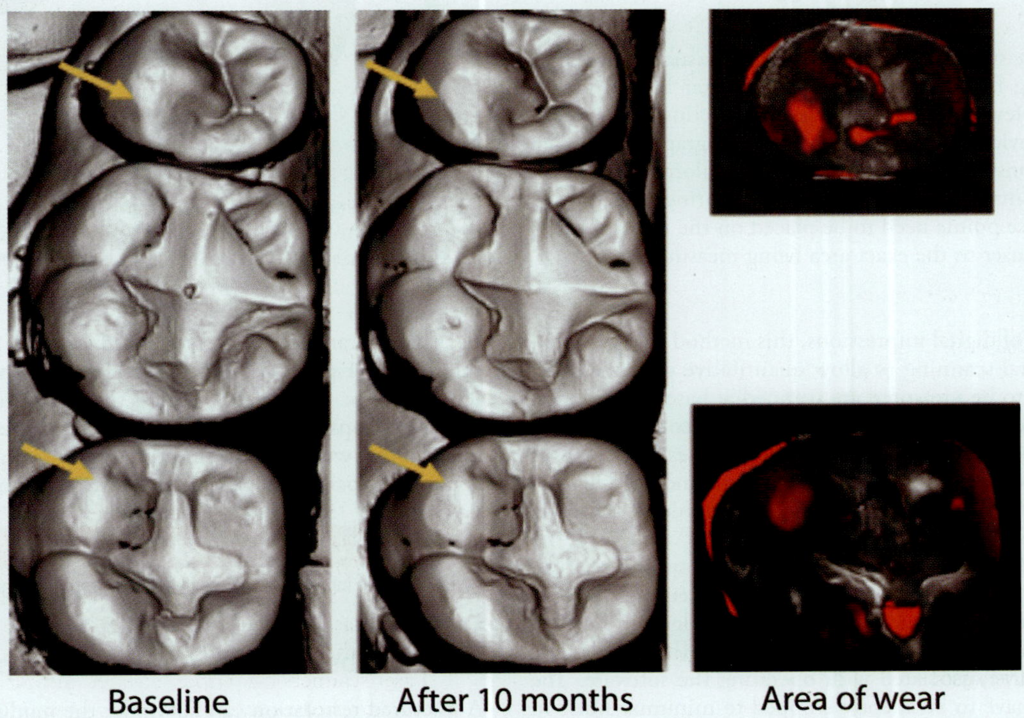

• **Fig. 18.1** Wear areas *(yellow arrows)* on teeth noted after 10 months of service on teeth opposing an all-ceramic fixed dental prosthesis. Comparison software on the far right reveals red areas indicating where wear occurred. (From Esquivel-Upshaw JF, et al.: In vivo wear of enamel by a lithia-disilicate core ceramic used for posterior FPDs: First-year result. *Int J Prosthodont* 19:391–396, 2006.)

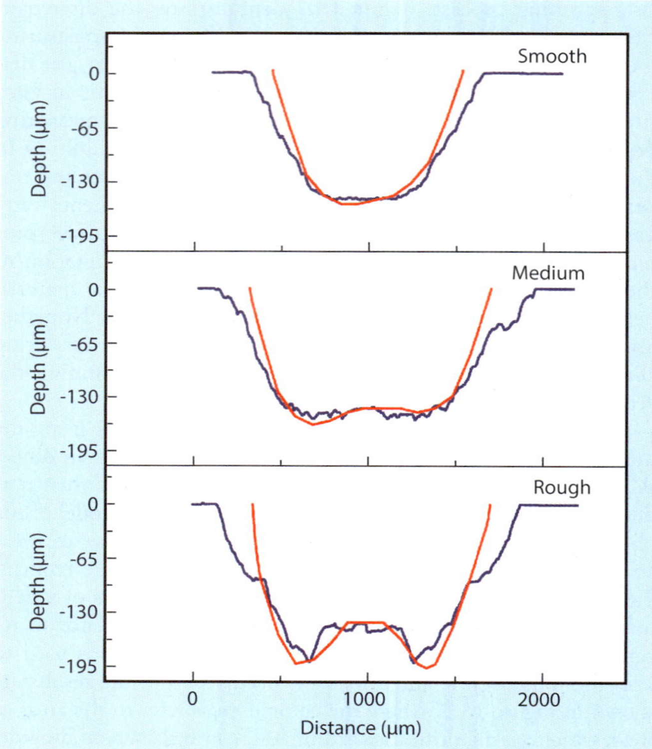

• **Fig. 18.2** Depth-profile comparison between laser scanner *(red)* and profilometer *(blue)* indicating major differences in depth and width of indentations caused by different grit diamond burs. Edge effect, artifact, and surface reflectance could be partially responsible for the inaccuracies. (From Hsu SM, et al.: Comprehensive analysis of laserscanner validity used for measurement of wear. *J Oral Rehabil* 46:503–510, 2019.)

light to probe the surface. The contact stylus is usually a metal or diamond ranging from 2 to 20 μm in diameter loaded with a contact load of few millinewtons while contacting the surface. The scan can provide a map of the surface topography. Although this method is considered precise for depth profilometry, the process is time-consuming. For this type of measuring device to be effective, reference points need to be placed on the teeth of interest to orient the user to the exact area being measured.

Direct Method

With the advent of digital impressions, this method uses the technology of intraoral scanning to allow quantitative wear measurement. The teeth to be measured are scanned at baseline and then again at periods of interest. These scans are then compared using comparison software that essentially superimposes both images and identifies the differences in depth and volume between the two. The process of intraoral scanning is technique sensitive. Some intraoral scanners use a powder spray of zinc oxide to minimize the reflection of enamel during the scanning process. The area being scanned has to be completely isolated so that saliva does not mix with the powder. The powdery sludge can become thick and cause an error in the scanning process. There is also the steep learning curve associated with operating the software. The scanned images have to be adeptly cropped to minimize noise in the superimposition. Figure 18.4 is an example of the direct method. Figure 18.4A and B depicts clinical images of two opposing quadrants, with the crown on the mandibular left molar being the area of interest and the opposing tooth on the maxillary. These

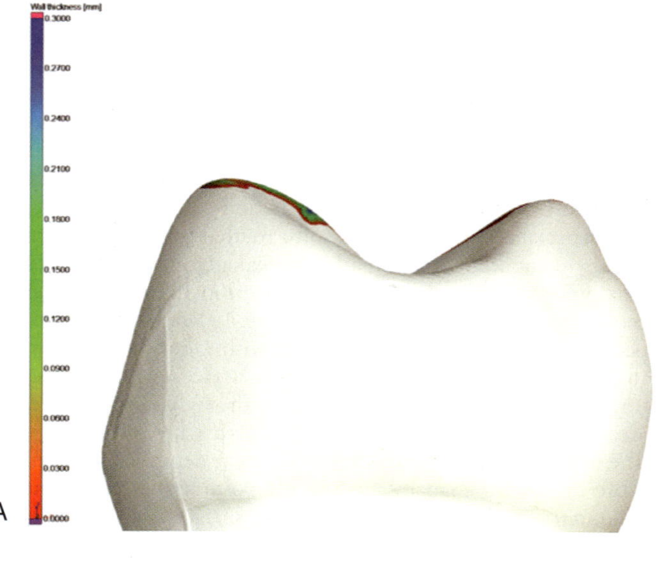

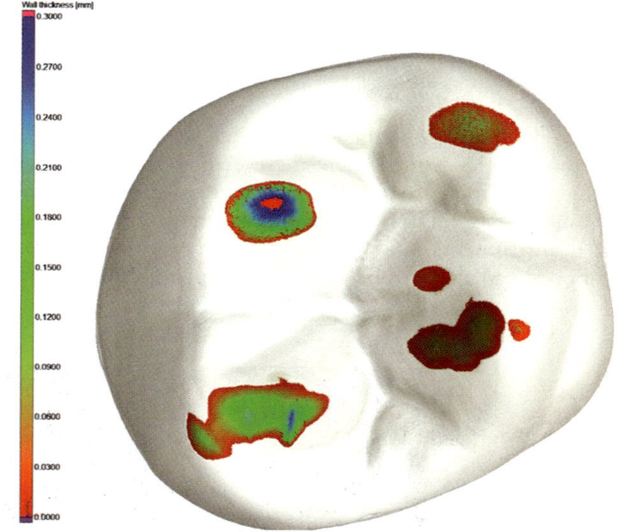

• **Fig. 18.3** Three-dimensional reconstructed image from micro-CT scan of a dentoform tooth demonstrating wear. **(A)** Mesial (or distal) aspect. **(B)** Occlusal surface. The color bar to the side reflects wear depth in millimeters.

teeth were scanned at baseline and then again at 6 months, and the images (Fig. 18.4C and D) demonstrate the amount of wear (color grid in millimeters) during this period of time. Although this is perhaps the most convenient and expedient method for quantifying wear, the technical sensitivity and the errors that could be associated with scanners have to be considered.

CRITICAL QUESTION

What forensic information can we ascertain from fractographic analyses?

Critical Observation and Fractographic Analysis

A fractured restoration can fall under the modified version of the USPHS under functional criteria. However, fracture surfaces often reveal information about how and why the fracture occurred. That is why the critical observation and analysis of fractures deserve a separate section in this chapter.

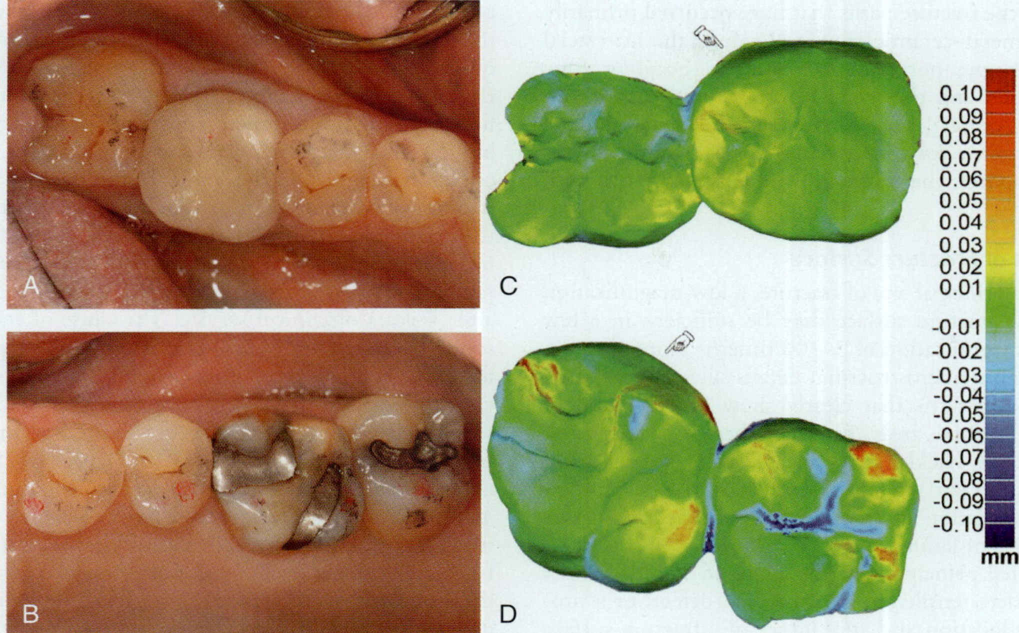

• **Fig. 18.4** Direct method of wear measurement using intraoral scanner. **(A)** A ceramic crown on mandibular left first molar. **(B)** Opposing left maxillary quadrant. **(C)** The result of superimposing baseline and 1-year scan to quantify the wear that occurred on the ceramic crown *(pointer)* by the comparison software using the adjacent second molar as the enamel control. The color bar to the side reflects wear depth on the ceramic restoration and the enamel control in millimeters. **(D)** The result of opposing maxillary first molar.

Characteristics of Fracture Surface

Fractography is the study of the fracture surfaces of materials. Through characteristics visible on the surface of these fractures, the origin of the fracture, the load and orientation of the fracture, and the progression of the failure can be determined for the particular material. There have been significant advances in the application of fractography to the understanding of fracture mechanics. Several works have identified the key parameters that are important to the understanding of why fractures occur. When a material fractures in a brittle manner, the fracture surface records the event in such a way that many important features are made clear. A schematic diagram of a typical crack in glass or ceramic is depicted in Figure 18.5. Some very prominent features of these cracks are the origin, mirror, mist, and hackle. These features, when visible by magnification, can usually give an indication as to the propagation direction of the fracture. The presence of any residual stresses can be determined from the fractured area and the stress at which fractures occur, which can be measured from the crack size.

Almost all mechanically induced cracks can be idealized as a semielliptical, sharp crack of depth a and half-width 2b (Fig. 18.5). If you consider the equation:

(1)

$$K_{Ic} = Y\sigma_f\sqrt{c} = \sqrt{2E\gamma_c}$$

where K_{Ic} is the critical stress intensity factor (fracture toughness), Y is a geometrical factor that accounts for the shape of the fracture-initiating crack, E is the elastic (Young's) modulus, c is the radius of an equivalent semicircular or semielliptical crack ($c = \sqrt{ab}$), and γ_c is the critical fracture energy (i.e., all the energy involved in fracture, including the creation of new surfaces). The small

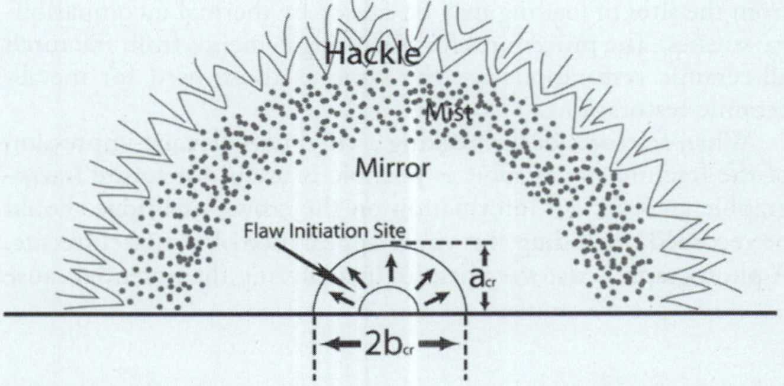

• **Fig. 18.5** Schematic diagram of crack in a brittle material with the critical flaw size and the different features that can enable calculation of stress and the direction of fracture.

semiellipse in Figure 18.5 represents the initial flaw size, and the large semiellipse is the critical flaw size that leads to fracture. Because the value of K_{Ic} can be obtained from testing standardized specimens, the level of stress causing the fracture can be calculated by the measurement of equivalent semielliptical crack, c. For further information on the process involved with fractographic analysis, the reader is referred to the fractographic books and articles mentioned at the end of this chapter.

Clinical fractures of metal–ceramic restorations, although rare, still occur, especially when a new alloy or veneering porcelain is being used or when a new technology has been adopted. As is generally true for all dental materials, there is a learning curve associated with the initial use of new products. Although there is an infinite number of fracture paths that may occur, three types are of particular importance in diagnosing the cause of fracture.

Figure 18.6 shows the fracture paths that have occurred primarily at three sites in a metal–ceramic crown: (1) along the interfacial region between opaque porcelain (P) and the bonding zone (I) between porcelain and the metal substrate (top), (2) within the bonding zone (center), and (3) between the metal and the bonding zone (bottom). For conventional metal–ceramic crowns made from cast copings, the bonding zone is synonymous with the metal oxide layer.

Characterization of Fracture Surface

To characterize the principal site of fracture, a low-magnification examination of the fracture surface may be sufficient in a few cases. However, a magnification of 3–100 times is more often required because minute microstructural details such as pores may reveal wake hackle patterns that clearly show the direction of crack propagation in these areas. Fractographers seek important crack features, such as hackle, twist hackle, wake hackle, arrest lines, and compression curl, to lead them toward the critical flaw or source of crack initiation and the possibility of identifying one or more mechanisms of failure.

Each of the three principal fracture paths in Figure 18.6 is indicative of excessive tensile stress, a material defect, or a processing factor. The location and appearance of a fracture surface are major factors used to determine the cause of fracture. For fractures that are confined to the occlusal surface of posterior crowns, a cone-crack type of fracture (apex of the cone at the fracture surface and the base of the cone extending into the veneer) suggests that localized loading at small contact areas may be the cause. Fractures that occur in the proximal occlusal area of the crowns may be caused by inadequate support of the veneer by the core framework material. Fractures that occur well away from the sites of loading may be caused by thermal incompatibility stresses. The procedures for obtaining evidence from fractured all-ceramic restorations are the same as those used for metal–ceramic restorations.

When fractures occur, making a vinyl polysiloxane impression of the fracture site as soon as possible is useful for future fractographic analysis. All information on the crown or bridge should be recorded, including the visual appearance of the fracture site. A photograph is also very helpful in analyzing the potential cause of fracture. The impression allows a replica of the fracture surface to be made from epoxy resin. The replica allows fractographic observations of the fracture surface to be made, and these models can then be examined by a fractography expert under low magnification using optical microscopy and stereomicroscopy, followed by scanning electron microscopy (SEM). The location of the critical flaw indicates the origin of the fracture. Fracture surface markings observed on the replica assist the expert in determining the origin and confirming the suspected cause of fracture. Shown in Figure 18.7A is a residual section of a fractured Procera AllCeram alumina-based crown with a glass-phase veneer that fractured after 4 years of clinical service. The cause of fracture can be assessed by visual inspection, characterization of principal fracture features, detailed examination of optical microscopy and stereomicroscopy images, and if necessary, SEM images. The stereomicroscopic analyses of the retrieved fractured segment revealed the fracture paths that are shown in Figure 18.7B. They include crack initiation (areas 1 and 3), crack propagation (areas 2 and 4), and completion of fracture (area 5). Area 3 illustrates the initiation of a cone crack that could have led to cone-type fracture discussed earlier but did not propagate far enough to cause the bulk fracture. This fracture analysis illustrates incidental surface damage in an area where crack propagation was localized only in the veneer ceramic. Figure 18.7C is the confirmation of five fracture surface features in the sketch by the SEM image. This forensic analysis of how the fracture progressed was made possible by the different landmarks that are prominent on fractured brittle surfaces.

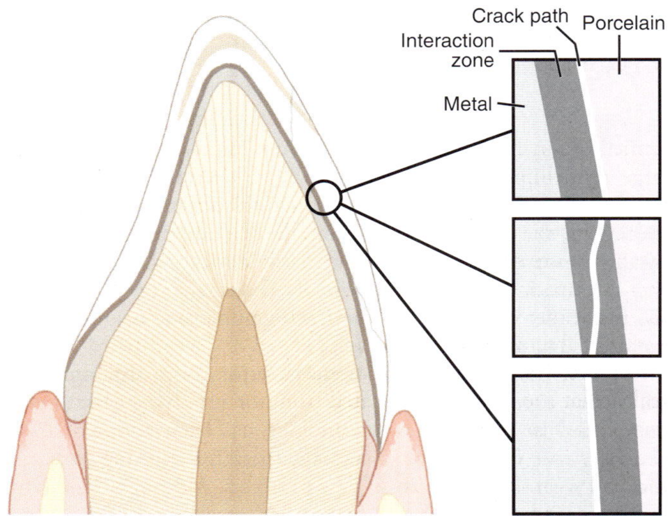

• **Fig. 18.6** Cross-sectional illustration of three principal types of interfacial zone fracture in a metal–ceramic crown.

The fractographic procedures described previously are based on the assumption that the prosthesis was free of cracks during try-in and during cementation. However, dentists are not typically trained to inspect prostheses received from the lab using fiberoptic transillumination. Examination under such lighting can reveal surface and subsurface cracks that may exist in the ceramic and metal–ceramic prostheses either before or after try-in for fit. Figure 18.8 shows a laboratory technician who is using a fiberoptic light source to inspect a ceramic prosthesis for cracks that may be hidden from typical fluorescent or incandescent light sources.

Many factors are associated with the fracture of all-ceramic prostheses. These factors fall into one of eight categories:

1. Inherent surface defects
2. Processing defects
3. Loading (bite force and load orientation)
4. Design
5. Material properties
6. Residual stress
7. Procedural errors
8. Diet

Within these categories, the following variables may contribute to crack initiation, crack propagation, chipping, and bulk fracture: surface treatment, excessive loading during try-in, bruxing loads, loading location, load distribution, load magnitude, transient cooling stresses, residual cooling stresses, inadequate tooth preparation, improper core framework design, inadequate crown thickness, inadequate core thickness, improper connector size, quality of the cement layer, bond quality of ceramic veneer to core ceramic, voids in the cement layer or at the cement/ceramic interface, and the elastic moduli of component and supporting substrate materials. To reduce the risk for ceramic fracture, sufficient tooth reduction, sufficient thickness of the ceramic, adequate prosthesis design, distributed vertical loading, and meticulous attention to the recommended manufacturers' procedures are required.

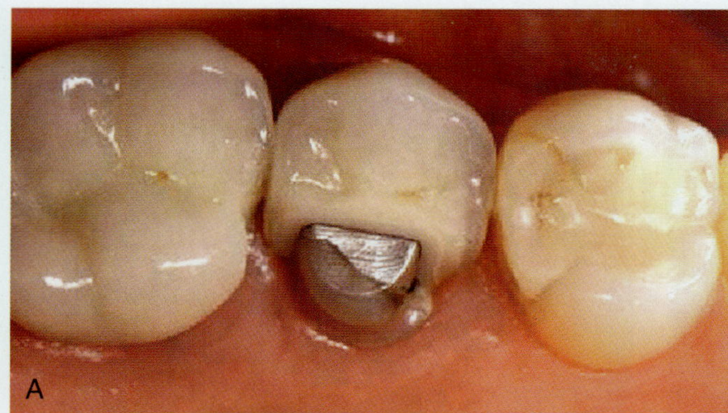

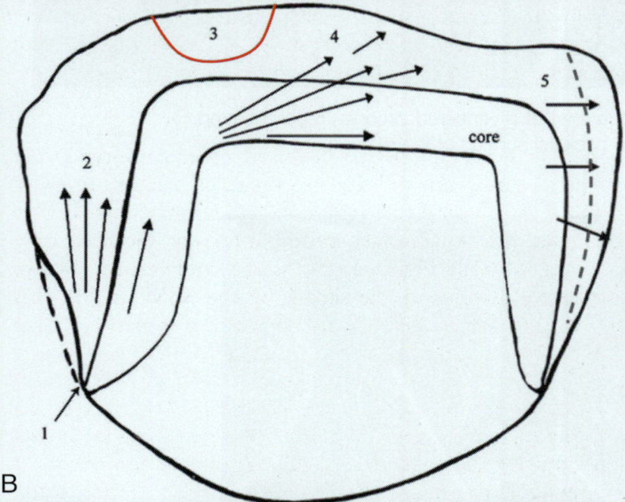

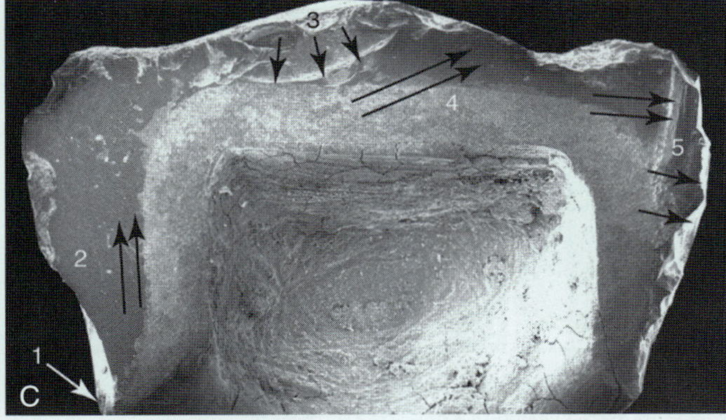

• **Fig. 18.7** Analysis of a fractured restoration. **(A)** Fractured Procera All-Ceram premolar crown. **(B)** Sketch of key findings after stereomicroscopic analyses of the retrieved fractured segment. The initiating crack occurred at the mesial margin (area 1) and propagated upward approximately 2 mm before crown fracture occurred in areas 2 and 4, terminating in the compression curl area 5. Area 3 represents contact damage within the occlusal veneering ceramic that does not extend into the alumina core ceramic. **(C)** Confirmation of the finding by scanning electron microscope image. (From Scherrer SS, et al.: Fractographic failure analysis of a Procera® AllCeram crown. Dent Mater 24:1107–1113, 2008. (Credit for part A photo): courtesy of Dr. U. Brodbeck, Zurich.)

Classification of Ceramic Restoration Fractures

Grading fractures of ceramic restorations has been recommended and is based loosely on the original USPHS criteria for grading restorations. Heinzte and Rousson introduced the classification in 2010, with class 1 being minor, no intervention required; class 2,

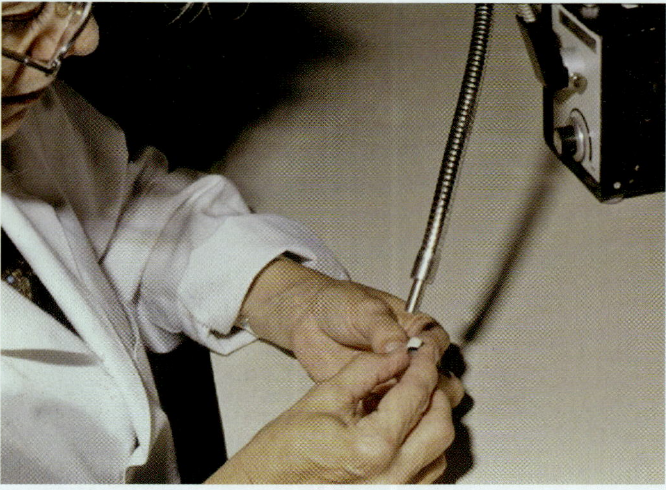

• **Fig. 18.8** Inspection for cracks using fiberoptic transillumination prior to cementation is important in improving the predictability of ceramic crowns.

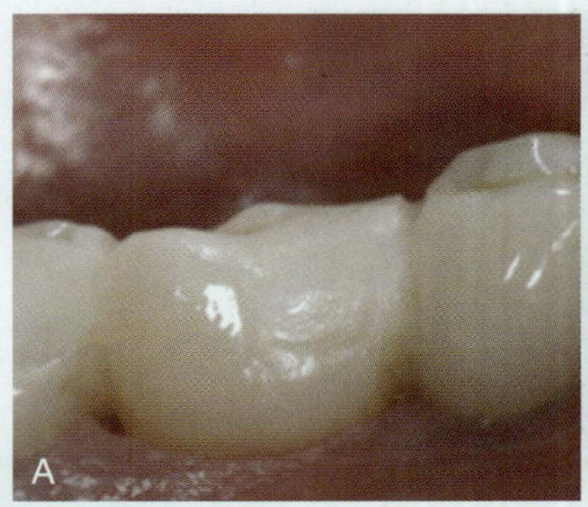

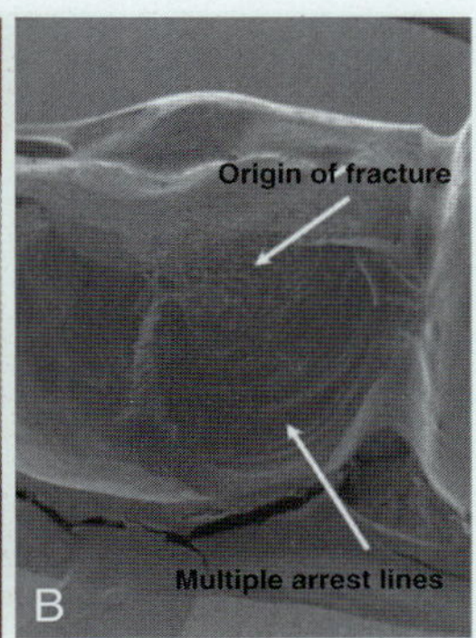

• **Fig. 18.9** Class 1 fracture. **(A)** Minor fracture on the lingual side of a ceramic–ceramic crown; no intervention required. **(B)** Scanning electron microscope identifies the fracture origin *(arrow)* on the occlusal surface and propagated gingivally, as shown by multiple arrest lines *(arrow).*

repair was needed; and class 3, replacement was required. Figures 18.9–18.11 illustrate three clinical scenarios of what these classes look like clinically. Figure 19.9A shows a veneered zirconia crown with a class 1 lingual fracture. The fracture was small enough that even the patient did not know there was anything wrong. SEM analysis (Fig. 18.9B) reveals the origin of the fracture to be on the occlusal surface of the crown. Figure 18.10A is a class 2 fracture of a veneered zirconia crown on the distal edge. Although the indication is to have this repaired because the fractured surface is substantial, these repairs made with composite resin and a silanating agent usually fail within a couple of years. Fractographic analysis (Fig. 18.10B) revealed that the fracture also originated from the occlusal surface of the prosthesis. Figure 18.11A and B is a class 3 fracture, also of a veneered zirconia crown. The fracture went through the veneer and fractured the core substructure. However, fractographic analysis (Fig. 18.11C–E) revealed that the fracture originated from the occlusal surface and propagated through a series of multiple fractures.

In summary, the performance of dental materials is best determined through clinical trials and observations because there are no in vitro tests that mimic the oral environment. However, there are limits to what can be measured intraorally, and interventions have to be ethical. The contributing factors to failure are very

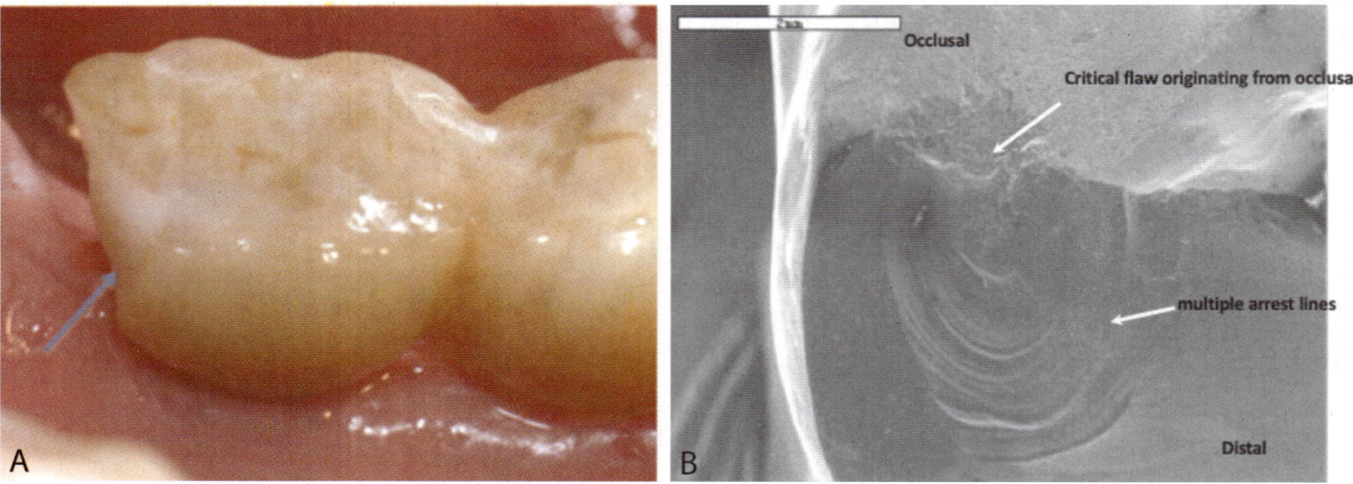

• **Fig. 18.10** Class 2 fracture. **(A)** Fracture at distal edge *(arrow)* of a veneered zirconia; repair needed. **(B)** Fractographic analysis identifies the critical flaw on the occlusal surface of the restoration.

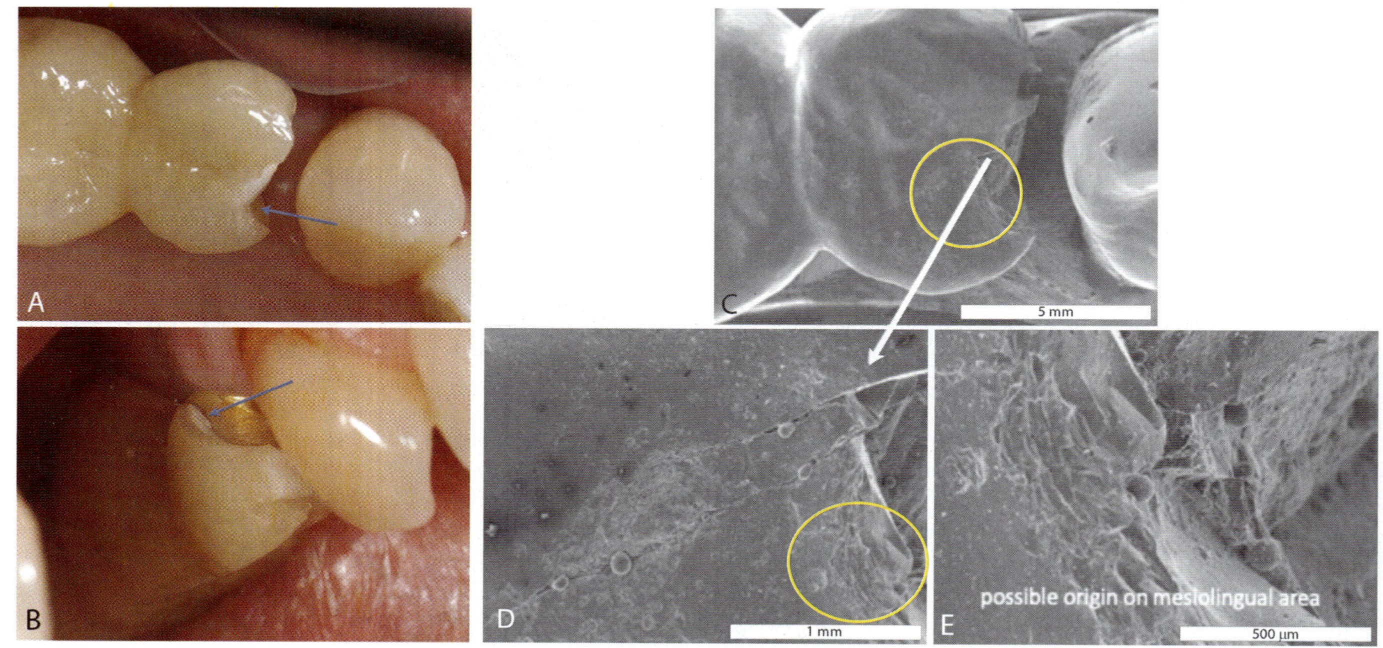

• **Fig. 18.11** Class 3 fracture. **(A)** Occlusal view of a fractured veneered zirconia; needs replacement. **(B)** Mesial-facial view showing fracture through the zirconia core. **(C–E)** Series of fractographic analysis demonstrates multiple fractures that propagated from one of the occlusal surfaces. Circles indicate the area expanded in the succeeding images.

difficult to ascertain without performing a systematic forensic analysis (such as in fractography). The biggest drawback is that these clinical tests, if done properly, are expensive and very time-consuming. By the time the results are released for a poorly performing material, the manufacturers might have already moved on to the promotion of another discovery. Thus, the feedback that should be gleaned to improve the next generation of materials is lost.

Summary

- Evidence-based dentistry—An approach to oral health care that requires the judicious integration of systematic assessments of clinically relevant scientific evidence, relating to the patient's oral and medical condition and history, with the dentist's clinical expertise and the patient's treatment needs and preferences.
- Different levels of evidence include:
  - Level 1—Evidence from a systematic review or meta-analysis of all relevant RCTs (randomized controlled trial) or evidence-based clinical practice guidelines based on systematic reviews of RCTs or three or more RCTs of good quality that have similar results.

- Level II—Evidence obtained from at least one well-designed RCT (e.g., large multisite RCT).
- Level III—Evidence obtained from well-designed controlled trials without randomization (i.e., quasiexperimental).
- Level IV—Evidence from well-designed case–control or cohort studies.
- Level V—Evidence from systematic reviews of descriptive and qualitative studies (metasynthesis).
- Level VI—Evidence from a single descriptive or qualitative study.
- Level VII—Evidence from the opinion of authorities and/or reports of expert committees.

- Case–control studies—Type of study that examines two groups at a point in time, usually groups with and without disease or intervention, and makes inferences from these.
- Prospective analysis study—Type of study that plans interventions, examines the results of these interventions over a period of time, and makes conclusions.
- Randomized controlled clinical trial—A prospective study that randomizes participants and employs a control group.
- Retrospective study—Type of study that examines past occurrences and interventions and deducts results and conclusions.
- Clinical evaluation of restorations
  - Perhaps the oldest and most important clinical assessment tool is the rating scale published by Cvar and Ryge in 1971.
  - The original parameters used for evaluating dental restorations were color match, marginal discoloration, marginal integrity, anatomical form, and the presence of dental caries.

Selected Readings

Esquivel JF, Kim MJ, Abdulhameed N, et al.: Randomized clinical study of wear of enamel antagonists against polished monolithic zirconia crowns, J Dent 68:19-27, 2018.

Esquivel-Upshaw JF, Clark AE, Shuster J, et al.: Randomized clinical trial of implant-supported ceramic-ceramic and metal-ceramic fixed dental prostheses: Preliminary results. J Prosthodont 23:73-82, 2014.

Esquivel-Upshaw JF, Ren F, Hsu SM, et al.: Novel testing for corrosion of glass-ceramics for dental applications, J Dent Res 97:296-302, 2018.

Esquivel-Upshaw JF, Rose WF, Barrett AA, et al.: In vivo wear of core ceramic, veneers, and enamel antagonists at three years. Dent Mater 28:615-621, 2012.

Esquivel-Upshaw JF, Rose WF, Oliveira ER, et al.: Randomized, controlled clinical trial of bilayer-ceramic and metal-ceramic crown performance. J Prosthodont 22:166-73, 2013.

Freiman SW, Mecholsky JJ: The Fracture of Brittle Materials: Testing and Analysis, Hoboken, New Jersey, John Wiley & Sons, Inc, 2012.

Hickel R, Peschke A, Tyas M, et al.: FDI World Dental Federation - clinical criteria for the evaluation of direct and indirect restorations. Update and clinical examples. J Adhes Dent 12:259-272, 2010.

McMurphy TB, Harris CA, Griggs JA: Accuracy and precision of fractal dimension measured on model surfaces. Dent Mater 30:302-307, 2014.

Mehl A, Gloger W, Kunzelmann K-H, et al.: A new optical 3-D device for the detection of wear. J Dent Res 76:1799-1807, 1997.

Schmalz G, Ryge G: Reprint of criteria for the clinical evaluation of dental restorative materials. Clin Oral Invest 9:215-232, 2005.

19

Emerging Technologies

CHAPTER OUTLINE

KEY TERMS

Bioactive—Having an effect on or eliciting a response from living tissue, an organism, or a cell, especially in inducing the formation of superficial hydroxyapatite.

Biomaterial—Any matter, surface, or construct that interacts with biological systems.

Biomimetics—Study of the formation, structure, or function of biologically produced substances and materials (e.g., silk or nacre) and biological mechanisms and processes (e.g., protein synthesis or mineralization) for the purpose of synthesizing similar products by artificial mechanisms that mimic natural structures.

CAD−CAM—*CAD* refers to computer-aided design technology, based on the use of computer software and systems to assist in the creation, modification, analysis, and optimization of two-dimensional or three-dimensional models of objects. Any computer program that embodies computer graphics and an application program that facilitates engineering functions in the design process can be classified as CAD software. The term *CAM* refers to computer-aided manufacturing of a restorative device using the CAD input file. CAM may be additive (buildup) or subtractive (machining of a device from a larger starting piece of material).

Cytology—The harvesting of disaggregated cells and related microscopic material for analysis of disease.

Nanotechnology—Technology that focuses on the atomic and molecular scale (<100 nm) of materials, devices, and other structures. On this scale, in which at least one dimension must be below 100 nm, quantum mechanics (quantum theory) controls material properties or behavior.

Osteoconductive—Capable of acting as a matrix or scaffold to facilitate new bone growth on its surface.

Self-assembling materials—Disordered materials that form an organized structure or pattern as a consequence of specific, local interactions among the components, without external direction.

Smart materials—Synthetic materials that interact with external stimuli, such as light, temperature, stress, moisture, pH, and electric/magnetic fields, in such a way as to alter specific properties in a controlled fashion and return to the original state after the stimulus has been removed.

Voxel—Volumetric picture element that represents a single sample, or data point, on a regularly spaced three-dimensional grid. It is analogous to how *pixel* defines a point in two-dimensional space.

Emerging applications of dental **biomaterials** are primarily focused on the prevention and treatment of tooth-related diseases, oral cancer, and tooth replacements. The materials being used currently are useful for treating and detecting such diseases, but they need further improvement. Caries prevention treatments have reduced the need for initial restorations, replacement restorations, and removable dentures. Minimally invasive dentistry concepts have led to sealing defective or leaking margins of restorations with sealing resins rather than performing restoration replacement procedures that can destroy healthy adjacent tissue (Mertz-Fairhurst et al., 1998).

The implementation of a cure for caries is likely to take at least 20 more years; therefore, most of the restorative materials in use today will likely remain in use for a decade or more. A cure for dental caries will have a dramatic impact on the use of restorative materials to repair the form and function of teeth with cavitated lesions. In the meantime, the use of dental amalgam will continue to decline, despite the durability of amalgam restorations, until it is eliminated because of the environmental restrictions on mercury release. Improved resin-based restorative materials will continue to supplant the use of amalgam. Before caries can be considered truly "curable," demand will remain high for remineralizing agents, **smart materials**, and durable repair and replacement materials that can avoid the need for repeated restorations of a tooth. The need for both repair and replacement will prevail due to the time-dependent failure or degradation of the presently available materials. The developed world has been leaders in promoting the use of high-cost esthetic restorations, even at the expense of limited durability. Many restorations are being placed for esthetic reasons and not for caries management, a trend that will continue well into the future. The choice of biomaterials for a given clinical situation will continue to be based on a comparative analysis of cost, benefits, and risks.

One should expect dentistry to continue its dependence on developments in materials science and technology. New dental biomaterials must satisfy the following perennial, requirements. They must:

1. Be nontoxic to human cells
2. Be toxic to microbes and fungi
3. Be able to provide an excellent seal between the oral cavity and the underlying tooth structure
4. Be sufficiently **bioactive** to stimulate in vivo repair of tissues that have been damaged by disease, trauma, or dental treatment
5. Have properties comparable to the tissue that is to be repaired or replaced
6. Exhibit handling properties that would allow ease of manipulation and promote optimal clinical performance
7. Exhibit an esthetically pleasing appearance

Over the past 30 years technology has advanced tremendously and has benefited dental materials science in a variety of ways, including laser applications, imaging technologies, composites technology, "smarter" and stronger ceramics, and minimally invasive dental procedures (Garcia & Tabak, 2009). **CAD−CAM** technology has reduced the need for impression materials and has also reduced the time required for fabricating and delivering both fixed and removable devices (Strub et al., 2006). At the time of this writing, it has been almost 12 years since Feitas (2000) predicted that the first micron-sized dental nanorobots would be constructed within 10–20 years. Such advances are very futuristic and may still not be realized for many decades. However, some of the other technologies foreseen at that time have made substantial progress, including those involving the use of **nanomaterials**, **biomimetics**, tissue engineering (TE), biotechnology, and regenerative dentistry. This chapter reviews technologies that have demonstrated their concept potential and have either been **recently** introduced but not yet clinically proven with long-term experiments. Several new materials that are certain to expand in use are also included.

In the following sections and subsections several technologies are discussed under various headings (**Nanotechnology**, Resin Restorative Materials, Tissue Engineering, Regenerative Dentistry, and so on). However, substantial overlap exists among these approaches to various oral health–related problems; therefore, any subcategorization is to a greater or lesser extent arbitrary. In the following discussions, the reader will often find that subject areas are overlapping. For example, a major thrust in developing restorative resin composites is to utilize ever smaller reinforcing filler particles. As explained in Chapter 5, this has led to the development of nanoparticle fillers, which overlaps with the field of nanotechnology. In another example, one of the major dental applications of regenerative dentistry uses stem cell biology to promote periodontal wound healing and tissue regeneration, which are also objectives of both biological delivery systems and TE. So, although TE does not always involve biological delivery systems or vice versa, it often does and is therefore, categorized separately.

Shown in Figure 19.1 is a flowchart of basic, translational, and clinical research links representing stages in the development and evaluation of emerging technologies and products. The farther to the right of the chart a technology or material is seen, the higher the probability that it will have a desirable clinical outcome.

Biomaterials

The term biomaterial is frequently encountered in modern scientific parlance and is associated with advanced medical treatment and replacement of body parts. It has a futuristic nuance attached to it. A biomaterial is designed to interact with living body or a biological environment. Biomaterial need not necessarily be biological or based on biorelated matter. In the present context only synthetically derived or highly processed nonsynthetic materials are considered. Biomaterial can be metal, plastic, or different types of composites. It can also be bioinspired or derived from nature. Most of the dental materials presently used in the dental clinics are designated biomaterials.

Nanotechnology

Nanotechnology uses nanosized particles and surface features with very high ratios of surface area to volume that are usually different in their bioactivity, solubility, and antimicrobial effects compared with larger particles of the same composition. Thus, changes in properties cannot be extrapolated by an inverse linear analysis of particle size but must be determined through in vitro and in vivo testing of the nanomaterials. In dentistry, nanotechnology had been focused on the development of nanoparticle fillers to improve dental composite esthetics. The use of nanotechnology today is more diverse.

In **biomimetics**, nanotechnology is being used to develop materials that promote hard tissue remineralization. Biomimetic materials and processes mimic those that occur in nature, particularly self-assembly of components to form, replace, or repair oral tissues. These concepts are discussed further later in this chapter.

For dental implants and related devices, nanoparticles are used to modify dental implant surfaces to influence the host response at the cellular and tissue levels. Electrophoretic sol–gel fabrication, pulsed laser deposition, sputter coating, and ion beam–assisted deposition are among the approaches used to develop nanotextured, thin-film, biocompatible coatings for implant surfaces. These technologies reduce the thickness of the coating layer and increase the specific surface area and reactivity to improve the interaction with the surrounding apical tissue.

Important nanoparticles include metals, such as silver, and ceramic powders, such as silica and titanium dioxide. In situ generated silver nanoparticles have been reported to be highly effective in restorative resins, bonding resins, and prosthetic resins for inhibiting a variety of biofilm-forming bacteria while not interfering with manipulation, curing, mechanical properties, or other performance properties. Silica nanoparticles already have wide use in dentistry, from toothpastes to composites. Titania nanoparticles are widely used for pigments in dental materials but lack the stronger antimicrobial effects of Ag.

Research stage	Basic research	Applied/transitional research		Clinical trials		Applicability to dental practices	
Technology classification	Emerging technology concepts	Nanotechnology advances	Nanotechnology validation	Established nanotechnology	Integrated nanotechnology and microtechnology	Spin-off technology	Cost-benefit demonstrated
Testing stage	Hypothesis testing	Product evaluation	Bridge between basic/applied and clinical practice	Pilot and retrospective studies	Randomized controlled trials	Performance appraisal	Refinement of technologies
Outcomes	Preliminary data	Comparative performance	Preliminary evidence	Validation of evidence	Promising treatment outcomes	Optimum treatment outcomes	Adoption by clinical practices or dental labs
Stage of technology development	Technologies are feasible		Technologies are imminent or validated		Further refinement needed	Technologies applied to health care tasks	Oral health care goals fully achieved
Level of evidence	Clinical simulation	Proof of concept	Probability of specific outcomes	Limited applicability of technology	Application of refined technology	Demonstrated benefits in lab and clinic tasks	Fully documented and well-established evidence
Level of success	Desirable technologies, materials, and devices		Possible future technologies, materials, and devices		Probable future technologies, materials, and devices	Likely future technologies, materials, and devices	Proven future technologies, materials, and devices

• **Fig. 19.1** Flowchart of basic, translational, and clinical research links to develop and evaluate emerging technologies and products.

Another recently introduced nanotechnology kills bacteria on contact on restoration surfaces. Infinix flowable composite (Nobio Ltd, Israel), which contains quaternary ammonium bound to silica (also known as *QASi*) was reported to significantly reduce *Enterococcus faecalis* on the surface of the material without affecting composite flexural strength, radiopacity, depth of cure, water sorption, or water solubility. After 6 and 12 months of use in vivo, there was a 50% reduction of live bacteria on Nobio QASi composites compared with control composites. An added advantage of the QASi-containing surfaces is that no "recharging" is needed, unlike the fluoride in glass ionomers that confers microbial resistance. Prevention of bacterial biofilm protects the integrity of the dental product restorations.

The introduction of microfill restoratives in the early 1970s ushered in the era of dental nanotechnology. As discussed in Chapter 5, microfilled composites contain silicone dioxide (SiO_2)-reinforcing particles about 40 nm in diameter that are dispersed in prepolymerized resins that have been ground to form so-called organic filler particles in the micron size range. Current microhybrid and nanofilled composites contain filler particles range from about 20 to 600 nm. This use of nanoparticle technology allows the formulation of dental materials with high translucency, excellent initial polish, and retention of gloss while maintaining mechanical properties and wear resistance equivalent to those of current clinically proven hybrid composites. Several 2- to 3-year clinical trials have investigated the nanohybrids performance in a variety of oral restorations and found that the nanohybrids show great promise for extending survival beyond the current 5–10 years. Currently, a variety of approaches designed to overcome the deficiencies of nanoparticle composites are in progress. None of these is likely to result in a breakthrough that will lead to a universal esthetic composite that can rival the durability of amalgam. However, there is a high likelihood that many will contribute incremental advantages that, when combined and optimized, will result in such a material by the next decade.

There is no doubt that recent developments in nanomaterials and nanotechnology will further advance dentistry and oral health care. One of the most stimulating perspectives for dental restorative nanomaterials is that nanotechnology can mimic the physicochemical-mechanical properties and the esthetic properties of dentin and enamel (biomimetics). Many dental materials have been generated through nanotechnology and are available for clinical application; such as resin composites and cements that can be used to restore tooth structures. Ceramics as well as silica-rich glass nanoparticles have been incorporated into commercially available resin composite to simulate the esthetic characteristics of tooth structure and to achieve excellent long-term physical and mechanical properties such as high strength, hardness, toughness, and wear resistance. However, in the selection of the appropriate restorative material, clinicians should take recourse to documented data available in long-term clinical studies.

Dental materials science may soon change significantly with better understanding of physical–chemical–biological concepts related to the phenomena manifested at the nanoscale. Newer nanomaterials may be created from materials such as sapphire or diamond and that would provide strength properties of unimaginable proportions. Future nanomaterials will also play an important role in the field of dental regeneration through knowledge acquired in the field of TE, developmental biology, and cell and molecular biology. Because of the limited regeneration capacity of dental tissues, the combination of stem cells and nanomaterials may facilitate the regeneration of dental tissues.

Resin Restorative Materials

Prolonging the service life of dental restorations is of great public health importance because it delays or avoids the need for repair or replacement of the restorations. The frontier for resin restorative materials continues to be the reduction of composite shrinkage, reduced porosity, improving the composite–dentin interface, reducing wear and attrition, and increasing the degree of conversion of resin monomers. Improvements in these characteristics are needed in order to increase the service life of resin-based restorations and thereby reduce the need to retreat the original restored teeth.

Longevity and survival studies have shown that dental resin composites available during the past 10 years or so have an average replacement time of 5.7 years.

The failures were mainly caused by three primary factors:

1. Surface loss due to two- and three-body wear.
2. Marginal deficiencies due to breakdown and/or gap formation.
3. Secondary marginal caries (secondary caries).

Although the relatively recent innovations discussed earlier ("Innovations in Dental Composites" in Chapter 5) have likely increased the service life of currently marketed resin composites, there is still an incomplete understanding of all factors that lead to failures. For example, there remains significant uncertainty on the interactions among several variables including bacterial biofilms, such as dental plaque and the mechanisms of wear, fatigue, fracture, and secondary caries. Current ongoing research is making progress to gain better insights into how interactions among physical and oral environmental factors and the composition of composites initiate and influence failure mechanisms (Petrovic et al., 2010). Future research should lead to developments that further extend durability and survivability, possibly rivaling that of amalgam.

Another factor that influences longevity is operator error. Materials that present difficult handling, curing, and other technique-related problems are inherently prone to mistakes that often lead to material defects (e.g., air inclusions and low degree of cure), which in turn hasten the onset of fatigue and other failure mechanisms. Here, too, substantial research and development effort is in progress that can be expected to lead to a series of ever more "technique insensitive" (forgiving), operator-friendly, resin-based materials that also maintain a balance of other required properties such as strength, wear resistance, and esthetics.

Two recently introduced novel flowable composites, G-aenial Universal Flo (GC America, Alsip, IL) and SureFil-SDR flow (Dentsply International, York, PA), among others, exemplify such operator-friendly materials. Both are highly translucent and offer flowable rheologies (i.e., consistencies) and easy handling together with a large depth and degree of conversion; they are marketed as bulk fill, universal restorative resins with exceptional ease of placement. Both exhibit low shrinkage and low shrinkage stress when tested in vitro, and early clinical trial results show that they have early-stage wear resistance and durability similar to those of current posterior resins.

G-aenial Universal Flo is based on 4,8-di(methacryloxy methylene)-tricyclodecane (TCDDMA), a bulky, space-filling dimethacrylate monomer. TCDDMA has a tricyclodecane three-ring central group that prevents monomers from aligning and thus offsets polymerization shrinkage. This "steric hindrance" effect slows the rate of polymerization and lengthens the time needed for the curing reaction to reach the point of solidification. This facilitates the ability of adjacent polymer chain segments to slip among themselves and relax stresses that develop before the resin paste solidifies.

SureFil-SDR flow utilizes what the company describes as a "polymerization modulator" in the backbone of the SDR resin monomer. This material (stress decreasing resin [SDR™] technology) is a new resin system that claims to allow internal reduction of the stress resulting from polymerization shrinkage. With SDR™ technology, a polymerization modulator was chemically embedded in the polymerizable resin backbone. Based on scientific evidence gathered to date, the polymerization modulator synergistically interacts with the camphorquinone photoinitiator to slow modulus development, allowing stress reduction without a reduction in the polymerization rate or conversion. A schematic of a dimethacrylate monomer—which appears to have a bulky, space-filling central group similar to that of TCDDMA—is shown in the company literature. Whatever the chemical structure, published results show that the material has flow and other handling characteristics, together with a high translucency, that promote a high degree and depth of cure. These features place it in the category of technique insensitive.

These two highly flowable composite products also contain a reinforcement filler loading on a par with highly loaded, nonflowable, even "packable" hybrids such as those described in Chapter 5. This high loading, together with low curing stress and a high level and depth of cure, account in large part for the expectation of their high durability and long service life.

Many such products are available in the market today and can be broadly classified into:

Low and High Viscosity

- Low-viscosity materials like Venus Bulk Fill (Heraus Kulzer; Hanau, Germany), Filtek Bulk Fill (3M ESPE), and SureFil SDR (Dentsply Caulk) are placed in 4 mm increments, have low viscosity and a higher wear rate.
- High-viscosity bulk placement materials such as Tetric EvoCeram Bulk Fill (Ivoclar Vivadent; Amherst, NY) and SonicFill (Kerr; Orange, CA) handle like highly filled composite resins, can be used to restore large preparations, and have 4 mm depths of cure depending upon the shade and curing light used.

Filtek Universal (3M ESPE, St Paul, MN) is a recent addition (2019) to the category of operator-friendly composites. The nanoparticle fillers in this composite provide superior shade matching and wear resistance. This composite contains two unique monomers: addition-fragmentation monomer (AFM) and aromatic urethane dimethacrylate (AUDMA). The AFM fragments and repolymerizes during curing, reducing curing stress and enhancing marginal integrity. The AUDMA decreases the number of reactive groups in the resin and increases polymer flexibility. Fewer reactive groups moderate the volumetric shrinkage, and the increased polymer flexibility reduces the stiffness of the polymer matrix before the matrix reaches the gelation point. Both of these contribute to decreased curing stress, improved marginal integrity, and ultimately, improved abrasive wear resistance.

Omnichroma (Tokuyama Dental America) is a single-shade, universal composite that matches every tooth shade, from A1 to D4.

The innovative material contains 260-nm spherical nanoparticles that can scatter red-to-yellow colors as ambient light impinges on and is reflected from the composite. The red-to-yellow scattering blends with the scattered light of the adjacent dentition to produce an esthetic color match and reduces operator sensitivity.

The depth of cure of these composites is by increasing composite translucency, adding additional camphorquinone, or by adding new photoinitiators like Ivocerin. Given the intensity of research and development, other products of this type can be expected and, with further improvements, significant progress toward the goal of ensuring reliably placed restorative resins with the durability and forgiveness of amalgam combined with the esthetics of porcelain can be expected in the near future.

Antimicrobial Materials

Although the clinical performance of dental resins has improved remarkably in terms of durability, bond strength, and esthetics, most resins lack antimicrobial properties. Consequently, the inclusion of bacteriostatic or bactericidal properties is greatly needed, especially since synthetic materials of all types readily facilitate bacterial colonization and biofilm formation. Such new, improved materials may be derived from formulas with better nanofiller or improved interphase bonding agents for the ceramic fillers and resins. Future composite restoratives may also arise from (1) new fluoride-containing monomers for the prevention of secondary caries (such as fluoride-releasing dimethacrylate monomer containing a ternary zirconium fluoride chelate), (2) antibacterial monomers (such as methacryloyloxy dodecylpyridinium bromide (MDPB), (3) antibacterial and fluoride-releasing monomers, (4) the use of a higher filler percentage with nanoparticles, and (5) **matrix metalloproteinase (MMP)**–inhibiting components incorporated in the composite. Continual fluoride uptake (recharging from food or periodic treatments) and release are desirable in restoratives to inhibit or prevent caries. Antimicrobial characteristics are desirable, but they must be sustained after polymerization. Silver and titanium particles continue to be considered for antimicrobial effects, alone or attached to polymers. Silica nanoparticles are already used in composites to improve polishability and translucency, but new nanoparticles may exhibit enhanced penetration into etched dentin to improve mechanical and adhesive properties. The MMP-inhibiting materials may deter degradation of the etched dentin that interfaces with a dental composite in the hybrid layer. Suppression of MMP by agents other than ethylenediaminetetraacetic acid (EDT) and chlorhexidine can also inhibit remineralization, which is a likely area of improvement for dentin-bonding agents.

The treatment and management of dental caries have always been fundamental parts of dentistry. Early discovery of the disease's demineralization process facilitates the ability to inhibit or arrest the caries process or to remineralize the lesion's tissue, which is of significant value to the patient. New nonfluoride-containing, antimicrobial monomers such as MDPB, may help to prevent secondary caries, whereas other more effective fluoride-containing/releasing resins may be invented for this purpose.

Endodontics has been dramatically changed by the introduction of hydraulic ceramic (water-setting) cements that create high-pH environments and thereby have antimicrobial properties. For example, the tricalcium silicates and calcium aluminates have enhanced endodontic and pulpal treatment with their antimicrobial properties and dimensional stability.

Antibiotics are being used as endodontic irrigation rinses, especially when they are combined with various acids or chemicals that quickly dissolve the dentinal smear layer created by endodontic instruments in a root canal. Combination devices containing a drug, bone morphogenic proteins (BMP), or amino acids are envisioned for endodontic and periodontal uses. Antimicrobial materials are needed for restoratives and other dental materials that have novel and improved properties compared with those that are now available. For instance, future materials may use the antimicrobial properties of the calcium silicates or calcium aluminates for enhanced endodontic and pulpal procedures necessitated by the adverse effects of bacterial action. Silver zeolite, triclosan, and modified (chlorinated) polyethylene or other polymers may satisfy applications where an antimicrobial material is needed.

Preventing and removing biofilms are especially important for periodontics and endodontics. Adjunctive liquids are needed that can quickly kill and remove bacterial colonies in biofilms during periodontal scaling. In endodontics, new irrigants are needed to better remove and deactivate smear layers containing remnant bacteria after root canal preparation. As with acid etching, the frontier for smear layer removal or biofilm dissolution continues to advance with faster, more effective treatment regimens.

Bioactive Materials

Most present-day dental materials do not induce dental tissue responses and are not bioactive. *Bioactivity* is defined in ISO 23317 as a property that elicits a specific biological response at the interface of the material, which results in the formation of a bond between tissue and material. As such, bioactivity incorporates antimicrobial, remineralizing, and bone-forming materials, as discussed in this section. Bioactive materials implanted in a living body form a thin layer rich in Ca and P on their surface. The material then connects to the living tissue through this apatite layer without a distinct boundary. Bioactive materials are useful for the healing of tissues, especially pulp and periapical tissues, and for supporting root development in immature teeth.

Bioactive materials available now include calcium hydroxide, bone grafts, bioglass particulates, and hydraulic (water-setting) ceramic powders. The calcium silicate powders are considered the gold standard for endodontic surgical procedures, pulpotomy, revascularization, and apexification procedures. The calcium aluminate–based powders, being more acid resistant, are being used with glass ionomers for supragingival cement for prosthodontics and have found limited use for restorative applications. Their acid resistance makes them useful for infected sites, which are generally acidic; as such, the aluminates may be used for the same indications as mineral trioxide aggregate (MTA) materials. Calcium phosphate cements are generally slower setting than the hydraulic cements but are being used for scaffolding purposes where the formation of hydroxyapatite (HAP) is necessary and porosity is acceptable.

Theobromine, a xanthine found in cocoa, promotes the formation of HAP mineral and increases the size of HAP crystals by upregulating osteogenesis, which would have numerous benefits. For instance, theobromine may remineralize adjacent tooth enamel and have the potential to close gaps between restoration and tooth, improve bond-strength durability associated with reduced bond degradation, and enhance bone integration with implant surfaces. The large crystallite size leads to resistance to dissolution via the decreased specific surface area available for acid dissolution. New bioactive materials are under development that, in general, will create a biomimetic "presence" in vivo that induces healing superior to those of many present-day dental materials.

Dental resins have been combined with bioactive TiO_2 nanoparticles to promote HAP formation, enhance mechanical strength, and act photocatalytically as a bactericidal agent. A dentin-bonding adhesive with TiO_2 nanoparticles can provide on-demand, photoinduced microbial inhibition and simultaneously fill marginal gaps via remineralization of adjacent dentin and enamel. This technology may reduce recurrent caries, improve tissue integration with implant surfaces, and prevent peri-implantitis or other infections at the tissue–implant interface. These results are intriguing and highly promising, but they have not yet been tested clinically.

The surface of materials is often what makes them bioactive. Titanium as an implant material is an example. Like chromium, titanium spontaneously reacts with oxygen to form a self-repairing, protective oxide layer (TiO_2), which makes the implant surface largely corrosion resistant, inert, and biocompatible. However, surface roughness and other aspects of surface topography, together with surface chemistry, are also known to strongly influence the early events in healing and osseointegration that follow implant placement. Interactions between proteins, cells, tissues, and implant surfaces play a role in determining the success or failure of all implanted materials and devices. The surface chemistry and topography-related mechanisms that control these events are poorly understood. Nevertheless, substantial research effort in dental implantology is currently directed at developing surfaces with controlled topography and chemistry at the nanoscale level to optimally promote protein adsorption and cell adhesion. Biomimetic calcium phosphate coatings for implants are under development to enhance **osteoconductive** properties and incorporate biological agents to accelerate bone healing in the peri-implant area. Overall, these research efforts to understand and control surfaces are showing great promise, and some are likely to lead to materials, processes, and/or procedures to enhance the reliability of placement, indications for use, and the success rate of dental implants.

CRITICAL QUESTION

What are the stages of research that will lead to the adoption of new remineralizing materials and processes for dental practices?

Remineralizing Agents and Materials

The remineralization of tooth surfaces with incipient lesions, prevention of secondary caries, and durable bonding to etched dentin are key areas of research for future dental materials (Donly et al., 1994; Lippert et al., 2004) because of their great public health importance in preventing sustained enamel demineralization and prolonging the service life of composite restorations without repair or replacement. In the future, nanoparticles of HAP may be helpful for remineralization because they are on the same crystalline scale as naturally occurring HAP crystals in teeth. A promising example of this approach was reported by Li et al. (2008) who found that 20 nm nanohydroxyapatite particles provided an anticaries repair effect while larger HAP particles did not.

New remineralizing dentin-bonding agents should ensure wetting and flow and preferably completely fill the demineralized zone created by etching prior to or simultaneous with bonding to the restorative material. For instance, new MTA-type products have been tested in the lab with polyacrylic acid and sodium tripolyphosphate as a dentin-bonding layer. When it was applied under a restorative material, the combined material infiltrated the demineralized collagen fibrils with precursors that restored the calcium phosphate at the interfaces of the dentin and the restorative material. These and other remineralizing materials are needed to move forward from the laboratory to clinical trials of new dental adhesives for composites. Incorporation of some of these technologies into primers and dentin-bonding agents is expected to both inhibit caries activity and increase the service life of composite restorations.

Low concentrations of fluoride are known to promote enamel and dentin remineralization (Gelhard & Arends, 1984). However, after treatments with topical fluoride gels, rinses, or dentifrices, salivary fluoride concentrations decrease exponentially to low concentrations within a few hours.

The appearance of secondary (recurrent) caries denotes a state of demineralization of the tooth tissues at the margin of a restoration. In today's dental practices, the margins of restorations are often placed in subgingival areas for the sake of enhanced esthetics, but this situation predisposes to increased plaque retention and secondary caries.

The clinical diagnosis of secondary caries is the most common reason for the replacement of restorations in general practice; this includes all types of restorations, such as those produced with amalgam, composite, and glass ionomer cement. Typically, 50%–60% of all replacements of directly placed restorations in general practice are associated with the diagnosis of secondary caries. Since 50%–75% of all restorations in adults are replacements of previously inserted restorations, the clinical diagnosis of secondary caries leads to billions of dollars of costs for patients. Therefore, it is important, in this context, to assess the scientific basis for the clinical diagnosis and prevention of secondary caries and to enhance the potential to remineralize previously demineralized enamel adjacent to restorations.

The dental literature reflects a strong demand for preventive and "healing" therapies for individuals at moderate risk for caries to prevent a shift to a high level of risk. For some of these individuals, the daily ingestion of fluoride from toothpaste, well water, and other fluoridated sources may be inadequate to prevent caries, especially when other risk factors are present. These factors include a reduced saliva flow rate, increased consumption of foods and beverages that contain fermentable carbohydrate (that is, cariogenic substances), and reduced tooth cleaning ability. Saliva analyses indicate that residual fluoride concentrations in the mouth after long periods between tooth brushing decrease from 1 ppm or more to a range between 0.02 and 0.08 ppm. Because of this reduction in fluoride, remineralization may not be possible, since the transfer of calcium and phosphate ions into enamel depends on a sufficient and sustainable supply of fluoride ions. Furthermore, because the concentration of calcium ions in saliva is also very low in healthy individuals (a maximum of approximately 60 ppm); remineralization may be further retarded without an additional source of calcium.

It is well known that low concentrations of fluoride have a beneficial effect on enamel and dentin remineralization. For treatments to be effective over periods longer than the brushing time and the subsequent time for salivary clearance, fluoride must be deposited and slowly released. Calcium fluoride or similar deposits act in such a way because of a surface covering of phosphate and/or proteins, which makes the CaF_2 less soluble under in vivo conditions than the pure form in inorganic solutions. Subsequently, in the presence of phosphate groups on the surface of calcium fluoride globules, fluoride is released with decreasing pH when the phosphate groups are protonated in dental plaque. Saliva alone has the ability to increase plaque pH with bicarbonates, although typically this process may take up to 2 hours. The susceptibility of apatite in enamel surface layers makes it critical to control the acidity of the plaque fluid and Ca^{2+} and PO_4^{3-} concentrations in saliva. The subsequent remineralization process is characterized by the reverse of this process. When the oral pH is restored to approximately 7, Ca^{2+} and PO_4^{3-} ions are incorporated into the depleted mineral layers of enamel as new apatite. The demineralized zones in the crystal lattice act as nucleation sites for new mineral deposition. In the presence of fluoride (at high concentrations), the original carbonated apatite (CAP) loses its remaining carbonate and is replaced by a hybrid of HAP and fluorapatite (FAP). This cycle is fundamentally dependent on enamel solubility and ion gradients. Essentially, the sudden drop in pH produces an undersaturation of these essential ions (Ca^{2+} and PO_4^{3-}) in plaque fluid with respect to tooth mineral following meals. This promotes the dissolution of enamel. At neutral pH, the ion supersaturation of plaque produces a reverse shift in the equilibrium, causing a mineral deposition within the tooth surface.

Emerging technologies and materials that promote remineralization at early and moderately advanced stages of caries will be developed more rapidly as soon as the primary factors that dominate the remineralization process can be controlled effectively. In addition, more sensitive imaging or measurement processes are needed to validate early stages of remineralization and to more effectively determine whether or not preventive therapies produce optimal outcomes.

Bone-Grafting Materials

Bone grafts are very often used in the treatment of deficits of the jaws which are attributed to accidents, surgical removal of benign lesions or malignant neoplasms, congenital abnormalities, periodontal inflammation, tooth abscess or dental extraction, and finally jaw atrophy due to advanced age or general debility. The bone defects require rehabilitation for a variety of reasons, for example, maintaining the normal anatomic outline, eliminating empty space, esthetic restoration, and for placing dental implants. Several surgical techniques are developed to treat bone deformities including bone grafting, guided bone regeneration, distraction osteogenesis, use of growth factors and stem cells.

According to the sourcing, bone grafts are categorized into the following types:

1. Autografts obtained from the patient itself, possessing no antigenic properties since the donor and the recipient are the same person.
2. Isografts derived from the same species and share the same antigenic properties (twins).
3. Allografts processed in an effort to eliminate antigenic properties since the donor and the recipient are different persons of the same species.
4. Xenografts obtained from different species.
5. Synthetic bone graft substitutes developed to mimic the natural bone tissue.
    - Autografts are considered the "gold standard" among the various available grafting materials due to their osteogenic properties, maintaining viable cells from the donor to the recipient site as well as osteoinductive characteristics since a variety of growth factors contribute to the differentiation of mesenchymal stem cells (MSCs) into osteoblasts.
    - Allografts derive from individuals of the same species but different genus, being selected, processed, and preserved in bone banks. The main types of these materials comprise: (1) fresh-frozen bone and (2) freeze-dried bone allograft.
    - Xenografts are derived from donors of a different species relative to the recipient. They possess osteoconductive features with limited resorptive potential and are often combined with growth factors or bone grafts of other origin. According to the source they can be classified as follows: Bovine (cow) substitutes, Equine (horse) substitutes, Porcine (pig) substitutes, and Algae (aquatic organisms) substitutes.
    - Alloplastic materials: Enormous progress in the field of biomaterials, the risk of infectious disease transmission, and efforts to reduce morbidity and cost have paved the way of research into the development of a variety of grafts of synthetic origin as alternatives. Alloplastic bone substitutes will be able to mimic the environment in which osteoblasts can grow naturally. These biomimetic materials characterized by osteoconductive, with no osteoinductive or osteogenic potential on their own, try to act as a three-dimensional (3-D) scaffold to support cell growth and bone formation. Presently used alloplastic materials include calcium phosphate, calcium carbonate, calcium sulfate, bioactive glasses, and polymers.

In addition to remineralizing small lesions, gross remineralizing treatments and bone grafts are increasingly needed for dentistry. Bone-grafting materials are necessary for various oral surgeries, such as alveolar ridge augmentation and sinus augmentation and for the placement of implants or to improve mandibular denture stability. Extraction socket grafting materials are gaining popularity to prevent the collapse of cortical bone and enable the placement of an implant. Also, patients prefer faster treatment with fewer surgeries, which is driving research toward single-stage implant procedures with immediate functional loading (IFL). Implants with nanotechnology coatings may increase the success and acceptability of the single-stage and IFL procedures, but before implant placement, grafts are often needed.

Graft materials are available containing allogeneic, xenogeneic, or synthetic HAP particles to act as a scaffold for gradual replacement by the patient's bone. These current bone grafts slowly resorb and the replacement bone densifies over months until a restorative denture or implant can be made. More rapid resorption and bone growth–stimulating materials are needed to meet the demand for faster implant placement after tooth extraction, even immediate placement. Some available grafting materials are designed for faster resorption and bone growth. For instance, PepGen P-15 (Dentsply Friadent, Mannheim Germany), an HAP product with an amino acid, is available for accelerating natural bone regeneration. Infuse (Medtronic, Minneapolis, MN), a collagen sponge with recombinant human bone morphogenetic protein-2 (rhBMP-2), is indicated for sinus augmentation and localized alveolar ridge augmentation. Bone morphogenetic proteins, also known as cytokines, represent a group of growth factors that can affect cell interactions and cell behavior. Perioglas and NovaBone Dental Putty (NovaBone Products, Jacksonville, FL) contain coarse (greater than 100 μm) bioglass particles for implantation as a resorbable scaffold for bone growth and periodontal grafting. Ostim-Paste (aap Biomaterials GmbH, Dieburg, Germany) is a nanocrystalline HAP paste that can be used to repair the intraoral bony defects that may result from cystectomies (a surgical procedure to remove a cyst), root tip resections, extractions, and surgical tooth removal and for augmentations in the areas of the alveolar processes and maxillary sinuses (sinus lift) as well as to fill periodontal defects. Clinical trials are needed to determine the success of each of these approaches and guide the development of future products.

New bioactive glasses are under development that contain more boron and silica than the original formulas of 45S5 bioglass (45 wt% SiO_2 and a 5:1 ratio of CaO to P_2O_5) for **osteogenesis**, and the new formulas may be resorbed more quickly with faster bone replacement. Copper or silver in these glasses may also enhance soft tissue deposition in other applications. Powders, fibers, or foams of the bioactive glasses may be used as scaffolds for use in the rapid replacement of bone or soft tissue. Scaffolds of bioactive glass are used for **osteoconductivity**, and they may also initiate **chondrogenesis**. The latter could be useful for **temporomandibular joint (TMJ)** treatments. Combinations of biodegradable polymers with bioactive glass particles may also enhance tissue replacement and serve as the basis for new grafting materials.

None of the currently available bone reconstruction material possesses all the desirable characteristics such a biomaterial should have viz. high osteoinductive and angiogenic potentials, biological safety, low patient morbidity, high volumetric stability, easy market availability, long shelf life, and reasonable production costs, further effort is required to make this objective feasible. Development of various bone regenerative materials in the form of hybrid ingredient products that include cells, growth factors, and/or gene-modifying drugs in combination with the aid of science, engineering, and nanotechnology will further open a new horizon in the field of bone regeneration. In future, the ideal bone graft material will most likely contain a combination of biomaterials with varying features that can control mechanical properties, pore morphology, interconnective pores, surface structure, release of active bone-promoting biomolecules, and controlled biodegradability, which ensures resorption during the tissue-remodeling process while maintaining the defect volume for bone ingrowth.

CRITICAL QUESTION

In which ways does the use of smart materials lead to improvement in the quality of oral health care?

Stimulus–Responsive "Smart" Materials

"Smart" materials are designed for interaction with external stimuli such as light, temperature change, stress, moisture, pH, or electric/magnetic fields (McCabe et al., 2009). Currently, these dental materials include:

(1) Zirconia ceramics that transform from a tetragonal to monoclinic crystal form when tensile stress is induced at crack tips, leading to an increase in crystal volume and compressive stress that tends to prevent propagation of the cracks.
(2) Composites designed for initiation of curing by irradiation with particular wavelengths of blue light or composite cements that change color when irradiated (for use in orthodontics).
(3) Glass ionomer cement that when desiccated, weakens the cement to make it easier to remove orthodontic bands.
(4) Glass ionomer restoratives that increase the release of fluoride when the pH in plaque fluid decreases (Ten Cate et al., 1995).

Nickel–titanium wires that soften when chilled below body temperature for bending are "smart" and very useful for threading together orthodontic brackets at the earliest treatment stages with the most misaligned teeth. Future smart materials may include cements that can be triggered to soften and allow debonding by a temperature change or irradiation process. Cements such as this would be very attractive for use with temporary crowns, orthodontics, and some implant restorations.

Emerging technologies and materials may also include smart hydrophilic resins that effectively seal moist microscopic crevices adjacent to defective restorations and release fluoride and/or other mineralizing agents when the pH of oral fluids decreases to a range of 4.0–5.5, that is, when enamel demineralization often occurs.

The use of sealants, varnishes, and composites that release fluoride is not new. However, most of the studies on these materials were based on commercial products whose compositions were not known precisely and whose ages at placement were unknown or not identified. In addition, few studies have analyzed the influence of particle composition, particle size, and particle size distribution, nor have they demonstrated the on-demand nature of "smart sealing materials."

Secondary caries and the unnecessary replacement of defective restorations can be prevented and adjacent enamel remineralized through one of the following preservative treatments: (1) sealing of marginal crevices adjacent to defective restorations with a hydrophilic resin; (2) sealing crevices with a smart resin capable of the controlled release of chlorhexidine or other antibacterial agent; (3) sealing crevices with a smart resin capable of the controlled release of fluoride; and (4) applying a sealing resin or varnish that can release xylitol or other caries management agents at specified concentrations over a specific period of time.

The rapid induction of anesthesia may be another future application for smart materials. For instance, particles or substances could be applied in the sulcus and an external trigger could start or stop the anesthetic reaction. Smart material concepts provide the clinician with better control, which will certainly suggest approaches for new products.

A recent innovation of Smart prep polymer burs (glass bead–reinforced polyamide) can selectively remove dentinal caries. This bur cannot cut hard healthy dentine. The hardness of dentine is 60–80 KHN whereas that of carious dentine is 30 KHN. The polymer bur (Smart Burs 2 SSWhite) has hardness of 50KHN. The bur is used at a speed of 500 rpm. The polymer bur can remove the carious dentine because it is softer than the bur. When it comes in contact with healthy dentine, it wears off because healthy dentine is harder than the bur. In minimally invasive practice, the smart burs have effective role.

Self-Assembling Materials

- Self-assembly is a process in which a disordered system of pre-existing components—be it molecules, polymers, colloids, or macroscopic particles—forms an organized structure or pattern as a consequence of specific, local interactions among the components themselves, without external direction.

Self-assembling material systems automatically construct prespecified assemblies. Viruses, cells, tissues, and whole organisms are examples of biological assemblies, whereas crystals are an example of nonbiological assemblies; both can be derived from polymers, metals, ceramics, or be composites of several types of components. Self-assembly occurs by orchestrated stages of initiation, propagation, and termination. Control systems for initiation and/or propagation may be templates (e.g., template polymerization of proteins, patterning of silica templates for electrical circuits), or they might depend simply on natural rules corresponding to energetically favorable physical, chemical, mechanical, and/or biological events (e.g., capillary forces, heterogeneous nucleation of crystallization, surface energy reduction, phase separation, micelle formation, and steric probabilities for molecular folding).

The bone or soft tissue scaffolding of graft materials can be considered to be self-assembling. The coarse particulate or spongy bone graft materials are designed to encourage biological tissue to respond and replace the structure where the scaffolding is placed. Future materials may include templates of proteins to encourage biological events, such as specific tissue (Fan et al., 2007). For example, the Stupp laboratory (Palmer et al., 2008; Webber et al., 2010) has developed a broad class of self-assembling peptide derivatives that offer exciting novel therapies of broad potential impact in regenerative medicine. These peptide amphiphiles (PAs) incorporate a short hydrophobic domain on one end of a hydrophilic oligopeptide sequence that also contains bioactive signaling sequences. Nanostructures can be designed from these peptides that, through self-assembly strategies and supramolecular chemistry, have the potential to combine biocompatibility with bioactivity and also offer broad engineering design flexibility for the development of multiple biomedical and biomaterials applications. This type of research has shown early-stage proof-of-concept results for some applications and is close to translation into clinical applications for others. However, for most applications (e.g., the regeneration of teeth), translation remains a distant but likely achievable target. Several of these possibilities also involve TE, biomimetics, and stem cell biology, which are discussed in greater detail below.

In future regenerative dental treatment might require materials under this class. Regenerative endodontics that aims at preserving the integrity of both the soft and hard tissues of the tooth will utilize self-assembling materials. Injectable biomaterials which can serve as stem cell carriers and supramolecular hydrogels will be used for regeneration of craniofacial and dental tissues, which consist of alveolar bone, temporomandibular joint, periodontal ligament, dentin, and pulp.

Self-Healing (Self-Repairing) Materials

Self-healing is an *autonomically* initiated response to damage or failure. In order to achieve this function, a self-healing material must be capable of (1) identifying and (2) repairing failures (Fischer, 2010).

Composite materials for restorations are subject to aging in situ, and all biomaterials typically have a limited lifetime; they gradually degrade because of physical, chemical, and/or biological phenomena such as creep, fatigue, unresolved internal stresses, corrosion, dissolution, erosion, or biodegradation. As a result, the material eventually fails at some stage, such as leakage at the resin–dentin bonded interface, fracture of resin composites, chipping of porcelain, or corrosion of amalgam. Nature manages to renew many biological materials. For example, bone continually remodels and can heal itself (self-repair) even after a major fracture. Nature's approach has inspired efforts to develop self-healing capabilities for synthetic materials. One of the first such materials, an epoxy system, is similar to resin-based dental materials. The self-healing system consists of microencapsulated dicyclopentadiene and Grubb's metathesis catalyst. If a crack occurs in the epoxy composite, some of the microcapsules are ruptured near the crack and release dicyclopentadiene, which subsequently fills the crack and reacts with the catalyst, resulting in polymerization of the dicyclopentadiene and repair of the crack. Such materials have been observed in laboratory tests to improve the recovery of composite fracture toughness after stress. Similar systems have exhibited a significantly longer service life under mechanical stress in situ compared with those without the potential for self-repair.

Another approach under investigation is a self-healing material that operates on the basis of a pH increase experienced by proteins during the maturation of a mussel byssus secretion to control catechol-Fe^{3+} interpolymer cross-linking via pH changes.

Although no biomaterials with such properties have been commercialized as yet, self-healing systems would be extremely useful for dental resins, as they would have significantly longer life cycles and improved clinical performance. They may very well perform better than those repaired with conventional macroscopic repair approaches, some of which have been shown *not* to lead to satisfactory mechanical properties of the repaired composite (Jandt & Sigusch, 2009).

These technologies are being intensively investigated at present and may well appear in dental products within a few years (Fischer, 2010).

Biological Materials

Biomaterials science is exploring new technologies and is increasingly shifting from materials science and engineering and replacement therapies to bioengineering and natural tissue repair or replacement therapies. Biological biomaterials lead to natural tissue restoration and rely heavily on TE, biomimetics, self-assembling systems, cell biology, regenerative dentistry, and other technologies.

Biomimetics

Biomimetics is an interdisciplinary field in which principles from engineering, chemistry, and biology are applied to the synthesis of materials, synthetic systems, or machines that have functions that mimic biological processes. Few examples are as follows:

- The aerodynamics of the famous Japanese Bullet train was inspired by the shape of a bird's beak.
- The first flying machine heavier than the air from the Wright brothers, in 1903, was inspired by flying pigeons.
- Velcro is born from the observation of the hooks implemented by some plants for the propagation of their seeds via animal's coat.

Biomimetic dentistry does not believe in invasive techniques and accepts the philosophy that natural tooth is the perfect structure as a result of its various properties including biology, function, esthetics, and biomechanics. This is a departure from the radical tooth preparation techniques which would eventually reduce the tooth structure to ensure retention and strength of the restorative material. Many a time the pulp vitality is endangered. Biomimetic dentistry uses materials which are more adhesive and at the same time tooth preparation is minimized and ensures pulp vitality.

Some of the advantages obtained through biomimetic dentistry are as follows:

- Increase the bond strength
- Preserve tooth structure with minimally invasive treatment approaches
- Minimize excessive preparation of teeth
- Minimize root canal treatments
- Prevent catastrophic failures
- Eliminate post-op pain and sensitivity
- Restore badly damaged teeth, otherwise considered unrestorable

(https://www.nejadinstitute.com/what-is-biomimetic-dentistry—accessed on January 5, 2021)

This field of research involves the study of the formation, structure, and function of biologically produced substances and materials (such as silk and conch shells) and biological mechanisms and processes (such as protein synthesis) for the purpose of synthesizing similar products by artificial mechanisms that mimic natural ones. Of particular interest here are those that involve self-assembly of components to form, replace, or repair oral tissues (Saunders, 2009; Fan et al., 2007).

An intriguing prospect for this approach is the use of self-assembling PAs that contain both a photopolymerizable group and the arginine–glycine–aspartic acid–serine (RGDS) cell adhesion sequence. The self-assembling nature of the PAs causes the formation of networks of prealigned nanofibers, mimicking natural fibers. These nanofibers can be formed into tissue-engineering scaffolds and used as substrates for **MSC** cultures. Topographical patterns produced from the aligned PA nanofibers were found to promote alignment of MSCs, which indicate that the cells sensed and responded to the nanoscale features of the scaffold surfaces. The aligned MSCs then differentiate to form bone-like tissue (Welch et al., 2010).

These technologies are under intensive investigation and development and will very likely be translated into clinically useful materials and treatments in the not too distant future. These and other biomimetic approaches and uses of tissues engineering scaffolds are discussed further in the sections headed "Tissue Engineering" and "Regenerative Dentistry."

Tissue Engineering

Tissue loss due to trauma, disease, or congenital abnormalities is a major health care problem especially when it happens in the craniofacial region. In regenerative medicine, there is a perceptible shift from using medical devices and whole tissue grafts, to specific bioactive, biodegradable synthetic or natural scaffolds combined with cells and/or biological molecules, to create a functional replacement tissue in a diseased or damaged site. Biomaterials are no more considered as mere nonfunctioning replacement tissue. They are specific materials, which will nurture, in three dimensions, a fully functioning and structurally acceptable regenerated tissue.

- TE is an interdisciplinary field that applies the principles of engineering and the life sciences toward the development of biological substitutes that restore, maintain, or improve tissue function.

According to the National Institutes of Health, TE is an emerging multidisciplinary field involving biology, medicine, and engineering that is likely to revolutionize health care and the quality of life for millions of people worldwide by restoring, maintaining, and enhancing tissue and organ function. The main requirements for producing an engineered tissue are the appropriate levels and sequencing of regulatory signals, the presence of responsive progenitor cells, an appropriate extracellular matrix or carrier construct (i.e., scaffold), and an adequate blood supply for oxygen and nutrients. Either biological or synthetic polymers are used to form the TE scaffolds. Recent advances in understanding growth factors and biodegradable polymer scaffolds have made possible the successful TE of cartilage, bone, and related tissues (Slavkin & Bartold, 2006). Nakashiwa and Reddi (2003) have summarized the remaining achievements required to develop the clinical techniques needed for the creation, substitution, and/or replacement of dental tissues. Among the many potential applications are fracture repair, dentin and periodontal ligament replacement, alveolar ridge augmentation, TMJ reconstruction, preosseointegration of dental implants, and partial or whole tooth regeneration.

Tooth loss is the most common organ failure. The regeneration of a tooth can include not only regrowth of the entire tooth complex as a complete biological organ but also regeneration of individual components, including enamel, dentin, pulp, cementum, and periodontal tissues (Yuan et al., 2011; Sonoyama et al., 2006). Currently there are two main lines of investigation regarding this possibility. The first deals with restoration of partial tooth damage and focuses on using the existing reparative capacities of the tooth and/or use of tooth-related **stem cells** for the repair of damaged tooth parts (Petrovic & Stefanovic, 2009). The second line of investigation focuses on whole-tooth regeneration by using stem cells and/or conventional TE techniques. The first successful bioengineering of entire tooth structures was reported in 2002 using cells from dissociated porcine third molar tooth buds seeded on biodegradable polymer scaffolds that were implanted in rat hosts for 20–30 weeks (Young et al., 2002).

Osteonecrosis is a new and serious dental disease that arises from bisphosphonates received intravenously or orally related to other medical conditions. More effective osteonecrosis treatments are also needed and biological solutions to this end may be found. Conventional debridement is ineffective; therefore, other treatment modalities are needed, to treat the condition, and to avoid the onset by dental events such as surgeries or extractions.

In periodontics, TE is being used to develop new therapies beyond those based solely on infection control. Chronic periodontitis is one of the most common oral diseases worldwide, after caries. TE strategies are currently being developed to serve as periodontal regenerative therapies for the restoration of lost alveolar bone, periodontal ligament, and root cementum. These strategies are based on the growth of new functional tissue rather than replacement of the periodontium. These studies have shown that regeneration of small- to moderate-sized periodontal defects using cell–scaffold constructs is feasible and that this technology may well evolve and become available for selected clinical scenarios in the near future (Chen & Jin, 2009; Chen et al., 2012). Yet even though TE has created the means for eventual predictable and optimal periodontal tissue regeneration, progress toward clinical studies and routine clinical periodontal regenerative medicine and clinical use remains in an early stage (Hollister & Murphy, 2011; Rosa et al., 2012).

A still greater challenge is major bone reconstruction after trauma or cancer, as well as augmentation following implants. There are formidable challenges for regenerating normal structure and restoring the functionality of tooth-supporting tissues. Future possibilities depend on a better understanding of the cellular and molecular mechanisms involved in periodontal tissue regeneration, the differentiation potential of stem cells, and the interactions among stem cells, scaffolds, and host tissues. Given the recent progress and intense research and development activities in these areas, it should soon be possible to place implants even under adverse anatomic or biological circumstances. Current findings also offer promise that TE will soon lead to the ability to reconstruct lost bone in bone deformities in a more effective and less traumatic way than that offered by the traditional autogenous bone transplantation approaches (Rosa et al., 2012).

At this time, it is difficult to predict the full impact of TE on the future of dentistry. However, it offers the ability to bring together advances in such disparate areas as materials science, genetics, molecular biology, and cell biology to develop new alternatives for the regeneration of both bone and soft tissues (Park et al., 2010) and for new restorative procedures to regenerate enamel.

An important consideration will be the cost of these procedures, at least initially. Not only is the cost of treatment important but also to be considered are the costs required to fully develop the technology, demonstrate clinical efficacy, overcome regulatory hurdles (Hollister & Murphy, 2011), and train clinicians in the use of these innovative techniques.

TE has changed the profile of therapeutic medicine and is progressing rapidly encompassing all the tissues of human body. Three decades ago, TE was just an idea and today it has become a potential therapy aiming for better predictability. A thorough understanding of embryonic development and stem cell biology is prerequisite for the development of newer products. Regeneration of oral tissues is a challenging task and requires understanding of the biological development of several tissues and interfaces. Stem cell therapy and engineering of irreversibly damaged tissues is no more a fiction but is actually progressing toward reality.

Delivery Systems for Biologicals

TE approaches that combine biomaterials with such biologicals as proteins (growth factors), genes, and cells (both differentiated and stem cells) are promising routes to the therapies discussed previously. Thus, they are a source of active ongoing research directed in part toward developing competent scaffolding materials capable of fulfilling application-specific requirements for biodegradation, biocompatibility, mechanical stability, biofunctionality, and processability (Hubbell, 2003; Lia et al., 2008).

The key attributes of any biological delivery system are controlled, sustained, and targeted release. Each of these attributes is fundamentally dependent on the ability to predictably generate a functionalized material (Tayalia & Mooney, 2009).

An example of a promising biological delivery strategy is to increase osseointegration of titanium implants by coating them with extracellular matrix components such as collagen, BMP, and other proteins known to improve healing, induce peri-implant bone formation, and enhance osseointegration. For this technology to advance, further development is required to learn how to orchestrate the release pattern, optimize the time that the active components remain bioactive, control degradation, optimize the extracellular matrix that forms on the implant surfaces, and achieve maximum bone formation at minimal concentrations. As these and other questions remain unanswered at present, this appears to be a viable approach but one likely to require 10 years or more before a version is available for general use in dental practice.

CRITICAL QUESTION

Why are engineered tooth roots more likely to have a greater impact on dentistry than the engineered whole teeth now under development?

Regenerative Dentistry

Restorative dentistry is only very gradually transitioning away from replacement therapies using synthetic materials toward biology-driven repair, replacement, and regenerative medicine therapies. As currently envisioned, regenerative dental treatments have three key requirements: (1) a scaffold structure (either biological or synthetic), (2) progenitor/stem cells, and (3) the presence of inductive morphogenetic signals. For these approaches, the mouth has special advantages compared with other locations owing to its minimally invasive access and ease of observation (Bayne, 2005).

For tooth regeneration, two major approaches have been taken, both of which utilize stem cells, the building blocks that can develop into various types of specialized cells. One approach uses scaffolds seeded with stem cells; the other uses stem cells without scaffolds. Significant progress has been made with both of these approaches (Zivkovic et al., 2010). The main characteristics of dental stem cells are their potential for multilineage differentiation and self-renewal.

Stem cells have been isolated from many tissues and organs, including dental tissues. Five types of dental stem cells have been established:

1. Dental pulp stem cells
2. Stem cells from exfoliated deciduous teeth (SHEDs)
3. Stem cells from apical papillae (SCAPs)
4. Periodontal ligament stem cells (PDLSCs)
5. Dental follicle progenitor cells

Dental stem cells can differentiate into odontoblasts, adipocytes, neuron-like cells, glial cells, osteoblasts, chondrocytes, melanocytes, myotubes, and endothelial cells. Possible application of these cells in various fields of medicine makes them good candidates for future research as a new, powerful tool for a variety of therapies, including those related to oral health (Petrovic & Stefanovic, 2009).

Although stem cells will eventually be used to grow replacement human teeth, the signaling processes that control the development of discrete dental morphologies for incisors, canines, premolars, and molars must be clearly understood before whole-tooth regeneration will become a practical goal. Although this goal remains speculative, substantial progress has been made in developing an understanding of the mechanisms and challenges involved, and several proof-of-concept investigations are leading the way (Koussoulakou et al., 2009; Yildirim et al., 2011; Duailibi et al., 2004; Galler et al., 2010).

The repair and regeneration of dental *tissues*, rather than whole-tooth regeneration, offer possibilities for earlier realization. Thus, intensive investigations are being directed toward the development of techniques and materials to regenerate dentin, pulp, periodontal ligaments, and even whole root structures.

The dentin–pulp complex offers a particularly attractive target for regeneration because the pulp chamber has a nearly ideal environment, and such an achievement would lay the foundation for eventual whole-tooth replacement (Sloan & Smith, 2007). For example, Huang et al. (2009) discovered that stem cells retrieved from dental pulp produce pulp-like tissue in an emptied human root canal, together with the deposition of dentin-like mineralized tissue on the canal walls. Yet another step toward regenerative endodontics was taken when SHEDs were observed to generate a dental pulp tissue when blended with nanofiber peptides as scaffold materials and injected into root canals. A similar approach by Galler et al. (2008) using the self-assembling PAs (discussed above) as scaffolds to encapsulate stem cells, taken from deciduous teeth, revealed that they proliferate and secrete a soft collagen matrix. Similarly, dental pulp stem cells differentiate into an osteoblast-like phenotype and deposit mineral when encapsulated. In addition to pulp and dentin, such a PA/dental stem cell biological delivery system also has potential as a treatment for dental caries by promoting the regeneration of mineralized as well as soft tissue. These examples demonstrate the feasibility of clinical regeneration of the dentin–pulp complex. At this time many challenges remain, and regeneration may never be applicable for all clinical circumstances. However, it is foreseeable in the relatively near term that stem cell/TE therapies will become available to stimulate pulp to deposit dentin and continue the natural developmental root growth of noninfected, accidentally injured immature teeth.

Regeneration of the tooth root represents yet another feasible near-term goal rather than the regeneration of the whole tooth. Arguably the adult tooth owes more of its biological vitality to the root than to the crown. This possibility was demonstrated by the transplantation of a root-shaped calcium phosphate mineral block loaded with swine SCAPs, which were coated with a resorbable gelatin-containing PDLSCs; it was placed into the extraction socket of a minipig lower incisor. This approach successfully generated a root/periodontal structure adequate for use in place of titanium or other implant material to attach a ceramic crown (Nakahara & Ide, 2007). SCAPs are easily accessible, since they can be isolated from human third molars. The development of a combination of SCAPs and PDLSCs encapsulated in a resorbable scaffold offers a relatively near-term means of clinically inducing a root form and connective tissue in alveolar bone for the attachment of an artificial crown.

Both biomaterials and biological materials are playing an indispensable role in progress toward regeneration of a tooth root, crown, pulp, dentin, enamel, or entire tooth. Repair occurs by the use of metals, ceramics, or synthetic resin materials, whereas regeneration is controlled by biological restoration. Tooth regeneration is an extension of concepts in the broad field of regenerative medicine to restore a tissue to its original form and function by biological mechanisms. Although substantial progress has been and is being made, whole-tooth regeneration remains a distant but achievable goal—one that would cause dentistry to undergo a paradigm shift from repair and replacement to regeneration.

Environmental Considerations

Green Dentistry

Oral health professionals who are concerned about the environmental impact of dental practices have coined the term "green dentistry" or "eco-friendly dentistry." The basic Rethink, Reduce, Reuse, and Recycle model forms the foundation of green dentistry. Some of the practices which are adopted are as follows:

- **Water conservation:** Dental instruments and equipment have to be cleaned meticulously and mouths rinsed thoroughly. Easy actions, like turning off the tap while washing hands or giving a patient a small amount to drink instead of a full cup, help save water.
- **Energy conservation:** Green dentists make good use of every modern technology that promises comfort, speed, and ease in the dentist's chair. But simple practices, like implementing motion sensors and turning off lights when not in use, can reduce energy usage.
- **Nontoxic products:** Instead of using amalgam fillings, green dentists opt for composite fillings, which are both safer and more natural looking. In an attempt to introduce green protocol, zirconium dental implants are introduced as an alternative to titanium dental implants because they are well tolerated in patients who are prone to metal sensitivity.
- **Reduction of waste:** Recycling is possible for so many areas of dentistry viz. paper drinking cups, paper bibs, plastic wrappers, magazines, etc. Cloth headrest covers that are washable, reusable cups and reusable metal suction tips are all tools that can be disinfected and reused and thereby minimizing waste.
- **Technology implementation:** Green dentists are converting to paper-free environments that include digitizing billing, patient data, and appointment reminders.

Dental offices flush gallons of clean drinking water down the drain every day and generate waste, and somehow get rid of huge amounts of other chemicals and disposable plastics. Green dentistry initiatives include installing amalgam separators, using digital X-ray imaging in place of photographic images, replacing disposable lab coats with washable coats, using suppliers that offer environmentally sound products and services, and installing energy-efficient lamps and other equipment. These changes have been found not only to substantially reduce environmental impact but also to lead to substantial cost savings and other benefits. Product suppliers now provide disinfectants for surfaces, immersion, and dental water lines that are not only environmentally safe but also have fast, clinically relevant kill times. Evacuation system detergents are developed that disinfect the tubing and also chelate mercury to enhance amalgam separation. Such products and other environmental initiatives are gaining acceptance and will quite likely become the standard of practice in the near future.

Green dentistry is new and it is evolving. As on today no one has perfected the art of eco-friendly dentistry but plenty of oral health professionals are making the effort.

https://earth911.com/living-well-being/is-green-dentistry-possible/

A broken tooth 6500 years ago was restored with a simple wax cap, the oldest recorded dental filling. A book with systematic description of dental diseases and their treatment existed in Roman Imperial times between 25 BCE and CE 50. Missing Roman teeth were restored with gold wire supporting a replacement human tooth with evidence that both steel and ivory were also used. There have been remarkable improvements in material choices and techniques over time. Perhaps the three most revolutionary modern advances are Buonocore's (1955) introduction to the feasibility of adhesive dentistry, Bowen's resin-based composites, and Branemark's understanding of the induction and management of osseointegration. Throughout the ages, dentistry has survived and flourished despite all these changes. Care and longevity of the teeth and the oral–facial complex has improved.

Digital dentistry has changed how dentists think and function. It has improved the patient's experience. It has created a distributed work flow to capitalize on the best expertise for different functions. Unquestionably, the impact of digital dentistry is disruptive—but in no way is it destructive.

As lines between physical, digital, and biological spheres blur, collaborations of computational design, additive manufacturing, materials science, and synthetic biology will unquestionably help shape the future. Opportunities for evolution and innovation in material science are exceptional.

Instruments and Processes

Diagnostic Devices and Techniques

As discussed in Chapter 15, various new and evolving modern diagnostic techniques have been introduced for caries, periodontal disease, oral cancer, herpes simplex infection, and candidiasis, as well as for incipient fractures and trauma. Promising technologies may produce images directly from the patient or use saliva or other biological specimens from the patient being treated. Diagnostic instruments have been based on radiographic, optical, laser fluorescence, ultrasound imaging, and electrical conductance technologies. A selected group of those that appear to be the more promising in the near term are discussed in the following sections.

Cone Beam Computed Tomography

In dentistry, cone beam computed tomography (CBCT) provides high-resolution, low-distortion, 3-D digital imaging of the hard tissues of the head. Thus, instead of pixels, the resolution is measured in **voxels**, and the images are often sharper than conventional CT images. The term *cone beam* refers to the cone shape of the X-ray beam used to create multiple thin slices instead of the fan-shaped beam in conventional CT. CBCT produces Panorex and cephalometric projections, which become 3-D images when the data are reformatted in a volume. The images that result can be manipulated with the instrument's visualization software from any point of view (e.g., in the axial, coronal, sagittal, and cross-sectional planes). Layers can be "peeled away" to show hidden underlying anatomical structures and defects. The slice thickness can be changed, and the structures can be tilted, zoomed, and highlighted. These new views can drastically change treatment decisions.

Swept-Source Optical Coherence Tomography

Swept-source optical coherence tomography (SS-OCT) is a CBCT-related technology that uses infrared laser optics rather than X-rays to generate high-resolution cross-sectional images of microstructures in biological systems. This technology has been under development for many years for various medical imaging tasks, including examination of the oral cavity. Recent progress indicates that a practical device may be available for dental applications within a few years. This nonionizing, real-time tomographic technology can detect structural flaws at a submicron scale for dental diagnostic tasks. For example, SS-OCT may be used to monitor the accuracy of composite restoration placement, the development of polymerization contraction gaps, the detection of vascular lesions, and the detection of occlusal caries.

Laser-Induced Fluorescence

Quantitative light-induced fluorescence (QLF; Inspektor Research Systems, Amsterdam, Netherlands) is a well-advanced technology, although it is not widely used in routine dental practice. QLF is a simple yet effective technique that detects and quantifies demineralization and remineralization of dental tissue and bacterial activity to reveal lesions in teeth before they become frank lesions or cavities. The QLF method is based on the autofluorescence of teeth and plaque microorganisms. When teeth are illuminated with high-intensity blue light, they fluoresce (re-emit) light in the green part of the spectrum; less light correlates with less mineral content in the enamel. Also, bacterial metabolic activity and plaque formation can be detected because they produce porphyrin-type biological pigments that fluoresce red light. This technique provides a measure of the degree of existing enamel demineralization via a small video sensor. A digital image of each tooth is collected, which can be analyzed for the amount of enamel loss. White spot lesions (early dental caries) can be detected and quantified, as can bacterial metabolic activity on and in the teeth. When lesions are identified at an early stage, the teeth can repair themselves if good oral hygiene practices are followed. This method also allows either the dentist or oral hygienist to provide the patient with immediate information and a direct incentive to monitor the quality of oral care procedures. The newer QLF-D BiLuminator collects white light and fluorescence images simultaneously to allow assessment of leaking restoration margins, secondary caries, occlusal and interproximal caries, sealant integrity and cariogenic activity under sealants, calculus, and gingivitis.

Laser Photothermal Radiometry

Laser photothermal radiometry (PTR) detects a small temperature rise modulated by thermal infrared (black-body) radiation emitted from hard dental tissue after absorption of the laser light and its nonradiative energy. In translucent materials such as enamel and dentin, depth information is obtained following optical-to-thermal energy conversion and transport of the incident laser power in two modes: (1) the heat conductivity from a near-surface distance (50–500 μm), controlled by the thermal diffusivity of enamel and radiatively through black-body emissions from several millimeter depths, owing to optical penetration of the diffusely scattered laser-induced optical field, and (2) partial infrared transparency (infrared "spectral windows") of the hard dental tissue, which allows the thermal photons to exit the enamel and register on the detector.

Two variations on this emerging nondestructive technology for exploiting the optothermophysical properties of teeth have been reported. Both take advantage of the effects that changes in porosity and the crystalline status of enamel have on the thermal and optical properties of hard tissues. As cariogenic demineralization and formation of subsurface lesions grow, optical scattering and absorption increase, whereas thermal conductivity and diffusivity decrease. The two detection modalities are called *infrared photothermal radiometry and modulated luminescence* (PTR-LUM) and *thermophotonic lock-in imaging* (TPLI).

PTR-LUM (The Canary System, Quantum Dental Technologies, Inc., Toronto, Canada) scans a tooth with a low-power pulsating (modulated) laser light. The light is scattered, absorbed by the tooth, and then re-emitted at a longer wavelength as luminescence, and heat is generated (<1°C). Simultaneously, heat (midinfrared) and light (near infrared) are measured to provide information on the presence and extent of decay up to a depth of a few millimeters below the surface.

TPLI uses a laser beam to illuminate the whole tooth and a midinfrared camera in the lock-in mode to produce images at a fixed frequency. TPLI is an extension of PTR into a full imaging modality. TPLI uses the same physical photothermal wave principles as PTR: increased light scattering and absorption by a carious lesion increase the thermal-wave amplitude and shift the thermal-wave centroid closer to the surface, producing contrast between a carious lesion and intact enamel in both amplitude and phase images. TPLI phase images are emissivity normalized (just as PTR phases are) and therefore are insensitive to the presence of surface stains. Amplitude images provide integrated information from deeper enamel regions because of the radiative contributions that overlap conductive heat transfer. TPLI imaging is noncontacting and is reported to have a higher sensitivity to very early demineralization than do dental radiographs.

Ultrasound Imaging

Better termed *ultrasonography*, this well-established medical diagnostic imaging technique has recently shown promise for high-resolution imaging with enhanced specificity and sensitivity for the early detection and monitoring of several oral pathologies. Ultrasonography is nonionizing and noninvasive, and with further development, handheld devices could become available for the detection of cracks, calculi, and periapical lesions, in addition to enamel and dentin demineralization caused by caries under and around existing restorations or on occlusal and interproximal surfaces.

Infrared Spectroscopy for Multiple Inflammatory Parameters

An optical spectroscopy instrument is under development to enhance the early detection and monitoring of peri-implant inflammation and thereby reduce the number of implant failures. The instrument uses visible, near-infrared spectroscopy to measure alterations in regional tissue hemodynamics in periodontal tissue. Tissue oxygenation at peri-implantitis sites is substantially reduced compared with healthy sites because of increases in deoxyhemoglobin and decreases in oxyhemoglobin at the peri-implantitis sites. To diagnose these changes, the instrument simultaneously measures tissue oxygenation, total tissue hemoglobin, deoxyhemoglobin, oxygenated hemoglobin, and tissue edema.

Salivary Genetic Testing

Genetic testing using saliva is a molecular biology–based analytical test particularly apropos for periodontal disease and oral cancer. Chairside salivary sampling can be analyzed by companies such as OralDNA Labs (Brentwood, TN) to identify patients who are genetically susceptible to periodontal disease. This genetic testing for the interleukin-1 (IL-1) gene cluster, a significant inflammatory mediator, complements other periodontal screening procedures and salivary bacterial DNA tests for specific oral pathogens. Saliva analysis is used to screen for oral human papillomavirus (HPV), especially the variants HPV-16 and HPV-18, as potential etiological agents in the development of squamous cell carcinoma of the head and neck. Diagnostic testing will continue to expand and enhance treatment modalities. Such tests can enhance patients' acceptance of treatment plans and improve their cooperation with the clinician to improve periodontal health.

Liquid-Based Cytology

Liquid-based **cytology** is a relatively new screening technique approved by the US Food and Drug Administration (FDA) for oral infections. It relies on the minimally invasive collection of transepithelial mucosal cells and other microbiological aspects for processing and evaluation. A clinician can request tests for several generalized oral conditions, such as herpes simplex infection and candidiasis, or suspicious areas of leukoplakia or erythroplakia (OralCDx, CDx Laboratories, Suffern, NY). Cytology provides the evidence needed to determine whether an immediate invasive full-thickness biopsy procedure should be performed.

Diagnostic technologies, such as CBCT, quantitative laser fluorescence (QLF), and salivary genetic testing, are at hand and growing. These and other techniques are expected to increase, with positive benefits for both clinicians and patients. Each technique varies with the mode of action and in its capability as a diagnostic aid. Differences in presentation and behavior among anatomical sites make it unlikely that any one diagnostic modality will have adequate sensitivity and specificity for all circumstances. Thus, a combination of diagnostic tools will continue to be needed to reliably diagnose oral diseases and conditions and to provide corrective or preventive treatment at a stage where these treatments can be most effective.

CRITICAL QUESTION

How does computer-aided design/computer-aided manufacturing (**CAD–CAM**) production of dental prostheses differ from the processes of stereolithography, robocasting, powder-bed ink-jet printing, and laser scanning?

Computer-Driven Fabrication Systems

The present dental CAD−CAM systems vary dramatically in their capabilities. Both copy-milling and true CAD−CAM systems have been developed. No equipment can acquire data directly in the mouth, but intraoral sensors are used to acquire data. Not every type of restoration can be created by CAD−CAM, although indications continue to expand. Both "additive" and "subtractive" systems are available. Temporary crowns can be made in the lab using either CAD or CAM systems. The additive systems use the programmed buildup of a design from a resin that is cured "voxel by voxel" to create the device. This requires resins that are cured in special computer-controlled lab equipment with ultraviolet light. Three-dimensional printing techniques have been developed for the formation of ceramic or resin composite restoratives (see Chapter 15). Three-dimensional printing techniques will continue to grow and use enhanced dental materials, especially for fixed prosthodontics. The 3-D printing techniques are beginning to be used to fabricate the metal framework of dental crowns and bridges. More advanced dental applications include the creation of bone graft scaffolds. Those developed to date are summarized in Figure 19.2. See Chapter 15 for a full discussion of these technologies.

Ceramic crowns, metal crowns, and metal superstructures (overdenture bars) have been made using the subtractive (machining) CAD−CAM method using blocks of zirconia, leucite-containing porcelain, filled resins, cobalt–chromium alloy, and titanium. Refinements and esthetic improvements are expected for all of the present systems.

Another emerging area is 3-D bioprinting. In 2019, Grigoryan et al. demonstrated the creation of blood vessel networks and organ-like topologies using biocompatible hydrogels with tartrazine, a yellow food color additive projection stereolithography. The technique involves polymerizing material using blue light, one thin layer at a time. To make the technique work, the light must be confined to a single layer so that it does not penetrate to previous layers and polymerize them in off-target geometries. Tartrazine absorbs blue light selectively so that intertwined vascular networks rapidly form in highly defined geometries.

These emerging technologies will dramatically expand the capabilities for 3-D printing, but they will also require a different set of dental and laboratory technical training skills.

This chapter has focused on technologies that are in the early stages of implementation and those that have not yet passed the proof-of-concept stage shown in the "level of evidence" section of Figure 19.1. Technologies that promote 3-D remineralization are needed by practicing dentists whose focus is on disease prevention, minimally invasive procedures, and improved methods for extending the survivability of restorations. Dentists, educators, and researchers will continue their search for improved technologies that detect early stages of lesion development. Improved monitoring of early carious lesions is essential to judge whether new methods and materials of disease management ensure remineralization to avoid surgical intervention. If successful, these technologies and diagnostic methods would satisfy the "proven technologies, materials, and devices" outcome of Figure 19.1.

Several innovative methods for prosthesis construction in lab settings have already emerged, and others are emerging. Technology improvements related to oral and maxillofacial reconstruction methods will continue to offer pathways to improve oral health care. Meanwhile, the search will continue for biological technologies that may allow "natural or organic" regeneration of lost or diseased tissues.

This chapter may serve as a platform from which further innovative technologies for oral and maxillofacial applications can evolve with the research of materials scientists, chemists, implantologists, molecular biologists, cell biologists, and geneticists. Sustained collaboration among researchers and clinicians is essential to expedite the development, evaluation, and adoption of new technologies for improving oral health outcomes.

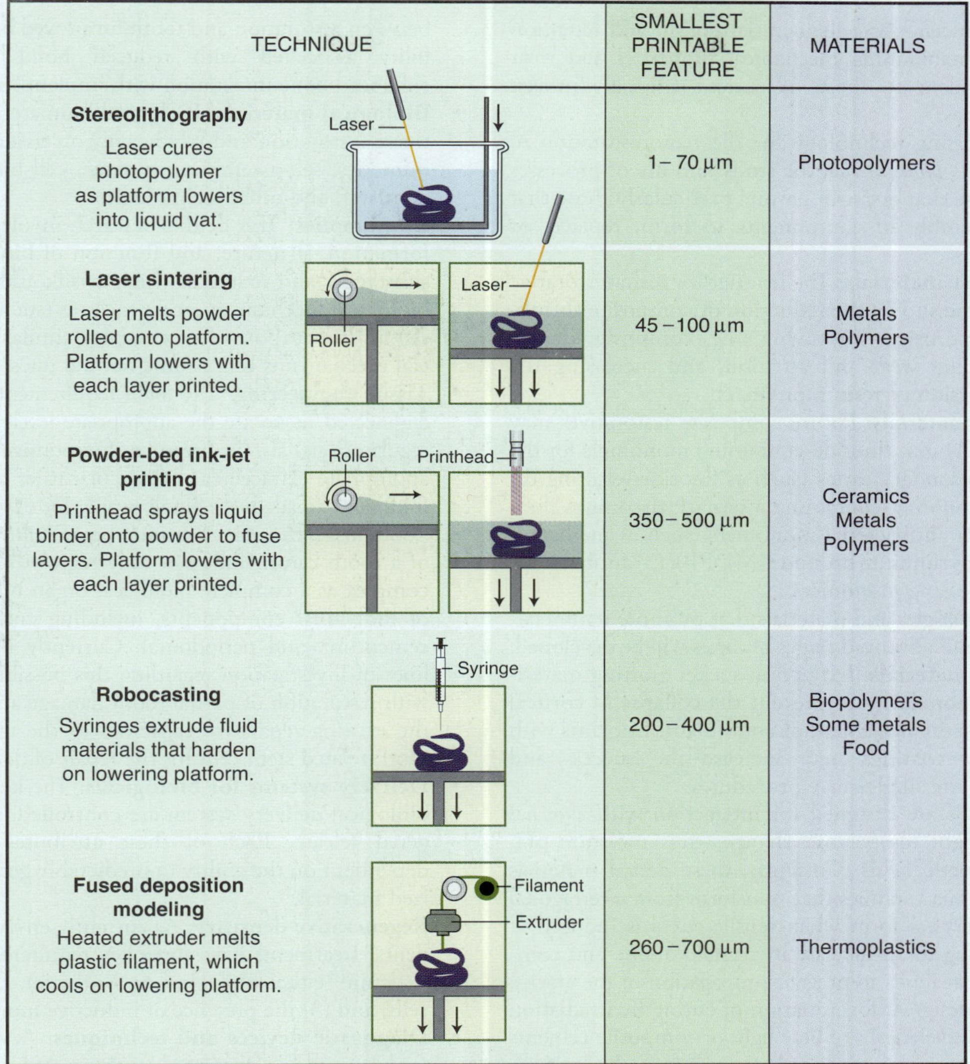

TECHNIQUE	SMALLEST PRINTABLE FEATURE	MATERIALS
Stereolithography Laser cures photopolymer as platform lowers into liquid vat.	1–70 µm	Photopolymers
Laser sintering Laser melts powder rolled onto platform. Platform lowers with each layer printed.	45–100 µm	Metals Polymers
Powder-bed ink-jet printing Printhead sprays liquid binder onto powder to fuse layers. Platform lowers with each layer printed.	350–500 µm	Ceramics Metals Polymers
Robocasting Syringes extrude fluid materials that harden on lowering platform.	200–400 µm	Biopolymers Some metals Food
Fused deposition modeling Heated extruder melts plastic filament, which cools on lowering platform.	260–700 µm	Thermoplastics

• **Fig. 19.2** The technologies available for three-dimensional printing. A variety of techniques can use various materials to build solid objects with different resolutions. (Adapted from Butscher A, Bohner M, Hofmann S, et al.: Structural and material approaches to bone tissue engineering in powder-based three-dimensional printing. *Acta Biomater* 7:907–920, 2011.)

Summary

- Minimally invasive dentistry concepts have led to sealing defective or leaking margins of restorations with sealing resins rather than destroying healthy adjacent tissue.
- Before caries can be considered truly "curable," demand will remain high for remineralizing agents, **smart materials**, and durable repair and replacement materials.
- New dental biomaterials must satisfy the following requirements. They must: (1) be nontoxic to human cells; (2) be toxic to microbes and fungi; (3) be able to form an excellent seal between the oral cavity and underlying tooth structure; (4) be sufficiently **bioactive** to stimulate in vivo repair of tissues that have been damaged by disease, trauma, or dental treatment; (5) have properties similar to the tissue that is to be repaired or replaced; (6) exhibit handling properties that allow ease of manipulation and promote optimal clinical performance; and (7) exhibit an esthetically pleasing appearance.
- **CAD–CAM** technology has reduced the need for impression materials and has also reduced the time required for fabricating and delivering both fixed and removable devices. Technologies that have made substantial progress are **nanomaterials, biomimetics**, tissue engineering, biotechnology, and regenerative dentistry.
- **Biomaterials**: Any matter, surface, or construct that interacts with biological systems is considered to be a biomaterial. In the present context only synthetically derived or highly processed nonsynthetic materials are discussed. In dentistry, these are also called dental materials.
- **Nanotechnology**: The introduction of microfill restoratives in the early 1970s ushered in the era of dental nanotechnology. Current microhybrid and nanofilled composites contain filler particles range from about 20 to 600 nm. This use of nanoparticle technology allows the formulation of dental materials

with high translucency, excellent initial polish, and retention of gloss while maintaining mechanical properties and wear resistance equivalent to those of current clinically proven hybrid composites.

- The most promising technology for the nanorestoration of tooth structure is *biomimetics*, the study and use of processes that mimic those that occur in nature, particularly those that involve self-assembly of components to form, replace, or repair oral tissues.
- **Resin restorative materials**: The frontier for resin restorative materials continues to be the reduction of composite shrinkage, reduced porosity, improving the composite–dentin interface, reducing wear and attrition, and increasing the degree of conversion of resin monomers.
- **Antimicrobial materials**: Future composite restoratives may also arise from (1) new fluoride-containing monomers for the prevention of secondary caries (such as fluoride-releasing dimethacrylate monomer containing a ternary zirconium fluoride chelate), (2) antibacterial monomers (such as methacryloyloxy dodecylpyridinium bromide (MDPB), (3) antibacterial and fluoride-releasing monomers.
- Emerging technologies and materials that promote remineralization at early and advanced stages of caries will be developed.
- **Bone-grafting materials**: Extraction socket grafting materials are gaining popularity to prevent the collapse of cortical bone and enable the placement of an implant. Implants with nanotechnology coatings may increase the success and acceptability of the single-stage procedures.
- "Smart" materials are designed for interaction with external stimuli such as light, temperature change, stress, moisture, pH, or electric/magnetic fields. Currently, these dental materials include (1) zirconia ceramics that transform from a tetragonal to monoclinic crystal form when tensile stress is induced at crack tips, leading to an increase in crystal volume and compressive stress that tends to prevent propagation of the cracks; (2) composites designed for initiation of curing by irradiation with particular wavelengths of blue light or composite cements that change color when irradiated (for use in orthodontics); (3) glass ionomer cement that when desiccated, weakens the cement to make it easier to remove orthodontic bands; and (4) glass ionomer restoratives that increase the release of fluoride when the pH in plaque fluid decreases. Nickel–titanium wires that soften when chilled below body temperature for bending are "smart" and very useful for threading together orthodontic brackets at the earliest treatment stages with the most misaligned teeth. Future smart materials may include cements that can be triggered to soften and allow debonding by a temperature change or irradiation process. Cements such as this would be very attractive for use with temporary crowns, orthodontics, and some implant restorations.
- **Bioactive materials**: Bioactive biomaterials with novel and improved properties are needed. For example, a bioactive material that promotes the formation of hydroxyapatite mineral. It would have numerous benefits, including remineralization of adjacent tooth substance, the potential to close gaps between restoration and tooth, improved bond strength durability associated with reduced bond degradation, and enhanced bone integration with implant surfaces.
- **Biological materials**: Biological biomaterials lead to natural tissue restoration and rely heavily on tissue engineering, biomimetics, self-assembling systems, cell biology, regenerative dentistry, and other technologies.
- **Biomimetics**: This field of research involves the study of the formation, structure, and function of biologically produced substances and materials (such as silk and conch shells) and biological mechanisms and processes (such as protein synthesis) for the purpose of synthesizing similar products by artificial mechanisms that mimic natural ones.
- **Tissue engineering**: The main requirements for producing an engineered tissue are the appropriate levels and sequencing of regulatory signals, the presence of responsive progenitor cells, an appropriate extracellular matrix or carrier construct (i.e., scaffold), and an adequate blood supply for oxygen and nutrients.
- Tooth loss is the most common organ failure. The regeneration of a tooth can include not only regrowth of the entire tooth complex as a complete biological organ but also regeneration of individual components, including enamel, dentin, pulp, cementum, and periodontal. Currently there are two main lines of investigation regarding this possibility. The first deals with restoration of partial tooth damage and focuses on using the existing reparative capacities of the tooth and/or use of tooth-related stem cells for the repair of damaged tooth parts.
- **Delivery systems for biologicals**: The key attributes of any biological delivery system are controlled, sustained, and targeted release. Each of these attributes is fundamentally dependent on the ability to predictably generate a functionalized material.
- **Regenerative dentistry**: As currently envisioned, regenerative dental treatments have three key requirements: (1) a scaffold structure (either biological or synthetic), (2) progenitor/stem cells, and (3) the presence of inductive morphogenetic signals.
- **Diagnostic devices and techniques**: A variety of new and evolving modern diagnostic techniques have been introduced in recent years for caries, periodontal disease, oral cancer, herpes simplex infection, and candidiasis as well as for incipient fractures and various other traumatic conditions.
- **Computer-driven fabrication systems**: Existing dental CAD−CAM systems vary dramatically in their capabilities. Both copy-milling and true CAD−CAM systems have been developed. Ceramic and metal crowns and metal superstructures (overdenture bars) have been made using subtractive (machining) of blocks of zirconia, leucite-containing porcelain, filled resins, cobalt–chromium alloy, and titanium. Temporary crowns can be made in the lab using CAD−CAM systems that are either "additive" or "subtractive."
- Three-dimensional printing techniques are being developed for the formation of ceramic or resin composite restoratives. Printing techniques will be a fruitful area where more sophisticated equipment and technologies can enable the use of enhanced dental materials, especially for fixed prosthodontics.

Review Questions

1. Write an essay on recent advances in dental materials.
2. Write notes on the following:
   - Use of nanotechnology in dentistry
   - Characteristics of biomaterials
   - Computer-driven fabrication systems
   - Regenerative dentistry
   - Bone-grafting materials.

Selected Readings

Amaechi B.T. Emerging technologies for diagnosis of dental caries: The road so far. J Appl Phys 105 102047 (2009)10.1063/1.3116632; The various technologies available to aid in detecting dental caries at the earliest stages are described, together with the associated diagnostic devices.

Bayne S.C. Dental biomaterials: Where are we and where are we going? J Dent Educ 69 (5) 571–585 (2005); The 2005 state of the art for restorative biomaterials is reviewed by examining the roles of truly biological biomaterials, traditional synthetic biomaterials, and performance outcomes for biomaterials. Biological biomaterials are discussed in terms of tissue engineering and stem cell research, self-assembling system opportunities, and nanotechniques or technologies. Future developments for major areas of synthetic biomaterials are considered for bonding systems, composites, visible light curing, ceramics, and cements. Performance outcomes are discussed for all biomaterials in terms of safety, efficacy, and longevity of materials.

Beuer F.; Schweiger J.; Edelhof D. Digital dentistry: An overview of recent developments for CAD/CAM generated restorations. Br Dent J 204 505–511 (2008)10.1038/sj.bdj.2008.350; This article gives an overview of CAD/CAM technologies and systems available in 2008.

Chen F.M.; Jin Y. Periodontal tissue engineering and regeneration: Current approaches and expanding opportunities. Tissue Eng Part B Rev 16 219–255 (2009).

Chen FM, Sun H-H, Lu H, Yu Q. Stem cell-delivery therapeutics for periodontal tissue regeneration. http://dx.doi.org/10.1016/j.biomaterials.2012.05.048.

Darvell B.W.; Wu R.C.T. "MTA"—An hydraulic silicate cement: Review update and setting reaction. Dent Mater (2011)10.1016/j.dental.2011.02.001.

de Josselin de Jong E.; Higham S.M.; Smith P.W.; et al. Quantified light-induced fluorescence, review of a diagnostic tool in prevention of oral disease. J Appl Phys 105 102031 (2009)10.1063/1.3116138.

Donly K.J.; Gomez C. In vitro de/remineralization of enamel caries at restoration margins utilizing fluoride releasing composite resin. Quintessence Int 25 355–358 (1994).

Duailibi M.T.; Duailibi S.T.; Young C.S.; et al. Bioengineered teeth from cultured rat tooth bud cells. J Dent Res 83 523–528 (2004).

E. Dianne Rekow, Digital dentistry: The new state of the art — Is it disruptive or destructive?

Dental Materials (Article in press)

Ensanya Ali Abou Neel, Wojciech Chrzanowski, Vehid M. Salih, Hae-Won Kim, Jonathan C. Knowles: Tissue engineering in dentistry, Journal of dentistry (2014), 42: 915–928

Fan C.; Chu L.; Rawls H.R.; et al. Development of an antimicrobial resin—a pilot study. Dent Mater 27 (4) 322–328 (2011)http://dx.doi.org/10.1016/j.dental.2010.11.008.

Fan Y.; Sun Z.; Wang R.; et al. Enamel inspired nanocomposite fabrication through amelogenin supramolecular assembly. Biomaterials 28 (19) 3034–3042 (2007).

Fischer H. Self-repairing material systems—a dream or a reality? Nat Sci 2 873–901 (2010)10.4236/ns.2010.28110; This review is an analysis of the underlying functional and constructional principles of existing natural and synthetic self-healing systems spanning a range of classes of materials; it leads to general rules and principles for the design of new and application-tailored self-healing material systems.

Freitas R.A. Jr: Nanodentistry, J Am Dent Assoc 131 (11) 1559–1565 (2000).

Galler K.M.; Cavender A.; Yuwono V.; et al. Self-assembling peptide amphiphile nanofibers as a scaffold for dental stem cells. Tissue Eng Part A 14 (12) 2051–2058 (2008)10.1089/ten.tea.2007.0413.

Galler K.M.; D'Souza R.N.; Hartgerink J.D. Biomaterials and their potential applications for dental tissue engineering. J Mater Chem 20 8730–8746 (2010)10.1039/C0JM01207F; A brief description is provided of oral anatomy and pathology, state-of-the-art treatment methods and their shortcomings, together with an overview of current strategies to fabricate bioactive matrices, with an emphasis on nanostructured materials. Design principles are suggested for scaffolding systems specifically tailored toward dental tissue regeneration. Future approaches are envisioned based on the emerging areas that rely on recent developments in tissue engineering and stem cell research.

Garcia I.; Tabak L.A. A view of the future: Dentistry and oral health in America. J Am Dent Assoc 140 (Suppl 1) 44S–48S (2009).

Gelhard T.B.; Arends J. Microradiography of in vivo remineralized lesions in human enamel. II. J Biol Buccale 12 59–65 (1984).

Ghorayeb S.R.; Bertoncini C.A.; Hinders M.K. Dental ultrasonography. IEEE Trans Ultrasound Ferroelect Freq Contr 55 (6) 1256–1266 (2008).

Håvard Jostein Haugen, Ståle Petter, Lyngstadaas, Filippo Rossi, Giuseppe Perale: Bone grafts: Which is the ideal biomaterial? *J Clin Periodontol.* 2019;46 (Suppl. 21):92-102., *DOI: 10.1111/jcpe.13058*

Helen A., Mandelis A., Finer Y., et al.: Quantitative evaluation of the kinetics of human enamel simulated caries using photothermal radiometry and modulated luminescence, J Biomed Opt 16(7): 071406-071401-071406-13, 2011. http://dx.doi.org/10.1117/1.3564909; This paper evaluates PTR-LUM, an emerging nondestructive technology, for its potential use for the characterization and quantification of early caries.

Hinders M.; Bertoncini C.; Ghoryeb S. Ultrasonographic detection of tooth flaws. Rev Prog Quant Nondestr Eval 29 1559–1565 (2010). AIP Press.

Hollister S.J.; Murphy W.L. Scaffold translation: Barriers between concept and clinic. Tissue Eng 17B (6) (2011)10.1089/ten.teb.2011.0251; This article reviews the technical, business, and philosophical barriers to the translation of scaffold-based bone tissue engineering therapies to clinical use. Enabling translation to clinical application requires both understanding the challenges and addressing the complete range of these challenges. Engineering scaffold designs as modular systems with a sliding scale of complexity is envisioned as an achievable approach for addressing the translational challenges.

Huang G.; Yamaza T.; Shea L.D.; et al. Stem/progenitor cell-mediated de novo regeneration of dental pulp with newly deposited continuous layer of dentin in an in vivo model. Tissue Eng Part A 16 605–615 (2009).

Hubbell J.A. Materials as morphogenetic guides in tissue engineering. Curr Opin Biotechnol 14 (5) 551–558 (2003).

Jandt Klaus D.; Sigusch Bernd W. Future perspectives of resin-based dental materials. Dent Mater 25 1001–1006 (2009); This outlook paper gives a view of selected potential future developments in the area of resin-based biomaterials with an emphasis on dental composites. A discussion of potential developments provides insights into future performance and application possibilities for these materials.

Koussoulakou D.S.; Margaritis L.H.; Koussoulakos S.L. A curriculum vitae of teeth: Evolution, generation, regeneration. Int J Biol Sci 5 226–243 (2009).

Le Guéhennec L.; Soueidan A.; Layrolle P. Surface treatments of titanium dental implants for rapid osseointegration. Dent Mater 23 (7) 844–854 (2007).

Li L.; Pan H.; Tao J.; et al. Repair of enamel by using hydroxyapatite nanoparticles as the building blocks. J Mater Chem 18 (34) 4079–4084 (2008).

Lippert F.; Parker D.M.; Jandt K.D. In situ remineralisation of surface softened human enamel studied with AFM nanoindentation. Surface Science 553 105–114 (2004).

Liu Y.; Ramanath H.S.; Wang D.A. Tendon tissue engineering using scaffold enhancing strategies. Trends Biotechnol 26 (4) 201–209 (2008).

McCabe J.F.; Yan Z.; Al Naimi O.T.; et al. Smart materials in dentistry—future prospects. Dent Mater J 28 (1) 37–43 (2009); Smart materials have properties that can be altered in a controlled fashion by, for example, stress, temperature, moisture, pH, and electric or magnetic fields. A key feature of smart behavior includes an ability to return to the original state after the stimulus has been removed.

McGlennen R.C. Salivary diagnostics: A catalyst for medical/dental collaboration. Comp Cont Educ Dent 32 (1) (2011).

Mertz-Fairhurst E.J.; Curtis J.W.; Ergle J.W.; et al. Ultraconservative and cariostatic sealed restorations: Results at year 10. J Am Dent Assoc 129 55–66 (1998); A classic study that demonstrated how effectively a sealing resin can penetrate defective margin gaps between either amalgam or composite restorations placed over carious dentin and prevent the progression of lesions.

Nakahara T.; Ide Y. Tooth regeneration: Implications for the use of bioengineered organs in first-wave organ replacement. Hum Cell 20 63–70 (2007).

Nakashiwa M.; Reddi H. The application of bone morphogenic proteins to dental tissue engineering. Nature Biotech 21 1025–1032 (2003); An overview of the current and potential uses of tissue engineering in dentistry and the role of bone morphogenic proteins (BMPs).

Nogueira-Filho G.; Xiang X.M.; Shibli J.A.; et al. On site noninvasive assessment of peri-implant inflammation by optical spectroscopy. J Periodont Res 46 382–388 (2011).

Nör J.E. Tooth regeneration in operative dentistry. Oper Dent 31 633–642 (2006).

Oei J.D.; Zhao W.W.; Chu L.; et al. Antimicrobial acrylic materials with in situ generated silver nanoparticles. J Biomed Mater Res Part B 100B 409–415 (2012); Resin biomaterials are described that can help prevent such problems as secondary caries and implant infections.

Otis L.L.; Everett M.J.; Sathyam U.S.; et al. Optical coherence tomography: A new imaging technology for dentistry. J Am Dent Assoc 131 511–514 (2000).

Palmer L.C.; Newcomb C.J.; Kaltz S.R.; et al. Biomimetic systems for hydroxyapatite mineralization inspired by bone and enamel. Chem Rev 108 4754–4783 (2008).

Park C.H.; Rios H.F.; Jin Q.; et al. Biomimetic hybrid scaffolds for engineering human tooth–ligament interfaces. Biomaterials 31 5945–5952 (2010).

Petrovic L.M.; Drobac M.R.; Stojanac I.L.; et al. A method of improving marginal adaptation by elimination of singular stress point in composite restorations during resin photo-polymerization. Dent Mater 26 (5) 449–455 (2010)10.1016/j.dental.2009.11.160.

Petrovic V.; Stefanovic V. Dental tissue—new source for stem cells. Sci World J 9 1167–1177 (2009)10.1100/tsw.2009.125; A review focusing on recent findings in the field of dental stem cell research and the potential for their therapeutic use.

Rhienmora P.; Haddawy P.; Suebnukarn S.; et al. Intelligent dental training simulator with objective skill assessment and feedback. Artif Intell Med 52(2) 115–121 (2011)http://dx.doi.org/10.1016/j.artmed.2011.04.003; A virtual reality dental training simulator is described together with methods for providing objective skill assessment and feedback. The simulator uses force feedback and can classify a particular operator as novice level or expert level and generate a report.

Rosa V, Della Bona A, Cavalcanti BN, et al: Tissue engineering: From research to dental clinics. Dent Mater. Available online 10 January 2012. http://dx.doi.org/10.1016/j.dental.2011.11.025; This review presents the principles underlying tissue engineering and the current challenges, perspectives, trends, and future applications of tissue engineering in dentistry.

Rugh J.D.; Hendricson W.D.; Glass B.J.; et al. Teaching evidence-based practice at the University of Texas Health Science Center San Antonio Dental School. Tex Dent J 128 (2) 187–190 (2011); The previous two articles describe the development and use of an online library of critically appraised topics, or "CATs," that present one-page summaries and critiques of the best available evidence on focused clinical questions. It provides an immediately available source for making evidence-based clinical dental decisions. http://cats.uthscsa.edu/

Rugh J.D.; Hendricson W.D.; Hatch J.P.; et al. The San Antonio CATs initiative. J Am Coll Dent 77 (2) 16–21 (2010).

Saunders S.A. Current practicality of nanotechnology in dentistry. Part 1: Focus on nanocomposite restoratives and biomimetics. Clin Cosm Invest Dent 1 47–61 (2009); This review discusses the current clinical utility of nanotechnology's most tangible contribution to dentistry to date: the restoration of tooth structure with nanocomposites. Characterized by filler-particle sizes of less than 100 nm, these materials can offer esthetic and strength advantages over conventional microfilled and hybrid resin-based composite (RBC) systems, primarily in terms of smoothness, polishability, and precision of shade characterization, plus flexural strength and microhardness similar to those of the better-performing posterior RBCs.

S. Titsinides, G. Agrogiannis, T. Karatzas: Bone grafting materials in dentoalveolar reconstruction: A comprehensive review, Japanese Dental Science Review 55 (2019) 26–32

Scheifele C.; Schmidt-Westhausen A.-M.; Dietrich T.; et al. The sensitivity and specificity of the OralCDx technique: Evaluation of 103 cases. Oral Oncol 40 (8) 824–828 (2004).

Seeman N.C. Nanotechnology and the double helix. Sci Am 290 92–99 (2004).

Shimada Y.; Sadr A.; Burrow M.F.; et al. Validation of swept-source optical coherence tomography (SS-OCT) for the diagnosis of occlusal caries. J Dent 38 (8) 655–665 (2010).

Slavkin H.C.; Bartold P.M. Challenges and potential in tissue engineering. Periodontol 41 9–15 (2006).

Sloan A.J.; Smith A.J. Stem cells and the dental pulp: Potential roles in dentine regeneration and repair. Oral Dis 13 151–157 (2007); This article explores tissue engineering alternatives for pulpcapping and root canal treatment using dental pulp progenitor/stem cells, morphogens, and biomaterial scaffolds. The potential of this approach as a clinical therapy is discussed and shown to require close control of the regenerative process, since uncontrolled regeneration can inadvertently lead to pulp obliteration and loss of tooth vitality.

Sonoyama W.; Liu Y.; Fang D.; et al. Mesenchymal stem cell-mediated functional tooth regeneration in swine. PLoS One 1 e79 (2006).

Strub J.R.; Rekow E.D.; Witkowski S. Computer-aided design and fabrication of dental restorations: Current systems and future possibilities. J Am Dent Assoc 137 (9) 1289–1296 (2006); Existing dental CAD/CAM systems are reviewed and found to vary dramatically in their capabilities. At present none can yet acquire data directly in the mouth and produce the full spectrum of restoration types that can be created by traditional techniques.

Subramani K.; Ahmed W. Emerging Nanotechnologies in Dentistry. Elsevier: St. Louis, MO; This book brings together an international team of experts from the fields of nanomaterials, biomedical engineering, and dentistry to cover the new materials and techniques with potential for intra- or extraoral use in the restoration, fixation, replacement, or regeneration of hard and soft tissues in and about the oral cavity and craniofacial region. New dental nanotechnologies include the use of advanced inorganic and organic materials, smart and biomimetic materials, tissue engineering, and drug delivery strategies.

Tabatabaei N.; Mandelis A.; Amaechi B.T. Thermophotonic lock-in imaging of early demineralized and carious lesions in human teeth. J Biomed Opt 16 071402 (2011)10.1117/1.3564890; A novel dental-imaging modality, thermophotonic lock-in imaging (TPLI), is described that uses photothermal wave technology and is capable of detecting early carious lesions and cracks on occlusal and approximal surfaces.

Tayalia P.; Mooney D.J. Controlled growth factor delivery for tissue engineering. Adv Mater 21 (32-33) 3269–3285 (2009).

ten Cate J.M.; van Duinen R.N. Hypermineralization of dentinal lesions adjacent to glass-ionomer cement restorations. J Dent Res 74 1266–1271 (1995).

Vorndran E.; Klammert U.; Ewald A.; et al. Simultaneous immobilization of bioactives during 3D powder printing of bioceramic drug-release matrices. Adv Funct Mater 20 (10) 1585–1591 (2010)10.1002/adfm.200901759; The combination of a degradable bioceramic scaffold and a drug delivery system in a single low temperature fabrication step is described for the reconstruction of bone defects. The production of calcium phosphate scaffolds by a multijet 3D printing system enables localized deposition of biologically active drugs and proteins with a spatial resolution of approximately 300 μm.

Webber M.J.; Kessler J.A.; Stupp S.I. Emerging peptide nanomedicine to regenerate tissues and organs (Review). J Intern Med 267 71–88 (2010) http://onlinelibrary.wiley.com/doi/10.1111/j.1365-2796.2009.021; The authors review their work on peptide nanostructures containing bioactive signals. These amphiphilic molecules are designed to self-assemble into biocompatible, bioactive biomaterials with the potential for use as novel therapies in a wide variety of regenerative medicine applications, including the repair of bone, dentin, and enamel and the regeneration of whole teeth.

Welch K.; Cai Y.; Engqvist H.; et al. Dental adhesives with bioactive and on-demand bactericidal properties. Dent Mater 26 (5) 491–499 (2010). ISSN 0109-5641, 10.1016/j.dental. 2010. 01.008.

Wolf L.F. Personal manufacturing. Chem Eng News 89 (46) 10–14 (2010); A review of CAD/CAM technologies and how they are being utilized for on-demand manufacturing of everything from medical devices such as those used in dentistry to food and consumer products.

Yildirim S.; Fu S.Y.; Kim K.; et al. Tooth regeneration: A revolution in stomatology and evolution in regenerative medicine. Int J Oral Sci 3 (3) 107–116 (2011); This review article explores existing and visionary approaches to tooth regeneration that represent a paradigm shift from repair by synthetic materials to regeneration by biological restoration to restore original form and function by biological substitutes.

Young C.S.; Terada S.; Vacanti J.P.; et al. Tissue engineering of complex tooth structures on biodegradable polymer scaffolds. J Dent Res 81 695–700 (2002).

Yuan Z.L.; Nie H.M.; Wang S.; et al. Biomaterial selection for tooth regeneration. Tissue Eng B-Rev 17 (5) 373–388 (2011); A critical review of current knowledge of biomaterial use in tooth regeneration is presented. The selection of native and/or synthetic polymers, three-dimensional scaffold fabrication, stem cell transplantation, and stem cell homing is discussed.

Zivkovic P.; Petrovic V.; Najman S.; et al. Stem cell–based dental tissue engineering. Sci World J: TSW Dev Embryol 10 901–916 (2010). http://dx.doi.org/10.1100/tsw.2010.81; This review focuses on the use of tissue engineering strategies in tooth regeneration using stem cells and stem cells/scaffold constructs. The authors point out that although whole tooth regeneration is still not possible, there are promising results.

Useful Websites (accessed February 2012)

The Inside Scoop. Interviews with Oral Health Researchers. A variety of subjects and technologies under development are reviewed via interviews with key scientists supported by the NIH National Institute of Dental and Craniofacial Research. Recent subjects include biomimetics, building a tooth, craniofacial research, dental composites, dental practice-based research networks, diagnostics, genes/genetics, head and neck cancer, health disparities, pain/inflammation, periodontal disease, research training experiences, salivary disorders/dry mouth and TMJ disorders. http://www.nidcr.nih.gov/Research/ResearchResults/InterviewsOHR/

Library of critically appraised topics related to clinical dental problems. The "CAT" library provides key word–searchable topics. Each topic is presented as a structured one-page summary and critique of the best available evidence on a focused question. The library is designed as a rapidly accessible source of evidence-based information for use in making clinical dental decisions. https://cats.uthscsa.edu/

The Eco-Dentistry Association. Information about the association and resources to develop "green" dental practices. http://www.ecodentistry.org/?page=AboutGreenDentistry

Dental Restorative Materials—A Pollution Prevention Perspective. Information regarding the health, safety, and environmental issues arising from the chemical ingredients used in dental restorative materials. http://wsppn.org/studies/dental-chemical-use/fact-sheets/restorative-materials/

Index

Page numbers followed by "f" indicate figures and "t" indicate tables, and "b" indicate boxes.

C

E

F

G

H

I

M

U

V

Z